D1520535

Drugs for the Geriatric Patient

Drugs for the Geriatric Patient

Ronald I. Shorr, M.D., M.S.
Ruth S. Jewett Professor of Geriatrics
Chief Division of Geriatric Medicine
Department of Aging and Geriatric Research, College of Medicine
Associate Director Institute on Aging, University of Florida
Director Education and Clinical Center (GRECC)
Malcom Randall Veteran's Affairs Medical Center
North Florida/South Georgia Veterans Health System
Gainesville, Florida

Angela B. Hoth, PharmD
Clinical Pharmacy Specialist
VA Medical Center
Iowa City, Iowa

Nathan Rawls, PharmD
Professor
Clinical Pharmacy
College of Pharmacy
University of Tennessee
Clinical Pharmacy Specialist
Pharmacy Service
Veterans Affairs Medical Center
Memphis, Tennessee

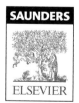

SAUNDERS

ELSEVIER

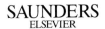

SAUNDERS
ELSEVIER

1600 John F. Kennedy Blvd.
Ste 1800
Philadelphia, PA 19103-2899

Drugs for the Geriatric Patient

ISBN-13: 978-1-4160-0208-6
ISBN-10: 1-4160-0208-1

Notice

Knowledge and best practice in this field are constantly changing. As new research and experience broaden our knowledge, changes in practice, treatment and drug therapy may become necessary or appropriate. Readers are advised to check the most current information provided (i) on procedures featured or (ii) by the manufacturer of each product to be administered, to verify the recommended dose or formula, the method and duration of administration, and contraindications. It is the responsibility of the practitioner, relying on their own experience and knowledge of the patient, to make diagnoses, to determine dosages and the best treatment for each individual patient, and to take all appropriate safety precautions. To the fullest extent of the law, neither the Publisher nor the Editors assume any liability for any injury and/or damage to persons or property arising out or related to any use of the material contained in this book.

The Publisher

Library of Congress Cataloging-in-Publication Data
Drugs for the geriatric patient / [edited by] Ronald I. Shorr, Angela B. Hoth, Nathan Rawls.
    p. ; cm.
    Includes bibliographical references and index.
    ISBN-13: 978-1-4160-0208-6
    ISBN-10: 1-4160-0208-1
  1. Geriatric pharmacology—Handbooks, manuals, etc. I. Shorr, Ronald I. II. Hoth, Angela B.
III. Rawls, Nathan.
    [DNLM: 1. Pharmaceutical Preparations—United States—Handbooks. 2. Aged—United States.
3. Drug Therapy—United States—Handbooks. QV 39 D7942 2007]
RC953.7.D795 2007
615.5'80846—dc22

2006051299

Acquisitions Editor: Rolla Couchman
Developmental Editor: Heather Krehling
Publishing Services Manager: Frank Polizzano
Design Direction: Karen O'Keefe Owens
Cover Photo by: Rebecca Brodwick

Printed in United States of America

Last digit is the print number: 9 8 7 6 5 4 2 1

To our families, patients, students and teachers, without whom this book would not be possible.

Table of Contents

Contribution by

Rebecca J. Beyth, M.D., M.Sc.
Associate Professor and Chief
Division of Career Development and Education
Department of Aging and Geriatrics
University of Florida
Associate Director
Rehabilitation and Outcomes Research Center
NFSGVHS (ISIB)
Gainesville, Florida

Introduction

Thank you for your interest in **Drugs for the Geriatric Patient**. We have designed this book to be used by providers of care to geriatric patients in a variety of settings. The material is accurate and easy to use. The sections are primarily self-explanatory and include such categories as brand names; a brief overview of clinical pharmacology; indications and dosages, including off-label uses in geriatric patients; and contraindications. Also included is a checklist entitled "Geriatric Side Effects at a Glance." Not all patients suffer side effects from medications, but we have identified some common side effects that providers should be aware of. Included also is regulatory information that applies to the use of certain drugs in long-term care settings in the United Sates and Food and Drug Administration black box information.

For drugs that are "OBRA regulated in U.S. Long-Term Care," we identified drugs that are explicitly regulated (e.g., antipsychotic agents) as well as those that are included in the interpretive guidelines for drug regimen review (e.g., drugs that are potentially inappropriate in the elderly). Interested parties should review the federal regulations for more specific information.

We hope this categorization scheme helps prescribers who are outside the United States. The patient and family education section may also be useful. For commonly used agents of special relevance to geriatric patients, we also include a narrative summary with relevant references.

Readers are encouraged to contact the editors with comments, concerns, and criticisms.

Acknowledgements

My thanks to Heather Krehling and Rolla Couchman for your patience and encouragement (and cheesesteak!)

Ron Shorr

Abbreviations

ABG	arterial blood gas
ac	before meals
ACE	angiotensin-converting enzyme
ACT	activated clotting time
ACTH	adrenocorticotropic hormone
AD	right ear
ADAS	Alzheimer's Disease Assessment Scale
ADH	antidiuretic hormone
ADHD	attention-deficit-hyperactivity disorder
ADP	adenosine diphosphate
aer	aerosol
AIDS	acquired immunodeficiency syndrome
alk	alkaline
ALS	amyotrophic lateral sclerosis
ALT	alanine aminotransferase, serum
AM, a.m.	ante meridiem
AMD	age-related macular degeneration
AMS	altered mental status
ANA	antinuclear antibody
ANC	absolute neutrophil count
APAP	acetaminophen
APL	acute promyelocytic leukemia
approx.	approximately
aPTT	activated partial thromboplastin time
ARB	angiotensin receptor blocker
ARDS	adult respiratory distress syndrome
AS	left ear
ASA	acetylsalicylic acid
5-ASA	5-aminosalicylic acid
AST	aspartate aminotransferase, serum
AT$_1$	angiotensin II receptor, type I
AT II	angiotensin II
ATP	adenosine triphosphate
AU	each ear
AUC	area under curve
AV	atrioventricular; arteriovenous
AZT	zidovudine
BB	beta-blocker, beta-blocking
bid	twice a day
BP	blood pressure
BPH	benign prostatic hyperplasia
BSA	body surface area
BUN	blood urea nitrogen
BZ	benzodiazepine
°C	degrees Celsius (centigrade)

Ca	calcium
CABG	coronary artery bypass grafting
CAD	coronary artery disease
cAMP	cyclic adenosine monophosphate
cap	capsule
cath	catheterize
CBC	complete blood count
cc	cubic centimeter
CDC	Centers for Disease Control and Prevention
CGMP	cyclic guanosine monophosphate
chew tab	tablet, chewable
CHF	congestive heart failure
Cl	chloride
cm	centimeter
CML	chronic myeloid leukemia
CMV	cytomegalovirus
CNS	central nervous system
CO_2	carbon dioxide
COMT	catechol-O-methyltransferase
COPD	chronic obstructive pulmonary disease
COX-2	cyclooxygenase-2
CPAP	continuous positive airway pressure
CPK	creatine phosphokinase
CR	creatine kinase
Cr	creatinine
CrCl	creatinine clearance
CRF	chronic renal failure
CRP	c-reactive protein
CRPS	complex regional pain syndrome
CSF	cerebrospinal fluid
CT	computer tomography
CTCL	cutaneous T-cell lymphoma
CV	cardiovascular
CVA	cerebrovascular accident
CVD	cardiovascular disease
CVP	central venous pressure
CXR	chest x-ray
D-C	discontinue
DCIS	ductal carcinoma in situ
DEA	Drug Enforcement Administration
DEXA	dual-energy x-ray absorptiometry
DHA	docosahexaenoic acid
DHE	dihydroergotamine
DHT	dihydrotestoserone
DIC	disseminated intravascular coagulation
dl	deciliter
D_LCO	diffusing capacity of carbon monoxide
DMARDs	disease-modifying antirheumatic drugs
DNA	deoxyribonucleic acid

DOPA	dihydroxyphenylalanine
DVT	deep vein thrombosis
D5W	5% dextrose in water
ECG	electrocardiogram
EDTA	ethylenediaminetetraacetic acid
EEG	electroencephalogram
EENT	eye, ear, nose, throat
EGFR	epidermal growth factor receptor
EIAED	enzyme-inducing antiepileptic drug
ELISA	enzyme-linked immunosorbent assay
elix	elixir
EPA	eicosapentaenoic acid
ESR	erythrocyte sedimentation rate
ESRD	end-stage renal disease
°F	degrees Fahrenheit
FDA	(U.S.) Food and Drug Administration
FEV$_1$	forced expiratory volume in 1 second
FSH	follicle-stimulating hormone
5-FU	5-fluorouracil
g	gram
GABA	gamma-aminobutyric acid
GAD	generalized anxiety disorder
GERD	gastroesophageal reflux disease
GFR	glomerular filtration rate
GGTP	gamma glutamyl transpeptidase
GI	gastrointestinal
GLP-1	glucagon-like peptide-1
GnRH	gonadotropin-releasing hormone
GP	glycoprotein
G6PD	glucose-6-phosphate dehydrogenase
gtt	drop
GU	genitourinary
H$_1$, H$_2$	histamine type 1, 2 receptors
HbA$_{1c}$	hemoglobin A$_{1c}$
HBV	hepatitis B virus
HCG	human chorionic gonadotropin
Hct	hematocrit
HCT, HCTZ	hydrochlorothiazide
HDL	high-density lipoprotein
Hgb	hemoglobin
5-HIAA	5-hydroxyindoleacetic acid
HIT	heparin-induced thrombocytopenia
HIV	human immunodeficiency virus
HIV-1, HIV-2	HIV types 1, 2
HMG CoA	3-hydroxy-3-methylglutaryl coenzyme A
H$_2$O	water
HPA	hypothalamic-pituitary-adrenal
hpf	high-powered field

hr	hour
hs	at bedtime
HSV	herpes simplex virus
HSV-1,	
HSV-2	HSV types 1, 2
5-HT	5-hydroxytryptamine
5-HT$_{1A}$,	
5-HT$_{2A}$,	
5-HT$_3$,	
5-HT$_4$	5-HT types 1A, 2A, 3, 4
HTN	hypertension
HUS	hemolytic uremic syndrome
IBS	irritable bowel syndrome
ICP	intracranial pressure
IgE	immunoglobulin E
IgG	immunoglobulin G
IL-1	interleukin-1
IM	intramuscular
INF	infusion
INH	inhalation; isonicotinic acid hydrazide (isoniazid)
inj	injection
INR	international normalized ratio
IO	intraosseous
IOP	intraocular pressure
IPPB	intermittent positive pressure breathing
iPTH	immunoreactive parathyroid hormone
ISA	intrinsic sympathomimetic activity
IU	international units
IV	intravenous
IVP	intravenous push
K	potassium
kg	kilogram
L	liter
LA	long acting
lb	pound
LBM	loose bowel movement
LDH	lactate dehydrogenase
LDL	low-density lipoprotein
LFTs	liver function tests
LH	luteinizing hormone
liq	liquid
LOC	level of consciousness
loz	lozenge
m	meter
m^2	square meter
MAC	*Mycobacterium avium* complex
MAO	monoamine oxidase
MAOI	monoamine oxidase inhibitor

MAP	mean arterial pressure
mcg	microgram
MDI	metered dose inhaler
mEq	milliequivalent
Mg	magnesium
mg	milligram
MI	myocardial infarction
min	minute
μl	microliter
ml	milliliter
mm	millimeter
mmol	millimole
MMSE	Mini-Mental Status Exam
mo	month
mRNA	messenger RNA
MRSA	methicillin-resistant *Staphylococcus aureus*
MS	musculoskeletal; multiple sclerosis
mu	milliunit
Na	sodium
neb	nebulizer
NK_1	neurokinin-1
NPO	nothing by mouth
NS	normal saline
NSAID	nonsteroidal anti-inflammatory drug
NYHA	New York Heart Association
O_2	oxygen
OBRA	Omnibus Reconciliation Act
OCD	obsessive-compulsive disorder
ONC	oncologic
oint	ointment
ophth	ophthalmic
OTC	over the counter
oz	ounce
P_i	inorganic phosphorus
PABA	para-aminobenzoic acid
$PaCO_2$	arterial partial pressure of carbon dioxide
PAF	paroxysmal atrial fibrillation
PAH	pulmonary arterial hypertension
PaO_2	arterial partial pressure of oxygen
PASI	psoriasis evaluation score
pc	after meals
PCA	patient-controlled analgesia
PCI	percutaneous coronary intervention
PCP	*Pneumocystis carinii* pneumonia
PCWP	pulmonary capillary wedge pressure
PDE-5	phosphodiesterase-5
PE	phenytoin equivalent

PEMA	phenylethylmalonamide
PFTs	pulmonary function tests
PID	pelvic inflammatory disease
PM, **pm**	post meridiem
PO	by mouth
PO$_4$	phosphate
postop	postoperative
PPH	primary pulmonary hypertension
pr	per rectum
prn	as needed
PSA	prostate-specific antigen
PSVT	paroxysmal supraventricular tachycardia
PT	prothrombin time
PTCA	percutaneous coronary transluminal angioplasty
PTH	parathyroid hormone
PTSD	post-traumatic stress disorder
PTT	partial thromboplastin time
PUD	peptic ulcer disease
PVC	premature ventricular contraction
PVR	peripheral vascular resistance
q	every
qAM	every morning
qday	every day
qh	every hour
qid	four times a day
qod	every other day
qPM	every night
q2h	every 2 hours
q3h	every 3 hours
q4h	every 4 hours
q6h	every 6 hours
q8h	every 8 hours
q12h	every 12 hours
RAIU	radioactive iodine uptake
RBC	red blood cell count
RDA	recommended daily allowance
rhPDGF	recombinant human platelet-derived growth factor
RIA	radioimmune assay
RLS	restless legs syndrome
RNA	ribonucleic acid
R-O	rule out
SA	sinoatrial
SC	subcutaneous
SCr	serum creatinine
sec	second
SGOT	serum glutamate oxaloacetate transaminase
SGPT	serum glutamate pyruvate transaminase
SIADH	syndrome of inappropriate antidiuretic hormone

SL	sublingual
SMX	sulfamethoxazole
SO_4	sulfate
sol	solution
SSRI	selective serotonin reuptake inhibitor
supp	suppository
susp	suspension
sust	sustained
SVR	systemic vascular resistance
SVT	supraventricular tachyarrythmias
syr	syrup
t1/2	half-time
T_3	triiodothyronine
T_4	thyroxine
tab	tablet
TB	tuberculosis, tuberculin
TCA	tricyclic antidepressant
temp	temperature
TEN	toxic epidermal necrolysis
TFTs	thyroid function test
TIA	transient ischemic attack
tid	three times a day
tinc	tincture
TK	tyrosine kinases
TMP	trimethoprim
TNF	tumor necrosis factor
top	topical
tPA	tissue plasminogen activator
TPN	total parenteral nutrition
TSH	thyroid stimulating hormone
TT	thrombin time
TTP	thrombotic thrombocytopenic purpura
U	unit
UA	urinalysis
ULN	upper limits of normal
UPDRS	United Parkinson Disease Rating Scale
URI	upper respiratory infection
UTI	urinary tract infection
UV	ultraviolet
UVA	ultraviolet A (long-wave)
vag	vaginal
Vd	volume of distribution
VEGF	vascular endothelial growth factor
VLDL	very low density lipoprotein
VMA	vanillylmandelic acid
vol	volume
VRE	vancomycin-resistant enterococcus
VREF	vancomycin-resistant Enterococcus faecium

VS	vital signs
w/	with
WBC	white blood cell count
wk	week
w/o	without
-XL, -XR	extended release preparations
yr	year

Medication use

Rebecca J. Beyth, M.D., M.Sc., and Ronald I. Shorr, M.D., M.S.

Summary Points

- In older persons, the relative increase in body fat and the decrease in lean body mass alter drug distribution so that fat-soluble drugs are distributed more widely and water-soluble drugs are distributed less widely.
- The cytochrome P450 (CYP) 3A hepatic metabolism of medications may result in a new medication causing a dangerous side effect of another medication, which was previously safely prescribed.
- An important pharmacokinetic change that occurs in persons of advanced age is that of reduced renal drug elimination.
- The sensitivity to drug effects may either increase or decrease with increasing age.
- The physician must carefully understand that protocol medicine may not be relevant to a heterogeneous older population.
- Nonadherence to medications is more common in older patients because they simply are prescribed more medications than younger patients.
- Poor communication with the prescribing physician, coupled with a decline in cognitive abilities, make older patients particularly vulnerable to misuse of medications.
- Older patients may attain adherence rates as high as 80% to 90% if they are given clear written and verbal instructions, a simple dosing schedule, and a reduced number of medications.
- Multiple comorbid conditions, environmental conditions, genetic variations, and the physiologic effects of aging all interact with each other to affect drug disposition in the elderly.
- Older patients are at increased risk of incurring adverse reactions from numerous classes of drugs.
- The incidence of adverse drug reactions in hospitalized patients increases with advanced age.
- Adverse drug reactions are often not recognized because the symptoms are nonspecific or mimic the symptoms of other illnesses.
- Polypharmacy correlates strongly with the incidence of adverse drug reactions.
- "Beers' list" of potentially inappropriate medications for seniors includes both older problematic medications and newer agents.

General issues in geriatric practice

Persons aged 65 and older compose only about 12% of the United States population, yet one third of all drugs are prescribed for them, and they consume more than 50% of over-the-counter medicines as well. Overall, more than 80% of all older people take at least one medication daily. Because an increasing number of patients are surviving to older ages and now account for such a large proportion of drug use, it is necessary for health care providers to understand the risks, benefits, and consequences of drug therapy in older patients. Several important pharmacologic and nonpharmacologic issues influence the safety and effectiveness of drug therapy in this population. This chapter focuses on these issues and attempts to offer practical suggestions to physicians who prescribe drugs for older patients.

Overview of clinical pharmacology
Pharmacokinetics
Pharmacokinetics, or the study of the action of a drug in the body over a period of time, changes with age. The physiologic changes that accompany aging affect the pharmacologic processes of absorption, distribution, metabolism, and excretion (Table 1). The effects of these age-related changes are variable and difficult to predict.[1] Some of these physiologic changes are related solely to aging, whereas others most likely are due to the combined effects of age, disease, and the environment. Although increasing age is often accompanied by reductions in the physiologic reserve of many organ systems independent of the effects of disease, these changes are not uniform. There is substantial variation from individual to individual, making some older patients more vulnerable than others. The alterations in pharmacokinetics and pharmacodynamics that occur with increasing age suggest a pharmacologic basis for concern about the vulnerability of the elderly to the effects of medications. Unfortunately, the results of epidemiologic studies that explore these relationships are unclear, in part because of the small number of older people included in premarketing studies relative to the patient population most likely to be exposed to the drug. The oldest old (i.e., those aged 80 or older) have generally not been included in clinical trials of investigational drugs, and those older subjects who do participate in such trials tend to be healthy "young-old" people. Thus, the results of these trials and the side effects reported often have limited application to the older patient with multiple illnesses who is taking several medications. In general, consideration of the individual patient, his or her physiologic status (i.e., hydration, nutrition, and cardiac output), and how this status affects the pharmacology of a particular drug are more important in prescribing that drug than any specific age-related changes.

Table 1 Age-related changes relevant to drug pharmacology

Pharmacologic process	Physiologic change	Clinical significance
Absorption	Decreased absorptive surface Decreased splanchnic blood flow Increased gastric pH Altered gastrointestinal motility	Little change in absorption with age
Distribution	Decreased total body water Decreased lean body mass Increased body fat Decreased serum albumin	Higher concentration of drugs that distribute in body fluids; increased distribution and often prolonged elimination half-lives of fat-soluble drugs
	Altered protein binding	Increased free fraction in plasma of some highly protein-bound acidic drugs
Metabolism	Reduced hepatic mass Reduced hepatic blood flow Decreased phase I metabolism	Often decreased first-pass metabolism and decreased rate of biotransformation of some drugs

Pharmacologic process	Physiologic change	Clinical significance
Elimination	Reduced renal plasma flow Reduced glomerular filtration rate Decreased tubular secretion function	Decreased renal elimination of drugs and metabolites; marked interindividual variation
Tissue sensitivity	Alterations in receptor number Alterations in receptor affinity Alterations in second-messenger function Alterations in cellular and nuclear responses	Patients are "more sensitive" or "less sensitive" to an agent

Absorption of drugs, which occurs mainly via passive diffusion, changes little with advancing age. The changes listed in Table 1 could potentially affect drug absorption. More important changes result from the concurrent administration of several medications. For example, antacids decrease the oral absorption of cimetidine, and alcohol accelerates the absorption of chloral hydrate.

Unlike absorption, drug distribution is affected by age in clinically meaningful ways. In older persons, the relative increase in body fat and the decrease in lean body mass alter drug distribution so that fat-soluble drugs are distributed more widely and water-soluble drugs are distributed less widely (Table 2). The increased distribution of fat-soluble drugs can delay elimination and may result in prolonged duration of action of a single dose. This effect is especially important for drugs such as hypnotics and analgesics, which are given in single doses on an intermittent basis. For example, the volume of distribution of diazepam is increased almost two-fold in older patients, and the elimination half-life is prolonged from 24 hours in young patients to approximately 90 hours in older patients.

Table 2 Volumes of distribution of commonly prescribed drugs

Increased volume*	Decreased volume*
Acetaminophen	Cimetidine
Chlordiazepoxide	Digoxin
Diazepam	Ethanol
Oxazepam	Gentamicin
Prazosin	Meperidine
Salicylates	Phenytoin
Thiopental	Quinine
Tolbutamide	Theophylline

*If the volume of distribution is decreased, drug levels tend to be higher.

In contrast, the volume of distribution of water-soluble compounds to reach a target plasma concentration is decreased. Likewise, due to the decreased volume of distribution, the loading dose of aminoglycosides is less in older patients.

For drugs that bind to serum proteins, equilibrium exists between the bound or ineffective portion and the unbound (free) or effective portion. For acidic drugs that are highly bound to albumin, the free plasma concentration may correlate best with pharmacologic effect. Although albumin levels decrease only slightly with age, they tend to decrease during periods of illness. This can result in elevated levels of free (unbound) acidic drugs in older persons during episodes of illness, and thus in an increased potential for toxicity. These changes can be significant for drugs such as thyroid hormone, digoxin, warfarin, and phenytoin.

Overall, changes in protein binding are an important consideration initially when a drug is being started, when the dosage is changed, when serum protein levels change, or when a drug displaces other protein-bound drugs. Because the free portion of the drug is generally smaller than the bound portion, the normal mechanisms of metabolism and excretion ultimately eliminate the free drug. If either hepatic or renal function is impaired due to age or disease, this elimination may be slowed.

Although in vitro studies of drug-metabolizing enzyme activity from human liver biopsy samples have not demonstrated any changes with aging, some investigators speculate that the decline in liver size with age may result in decreased metabolic capacity. A significant decline in liver blood flow occurs with age, with reductions of 25% to 47% being reported in persons between the ages of 25 and 90. This decrease in hepatic blood flow is clinically important because hepatic metabolism is the rate-limiting step that determines the clearance of most metabolized drugs. This change is especially relevant for drugs that undergo rapid hepatic metabolism (e.g., propranolol). Also, drugs that undergo extensive first-pass metabolism are likely to reach higher blood levels if hepatic blood flow is decreased.

The liver metabolizes drugs through two distinct systems. Phase I metabolism involves drug oxidation, reduction, and hydrolysis, and phase II metabolism involves glucuronidation, sulfation, acetylation, and methylation. Phase I metabolism is catalyzed primarily by the cytochrome P450 (CYP) system in the smooth endoplasmic reticulum of hepatocytes. CYP enzymes are a superfamily of microsomal drug-metabolizing enzymes that are important in the biosynthesis and degradation of endogenous compounds such as steroids, lipids, and vitamins, as well as the metabolism of most commonly used drugs. Phase I metabolism activity decreases substantially with age. Drugs that are metabolized through phase I enzymatic activity have prolonged half-lives. Examples of drugs whose metabolism is slowed because of these age-related changes in hepatic metabolism are listed in Box 1.

BOX 1
Commonly prescribed drugs with prolonged hepatic metabolism

- Acetaminophen
- Amitriptyline
- Barbiturates
- Chlordiazepoxide
- Diazepam
- Diphenhydramine
- Flurazepam
- Ibuprofen
- Labetalol
- Lidocaine
- Meperidine
- Nortriptyline
- Phenytoin
- Prazosin
- Propranolol
- Quinidine
- Salicylates
- Theophylline
- Tolbutamide
- Warfarin

Age-related changes in phase I metabolism coupled with the use of multiple medications place older patients at increased risk for adverse drug reactions. Adverse drug reactions occur due to either inhibition or induction of CYP enzymes, especially CYP3A, which is believed to be involved in the metabolism of more than one half of the currently prescribed drugs.[2,3] Clinical outcomes are determined by the potency of the CYP3A inhibitor (moderate versus potent), the availability of alternative pathways, and the seriousness of the symptoms. A drug is considered a potent CYP3A inhibitor if it causes more than a fivefold increase in the plasma concentration of another drug that is primarily dependent on CYP3A for its metabolism.[4] Examples of CYP3A inhibitors and inducers are listed in Table 3. Thus, clinicians should be cogent of potential drug interactions when they prescribe drugs from classes that include potent or moderate inhibitors of CYP3A. If a potent CYP3A inhibitor or inducer and substrate must be taken together, dosage adjustment and close clinical monitoring are warranted to avoid adverse reactions. Because the number of drug-drug interactions related to the CYP system is large, the interested reader is referred to tables at a Website of the Indiana University School of Medicine (http://medicine.iupui.edu/flockhart/clinlist.htm).

Table 3 Common drug substrates, inhibitors, and inducers of CYP3A, according to drug class*

CYP3A substrates	CYP3A inhibitors	CYP3A inducers
Calcium channel blockers	Calcium channel blockers	Rifamycins
Diltiazem	Diltiazem	Rifabutin
Felodipine	Verapamil	Rifampin
Nifedipine		Rifapentine
Verapamil	Azole antifungal agents	
	Itraconazole	Anticonvulsant agents
Immunosuppressant agents	Ketoconazole	Carbamazepine
Cyclosporine		Phenobarbital
Tacrolimus	Macrolide antibiotics	Phenytoin
	Clarithromycin	
Benzodiazepines	Erythromycin	Anti-HIV agents
Alprazolam	Troleandomycin	Efavirenz
Midazolam	(not azithromycin)	Nevirapine
Triazolam		
	Anti-HIV agents	Other
Statins	Delavirdine	St. John's wort
Atorvastatin	Indinavir	
Lovastatin	Ritonavir	
(not pravastatin)	Saquinavir	
Macrolide antibiotics	Others	
Clarithromycin	Grapefruit juice	
Erythromycin	Mifepristone	
	Nefazodone	
Anti-HIV agents		
Indinavir		
Nelfinavir		
Ritonavir		
Saquinavir		
Others		
Losartan		
Sildenafil		

*These inhibitors and inducers can interact with any CYP3A substrate and may have important clinical consequences. HIV, human immunodeficiency virus.
From Wilkinson GR: Drug metabolism and variability among patients in drug response. N. Engl J Med 2005; 352:2217.

Phase II hepatic metabolism involves the conjugation of drugs or their metabolites to organic substrates. The elimination of drugs that undergo phase II metabolism by conjugation (i.e., acetylation, glucouronidation, sulfation, and glycine conjugation) is generally altered less with age. Thus, drugs that require only phase II metabolism for excretion (e.g., triazolam) do not have a prolonged half-life in older people. These drugs contrast with drugs such as diazepam that undergo both phases of metabolism and have active intermediate metabolites. Although the effect of aging on hepatic drug metabolism is variable, phase I metabolism is the process that is most likely to decrease in older persons.

The apparent variable effect of age on drug metabolism is probably due to the fact that age is only one of many factors that affect drug metabolism. For example, cigarette smoking, alcohol intake, dietary modification, drugs, viral illness, caffeine intake, and other unknown factors also affect the rate of drug metabolism.

Induction of drug metabolism can occur in older persons. The rate of elimination of theophylline is increased by smoking and by phenytoin in both young and older persons alike.[1] Thus, this adaptive response is preserved with age. Not all metabolizing isoenzymes are induced equally in the young and the old. For example, antipyrine elimination is increased after pretreatment with dichlorolphenazone in younger patients but not in older patients.

An important pharmacokinetic change that occurs in persons of advanced age is that of reduced renal drug elimination (Box 2). This change results from the age-related decline in both glomerular filtration rate and tubular function. Drugs that depend on glomerular function (e.g., gentamicin) and drugs that depend on tubular secretion (e.g., penicillin) for elimination both exhibit reduced excretion in older patients. Because drug elimination is correlated with creatinine clearance, measurement of creatinine clearance is helpful in determining the maintenance dose. In the kidney, the average creatinine clearance declines by 50% from age 25 to age 85 despite a serum creatinine level that remains unchanged at approximately 1.0 mg/dL. Because the serum creatinine (Cr) tends to overestimate the actual creatinine clearance in older persons, the commonly cited formula devised by Cockroft and Gault may be used to estimate creatinine clearance (CrCl) in older adults:

$$CrCl = \frac{(140 - age) \times wt\ (kg)}{7.2 \times serum\ Cr\ (mg/dl)}$$

BOX 2
Drugs with decreased renal elimination in older persons

- Amantadine
- Ampicillin
- Atenolol
- Ceftriaxone
- Cephradine
- Cimetidine
- Digoxin
- Doxycycline
- Furosemide
- Gentamicin
- Hydrochlorothiazide
- Kanamycin
- Lithium
- Pancuronium
- Penicillin
- Phenobarbital
- Procainamide
- Ranitidine
- Sotalol
- Triamterene

In women, the estimated value is 85% of the calculated value at the same weight and serum creatinine concentration. Although this equation is useful in adjusting for age, weight, and the measured serum creatinine level, it does not account for individual variation. This formula has been validated in ambulatory and hospitalized patients, but some studies suggest that it may not be accurate when applied to frail nursing home patients.[5]

Altered renal clearance leads to two clinically relevant consequences: (1) the half-lives of renally excreted drugs are prolonged, and (2) the serum levels of these drugs are increased. For drugs with large therapeutic indexes (e.g., penicillin), this is of little clinical importance, but for drugs with a narrower therapeutic index (e.g., digoxin, cimetidine, aminoglycosides), side effects may occur in older patients if dose reductions are not made. Thus, it is not surprising that digoxin is the drug that most often causes side effects in the elderly, especially if the dose exceeds 0.125 mg/day.[6]

To further define dose requirements, therapeutic drug monitoring should also be performed for drugs with a low therapeutic index.

Pharmacodynamics

In addition to the factors that determine the drug concentration at the site of action (pharmacokinetics), the effect of a drug also depends on the sensitivity of the target organ to the drug. The biochemical and physiologic effects of drugs and their mechanisms of action (pharmacodynamics) and the effects of aging are not clearly known. Pharmacodynamics has been even less extensively studied in older patients than pharmacokinetics. Generalizations are not straightforward, and the effect of age on sensitivity to drugs varies with the drug studied and the response measured. These differences in sensitivity occur in the absence of marked reductions in the metabolism of the drug and its related compounds. Thus, sensitivity to drug effects may either increase or decrease with increasing age.

For example, older patients seem to be more sensitive to the sedative effects of given blood levels of benzodiazepine drugs (e.g., diazepam) but less sensitive to the effects of drugs mediated by β-adrenergic receptors (e.g., isoproterenol, propranolol). Although an age-related decline in hormone receptor affinity or number (e.g., in β-adrenergic receptors) is suspected, definitive data demonstrating such an alteration are sparse. Other possible explanations offered for these differences are alterations in second-messenger function and alterations in cellular and nuclear responses.

Because the response of older patients to any given medication is variable and cannot be foreseen, all drugs should be used appropriately but judiciously in older patients, and the physician should resist the temptation to apply protocol medicine. In general, knowledge of the pharmacology of the drugs prescribed, limits on the number of drugs used, determination of the preparation and dosage of the drug based on the patient's general condition and ability to handle the drug, combined with downward adjustment of the dose in the presence of known hepatic or renal impairment, and surveillance for untoward effects will minimize the risks of medication use in the elderly.

Therapeutic risks: Special considerations in the elderly
Adherence to drug therapy

Despite consideration by the clinician of age-related changes and possible drug-drug and drug-disease interactions, the full benefit of a drug may not be seen if the patient does not take the drug as prescribed. Adherence is the extent to which a patient's behavior concurs with the directions provided by his or her physician. Nonadherence with medication prescriptions is a problem common in patients of all ages and is not unique to older patients.[7] But because older patients use more medications than younger patients, and nonadherence increases in proportion to the number of medications used, nonadherence is more common in older patients.

Nonadherence with drug therapy is reported to occur in one third to one half of older patients. Approximately one in five prescriptions is not filled, and between one third and two thirds of patients who do fill their prescriptions use the medication in a manner different from that intended. Several causes of nonadherence have been identified and are listed in Table 4.

Table 4 Factors influencing adherence

Factor	Effect on adherence
Age	None
Sex	None
Education level	None
Ethnicity	None
Financial status	None
Actual severity of disease	None
Actual effectiveness or toxicity of drug	None
Belief by the patient that the disease being treated is serious	None
Belief by the patient that the medication will treat or prevent the disease or condition	Increase
Careful explanation by the doctor of the purpose of the medication	Increase
Number of drugs used	Decrease
Long duration of therapy	Decrease
Complex scheduling	Decrease
Safety closure bottles	Decrease

The cost of medication and insurance coverage can affect adherence in various ways. Patients may not purchase drugs if they cannot afford the out-of-pocket cost. On the other hand, expensive medications are sometimes perceived as being more powerful and therefore more beneficial. If patients do not pay for their medications because of their insurance benefits, adherence with the more expensive medications may be increased.

Among the causes of adherence, careful explanation by the physician of the purpose of the medication is especially important for older patients.[8] Poor communication with the prescribing physician, coupled with a decline in cognitive abilities, make older patients particularly vulnerable to misuse of medications. Persons with mild dementia may forget to take medications even though they are otherwise capable of living in an unsupervised environment. In fact, most or 90% of instances of nonadherence take the form of underadherence or taking too little of a prescribed medication.[9] Devices that sound a buzzer to remind patients to take a medication, reminder calls from a family member or friend, and the act of laying out medications daily are helpful aids in improving adherence. If possible, it is helpful to prescribe medications that can be taken less frequently. In fact, older patients may attain adherence rates as high as 80% to 90% if they are given clear written and verbal instructions, a simple dosing schedule, and a reduced number of medications.[10]

Serious complications can arise if the prescriber incorrectly assumes that the patient has adhered to the therapy. When a medication appears to be ineffective, the prescriber often increases the dose or prescribes a more powerful drug. A change in circumstance, such as increased supervision from a home nursing agency or family member or hospitalization, can then lead to toxicity.

Another kind of problem with adherence is exemplified by the role of diet in the adjustment of diuretics and oral hypoglycemic agents. The dosages of these medications are often prescribed initially in the hospital, where the patient's diet is strictly controlled. However, when the patient is discharged to a less controlled environment where he or she does not adhere to salt or carbohydrate restrictions, readmission for congestive heart failure or hyperglycemia may result. This type of adverse outcome might be avoided if the medication were adjusted to a more realistic diet while the patient is still in the hospital.

Knowledge base of safety and efficacy

Drug therapy in elderly persons is complicated by many factors that are unique to this age group. Multiple comorbid conditions, environmental conditions, genetic variations, and the physiologic effects of aging all interact with each other to affect drug disposition in the elderly. Although a judicious use of medications can profoundly affect the mortality and morbidity of many diseases in the elderly, appropriate use of medications is hampered by a lack of data. There are few data on the effects of age at the site of drug action, and likewise, there is insufficient information about drug disposition and response in the very elderly, those over 85 years of age.[11] These older patients, who are often the intended targets of new drug therapies, are usually not recruited to participate in clinical drug trials, so extrapolations on dosage and possible side effects of drugs may or may not be appropriate.

Risk of adverse drug reactions

An adverse drug reaction is defined as harm directly caused by a drug. Older patients are at increased risk of incurring adverse reactions from certain classes of drugs. *Primum non nocere* ("first do no harm") is a phrase that is especially applicable when prescribing drugs for the elderly. Adverse drug reactions are the most common form of iatrogenic illness. The incidence of adverse drug reactions in hospitalized patients increases from about 10% in 40- to 50-year-old patients to 25% in patients older than 80. In the ambulatory setting, Gurwitz and associates[12] found that the overall rate of adverse drug events was 50.1 per 1000 person-years, with a rate of 13.8 preventable adverse drug events per 1000 person-years. Of the adverse drug events, 578 (38.0%) were categorized as serious, life-threatening, or fatal; 244 (42.2%) of these more severe events were deemed preventable. Errors associated with preventable adverse drug events occurred most often at the stages of prescribing and monitoring, but adverse drug events related to patient adherence also were common. Cardiovascular medications, diuretics, nonopioid analgesics, hypoglycemics, and anticoagulants were the most common medication categories associated with preventable adverse drug events. In nursing homes, Gurwitz and colleagues[13] found that the overall rate of adverse drug events was 9.8 per 100 resident-months, with a rate of 4.1 preventable adverse drug events per 100 resident-months. Errors associated with preventable events occurring most often at the stages of ordering and monitoring were observed.

Many drugs commonly prescribed for older patients result in potentially life-threatening or disabling adverse reactions (Table 5). Cardiovascular and psychotropic drugs are the agents most commonly associated with serious adverse reactions in the elderly. This fact results from a combination of their narrow therapeutic-toxic window, age-related changes such as reduced renal excretion and a prolonged duration of action, which predispose the older patient to adverse reactions. Because clinical drug trials generally do not require drugs to be tested in the population that will ultimately receive them (i.e., older patients with one or more serious illnesses), the risk-versus-benefit ratio of most drugs is not clearly known for older patients. Adverse drug reactions are often not recognized because the symptoms are nonspecific or mimic the symptoms of other illnesses. Often another drug is prescribed to treat these symptoms, resulting in polypharmacy and further increasing the likelihood of an adverse drug reaction. This effect may be compounded when patients visit multiple physicians who prescribe drugs independently of each other. Drugs that are commonly prescribed for older patients that can interact with each other are described in Table 6.

Table 5 Examples of adverse drug reactions

Type of drug	Common adverse reactions
Aminoglycosides	Renal failure, hearing loss
Antiarrhythmics	Diarrhea (quinidine); urinary retention (disopyramide)
Anticholinergics	Dry mouth, constipation, urinary retention, delirium
Antipsychotics	Delirium, sedation, hypotension, extrapyramidal movement disorders
Diuretics	Dehydration, hyponatremia, hypokalemia, incontinence
Narcotics	Constipation
Sedative-hypnotics	Excessive sedation, delirium, gait disturbances

Table 6 Examples of potentially important drug-drug interactions

Example	Interaction	Potential effects
Antacids with digoxin, isoniazid (INH), and antipsychotics	Interference with drug absorption	Decreased drug effectiveness
Cimetidine with propranolol, theophylline, phenytoin (Dilantin)	Altered metabolism	Decreased drug clearance, increased risk of toxicity
Lithium with diuretics	Altered excretion	Increased risks of toxicity and electrolyte imbalance
Warfarin with oral hypoglycemics, aspirin, chloral hydrate	Displacement from binding proteins	Increased effects and risk of toxicity

Despite the association of increased adverse drug reactions with older age, many studies have failed to show an effect independent of age. What is known is that polypharmacy correlates strongly with the incidence of adverse drug reactions and, as noted earlier, older patients are prescribed more drugs than their younger counterparts. Older patients also have other characteristics that further predispose them to adverse drug reactions. These include a greater severity of illness, multiple comorbidities, smaller body size, changes in hepatic and renal metabolism and excretion, and prior drug reactions. The more common types of potential adverse drug interactions in older patients are drug displacement from protein-binding sites by other highly protein-bound drugs, induction or suppression of the metabolism of other drugs, and the additive effects of different drugs on blood pressure and mental function. Additionally, several drugs also interact adversely with underlying medical conditions in older patients creating "drug-disease" interactions (Table 7). Health care providers should not only have a thorough knowledge of the more common drug side effects, adverse drug reactions, and potential drug interactions in older patients; they should also question patients about common side effects when they review drug regimens.

Table 7 Some important drug-disease interactions in older patients

Disease	Drug	Adverse effects
Cardiac conduction disorders	Tricyclic antidepressants	Heart block
Chronic obstructive pulmonary disease	β-Blockers, opiates	Bronchoconstriction, respiratory depression
Chronic renal impairment	NSAIDs, contrast agents, aminoglycosides	Acute renal failure
Congestive heart failure	β-Blockers, verapamil	Acute cardiac decompensation
Dementia	Psychotropic drugs, levodopa, antiepileptic agents	Increased confusion, delirium
Depression	β-Blockers, centrally acting antihypertensives, alcohol, benzodiazepines, corticosteroids	Precipitation or exacerbation of depression
Diabetes mellitus	Diuretics, prednisone	Hyperglycemia
Glaucoma	Antimuscarinic drugs	Acute glaucoma
Hypertension	NSAIDs	Increase in blood pressure
Hypokalemia	Digoxin	Cardiac arrhythmias
Peptic ulcer disease	NSAIDs, anticoagulants	Gastrointestinal hemorrhage
Peripheral vascular disease	β-blockers	Intermittent claudication
Prostatic hyperplasia	Antimuscarinic agents	Urinary retention

"Appropriate" drug therapy in older adults

In 1991, Beers and colleagues developed a list of medications identified by a multidisciplinary group of experts to be inappropriate for routine use in older adults. These medications, sometimes known as the "Beers' list" have evolved as new agents have been identified as potentially problematic in older patients[14] (Table 8). Agents identified as potentially inappropriate include certain pain relievers, long-acting benzodiazepines, anticholinergic agents, and antihypertensive agents. Individual patients may tolerate one or more of these agents, especially in the setting of long-term use; however, if new drug therapy is initiated in older adults, the Beers' list can help to identify agents to avoid as first-line therapy.

Table 8 2002 criteria for potentially inappropriate medication use in older adults: independent of diagnoses or conditions

Drug	Concern	Severity Rating (high or low)
Propoxyphene (Darvon) and combination products (Darvon with ASA, Darvon-N, and Darvocet-N)	Offers few analgestic advantages over acetaminophen, yet has the adverse effects of other narcotic drugs.	Low
Indomethacin (Indocin and Indocin SR)	Of all available nonsteroidal anti-inflammatory drugs, this drug produces the most CNS adverse effects.	High

Drug	Concern	Severity Rating (high or low)
Pentazocine (Talwin)	Narcotic analgesic that causes more CNS adverse effects, including confusion and hallucinations, more commonly than other narcotic drugs. Additionally, it is a mixed agonist and antagonist.	High
Trimethobenzamide (Tigan)	One of the least effective antiemetic drugs, yet it can cause extrapyramidal adverse effects.	High
Muscle relaxants and antispasmodics: methocarbamol (Robaxin), carisoprodol (Soma), chlorzoxazone (Paraflex), metaxalone (Skelaxin), cyclobenzaprine (Flexeril), and oxybutynin (Ditropan) Do not consider the extended-release Ditropan XL	Most muscle relaxants and antispasmodic drugs are poorly tolerated by elderly patients, because these cause anticholinergic adverse effects, sedation, and weakness. Additionally, their effectiveness at doses tolerated by elderly patients is questionable.	High
Flurazepam (Dalmane)	This benzodiazepine hypnotic has an extremely long half-life in elderly patients (often days), producing prolonged sedation and increasing the incidence of falls and fracture. Medium- or short-acting benzodiazepines are preferable.	High
Amitriptyline (Elavil), chlordiazepoxide-amitriptyline (Limbitrol), and perphenazine-amitriptyline (Triavil)	Because of its strong anticholinergic and sedation properties, amitriptyline is rarely the antidepressant of choice for elderly patients.	High
Doxepin (Sinequan)	Because of its strong anticholinergic and sedating properties, doxepin is rarely the antidepressant of choice for elderly patients.	High
Meprobamate (Miltown and Equanil)	This is a highly addictive and sedating anxiolytic. Those using meprobamate for prolonged periods may become addicted and may need to be withdrawn slowly.	High

Drug	Concern	Severity Rating (high or low)
Doses of short-acting benzodiazepines: doses greater than lorazepam (Ativan) 3 mg; oxazepam (Serax), 60 mg; alprazolam (Xanax), 2 mg: temazepam (Restoril), 15 mg; and triazolam (Halcion), 0.25 mg	Because of increased sensitivity to benzoadiazepines in elderly patients, smaller doses may be effective as well as safer. Total daily doses should rarely exceed the suggested maximums.	High
Long-acting benzodiazepines: chlordiazepoxide (Librium) chlordiazepoxide amitriptyline (Limbitrol) clidinium-chlordiazepoxide (Librax), diazepam (Valium), quazepam (Doral), halazepam (Paxipam), and chlorazepate (Tranxene)	These drugs have a long half-life in elderly patients (often several days), producing prolonged sedation and increasing the risk of falls and fractures. Short- and intermediate-acting benzodiazepines are preferred if a benzodiazepine is required.	High
Disopyramide (Norpace and Norpace OR)	Of all antiarrhythmic drugs, this is the most potent negative inotrope and therefore may induce heart failure in elderly patients. It is also strongly anticholinergic. Other antiarrhythmic drugs should be used.	High
Digoxin (Lanoxin) (should not exceed 125 mg/d except when treating atrial arrhythmias)	Decreased renal clearance may lead to increased risk of toxic effects.	Low
Short-acting dipyridamole (Persantine). Do not consider the long-acting dipyridamole (which has better properties than the short-acting in older adults) except with patients with artificial heart valves	May cause orthostatic hypotension	Low
Methyldopa (Aldomet) and methyldopa-hydrochlorothiazide (Aldoril)	May cause bradycardia, and exacerbate depression in elderly patients.	High
Reserpine at doses 0.25 mg	May induce depression, impotence, sedation, and orthostatic hypotension.	Low
Chlorpropamide (Diabinese)	It has a prolonged half-life in elderly patients and could cause prolonged hypoglycemia. Additionally, it is the only oral hypoglycemic agent that causes SIADH.	High

Drug	Concern	Severity Rating (high or low)
Gastrointestinal antispasmodic drugs: dicyclomine (Bentyl), hyoscyamine (Levsin and Levsinex), propantheline (Pro-Banthine) belladonna alkaloids (Donnatal and others), and clidinium-chlordiazepoxide (Librax)	GI antispasmodic drugs are highly anticholinergic and have uncertain effectiveness. These drugs should be avoided (especially for long-term use).	High
Anticholinergics and antihistamines: chlorpheniramine (Chlor-Trimeton), diphenhydramine (Benadryl), hydroxyzine (Vistaril and Atarax), cyproheptadine (Periactin), promethazine (Phenergan), dexchlorpheniramine (Polaramine)	All nonprescription and many prescription antihistamines may have potent anticholinergic properties. Nonanticholinergic antihistamines are preferred in elderly patients when treating allergic reactions.	High
Diphenhydramine (Benadryl)	May cause confusion and sedation. Should not be used as a hypnotic, and when used to treat emergency allergic reactions, it should be used in the smallest possible dose.	High
Ergot mesyloids (Hydergine) and cyclandelate (Cyclospasmol)	Have not been shown to be effective in the doses studied.	Low
Ferrous sulfate >325 mg/d	Doses >325 mg/d do not dramatically increase the amount absorbed but greatly increase the incidence of constipation.	Low
All barbiturates (except phenobarbital) except when used to control seizures	Are highly addictive and cause more adverse effects than most sedative or hypnotic drugs in elderly patients.	High
Meperidine (Demerol)	Not an effective oral analgesic in doses commonly used. May cause confusion and has many disadvantages over other narcotic drugs.	High
Ticlopidine (Ticlid)	Has been shown to be no better than aspirin in preventing clotting and may be considerably more toxic. Safer, more effective alternatives exist.	High

Drug	Concern	Severity Rating (high or low)
Ketorolac (Toradol)	Immediate and long-term use should be avoided in older persons, because a significant number have asymptomatic GI pathologic conditions.	High
Amphetamines and anorexic agents	These drugs have potential for causing dependence, hypertension, angina, and myocardial infarction.	High
Long-term use of full dosage, longer half-life, non–COX-selective NSAIDs: naproxen (Naprosyn, Avaprox, and Aleve), oxaprozin (Daypro), and piroxicam (Feldene)	Have the potential to produce GI bleeding, renal failure, high blood pressure, and heart failure.	High
Daily fluoxetine (Prozac)	Long half-life of drug and risk of producing excessive CNS stimulation, sleep disturbances, and increasing agitation. Safer alternatives exist.	High
Long-term use of stimulant laxatives: bisacodyl (Dulcolax), cascara sagrada, and Neoloid except in the presence of opiate analgesic use	May exacerbate bowel dysfunction.	High
Amiodarone (Cordarone)	Associated with QT interval problems and risk of provoking torsades de pointes. Lack of efficacy in older adults.	High
Orphenadrine (Norflex)	Causes more sedation and anticholinergic adverse effects than safer alternatives.	High
Guanethidine (Ismelin)	May cause orthostatic hypotension. Safer alternatives exist.	High
Guanadrel (Hylorel)	May cause orthostatic hypotension.	High
Cyclandetate (Cyclospasmol)	Lack of efficacy.	Low
Isoxsurpine (Vasodilan)	Lack of efficacy.	Low
Nitrofurantoin (Macrodantin)	Potential for renal impairment. Safer alternatives available.	High
Doxazosin (Cardura)	Potential for hypotension, dry mouth, and urinary problems.	Low

Drug	Concern	Severity Rating (high or low)
Methyltestosterone (Android, Virilon, and Testrad)	Potential for prostatic hypertrophy and cardiac problems.	High
Thioridazine (Mellaril)	Greater potential for CNS and extrapyramidal adverse effects.	High
Mesoridazine (Serentil)	CNS and extrapyramidal adverse effects.	High
Short-acting nifedipine (Procardia and Adalat)	Potential for hypotension and constipation.	High
Clonidine (Catapres)	Potential for orthostatic hypotension and CNS adverse effects.	Low
Mineral oil	Potential for aspiration and adverse effects. Safer alternatives available.	High
Cimetidine (Tagamet)	CNS adverse effects, including confusion.	Low
Ethacrynic acid (Edecrin)	Potential for hypertension and fluid imbalances. Safer alternatives available.	Low
Desiccated thyroid	Concern about cardiac effects. Safer alternatives available.	High
Amphetamines (excluding methylphenidate hydrochloride and anorexics)	Stimulate adverse CNS effects.	High
Estrogens only (oral)	Evidence of the carcinogenic (breast and endometrial cancers) potential of these agents and lack of cardioprotective effect in older women.	Low

Abbreviations: CNS, central nervous system; COX, cyclooxygenase; GI, gastrointestinal; NSAIDs, nonsteroidal anti-inflammatory drugs; SIADH, syndrome of inappropriate antidiuretic hormone secretion. From Fick DM, Cooper JW, Wade WE, et al: Updating the Beers criteria for potentially inappropriate medication use in older adults: Results of a U.S. consensus panel of experts. Arch Intern Med 2003; 163:2716.

Complementary and alternative medications

The prevalence of complementary and alternative medication (CAM) is increasing among older adults. In a recent report, nearly two thirds of ambulatory elderly used at least one form of CAM, but much of CAM use was unrecognized by physicians. CAMs have been associated with adverse events (Table 9) and important drug interactions between CAMs and conventional drug therapies have been described (Table 10). A complete medication history in older adults should include an inquiry into the use of CAMs.[15,16]

Table 9 Potential adverse effects of herbal remedies and their major constituents*

Cardiotoxicity	Neurotoxicity or convulsions
Aconite root tuber	Aconite root tuber
Herbs rich in cardioactive glycosides	*Alocasia macrorrhiza* root tuber†
Herbs rich in colchicine	Artemisia species rich in santonin
Leigongteng	Essential oils rich in ascaridole
Licorice root	Essential oils rich in thujone
Mahuang	Ginkgo seed or leaf‡
Pokeweed leaf or root	Herbs rich in colchicine
Scotch broom†	Herbs rich in podophyllotoxin
Squirting cucumber†	Indian tobacco herb
Hepatotoxicity	Kava rhizome†
Certain herbs rich in anthranoids	Mahuang
Certain herbs rich in protoberberine alkaloids	Nux vomica
Chapparal leaf or stem	Pennyroyal oil
Germander species	Star fruit
Green-tea leaf†	Yellow jessamine rhizome
Herbs rich in coumarin	**Renal toxicity**
Herbs rich in podophyllotoxin	β-Aescin (saponin mixture from horse-chestnut seed)
Herbs rich in toxic pyrrolizidine alkaloids	Cape aloes†
Impila root	Cat's claw†
Kava rhizome	Certain essential oils
Kombucha	Chaparral leaf or stem†
Mahuang	Chinese yew
Pennyroyal oil	Herbs rich in aristolochic acids
Skullcap	Impila root
Soy phytoestrogens†	Jering fruit
	Pennyroyal oil
	Squirting cucumber†
	Star fruit

*The full version of this table is available from the National Auxiliary Publications Service (NAPS). (See NAPS document no. 05609 for 33 pages of supplementary material. To order, contact NAPS, c/o Microfiche Publications, 248 Hempstead Tpke., West Hempstead, NY 11552.) Adverse effects of multiple-herb therapies are not included. Case reports do not always provide adequate evidence that the remedy in question was labeled correctly. As a result, it is possible that some of the adverse events reported for a specific herb were actually due to a different, unidentified botanical or another adulterant or contaminant.

†A single case was reported without reference to previous cases.

‡Convulsions have been observed after large doses of yinguo (ginkgo seed), a traditional Asian food and medicine, which contains the convulsive agent 4'-O-methylpyridoxine (MPN).[12,13] Recently, anecdotal reports have associated ginkgo-containing preparations available on the Western market with seizures,[14] and these adverse events have also been reported in patients with seizure disorders stabilized by valproate.[15] How Western ginkgo preparations might induce seizures is still unclear. MPN has been detected in ginkgo leaf and preparations that contain it, but usually at subtoxic levels.[16]

From de Smet PA: Herbal remedies. N Engl J Med 2002; 347:2047.

Table 10 Potential interactions between herbs and conventional drugs*

Herb	Conventional drug	Comments
Ginkgo leaf	Acetylsalicylic acid Rofecoxib Warfarin Trazodone	Ginkgo combined with acetylsalicylic acid,† rofecoxib,† or warfarin† has been associated with bleeding reactions; ginkgo alone has also been associated with bleeding (case reports). Coma was reported in a patient with Alzheimer's disease who took ginkgo leaf with trazodone.†
Hawthorn leaf or flower	Digitalis glycosides	Because hawthorn may exert digitalis-like inotropic effects, it is prudent to monitor persons taking this herb in addition to digitalis glycosides closely.
St. John's wort	5-Aminolevulinic acid Amitriptyline Cyclosporine Digoxin Indianavir Midazolam Nefazodone Nevirapine Oral contraceptives Paroxetine Phenprocoumon Sertraline Simvastatin Tacrolimus Theophylline Warfarin	A phototoxic reaction occurred in a patient simultaneously exposed to 5-aminolevulinic acid and St. John's wort†; in clinical studies, pretreatment with St. John's wort decreased the area under the curve for amitriptyline (and its active metabolite nortriptyline), digoxin, indinavir, midazolam, phenprocoumon, and the active metabolite of simvastatin (simvastatin hydroxy acid)‡; case reports have associated St. John's wort with reduced levels of cyclosporine (sometimes with transplant rejection), tacrolimus†, and theophylline†; with increased oral clearance of nevirapine; with intermenstrual bleeding or altered menstrual bleeding in users of oral contraceptives; and with reduced effects of phenprocoumon† and warfarin; lethargy and grogginess were reported in a patient taking St. John's wort and paroxetine†, and the serotonin syndrome has been reported in users of nefazodone† or sertraline (case reports); St. John's wort alone has been associated with serotonin syndrome–like events (case reports).
Asian ginseng root	Phenelzine	Mania has been reported in a patient taking ginseng and phenelzine†; Asian ginseng alone has also been associated with mania.†
	Warfarin	A patient taking ginseng and warfarin had a decreased international normalized ratio.†
Garlic bulb	Ritonavir	Two brief case reports describe gastrointestinal toxic effects in patients taking garlic and ritonavir.
	Saquinavir	In a clinical study, the area under the curve for saquinavir decreased by 51% in patients taking garlic for 20 days; it returned to 65% of baseline after a 10-day washout period.
	Warfarin	A brief case report described an increased clotting time in two patients taking warfarin and garlic; garlic alone has also been associated with bleeding (case reports).

Herb	Conventional drug	Comments
Kava rhizome	Alprazolam Cimetidine Terazosin	Lethargy and disorientation were reported in a patient receiving this triple-drug regimen.†
Yohimbe bark	Centrally active antihypertensive agents	Yohimbine (a major alkaloid in yohimbe bark) may antagonize guanabenz and the methyldopa metabolite through its α_2-adrenoceptor antagonistic properties.
	Tricyclic antidepressants	In clinical studies, tricyclic antidepressants increased the sensitivity to the autonomic and central adverse effects of yohimbine (major alkaloid in yohimbine bark).

*The full version of this table is available from the National Auxilliary Publications Service (NAPS). (See NAPS document no. 05609 for 33 pages of supplementary material. To order, contact NAPS, c/o Microfiche Publications, 248 Hempstead Tpke., West Hempstead, NY 11552.) Interactions associated with multiple-herb therapies are not included. Case reports do not always provide adequate evidence that the remedy in question was labeled correctly. As a result, it is possible that some of the interactions reported for a specific herb were actually due to a different, unidentified bontanical or to another adulterant or contaminant.

†A single case was reported without reference to previous cases.

‡With the exception of phenprocoumon, these drugs are all substrates for cytochrome P-4503A, P-glycoprotein, or both.

From de Smet PA: Herbal remedies. N Engl J Med 2002; 347:2048.

Prescribing in the nursing home

Federal legislation has been implemented to limit the use of psychoactive drugs in nursing home residents. The Nursing Home Reform Amendments of the Omnibus Budget Reconciliation Act of 1987 (OBRA) require regulation of the use of psychoactive medications in Medicare- and Medicaid-certified nursing homes in the form of explicit documentation in the medical record to justify the need for such drugs, as well as close monitoring and periodic withdrawal of these antipsychotic medications. Guidelines for antipsychotics, anxiolytics, and sedatives were developed and implemented. Although the effects of these guidelines on the use of anxiolytics and sedatives have not been determined, the use of antipsychotic drugs in nursing homes has been shown to be reduced.[17]

The effectiveness of psychotropic drugs in the management of behavioral disturbances related to dementia has not been established.[18] Often, nonpharmacologic interventions may be just as effective with less risk in managing some of the behaviors seen in elderly nursing home residents.[19,20] Examples include increased tolerance from staff members for repetitive requests, specially designed facilities to accommodate freedom of movement and supervision, more personal attention and support, avoidance of caffeine at night, regular exercise, and later bedtimes.

Medicare Prescription Drug Improvement and Modernization Act

In 2003, the U.S. congress passed the Medicare Prescription Drug Improvement and Modernization Act (Medicare Part D), which provides Medicare beneficiaries the opportunity to receive prescription drugs with financial assistance from Medicare. In each U.S. state, beneficiaries select from a myriad of individual plans, each with a different formulary, deductible, and copayment structure. With a Medicare number, and a list of currently prescribed medications, individual patients can identify a plan with the lowest annual out-of-pocket expenses. Providers and pa-

tients are referred to the following Website: http://www.medicare.gov/medicarere
form/partdprototype.asp. Several classes of medicines are excluded from Medicare Part D: benzodiazepines, barbiturates, nonprescription drugs, most prescription vitamin and mineral products, drugs for weight loss or weight gain, and drugs
for the symptomatic relief of coughs or colds. Medicare Part D allows states,
through Medicaid, to pay for these agents for Medicare enrollees who are enrolled
in both programs.

Summary

It is important for health care providers to be aware of the issues involved in using
drug therapies in older patients, because older patients are most vulnerable to the
adverse effects of drugs. Although more data are needed to guide clinical decision
making in prescribing drugs for older patients, some simple considerations can
make drug use safer and more effective. Careful, compassionate attention to these
factors can have a profound effect on improving the quality of life, medication use,
and the overall cost of health care in this vulnerable population.

References

1. Cusack BJ: Pharmacokinetics in older persons. Am J Geriatr Pharmacother 2004;2:274-302.
2. Wilkinson GR: Drug metabolism and variability among patients in drug response. N Engl J Med 2005;352:2211-2221.
3. Ray WA, Murray KT, Meredith S, et al: Oral erythromycin and the risk of sudden death from car-diac causes. N Engl J Med 2004;351:1089-1096.
4. CYP3A and drug interactions. Med Lett Drugs Ther 2005;47:54-55.
5. Drusano GL, Munice HL Jr, Hoopes JM, et al: Commonly used methods of estimating creatinine clearance are inadequate for elderly debilitated nursing home patients. J Am Geriatr Soc 1988;36:437-441.
6. Nolan L, O'Malley K: Prescribing for the elderly. Part I: Sensitivity of the elderly to adverse drug reactions. J Am Geriatr Soc 1988;36:142-149.
7. Osterberg L, Blaschke T: Adherence to medication. N Engl J Med 2005;353:487-497.
8. Becker MH: Patient adherence to prescribed therapies. Med Care 1985;23:539-555.
9. Cooper JK, Love DW, Raffoul PR: Intentional prescription nonadherence (noncompliance) by the elderly. J Am Geriatr Soc 1982;30:329-333.
10. Black DM, Brand RJ, Greenlick M, et al: Compliance to treatment for hypertension in elderly pa-tients: The SHEP pilot study. Systolic Hypertension in the Elderly Program. J Gerontol 1987;42:552-557.
11. Gurwitz JH, Col NF, Avorn J: The exclusion of the elderly and women from clinical trials in acute myocardial infarction. JAMA 1992;268:1417-1422.
12. Gurwitz JH, Field TS, Harrold LR, et al: Incidence and preventability of adverse drug events among older persons in the ambulatory setting. JAMA 2003;289:1107-1116.
13. Gurwitz JH, Field TS, Judge J, et al: The incidence of adverse drug events in two large academic long-term care facilities. Am J Med 2005;118:251-258.
14. Fick DM, Cooper JW, Wade WE, et al: Updating the Beers criteria for potentially inappropriate medication use in older adults: Results of a U.S. consensus panel of experts. Arch Intern Med 2003;163:2716-2724.
15. Cohen RJ, Ek K, Pan CX: Complementary and alternative medicine (CAM) use by older adults: A comparison of self-report and physician chart documentation. J Gerontol A Biol Sci Med Sci 2002;57:M223-M227.
16. de Smet PA: Herbal remedies. N Engl J Med 2002;347:2046-2056.
17. Shorr RI, Fought RL, Ray WA: Changes in antipsychotic drug use in nursing homes during imple-mentation of the OBRA-87 regulations. JAMA 1994;271:358-362.
18. Sink KM, Holden KF, Yaffe K: Pharmacological treatment of neuropsychiatric symptoms of de-mentia: A review of the evidence. JAMA 2005;293:596-608.
19. Avorn J, Soumerai SB, Everitt DE, et al: A randomized trial of a program to reduce the use of psy-choactive drugs in nursing homes. N Engl J Med 1992;327:168-173.
20. Avorn J, Gurwitz JH: Drug use in the nursing home. Ann Intern Med 1995;123:195-204.

abacavir sulfate

(a-ba-ka'-vir sul'-fate)

■ **Brand Name(s):** Ziagen

> Combinations
> **Rx:** with lamivudine (Epzicom); with zidovudine and lamivudine (Trizivir)
> **Chemical Class:** Nucleoside analog

■ **Clinical Pharmacology:**
> **Mechanism of Action:** An antiretroviral that inhibits the activity of HIV-1 reverse transcriptase by competing with the natural substrate deoxyguanosine-5'-triphosphate (dGTP) and by its incorporation into viral DNA. **Therapeutic Effect:** Inhibits viral DNA growth.
> **Pharmacokinetics:** Rapidly and extensively absorbed after PO administration. Protein binding: 50%. Widely distributed, including to CSF and erythrocytes. Metabolized in the liver to inactive metabolites. Primarily excreted in urine. Unknown if removed by hemodialysis. **Half-life:** 1.5 hr.

■ **Available Forms:**
> • *Tablets*: 300 mg.
> • *Oral Solution*: 20 mg/ml.

■ **Indications and Dosages:**
> **HIV infection (in combination with other ID-antiretrovirals):** PO 300 mg twice a day or 600 mg once daily.
> **Dosage in hepatic impairment:** *Mild impairment*: 200 mg twice a day. *Moderate to severe impairment*: Not recommended.

■ **Contraindications:** Moderate or severe hepatic impairment

■ **Side Effects**
> **Frequent**
> Nausea (47%), nausea with vomiting (16%), diarrhea (12%), decreased appetite (11%)
> **Occasional**
> Insomnia (7%)

■ **Serious Reactions**
> • A hypersensitivity reaction may be life-threatening. Signs and symptoms include fever, rash, fatigue, intractable nausea and vomiting, severe diarrhea, abdominal pain, cough, pharyngitis, and dyspnea.
> • Life-threatening hypotension may occur.
> • Lactic acidosis and severe hepatomegaly may occur.

Special Considerations
> • Always check updated treatment guidelines before initiating or changing antiretroviral therapy. (http://AIDSinfo.nih.gov)

Patient/Family Education
- May administer without regard for food
- If you miss a dose: take the missed dose as soon as you remember, then go back to your normal dosing schedule; skip the missed dose if it is time for your next dose; do not take 2 doses at the same time
- Do not take any other medication, including OTC drugs, without consulting the physician
- Abacavir is not a cure for HIV infection, nor does it reduce the risk of transmitting HIV to others

Monitoring Parameters
- CBC, metabolic panel, CD4 lymphocyte count, HIV RNA level
- Pattern of daily bowel activity and stool consistency
- Weight

Geriatric side effects at a glance:
❏ CNS ☑ Bowel Dysfunction ❏ Bladder Dysfunction ❏ Falls

U.S. Regulatory Considerations
☑ FDA Black Box

Hypersensitivity Reactions: severe and fatal reactions associated with therapy. This drug should never be restarted after suspected hypersensitivity reaction as more severe symptoms can occur within hours and may include life-threatening hypotension and death. Severe or fatal reaction may occur within hrs after reintroduction of drug in patients with unrecognized symptoms of hypersensitivity.

❏ OBRA regulated in U.S. Long Term Care

abciximab

(ab-siks'-ih-mab)

Brand Name(s): ReoPro
Chemical Class: Glycoprotein (GP) IIb/IIIa inhibitor

Clinical Pharmacology:
Mechanism of Action: A glycoprotein IIb/IIIa receptor inhibitor that rapidly inhibits platelet aggregation by preventing the binding of fibrinogen to GP IIb/IIIa receptor sites on platelets. **Therapeutic Effect:** Prevents closure of treated coronary arteries. Prevents acute cardiac ischemic complications.

Pharmacokinetics: Rapidly cleared from plasma. Initial-phase half-life is less than 10 min; second-phase *half-life* is 30 min. Platelet function generally returns within 48 hr.

Available Forms:
- Injection: 2 mg/ml (5-ml vial).

Indications and Dosages:
Percutaneous coronary intervention (PCI): IV Bolus 0.25 mg/kg 10-60 min before angioplasty or atherectomy, then 12-hr IV infusion of 0.125 mcg/kg/min. Maximum: 10 mcg/min.

PCI (*unstable angina*): IV Bolus 0.25 mg/kg, followed by 18- to 24-hr infusion of 10 mcg/min, ending 1 hr after procedure.

■ **Contraindications:** Active internal bleeding, arteriovenous malformation or aneurysm, cerebrovascular accident (CVA) with residual neurologic defect, history of CVA (within the past 2 yr) or oral anticoagulant use within the past 7 days unless PT is less than 1.2 × control, history of vasculitis, hypersensitivity to murine proteins, intracranial neoplasm, prior IV dextran use before or during percutaneous transluminal coronary angioplasty (PTCA), recent surgery or trauma (within the past 6 wk), recent (within the past 6 wk or less) GI or GU bleeding, thrombocytopenia (less than 100,000 cells/μl), and severe uncontrolled hypertension

■ **Side Effects**
Frequent
Nausea (16%), hypotension (12%)
Occasional (9%)
Vomiting
Rare (3%)
Bradycardia, confusion, dizziness, pain, peripheral edema, urinary tract infection

■ **Serious Reactions**
- Major bleeding complications may occur. If complications occur, stop the infusion immediately.
- Hypersensitivity reaction may occur.
- Atrial fibrillation or flutter, pulmonary edema, and complete AV block occur occasionally.

Special Considerations

- Fab fragment of the chimeric human-murine monoclonal antibody 7E3
- Intended to be used with aspirin and heparin
- Discontinue if bleeding occurs that is not controlled by compression
- Discontinue if PTCA fails
- Eptifibatide, tirofiban, and abciximab can all decrease the incidence of cardiac events associated with acute coronary syndromes; direct comparisons are needed to establish which, if any, is superior; for angioplasty, until more data become available, abciximab appears to be the drug of choice

■ **Patient/Family Education**
- Use an electric razor and soft toothbrush to prevent bleeding
- Report signs of bleeding, including black or red stool, coffee-ground emesis, red or dark urine, or red-speckled mucus from cough

■ **Monitoring Parameters**
- Baseline platelet count, prothrombin time, aPTT; during INF closely monitor platelet count and aPTT (heparin therapy)
- Stop abciximab and heparin infusion if serious bleeding uncontrolled by pressure occurs
- Assess skin for ecchymosis and petechiae; also, assess for GI, GU, and retroperitoneal bleeding and for bleeding at all puncture sites
- Assess for signs and symptoms of hemorrhage, including a decrease in blood pressure, increase in pulse rate, abdominal or back pain, and severe headache
- Assess urine for hematuria

- **Geriatric side effects at a glance:**
  - ☐ CNS   ☐ Bowel Dysfunction   ☐ Bladder Dysfunction   ☐ Falls

- **U.S. Regulatory Considerations**
  - ☑ FDA Black Box
  Hypersensitivity reaction to this drug is a multi-organ clinical syndrome usually characterized by a sign or symptom in 2 or more of the following groups: 1) fever, 2) rash, 3) gastrointestinal (including nausea, vomiting, diarrhea, or abdominal pain), 4) constitutional (e.g., generalized malaise, fatigue, or achiness), and 5) respiratory (e.g., dyspnea, cough, or pharyngitis).
  - ☐ OBRA regulated in U.S. Long Term Care

acamprosate calcium

(ah-camp'-ro-sate kal'-see-um)

- **Brand Name(s):** Campral
  Chemical Class: Amino acid derivative

- **Clinical Pharmacology:**
  Mechanism of Action: An alcohol abuse deterrent that appears to interact with glutamate and gamma-aminobutyric acid neurotransmitter systems centrally, restoring their balance. **Therapeutic Effect:** Reduces alcohol dependence.
  Pharmacokinetics: Slowly absorbed from the GI tract. Steady-state plasma concentrations are reached within 5 days. Does not undergo metabolism. Excreted in urine.
  Half-life: 20-33 hr.

- **Available Forms:**
  - *Tablets*: 333 mg.

- **Indications and Dosages:**
  Maintenance of alcohol abstinence in alcohol-dependent patients who are abstinent at initiation of treatment: PO Two tablets 3 times a day.
  Dosage in renal impairment: For patients with creatinine clearance of 30-49 ml/min, dosage is decreased to 1 tablet 3 times a day.

- **Contraindications:** Severe renal impairment (creatinine clearance of 30 ml/min or less)

- **Side Effects**
  Frequent (17%)
  Diarrhea
  Occasional (6%-4%)
  Insomnia, asthenia, fatigue, anxiety, flatulence, nausea, depression, pruritus
  Rare (3%-1%)
  Dizziness, anorexia, paresthesia, diaphoresis, dry mouth

■ **Serious Reactions**
  • Acute renal failure has been reported.

Special Considerations
  • Does not cause disulfiram-like reaction with ingestion of alcohol
  • Higher doses appear to be more effective for maintaining abstinence
  • The optimal time to initiate therapy has not been identified

■ **Patient/Family Education**
  • Use caution operating hazardous machinery, including automobiles, until there is reasonable certainty that acamprosate will not affect ability to engage in such activities
  • Continue use even in the event of a relapse and discuss any renewed drinking with prescriber
  • To be used as part of a treatment program that includes psychosocial support

■ **Monitoring Parameters**
  • Maintenance of alcohol abstinence
  • Pattern of daily bowel activity and stool consistency

■ **Geriatric side effects at a glance:**
  ❏ CNS ❏ Bowel Dysfunction ❏ Bladder Dysfunction ❏ Falls

■ **U.S. Regulatory Considerations**
  ❏ FDA Black Box ❏ OBRA regulated in U.S. Long Term Care

acarbose

(ay'-car-bose)

■ **Brand Name(s):** Precose
  Chemical Class: α-Amylase inhibitor; α-glucosidase inhibitor

■ **Clinical Pharmacology:**
  Mechanism of Action: An alpha-glucosidase inhibitor that delays glucose absorption and digestion of carbohydrates, resulting in a smaller rise in blood glucose concentration after meals. **Therapeutic Effect:** Lowers postprandial hyperglycemia.
  Pharmacokinetics: Low absorption within the GI tract. Extensive metabolism in the intestinal wall. Degraded in the intestine by bacterial and digestive enzymes. Excreted in feces and urine. **Half-life:** 2 hr.

■ **Available Forms:**
  • *Tablets*: 25 mg, 50 mg, 100 mg.

■ **Indications and Dosages:**
  Diabetes mellitus: PO Initially, 25 mg 3 times a day with first bite of each main meal. May increase at 4- to 8-wk intervals. Maximum: For patients weighing more than 60 kg, 100 mg 3 times a day; for patients weighing 60 kg or less, 50 mg 3 times a day.

■ **Contraindications:** Chronic intestinal diseases associated with marked disorders of digestion or absorption, cirrhosis, colonic ulceration, conditions that may deteriorate as a result of increased gas formation in the intestine, diabetic ketoacidosis, hypersensitivity to acarbose, inflammatory bowel disease, partial intestinal obstruction or predisposition to intestinal obstruction, significant renal dysfunction (serum creatinine level greater than 2 mg/dl)

■ **Side Effects**
Side effects diminish in frequency and intensity over time.
Frequent
Transient GI disturbances: flatulence (77%), diarrhea (33%), abdominal pain (21%)

■ **Serious Reactions**
- None known.

Special Considerations
- Does not cause hypoglycemia
- Reduces HbA_{1c} 0.5%-1%
- Blood glucose; HbA_{1c} 3-6 mo
- Consider ALT/AST during first yr

■ **Patient/Family Education**
- Take glucose rather than complex carbohydrates to abort hypoglycemic episodes
- Decrease adverse GI effects by reducing dietary starch content
- Do not skip or delay meals
- Avoid alcohol
- Consult the physician when glucose demands are altered (such as with fever, heavy physical activity, infection, stress, trauma)
- Exercise, good personal hygiene (including foot care), not smoking, and weight control are essential parts of therapy

■ **Monitoring Parameters**
- Food intake and blood glucose, glycosylated hemoglobin, and AST levels
- Assess for signs and symptoms of hypoglycemia (anxiety, cool wet skin, diplopia, dizziness, headache, hunger, numbness in mouth, tachycardia, tremors) or hyperglycemia (deep rapid breathing, dim vision, fatigue, nausea, polydipsia, polyphagia, polyuria, vomiting)
- Be alert to conditions that alter glucose requirements, including fever, increased activity or stress, or a surgical procedure

■ **Geriatric side effects at a glance:**
  ❑ CNS ☑ Bowel Dysfunction ❑ Bladder Dysfunction ❑ Falls
  Other: None

■ **Use with caution in older patients with:** Impaired renal function

■ **U.S. Regulatory Considerations**
  ❑ FDA Black Box ❑ OBRA regulated in U.S. Long Term Care

■ **Other Uses in Geriatric Patient:** None

- **Side Effects:**
  Of particular importance in the geriatric patient: Flatulence, abdominal discomfort, diarrhea

- **Geriatric Considerations - Summary:** GI effects may be even more prevalent in older adults. Not associated with hypoglycemia when used as monotherapy. If hypoglycemia occurs in a patient taking acarbose, use oral glucose for treatment as acarbose may prevent the absorption of other complex carbohydrates. Avoid in older adults with SCr > 2 mg/dl.

- **References:**
  1. Haas L. Management of diabetes mellitus medications in the nursing home. Drugs & Aging 2005;22:209-218.
  2. Rosenstock J. Management of type 2 diabetes mellitus in the elderly: special considerations. Drugs & Aging 2001;18:31-44.

acebutolol hydrochloride

(a-se-byoo'-toe-lole hye-droe-klor'-ide)

- **Brand Name(s):** Sectral
  Chemical Class: β_1-Adrenergic blocker, cardioselective

- **Clinical Pharmacology:**
  Mechanism of Action: A beta$_1$-adrenergic blocker that competitively blocks beta$_1$-adrenergic receptors in cardiac tissue. Reduces the rate of spontaneous firing of the sinus pacemaker and delays AV conduction. **Therapeutic Effect:** Slows heart rate, decreases cardiac output, decreases BP, and exhibits antiarrhythmic activity.
  Pharmacokinetics:

Route	Onset	Peak	Duration
PO (hypotensive)	1-1.5 hr	2-8 hr	24 hr
PO (antiarrhythmic)	1 hr	4-6 hr	10 hr

  Well absorbed from the GI tract. Protein binding: 26%. Undergoes extensive first-pass liver metabolism to active metabolite. Eliminated via bile, secreted into GI tract via intestine, and excreted in urine. Removed by hemodialysis. **Half-life:** 3-4 hr; metabolite, 8-13 hr.

- **Available Forms:**
  - *Capsules:* 200 mg, 400 mg.

- **Indications and Dosages:**
  Mild to moderate hypertension: PO Initially, 400 mg/day in 12 divided doses. Range: Up to 1200 mg/day in 2 divided doses. Maintenance: 400-800 mg/day.
  Ventricular arrhythmias: PO Initially, 200-400 mg/day. Maximum: 800 mg/day.
  Dosage in renal impairment: Dosage is modified based on creatinine clearance.

Creatinine Clearance	% of Usual Dosage
less than 50 ml/min	50
less than 25 ml/min	25

- ■ **Unlabeled Uses:** Treatment of anxiety, chronic angina pectoris, hypertrophic cardio-myopathy, MI, pheochromocytoma, syndrome of mitral valve prolapse, thyrotoxico-sis, tremors

- ■ **Contraindications:** Cardiogenic shock, heart block greater than first degree, overt heart failure, severe bradycardia

- ■ **Side Effects**
  Frequent
  Hypotension manifested as dizziness, nausea, diaphoresis, headache, cold extremi-ties, fatigue, constipation, or diarrhea
  Occasional
  Insomnia, urinary frequency, impotence or decreased libido
  Rare
  Rash, arthralgia, myalgia, confusion, altered taste

- ■ **Serious Reactions**
  - Overdose may produce profound bradycardia and hypotension.
  - Abrupt withdrawal may result in diaphoresis, palpitations, headache, and tremors.
  - Acebutolol administration may precipitate CHF or MI in patients with heart dis-ease; thyroid storm in those with thyrotoxicosis; or peripheral ischemia in those with existing peripheral vascular disease.
  - Hypoglycemia may occur in patients with previously controlled diabetes.
  - Signs of thrombocytopenia, such as unusual bleeding or bruising, occur rarely.

Special Considerations
  - Fewer CNS and bronchospastic effects than other beta-blockers

- ■ **Monitoring Parameters**
  - Heart rate, blood pressure
  - ECG for arrhythmias
  - Stool frequency and consistency, urine output
  - Signs and symptoms of CHF

- ■ **Patient/Family Education**
  - Do not discontinue abruptly; may require taper; rapid withdrawal may produce re-bound hypertension or angina
  - Report excessive fatigue, headache, prolonged dizziness, shortness of breath, or weight gain
  - Do not use nasal decongestants or OTC cold preparations (stimulants) without physician approval
  - Restrict salt and alcohol intake

- ■ **Geriatric side effects at a glance:**
  ❏ CNS ❏ Bowel Dysfunction ❏ Bladder Dysfunction ❏ Falls

- ■ **U.S. Regulatory Considerations**
  ☑ FDA Black Box
  In patients using orally administered beta-blockers, abrupt withdrawal may precipi-tate angina or lead to myocardial infarction or ventricular arrhythmias.
  ❏ OBRA regulated in U.S. Long Term Care

acetaminophen

(ah-seet'-ah-min-oh-fen)

■ **Brand Name(s):**
   OTC: Acephen, Apacet, Arthritis Pain Formula, Aspirin-Free Pain Relief, Feverall, Genapap, Liquiprin, Neopap, Panadol, Tapanol, Tempra, Tylenol

   Combinations
   Rx: with butalbital (Phrenilin); with butalbital and caffeine (Fioricet, Esgic, Isocet); with butalbital, caffeine, and codeine (Amaphen, Fioricet w/codeine); with codeine (Tylenol, Phenaphen No. 2,3,4); with dichloralphenazone and isometheptene (Midrin, Midchlor); with hydrocodone (Vicodin, Lorcet, Lortab); with oxycodone (Percocet, Roxicet, Tylox); with pentazocine (Talacen); with propoxyphene (Wygesic, Darvocet-N)
   OTC: with pamabrom + pyrilamine (Midol PMS, Pamprin); with antihistamine and decongestant (Actifed Plus, Drixoral Cold & Flu, Benadryl Sinus, Sine-Off, Sinarest); with decongestant, antihistamine, dextromethorphan (Nyquil)
   Chemical Class: Para-aminophenol derivative

■ **Clinical Pharmacology:**
   Mechanism of Action: A central analgesic whose exact mechanism is unknown, but appears to inhibit prostaglandin synthesis in the CNS and, to a lesser extent, block pain impulses through peripheral action. Acetaminophen acts centrally on hypothalamic heat-regulating center, producing peripheral vasodilation (heat loss, skin erythema, sweating). **Therapeutic Effect:** Results in antipyresis. Produces analgesic effect. Results in antipyresis.
   Pharmacokinetics:

Route	Onset	Peak	Duration
PO	15-30 min	1-1.5 hr	4-6 hr

   Rapidly, completely absorbed from GI tract; rectal absorption variable. Protein binding: 20%-50%. Widely distributed to most body tissues. Metabolized in liver; excreted in urine. Removed by hemodialysis. **Half-life:** 1-4 hr (half-life is increased in those with liver disease, elderly).

■ **Available Forms:**
   • *Caplet (Genapap, Tylenol)*: 500 mg.
   • *Caplet, extended release (Mapap, Tylenol Arthritis Pain)*: 650 mg.
   • *Capsule (Mapap)*: 500 mg.
   • *Elixir*: 160 mg/5 ml.
   • *Liquid, oral (Tylenol Extra Strength)*: 500 mg/15 ml.
   • *Suppository, rectal*: 80 mg (Acephen, Feverall), 120 mg (Feverall), 325 mg (Feverall), 650 mg (Feverall).
   • *Tablet (Genapap, Mapap, Tylenol)*: 325 mg, 500 mg.
   • *Tablet, chewable (Genapap, Mapap, Tylenol)*: 80 mg.

■ **Indications and Dosages:**
   Analgesia and antipyresis: PO 325-650 mg q4-6h or 1g 3-4 times/day. Maximum: 4 g/day. Rectal 650 mg q4-6h. Maximum: 6 doses/24 hr.

9

Dosage in renal impairment:

Creatinine Clearance	Frequency
10-50 ml/min	q6h
Less than 10 ml/min	q8h

■ **Contraindications:** Active alcoholism, liver disease, or viral hepatitis, all of which increase the risk of hepatotoxicity

■ **Side Effects**
Rare
Hypersensitivity reaction

■ **Serious Reactions**
- Acetaminophen toxicity is the primary serious reaction.
- Early signs and symptoms of acetaminophen toxicity include anorexia, nausea, diaphoresis, and generalized weakness within the first 12-24 hr.
- Later signs of acetaminophen toxicity include vomiting, right upper quadrant tenderness, and elevated liver function tests within 48-72 hr after ingestion.
- The antidote to acetaminophen toxicity is acetylcysteine.

■ **Patient/Family Education**
- Many OTC drugs contain acetaminophen; additive dosage may exceed 4 g/day maximum and increase risk of hepatotoxicity
- Consult with physician before using acetaminophen more than 10 days or for a fever lasting more than 3 days

■ **Geriatric side effects at a glance:**
❑ CNS ❑ Bowel Dysfunction ❑ Bladder Dysfunction ❑ Falls
☑ Other: Elevated liver function studies

■ **Use with caution in older patients with:** Hepatic impairment, daily alcohol use > 3 drinks per day

■ **U.S. Regulatory Considerations**
❑ FDA Black Box ❑ OBRA regulated in U.S. Long Term Care

■ **Other Uses in Geriatric Patient:** None

■ **Side Effects:**
Of particular importance in the geriatric patient: None

■ **Geriatric Considerations - Summary**
Preferred analgesic for mild to moderate pain in older adults due to safety profile. More effective in chronic pain when used on a scheduled basis. The extended-release product allows for q8h dosing, which may enhance compliance in patients taking acetaminophen for chronic pain.

■ **Reference:**
1. Acetaminophen safety. Med Lett Drugs Ther 2002;44:91-93.

acetaminophen; dichloralphenazone; isometheptene mucate

(ah-seet'-ah-min-oh-fen; dye-klor-al-fen'-a-zone; i-so-meh-thep'-tene)

■ **Brand Name(s):** I.D.A, Midrin, Migratine, Migrin-A
   Chemical Class: Sympathomimetic amine

■ **Clinical Pharmacology:**
   Mechanism of Action: Acetaminophen: A central analgesic whose exact mechanism is unknown, but appears to inhibit prostaglandin synthesis in the CNS and, to a lesser extent, block pain impulses through peripheral action. Acetaminophen acts centrally on hypothalamic heat-regulating center, producing peripheral vasodilation (heat loss, skin erythema, sweating). Isometheptene: An indirect-acting sympathomimetic agent with vasoconstricting activity whose exact mechanism is unknown, but appears to constrict cerebral blood vessels and reduce pulsation in cerebral arteries that may be responsible for the pain of migraine headaches. Dichloralphenazone: A complex of chloral hydrate and antipyrine that acts as a mild sedative and relaxant. **Therapeutic Effect:** Relieves migraine headaches.
   Pharmacokinetics: Rapidly, completely absorbed from GI tract; rectal absorption variable. Widely distributed to most body tissues. Acetaminophen is metabolized in liver; excreted in urine. Dichloralphenazone is hydrolyzed to active compounds chloral hydrate and antipyrine. Chloral hydrate is metabolized in the liver and erythrocytes to the active metabolite trichloroethanol, which may be further metabolized to inactive metabolite. It is also metabolized in the liver and kidneys to inactive metabolites. The pharmacokinetics of isometheptene is not reported. Removed by hemodialysis. **Half-life:** Acetaminophen: 1-4 hr (half-life is increased in those with liver disease, elderly, neonates; decreased in children).

■ **Available Forms:**
   • *Capsules*: Acetaminophen 325 mg, isometheptene mucate 65 mg, dichloralphenazone 100 mg (I.D.A, Midrin, Migrin-A).

■ **Indications and Dosages:**
   Migraine headache: PO Initially, 2 capsules, followed by 1 capsule every hour until relief is obtained. Maximum: 5 capsules/12 hr.
   Tension headache: PO 1-2 capsules q4h. Maximum: 8 capsules/24 hr.

■ **Contraindications:** Glaucoma, hypersensitivity to acetaminophen, isometheptene, dichloralphenazone, or any component of the formulation, hepatic disease, hypertension, organic heart disease, MAO inhibitor therapy, severe renal disease

■ **Side Effects**
   Occasional
   Transient dizziness

Rare
Hypersensitivity reaction

- **Serious Reactions**
  - Acetaminophen toxicity is the primary serious reaction.
  - Early signs and symptoms of acetaminophen toxicity include anorexia, nausea, diaphoresis, and generalized weakness within the first 12 to 24 hr.
  - Later signs of acetaminophen toxicity include vomiting, right upper quadrant tenderness, and elevated liver function tests within 48 to 72 hr after ingestion.
  - The antidote to acetaminophen toxicity is acetylcysteine.

- **Geriatric side effects at a glance:**
  ❏ CNS ❏ Bowel Dysfunction ❏ Bladder Dysfunction ❏ Falls

- **U.S. Regulatory Considerations**
  ❏ FDA Black Box ❏ OBRA regulated in U.S. Long Term Care

acetazolamide

(a-seat-a-zole'-a-mide)

- **Brand Name(s):** Dazamide, Diamox, Diamox Sequels
  Chemical Class: Carbonic anhydrase inhibitor; sulfonamide derivative

- **Clinical Pharmacology:**
  Mechanism of Action: A carbonic anhydrase inhibitor that reduces formation of hydrogen and bicarbonate ions from carbon dioxide and water by inhibiting, in proximal renal tubule, the enzyme carbonic anhydrase, thereby promoting renal excretion of sodium, potassium, bicarbonate, and water. Ocular: Reduces rate of aqueous humor formation, lowers intraocular pressure. **Therapeutic Effect:** Produces anticonvulsant activity.
  Pharmacokinetics: Rapidly absorbed. Protein binding: 95%. Widely distributed throughout body tissues including erythrocytes, kidneys, and blood-brain barrier. Not metabolized. Excreted unchanged in urine. Removed by hemodialysis. **Half-life:** 2.4-5.8 hr.

- **Available Forms:**
  - *Capsules, sustained release*: 500 mg (Diamox Sequels).
  - *Powder for reconstitution*: 500 mg.
  - *Tablets*: 125 mg, 250 mg (Diamox).

- **Indications and Dosages:**
  Glaucoma: PO 250 mg 1-4 times/day. Extended-Release: 500 mg 1-2 times/day usually given in morning and evening.
  Secondary glaucoma, preop treatment of acute congestive glaucoma: PO/IV 250 mg q4h, 250 mg q12h; or 500 mg, then 125-250 mg q4h.
  Edema: IV 25-375 mg once daily.
  Epilepsy: Oral 375-1000 mg/day in 1-4 divided doses.

Acute mountain sickness: PO 500-1000 mg/day in divided doses. If possible, begin 24-48 hr before ascent; continue at least 48 hr at high altitude. Initially, 250 mg 2 times/day; use lowest effective dose.

Dosage in renal impairment:

Creatinine Clearance	Dosage Interval
10-50 ml/min	q12h
Less than 10 ml/min	avoid use

■ **Unlabeled Uses:** Urine alkalinization, respiratory stimulant in COPD

■ **Contraindications:** Severe renal disease, adrenal insufficiency, hypochloremic acidosis, hypersensitivity to acetazolamide, to any component of the formulation, or to sulfonamides.

■ **Side Effects**

Frequent

Unusually tired/weak, diarrhea, increased urination/frequency, decreased appetite/weight, altered taste (metallic), nausea, vomiting, numbness in extremities, lips, mouth

Occasional

Depression, drowsiness

Rare

Headache, photosensitivity, confusion, tinnitus, severe muscle weakness, loss of taste

■ **Serious Reactions**
• Long-term therapy may result in acidotic state.
• Nephrotoxicity/hepatotoxicity occurs occasionally, manifested as dark urine/stools, pain in lower back, jaundice, dysuria, crystalluria, renal colic/calculi.
• Bone marrow depression may be manifested as aplastic anemia, thrombocytopenia, thrombocytopenic purpura, leukopenia, agranulocytosis, hemolytic anemia.

■ **Patient/Family Education**
• Carbonated beverages taste flat
• If GI symptoms occur, take with food

■ **Monitoring Parameters**
• Serum electrolytes, creatinine

■ **Geriatric side-effects at a glance:**
☑ CNS ☐ Bowel Dysfunction ☐ Bladder Dysfunction ☐ Falls

■ **U.S. Regulatory Considerations**
☐ FDA Black Box ☐ OBRA regulated in U.S. Long Term Care

acetic acid

(a-cee'-tik as'-id)

■ **Brand Name(s):** Acetasol, Acidic Vaginal Jelly, Acid Jelly, Aci-Jel, Borofair, Fem pH, Relagard, Vasotate, Vosol

Combinations
Rx: with hydrocortisone (VoSol HC Otic, AA HC Otic, Acetasol HC); with oxyquinoline (Aci-Jel)
Chemical Class: Organic acid

■ **Clinical Pharmacology:**
Mechanism of Action: The mechanism by which acetic acid exerts its antibacterial and antifungal actions is unknown. **Therapeutic Effect:** Antibacterial and antifungal.
Pharmacokinetics: Unknown.

■ **Available Forms:**
- *Solution (irrigation)*: 0.25%
- *Solution (otic)*: 2%
- *Gel (vaginal)*: 0.92%

■ **Indications and Dosages:**
Superficial infections of the external auditory canal: Topical Carefully remove all cerumen and debris to allow acetic acid to contact infected surfaces directly. Instill 4-6 drops of otic solution in the affected ear q2-3h. Lie on side with the affected ear uppermost; instill drops and remain on side for 5 min.

■ **Contraindications:** Hypersensitivity to acetic acid or any of the ingredients. Perforated tympanic membrane is frequently considered a contraindication to the use of any medication in the external ear canal.

■ **Side Effects**
Occasional
Stinging or burning
Rare
Local irritation, superinfection

■ **Serious Reactions**
- Superinfection with prolonged use
- *Alert* Discontinue promptly if sensitization or irritation occurs.

■ **Patient/Family Education**
- When administering the otic solution, lie on the side with the affected ear uppermost; instill drops and remain on side for 5 min.

■ **Geriatric side effects at a glance:**
    ❑ CNS   ❑ Bowel Dysfunction   ❑ Bladder Dysfunction   ❑ Falls

■ **U.S. Regulatory Considerations**
   ❑ FDA Black Box   ❑ OBRA regulated in U.S. Long Term Care

acetylcysteine

(a-se-teel-sis'-tay-een)

■ **Brand Name(s):** Acetadote, Mucomyst
   Chemical Class: Amino acid, L-cysteine

■ **Clinical Pharmacology:**
   Mechanism of Action: An intratracheal respiratory inhalant that splits the linkage of mucoproteins, reducing the viscosity of pulmonary secretions. **Therapeutic Effect:** Facilitates the removal of pulmonary secretions by coughing, postural drainage, mechanical means. Protects against acetaminophen overdose–induced hepatotoxicity. **Pharmacokinetics:** Protein binding: 83% (injection). Rapidly and extensively metabolized in liver. Deacetylated by the liver to cysteine and subsequently metabolized. Excreted in urine. **Half-life:** 5.6 hr (injection).

■ **Available Forms:**
   • *Injection* (*Acetadote*): 20% (200 mg/ml).
   • *Inhalation Solution* (*Mucomyst*): 10% (100 mg/ml), 20% (200 mg/ml).

■ **Indications and Dosages:**
   Adjunctive treatment of viscid mucus secretions from chronic bronchopulmonary disease and for pulmonary complications of cystic fibrosis: Nebulization *Alert* Bronchodilators should be given 15 min before acetylcysteine. 3-5 ml (20% solution) 3-4 times a day or 6-10 ml (10% solution) 3-4 times a day. Range: 1-10 ml (20% solution) q2-6h or 2-20 ml (10% solution) q2-6h .
   Treatment of viscid mucus secretions in patients with a tracheostomy: Intratracheal 1-2 ml of 10% or 20% solution instilled into tracheostomy q1-4h.
   Acetaminophen overdose: PO (Oral solution 5%) Loading dose of 140 mg/kg, followed in 4 hr by maintenance dose of 70 mg/kg q4h for 17 additional doses (unless acetaminophen assay reveals nontoxic level). Repeat dose if emesis occurs within 1 hr of administration. Continue until all doses are given, even if acetaminophen plasma level drops below toxic range. IV 150 mg/kg infused over 15 min, then 50 mg/kg infused over 4 hr, then 100 mg/kg infused over 16 hr. See administration and handling.
   Prevention of renal damage from dyes used during certain diagnostic tests: PO (Oral solution 5%) 600 mg twice a day for 4 doses starting the day before the procedure.

■ **Unlabeled Uses:** Prevention of renal damage from dyes given during certain diagnostic tests (such as CT scans)

■ **Contraindications:** None known.

■ **Side Effects**
   Frequent
   Inhalation: Stickiness on face, transient unpleasant odor

Occasional
Inhalation: Increased bronchial secretions, throat irritation, nausea, vomiting, rhinorrhea
Rare
Inhalation: Rash
Oral: Facial edema, bronchospasm, wheezing

■ **Serious Reactions**
  • Large doses may produce severe nausea and vomiting.

Special Considerations
  • Disagreeable odor may be noted
  • Solution in opened bottle may change color; of no significance

■ **Monitoring Parameters**
  • Respiratory rate, depth, and rhythm before treatment
  • Check color, consistency, and amount of sputum

■ **Patient/Family Education**
  • Drink plenty of fluids

■ **Geriatric side effects at a glance:**
  ❑ CNS ❑ Bowel Dysfunction ❑ Bladder Dysfunction ❑ Falls

■ **U.S. Regulatory Considerations**
  ❑ FDA Black Box ❑ OBRA regulated in U.S. Long Term Care

acitretin

(a-si-tre'-tin)

■ **Brand Name(s):** Soriatane
  Chemical Class: Retinoid analog

■ **Clinical Pharmacology:**
  Mechanism of Action: A second-generation retinoid that adjusts factors influencing epidermal proliferation, RNA/DNA synthesis, controls glycoprotein, and governs immune response. **Therapeutic Effect:** Regulates keratinocyte growth and differentiation.
  Pharmacokinetics: Well absorbed from the GI tract. Food increases rate of absorption. Protein binding: greater than 99%. Metabolized in liver. Excreted in bile and urine. Not removed by hemodialysis. **Half-life:** 49 hr.

■ **Available Forms:**
  • *Capsules*: 10 mg, 25 mg (Soriatane).

- **Indications and Dosages:**
  Psoriasis: PO 25-50 mg/day as a single dose with main meal. May increase to 75 mg/day if necessary and dose tolerated. Maintenance: 25-50 mg/day after the initial response is noted. Continue until lesions have resolved.

- **Contraindications:** Severely impaired liver or kidney function, chronic abnormal elevated lipid levels, concomitant use of methotrexate or tetracyclines, hypersensitivity to acitretin, etretinate, or other retinoids, sensitivity to parabenz (used as preservative in gelatin capsule)

- **Side Effects**
  Frequent
  Lip inflammation, alopecia, skin peeling, shakiness, dry eyes, rash, hyperesthesia, paresthesia, sticky skin, dry mouth, epistaxis, dryness/thickening of conjunctiva
  Occasional
  Eye irritation, brow and lash loss, sweating, chills, sensation of cold, flushing, edema, blurred vision, diarrhea, nausea, thirst

- **Serious Reactions**
  - Benign intracranial hypertension (pseudotumor cerebri) occurs rarely.

- **Patient/Family Education**
  - Avoid exposure to sun and sunlamps

- **Monitoring Parameters**
  - Transaminase levels monthly for first 6 mo then every 3 mo
  - Lipid levels monthly for first 4 mo then every 2-3 mo
  - Yearly radiographs to monitor for drug-induced vertebral abnormalities

- **Geriatric side effects at a glance:**
  ❑ CNS ❑ Bowel Dysfunction ❑ Bladder Dysfunction ❑ Falls

- **U.S. Regulatory Considerations**
  ☑ FDA Black Box
  Although not relevant to the geriatric patient, the drug is associated with a teratogenicity risk in females.
  ❑ OBRA regulated in U.S. Long Term Care

acyclovir

(ay-sye'-kloe-veer)

- **Brand Name(s):** Zovirax, Zovirax Topical
  Chemical Class: Acyclic purine nucleoside analog

■ Clinical Pharmacology:

Mechanism of Action: A synthetic nucleoside that converts to acyclovir triphosphate, becoming part of the DNA chain. **Therapeutic Effect:** Interferes with DNA synthesis and viral replication. Virustatic.

Pharmacokinetics: Poorly absorbed from the GI tract; minimal absorption following topical application. Protein binding: 9%-36%. Widely distributed. Partially metabolized in liver. Excreted primarily in urine. Removed by hemodialysis. **Half-life:** 2.5 hr (increased in impaired renal function).

■ Available Forms:

- *Capsules:* 200 mg.
- *Tablets:* 400 mg, 800 mg.
- *Injection Solution:* 50 mg/ml.
- *Oral Suspension:* 200 mg/5 ml.
- *Powder for Injection:* 500 mg, 1000 mg.
- *Ointment:* 5%.

■ Indications and Dosages:

Genital herpes (initial episode): IV 5 mg/kg q8h for 5 days. PO 200 mg q4h 5 times a day

Genital herpes (recurrent): PO (Less than 6 episodes per year) 200 mg q4h 5 times a day for 5 days PO (6 episodes or more per year) 400 mg 2 times a day or 200 mg 3-5 times a day for up to 12 mo.

Herpes simplex mucocutaneous: IV 5 mg/kg/dose q8h for 7 days

Herpes simplex encephalitis: IV 10 mg/kg q8h for 10 days

Herpes zoster (caused by varicella): IV 10 mg/kg q8h for 7 days.

Herpes zoster (shingles): PO 800 mg q4h 5 times a day for 7-10 days. Topical Apply to affected area 3-6 times a day for 7 days

Varicella (chickenpox): PO 800 mg 4 times a day for 5 days.

Dosage in renal impairment: Dosage and frequency are modified based on severity of infection and degree of renal impairment.

PO, Normal dose 200 mg q4h:

Creatinine clearance greater than 10 ml/min : Give usual dose and at normal interval, 200 mg q4h.

Creatinine clearance 10 ml/min and less: 200 mg q12h.

PO, Normal dose 400 mg q12h

Creatinine clearance greater than 10 ml/min: Give usual dose and at normal interval, 400 mg q12h.

Creatinine clearance 10 ml/min and less: 200 mg q12h.

PO, Normal dose 800 mg q4h

Creatinine clearance greater than 25 ml/min: Give usual dose and at normal interval, 800 mg q4h.

Creatinine clearance 10-25 ml/min: 800 mg q8h.

Creatinine clearance less than 10 ml/min: 800 mg q12h.

IV

Creatinine Clearance	Dosage Percent	Dosage Interval
greater than 50 ml/min	100	8 hr
25-50 ml/min	100	12 hr
10-24 ml/min	100	24 hr
less than 10 ml/min	50	24 hr

■ Unlabeled Uses:
Oral, parenteral: Prophylaxis of herpes simplex and herpes zoster infections, infectious mononucleosis.

Topical: Treatment adjunct for herpes zoster infections.

■ **Contraindications:** None known.

■ **Side Effects**
  Frequent
  Parenteral (9%-7%): Phlebitis or inflammation at IV site, nausea, vomiting
  Topical (28%): Burning, stinging
  Occasional
  Oral (12%-6%): Malaise, nausea
  Parenteral (3%): Pruritus, rash, urticaria
  Topical (4%): Pruritus
  Rare
  Oral (3%-1%): Vomiting, rash, diarrhea, headache
  Parenteral (2%-1%): Confusion, hallucinations, seizures, tremors
  Topical (*less than* 1%): Rash

■ **Serious Reactions**
  • Rapid parenteral administration, excessively high doses, or fluid and electrolyte imbalance may produce renal failure exhibited by such signs and symptoms as abdominal pain, decreased urination, decreased appetite, increased thirst, nausea, and vomiting.
  • Toxicity has not been reported with oral or topical use.

Special Considerations

  • In recurrent herpes genitalis and herpes labialis in non-immunocompromised patients, no evidence of clinical benefit from topical acyclovir

■ **Patient/Family Education**
  • Drink adequate fluids during therapy
  • Do not touch lesions to prevent spreading the infection to new sites
  • Space doses evenly around the clock and continue taking acyclovir for the full course of treatment
  • Use a finger cot or rubber glove when applying the ointment
  • Avoid sexual intercourse while lesions are visible to prevent infecting the partner

■ **Geriatric side effects at a glance:**
  ☑ CNS   ☐ Bowel Dysfunction   ☐ Bladder Dysfunction   ☐ Falls

■ **U.S. Regulatory Considerations**
  ☐ FDA Black Box   ☐ OBRA regulated in U.S. Long Term Care

adalimumab

(a-dal-aye'-mu-mab)

■ **Brand Name(s):** Humira
  Chemical Class: Monoclonal antibody

- **Clinical Pharmacology:**
  Mechanism of Action: A monoclonal antibody that binds specifically to tumor necrosis factor (TNF) alpha, blocking its interaction with cell surface TNF receptors. **Therapeutic Effect:** Reduces inflammation, tenderness, and swelling of joints; slows or prevents progressive destruction of joints in rheumatoid arthritis.
  Pharmacokinetics: Half-life: 10-20 days.

- **Available Forms:**
  - *Injection*: 40 mg/0.8 ml in prefilled syringes.

- **Indications and Dosages:**
  Rheumatoid arthritis, psoriatic arthritis: Subcutaneous 40 mg every other week. Dose may be increased to 40 mg/wk in those not taking methotrexate.

- **Contraindications:** Active infections

- **Side Effects**
  Frequent (20%)
  Injection site, erythema, pruritus, pain, and swelling
  Occasional (12%-9%)
  Headache, rash, sinusitis, nausea
  Rare (7%-5%)
  Abdominal or back pain, hypertension

- **Serious Reactions**
  - Rare reactions include hypersensitivity reactions, malignancies, respiratory tract infections, bronchitis, UTIs, and more serious infections (such as pneumonia, tuberculosis, cellulitis, pyelonephritis, and septic arthritis).

Special Considerations

- Evaluate for latent tuberculosis infection with a tuberculin skin test before initiation of therapy
- Adalimumab does not contain preservatives — unused portions of drug should be discarded

- **Patient/Family Education**
  - Injection sites should be rotated and injections should never be given into areas where the skin is tender, bruised, red, or hard
  - Intended for use under the guidance and supervision of the clinician; patients may self-inject if appropriate and with medical follow-up, after proper training in injection technique, including proper syringe and needle disposal
  - Injection site reactions generally occur in the first month of treatment and decrease with continued therapy
  - Avoid receiving live vaccines during adalimumab treatment

- **Monitoring Parameters**
  - *Therapeutic*: Rheumatoid arthritis signs and symptoms (joint stiffness, pain, swollen/tender joints), mobility, quality of life, radiographs of affected joints, ESR, CRP
  - *Toxicity*: Temperature, blood pressure periodically, signs and symptoms of respiratory infection, including tuberculosis, hypersensitivity, anti-adalimumab antibodies (ELISA) at least once during therapy, anti-dsDNA antibody determinations in patients presenting with lupus-like symptoms (e.g., tiredness, rash, bone pain), CBC, routine blood chemistry periodically during long-term therapy

- **Geriatric side effects at a glance:**
  - ☐ CNS ☐ Bowel Dysfunction ☐ Bladder Dysfunction ☐ Falls

- **U.S. Regulatory Considerations**
  - ☑ FDA Black Box
  Risk of Infection: Cases of tuberculosis (frequently disseminated or extrapulmonary) have been reported during therapy
  - ☐ OBRA regulated in U.S. Long Term Care

adefovir dipivoxil

(a-def'-o-veer)

- **Brand Name(s):** Hepsera
  Chemical Class: Nucleotide analog

- **Clinical Pharmacology:**
  Mechanism of Action: An antiviral that inhibits the enzyme DNA polymerase, causing DNA chain termination after its incorporation into viral DNA. **Therapeutic Effect:** Prevents cell replication of viral DNA.
  Pharmacokinetics: Binds to proteins after PO administration. Protein binding: less than 4%. Excreted in urine. **Half-life:** 7 hr (increased in impaired renal function).

- **Available Forms:**
  - *Tablets:* 10 mg.

- **Indications and Dosages:**
  Chronic hepatitis B in patients with normal renal function: PO 10 mg once a day.
  Chronic hepatitis B in patients with impaired renal function: *Creatinine clearance 20-49 ml/min.* 10 mg q48h. *Creatinine clearance 10-19 ml/min.* 10 mg q72h. *On hemodialysis.* 10 mg every 7 days following dialysis.

- **Contraindications:** None known.

- **Side Effects**
  Frequent (13%)
  Asthenia
  Occasional (9%-4%)
  Headache, abdominal pain, nausea, flatulence
  Rare (3%)
  Diarrhea, dyspepsia

- **Serious Reactions**
  - Nephrotoxicity characterized by increased serum creatinine and decreased serum phosphorus levels is a treatment-limiting toxicity of adefovir therapy.
  - Lactic acidosis and severe hepatomegaly occur rarely, particularly in female patients.

- Offer HIV testing before treatment
- Effective in patients with HBV resistant to lamivudine
- Histologic improvement seen in 60% of treated patients, but long-term effect unknown
- Always check updated treatment guidelines before initiating or changing antiretroviral therapy. (http://AIDSinfo.nih.gov)

■ **Patient/Family Education**
- Avoid behavior that may cause exposure to HIV
- Comply with follow-up laboratory testing; tests will help monitor kidney and liver function and hepatitis B virus levels
- Immediately notify the physician if unusual muscle pain, abdominal pain with nausea and vomiting, a cold feeling in arms and legs, and dizziness occurs; these signs and symptoms may signal the onset of lactic acidosis
- Continue to take adefovir as prescribed because a very serious form of hepatitis may develop if the drug is stopped
- Notify the physician of yellow skin color or whites of the eyes or other unusual signs or symptoms; it may indicate serious liver problems

■ **Monitoring Parameters**
- ALT, AST, bilirubin, HBV DNA level, INR, renal function
- Intake and output
- Closely monitor for serious reactions, especially in patients taking other drugs that are excreted by the kidneys or are known to affect renal function

■ **Geriatric side effects at a glance:**
   ❏ CNS ❏ Bowel Dysfunction ❏ Bladder Dysfunction ❏ Falls

■ **U.S. Regulatory Considerations**
   ☑ FDA Black Box
   Severe acute exacerbations of hepatitis reported once anti-hepatitis B therapy discontinued. Monitor hepatic function closely post therapy.
   ❏ OBRA regulated in U.S. Long Term Care

adenosine

(ah-den'-oh-seen)

■ **Brand Name(s):** Adenocard, Adenojec, Adenoscan, My-O-Den
   Chemical Class: Endogenous nucleoside

■ **Clinical Pharmacology:**
   Mechanism of Action: A cardiac agent that slows impulse formation in the SA node and conduction time through the AV node. Adenosine also acts as a diagnostic aid in myocardial perfusion imaging or stress echocardiography. **Therapeutic Effect:** Depresses left ventricular function and restores normal sinus rhythm.

Pharmacokinetics: Rapidly cleared from the circulation via cellular uptake, primarily by erythrocytes and vascular endothelial cells. Extensively distributed and rapidly metabolized either via phosphorylation to adenosine monophosphate by adenosine kinase, or via deamination to inosine by adenosine deaminase in the cytosol. **Half-life:** 10 sec.

- **Available Forms:**
  - Injection (*Adenocard*): 3 mg/ml in 2-ml, 4-ml syringes.
  - Injection (*Adenoscan*): 3 mg/ml in 20-ml, 30-ml vials.

- **Indications and Dosages:**
  Paroxysmal supraventricular tachycardia **(PSVT):** Rapid IV bolus Initially, 6 mg given over 1-2 sec. If first dose does not convert within 1-2 min, give 12 mg; may repeat 12-mg dose in 1-2 min if no response has occurred
  Diagnostic testing: IV infusion 140 mcg/kg/min for 6 min.

- **Contraindications:** Atrial fibrillation or flutter, second- or third-degree AV block or sick sinus syndrome (with functioning pacemaker), ventricular tachycardia

- **Side Effects**
  Frequent (18%-12%)
  Facial flushing, dyspnea
  Occasional (7%-2%)
  Headache, nausea, light-headedness, chest pressure
  Rare (less than or equal to 1%)
  Numbness or tingling in arms; dizziness; diaphoresis; hypotension; palpitations; chest, jaw, or neck pain

- **Serious Reactions**
  - May produce short-lasting heart block.

- **Patient/Family Education**
  - Report unusual signs and symptoms, including chest pain, chest pounding or palpitations, or difficulty breathing or shortness of breath
  - Facial flushing, headache, and nausea may occur but these symptoms will resolve

- **Monitoring Parameters**
  - Heart rate and rhythm, blood pressure, intake and output, electrolyte levels

- **Geriatric side effects at a glance:**
  ☐ CNS ☐ Bowel Dysfunction ☐ Bladder Dysfunction ☐ Falls

- **U.S. Regulatory Considerations**
  ☑ FDA Black Box
  Nephrotoxicity associated with chronic therapy. Monitor renal function during therapy.
  ☐ OBRA regulated in U.S. Long Term Care

albendazole

(al-ben'-da-zole)

■ **Brand Name(s):** Albenza
Chemical Class: Benzimidazole derivative

■ **Clinical Pharmacology:**
Mechanism of Action: A benzimidazole carbamate anthelmintic that degrades parasite cytoplasmic microtubules, irreversibly blocks cholinesterase secretion, glucose uptake in helminth and larvae (depletes glycogen, decreases ATP production, depletes energy). Vermicidal. **Therapeutic Effect:** Immobilizes and kills worms.
Pharmacokinetics: Poorly and variably absorbed from GI tract. Widely distributed, cyst fluid and including cerebrospinal fluid (CSF). Protein binding: 70%. Extensively metabolized in liver. Primarily excreted in urine and bile. Not removed by hemodialysis. **Half-life:** 8-12 hr.

■ **Available Forms:**
• *Tablets*: 200 mg (Albenza).

■ **Indications and Dosages:**
Neurocysticercosis: PO *Weight more than 60 kg.* 400 mg 2 times/day. Continue for 28 days, rest 14 days, repeat cycle 3 times. *Weight less than 60 kg.* 15 mg/kg/day. Continue for 28 days, rest 14 days, repeat cycle 3 times.
Cystic hydatid: PO *Weight more than 60 kg.* 400 mg 2 times/day. Continue for 8-30 days. *Weight less than 60 kg.* 15 mg/kg/day. Continue for 8-30 days.

■ **Unlabeled Uses:** Angiostrongyliasis, cysticercosis, gnathostomiasis, liver flukes, trichuriasis

■ **Contraindications:** Hypersensitivity to albendazole or any component of the formulation

■ **Side Effects**
Frequent
Neurocysticercosis: Nausea, vomiting, headache
Hydatid: Abnormal liver function tests, abdominal pain, nausea, vomiting
Occasional
Neurocysticercosis: Increased intracranial pressure, meningeal signs
Hydatid: Headache, dizziness, alopecia, fever

■ **Serious Reactions**
• Pancytopenia occurs rarely.
• In presence of cysticercosis, drug may produce retinal damage in presence of retinal lesions.

Special Considerations
• For appropriate infections, retest stool 3 wk after treatment to detect residual ova

24

- Patients treated for neurocysticercosis should receive steroid and anticonvulsant therapy

■ **Patient/Family Education**
  - Notify the physician if fever, chills, sore throat, or unusual bleeding occurs

■ **Monitoring Parameters**
  - CBC and liver function

■ **Geriatric side effects at a glance:**
  ❏ CNS ❏ Bowel Dysfunction ❏ Bladder Dysfunction ❏ Falls

■ **U.S. Regulatory Considerations**
  ❏ FDA Black Box ❏ OBRA regulated in U.S. Long Term Care

albuterol

(al-byoo'-ter-ole)

■ **Brand Name(s):** AccuNeb, Proventil, Proventil HFA, Proventil Repetabs, Ventolin, Ventolin HFA, Ventolin Rotacaps, Volmax, VoSpire ER

  Combinations
  Rx: with ipratropium (Combivent)
  Chemical Class: Sympathomimetic amine; β_2-adrenergic agonist

■ **Clinical Pharmacology:**
  Mechanism of Action: A sympathomimetic that stimulates beta$_2$-adrenergic receptors in the lungs, resulting in relaxation of bronchial smooth muscle. **Therapeutic Effect:** Relieves bronchospasm and reduces airway resistance.
  Pharmacokinetics:

Route	Onset	Peak	Duration
PO	15-30 min	2-3 hr	4-6 hr
PO (extended-release)	30 min	2-4 hr	12 hr
Inhalation	5-15 min	0.5-2 hr	2-5 hr

  Rapidly, well absorbed from the GI tract; gradually absorbed from the bronchi after inhalation. Metabolized in the liver. Primarily excreted in urine. **Half-life:** 2.7-5 hr (PO); 3.8 hr (inhalation).

■ **Available Forms:**
  - *Syrup*: 2 mg/5 ml.
  - *Tablets (Proventil, Ventolin)*: 2 mg, 4 mg.
  - *Tablets (Extended-Release)*: 4 mg (Proventil Repetabs, Volmax, VoSpire ER), 8 mg (Volmax, VoSpire ER).
  - *Inhalation Aerosol (Proventil, Ventolin)*: 90 mcg/spray.
  - *Inhalation Solution (AccuNeb)*: 0.75 mg/3 ml (0.63 mg/3 ml albuterol), 1.5 mg/3 ml (1.25 mg/3 ml albuterol).
  - *Inhalation Solution*: 0.083% (Proventil), 0.5% (Proventil, Ventolin).

■ Indications and Dosages:

Acute bronchospasm: Inhalation 4-8 puffs q20min up to 4 hr, then q1-4h as needed. Nebulization 2.5-5 mg q20min for 3 doses, then 2.5-10 mg q1-4h or 10-15 mg/hr continuously.

Bronchospasm: PO 2 mg 3-4 times a day. Maximum: 8 mg 4 times a day. PO (Extended-Release) 4-8 mg q12h. Nebulization 2.5 mg 3-4 times a day over 5-15 min.

Chronic bronchospasm: Inhalation 1-2 puffs q4-6h. Maximum: 12 puffs per day.

Exercise-induced bronchospasm: Inhalation 2 puffs 15-30 min before exercise.

■ Contraindications: History of hypersensitivity to sympathomimetics

■ Side Effects

Frequent

Headache (27%); nausea (15%); restlessness, nervousness, tremors (20%); dizziness (less than 7%); throat dryness and irritation, pharyngitis (less than 6%); BP changes, including hypertension (5%-3%); heartburn, transient wheezing (less than 5%)

Occasional (3%-2%)

Insomnia, asthenia, altered taste

Inhalation: Dry, irritated mouth or throat; cough; bronchial irritation

Rare

Somnolence, diarrhea, dry mouth, flushing, diaphoresis, anorexia

■ Serious Reactions

- Excessive sympathomimetic stimulation may produce palpitations, extrasystole, tachycardia, chest pain, a slight increase in BP followed by a substantial decrease, chills, diaphoresis, and blanching of skin.
- Too-frequent or excessive use may lead to decreased bronchodilating effectiveness and severe, paradoxical bronchoconstriction.

Special Considerations

- Inhalation technique critical
- Consider spacer devices
- Rinse mouth immediately after inhalation
- Avoid excessive use of caffeine

■ Monitoring Parameters

- 12-lead ECG, ABG determinations, pulse rate, respirations, serum potassium levels

■ Patient/Family Education

- See clinician if using ≥4 inhalations/day on regular basis or >1 canister (200 inhalations) in 8 wk

■ Geriatric side effects at a glance:

☑ CNS ❑ Bowel Dysfunction ❑ Bladder Dysfunction ❑ Falls

Other: Tachycardia, Tremor

■ Use with caution in older patients with: Cardiovascular disease, especially angina, arrhythmias, or CHF; Parkinsonism, Essential Tremor, Hyperthyroidism, Anxiety

■ U.S. Regulatory Considerations

☑ FDA Black Box

Lactic acidosis and severe hepatomegaly with steatosis (including fatal cases) have been reported with the use of nucleoside analogs alone or in combination with other antiretrovirals.

☑ OBRA regulated in U.S. Long Term Care

■ **Other Uses in Geriatric Patient:** None

■ **Side Effects:**
Of particular importance in the geriatric patient: Tachycardia, palpitations, CNS stimulation, anxiety, nervousness, dizziness, tremor, cough, hypokalemia (dose-dependent)

■ **Geriatric Considerations - Summary:** Ensure that the older adult can adequately use the inhalation device. A spacer may be beneficial in those unable to coordinate device operation and inhalation. Spacer devices improve drug delivery to the lungs, therefore monitor closely as the patient may also experience increased systemic side effects with improved exposure to albuterol. Monitor cardiac status.

■ **References:**
1. Salpeter SR. Cardiovascular safety of beta 2-adrenoceptor agonist use in patients with obstructive airway disease: a systematic review. Drugs & Aging 2004;21:405-414.
2. Newnham DM. Asthma medications and their potential adverse effects in the elderly: recommendations for prescribing. Drug Safety 2001;24:1065-1080.

alclometasone dipropionate

(al-kloe-met'-a-sone di-pro'-pee-on-ate)

■ **Brand Name(s):** Aclovate
Chemical Class: Corticosteroid, synthetic

■ **Clinical Pharmacology:**
Mechanism of Action: Topical corticosteroids exhibit anti-inflammatory, antipruritic, and vasoconstrictive properties. Clinically, these actions correspond to decreased edema, erythema, pruritus, plaque formation, and scaling of the affected skin.
Pharmacokinetics: Approximately 3% is absorbed during an 8-hr period. Metabolized in the liver. Excreted in the urine.

■ **Available Forms:**
- *Cream*: (Aclovate)
- *Ointment*: (Aclovate)

■ **Indications and Dosages:**
Atopic dermatitis, contact dermatitis, dermatitis, discoid lupus erythematosus, eczema, exfoliative dermatitis, granuloma annulare, lichen planus, lichen simplex, polymorphous light eruption, pruritus, psoriasis, Rhus dermatitis, seborrheic dermatitis, xerosis: Topical Apply a thin film to the affected area 2-3 times a day.

■ **Contraindications:** Hypersensitivity to alclometasone, other corticosteroids, or any of its components.

■ **Side Effects**
Frequent
Burning, erythema, maculopapular rash, pruritus, skin irritation, xerosis
Occasional
Acneiform rash, contact dermatitis, folliculitis, glycosuria, growth inhibition, headache, hyperglycemia, infection, miliaria, papilledema, skin atrophy, skin hypopigmentation, skin ulcer, striae, telangiectasia
Rare
Adrenolcortical insufficiency, increased intracranial pressure, pseudotumor cerebri, impaired wound healing, Cushing's syndrome, HPA suppression, skin ulcers, tolerance, withdrawal, visual impairment, ocular hypertension, cataracts

■ **Patient/Family Education**
• Apply sparingly only to affected area
• Avoid contact with the eyes
• Do not put bandages or dressings over treated area unless directed by clinician
• Discontinue drug, notify clinician if local irritation or fever develops
• Do not use on weeping, denuded, or infected areas

■ **Geriatric side effects at a glance:**
❑ CNS ❑ Bowel Dysfunction ❑ Bladder Dysfunction ❑ Falls

■ **U.S. Regulatory Considerations**
❑ FDA Black Box ❑ OBRA regulated in U.S. Long Term Care

alefacept

(a-la-fa'-cept)

■ **Brand Name(s):** Amevive
Chemical Class: Dimeric fusion protein

■ **Clinical Pharmacology:**
Mechanism of Action: An immunologic agent that interferes with the activation of T-lymphocytes by binding to the lymphocyte antigen, thus reducing the number of circulating T-lymphocytes. **Therapeutic Effect:** Prevents T cells from becoming overactive, which may help reduce symptoms of chronic plaque psoriasis.
Pharmacokinetics: Half-life: 270 hr.

■ **Available Forms:**
• *Powder for Injection:* 7.5 mg for IV administration, 15 mg for IM administration.

■ Indications and Dosages:

Plaque psoriasis: IV 7.5 mg once weekly for 12 wk. IM 15 mg once weekly for 12 wk.

■ Contraindications:
History of systemic malignancy, concurrent use of immunosuppressive agents or phototherapy

■ Side Effects
Frequent (16%)
Injection site pain and inflammation (with IM administration)
Occasional (5%)
Chills
Rare (2% or less)
Pharyngitis, dizziness, cough, nausea, myalgia

■ Serious Reactions
- Rare reactions include hypersensitivity reactions, lymphopenia, malignancies, and serious infections requiring hospitalization (such as abscess, pneumonia, and postoperative wound infection).
- Coronary artery disease and MI occur in less than 1% of patients.

■ Patient/Family Education
- Inform patients of the need for monitoring of lymphocyte counts during therapy; increased risk of infection or a malignancy
- Avoid contact with infected individuals and situations that might place him or her at risk for infection

■ Monitoring Parameters
- *Efficacy*: Psoriasis Area and Severity Index (PASI)—extent of area affected and severity of erythema, scaling, and thickness of plaques
- *Toxicity*: CD4+ lymphocyte counts weekly during 12-wk course; withhold therapy if counts below 250 cells/μl

■ Geriatric side effects at a glance:
❏ CNS   ❏ Bowel Dysfunction   ❏ Bladder Dysfunction   ❏ Falls

■ U.S. Regulatory Considerations
❏ FDA Black Box   ❏ OBRA regulated in U.S. Long Term Care

alendronate sodium

(a-len-droe'-nate soe'-dee-um)

- **Brand Name(s):** Fosamax
  Chemical Class: Pyrophosphate analog

- **Clinical Pharmacology:**
  Mechanism of Action: A bisphosphonate that inhibits normal and abnormal bone resorption, without retarding mineralization. **Therapeutic Effect:** Leads to significantly increased bone mineral density; reverses the progression of osteoporosis.
  Pharmacokinetics: Poorly absorbed after oral administration. Protein binding: 78%. After oral administration, rapidly taken into bone, with uptake greatest at sites of active bone turnover. Excreted in urine. **Terminal half-life:** Greater than 10 yr (reflects release from skeleton as bone is resorbed).

- **Available Forms:**
  - *Tablets:* 5 mg, 10 mg, 35 mg, 40 mg, 70 mg.
  - *Oral Solution:* 70 mg/75 ml.

- **Indications and Dosages:**
  Osteoporosis (in men): PO 10 mg once a day in the morning or 70 mg weekly.
  Glucocorticoid-induced osteoporosis: PO *Elderly.* 5 mg once a day in the morning. *Postmenopausal women not receiving estrogen.* 10 mg once a day in the morning.
  Postmenopausal osteoporosis: PO (treatment) 10 mg once a day in the morning or 70 mg weekly. PO (prevention) 5 mg once a day in the morning or 35 mg weekly.
  Paget's disease: PO 40 mg once a day in the morning for 6 mo.

- **Contraindications:** GI disease, including dysphagia, frequent heartburn, gastrointestinal reflux disease, hiatal hernia, and ulcers; inability to stand or sit upright for at least 30 minutes; renal impairment; sensitivity to alendronate

- **Side Effects**
  Frequent (8%-7%)
  Back pain, abdominal pain
  Occasional (3%-2%)
  Nausea, abdominal distention, constipation, diarrhea, flatulence
  Rare (less than 2%)
  Rash, severe bone, joint, muscle pain, osteonecrosis of the jaw

- **Serious Reactions**
  - Overdose causes hypocalcemia, hypophosphatemia, and significant GI disturbances.
  - Esophageal irritation occurs if alendronate is not given with 6-8 oz of plain water or if the patient lies down within 30 min of drug administration.

Special Considerations
  - A dental examination with appropriate preventive dentistry should be considered prior to treatment with bisphosphonates in patients with concomitant risk factors (e.g., cancer, chemotherapy, corticosteroid use, poor oral hygiene). While on bis-

phosphonate treatment, patients with concomitant risk factors should avoid invasive dental procedures if possible. For patients who develop osteonecrosis of the jaw while on bisphosphonate therapy, dental surgery may exacerbate the condition. For patients requiring dental procedures, there is no data available to suggest whether discontinuation of bisphosphonate treatment reduces the risk of osteonecrosis of the jaw.

■ **Patient/Family Education**
- Patients should receive supplemental calcium and vitamin D if dietary intake is inadequate
- Administer 30 min before the first food/beverage/medication of the day with 6-8 oz plain water; avoid lying down for at least 30 min
- Weekly administration may be an advantage
- Some experts recommend cessation of therapy after 5 yr due to theoretical concerns of poor quality bone formation with prolonged therapy
- Consider beginning weight-bearing exercises and modifying behavioral factors, such as reducing alcohol consumption and stopping cigarette smoking
- Inform your dentist if you are taking this drug.
- If you develop jaw pain, loose teeth, or signs of oral infection, immediately inform your doctor.

■ **Monitoring Parameters**
- Serum electrolytes, including serum alkaline phosphatase and serum calcium levels

■ **Geriatric side effects at a glance:**
❑ CNS ☑ Bowel Dysfunction ❑ Bladder Dysfunction ❑ Falls

■ **U.S. Regulatory Considerations**
❑ FDA Black Box ❑ OBRA regulated in U.S. Long Term Care

alfuzosin hydrochloride

(ale-fyoo-zoe'-sin)

■ **Brand Name(s):** Uroxatral
   Chemical Class: Quinazoline

■ **Clinical Pharmacology:**
   Mechanism of Action: An alpha$_1$ antagonist that targets receptors around bladder neck and prostate capsule. **Therapeutic Effect:** Relaxes smooth muscle and improves urinary flow and symptoms of prostatic hyperplasia.
   Pharmacokinetics: Rapidly absorbed and widely distributed. Protein binding: 90%. Extensively metabolized in the liver. Primarily excreted in urine. **Half-life:** 3-9 hr.

■ **Available Forms:**
- *Tablets (Extended-Release)*: 10 mg.

■ **Indications and Dosages:**
Benign prostatic hyperplasia: PO 10 mg once a day, approximately 30 min after same meal each day.

■ **Contraindications:** Hepatic disease, concomitant use of ketoconazole, itraconazole, ritonavir

■ **Side Effects**
Frequent (7%-6%)
Dizziness, headache, malaise
Occasional (4%)
Dry mouth
Rare (3%-2%)
Nausea, dyspepsia (such as heartburn, and epigastric discomfort), diarrhea, orthostatic hypotension, tachycardia, drowsiness

■ **Serious Reactions**
• Ischemia-related chest pain may occur rarely.
• Priapism has been reported.

Special Considerations
• In clinical trials, peak flow rates increase from a baseline of 10 ml/sec to 12 ml/sec; American Urological Association (AUA) scores decreased by 4-7 points from a baseline of 18

■ **Patient/Family Education**
• Take immediately after the same meal each day
• Hypotension or postural hypotension may occur with first doses
• Avoid performing tasks that require mental alertness or motor skills until response to the drug has been established
• Notify the physician if headache occurs
• Do not chew or crush extended-release tablets

■ **Monitoring Parameters**
• Liver function

■ **Geriatric side effects at a glance:**
☑ CNS ☐ Bowel Dysfunction ☐ Bladder Dysfunction ☑ Falls
Other: Orthostatic Hypotension, Worsening of urge or mixed urinary incontinence

■ **Use with caution in older patients with:** Congestive heart failure, patients taking medications for impotence (e.g., vardenafil, sildenafil, or tadalafil)

■ **U.S. Regulatory Considerations**
☐ FDA Black Box ☐ OBRA regulated in U.S. Long Term Care

■ **Side Effects:**
Of particular importance in the geriatric patient: Orthostatic Hypotension, Worsening of urge or mixed urinary incontinence

- **Geriatric Considerations - Summary:** Alpha-adrenergic blockers are modestly effective alone, and in combination with 5-alpha reductase inhibitors (e.g., finasteride) in the treatment of urinary obstructive symptoms related to benign prostatic hyperplasia. Alfuzosin is a "uroselective" alpha-blocker which appears to cause less orthostatic hypotension than nonselective alpha-blockers such as terazosin, prazosin, and doxazosin.

- **References:**
  1. McConnell JD, Roehrborn CG, Bautista OM, et al. The long-term effect of doxazosin, finasteride, and combination therapy on the clinical progression of benign prostatic hyperplasia. N Engl J Med 2003;349:2387-2398.
  2. Lowe FC. Role of the newer alpha$_1$-adrenergic-receptor antagonists in the treatment of benign prostatic hyperplasia-related lower urinary tract symptoms. Clin Ther 2004;26:1701-1713.
  3. Alfuzosin (uroxatral)—another alpha1-blocker for benign prostatic hyperplasia. Med Lett Drugs Ther 2004;46:1-2.

allopurinol

(al-oh-pure'-i-nole)

- **Brand Name(s):** Aloprim, Zyloprim
  Chemical Class: Hypoxanthine isomer; xanthine oxidase inhibitor

- **Clinical Pharmacology:**
  Mechanism of Action: A xanthine oxidase inhibitor that decreases uric acid production by inhibiting xanthine oxidase, an enzyme. **Therapeutic Effect:** Reduces uric acid concentrations in both serum and urine.
  Pharmacokinetics:

Route	Onset	Peak	Duration
PO/IV	2-3 days	1-3 wk	1-2 wk

  Well absorbed from the GI tract. Widely distributed. Metabolized in the liver to active metabolite. Excreted primarily in urine. Removed by hemodialysis. **Half-life:** 1-3 hr; metabolite, 12-30 hr.

- **Available Forms:**
  - *Tablets* (*Zyloprim*): 100 mg, 300 mg.
  - *Powder for Injection* (*Aloprim*): 500 mg.

- **Indications and Dosages:**
  Chronic gouty arthritis: PO Initially, 100 mg/day; may increase by 100 mg/day at weekly intervals. Maximum: 800 mg/day. Maintenance: 100-200 mg 2-3 times a day or 300 mg/day.
  To prevent uric acid nephropathy during chemotherapy: PO Initially, 600-800 mg/day starting 2-3 days before initiation of chemotherapy or radiation therapy. IV 200-400 mg/m^2/day beginning 24-48 hr before initiation of chemotherapy. **Alert** Maintenance dosage is based on serum uric acid levels. Discontinue following the period of tumor regression.

Prevention of uric acid calculi: PO 100-200 mg 1-4 times a day or 300 mg once a day.
Recurrent calcium oxalate calculi: PO Initially, 100 mg/day, gradually increased until optimal uric acid level is reached.
Dosage in renal impairment: Dosage is modified based on creatinine clearance.

Creatinine Clearance	Dosage Adjustment
10-20 ml/min	200 mg/day
3-9 ml/min	100 mg/day
less than 3 ml/min	100 mg at extended intervals

■ **Unlabeled Uses:** In mouthwash following fluorouracil therapy to prevent stomatitis

■ **Contraindications:** Acute gout

■ **Side Effects**
   Occasional
   Oral: Somnolence, unusual hair loss
   IV: Rash, nausea, vomiting
   Rare
   Diarrhea, headache

■ **Serious Reactions**
   • Pruritic maculopapular rash possibly accompanied by malaise, fever, chills, joint pain, nausea, and vomiting should be considered a toxic reaction.
   • Severe hypersensitivity may follow appearance of rash.
   • Bone marrow depression, hepatic toxicity, peripheral neuritis, and acute renal failure occur rarely.

Special Considerations
   • Increased acute attacks of gout during early stages of allopurinol administration—cover with colchicine
   • Maintenance doses of colchicine (0.6 mg qd-bid) should be given prophylactically along with starting with low doses of allopurinol
   • To reduce risk of flare, begin with 100 mg qd and increase by 100 mg qwk until serum uric acid is 6 mg/dl or less.
   • Parenteral formulation available as orphan drug and in Canada

■ **Patient/Family Education**
   • It may take 1 wk or longer of administration of the drug for it to reach full therapeutic effect
   • Drink 10-12 eight-ounce glasses of fluid daily while taking medication
   • Avoid tasks that require mental alertness or motor skills until response to the drug is established

■ **Monitoring Parameters**
   • Serum uric acid; can usually be achieved in 1-3 wk

■ **Geriatric side effects at a glance:**
   ❑ CNS ❑ Bowel Dysfunction ❑ Bladder Dysfunction ❑ Falls
   Other: Rash, Hypersensitivity Reactions

■ **Use with caution in older patients with:** Renal impairment, Dehydration

U.S. Regulatory Considerations
❑ FDA Black Box ❑ OBRA regulated in U.S. Long Term Care

Other Uses in Geriatric Patient: Nonbacterial Prostatitis, Prevention of Tumor Lysis Syndrome

Side Effects:
Of particular importance in the geriatric patient: Drowsiness, malaise, headache, nausea, diarrhea, maculopapular rash, hypersensitivity reactions—fever, exfoliative dermatitis, liver function abnormalities, renal impairment, eosinophilia

Geriatric Considerations - Summary: Adjust allopurinol dose based on creatinine clearance. Do not initiate during acute gout attack. Monitor fluid intake to maintain urinary output. Allopurinol metabolism to oxipurinol (potent inhibitor of xanthine oxidase) is not reduced by age, but renal excretion of oxipurinol is significantly reduced in healthy older adults. Metabolism and excretion of both allopurinol and oxipurinol may be further reduced in older adults with chronic disease. Increased oxipurinol serum concentrations are associated with toxicities seen with increasing age. Serum uric acid levels generally normalize within 14 days of starting allopurinol, gout attacks subside within 3-6 mo, but tophi dissolution may take up to 1 yr or longer.

References:
1. Turnheim K, Krivanek P, Oberbauer R. Pharmacokinetics and pharmacodynamics of allopurinol in elderly and young subjects. Br J Clin Pharmacol 1999;48:501-509.
2. Fam AG. Gout in the elderly: clinical presentation and treatment. Drugs & Aging 1998;13:229-243.
3. Persson B, Ronquist G, Ekblom M: Ameliorative effect of allopurinol on nonbacterial prostatitis: a parallel double-blind controlled study. J Urol 1996;155:961-964.

almotriptan malate

(al-moh-trip'-tan mal'-ate)

Brand Name(s): Axert
Chemical Class: Serotonin derivative

Clinical Pharmacology:
Mechanism of Action: A serotonin receptor agonist that binds selectively to vascular receptors, producing a vasoconstrictive effect on cranial blood vessels. *Therapeutic Effect:* Produces relief of migraine headache.
Pharmacokinetics: Well absorbed after PO administration. Metabolized by the liver, excreted in urine. *Half-life:* 3-4 hr.

Available Forms:
• *Tablets:* 6.5 mg, 12.5 mg.

Indications and Dosages:
Migraine headache: PO Initially, 6.25-12.5 mg as a single dose. If headache improves but then returns, dose may be repeated after 2 hr. Maximum: 2 doses/24 hr.

Dosage in renal impairment: Recommended initial dose is 6.25 mg and maximum daily dose is 12.5 mg.

■ **Contraindications:** Arrhythmias associated with conduction disorders, hemiplegic or basilar migraine, ischemic heart disease (including angina pectoris, history of MI, silent ischemia, and Prinzmetal's angina), uncontrolled hypertension, use within 24 hr of ergotamine-containing preparation or another serotonin receptor antagonist, use within 14 days of MAOIs, Wolff-Parkinson-White syndrome

■ **Side Effects**
   Frequent
   Nausea, dry mouth, paresthesia, flushing
   Occasional
   Changes in temperature sensation, asthenia, dizziness

■ **Serious Reactions**
   • Excessive dosage may produce tremor, red extremities, reduced respirations, cyanosis, seizures, and chest pain.
   • Serious arrhythmias occur rarely, particularly in patients with hypertension or diabetes, obese patients, smokers, and those with a strong family history of coronary artery disease.

Special Considerations
   • Safety of treating, on average, more than 4 headaches in a 30-day period has not been established
   • Controlled trials have not adequately established the effectiveness of a second dose if the initial dose is ineffective
   • Superiority over other triptan migraine headache agents has not been demonstrated

■ **Patient/Family Education**
   • Use only to treat migraine headache, not for prevention
   • Take a single dose of almotriptan as soon as migraine symptoms appear
   • Lie down in a quiet, dark room for additional benefit after taking this drug
   • Avoid tasks that require mental alertness or motor skills until response to the drug has been established
   • Notify the physician immediately if palpitations, pain or tightness in the chest or throat, or pain or weakness in the extremities occurs

■ **Monitoring Parameters**
   • Evaluate for relief of migraines and associated symptoms, including nausea and vomiting, photophobia, and phonophobia (sound sensitivity)

■ **Geriatric side effects at a glance:**
   ❑ CNS   ❑ Bowel Dysfunction   ❑ Bladder Dysfunction   ❑ Falls

■ **U.S. Regulatory Considerations**
   ❑ FDA Black Box   ❑ OBRA regulated in U.S. Long Term Care

alprazolam

(al-pray'-zoe-lam)

- **Brand Name(s):** Xanax, Niravam, Xanax, Xanax XR
  Chemical Class: Benzodiazepine
  DEA Class: Schedule IV

- **Clinical Pharmacology:**
  Mechanism of Action: A benzodiazepine that enhances the action of the inhibitory neurotransmitter gamma-aminobutyric acid in the brain. **Therapeutic Effect:** Produces sedative effect from its CNS depressant action.
  Pharmacokinetics: Well absorbed from GI tract. Protein binding: 80%. Metabolized in the liver. Primarily excreted in urine. Minimal removal by hemodialysis. **Half-life:** 11-16 hr.

- **Available Forms:**
  - *Oral Solution (Alprazolam Intensol):* 1 mg/ml.
  - *Tablets (Xanax):* 0.25 mg, 0.5 mg, 1 mg, 2 mg.
  - *Tablets (Extended-Release [Xanax XR]):* 0.5 mg, 1 mg, 2 mg, 3 mg.
  - *Tablets (Orally Disintegrating [Niravam]):* 0.25 mg, 0.5 mg, 1 mg, 2 mg.

- **Indications and Dosages:**
  Anxiety disorders: PO (Immediate-Release) Initially, 0.25 mg 2-3 times a day. Gradually increase to optimum therapeutic response. **Debilitated patients, Patients with hepatic disease or low serum albumin.** Initially, 0.25 mg 2-3 times a day. Gradually increase to optimum therapeutic response. PO (Orally Disintegrating) 0.25-0.5 mg 3 times a day. Maximum: 4 mg/day in divided doses.
  Anxiety with depression: PO 2.5-3 mg/day in divided doses.
  Panic disorder: PO (Immediate-Release) Initially, 0.125-0.25 mg twice a day. May increase in 0.125-mg increments until desired effect attained. PO (Extended-Release) Alert To switch from immediate-release to extended-release form, give total daily dose (immediate-release) as a single daily dose of extended-release form. Initially, 0.5 mg once daily. May titrate at 3- to 4- day intervals. Range: 3-6 mg/day. Maximum: 10 mg/day. PO (Orally Disintegrating) Initially, 0.5 mg 3 times a day. May increase at 3- to 4-day intervals. Range: 5-6 mg/day. Maximum: 10 mg/day.

- **Unlabeled Uses:** Management of agitation and insomnia in dementia patients

- **Contraindications:** Acute alcohol intoxication with depressed vital signs, acute angle-closure glaucoma, concurrent use of itraconazole or ketoconazole, myasthenia gravis, severe COPD

- **Side Effects**
  Frequent
  Ataxia; light-headedness; transient, mild somnolence; slurred speech (particularly in elderly or debilitated patients)
  Occasional
  Confusion, depression, blurred vision, constipation, diarrhea, dry mouth, headache, nausea

Rare
Behavioral problems such as anger, impaired memory, paradoxical reactions such as insomnia, nervousness, or irritability

■ **Serious Reactions**
- Abrupt or too rapid withdrawal may result in pronounced restlessness, irritability, insomnia, hand tremors, abdominal and muscle cramps, diaphoresis, vomiting, and seizures.
- Overdose results in somnolence, confusion, diminished reflexes, and coma.
- Blood dyscrasias have been reported rarely.

■ **Patient/Family Education**
- Not for "everyday" stress or longer than 3 mo; avoid driving, activities that require alertness
- Caution when medication discontinued abruptly after long-term (>4 wk) use—may precipitate withdrawal syndrome
- Avoid tasks that require mental alertness or motor skills until response to the drug is established
- Smoking reduces alprazolam's effectiveness

■ **Geriatric side effects at a glance:**
☑ CNS   ❑ Bowel Dysfunction   ❑ Bladder Dysfunction   ☑ Falls
Other: Withdrawal symptoms after long-term use

■ **Use with caution in older patients with:** Concurrent treatment with potent CYP 3A4 inhibitors (e.g., itraconazole) leads to increased plasma concentrations of alprazolam; COPD; Untreated sleep apnea

■ **U.S. Regulatory Considerations**
❑ FDA Black Box   ☑ OBRA regulated in U.S. Long Term Care

■ **Other Uses in Geriatric Patient:** Anxiety symptoms and related disorders, Dementia-related behavioral problems, Skeletal muscle strain

■ **Side Effects:**
Of particular importance in the geriatric patient: Sedation, withdrawal symptoms when abruptly discontinued (e.g., during hospitalization) rather than tapered

■ **Geriatric Considerations - Summary:** Benzodiazepines are effective anxiolytic agents, and hypnotics. These drugs should be reserved for short-term use. SSRIs are preferred for long-term management of anxiety disorders in older adults, and sedating antidepressants (e.g., trazodone) or eszopiclone are preferred for long-term management of sleep problems. Long-acting benzodiazepines, including flurazepam, chlordiazepoxide, clorazepate, diazepam, clonazepam, and quazepam should generally be avoided in older adults as these agents have been associated with oversedation. On the other hand, short acting benzodiazepines (e.g., triazolam) have been associated with a higher risk of withdrawal symptoms. When initiating therapy, benzodiazepines should be titrated carefully to avoid oversedation. In addition, many of the drugs in this class have been associated with severe withdrawal symptoms (e.g., anxiety and/or agitation, seizures) when discontinued abruptly.

■ **References:**
1. Leipzig RM, Cumming RG, Tinetti ME. Drugs and falls in older people: a systematic review and meta-analysis: I. Psychotropic drugs. J Am Geriatr Soc 1999;47:30-39.
2. Shorr RI, Robin DW. Rational use of benzodiazepines in the elderly. Drugs Aging 1994;4:9-20.
3. Shader RI, Greenblatt DJ. Use of benzodiazepines in anxiety disorders. N Engl J Med 1993;328:1398-1405.

alprostadil (prostaglandin E_1, PGE_1)

(al-pros'-ta-dil)

■ **Brand Name(s):** Caverject, Edex, Muse
  Chemical Class: Prostaglandin E_1

■ **Clinical Pharmacology:**
  Mechanism of Action: A prostaglandin that directly affects vascular and ductus arteriosus smooth muscle and relaxes trabecular smooth muscle. **Therapeutic Effect:** Causes vasodilation; dilates cavernosal arteries, allowing blood flow to and entrapment in the lacunar spaces of the penis.
  Pharmacokinetics: Absorption occurs from the urethral lining when inserted as a urethral suppository. Protein binding: 81%-99% (injection). Rapidly metabolized. Excreted in urine and lung. **Half-life:** 5-10 min (injection).

■ **Available Forms:**
  • Urethral Pellet (Muse): 125 mcg, 250 mcg, 500 mcg, 1000 mcg.

■ **Indications and Dosages:**
  Impotence: Pellet, Intracavernosal Dosage is individualized.

■ **Unlabeled Uses:** Treatment of atherosclerosis, gangrene, pain due to severe peripheral arterial occlusive disease, pulmonary hypertension

■ **Contraindications:** Conditions predisposing to anatomic deformation of penis, penile implants, priapism
  Alert: Patient should not have intercourse with pregnant sexual partners unless a condom is used.

■ **Side Effects**
  Frequent
  Intracavernosal (4%-1%): Penile pain (37%), prolonged erection, hypertension, localized pain, penile fibrosis, injection site hematoma or ecchymosis, headache, respiratory infection, flu-like symptoms
  Intraurethral (3%): Penile pain (36%), urethral pain or burning, testicular pain, urethral bleeding, headache, dizziness, respiratory infection, flu-like symptoms

39

Systemic (greater than 1%): Fever, flushing, bradycardia, hypotension, tachycardia, diarrhea

Occasional

Intracavernosal (less than 1%): Hypotension, pelvic pain, back pain, dizziness, cough, nasal congestion

Intraurethral (less than 3%): Fainting, sinusitis, back and pelvic pain

Systemic (less than 1%): Anxiety, lethargy, myalgia, arrhythmias, respiratory depression, anemia, bleeding, hematuria

■ Serious Reactions

- Overdose is manifested as apnea, flushing of the face and arms, and bradycardia.
- Cardiac arrest and sepsis occur rarely.
- Seizures, apnea, sepsis, and thrombocytopenia occur rarely.
- Priapism occurs in 0.4% of patients receiving alprostadil injection and in less than 0.1% of patients receiving the drug intraurethrally.

Special Considerations

- For intracavernosal use administer first dose under medical supervision. Use ½-inch 27-30 gauge needle along dorsolateral aspect of proximal third of penis. Alternate sides
- Urinate prior to intraurethral use to disperse pellet
- Use lowest dose allowing satisfactory erection lasting 1 hr or longer

■ Patient/Family Education

- Proper use of injection
- Proper use of suppository
- Store unopened foil pouches in the refrigerator; medicine is good for 14 days at room temperature

■ Monitoring Parameters

- Efficacy and side effects

■ Geriatric side effects at a glance:

❑ CNS ❑ Bowel Dysfunction ❑ Bladder Dysfunction ❑ Falls

■ U.S. Regulatory Considerations

☑ FDA Black Box

Apnea in neonates

❑ OBRA regulated in U.S. Long Term Care

alteplase, recombinant

(al-teep'-lase)

- **Brand Name(s):** Activase, Cathflo Activase
  Chemical Class: Tissue plasminogen activator (tPA)

- **Clinical Pharmacology:**
  Mechanism of Action: A tissue plasminogen activator that acts as a CV-thrombolytic by binding to the fibrin in a thrombus and converting entrapped plasminogen to plasmin. This process initiates fibrinolysis. **Therapeutic Effect:** Degrades fibrin clots, fibrinogen, and other plasma proteins.
  Pharmacokinetics: Rapidly metabolized in the liver. Primarily excreted in urine. **Half-life:** 35 min.

- **Available Forms:**
  - *Powder for Injection:* 2 mg (Cathflo Activase), 50 mg (Activase), 100 mg (Activase).

- **Indications and Dosages:**
  Acute MI: IV Infusion *Weight greater than 67 kg.* 100 mg over 90 min, starting with 15-mg bolus over 1-2 min, then 50 mg over 30 min, then 35 mg over 60 min. Or a 3-hr infusion, giving 60 mg over first hr (6-10 mg as bolus over 1-2 min), 20 mg over second hr, and 20 mg over third hr. *Weight 67 kg or less:* 100 mg over 90 min, starting with 15-mg bolus, then 0.75 mg/kg over 30 min (maximum: 50 mg), then 0.5 mg/kg over 60 min (maximum: 35 mg). Or 3-hr infusion of 1.25 mg/kg giving 60% of dose over first hr (6%-10% as 1- to 2-min bolus), 20% over second hr, and 20% over third hr.
  Acute pulmonary emboli: IV Infusion 100 mg over 2 hr. Institute or reinstitute heparin near end or immediately after infusion when aPTT or thrombin time (TT) returns to twice normal or less.
  Acute ischemic stroke: IV Infusion 0.9 mg/kg over 60 min (load with 0.09 mg/kg [10% of 0.9 mg/kg dose] as IV bolus over 1 min). **Alert** Dose should be given within the first 3 hr of onset of symptoms.
  Central venous catheter clearance: IV 2 mg; may repeat after 2 hr.

- **Unlabeled Uses:** Acute peripheral occlusive disease, basilar artery occlusion, cerebral infarction, deep vein thrombosis, femoropopliteal artery occlusion, mesenteric or subclavian vein occlusion, pleural effusion (parapneumonic)

- **Contraindications:** Active internal bleeding, AV malformation or aneurysm, bleeding diathesis, intracranial neoplasm, intracranial or intraspinal surgery or trauma, recent (within past 2 mo) cerebrovascular accident, severe uncontrolled hypertension

- **Side Effects**
  Frequent
  Superficial bleeding at puncture sites, decreased BP
  Occasional
  Allergic reaction, such as rash or wheezing; bruising

- **Serious Reactions**
  - Severe internal hemorrhage may occur.
  - Lysis of coronary thrombi may produce atrial or ventricular arrhythmias or stroke.

- Heparin (in doses sufficient to prolong the aPTT to 1.5-2 times control value) is usually administered in conjunction with thrombolytic therapy; aspirin may also be administered to inhibit platelet aggregation during and/or following post-thrombolytic therapy
- Compress arterial puncture sites at least 30 min

Monitoring Parameters
- Prior to initiation of therapy: coagulation tests, hematocrit, platelet count
- Blood pressure

Geriatric side effects at a glance:
❑ CNS ❑ Bowel Dysfunction ❑ Bladder Dysfunction ❑ Falls

U.S. Regulatory Considerations
❑ FDA Black Box ❑ OBRA regulated in U.S. Long Term Care

aluminum chloride hexahydrate

(a-loo'-mi-num klor'-ide hexa-hye'-drate)

Brand Name(s): Drysol, Xerac AC
OTC: Powder, solution
Chemical Class: Trivalent cation

Clinical Pharmacology:
Mechanism of Action: Aluminum salts cause an obstruction of the distal sweat gland. This obstruction causes metal ions to precipitate with mucopolysaccharides, damaging epithelial cells along the lumen of the duct, and forming a plug to block sweat output. **Therapeutic Effect:** Results in decreased secretion of the sweat glands. **Pharmacokinetics:** Not known.

Available Forms:
- *Topical Solution*: 6.25% (Xerac AC), 20% (Drysol).

Indications and Dosages:
Antiperspirant: Topical Apply to each underarm once a day, at bedtime.
Hyperhidrosis: Topical Apply to affected areas once a day, at bedtime.

Contraindications: Hypersensitivity to aluminum chloride or any one of its components.

Side Effects
Frequent
Itching, burning, tingling sensation

Occasional
Rash

■ **Serious Reactions**
- Hypersensitivity reaction, such as rash may occur.

■ **Patient/Family Education**
- Do not apply to broken or irritated skin
- For maximum effect, cover treated area with Saran wrap held in place by snug-fitting shirt, mitten, or sock (never hold Saran wrap in place with tape)
- Avoid contact with eyes
- May be harmful to cotton fibers or certain metals
- Do not apply other deodorants or antiperspirants while using this drug

■ **Geriatric side effects at a glance:**
❑ CNS ❑ Bowel Dysfunction ❑ Bladder Dysfunction ❑ Falls

■ **U.S. Regulatory Considerations**
❑ FDA Black Box ❑ OBRA regulated in U.S. Long Term Care

aluminum salts group

■ **Brand Name(s):**

Combinations
OTC: Aluminum acetate and acetic acid (Otic Domeboro); aluminum hydroxide and magnesium carbonate (Gaviscon Extra Strength, Gaviscon Liquid); aluminum hydroxide and magnesium trisilicate (Gaviscon); aluminum hydroxide, magnesium hydroxide, and simethicone (Maalox Fast Release Liquid, Maalox Max, Mylanta Extra Strength Liquid, Mylanta Liquid); aluminum sulfate and calcium acetate (Bluboro, Domeboro, Pedi-Boro)
Chemical Class: Trivalent cation

■ **Clinical Pharmacology:**
Mechanism of Action: An antacid that reduces gastric acid by binding with phosphate in the intestine, and then is excreted as aluminum carbonate in feces. Aluminum carbonate may increase the absorption of calcium due to decreased serum phosphate levels. The drug also has astringent and adsorbent properties. *Therapeutic Effect:* Neutralizes or increases gastric pH; reduces phosphates in urine, preventing formation of phosphate urinary stones; reduces serum phosphate levels; decreases fluidity of stools.
Pharmacokinetics: Varies in each formulation.

■ **Available Forms:**
Aluminum hydroxide:
- *Capsules:* 400 mg (Alu-Cap), 500 mg (Dialume).
- *Liquid:* 600 mg/5 mg (ALternaGEL).
- *Suspension:* 320 mg/5 ml (Amphojel), 450 mg/5 ml, 675 mg/ 5 ml.

- *Tablets*: 300 mg (Amphojel), 500 mg (Alu-Tab), 600 mg (Amphojel).

Aluminum acetate & acetic acid:
- *Otic solution*: 2% acetic acid and aluminum acetate (Otic Domeboro).

Aluminum hydroxide and magnesium carbonate:
- *Liquid*: 31.7 mg aluminum hydroxide and 119.3 mg magnesium carbonate/5 ml (Gaviscon Liquid); 84.6 mg aluminum hydroxide and 79.1 mg magnesium carbonate/5 ml (Gaviscon Extra Strength).
- *Tablets, chewable*: 160 mg aluminum hydroxide and 1.5 mg magnesium carbonate (Gaviscon Extra Strength Relief).

Aluminum hydroxide & magnesium hydroxide:
- *Suspension*: 225 mg aluminum hydroxide and 200 mg magnesium hydroxide/5 ml (Maalox).
- *Suspension*: 600 mg aluminum hydroxide and 300 mg magnesium hydroxide/5 ml (Maalox TC).

Aluminum hydroxide & magnesium trisilicate:
- *Tablets, chewable*: 80 mg aluminum hydroxide and 20 mg magnesium hydroxide (Gaviscon).

Aluminum hydroxide, magnesium hydroxide, & simethicone:
- *Liquid*: 200 mg aluminum hydroxide, 200 mg magnesium hydroxide, and 20 mg simethicone/5 ml (Mylanta); 400 mg aluminum hydroxide, 400 mg magnesium hydroxide, and 40 mg simethicone/5 ml (Maalox Max); 500 mg aluminum hydroxide, 450 mg magnesium hydroxide, and 20 mg simethicone/5 ml (Maalox Fast Release); 400 mg aluminum hydroxide, 400 mg magnesium hydroxide, and 40 mg simethicone/5 ml (Mylanta Extra Strength).

Aluminum sulfate & calcium acetate:
- *Powder, for topical solution*: packets (Bluboro, Domeboro, Pedi-Boro).
- *Tablets, effervescent, for topical solution*: effervescent tablets (Domeboro).

■ **Indications and Dosages:**

Aluminum hydroxide:
Peptic ulcer disease:
PO
5-15 ml as above. 15-45 ml q3-6h or 1 and 3 hr after meals and at bedtime.
Antacid:
PO
30 ml 1 and 3 hr after meals and at bedtime.
Gastrointestinal (GI) bleeding prevention:
PO
30-60 ml/hr.
Hyperphosphatemia:
PO
500-1800 mg 1 and 3 hr after meals and at bedtime.

Aluminum acetate & acetic acid:
Superficial infections of the external auditory canal:
Otic
Instill 4-6 drops in ear(s) q2-3h.

Aluminum hydroxide & magnesium carbonate:
Antacid:
PO
15-30 ml 4 times/day of the liquid; chew 2-4 tablets 4 times/day.

Aluminum hydroxide & magnesium hydroxide:
Antacid:
PO
5-10 ml 4-6 times/day.

Aluminum hydroxide & magnesium trisilicate:
Antacid:
PO
Chew 2-4 tablets 4 times/day or as directed.
Aluminum hydroxide, magnesium hydroxide, and simethicone:
Antacid (with flatulence):
PO
10-20 ml or 2-4 tablets 4-6 times/day.
Aluminum sulfate & calcium acetate:
Inflammatory skin conditions with weeping that occurs in dermatitis:
Topical
Soak affected area in solution 2-4 times/day for 15-30 min or apply wet dressing soaked in solution 2-4 times/day for 30-min treatment periods. Domeboro: Saturate dressing and apply to affected area and saturate every 15-30 min; or soak for 15-30 min 3 times/day.

■ **Contraindications:** Intestinal obstruction, hypersensitivity to aluminum or any component of the formulation

■ **Side Effects**
Frequent
PO: Chalky taste, mild constipation, stomach cramps
Topical: Burning, itching
Occasional
PO: Nausea, vomiting, speckling or whitish discoloration of stools
Otic: Burning or stinging in ear
Topical: New or continued redness, skin dryness
Rare
Otic: Skin rash, redness, swelling or pain in ear

■ **Serious Reactions**
• Prolonged constipation may result in intestinal obstruction.
• Excessive or chronic use may produce hypophosphatemia manifested as anorexia, malaise, muscle weakness, or bone pain and resulting in osteomalacia and osteoporosis.
• Prolonged use may produce urinary calculi.

■ **Patient/Family Education**
• Thoroughly chew chewable tablets before swallowing, follow with a glass of water
• May impair absorption of many drugs; do not take other drugs within 1 hr before or 4 hr after aluminum hydroxide administration
• Stools may appear white or speckled
• Maintain adequate fluid intake

■ **Monitoring Parameters**
• Consider monitoring for hypophosphatemia
• Daily bowel activity and stool consistency

■ **Geriatric side effects at a glance:**
❏ CNS ☑ Bowel Dysfunction ❏ Bladder Dysfunction ❏ Falls

■ **U.S. Regulatory Considerations**
❏ FDA Black Box ❏ OBRA regulated in U.S. Long Term Care

amantadine hydrochloride

(a-man'-ta-deen hye-droe-klor'-ide)

- **Brand Name(s):** Symmetrel
  Chemical Class: Adamantane derivative; tricyclic amine

- **Clinical Pharmacology:**
  Mechanism of Action: A dopaminergic agonist that blocks the uncoating of influenza A virus, preventing penetration into the host and inhibiting M2 protein in the assembly of progeny virions. Amantadine also blocks the reuptake of dopamine into presynaptic neurons and causes direct stimulation of postsynaptic receptors. **Therapeutic Effect:** Antiviral and antiparkinsonian activity.
  Pharmacokinetics: Rapidly and completely absorbed from the GI tract. Protein binding: 67%. Widely distributed. Primarily excreted in urine. Minimally removed by hemodialysis. **Half-life:** 11-15 hr (increased in the elderly, decreased in impaired renal function).

- **Available Forms:**
  - *Capsules*: 100 mg.
  - *Syrup*: 50 mg/5 ml.
  - *Tablets*: 100 mg.

- **Indications and Dosages:**
  Treatment of influenza A : PO 100 mg a day. Initiate within 24-48 hr after onset of symptoms; discontinue as soon as possible based on clinical response.
  Prevention of infuenza A: PO 100 mg twice a day.
  Parkinson's disease, extrapyramidal symptoms: PO 100 mg twice a day. May increase up to 400 mg/day in divided doses.
  Dosage in renal impairment: Dose and frequency are modified based on creatinine clearance.

Creatinine Clearance	Dosage
30-50 ml/min	200 mg first day; 100 mg/day thereafter
15-29 ml/min	200 mg first day; 100 mg on alternate days
less than 15 ml/min	200 mg every 7 days

- **Unlabeled Uses:** Fatigue associated with multiple sclerosis

- **Contraindications:** None known.

- **Side Effects**
  Frequent (10%-5%)
  Nausea, dizziness, poor concentration, insomnia, nervousness
  Occasional (5%-1%)
  Orthostatic hypotension, anorexia, headache, livedo reticularis (reddish blue, netlike blotching of skin), blurred vision, urine retention, dry mouth or nose
  Rare
  Vomiting, depression, irritation or swelling of eyes, rash

Serious Reactions
- CHF, leukopenia, and neutropenia occur rarely.
- Hyperexcitability, seizures, and ventricular arrhythmias may occur.

Patient/Family Education
- Administer at least 4 hr before bedtime to prevent insomnia
- Take with meals for better absorption and to decrease GI symptoms
- Arise slowly from a reclining position; avoid hazardous activities if dizziness or blurred vision occurs
- Do not discontinue abruptly in Parkinson's disease

Monitoring Parameters
- Renal function
- Intake and output
- Clinical reversal of symptoms

Geriatric side effects at a glance:
☑ CNS   ☐ Bowel Dysfunction   ☐ Bladder Dysfunction   ☐ Falls

U.S. Regulatory Considerations
☐ FDA Black Box   ☐ OBRA regulated in U.S. Long Term Care

ambenonium chloride

(am-be-noe'-nee-um klor'-ide)

Brand Name(s): Mytelase
Chemical Class: Cholinesterase inhibitor; quaternary ammonium compound

Clinical Pharmacology:
Mechanism of Action: A cholinesterase inhibitor that enhances and prolongs cholinergic function by increasing the concentration of acetylcholine through inhibition of the hydrolysis of acetylcholine. **Therapeutic Effect:** Increases muscle strength in myasthenia gravis.
Pharmacokinetics: Poorly absorbed after PO administration.

Available Forms:
- *Tablets*: 10 mg (Mytelase).

Indications and Dosages:
Myasthenia gravis: PO 5-25 mg 3 or 4 times a day. If well tolerated, after 1 or 2 days, may increase to 50-75 mg 3 times a day. Range: 5-200 mg/day in divided doses.

- **Contraindications:** Not recommended in patients receiving routine administration of atropine or other belladonna derivatives. Not recommended in patients receiving mecamylamine.

- **Side Effects**
    Frequent
    Abdominal pain, diarrhea, increased salivation, miosis, sweating, and vomiting
    Occasional
    Anxiety, blurred vision, and urinary urgency
    Rare
    Trembling, difficulty moving or controlling movement of the tongue, neck, or arms

- **Serious Reactions**
    - Overdosage may result in cholinergic crisis, characterized by severe nausea, vomiting, diarrhea, increased salivation, diaphoresis, bradycardia, hypotension, flushed skin, stomach pain, respiratory depression, seizures, and paralysis of muscles.
    - Increasing muscle weakness of myasthenia gravis may occur. Antidote: 0.5-1mg IV atropine sulfate with other supportive treatment.

- **Patient/Family Education**
    - Notify clinician of nausea, vomiting, diarrhea, sweating, increased salivation, irregular heartbeat, muscle weakness, severe abdominal pain or difficulty in breathing
    - Administer on an empty stomach

- **Monitoring Parameters**
    - Narrow margin between 1st appearance of side effects and serious toxicity
    - Symptoms of increasing muscle weakness may be due to cholinergic crisis (overdosage) or myasthenic crisis (increased disease severity); if crisis is myasthenia, patient will improve after 1-2 mg edrophonium; if cholinergic, withdraw ambenonium and administer atropine

- **Geriatric side effects at a glance:**
    ❑ CNS ❑ Bowel Dysfunction ❑ Bladder Dysfunction ❑ Falls

- **U.S. Regulatory Considerations**
    ❑ FDA Black Box ❑ OBRA regulated in U.S. Long Term Care

amcinonide

(am-sin'-oh-nide)

■ **Brand Name(s):** Cylocort
  Chemical Class: Corticosteroid, synthetic

■ **Clinical Pharmacology:**
  Mechanism of Action: Topical corticosteroids have anti-inflammatory, antipruritic, and vasoconstrictive properties. The exact mechanism of the anti-inflammatory process is unclear. **Therapeutic Effect:** Reduces or prevents tissue response to inflammatory process.
  Pharmacokinetics: Well absorbed systemically. Large variation in absorption among sites: forearm 1%; scalp 4%, forehead 7%, scrotum 36%. Greatest penetration occurs at groin, axillae, and face. Protein binding in varying degrees. Metabolized in liver. Primarily excreted in urine.

■ **Available Forms:**
  • *Lotion*: 0.1% (Cylocort).
  • *Cream*: 0.1% (Cylocort).
  • *Ointment*: 0.1% (Cylocort).

■ **Indications and Dosages:**
  Dermatoses: Topical Apply sparingly 2-3 times/day.

■ **Contraindications:** History of hypersensitivity to amcinonide or other corticosteroids.

■ **Side Effects**
  Frequent
  Itching, redness, irritation, burning
  Occasional
  Dryness, folliculitis, hypertrichosis, acneiform eruptions, hypopigmentation, perioral dermatitis
  Rare
  Allergic contact dermatitis, maceration of the skin, secondary infection, skin atrophy.

■ **Serious Reactions**
  • The serious reactions of long-term therapy (greater than 2 weeks) and the addition of occlusive dressings are reversible hypothalamic-pituitary-adrenal (HPA) axis suppression, manifestations of Cushing's syndrome, hyperglycemia, and glucosuria.
  • Abruptly withdrawing the drug after long-term therapy may require supplemental systemic corticosteroids.

■ **Patient/Family Education**
  • Apply sparingly only to affected area
  • Avoid contact with eyes

- Do not put bandages or dressings over treated area unless directed by clinician
- Do not use on weeping, denuded, or infected areas

■ **Monitoring Parameters**
- Blood glucose levels, blood pressure, electrolytes

■ **Geriatric side effects at a glance:**
❑ CNS ❑ Bowel Dysfunction ❑ Bladder Dysfunction ❑ Falls

■ **U.S. Regulatory Considerations**
❑ FDA Black Box ❑ OBRA regulated in U.S. Long Term Care

amikacin sulfate

(am-i-kay'-sin sul'-fate)

■ **Brand Name(s):** Amikin
Chemical Class: Aminoglycoside

■ **Clinical Pharmacology:**
Mechanism of Action: An aminoglycoside antibacterial that irreversibly binds to protein on bacterial ribosomes. **Therapeutic Effect:** Interferes with protein synthesis of susceptible microorganisms.
Pharmacokinetics: Rapid, complete absorption after IM administration. Protein binding: 0%-10%. Widely distributed (doesn't cross the blood-brain barrier, low concentrations in CSF). Excreted unchanged in urine. Removed by hemodialysis. **Half-life:** 2-4 hr (increased in impaired renal function; decreased in cystic fibrosis and burn or febrile patients).

■ **Available Forms:**
- **Injection:** 62.5 mg/ml, 250 mg/ml.

■ **Indications and Dosages:**
UTIs: IV, IM 250 mg q12h.
Moderate to severe infections: IV, IM 15 mg/kg/day in divided doses q8-12h. Maximum 1.5 g/day.
Dosage in renal impairment: Dosage and frequency are modified based on the degree of renal impairment and serum drug concentration. After a loading dose of 5-7.5 mg/kg, the maintenance dose and frequency are based on serum creatinine levels and creatinine clearance.

■ **Contraindications:** Hypersensitivity to amikacin, or other aminoglycosides (cross-sensitivity), or their components.

■ **Side Effects**
Frequent
IM: Pain, induration
IV: Phlebitis, thrombophlebitis

Occasional

Hypersensitivity reactions (rash, fever, urticaria, pruritus)

Rare

Neuromuscular blockade (difficulty breathing, drowsiness, weakness)

■ **Serious Reactions**

- Serious reactions may include nephrotoxicity (as evidenced by increased thirst, decreased appetite, nausea, vomiting, increased BUN and serum creatinine levels, and decreased creatinine clearance); neurotoxicity (manifested as muscle twitching, visual disturbances, seizures, and tingling); and ototoxicity (as evidenced by tinnitus, dizziness, and loss of hearing).

■ **Monitoring Parameters**

- Urine output, serum creatinine
- Serum peak, drawn 30-60 min after IV INF or 60 min after IM inj; trough level drawn just before next dose; adjust dosage per levels (usual therapeutic plasma levels; peak 20-35 mg/L, trough 10 mg/L or less)
- Skin for rash

■ **Geriatric side effects at a glance:**

❑ CNS   ❑ Bowel Dysfunction   ❑ Bladder Dysfunction   ❑ Falls

■ **U.S. Regulatory Considerations**

☑ FDA Black Box

Risk for neurotoxicity (auditory and vestibular ototoxicity) and nephrotoxicity. Risk is greater in patients with impaired renal function and in those who receive high doses or prolonged therapy.

❑ OBRA regulated in U.S. Long Term Care

amiloride hydrochloride

(a-mill'-oh-ride hye-droe-klor'-ide)

■ **Brand Name(s):** Midamor

Combinations
Rx: with hydrochlorothiazide (Moduretic)
Chemical Class: Pyrazine

■ **Clinical Pharmacology:**

Mechanism of Action: A guanidine derivative that acts as a potassium-sparing diuretic, antihypertensive, and antihypokalemic by directly interfering with sodium reabsorption in the distal tubule. **Therapeutic Effect:** Increases sodium and water excretion and decreases potassium excretion.

Pharmacokinetics:

Route	Onset	Peak	Duration
PO	2 hr	6-10 hr	24 hr

Incompletely absorbed from the GI tract. Protein binding: Minimal. Primarily excreted in urine; partially eliminated in feces. **Half-life:** 6-9 hr.

■ **Available Forms:**
- *Tablets*: 5 mg.

■ **Indications and Dosages:**
To counteract potassium loss induced by other diuretics: PO Initially, 5 mg/day or every other day.
Dosage in renal impairment:

Creatinine Clearance	Dosage
10-50 ml/min	50% of normal
less than 10 ml/min	avoid use

■ **Unlabeled Uses:** Treatment of edema associated with CHF, liver cirrhosis, and nephrotic syndrome; treatment of hypertension; reduces lithium-induced polyuria, slows pulmonary function reduction in cystic fibrosis

■ **Contraindications:** Acute or chronic renal insufficiency, anuria, diabetic nephropathy, patients on other potassium-sparing diuretics, serum potassium greater than 5.5 mEq/L

■ **Side Effects**
Frequent (8%–3%)
Headache, nausea, diarrhea, vomiting, decreased appetite
Occasional (3%–1%)
Dizziness, constipation, abdominal pain, weakness, fatigue, cough, impotence
Rare (less than 1%)
Tremors, vertigo, confusion, nervousness, insomnia, thirst, dry mouth, heartburn, shortness of breath, increased urination, hypotension, rash

■ **Serious Reactions**
- Severe hyperkalemia may produce irritability, anxiety, a feeling of heaviness in the legs, paresthesia of hands, face, and lips, hypotension, bradycardia, tented T waves, widening of QRS, and ST depression.

■ **Patient/Family Education**
- Notify clinician of muscle weakness, fatigue, flaccid paralysis
- Take with food or milk for GI symptoms
- Take early in day to prevent nocturia
- Avoid large quantities of potassium-rich foods: oranges, bananas, salt substitutes

■ **Monitoring Parameters**
- Electrolytes

■ **Geriatric side effects at a glance:**
  ❏ CNS ❏ Bowel Dysfunction ❏ Bladder Dysfunction ❏ Falls

   ☑ FDA Black Box
   Hyperkalemia, if uncorrected, is potentially fatal
   ❑ OBRA regulated in U.S. Long Term Care

aminocaproic acid

(a-mee-noe-ka-proe'-ik as'-id)

■ **Brand Name(s):** Amicar
   Chemical Class: Monoaminocarboxylic acid, synthetic

■ **Clinical Pharmacology:**
   Mechanism of Action: A systemic hemostatic that acts as an antifibrinolytic and antihemorrhagic by inhibiting the activation of plasminogen activator substances. **Therapeutic Effect:** Prevents formation of fibrin clots.
   Pharmacokinetics: Rapidly absorbed following PO administration. Does not appear to bind to plasma protein. Excreted rapidly in urine, mostly unchanged. **Half-life:** 2 hr.

■ **Available Forms:**
   • *Syrup*: 250 mg/ml.
   • *Tablets*: 500 mg.
   • *Injection*: 250 mg/ml.

■ **Indications and Dosages:**
   Acute bleeding: PO, IV Infusion 4-5g over first hr; then 1-1.25 g/hr. Continue for 8 hr or until bleeding is controlled. Maximum: 30 g/24 hr.
   Dosage in renal impairment: Decrease dose to 25% of normal.

■ **Unlabeled Uses:** Control of bleeding in thrombocytopenia, control of oral bleeding in congenital and acquired coagulation disorders, prevention of recurrence of subarachnoid hemorrhage, prevention of hemorrhage in hemophiliacs following dental surgery, treatment of traumatic hyphema

■ **Contraindications:** Evidence of active intravascular clotting process, disseminated intravascular coagulation without concurrent heparin therapy, hematuria of upper urinary tract origin (unless benefit outweighs risk);

■ **Side Effects**
   Occasional
   Nausea, diarrhea, cramps, decreased urination, decreased BP, dizziness, headache, muscle fatigue and weakness, myopathy, bloodshot eyes

■ **Serious Reactions**
   • Too rapid IV administration produces tinnitus, rash, arrhythmias, unusual fatigue, and weakness.

- Rarely, a grand mal seizure occurs, generally preceded by weakness, dizziness, and headache.

■ **Patient/Family Education**
- Report any signs of bleeding or myopathy
- Change position slowly to decrease orthostatic hypotension
- No need to adjust INR in warfarin anticoagulated patients with topical hemostatic mouthwash use

■ **Monitoring Parameters**
- Do not administer without a definite diagnosis and laboratory findings indicative of hyperfibrinolysis
- Blood studies including coagulation factors, platelets, fibrinolysin; CPK, urinalysis
- Blood pressure, heart rate

■ **Geriatric side effects at a glance:**
  ❏ CNS ❏ Bowel Dysfunction ❏ Bladder Dysfunction ❏ Falls

■ **U.S. Regulatory Considerations**
  ❏ FDA Black Box ❏ OBRA regulated in U.S. Long Term Care

aminophylline/theophylline

(am-in-off'-i-lin; thee-off'-i-lin)

■ **Brand Name(s):** (aminophylline) Phyllocontin, (theophylline) Elixophyllin, Quibron-T, Quibron-T/SR, Slo-bid Gyrocaps, Theo-24, Theochron, Theodur, Theolair, Theolair-SR, T-Phyl, Uniphyl
  Chemical Class: Ethylenediamine derivative

■ **Clinical Pharmacology:**
  Mechanism of Action: A xanthine derivative that acts as a bronchodilator by directly relaxing smooth muscle of the bronchial airways and pulmonary blood vessels. **Therapeutic Effect:** Relieves bronchospasm and increases vital capacity.
  Pharmacokinetics: Rapidly and well absorbed. Protein binding: Moderate (to albumin). Extensively metabolized in liver. Partially excreted in urine. **Half-life:** 6-12 hr (varies).

■ **Available Forms:**
- *Capsules (Extended-Release [Theo-24]):* 100 mg, 200 mg, 300 mg, 400 mg.
- *Elixir (Elixophyllin):* 80 mg/15 ml.
- *Oral Solution:* 80 mg/15 ml.

- *Tablets (Controlled-Release [Theochron]):* 100 mg (Theochron, T-Phyl), 200 mg (Theochron, T-Phyl), 300 mg (Quibron-T/SR, Theochron, Theolair-SR), 400 mg (Uniphyl), 500 mg (Theolair-SR), 600 mg (Uniphyl).
- *Infusion (theophylline):* 0.8 mg/ml, 1.6 mg/ml, 2 mg/ml, 3.2 mg/ml, 4 mg/ml.
- *Injection (aminophylline):* 25 mg/ml.

■ Indications and Dosages:
Asthma: IV 5 mg/kg bolus, then 0.2 mg/kg/hr continuous infusion. PO Initially, 5 mg/kg, then 2 mg/kg q8h. PO (Controlled-Release 12-Hour Formulations) Initially, 300 mg/day in 2 divided doses. May increase in 3 days to 400 mg/day in 2 divided doses. May increase in 3 days to 600 mg/day in 2 divided doses. PO (Extended-Release 24-Hour Formulations) Initially, 300-400 mg/day. May increase in 3 days to 400-600 mg/day. May then titrate according to blood level.

■ Contraindications: History of hypersensitivity to caffeine or xanthine

■ Side Effects
Frequent
Altered smell (during IV administration), restlessness, tachycardia, tremor
Occasional
Heartburn, vomiting, headache, mild diuresis, insomnia, nausea

■ Serious Reactions
- Too-rapid IV administration may produce marked hypotension with accompanying faintness, light-headedness, palpitations, tachycardia, hyperventilation, nausea, vomiting, angina-like pain, seizures, ventricular fibrillation, and cardiac standstill.

■ Patient/Family Education
- Avoid large amounts of caffeine-containing products
- If GI upset occurs, take with 8 oz water
- Notify clinician if nausea, vomiting, insomnia, jitteriness, headache, rash, palpitations occur

■ Monitoring Parameters
- Serum theophylline concentrations every 6-12 mo or with status changes (therapeutic level is 10-20 mcg/ml); toxicity may occur with small increase above 20 mcg/ml, especially in the elderly
- Serious side effects (ventricular dysrhythmias, seizures, death) may occur without preceding signs of less serious toxicity (nausea, restlessness)
- Arterial blood gases (ABGs)

■ Geriatric side effects at a glance:
☑ CNS   ☐ Bowel Dysfunction   ☐ Bladder Dysfunction   ☐ Falls
Other: Tachycardia, Psychosis, Tremor

■ Use with caution in older patients with: Cardiovascular disease (CVD), especially angina, arrhythmias, or CHF, Cor Pulmonale, Hepatic dysfunction, Active peptic ulcer disease, GERD, Anxiety, Seizure disorders, Migraine headaches, Hyperthyroidism

■ U.S. Regulatory Considerations
☐ FDA Black Box   ☑ OBRA regulated in U.S. Long Term Care

■ Other Uses in Geriatric Patient: None

- **Side Effects:**
  Of particular importance in the geriatric patient: Confusion, nervousness, tachycardia, palpitations, PVCs, tremor, nausea, loss of appetite, hyperuricemia

- **Geriatric Considerations - Summary:** 100 mg aminophylline = 79 mg theophylline. Same pharmacokinetic and monitoring parameters as for theophylline. Increased risk of side effects in patients with CVD and hepatic dysfunction. Theophylline (aminophylline) has a narrow therapeutic index and is associated with numerous drug interactions. Target serum concentrations are 5-20 mg/l, with adverse effects increasing above 10 mg/l. Hepatic metabolism and renal excretion decline with age and the half-life of theophylline increases by 3 to 9 hr in older adults. Smoking induces theophylline (aminophylline) metabolism; therefore, if a patient stops smoking, empiric dosage reduction may be indicated and follow serum concentrations closely.

- **References:**
  1. Tune LE. Anticholinergic effects of medication in elderly patients. J Clin Psychiatry 2001;62(suppl 21):11-14.
  2. Ohnishi A, Kato M, Kojima J, et. al. Differential pharmacokinetics of theophylline in elderly patients. Drugs & Aging 2003;20:71-84.
  3. Newnham DM. Asthma medications and their potential adverse effects in the elderly: recommendations for prescribing. Drug Saf 2001;24:1065-1080.

aminosalicylic acid

(a-mee-noe-sal-i-si-lik as-id)

- **Brand Name(s):** Paser
  Chemical Class: Salicylate derivative

- **Clinical Pharmacology:**
  Mechanism of Action: An antitubercular agent active against *Mycobacterium tuberculosis*. Thought to exhibit competitive antagonism of folic acid synthesis. **Therapeutic Effect:** Bacteriostatic activity in susceptible microorganisms.
  Pharmacokinetics: Readily absorbed from the gastrointestinal (GI) tract. Protein binding: 50%-60%. Widely distributed (including cerebrospinal fluid [CSF]). Metabolized in liver. Primarily excreted in urine. Removed by hemodialysis. **Half-life:** 1.1-1.62 hr.

- **Available Forms:**
  - *Packet Granules:* 4 g/packet granules (Paser).
  - *Tablets, Enteric-coated:* 7.7 grains (Paser).
  - *Tablets, Sustained-release:* 500 mg (Paser).

- **Indications and Dosages:**
  Tuberculosis: PO 4g in divided doses 3 times/day.

- **Unlabeled Uses:** Crohn's disease, hyperlipidemia, ulcerative colitis

- **Contraindications:** End-stage renal disease, hypersensitivity to aminosalicylic acid products

- **Side Effects**
  Occasional
  Abdominal pain, diarrhea, nausea, vomiting
  Rare
  Hypersensitivity reactions, hepatotoxicity, thrombocytopenia

- **Serious Reactions**
  - Liver toxicity and hepatitis, blood dyscrasias occur rarely.
  - Agranulocytosis, methemoglobinemia, thrombocytopenia have been reported.

Special Considerations
  - If recognized promptly, drug-induced hepatitis resolves quickly; 21% mortality if the reaction is unrecognized
  - Desensitization has been accomplished with 10 mg aminosalicylic acid given as a single dose; double the dose q2 days until total of 1 g then follow the regular schedule of administration; if a mild temperature rise or skin reaction develops, drop back one level or hold the progression for one cycle; reactions are rare after a total dosage of 1.5 g

- **Patient/Family Education**
  - Sprinkle granules on applesauce or yogurt or add to acidic juice such as orange, tomato, grape, apple, grapefruit, or cranberry; swirl well, granules sink
  - Protect from moisture, light, and extremes of temperature; do not use if packets are swollen or if granules turn dark brown or purple
  - Notify clinician if fever, sore throat, unusual bleeding, bruising, or skin rashes occur
  - The skeleton of the granules may be seen in the stool
  - Avoid crowds or those with known infection

- **Monitoring Parameters**
  - Monitor carefully in first 3 mo of therapy for signs of intolerance/drug-induced hepatitis (rash, fever, jaundice, hepatomegaly)
  - Liver function

- **Geriatric side effects at a glance:**
  ❑ CNS ❑ Bowel Dysfunction ❑ Bladder Dysfunction ❑ Falls

- **U.S. Regulatory Considerations**
  ❑ FDA Black Box ❑ OBRA regulated in U.S. Long Term Care

amiodarone hydrochloride

(a-mee'-oh-da-rone hye-droe-klor'-ide)

- **Brand Name(s):** Cordarone, Cordarone IV, Pacerone
  Chemical Class: Iodinated benzofuran derivative

- **Clinical Pharmacology:**
  Mechanism of Action: A cardiac agent that prolongs duration of myocardial cell action potential and refractory period by acting directly on all cardiac tissue. Decreases AV and sinus node function. **Therapeutic Effect:** Suppresses arrhythmias.
  Pharmacokinetics:

Route	Onset	Peak	Duration
PO	3 days-3 wk	1 wk-5 mo	7-50 days after discontinuation

  Slowly, variably absorbed from GI tract. Protein binding: 96%. Extensively metabolized in the liver to active metabolite. Excreted via bile; not removed by hemodialysis.
  Half-life: 26-107 days; metabolite, 61 days.

- **Available Forms:**
  - *Tablets:* 100 mg (Pacerone), 200 mg (Cordarone, Pacerone), 400 mg (Pacerone).
  - *Injection (Cordarone* IV): 50 mg/ml.

- **Indications and Dosages:**
  Life-threatening recurrent ventricular fibrillation or hemodynamically unstable ventricular tachycardia: PO Initially, 800-1600 mg/day in 2-4 divided doses for 1-3 wk. After arrhythmia is controlled or side effects occur, reduce to 600-800 mg/day for about 4 wk. Maintenance: 200-600 mg/day. IV Infusion Initially, 1050 mg over 24 hr; 150 mg over 10 min, then 360 mg over 6 hr; then 540 mg over 18 hr. May continue at 0.5 mg/min for up to 2-3 wk regardless of age or renal or left ventricular function.

- **Unlabeled Uses:** Control of hemodynamically stable ventricular tachycardia, control of rapid ventricular rate due to accessory pathway conduction in preexcited atrial arrhythmias, conversion of atrial fibrillation to normal sinus rhythm, in cardiac arrest with persistent ventricular tachycardia or ventricular fibrillation, paroxysmal supraventricular tachycardia, polymorphic ventricular tachycardia or wide complex tachycardia of uncertain origin, prevention of postoperative atrial fibrillation

- **Contraindications:** Bradycardia-induced syncope (except in the presence of a pacemaker), second- and third-degree AV block, severe hepatic disease, severe sinus-node dysfunction

- **Side Effects**
  Expected
  Corneal microdeposits are noted in almost all patients treated for more than 6 mo (can lead to blurry vision).
  Frequent (greater than 3%)
  Parenteral: Hypotension, nausea, fever, bradycardia.
  Oral: Constipation, headache, decreased appetite, nausea, vomiting, paresthesias, photosensitivity, muscular incoordination.

Occasional (less than 3%)
Oral: Bitter or metallic taste; decreased libido; dizziness; facial flushing; blue-gray coloring of skin (face, arms, and neck); blurred vision; bradycardia; asymptomatic corneal deposits.
Rare (less than 1%)
Oral: Rash, vision loss, blindness.

▪ Serious Reactions
- Serious, potentially fatal pulmonary toxicity (alveolitis, pulmonary fibrosis, pneumonitis, acute respiratory distress syndrome) may begin with progressive dyspnea and cough with crackles, decreased breath sounds, pleurisy, CHF, or hepatotoxicity.
- Amiodarone may worsen existing arrhythmias or produce new arrhythmias (called proarrhythmias).

Special Considerations
- Should be administered only by clinicians experienced in treatment of life-threatening dysrhythmias who are thoroughly familiar with the risks and benefits of amiodarone therapy

▪ Patient/Family Education
- Take with food and/or divide doses if GI intolerance occurs, do not take oral form with grapefruit juice
- Use sunscreen or stay out of sun to prevent burns
- Report side effects immediately
- Skin discoloration is usually reversible

▪ Monitoring Parameters
- Chest x-ray, ophth referral, and PFTs (baseline and q3 mo)
- Electrolytes
- LFTs
- ECG; QT interval prolongation of 10%-15% suggests therapeutic effect
- TFTs
- CNS symptoms

▪ Geriatric side effects at a glance:
❑ CNS   ❑ Bowel Dysfunction   ❑ Bladder Dysfunction   ❑ Falls

▪ U.S. Regulatory Considerations
☑ FDA Black Box
Potentially fatal pulmonary toxicity (hypersensitivity pneumonitis or interstitial/alveolar pneumonitis); hepatotoxicity; proarrhythmic effects
❑ OBRA regulated in U.S. Long Term Care

amitriptyline hydrochloride

(a-mee-trip'-ti-leen hye-droe-klor'-ide)

■ **Brand Name(s):** Elavil

    Combinations
    Rx: with chlordiazepoxide (Limbitrol); with perphenazine (Triavil)
    Chemical Class: Dibenzocycloheptene derivative; tertiary amine

■ **Clinical Pharmacology:**
    Mechanism of Action: A tricyclic antidepressant that blocks the reuptake of neurotransmitters, including norepinephrine and serotonin, at presynaptic membranes, thus increasing their availability at postsynaptic receptor sites. Also has strong anticholinergic activity. **Therapeutic Effect:** Relieves depression.
    Pharmacokinetics: Rapidly and well absorbed from the GI tract. Protein binding: 90%. Undergoes first-pass metabolism in the liver. Primarily excreted in urine. Minimal removal by hemodialysis. **Half-life:** 10-26 hr.

■ **Available Forms:**
- *Tablets* (Elavil): 10 mg, 25 mg, 50 mg, 75 mg, 100 mg, 150 mg.
- *Injection* (Elavil): 10 mg/ml.

■ **Indications and Dosages:**
    Depression: PO Initially, 10-25 mg at bedtime. May increase by 10-25 mg at weekly intervals. Range: 25-150 mg/day. IM 20-30 mg 4 times a day.
    Pain management: PO 25-100 mg at bedtime.

■ **Unlabeled Uses:** Relief of neuropathic pain, such as that experienced by patients with diabetic neuropathy or postherpetic neuralgia; treatment of anxiety, bulimia nervosa, migraine, nocturnal enuresis, panic disorder, peptic ulcer, phantom limb pain

■ **Contraindications:** Acute recovery period after MI, use within 14 days of MAOIs

■ **Side Effects**
    Frequent
    Dizziness, somnolence, dry mouth, orthostatic hypotension, headache, increased appetite, weight gain, nausea, unusual fatigue, unpleasant taste
    Occasional
    Blurred vision, confusion, constipation, hallucinations, delayed micturition, eye pain, arrhythmias, fine muscle tremors, parkinsonian syndrome, anxiety, diarrhea, diaphoresis, heartburn, insomnia
    Rare
    Hypersensitivity, alopecia, tinnitus, breast enlargement, photosensitivity

■ **Serious Reactions**
- Overdose may produce confusion, seizures, severe somnolence, arrhythmias, fever, hallucinations, agitation, dyspnea, vomiting, and unusual fatigue or weakness.
- Abrupt discontinuation after prolonged therapy may produce headache, malaise, nausea, vomiting, and vivid dreams.

- Blood dyscrasias and cholestatic jaundice occur rarely.

■ Patient/Family Education
- Therapeutic effects may take 3-6 wk
- Use caution in driving or other activities requiring alertness
- Avoid rising quickly from sitting to standing
- Avoid alcohol ingestion, other CNS depressants
- Do not discontinue abruptly after long-term use
- Wear sunscreen or large hat to prevent photosensitivity
- Increase fluids, bulk in diet if constipation occurs
- Gum, hard sugarless candy, or frequent sips of water for dry mouth

■ Monitoring Parameters
- Mental status: mood, sensorium, affect, suicidal tendencies
- Determination of amitriptyline plasma concentrations is not routinely recommended but may be useful in identifying toxicity, drug interactions, or noncompliance (adjustments in dosage should be made according to clinical response not plasma concentrations)
- Though not used clinically, therapeutic plasma levels 125-250 mcg/l (including active metabolites)
- Blood pressure, pulse

■ Geriatric side effects at a glance:
☑ CNS   ☑ Bowel Dysfunction   ☑ Bladder Dysfunction   ☑ Falls
Other: Orthostatic hypotension, cardiac conduction disturbances, anticholinergic side effects.

■ Use with caution in older patients with: Cardiovascular disease, prostatic hyptertrophy or other conditions which increase the risk of urinary retention

■ U.S. Regulatory Considerations
☑ FDA Black Box
- Because there is an increased risk of suicide in children and adolescents, older adults should also be closely monitored for suicide ideation.
☑ OBRA regulated in U.S. Long Term Care

■ Other Uses in Geriatric Patient: Neuropathic pain, urge urinary incontinence

■ Side Effects:
Of particular importance in the geriatric patient: Anticholinergic effects, extrapyramidal symptoms, high doses (greater than 100 mg) may increase risk of sudden death

■ Geriatric Considerations - Summary: Although tricyclic antidepressants are effective in the treatment of major depression in older adults, the side-effect profile and low toxic-to-therapeutic ratio relegate them to second-line agents (after serotonin reuptake inhibitors) for most older patients. These agents are effective in the treatment of urge urinary incontinence and neuropathic pain, but must be monitored closely. Of the tricyclic antidepressants, imipramine and amitryptiline have the highest anticholinergic activity and may be useful for management of incontinence, but should otherwise be avoided.

■ **References:**
  1. Leipzig RM, Cumming RG, Tinetti ME. Drugs and falls in older people: a systematic review and meta-analysis: I. Psychotropic drugs. J Am Geriatr Soc 1999;47:30-39.
  2. Cadieux RJ. Antidepressant drug interactions in the elderly. Understanding the P-450 system is half the battle in reducing risks. Postgrad Med 1999;106:231-240, 245.
  3. Ray WA, Meredith S, Thapa PB, et al. Cyclic antidepressants and the risk of sudden cardiac death. Clin Pharmacol Ther 2004;75:234-241.
  4. Roose SP, Laghrissi-Thode F, Kennedy JS, et al. Comparison of paroxetine and nortriptyline in depressed patients with ischemic heart disease. JAMA 1998;279:287-291.

amlexanox

(am-lex'-an-ox)

■ **Brand Name(s):** Aphthasol
  Chemical Class: Benzopyrano-bipyridine carboxylic acid derivative

■ **Clinical Pharmacology:**
  Mechanism of Action: A mouth agent that has anti-allergic and anti-inflammatory properties. Appears to inhibit formation and/or release of inflammatory mediators (e.g., histamine) from mast cells, neutrophils, mononuclear cells. **Therapeutic Effect:** Alleviates signs and symptoms of aphthous ulcers.
  Pharmacokinetics: After topical application, most systemic absorption occurs from the GI tract. Metabolized to inactive metabolite. Excreted in urine. **Half-life:** 3.5 hr.

■ **Available Forms:**
  • *Paste*: 5% (Aphthasol).

■ **Indications and Dosages:**
  Aphthous ulcers: Topical Administer ¼ inch directly to ulcers 4 times/day (after meals and at bedtime) following oral hygiene.

■ **Contraindications:** Hypersensitivity to amlexanox or any component of the formulation

■ **Side Effects**
  Rare
  Stinging, burning at administration site, transient pain, rash

■ **Serious Reactions**
  • Ingestion of a full tube would result in nausea, vomiting, and diarrhea.

■ **Patient/Family Education**
  • Discontinue if rash develops
  • Apply after oral hygiene

- **Monitoring Parameters**
  - Therapeutic response to therapy

- **Geriatric side effects at a glance:**
  - ❑ CNS ❑ Bowel Dysfunction ❑ Bladder Dysfunction ❑ Falls

- **U.S. Regulatory Considerations**
  - ❑ FDA Black Box ❑ OBRA regulated in U.S. Long Term Care

amlodipine besylate

(am-loe'-di-peen be'-si-late)

- **Brand Name(s):** Norvasc

  Combinations
  Rx: with atorvastatin (Caduet); with benazepril (Lotrel)
  Chemical Class: Dihydropyridine

- **Clinical Pharmacology:**
  Mechanism of Action: An antihypertensive that inhibits calcium movement across cardiac and vascular smooth-muscle cell membranes. **Therapeutic Effect:** Relieves angina by dilating coronary arteries, peripheral arteries, and arterioles. Decreases total peripheral vascular resistance and BP by vasodilation.
  Pharmacokinetics:

Route	Onset	Peak	Duration
PO	0.5-1 hr	6-12 hr	24 hr

  Slowly absorbed from the GI tract. Protein binding: 93%. Undergoes first-pass metabolism in the liver. Excreted primarily in urine. Not removed by hemodialysis. **Half-life:** 30-50 hr (increased in the elderly and those with liver cirrhosis).

- **Available Forms:**
  - *Tablets:* 2.5 mg, 5 mg, 10 mg.

- **Indications and Dosages:**
  Hypertension: PO Initially, 5 mg/day as a single dose. Maximum: 10 mg/day. *Small-Frame, Fragile, Elderly.* Initially, 2.5 mg/day as a single dose.
  Angina (chronic stable or vasospastic): PO 5 mg/day as a single dose. *Patients with hepatic insufficiency.* 5 mg/day as a single dose.
  Dosage in renal impairment: (Hypertension) 2.5 mg/day. (Angina) 5 mg/day.

- **Contraindications:** Severe hypotension

- **Side Effects**
  Frequent (greater than 5%)
  Peripheral edema, headache, flushing
  Occasional (less than 5%)
  Dizziness, palpitations, nausea, unusual fatigue or weakness (asthenia)

Rare (less than 1%)
Chest pain, bradycardia, orthostatic hypotension

■ **Serious Reactions**
  • Overdose may produce excessive peripheral vasodilation and marked hypotension with reflex tachycardia.

■ **Patient/Family Education**
  • Notify clinician of irregular heartbeat, shortness of breath, swelling of feet and hands, pronounced dizziness, hypotension
  • Do not abruptly discontinue amlodipine; compliance with therapy is essential to control hypertension
  • Avoid tasks that require alertness and motor skills until response to the drug has been established
  • Avoid drinking grapefruit juice while taking this drug

■ **Monitoring Parameters**
  • Blood pressure—if the patient's systolic BP is less than 90 mm Hg, withhold the medication and notify the physician
  • Assess skin for flushing and peripheral edema, especially behind the medial malleolus and the sacral area

■ **Geriatric side effects at a glance:**
  ❑ CNS ❑ Bowel Dysfunction ❑ Bladder Dysfunction ❑ Falls

■ **U.S. Regulatory Considerations**
  ❑ FDA Black Box ❑ OBRA regulated in U.S. Long Term Care

ammonium lactate

(ah-moe'-nee-um lack'-tate)

■ **Brand Name(s):** AmLactin, Lac-Hydrin, Lac-Hydrin Five, Lac-Lotion
  Chemical Class: Alpha-hydroxy acid

■ **Clinical Pharmacology:**
  Mechanism of Action: Lactic acid is an alpha-hydroxy acid that influences hydration, decreases corneocyte cohesion, reduces excessive epidermal keratinization in hyperkeratotic conditions, and induces synthesis of mucopolysaccharides and collagen in photodamaged skin. The exact mechanism is not known. *Therapeutic Effect:* Increases hydration of the skin.
  Pharmacokinetics: Not known.

■ **Available Forms:**
  • *Cream:* 12% (Amlactin).
  • *Lotion:* 5% (Lac-Hydrin Five), 12% (Amlactin, Lac-Hydrin. Lac-Lotion).

- **Indications and Dosages:**
  Treatment of ichthyosis vulgaris and xerosis: PO Apply sparingly and rub into area thoroughly q12h.

- **Contraindications:** Hypersensitivity to ammonium lactate.

- **Side Effects**
  Occasional (15%-2%)
  Burning, stinging, rash, dry skin

Special Considerations

- Side effects greater in fair-skinned individuals, if applied to abraded or inflamed areas, and in ichthyosis (where incidence of burning, stinging, and erythema is 10%)

- **Patient/Family Education**
  - For external use only
  - Avoid exposure to sunlight

- **Geriatric side effects at a glance:**
  ❑ CNS ❑ Bowel Dysfunction ❑ Bladder Dysfunction ❑ Falls

- **U.S. Regulatory Considerations**
  ❑ FDA Black Box ❑ OBRA regulated in U.S. Long Term Care

amobarbital sodium

(am-oh-bar'-bi-tal soe'-dee-um)

- **Brand Name(s):** Amytal sodium

  Combinations
  Rx: with secobarbital (Tuinal)
  Chemical Class: Barbituric acid derivative

  DEA Class: Schedule II

- **Clinical Pharmacology:**
  Mechanism of Action: A barbiturate that depresses the sensory cortex, decreases motor activity, and alters cerebellar function. **Therapeutic Effect:** Produces drowsiness, sedation, and hypnosis.
  Pharmacokinetics: Readily absorbed from the GI tract and distributed. Protein binding: 60%. Metabolized in liver primarily by the hepatic microsomal enzyme system. Primarily excreted in urine. **Half-life:** 16-40 hr.

- **Available Forms:**
  - *Powder for Injection*: 500 mg (Amytal sodium).

■ Indications and Dosages:

Hypnotic: IM, IV 65-200 mg at bedtime. **IM:** Administer deeply into a large muscle. Do not use more than 5 ml at any single site (may cause tissue damage). Maximum: 500 mg. **IV:** Use only when IM administration is not feasible. Administer by slow IV injection. Maximum: 50 mg/min.

Preanesthetic: IM, IV 65-500 mg at bedtime.

Sedative: IV 30-50 mg given 2 or 3 times/day.

■ Unlabeled Uses: Anticonvulsant

■ Contraindications: History of manifest or latent porphyria, marked liver dysfunction, marked respiratory disease in which dyspnea or obstruction is evident, and hypersensitivity to amobarbital products.

■ Side Effects

Frequent

Somnolence, headache, confusion, dizziness

Occasional

Nausea, vomiting, visual abnormalities, such as spots before eyes, difficulty focusing, blurred vision, dry mouth or pharynx, tongue irritation, water retention, increased sweating, constipation, or diarrhea

■ Serious Reactions

- Overdosage results in severe respiratory depression, skeletal muscle flaccidity, bronchospasm, cardiovascular disturbances, such as CHF, hypotension or hypertension, arrhythmias, cold and clammy skin, cyanosis, and coma.
- Tolerance may occur with repeated use.

■ Patient/Family Education

- Indicated only for short-term treatment of insomnia; probably ineffective after 2 wk; physical dependency may result when used for extended time (45-90 days depending on dose)
- Avoid driving or other activities requiring alertness
- Avoid alcohol ingestion or CNS depressants
- Do not discontinue medication abruptly after long-term use

■ Monitoring Parameters

- Serum folate, vitamin D (if on long-term therapy)
- PT in patients receiving anticoagulants
- Blood pressure, pulse

■ Geriatric side effects at a glance:

☑ CNS   ☐ Bowel Dysfunction   ☐ Bladder Dysfunction   ☑ Falls

Other: Withdrawal symptoms after long-term use

■ Use with caution in older patients with: Not recommended for use in older adults.

■ U.S. Regulatory Considerations

☐ FDA Black Box   ☑ OBRA regulated in U.S. Long Term Care

■ Other Uses in Geriatric Patient: Anxiety disorders, sleep disorders, seizure disorders

- **Side Effects:**
  Of particular importance in the geriatric patient: Sedation, withdrawal symptoms when abruptly discontinued (e.g., during hospitalization) rather than tapered

- **Geriatric Considerations - Summary:** Because barbiturates have a low therapeutic window, a wide range of drug interactions and rapid development of tolerance, great potential for abuse and dependence, these agents are not recommended for use in older adults.

- **Reference:**
  1. Hypnotic drugs. Med Lett Drugs Ther 2000;42:71-72.

amoxapine

(a-mox'-a-peen)

- **Brand Name(s):** Asendin
  Chemical Class: Dibenzocycloheptene derivative; secondary amine

- **Clinical Pharmacology:**
  Mechanism of Action: A tricyclic antidepressant that blocks the reuptake of neurotransmitters, such as norepinephrine and serotonin, at CNS presynaptic membranes, increasing their availability at postsynaptic receptor sites. The metabolite, 7-OH-amoxapine has significant dopamine receptor blocking activity similar to haloperidol. **Therapeutic Effect:** Produces antidepressant effects.
  Pharmacokinetics: Rapidly, well absorbed from the GI tract. Protein binding: 90%. Metabolized in liver. Excreted in urine and feces. **Half-life:** 8 hr.

- **Available Forms:**
  - *Tablets*: 25 mg, 50 mg, 100 mg, 150 mg (Asendin).

- **Indications and Dosages:**
  Depression: PO Initially, 25 mg at bedtime. May increase by 25 mg/day q3-7 days. Maximum: 400 mg/day (outpatient), 600 mg/day (inpatient).

- **Unlabeled Uses:** Panic disorder

- **Contraindications:** Acute recovery period following myocardial infarction (MI), within 14 days of MAOI ingestion, hypersensitivity to dibenzoxazepine compounds

- **Side Effects**
  Frequent
  Drowsiness, fatigue, xerostomia, constipation, weight gain
  Occasional
  Nausea, dizziness, headache, confusion, nervousness, restlessness, insomnia, edema, tremor, blurred vision, aggressiveness, muscle weakness

Rare
Paradoxical reactions (agitation, restlessness, nightmares, insomnia, extrapyramidal symptoms, particularly fine hand tremor), laryngitis, seizures

■ Serious Reactions
- High dosage may produce cardiovascular effects, including severe postural hypotension, dizziness, tachycardia, palpitations, and arrhythmias, and seizures. High dosage may also result in altered temperature regulation, such as hyperpyrexia or hypothermia.
- Abrupt withdrawal from prolonged therapy may produce headache, malaise, nausea, vomiting, and vivid dreams.

■ Patient/Family Education
- Therapeutic effects may take 2-3 wk
- Use caution in driving or other activities requiring alertness
- Avoid rising quickly from sitting to standing
- Avoid alcohol ingestion, other CNS depressants
- Do not discontinue abruptly after long-term use
- Wear sunscreen or large hat to prevent photosensitivity
- Increase fluids, bulk in diet if constipation occurs
- Use gum, hard sugarless candy, or frequent sips of water for dry mouth
- Potential for tardive dyskinesia

■ Monitoring Parameters
- Blood pressure, pulse

■ Geriatric side effects at a glance:
☑ CNS ☑ Bowel Dysfunction ☑ Bladder Dysfunction ☑ Falls

Other: Orthostatic hypotension, cardiac conduction disturbances, anticholinergic side effects

■ Use with caution in older patients with: Cardiovascular disease, prostatic hypertrophy or other conditions which increase the risk of urinary retention

■ U.S. Regulatory Considerations
☑ FDA Black Box
- Because there is an increased risk of suicide in children and adolescents, older adults should also be closely monitored for suicide ideation.

☑ OBRA regulated in U.S. Long Term Care

■ Other Uses in Geriatric Patient: Neuropathic pain, urge urinary incontinence

■ Side Effects:
Of particular importance in the geriatric patient: Anticholinergic effects, extrapyramidal symptoms, high doses (greater than 100 mg) may increase risk of sudden death

■ Geriatric Considerations - Summary: Although tricyclic antidepressants are effective in the treatment of major depression in older adults, the side-effect profile and low toxic-to-therapeutic ratio relegate them to second-line agents (after serotonin reuptake inhibitors) for most older patients. These agents are effective in the treatment

of urge urinary incontinence and neuropathic pain, but must be monitored closely. Of the tricyclic antidepressants, imipramine and amitryptyline have the highest anticholinergic activity and may be useful for management of incontinence, but should otherwise be avoided.

References:

1. Leipzig RM, Cumming RG, Tinetti ME. Drugs and falls in older people: a systematic review and meta-analysis: I. Psychotropic drugs. J Am Geriatr Soc 1999;47:30-39.
2. Cadieux RJ. Antidepressant drug interactions in the elderly. Understanding the P-450 system is half the battle in reducing risks. Postgrad Med 1999;106:231-240, 245.
3. Ray WA, Meredith S, Thapa PB, et al. Cyclic antidepressants and the risk of sudden cardiac death. Clin Pharmacol Ther 2004;75:234-241.
4. Roose SP, Laghrissi-Thode F, Kennedy JS, et al. Comparison of paroxetine and nortriptyline in depressed patients with ischemic heart disease. JAMA 1998;279:287-291.

amoxicillin

(a-mox-i-sil'-in)

■ **Brand Name(s):** Amoxicot, Amoxil, Biomox, DisperMox, Moxilin, Polymox, Trimox, Wymox)
  Chemical Class: Penicillin derivative, aminopenicillin

■ **Clinical Pharmacology:**
  Mechanism of Action: A penicillin that inhibits bacterial cell wall synthesis. **Therapeutic Effect:** Bactericidal in susceptible microorganisms.
  Pharmacokinetics: Well absorbed from the GI tract. Protein binding: 20%. Partially metabolized in the liver. Primarily excreted in urine. Removed by hemodialysis. **Half-life:** 1-1.3 hr (increased in impaired renal function).

■ **Available Forms:**
  • *Capsules:* 250 mg (Amoxil, Biomox, Trimox, Wymox), 500 mg (Amoxil, Biomox, Trimox).
  • *Powder for Reconstitution:* 50 mg/ml (Trimox), 125 mg/5 ml (Amoxil, Trimox), 200 mg/ml (Amoxil), 250 mg/ml (Amoxil, Biomox, Trimox), 400 mg/ml (Amoxil).
  • *Tablets (Amoxil):* 500 mg, 875 mg.

■ **Indications and Dosages:**
  Susceptible infections: PO 250-500 mg q8h or 500-875 mg q12h.
  Lower respiratory tract infection: PO 500 mg q8h or 875 mg q12h.
  H. pylori infection: PO 1 g twice a day in combination with clarithromycin and lansoprazole for 14 days.
  Gonorrhea: PO 3 g as a single dose.
  Endocarditis prophylaxis: PO 2 g 1 hr before procedure.
  Dosage in renal impairment: Dosage interval is modified based on creatinine clearance. Creatinine clearance 10-30 ml/min. Usual dose q12h. Creatinine clearance less than 10 ml/min. Usual dose q24h.

- **Unlabeled Uses:** Treatment of Lyme disease and typhoid fever

- **Contraindications:** Hypersensitivity to any penicillin, infectious mononucleosis

- **Side Effects**
  Frequent
  GI disturbances (mild diarrhea, nausea, or vomiting), headache, oral or vaginal candidiasis
  Occasional
  Generalized rash, urticaria

- **Serious Reactions**
  - Antibiotic-associated colitis and other superinfections may result from altered bacterial balance.
  - Severe hypersensitivity reactions, including anaphylaxis and acute interstitial nephritis occur rarely.

Special Considerations
  - Individualize treatment based on local susceptibility patterns.
  - High rates of rash in patients on allopurinol, with mononucleosis, or lymphocytic leukemia

- **Patient/Family Education**
  - May administer on a full or empty stomach
  - Administer at even intervals and continue therapy for the full course of treatment

- **Geriatric side effects at a glance:**
  ☐ CNS ☑ Bowel Dysfunction ☐ Bladder Dysfunction ☐ Falls

- **U.S. Regulatory Considerations**
  ☐ FDA Black Box ☐ OBRA regulated in U.S. Long Term Care

amoxicillin/clavulanate potassium

(a-mox-i-sil'-in clav-u-lan'-ate)

- **Brand Name(s):** Augmentin, Augmentin ES-600, Augmentin XR
  Chemical Class: Penicillin derivative, aminopenicillin; β-lactamase inhibitor (clavulanate)

- **Clinical Pharmacology:**
  Mechanism of Action: Amoxicillin inhibits bacterial cell wall synthesis, while clavulanate inhibits bacterial beta-lactamase. **Therapeutic Effect:** Amoxicillin is bactericidal in susceptible microorganisms. Clavulanate protects amoxicillin from enzymatic degradation.

Pharmacokinetics: Well absorbed from the GI tract. Protein binding: 20%. Partially metabolized in the liver. Primarily excreted in urine. Removed by hemodialysis. **Half-life:** 1-1.3 hr (increased in impaired renal function).

■ **Available Forms:**
- *Tablets* (*Augmentin*): 250 mg-125 mg, 500 mg-125 mg, 875 mg-125 mg.
- *Tablets* (*Extended-Release* [*Augmentin* XR]): 1000 mg-62.5 mg.

■ **Indications and Dosages:**
Mild to moderate infections: PO 500 mg q12h or 250 mg q8h.
Severe infections, respiratory tract infections: PO 875 mg q12h or 500 mg q8h.
Community-acquired pneumonia, sinusitis: PO 2 g (extended-release tablets) q12h for 7-10 days.
Sinusitis: PO 2 g (extended-release tablets) q12h for 7-10 days.
Dosage in renal impairment: Dosage and frequency are modified based on creatinine clearance. *Creatinine clearance 10-30 ml/min.* 250-500 mg q12h. *Creatinine clearance less than 10 ml/min.* 250-500 mg q24h.

■ **Unlabeled Uses:** Treatment of bronchitis and chancroid

■ **Contraindications:** Hypersensitivity to any penicillins, infectious mononucleosis

■ **Side Effects**
Frequent
GI disturbances (mild diarrhea, nausea, vomiting), headache, oral or vaginal candidiasis
Occasional
Generalized rash, urticaria

■ **Serious Reactions**
- Antibiotic-associated colitis and other superinfections may result from altered bacterial balance.
- Severe hypersensitivity reactions, including anaphylaxis and acute interstitial nephritis occur rarely.

Special Considerations
- Augmentin XR indicated for treatment of community-acquired pneumonia or bacterial sinusitis due to beta-lactamase-producing strains with reduced penicillin susceptibility
- High rates of rash in patients on allopurinol, with mononucleosis, or lymphocytic leukemia
- Individualize treatment based on local susceptibility patterns.

■ **Patient/Family Education**
- Administer with food to decrease GI side effects and enhance absorption
- Administer at even intervals and continue therapy for the full course of treatment

■ **Geriatric side effects at a glance:**
❑ CNS ☑ Bowel Dysfunction ❑ Bladder Dysfunction ❑ Falls

■ **U.S. Regulatory Considerations**
❑ FDA Black Box ❑ OBRA regulated in U.S. Long Term Care

amphetamine sulfate

(am-fet'-ah-meen sul'-fate)

■ **Brand Name(s)**

Combinations
Rx: with dextroamphetamine: (Adderall, Adderall XR)
Chemical Class: β-phenylisopropylamine (racemic)

DEA Class: Schedule II

■ **Clinical Pharmacology:**
Mechanism of Action: A sympathomimetic amine that produces CNS and respiratory stimulation, mydriasis, bronchodilation, a pressor response, and contraction of the urinary sphincter. Directly effects alpha and beta receptor sites in peripheral system. Enhances release of norepinephrine by blocking reuptake, inhibiting monoamine oxidase. **Therapeutic Effect:** Increases motor activity, mental alertness; decreases drowsiness, fatigue.
Pharmacokinetics: Well absorbed from the GI tract. Protein binding: 20%. Widely distributed (including CSF). Metabolized in liver. Excreted in urine. Unknown if removed by hemodialysis. **Half-life:** 7-31 hr.

■ **Available Forms:**
  • *Tablets:* 5 mg, 10 mg.

■ **Indications and Dosages:**
Attention-deficit hyperactivity disorder (ADHD), narcolepsy: PO 5-20 mg 1-3 times/day. Initially, 5 mg twice a day. Increase by 10 mg at weekly intervals until therapeutic response is achieved.

■ **Unlabeled Uses:** Depression, obsessive-compulsive disorder

■ **Contraindications:** Advanced arteriosclerosis, agitated states, glaucoma, history of drug abuse, history of hypersensitivity to sympathomimetic amines, hyperthyroidism, moderate to severe hypertension, symptomatic cardiovascular disease, within 14 days following discontinuation of an MAOI

■ **Side Effects**
Frequent
Irregular pulse, increased motor activity, talkativeness, nervousness, mild euphoria, insomnia
Occasional
Headache, chills, dry mouth, GI distress, worsening depression in patients who are clinically depressed, tachycardia, palpitations, chest pain

■ **Serious Reactions**
  • Overdose may produce skin pallor or flushing, arrhythmias, and psychosis.
  • Abrupt withdrawal following prolonged administration of high dosage may produce lethargy (may last for weeks).
  • Prolonged administration to children with ADHD may produce a temporary suppression of normal weight and height patterns.

■ **Patient/Family Education**
- Take early in the day
- Do not discontinue abruptly
- Avoid hazardous activities until stabilized on medication
- Sip tepid water and sugarless gum to relieve dry mouth

■ **Monitoring Parameters**
- Heart rate, pulse
- Weight

■ **Geriatric side effects at a glance:**
☑ CNS ☐ Bowel Dysfunction ☐ Bladder Dysfunction ☐ Falls

■ **U.S. Regulatory Considerations**
☑ FDA Black Box
- CNS stimulant use has a high abuse potential with the risk of dependence.
- Misuse may cause sudden death and serious cardiovascular adverse events.
☐ OBRA regulated in U.S. Long Term Care

amphotericin B / amphotericin B cholesteryl / amphotericin B lipid complex / liposomal amphotericin B

(am-foe-ter′-i-sin bee)

■ **Brand Name(s):** Abelcet (ABLC); AmBisome, Amphotec, Fungizone (IV and topical)
Chemical Class: Amphoteric polyene lipid complex (ABLC)

■ **Clinical Pharmacology:**
Mechanism of Action: The amphotericin B group is an antifungal and antiprotozoal and generally fungistatic but may become fungicidal with high dosages or very susceptible microorganisms. This drug binds to sterols in the fungal cell membrane.
Therapeutic Effect: Increases fungal cell-membrane permeability, allowing loss of potassium and other cellular components.
Pharmacokinetics: Protein binding: 90%. Widely distributed. Metabolic fate unknown. Cleared by nonrenal pathways. Minimal removal by hemodialysis. Amphotec and Abelcet are not dialyzable. Amphotec **Half-life:** 26-28 hr. Abelcet **Half-life:** 7.2 days. AmBisome **Half-life:** 100-153 hr.

■ **Available Forms:**
- Injection: 50 mg, 50 mg (Fungizone), 100 mg (Amphotec), 50 mg (AmBisome).
- *Suspension for Injection*: 5 mg/ml (Amphotericin B lipid complex, Abelcet).
- *Cream, Lotion, Ointment*: 3% (Fungizone).

■ **Indications and Dosages:**
Invasive fungal infections unresponsive or intolerant to Fungizone (Abelcet): IV Infusion 5 mg/kg at rate of 2.5 mg/kg/hr.

Empiric treatment for fungal infection in patients with febrile neutropenia; for aspergillus, candida, or cryptococcus infections unresponsive to Fungizone; or for patients with renal impairment or toxicity from Fungizone (AmBisome): IV Infusion 3-5 mg/kg over 1 hr.

Invasive aspergillus in patients with renal impairment, renal toxicity, or treatment failure with Fungizone (Amphotec): IV Infusion 3-4 mg/kg over 2-4 hr.

Cutaneous and mucocutaneous infections caused by Candida albicans, such as paronychia, oral thrush, and intertriginous candidiasis (Topical): Apply liberally to the affected area and rub in 2-4 times/day.

Cryptococcosis; blastomycosis; systemic candidiasis; disseminated forms of moniliasis, coccidioidomycosis, and histoplasmosis; zygomycosis; sporotrichosis; and aspergillosis (Fungizone): IV Infusion Dosage based on patient tolerance, severity of infection. Initially, 1-mg test dose is given over 20-30 min. If test dose is tolerated, 5-mg dose may be given the same day. Subsequently, increases of 5 mg/dose are made q12-24h until desired daily dose is reached. Alternatively, if test dose is tolerated, a dose of 0.25 mg/kg is given same day; increased to 0.5 mg/kg the second day. Dose increased until desired daily dose reached. Total daily dose: 1 mg/kg/day up to 1.5 mg/kg every other day. Do not exceed maximum total daily dose of 1.5 mg/kg.

■ **Contraindications:** Hypersensitivity to amphotericin B, sulfite

■ **Side Effects**
Frequent (greater than 10%)
Abelcet: Chills, fever, increased serum creatinine, multiple organ failure
AmBisome: Hypokalemia, hypomagnesemia, hyperglycemia, hypocalcemia, edema, abdominal pain, back pain, chills, chest pain, hypotension, diarrhea, nausea, vomiting, headache, fever, rigors, insomnia, dyspnea, epistaxis, increased liver/renal function test results
Amphotec: Chills, fever, hypotension, tachycardia, increased creatinine, hypokalemia, bilirubinemia
Fungizone: Fever, chills, headache, anemia, hypokalemia, hypomagnesemia, anorexia, malaise, generalized pain, nephrotoxicity
Topical: Local irritation, dry skin
Rare
Topical: Skin rash

■ **Serious Reactions**
- Cardiovascular toxicity as evidenced by hypotension and ventricular fibrillation and anaphylaxis occurs rarely.
- Vision and hearing alterations, seizures, liver failure, coagulation defects, multiple organ failure, and sepsis may be noted.

■ **Patient/Family Education**
- Long-term therapy may be needed to clear infection (2 wk-3 mo depending on type of infection)

- Fever reaction may decrease with continued therapy
- Muscle weakness may occur from drug-related loss of potassium

■ **Monitoring Parameters**
- BUN, serum creatinine; if BUN exceeds 40 mg/dl or serum creatinine exceeds 3 mg/dl, discontinue the drug or reduce dosage until renal function improves
- Regular monitoring of CBC, K, Na, Mg, LFTs
- Total dosage
- Blood pressure, pulse, respirations, and temperature every 15 min, then every 30 min for the first 4 hr of the infusion to assess for adverse reactions. Adverse reactions include abdominal pain, anorexia, chills, fever, nausea, vomiting, and tremors. If adverse reactions occur, slow the infusion rate and give prescribed drugs to provide symptomatic relief. For patients with a severe reaction and those without orders for symptomatic relief, stop the infusion and notify the physician.

■ **Geriatric side effects at a glance:**
❑ CNS ☑ Bowel Dysfunction ❑ Bladder Dysfunction ❑ Falls

■ **U.S. Regulatory Considerations**
☑ FDA Black Box
Amphotericin (nonliposomal) - Do not use to treat noninvasive forms of fungal diseases. Exercise caution to prevent inadvertent overdose.
❑ OBRA regulated in U.S. Long Term Care

ampicillin

(am-pi-sill'-in)

■ **Brand Name(s):** Amficot, Omnipen, Omnipen-N, Polycillin, Polycillin-N, Principen, Totacillin, Totacillin-N

Combinations
Rx: with probenecid (Polycillin PRB, Probampicin)
Chemical Class: Penicillin derivative, aminopenicillin

■ **Clinical Pharmacology:**
Mechanism of Action: A penicillin that inhibits cell wall synthesis in susceptible microorganisms. *Therapeutic Effect:* Produces bactericidal effect.
Pharmacokinetics: Moderately absorbed from the GI tract. Protein binding: 28%. Widely distributed. Partially metabolized in liver. Primarily excreted in urine. Removed by hemodialysis. *Half-life:* 1-1.9 hr (half-life increased in impaired renal function).

■ **Available Forms:**
- *Capsules:* 250 mg (Amficot), 500 mg (Omnipen, Principen, Totacillin).
- *Powder for Injection:* 125 mg (Omnipen-N, Polycillin-N), 250 mg (Omnipen-N, Polycillin-N, Totacillin-N), 500 mg (Omnipen-N, Polycillin-N, Totacillin-N), 1 g (Omnipen-N, Polycillin-N, Totacillin-N), 2 g (Omnipen-N, Polycillin-N, Totacillin-N), 10 g (Omnipen-N, Polycillin-N).

■ **Indications and Dosages:**
Respiratory tract, skin/skin-structure infections: PO 250-500 mg q6h. IM, IV 250-500 mg q6h.
Bacterial meningitis, septicemia: IM, IV 2g q4h or 3g q6h.
Gonococcal infections: PO 3.5g one time with 1g probenecid.
Perioperative prophylaxis: IM, IV 2g 30 min before procedure. May repeat in 8 hr.

■ **Contraindications:** Hypersensitivity to any penicillin, infectious mononucleosis

■ **Side Effects**
Frequent
Pain at IM injection site, GI disturbances, including mild diarrhea, nausea, or vomiting, oral or vaginal candidiasis
Occasional
Generalized rash, urticaria, phlebitis, thrombophlebitis with IV administration, headache
Rare
Dizziness, seizures, especially with IV therapy

■ **Serious Reactions**
• Altered bacterial balance may result in potentially fatal superinfections and antibacterial-associated colitis as evidenced by abdominal cramps, watery or severe diarrhea, and fever.
• Severe hypersensitivity reactions, including anaphylaxis and acute interstitial nephritis, occur rarely.

Special Considerations
• Individualize treatment based on local susceptibility patterns.
• High rates of rash in patients on allopurinol, with mononucleosis, lymphatic leukemia
• Amoxicillin is better oral choice given greater ease of dosing and lower incidence of diarrhea

■ **Patient/Family Education**
• Administer on an empty stomach
• Administer at even intervals and continue therapy for the full course of treatment

■ **Geriatric side effects at a glance:**
❑ CNS ☑ Bowel Dysfunction ❑ Bladder Dysfunction ❑ Falls

■ **U.S. Regulatory Considerations**
❑ FDA Black Box ❑ OBRA regulated in U.S. Long Term Care

ampicillin/sulbactam sodium

(am-pi-sill'-in/sul-bac'-tam)

■ **Brand Name(s):** Unasyn
  Chemical Class: Penicillin derivative, aminopenicillin; penicillinate (sulbactam)

■ **Clinical Pharmacology:**
  Mechanism of Action: Ampicillin inhibits bacterial cell wall synthesis, while sulbactam inhibits bacterial beta-lactamase. **Therapeutic Effect:** Ampicillin is bactericidal in susceptible microorganisms. Sulbactam protects ampicillin from enzymatic degradation
  Pharmacokinetics: Protein binding: 28%-38%. Widely distributed. Partially metabolized in the liver. Primarily excreted in urine. Removed by hemodialysis. **Half-life:** 1 hr (increased in impaired renal function).

■ **Available Forms:**
  • *Powder for Injection*: 1.5 g (ampicillin 1 g/sulbactam 500 g), 3 g (ampicillin 2 g/sulbactam 1g).

■ **Indications and Dosages:**
  Skin and skin-structure, intra-abdominal, and gynecologic infections: IV, IM 1.5 g (1g ampicillin/500 mg sulbactam) to 3 g (2 g ampicillin/1 g sulbactam) q6h.
  Dosage in renal impairment: Dosage and frequency are modified based on creatinine clearance and the severity of the infection.

Creatinine Clearance	Dosage
greater than 30 ml/min	0.5-3 g q6-8h
15-29 ml/min	1.5-3 g q12h
5-14 ml/min	1.5-3 g q24h
less than 5 ml/min	Not recommended

■ **Contraindications:** Hypersensitivity to any penicillin or sulbactam, infectious mononucleosis

■ **Side Effects**
  Frequent
  Diarrhea and rash (most common), urticaria, pain at IM injection site, thrombophlebitis with IV administration, oral or vaginal candidiasis
  Occasional
  Nausea, vomiting, headache, malaise, urine retention

■ **Serious Reactions**
  • Severe hypersensitivity reactions, including anaphylaxis, acute interstitial nephritis, and blood dyscrasias may occur.
  • Antibiotic-associated colitis and other superinfections may result from altered bacterial balance.
  • Overdose may produce seizures.

- Individualize treatment based on local susceptibility patterns.

■ **Geriatric side effects at a glance:**
   ❑ CNS   ☑ Bowel Dysfunction   ❑ Bladder Dysfunction   ❑ Falls

■ **U.S. Regulatory Considerations**
   ❑ FDA Black Box   ❑ OBRA regulated in U.S. Long Term Care

amprenavir

(am-pren'-a-veer)

■ **Brand Name(s):** Agenerase
   Chemical Class: Protease inhibitor, HIV

■ **Clinical Pharmacology:**
   Mechanism of Action: An antiretroviral that inhibits HIV-1 protease by binding to the enzyme's active site, thus preventing processing of viral precursors and resulting in the formation of immature, noninfectious viral particles. **Therapeutic Effect:** Impairs HIV replication and proliferation.
   Pharmacokinetics: Rapidly absorbed after PO administration. Protein binding: 90%. Metabolized in the liver. Primarily excreted in feces. **Half-life:** 7.1-10.6 hr.

■ **Available Forms:**
   - *Capsules*: 50 mg.
   - *Oral Solution*: 15 mg/ml.

■ **Indications and Dosages:**
   HIV-1 infection (in combination with other ID-antiretrovirals): PO 1200 mg twice a day. Oral solution 1400 mg twice a day.
   Dosage in hepatic impairment: Dosage and frequency are modified based on the Child-Pugh score.

Child-Pugh Score	Capsules	Oral Solution
5-8	450 mg bid	513 mg bid
9-12	300 mg bid	342 mg bid

■ **Contraindications:** None known.

■ **Side Effects**
   Frequent
   Diarrhea or loose stools (56%), nausea (38%), oral paresthesia (30%), rash (25%), vomiting (20%)
   Occasional
   Peripheral paresthesia (12%), depression (4%)

■ **Serious Reactions**
  • Severe hypersensitivity reactions or Stevens-Johnson syndrome as evidenced by blisters, peeling of the skin, loosening of skin and mucous membranes, and fever may occur.

Special Considerations
  • Always check updated treatment guidelines before initiating or changing antiretroviral therapy. (http://AIDSinfo.nih.gov)

■ **Patient/Family Education**
  • May take with or without food, but do not take with a high-fat meal
  • Do not take supplemental vitamin E; capsule and liquid forms have vitamin E in them
  • Amprenavir is not a cure for HIV infection, nor does it reduce the risk of transmitting HIV to others

■ **Monitoring Parameters**
  • CBC, metabolic panel, hepatic function panel, CD4 lymphocyte count, HIV RNA level
  • Skin for rash
  • Pattern of daily bowel activity and stool consistency

■ **Geriatric side effects at a glance:**
  ❑ CNS ☑ Bowel Dysfunction ❑ Bladder Dysfunction ❑ Falls

■ **U.S. Regulatory Considerations**
  ☑ FDA Black Box ❑ OBRA regulated in U.S. Long Term Care

amyl nitrite

(am'-il nye'-trite)

■ **Brand Name(s):** Amyl nitrite
  Chemical Class: Nitrate, organic

■ **Clinical Pharmacology:**
  Mechanism of Action: A nitrite vasodilator that relaxes smooth muscles. Reduces afterload and improves vascular supply to the myocardium. **Therapeutic Effect:** Dilates coronary arteries, improves blood flow to ischemic areas within myocardium. Following inhalation, systemic vasodilation occurs.
  Pharmacokinetics: The vapors are absorbed rapidly through the pulmonary alveoli and metabolized rapidly. Partially excreted in the urine.

■ **Available Forms:**
  • *Solution*: 0.3 ml (Amyl nitrite).

Indications and Dosages:

Acute relief of angina pectoris: Nasal inhalation Place crushed capsule to nostrils for 0.18-0.3 ml inhalation of vapors. Repeat at 5-10 min intervals. No more than 3 doses in 15-30 min period.

Unlabeled Uses: Cyanide toxicity

Contraindications: Closed-angle glaucoma, severe anemia, head injury, postural hypotension, hypersensitivity to nitrates

Side Effects

Frequent

Headache (may be severe) occurs mostly in early therapy, diminishes rapidly in intensity, usually disappears during continued treatment; transient flushing of face and neck; dizziness (especially if patient is standing immobile or is in a warm environment); weakness; postural hypotension

Occasional

Nausea, rash, vomiting

Rare

Involuntary passage of urine and feces, restlessness, weakness

Serious Reactions
- Large doses may produce hemolytic anemia or methemoglobinemia.
- Severe postural hypotension manifested by fainting, pulselessness, cold or clammy skin, and profuse sweating may occur.
- Tolerance may occur with repeated, prolonged therapy.
- High dose tends to produce severe headache.

Special Considerations
- Volatile nitrites abused for sexual stimulation; transient dizziness, weakness, or other signs of cerebral hypoperfusion may develop following inhalation

Patient/Family Education
- Drug should be inhaled while the patient is seated or lying down
- Taking after drinking alcohol may worsen side effects
- Alert to probable headache, dizziness, or flushing side effects
- Amyl nitrite is very flammable
- Tolerance may develop with repeated use

Monitoring Parameters
- Blood pressure, pulse
- Onset, type, location, intensity, and duration of anginal pain

Geriatric side effects at a glance:
❏ CNS   ❏ Bowel Dysfunction   ❏ Bladder Dysfunction   ❏ Falls

U.S. Regulatory Considerations
❏ FDA Black Box   ❏ OBRA regulated in U.S. Long Term Care

anagrelide

(an-ag'-gre-lide)

■ **Brand Name(s):** Agrylin
Chemical Class: Quinazoline derivative

■ **Clinical Pharmacology:**
Mechanism of Action: A hematologic agent that reduces platelet production and prevents platelet shape changes caused by platelet aggregating agents. **Therapeutic Effect:** Inhibits platelet aggregation.
Pharmacokinetics: After oral administration, plasma concentration peaks within 1 hr. Extensively metabolized. Primarily excreted in urine. **Half-life:** About 3 days.

■ **Available Forms:**
- *Capsules*: 0.5 mg, 1 mg.

■ **Indications and Dosages:**
Thrombocythemia: PO Initially, 0.5 mg 4 times a day or 1 mg twice a day. Adjust to lowest effective dosage, increasing by up to 0.5 mg/day or less in any 1 wk. Maximum: 10 mg/day or 2.5 mg/dose.

■ **Contraindications:** Severe hepatic impairment

■ **Side Effects**
Frequent (5% or more)
Headache, palpitations, diarrhea, abdominal pain, nausea, flatulence, bloating, asthenia, pain, dizziness
Occasional (less than 5%)
Tachycardia, chest pain, vomiting, paresthesia, peripheral edema, anorexia, dyspepsia, rash
Rare
Confusion, insomnia .

■ **Serious Reactions**
- Angina, heart failure, and arrhythmias occur rarely.

■ **Patient/Family Education**
- Platelet count should respond within 7-14 days of beginning therapy

■ **Monitoring Parameters**
- Platelet count q2 days during first wk, then weekly thereafter until maintenance dose reached
- BUN and serum creatinine levels and hepatic enzyme test
- Assess the patient with suspected heart disease for tachycardia, palpitations, and signs and symptoms of CHF, such as dyspnea

- Assess skin for bruises or petechiae, and inspect catheter and needle insertion sites for bleeding; also assess for signs and symptoms of GI bleeding

■ **Geriatric side effects at a glance:**
  ❑ CNS ❑ Bowel Dysfunction ❑ Bladder Dysfunction ❑ Falls

■ **U.S. Regulatory Considerations**
  ❑ FDA Black Box ❑ OBRA regulated in U.S. Long Term Care

anakinra

(an-a-kin'-ra)

■ **Brand Name(s):** Kineret
  Chemical Class: Recombinant interleukin receptor antagonist (IL-1Ra)

■ **Clinical Pharmacology:**
  Mechanism of Action: An interleukin-1 (IL-1) receptor antagonist that blocks the binding of IL-1, a protein that is a major mediator of joint disease and is present in excess amounts in patients with rheumatoid arthritis. **Therapeutic Effect:** Inhibits the inflammatory response.
  Pharmacokinetics: No accumulation of anakinra in tissues or organs was observed after daily subcutaneous doses. Excreted in urine. **Half-life:** 4-6 hr.

■ **Available Forms:**
  - *Solution*: 100-mg syringe.

■ **Indications and Dosages:**
  Rheumatoid arthritis: Subcutaneous 100 mg/day, given at same time each day.

■ **Contraindications:** Known hypersensitivity to *Escherichia coli*–derived proteins, serious infection

■ **Side Effects**
  Occasional
  Injection site ecchymosis, erythema, and inflammation
  Rare
  Headache, nausea, diarrhea, abdominal pain

■ **Serious Reactions**
  - Infections, including upper respiratory tract infection, sinusitis, flu-like symptoms, and cellulitis, have been noted.
  - Neutropenia may occur, particularly when anakinra is used in combination with tumor necrosis factor-blocking agents.

Special Considerations
  - Currently recommended for management of rheumatoid arthritis after failure of other DMARD agents

- **Patient/Family Education**
  - Signs and symptoms of allergic reactions, injection site reactions, and infections and advised of appropriate actions
  - Proper disposal of needles, syringes

- **Monitoring Parameters**
  - Patient reported outcomes (disability index, patient global assessment), physician assessments (tender/painful/swollen joints, physician's global assessment), objective measures (ESR, CRP); neutrophil counts baseline, q3mo, then quarterly qyr

- **Geriatric side effects at a glance:**
  ❑ CNS   ❑ Bowel Dysfunction   ❑ Bladder Dysfunction   ❑ Falls

- **U.S. Regulatory Considerations**
  ❑ FDA Black Box   ❑ OBRA regulated in U.S. Long Term Care

anastrozole

(an-as'-troe-zole)

- **Brand Name(s):** Arimidex
  Chemical Class: Benzyltriazole derivative

- **Clinical Pharmacology:**
  Mechanism of Action: Decreases the circulating estrogen level by inhibiting aromatase, the enzyme that catalyzes the final step in estrogen production. **Therapeutic Effect:** Inhibits the growth of breast cancers that are stimulated by estrogens.
  Pharmacokinetics: Well absorbed into systemic circulation (absorption not affected by food). Protein binding: 40%. Extensively metabolized in the liver. Eliminated by biliary system and, to a lesser extent, kidneys. **Mean half-life:** 50 hr in postmenopausal women. Steady-state plasma levels reached in about 7 days.

- **Available Forms:**
  - *Tablets:* 1 mg.

- **Indications and Dosages:**
  Breast cancer: PO 1 mg once a day.

- **Contraindications:** None known.

- **Side Effects**
  Frequent (16%-8%)
  Asthenia, nausea, headache, hot flashes, back pain, vomiting, cough, diarrhea
  Occasional (6%-4%)
  Constipation, abdominal pain, anorexia, bone pain, pharyngitis, dizziness, rash, dry mouth, peripheral edema, pelvic pain, depression, chest pain, paresthesia

Rare (2%-1%)
Weight gain, diaphoresis

■ **Serious Reactions**
  • Thrombophlebitis, anemia, leukopenia, and vaginal hemorrhage occur rarely.

Special Considerations
  • No difference between doses of 1-10 mg qd
  • Objective response in 10% of patients
  • Usually ineffective in estrogen receptor negative patients and those unresponsive to prior tamoxifen

■ **Patient/Family Education**
  • Notify the physician if asthenia, hot flashes, and nausea become unmanageable

■ **Monitoring Parameters**
  • Body weight, edema
  • Thromboembolic events
  • CBC, blood chemistry, LFTs, serum lipids

■ **Geriatric side effects at a glance:**
  ❑ CNS   ❑ Bowel Dysfunction   ❑ Bladder Dysfunction   ❑ Falls

■ **U.S. Regulatory Considerations**
  ❑ FDA Black Box   ❑ OBRA regulated in U.S. Long Term Care

anthralin

(an'-thra-lin)

■ **Brand Name(s):** A-Fil, Anthra-Derm, Drithocreme, Dritho-Scalp, Micanol, Psoriatec
  OTC: (capsules, tablets, chewable tablets, syrup, elixir, cream, spray)
  Chemical Class: Anthratriol derivative

■ **Clinical Pharmacology:**
  Mechanism of Action: A topical agent that binds DNA, inhibiting synthesis of nucleic protein, and reduces mitotic activity. **Therapeutic Effect:** Results in damage to DNA sugar and enhances membrane lipid peroxidation, which may play a critical role in the antipsoriatic action.
  Pharmacokinetics: Poorly absorbed systemically, but excellent epidermal absorption. Auto-oxidized to inactive metabolites – danthrone and dianthrone. Rapid urinary excretion, so significant levels do not accumulate in the blood or other tissues.
  Half-life: 6 hr.

■ **Available Forms:**
  • **Cream:** 0.1% (Drithocreme), 0.25% (Drithocreme, Dritho-Scalp), 0.5% (Drithocreme, Dritho-Scalp), 1% (Anthra-Derm).

- *Ointment*: 0.1% (Anthra-Derm), 0.25% (Anthra-Derm), 0.5% (Anthra-Derm), 1% (Micanol, Psoriatec).

■ **Indications and Dosages:**
Psoriasis: Topical Apply in a thin layer to affected areas q12h or q24h.

■ **Unlabeled Uses:** Inflammatory linear verrucous epidermal nevus

■ **Contraindications:** Acute psoriasis where inflammation is present, erythroderma, hypersensitivity to anthralin

■ **Side Effects**
Frequent
Irritation
Rare
Neutrophilia, proteinuria, staining of the skin

■ **Serious Reactions**
- Patients with renal disease should have routine urine tests for albuminuria.
- Hypersensitivity reaction, such as burning, erythema, and dermatitis, may occur.

■ **Patient/Family Education**
- Use plastic gloves for application and wear a plastic cap over treated scalp at bedtime to avoid staining
- Apply a protective film of petrolatum to areas surrounding plaque
- May stain fabrics
- Notify the physician if severe irritation or edema occurs

■ **Geriatric side effects at a glance:**
❑ CNS ❑ Bowel Dysfunction ❑ Bladder Dysfunction ❑ Falls

■ **U.S. Regulatory Considerations**
❑ FDA Black Box ❑ OBRA regulated in U.S. Long Term Care

apraclonidine hydrochloride

(a-pra-klon'-i-deen hye-droe-klor'-ide)

■ **Brand Name(s):** Lodipine
Chemical Class: α_2-Adrenergic agonist

■ **Clinical Pharmacology:**
Mechanism of Action: An ocular alpha-adrenergic agent that is a relatively selective alpha$_2$ receptor agonist. **Therapeutic Effect:** Reduces intraocular pressure.

Pharmacokinetics: Onset of action occurs within 1 hr. The duration of a single dose is about 12 hr. **Half-life:** 8 hr.

■ **Available Forms:**
- *Ophthalmic Solution*: 0.5%, 1% (Lodipine).

■ **Indications and Dosages:**
Glaucoma: Ophthalmic Instill 1 drop of 0.5% solution to affected eye(s) 3 times daily.
Intraocular hypertension, post laser surgery: Ophthalmic Instill 1 drop of 1% solution in operative eye(s) 1 hr before surgery and 1 drop postoperatively.

■ **Unlabeled Uses:** Postcycloplegic intraocular pressure spikes, intraocular pressure from postcataract surgery.

■ **Contraindications:** Hypersensitivity to apraclonidine or clonidine or any component of the formulation.

■ **Side Effects**
Frequent
Eye discomfort, dry mouth.
Occasional
Headache, constipation, redness around eye, conjunctivitis, changes in visual acuity, mydriasis, ocular inflammation.
Rare
Nasal decongestion.

■ **Serious Reactions**
- Allergic reaction occurs rarely.
- Peripheral edema and arrhythmias have been reported

■ **Geriatric side effects at a glance:**
❑ CNS ❑ Bowel Dysfunction ❑ Bladder Dysfunction ❑ Falls

■ **U.S. Regulatory Considerations**
❑ FDA Black Box ❑ OBRA regulated in U.S. Long Term Care

aprepitant

(ap-re'-pi-tant)

■ **Brand Name(s):** Emend, Emend 3-Day
Chemical Class: Triazolone derivative

■ **Clinical Pharmacology:**
Mechanism of Action: A selective human substance P and neurokinin-1 (NK$_1$) receptor antagonist that inhibits chemotherapy-induced nausea and vomiting centrally in the

chemoreceptor trigger zone. **Therapeutic Effect:** Prevents the acute and delayed phases of chemotherapy-induced emesis, including vomiting caused by high-dose cisplatin.

Pharmacokinetics: Crosses the blood-brain barrier. Extensively metabolized in the liver. Eliminated primarily by liver metabolism (not excreted renally). **Half-life:** 9-13 hr.

■ **Available Forms:**
- *Capsules (Emend):* 80 mg, 125 mg.
- *Kit (Emend 3-Day):* 125 mg-80 mg.

■ **Indications and Dosages:**
Prevention of chemotherapy-induced nausea and vomiting: PO 125 mg 1 hr before chemotherapy on day 1 and 80 mg once a day in the morning on days 2 and 3.

■ **Contraindications:** Concurrent use of astemizole, cisapride, pimozide, or terfenadine

■ **Side Effects**
Frequent (17%–10%)
Fatigue, nausea, hiccups, diarrhea, constipation, anorexia
Occasional (8%–4%)
Headache, vomiting, dizziness, dehydration, heartburn
Rare (3% or less)
Abdominal pain, epigastric discomfort, gastritis, tinnitus, insomnia

■ **Serious Reactions**
- Neutropenia and mucous membrane disorders occur rarely.

Special Considerations
- Augments the antiemetic activity of the 5-HT$_3$-receptor antagonist ondansetron and the corticosteroid dexamethasone and inhibits both the acute and delayed phases of cisplatin-induced emesis

■ **Patient/Family Education**
- Nausea and vomiting should be relieved shortly after drug administration
- Notify the physician if headache or persistent vomiting occurs

■ **Monitoring Parameters**
- Assess pattern of daily bowel activity and stool consistency; also auscultate bowel sounds for peristalsis and record time of evacuation

■ **Geriatric side effects at a glance:**
❑ CNS ❑ Bowel Dysfunction ❑ Bladder Dysfunction ❑ Falls

■ **U.S. Regulatory Considerations**
❑ FDA Black Box ❑ OBRA regulated in U.S. Long Term Care

argatroban

(ar-gat'-tro-ban)

■ **Brand Name(s):** Acova
  Chemical Class: L-Arginine derivative; thrombin inhibitor

■ **Clinical Pharmacology:**
  Mechanism of Action: A direct thrombin inhibitor that reversibly binds to thrombin-active sites. Inhibits thrombin-catalyzed or thrombin-induced reactions, including fibrin formation, activation of coagulant factors V, VIII, and XIII; also inhibits protein C formation, and platelet aggregation. **Therapeutic Effect:** Produces anticoagulation.
  Pharmacokinetics: Following IV administration, distributed primarily in extracellular fluid. Protein binding: 54%. Metabolized in the liver. Primarily excreted in the feces, presumably through biliary secretion. **Half-life:** 39-51 min.

■ **Available Forms:**
  • Injection: 100 mg/ml.

■ **Indications and Dosages:**
  To prevent and treat heparin-induced thrombocytopenia: IV Infusion Initially, 2 mcg/kg/min administered as a continuous infusion. After initial infusion, dose may be adjusted until steady-state aPTT is 1.5-3 times initial baseline value, not to exceed 100 sec.
  Percutaneous coronary intervention: IV Infusion Initially, 25 mcg/kg/min and administer bolus of 350 mcg/kg over 3-5 min. ACT (activated clotting time) checked in 5-10 min following bolus. If ACT is less than 300 sec, give additional bolus 150 mcg/kg, increase infusion to 30 mcg/kg/min. If ACT is greater than 450 sec, decrease infusion to 15 mcg/kg/min. Once ACT of 300-450 sec achieved, proceed with procedure.
  Dosage in hepatic impairment: Initially, 0.5 mcg/kg/min.

■ **Unlabeled Uses:** Cerebral thrombosis, MI

■ **Contraindications:** Overt major bleeding

■ **Side Effects**
  Frequent (8%–3%)
  Dyspnea, hypotension, fever, diarrhea, nausea, pain, vomiting, infection, cough

■ **Serious Reactions**
  • Ventricular tachycardia and atrial fibrillation occur occasionally.
  • Major bleeding and sepsis occur rarely.

Special Considerations
  • Discontinue all parenteral anticoagulants prior to administration
  • Recognize the potential for combined effects on INR with co-administration of argatroban and warfarin; an INR should be measured daily while argatroban and warfarin are co-administered; in general, with doses of argatroban up to 2 mcg/kg/min, argatroban can be discontinued when the INR is greater than 4 on combined therapy; after argatroban is discontinued, repeat the INR measurement in 4-6 hr; re-

sume the argatroban infusion if the repeat INR is below the desired therapeutic range; repeat this procedure daily until the desired therapeutic range on warfarin alone is reached; for argatroban doses greater than 2 mcg/kg/min, temporarily reduce the dose of argatroban to a dose of 2 mcg/kg/min; repeat the INR on argatroban and warfarin 4-6 hr after reduction of the argatroban dose and follow the process outlined above for administering argatroban at doses up to 2 mcg/kg/min

■ **Patient/Family Education**
- Use an electric razor and soft toothbrush to prevent bleeding
- Report black or red stool, coffee-ground vomitus, red or dark urine, or blood-tinged mucus from cough

■ **Monitoring Parameters**
- aPTT, hemoglobin, hematocrit, platelet count
- Monitor for any complaints of abdominal or back pain, a decrease in blood pressure, increase in pulse rate, and severe headache, which indicates hemorrhage

■ **Geriatric side effects at a glance:**
❑ CNS ❑ Bowel Dysfunction ❑ Bladder Dysfunction ❑ Falls

■ **U.S. Regulatory Considerations**
❑ FDA Black Box ❑ OBRA regulated in U.S. Long Term Care

aripiprazole

(ay-ri-pip'-ray-zole)

■ **Brand Name(s):** Abilify
Chemical Class: Quinolinone derivative

■ **Clinical Pharmacology:**
Mechanism of Action: An antipsychotic agent that provides partial agonist activity at dopamine and serotonin (5-HT_{1A}) receptors and antagonist activity at serotonin (5-HT_{2A}) receptors. **Therapeutic Effect:** Diminishes schizophrenic behavior.
Pharmacokinetics: Well absorbed through the GI tract. Protein binding: 99% (primarily albumin). Reaches steady levels in 2 wk. Metabolized in the liver. Eliminated primarily in feces and, to a lesser extent, in urine. Not removed by hemodialysis. **Half-life:** 75 hr.

■ **Available Forms:**
- *Tablets:* 5 mg, 10 mg, 15 mg, 20 mg, 30 mg.
- *Oral Solution:* 1 mg/ml.

■ **Indications and Dosages:**
Schizophrenia: PO Initially, 10-15 mg once a day. May increase up to 30 mg/day.
Bipolar disorder: PO 30 mg once a day. May decrease to 15 mg/day based on patient tolerance.

■ **Unlabeled Uses:** Schizoaffective disorder

■ **Contraindications:** None known.

■ **Side Effects**
Frequent (11%–5%)
Weight gain, headache, insomnia, vomiting
Occasional (4%–3%)
Light-headedness, nausea, akathisia, somnolence
Rare (2% or less)
Blurred vision, constipation, asthenia or loss of energy and strength, anxiety, fever, rash, cough, rhinitis, orthostatic hypotension

■ **Serious Reactions**
- Extrapyramidal symptoms and neuroleptic malignant syndrome occur rarely.
- Prolonged QT interval occurs rarely.

Special Considerations
- Reports of efficacy in acutely relapsed schizophrenia and schizoaffective disorder, and has an improved tolerability profile compared to haloperidol

■ **Patient/Family Education**
- Understanding of potential interference with cognitive and motor performance, potential for drug interactions, and risk factors for neuroleptic malignant syndrome (overheating, dehydration)
- Avoid alcohol
- Avoid tasks that require mental alertness or motor skills until response to the drug has been established

■ **Monitoring Parameters**
- Improvement of both positive and negative schizophrenic symptoms; periodic BP and heart rate; abnormal movement monitoring; weight

■ **Geriatric side effects at a glance:**
☑ CNS ☑ Bowel Dysfunction ☐ Bladder Dysfunction ☑ Falls
Other: Weight gain, glucose intolerance, diabetes, orthostatic hypotension, extrapyramidal symptoms

■ **Use with caution in older patients with:** Diabetes, glucose intolerance, cardiovascular disease

■ **U.S. Regulatory Considerations**
☑ FDA Black Box
There is an increased risk of death in older patients with dementia. Although the causes of death were varied, most of the deaths appeared to be either cardiovascular (e.g., heart failure, sudden death) or infectious (e.g., pneumonia) in nature. This drug is not approved for treatment of patients with dementia-related psychosis.
☑ OBRA regulated in U.S. Long Term Care

■ **Other Uses in Geriatric Patient:** Behavior disturbances in the setting of dementia

■ **Side Effects:**
   Of particular importance in the geriatric patient: Weight gain, glucose intolerance, diabetes, increased risk of death

■ **Geriatric Considerations - Summary:** Direct comparisons between older and newer antipsychotic drugs in demented elderly persons are scarce. Newer agents have the theoretical advantage of a lower incidence of tardive dyskinesia but may cause weight gain, impaired glycemic control, and increased risk for cardiovascular events. These agents should be used with caution in demented elderly persons, with frequent monitoring for side effects and a low threshold for discontinuing use. Indeed, the Food and Drug Administration has recently released an advisory about these medications outlining the risk for increased mortality.

■ **References:**
   1. Sink KM, Holden KF, Yaffe K. Pharmacological treatment of neuropsychiatric symptoms of dementia: a review of the evidence. JAMA 2005;293:596-608.
   2. Alexopoulos GS, Streim J, Carpenter D, Docherty JP. Using antipsychotic agents in older patients. J Clin Psychiatry 2004;65 (Suppl 2):5-99.
   3. Cohen D. Atypical antipsychotics and new onset diabetes mellitus. An overview of the literature. Pharmacopsychiatry 2004;37:1-11.
   4. Deaths with antipsychotics in elderly patients with behavioral disturbances. Available at: www.fda.gov/cder/drug/advisory/antipsychotics.htm.
   5. Katz IR. Optimizing atypical antipsychotic treatment strategies in the elderly. J Am Geriatr Soc 2004;52:S272-S277.

ascorbic acid

(a-skor'-bic)

■ **Brand Name(s):** Ascor L 500, CEE-500, Cenolate, Mega-C/A Plus
   OTC: Ascorbicap, Cebid Timecelles, Cecon, Cevi-Bid, Ce-Vi-Sol, C-Crystals, Dull-C, Flavorcee
   Chemical Class: NUTR-vitamin, water soluble

■ **Clinical Pharmacology:**
   Mechanism of Action: Assists in collagen formation and tissue repair and is involved in oxidation reduction reactions and other metabolic reactions. **Therapeutic Effect:** Involved in carbohydrate use and metabolism, as well as synthesis of carnitine, lipids, and proteins. Preserves blood vessel integrity.
   Pharmacokinetics: Readily absorbed from the GI tract. Protein binding: 25%. Metabolized in the liver. Excreted in urine. Removed by hemodialysis.

■ **Available Forms:**
   • *Capsules (Controlled-Release):* 500 mg.
   • *Liquid:* 500 mg/5 ml.

- *Oral Solution*: 500 mg/5 ml.
- *Tablets*: 100 mg, 250 mg, 500 mg, 1 g.
- *Tablets (Chewable)*: 100 mg, 250 mg, 500 mg.
- *Tablets (Controlled-Release)*: 500 mg, 1 g, 1,500 mg.
- *Injection*: 222 mg/ml (Mega-C/A Plus, Vitamin C), 250 mg/ml (Cenolate), 500 mg/ml (Ascor L 500, Cee-500, Cenolate, Vitamin C).

■ Indications and Dosages:
Dietary supplement (RDA - elemental calcium): PO Males: 90 mg/day. Maximum: 2,000 mg/day. *Females*: 75 mg/day. Maximum: 2,000 mg/day.
Acidification of urine: PO 4-12 g/day in 3-4 divided doses.
Scurvy: PO 100-250 mg 1-2 times a day.
Prevention and reduction of severity of colds: PO 1-3 g/day in divided doses.

■ Unlabeled Uses:
Chronic iron toxicity, control of idiopathic methemoglobinemia, macular degeneration, prevention of common cold, urine acidifier

■ Contraindications:
None known.

■ Side Effects
Rare
Abdominal cramps, nausea, vomiting, diarrhea, increased urination with doses exceeding 1 g
Parenteral: Flushing, headache, dizziness, sleepiness or insomnia, soreness at injection site.

■ Serious Reactions
- Ascorbic acid may acidify urine, leading to crystalluria.
- Large doses of IV ascorbic acid may lead to deep vein thrombosis.
- Abrupt discontinuation after prolonged use of large doses may produce rebound ascorbic acid deficiency.

■ Patient/Family Education
- Reduce ascorbic acid dosage gradually because abrupt discontinuation may produce rebound deficiency

■ Reference:
1. Dietary Reference Intakes, www.nap.edu

■ Geriatric side effects at a glance:
❑ CNS   ❑ Bowel Dysfunction   ❑ Bladder Dysfunction   ❑ Falls

■ U.S. Regulatory Considerations
❑ FDA Black Box   ❑ OBRA regulated in U.S. Long Term Care

aspirin/acetylsalicylic acid/ASA

(as'-pir-in)

- **Brand Name(s):** Entaprin, Halfprin, St. Joseph, YSP Aspirin, Zero-Order Release, ZOR-prin
  OTC: Ascriptin, Aspergum, Bayer, Ecotrin, Ecotrin Maximum Strength, 8-Hour Bayer Extended Release, Empirin, Maximum Bayer, Norwich

  Combinations
  Rx: with butalbital (Fiorinal); with codeine (Empirin); with dihydrocodeine and caffeine (Synalgos DC); with dipyridamole (Aggrenox); with oxycodone (Percodan); with propoxyphene (Darvon)
  OTC: with antacids (Ascriptin, Bufferin, Magnaprin)
  Chemical Class: Salicylate derivative

- **Clinical Pharmacology:**
  Mechanism of Action: A nonsteroidal salicylate that inhibits prostaglandin synthesis, acts on the hypothalamus heat-regulating center, and interferes with the production of thromboxane A, a substance that stimulates platelet aggregation. **Therapeutic Effect:** Reduces inflammatory response and intensity of pain; decreases fever; inhibits platelet aggregation.
  Pharmacokinetics:

Route	Onset	Peak	Duration
PO	1 hr	2-4 hr	4-6 hr

  Rapidly and completely absorbed from GI tract; enteric-coated absorption delayed; rectal absorption delayed and incomplete. Protein binding: High. Widely distributed. Rapidly hydrolyzed to salicylate. **Half-life:** 15-20 min (aspirin); 2-3 hr (salicylate at low dose); more than 20 hr (salicylate at high dose).

- **Available Forms:**
  - *Tablets:* 162 mg (Halfprin), 325 mg (Bayer), 500 mg (Bayer).
  - *Tablets (Chewable [Bayer, St. Joseph]):* 81 mg.
  - *Tablets (Enteric-Coated [Bayer, Ecotrin, St. Joseph]):* 81 mg, 325 mg, 500 mg, 650 mg.
  - *Caplets (Bayer):* 81 mg, 325 mg, 500 mg.
  - *Gelcaps (Bayer):* 325 mg, 500 mg.
  - *Suppositories:* 60 mg, 120 mg, 125 mg, 200 mg, 325 mg, 600 mg, 650 mg.

- **Indications and Dosages:**
  Analgesia, fever: PO, Rectal 325-1000 mg q4-6h
  Anti-inflammatory: PO Initially, 2.4-3.6 g/day in divided doses; then 3.6-5.4 g/day.
  Platelet aggregation inhibitor: PO 80-325 mg/day.

- **Unlabeled Uses:** Acute ischemic stroke, MI (prophylaxis), prevention of thromboembolism, rheumatic fever

- **Contraindications:** Allergy to tartrazine dye, bleeding disorders, GI bleeding or ulceration, hepatic impairment, history of hypersensitivity to aspirin or NSAIDs

■ **Side Effects**
Occasional
GI distress (including abdominal distention, cramping, heartburn, and mild nausea); allergic reaction (including bronchospasm, pruritus, and urticaria)

■ **Serious Reactions**
- High doses of aspirin may produce GI bleeding and gastric mucosal lesions.
- Low-grade toxicity characterized by tinnitus, generalized pruritus (possibly severe), headache, dizziness, flushing, tachycardia, hyperventilation, diaphoresis, and thirst.
- Marked toxicity is characterized by hyperthermia, restlessness, seizures, abnormal breathing patterns, respiratory failure, and coma.

Special Considerations
- 81 mg qd may be as effective as higher doses in primary and secondary MI prevention

■ **Patient/Family Education**
- Administer with food
- Do not exceed recommended doses
- Read label on other OTC drugs, many contain aspirin
- Therapeutic response may take 2 wk (arthritis)
- Avoid alcohol ingestion, GI bleeding may occur
- Do not crush or chew enteric-coated or extended-release tablets
- Report ringing in ears or resistant abdominal pain

■ **Monitoring Parameters**
- AST, ALT, bilirubin, creatinine, CBC, hematocrit if patient is on long-term therapy
- Urine pH for signs of sudden acidification

■ **Geriatric side effects at a glance:**
❏ CNS ❏ Bowel Dysfunction ❏ Bladder Dysfunction ❏ Falls

■ **U.S. Regulatory Considerations**
❏ FDA Black Box ❏ OBRA regulated in U.S. Long Term Care

atazanavir sulfate

(at-a-za-na'-veer sul'-fate)

■ **Brand Name(s):** Reyataz
Chemical Class: Protease inhibitor, HIV

■ **Clinical Pharmacology:**
Mechanism of Action: An antiviral that acts as an HIV-1 protease inhibitor, selectively preventing the processing of viral precursors found in cells infected with HIV-1. **Therapeutic Effect:** Prevents the formation of mature HIV cells.

Pharmacokinetics: Rapidly absorbed after PO administration. Protein binding: 86%. Extensively metabolized in the liver. Excreted primarily in urine and, to a lesser extent, in feces. **Half-life:** 5-8 hr.

■ **Available Forms:**
  • *Capsules:* 100 mg, 150 mg, 200 mg.

■ **Indications and Dosages:**
  HIV-1 infection: PO *Antiretroviral-naive.* 400 mg (2 capsules) once a day with food. *Antiretroviral-experienced.* 300 mg and ritonavir (Norvir) 100 mg once a day.
  HIV-1 infection (concurrent therapy with efavirenz): PO 300 mg atazanavir, 100 mg ritonavir, and 600 mg efavirenz as a single daily dose with food.
  HIV-1 infection (concurrent therapy with didanosine): PO Give atazanavir with food 2 hr before or 1 hr after didanosine.
  HIV-1 infection (concurrent therapy with tenofovir): PO 300 mg atazanavir and 100 mg ritonavir and 300 mg tenofovir given as a single daily dose with food.
  HIV-1 infection in patients with mild to moderate hepatic impairment: PO Alert Avoid use in patients with severe hepatic impairment. 300 mg once a day with food.

■ **Contraindications:** Concurrent use with ergot derivatives, midazolam, pimozide, or triazolam; severe hepatic insufficiency

■ **Side Effects**
  Frequent (16%-14%)
  Nausea, headache
  Occasional (9%-4%)
  Rash, vomiting, depression, diarrhea, abdominal pain, fever
  Rare (3% or less)
  Dizziness, insomnia, cough, fatigue, back pain

■ **Serious Reactions**
  • A severe hypersensitivity reaction (marked by angioedema and chest pain) and jaundice may occur.

Special Considerations

  • Reduced susceptibility to atazanavir is conferred by the following mutations of the HIV protease gene: N88S, I50L, I84V, A71V, and M46I
  • In patients with no prior antiretroviral therapy, a randomized trial found atazanavir equivalent to efavirenz when both were part of a 3 drug combination including zidovudine and lamivudine; another trial found atazanavir equivalent to nelfinavir when both were part of a 3 drug combination including lamivudine and stavudine
  • In patients with prior antiretroviral therapy, a randomized trial found that viral suppression rates for atazanavir were lower than with lopinavir/ritonavir (HIV RNA <400 copies/ml after 24 weeks of therapy: 54% vs 75%; HIV RNA <50 copies/ml after 24 wk of therapy: 34% vs 50%; CD4 count change after 24 wk of therapy: +101 cells/mm^3 vs 121 cells/mm^3
  • Always check updated treatment guidelines before initiating or changing antiretroviral therapy (http://AIDSinfo.nih.gov)

■ **Patient/Family Education**
  • Antacids or buffered medications reduce absorption of atazanavir; take atazanavir 2 hr before or 1 hr after antacids or buffered medications
  • Any medications that reduce stomach acid also reduce absorption of atazanavir; consult prescriber before using

- Take with food; eating small, frequent meals may offset the drug's side effects of nausea and vomiting
- Atazanavir is not a cure for HIV infection, nor does it reduce the risk of transmitting HIV to others

■ **Monitoring Parameters**
  - CBC, ALT, AST, bilirubin, HIV RNA, CD4 count
  - Pattern of daily bowel activity and stool consistency
  - Skin for rash
  - Monitor for onset of depression
  - Determine if the patient experiences headache

■ **Geriatric side effects at a glance:**
  ❑ CNS ❑ Bowel Dysfunction ❑ Bladder Dysfunction ❑ Falls

■ **U.S. Regulatory Considerations**
  ❑ FDA Black Box ❑ OBRA regulated in U.S. Long Term Care

atenolol

(a-ten'-oh-lol)

■ **Brand Name(s):** Tenormin

> Combinations
> **Rx:** with chlorthalidone (Tenoretic)
> **Chemical Class:** β_1-Adrenergic blocker, cardioselective

■ **Clinical Pharmacology:**
  Mechanism of Action: A beta$_1$-adrenergic blocker that acts as an antianginal, antiarrhythmic, and CV-antihypertensive-BB agent by blocking beta$_1$-adrenergic receptors in cardiac tissue. **Therapeutic Effect:** Slows sinus node heart rate, decreasing cardiac output and BP. Decreases myocardial oxygen demand.
  Pharmacokinetics:

Route	Onset	Peak	Duration
PO	1 hr	2-4 hr	24 hr

  Incompletely absorbed from the GI tract. Protein binding: 6%-16%. Minimal liver metabolism. Primarily excreted unchanged in urine. Removed by hemodialysis. **Half-life:** 6-7 hr (increased in impaired renal function).

■ **Available Forms:**
  - *Tablets*: 25 mg, 50 mg, 100 mg.
  - *Injection*: 5 mg/10 ml.

■ **Indications and Dosages:**
  Hypertension: PO Usual initial dose, 25 mg a day.
  Angina pectoris: PO Usual initial dose, 25 mg a day.

Acute MI: IV Give 5 mg over 5 min; may repeat in 10 min. In those who tolerate full 10-mg IV dose, begin 50-mg tablets 10 min after last IV dose followed by another 50-mg oral dose 12 hr later. Thereafter, give 100 mg once a day or 50 mg twice a day for 6-9 days. Or, for those who do not tolerate full IV dose, give 50 mg orally twice a day or 100 mg once a day for at least 7 days.

Dosage in renal impairment: Dosage interval is modified based on creatinine clearance.

Creatinine Clearance	Dosage Interval
15-35 ml/min	50 mg a day
less than 15 ml/min	50 mg every other day

- ■ **Unlabeled Uses:** Acute alcohol withdrawal, arrhythmia (especially supraventricular and ventricular tachycardia), improved survival in diabetics with heart disease, mild to moderately severe CHF (adjunct); prevention of migraine, thyrotoxicosis, tremors; treatment of hypertrophic cardiomyopathy, pheochromocytoma, and syndrome of mitral valve prolapse

- ■ **Contraindications:** Cardiogenic shock, overt heart failure, second- or third-degree heart block, severe bradycardia

- ■ **Side Effects**

    Atenolol is generally well tolerated, with mild and transient side effects.

    Frequent

    Hypotension manifested as cold extremities, constipation or diarrhea, diaphoresis, dizziness, fatigue, headache, and nausea

    Occasional

    Insomnia, flatulence, urinary frequency, impotence or decreased libido, depression

    Rare

    Rash, arthralgia, myalgia, confusion, altered taste

- ■ **Serious Reactions**
    - Overdose may produce profound bradycardia and hypotension.
    - Abrupt atenolol withdrawal may result in diaphoresis, palpitations, headache, and tremors.
    - Atenolol administration may precipitate CHF or MI in patients with cardiac disease; thyroid storm in those with thyrotoxicosis; and peripheral ischemia in those with existing peripheral vascular disease.
    - Thrombocytopenia, manifested as unusual bruising or bleeding, occurs rarely.

Special Considerations

- Properties of low lipid solubility and competitive cardioselectivity yield less CNS and bronchospastic adverse effects than propranolol

- ■ **Patient/Family Education**
    - Do not discontinue abruptly, may precipitate angina
    - Report bradycardia, dizziness, confusion, depression, fever, shortness of breath, swelling of the extremities
    - Take pulse at home, notify clinician if less than 50 beats/min
    - Avoid hazardous activities if dizziness, drowsiness, light-headedness are present
    - May mask the symptoms of hypoglycemia, except for sweating, in diabetic patients
    - Restrict alcohol and salt intake

■ **Monitoring Parameters**
- Blood pressure, heart rate
- Pattern of daily bowel activity and stool consistency
- Intake and output
- Weight

■ **Geriatric side effects at a glance:**
☐ CNS ☐ Bowel Dysfunction ☐ Bladder Dysfunction ☐ Falls

■ **U.S. Regulatory Considerations**
☑ FDA Black Box
In patients using orally administered beta blockers, abrupt withdrawal may precipitate angina or lead to myocardial infarction or ventricular arrhythmias.
☐ OBRA regulated in U.S. Long Term Care

atomoxetine hydrochloride

(at'-oh-mox-e-teen hye-droe-klor'-ide)

■ **Brand Name(s):** Strattera
Chemical Class: Propylamine derivative

■ **Clinical Pharmacology:**
Mechanism of Action: A norepinephrine reuptake inhibitor that enhances noradrenergic function by selective inhibition of the presynaptic norepinephrine transporter. **Therapeutic Effect:** Improves symptoms of attention-deficit hyperactivity disorder (ADHD).
Pharmacokinetics: Rapidly absorbed after PO administration. Protein binding: 98% (primarily to albumin). Eliminated primarily in urine and, to a lesser extent, in feces. Not removed by hemodialysis. **Half-life:** 4-5 hr in general population, 22 hr in 7% of Caucasians and 2% of African-Americans; increased in moderate to severe hepatic insufficiency.

■ **Available Forms:**
- *Capsules*: 10 mg, 18 mg, 25 mg, 40 mg, 60 mg, 80 mg, 100 mg.

■ **Indications and Dosages:**
ADHD: PO 40 mg once a day. May increase after at least 3 days to 80 mg as a single daily dose or in divided doses. Maximum: 100 mg.
Dosage in hepatic impairment: Expect to administer 50% of normal atomoxetine dosage to patients with moderate hepatic impairment and 25% of normal dosage to those with severe hepatic impairment.

■ **Unlabeled Uses:** Treatment of depression.

■ **Contraindications:** Angle-closure glaucoma, use within 14 days of MAOIs

■ **Side Effects**
Frequent
Headache, dyspepsia, nausea, vomiting, fatigue, decreased appetite, dizziness, altered mood
Occasional
Tachycardia, hypertension, weight loss, irritability
Rare
Insomnia, sexual dysfunction in adults, fever

■ **Serious Reactions**
- Urine retention or urinary hesitance may occur.
- In overdose, gastric emptying and repeated use of activated charcoal may prevent systemic absorption.
- Severe hepatic injury occurs rarely.

Special Considerations
- Promoted as a "milder" but equally efficacious agent; inadequate comparisons available — should not be considered over conventional therapy

■ **Patient/Family Education**
- Take the last daily dose of atomoxetine early in the evening to avoid insomnia
- Avoid tasks that require mental alertness and motor skills until response to the drug has been established
- Notify the physician if fever, irritability, palpitations, or vomiting occurs

■ **Monitoring Parameters**
- Pretreatment blood samples for PCR-CYP2D6 genotyping (poor-metabolizer alleles) in selected patients (e.g., those with a history of super sensitivity/marked clinical response to other medications)
- History: Improvement of ADHD symptoms such as inattentiveness, hyperactivity, anxiety, impaired academic/social functioning; interviewing via ADHD Rating Scale-IV (parent version); routine blood chemistry periodically during prolonged administration; BP, pulse rate, body weight periodically during prolonged administration; signs and symptoms of toxicity

■ **Geriatric side effects at a glance:**
☑ CNS ☐ Bowel Dysfunction ☐ Bladder Dysfunction ☐ Falls

■ **U.S. Regulatory Considerations**
☑ FDA Black Box
- CNS stimulant use has a high abuse potential with the risk of dependence.
- Misuse may cause sudden death and serious cardiovascular adverse events.
- Although not relevant to geriatric patients, this drug may produce suicidal ideation in children and adolescents.
☐ OBRA regulated in U.S. Long Term Care

atorvastatin calcium

(a-tore'-va-sta-tin kal'-see-um)

■ **Brand Name(s):** Lipitor

> Combinations
> **Rx:** with amlodipine (Caduet)
> **Chemical Class:** Substituted hexahydronaphthalene

■ **Clinical Pharmacology:**
> **Mechanism of Action:** An antihyperlipidemic that inhibits hydroxymethylglutaryl-CoA (HMG-CoA) reductase, the enzyme that catalyzes the early step in cholesterol synthesis. **Therapeutic Effect:** Decreases LDL and VLDL cholesterol, and plasma triglyceride levels; increases HDL cholesterol concentration.
> **Pharmacokinetics:** Poorly absorbed from the GI tract. Protein binding: greater than 98%. Metabolized in the liver. Minimally eliminated in urine. Plasma levels are markedly increased in chronic alcoholic hepatic disease, but are unaffected by renal disease. **Half-life:** 14 hr.

■ **Available Forms:**
> • *Tablets*: 10 mg, 20 mg, 40 mg, 80 mg.

■ **Indications and Dosages:**
> **Prevention of cardiovascular disease (CVD):** PO 10 mg once daily.
> **Hyperlipidemias:** PO Initially, 10-20 mg/day (40 mg in patients requiring greater than 45% reduction in LDL-C). Range: 10-80 mg/day.

■ **Unlabeled Uses:** Secondary prevention of ischemia in patients with CHF

■ **Contraindications:** Active hepatic disease, unexplained elevated liver function test results

■ **Side Effects**
> Atorvastatin is generally well tolerated. Side effects are usually mild and transient.
> **Frequent (16%)**
> Headache
> **Occasional (5%–2%)**
> Myalgia, rash or pruritus, allergy
> **Rare (2%-1%)**
> Flatulence, dyspepsia

■ **Serious Reactions**
> • Cataracts may develop, and photosensitivity may occur.

Special Considerations
> • Base statin selection on lipid-lowering potency, cost, and availability
> • Potency and ability to lower serum triglycerides are unique among the HMG-CoA reductase inhibitors. However, no outcome data available

Patient/Family Education
- Report symptoms of myalgia, muscle tenderness, or weakness
- Take daily doses in the evening for increased effect
- Follow prescribed diet
- Periodic laboratory tests are an essential part of therapy
- Do not take other medications without physician approval

Monitoring Parameters
- Cholesterol (maximum therapeutic response 4-6 wk)
- LFTs (AST, ALT) at baseline and at 12 wk of therapy: if no change, no further monitoring necessary (discontinue if elevations persist at >3 × upper limit of normal)
- CPK in patients complaining of diffuse myalgia, muscle tenderness, or weakness
- Assess skin for rash

Geriatric side effects at a glance:
❑ CNS   ❑ Bowel Dysfunction   ❑ Bladder Dysfunction   ❑ Falls

U.S. Regulatory Considerations
❑ FDA Black Box   ❑ OBRA regulated in U.S. Long Term Care

atovaquone

(a-toe'-va-kwone)

Brand Name(s): Mepron

Combinations
Rx: with proguanil (Malarone)
Chemical Class: Hydroxynaphthoquinone derivative

Clinical Pharmacology:
Mechanism of Action: A systemic anti-infective that inhibits the mitochondrial electron-transport system at the cytochrome bc1 complex (Complex III), which interrupts nucleic acid and adenosine triphosphate synthesis. **Therapeutic Effect:** Antiprotozoal and antipneumocystic activity.

Pharmacokinetics: Absorption increased with a high-fat meal. Protein binding: greater than 99%. Metabolized in liver. Primarily excreted in feces. **Half-life:** 2-3 days.

Available Forms:
- *Oral Suspension:* 750 mg/5 ml.

Indications and Dosages:
Pneumocystis carinii pneumonia (PCP): PO 750 mg twice a day with food for 21 days.
Prevention of PCP: PO 1500 mg once a day with food.

Contraindications: Development or history of potentially life-threatening allergic reaction to the drug

Side Effects
Frequent (greater than 10%)
Rash, nausea, diarrhea, headache, vomiting, fever, insomnia, cough
Occasional (less than 10%)
Abdominal discomfort, thrush, asthenia, anemia, neutropenia

Serious Reactions
- None known.

Special Considerations
- Plasma concentrations have been shown to correlate with the likelihood of successful treatment and survival

Patient/Family Education
- Take for the full course of treatment
- Do not take any other medications without first notifying the physician
- Notify the physician if diarrhea, rash, or other new symptoms occur

Monitoring Parameters
- Pattern of daily bowel activity and stool consistency
- Skin for rash
- Hgb levels, intake and output, and renal function test results
- Monitor patients closely because of age-related cardiac, hepatic, and renal impairment

Geriatric side effects at a glance:
☐ CNS ☑ Bowel Dysfunction ☐ Bladder Dysfunction ☐ Falls

U.S. Regulatory Considerations
☐ FDA Black Box ☐ OBRA regulated in U.S. Long Term Care

atropine sulfate

(a'-troe-peen sul'-fate)

■ **Brand Name(s):** AtroPen Autoinjector, Atropine Care, Atropisol, Atrosulf-1, Isopto Atropine, Ocu-Tropine, Sal-Tropine
Chemical Class: Belladonna alkaloid

■ **Clinical Pharmacology:**
Mechanism of Action: An acetylcholine antagonist that inhibits the action of acetylcholine by competing with acetylcholine for common binding sites on muscarinic receptors, which are located on exocrine glands, cardiac and smooth-muscle ganglia, and intramural neurons. This action blocks all muscarinic effects. **Therapeutic Effect:** Decreases GI motility and secretory activity, and GU muscle tone (ureter, bladder); produces ophthalmic cycloplegia, and mydriasis.

Pharmacokinetics: AtroPen Autoinjector: Rapidly and well absorbed after IM administration. Much of the drug is destroyed by enzymatic hydrolysis, particularly in the liver. Partially excreted unchanged in urine.

■ **Available Forms:**
- *Injection:* 0.05 mg/ml, 0.1 mg/ml, 0.4 mg/0.5 ml, 0.4 mg/ml, 0.5 mg/ml, 1 mg/ml.
- *IM Injection (AtroPen):* 0.25 mg, 0.5 mg, 1 mg, 2 mg.
- *Ophthalmic Ointment:* 0.5%, 1%.
- *Ophthalmic Solution:* 0.5% (Isopto Atropine), 1% (Atropisol, Isopto Atropine), 2% (Atropisol).

■ **Indications and Dosages:**
Asystole, slow pulseless electrical activity: IV 1 mg; may repeat q3-5min up to total dose of 0.04 mg/kg.
Pre-anesthetic: IV, IM, Subcutaneous 0.4-0.6 mg 30-60 min pre-op.
Bradycardia: IV 0.5-1 mg q5min not to exceed 2 mg or 0.04 mg/kg.
Cycloplegic refraction, postoperative mydriasis, uveitis: Ophthalmic Solution Instill 1 drop of 1% or 2% solution in affected eye(s) up to 4 times a day. Ophthalmic Ointment Apply ointment several hours prior to examination when used for refraction.
Poisoning by susceptible organophosphorous nerve agents having cholinesterase activity, organophosphorous or carbamate insecticides: IM AtroPen 2 mg (green).

■ **Unlabeled Uses:** Malignant glaucoma

■ **Contraindications:** Bladder neck obstruction due to prostatic hypertrophy, cardiospasm, intestinal atony, myasthenia gravis in those not treated with neostigmine, narrow-angle glaucoma, obstructive disease of the GI tract, paralytic ileus, severe ulcerative colitis, tachycardia secondary to cardiac insufficiency or thyrotoxicosis, toxic megacolon, unstable cardiovascular status in acute hemorrhage

■ **Side Effects**
Frequent
Dry mouth, nose, and throat that may be severe; decreased sweating, constipation, irritation at subcutaneous or IM injection site
Occasional
Swallowing difficulty, blurred vision, bloated feeling, impotence, urinary hesitancy
Ophthalmic: Mydriasis, blurred vision, photophobia, decreased visual acuity, tearing, dry eyes or dry conjunctiva, eye irritation, crusting of eyelid
Rare
Allergic reaction, including rash and urticaria; mental confusion or excitement, fatigue

■ **Serious Reactions**
- Overdosage may produce tachycardia, palpitations, hot, dry or flushed skin, absence of bowel sounds, increased respiratory rate, nausea, vomiting, confusion, somnolence, slurred speech, dizziness, and CNS stimulation.
- Overdosage may also produce psychosis as evidenced by agitation, restlessness, rambling speech, visual hallucinations, paranoid behavior, and delusions, followed by depression.
- Increased intraocular pressure occurs rarely with the use of the ophthalmic form.

■ **Patient/Family Education**
- Warm, dry, flushing feeling may occur upon administration

■ Monitoring Parameters
- Blood pressure, heart rate, temperature
- Skin turgor and mucous membranes to evaluate hydration status
- Bowel sounds for presence of peristalsis
- Intake and output

■ Geriatric side effects at a glance:
☑ CNS ☐ Bowel Dysfunction ☑ Bladder Dysfunction ☐ Falls

■ U.S. Regulatory Considerations
☐ FDA Black Box ☐ OBRA regulated in U.S. Long Term Care

atropine sulfate; diphenoxylate hydrochloride

(a'-troe-peen sul'-fate; dye-fen-ox'-i-late hye-droe-klor'-ide)

■ Brand Name(s): Lomocot, Lomotil, Lonox, Vi-Atro
Chemical Class: Meperidine analog

DEA Class: Schedule V

■ Clinical Pharmacology:
Mechanism of Action: A meperidine derivative that acts locally and centrally on gastric mucosa. **Therapeutic Effect:** Reduces intestinal motility.
Pharmacokinetics: Well absorbed from the GI tract. Metabolized in the liver to active metabolite. Primarily eliminated in feces. **Half-life:** 2.5 hr; metabolite, 12-24 hr.

■ Available Forms:
- *Tablets* (*Lomotil, Lonox*): 2.5 mg diphenoxylate/0.025 mg atropine.
- *Liquid* (*Lomotil*): 2.5 mg/5 ml.

■ Indications and Dosages:
Diarrhea: PO Initially, 15-20 mg/day in 3-4 divided doses; then 5-15 mg/day in 2-3 divided doses.

■ Contraindications: Dehydration, jaundice, narrow-angle glaucoma, severe hepatic disease

■ Side Effects
Frequent
Somnolence, light-headedness, dizziness, nausea
Occasional
Headache, dry mouth
Rare
Flushing, tachycardia, urine retention, constipation, paradoxical reaction (marked by restlessness and agitation), blurred vision

■ Serious Reactions
- Dehydration may predispose to diphenoxylate toxicity.
- Paralytic ileus and toxic megacolon (marked by constipation, decreased appetite, and stomach pain with nausea or vomiting) occur rarely.
- Severe anticholinergic reaction, manifested by severe lethargy, hypotonic reflexes, and hyperthermia, may result in severe respiratory depression and coma.

Special Considerations
- Equally effective as codeine or loperamide

■ Patient/Family Education
- Prolonged use not recommended
- Drowsiness or dizziness may occur; use caution when driving or operating dangerous machinery
- Avoid alcohol

■ Monitoring Parameters
- Bowel sounds and bowel activity

■ Geriatric side effects at a glance:
☑ CNS ☑ Bowel Dysfunction ☑ Bladder Dysfunction ☐ Falls
Other: Constipation, euphoria, dry mouth, blurred vision

■ Use with caution in older patients with: Urinary Incontinence, Psychosis

■ U.S. Regulatory Considerations
☐ FDA Black Box ☑ OBRA regulated in U.S. Long Term Care

■ Other Uses in Geriatric Patient: None

■ Side Effects:
Of particular importance in the geriatric patient: Anticholinergic effects

■ Geriatric Considerations - Summary: Diphenoxylate is an analog of meperidine and can cause opiate adverse effects. When discontinued, physical dependence and withdrawal symptoms can occur. Adverse GI effects such as constipation, nausea/vomiting, and abdominal pain may result from normal doses. Atropine is added to discourage abuse but can cause anticholinergic adverse effects in the older adult. The benefits of this drug combination for older adults are limited by the risk of adverse effects.

auranofin/aurothioglucose

(au-rane'-oh-fin/aur-oh-thye-oh-gloo'-kose)

■ **Brand Name(s):** Ridaura, Solganal
  Chemical Class: Gold compound

■ Clinical Pharmacology:

Mechanism of Action: Gold compounds that alter cellular mechanisms, collagen biosynthesis, enzyme systems, and immune responses. **Therapeutic Effect:** Suppress synovitis in the active stage of rheumatoid arthritis.

Pharmacokinetics: Auranofin (29% gold): Moderately absorbed from the GI tract. Protein binding: 60%. Rapidly metabolized. Primarily excreted in urine. **Half-life:** 21-31 days. Aurothioglucose (50% gold): Slowly and erratically absorbed after IM administration. Protein binding: 95%-99%. Primarily excreted in urine. **Half-life:** 3-27 days (increased with increased number of doses).

■ Available Forms:

- *Capsules (Ridaura):* 3 mg.
- *Injection (Solganal):* 50-mg/ml suspension.

■ Indications and Dosages:

Rheumatoid arthritis: PO 6 mg/day as a single or 2 divided doses. If there is no response in 6 mo, may increase to 9 mg/day in 3 divided doses. If response is still inadequate, discontinue. IM Initially, 10 mg, followed by 25 mg for 2 doses, then 50 mg weekly until total dose of 0.8-1g has been given. If patient has improved and shows no signs of toxicity, may give 50 mg q3-4wk for many months.

■ Unlabeled Uses: Treatment of pemphigus, psoriatic arthritis

■ Contraindications: Bone marrow aplasia, history of gold-induced pathologies (including blood dyscrasias, exfoliative dermatitis, necrotizing enterocolitis, and pulmonary fibrosis), severe blood dyscrasias

■ Side Effects

Frequent

Auranofin: Diarrhea (50%), pruritic rash (26%), abdominal pain (14%), stomatitis (13%), nausea (10%)

Aurothioglucose: Rash (39%), stomatitis (19%), diarrhea (13%).

Occasional

Aurothioglucose: Nausea, vomiting, anorexia, abdominal cramps

■ Serious Reactions

- Signs and symptoms of gold toxicity, the primary serious reaction, include decreased Hgb level, decreased granulocyte count (less than 150,000/mm^3), proteinuria, hematuria, stomatitis, blood dyscrasias (anemia, leukopenia [WBC count less than 4000/mm^3], thrombocytopenia, and eosinophilia), glomerulonephritis, nephrotic syndrome, and cholestatic jaundice.

Special Considerations

- Pruritus is a warning sign for development of cutaneous reactions
- Metallic taste may be a warning sign of stomatitis development

■ Monitoring Parameters

- CBC, platelet count, urinalysis, renal function, and LFTs before treatment
- CBC, platelet count, urinalysis every mo during therapy
- Gold toxicity

■ Geriatric side effects at a glance:

❑ CNS   ❑ Bowel Dysfunction   ❑ Bladder Dysfunction   ❑ Falls

aurothioglucose/gold sodium thiomalate

(aur-oh-thye-oh-gloo'kose/gold sodium thye-oh-maa'late)

■ **Brand Name(s):** Solganal; Myochrysine
Chemical Class: Heavy metal, active gold compound (50%)

■ **Clinical Pharmacology:**
Mechanism of Action: *Aurothioglucose:* A gold compound that alters cellular mechanisms, collagen biosynthesis, enzyme systems, and immune responses. **Therapeutic Effect:** Suppresses synovitis of the active stage of rheumatoid arthritis.: *Gold sodium thiomalate:* A gold compound whose mechanism of action is unknown. May decrease prostaglandin synthesis or alter cellular mechanisms by inhibiting sulfhydryl systems. **Therapeutic Effect:** Decreases synovial inflammation, retards cartilage and bone destruction, suppresses or prevents but does not cure, arthritis, synovitis.
Pharmacokinetics: *Aurothioglucose (50% gold):* Slow, erratic absorption after IM administration. Protein binding: 95%-99%. Primarily excreted in urine. **Half-life:** 3-27 days (half-life increased with increased number of doses).: *Gold sodium thiomalate:* Well absorbed. Protein binding: 95%. Widely distributed. Metabolized in liver. Excreted in urine and feces. Not removed by hemodialysis. **Half-life:** 5 days.

■ **Available Forms:**
Aurothioglucose:
• *Injection:* 50 mg/ml suspension (Solganal).
Gold sodium thiomalate:
• *Injection:* 50 mg/ml (Myochrysine).

■ **Indications and Dosages:**
Rheumatoid arthritis (aurothioglucose): IM Initially, 10 mg, then 25 mg for 2 doses, then 50 mg weekly thereafter until total dose of 0.8-1 g given. If patient is improved and there are no signs of toxicity, may give 50 mg at 3- to 4-wk intervals for many months.
Rheumatoid arthritis (gold sodium thiomalate): IM Initially, 10 mg, then 25 mg for 2nd dose. Follow with 25-50 mg/wk until improvement noted or total of 1 g administered. Maintenance: 25-50 mg q2wk for 2-20 wk; if stable, may increase to q3-4wk intervals.
Dosage in renal impairment:

Creatinine Clearance	Dosage
50-80 ml/min	50% of usual dosage
less than 50 ml/min	not recommended

■ **Unlabeled Uses:** Treatment of pemphigus, psoriatic arthritis

■ **Contraindications:** *Aurothioglucose*
Bone marrow aplasia, history of gold-induced pathologies, including blood dyscrasias, exfoliative dermatitis, necrotizing enterocolitis, and pulmonary fibrosis, serious adverse effects with previous gold therapy, severe blood dyscrasias

Gold sodium thiomalate
Colitis, concurrent use of antimalarials, immunosuppressive agents, penicillamine, or phenylbutazone, congestive heart failure (CHF), exfoliative dermatitis, history of blood dyscrasias, severe liver or renal impairment, systemic lupus erythematosus

■ Side Effects
Frequent
Aurothioglucose: Rash, stomatitis, diarrhea
Gold sodium thiomalate: Pruritic dermatitis, stomatitis, marked by erythema, redness, shallow ulcers of oral mucous membranes, sore throat, and difficulty swallowing, diarrhea or loose stools, abdominal pain, nausea
Occasional
Aurothioglucose: Nausea, vomiting, anorexia, abdominal cramps
Gold sodium thiomalate: Vomiting, anorexia, flatulence, dyspepsia, conjunctivitis, photosensitivity
Rare
Gold sodium thiomalate: Constipation, urticaria, rash

■ Serious Reactions
- Gold toxicity is the primary serious reaction. Signs and symptoms of gold toxicity include decreased Hgb, leukopenia (WBC count less than 4000/mm^3), reduced granulocyte counts (less than 150,000/mm^3), proteinuria, hematuria, stomatitis (sores, ulcers, and white spots in the mouth and throat), blood dyscrasias (anemia, leukopenia, thrombocytopenia, and eosinophilia), glomerulonephritis, nephritic syndrome, and cholestatic jaundice.

Special Considerations
- Administer in gluteal muscle with patient recumbent for 10 min after injection
- Pruritus is a warning sign for development of cutaneous reactions
- Metallic taste may be a warning sign of stomatitis development

■ Patient/Family Education
- Avoid exposure to sunlight because it may cause a gray to blue pigment to appear on the skin
- Maintain diligent oral hygiene to prevent stomatitis

■ Monitoring Parameters
- CBC, platelet count, urinalysis, renal function, and LFTs before treatment
- CBC, platelet count, urinalysis every mo during therapy
- Gold toxicity

■ Geriatric side effects at a glance:
❑ CNS   ❑ Bowel Dysfunction   ❑ Bladder Dysfunction   ❑ Falls

■ U.S. Regulatory Considerations
❑ FDA Black Box   ❑ OBRA regulated in U.S. Long Term Care

azathioprine

(ay-za-thye'-oh-preen)

- **Brand Name(s):** Azasan, Azathioprine Sodium, Imuran
  Chemical Class: 6-Mercaptopurine derivative; purine analog

- **Clinical Pharmacology:**
  Mechanism of Action: An immunologic agent that antagonizes purine metabolism and inhibits DNA, protein, and RNA synthesis. **Therapeutic Effect:** Suppresses cell-mediated hypersensitivities; alters antibody production and immune response in transplant recipients; reduces the severity of arthritis symptoms.
  Pharmacokinetics: Well absorbed from the GI tract following PO administration. Protein binding: 30%. Metabolized in liver. Excreted in urine. **Half-life:** 5 hr.

- **Available Forms:**
  - *Tablets*: 25 mg (Azasan), 50 mg (Azasan, Imuran), 75 mg (Azasan), 100 mg (Azasan).
  - *Injection* (**Imuran**): 100-mg vial.

- **Indications and Dosages:**
  Adjunct in prevention of renal allograft rejection: PO, IV 2-5 mg/kg/day on day of transplant, then 1-3 mg/kg/day as maintenance dose.
  Rheumatoid arthritis: PO Initially, 1 mg/kg/day (50-100 mg); may increase by 25 mg/day until response or toxicity.
  Dosage in renal impairment: Dosage is modified based on creatinine clearance.

Creatinine Clearance	Dose
10-50 ml/min	75% of usual dose
less than 10 ml/min	50% of usual dose

- **Unlabeled Uses:** Treatment of biliary cirrhosis, chronic active hepatitis, glomerulonephritis, inflammatory bowel disease, inflammatory myopathy, multiple sclerosis, myasthenia gravis, nephrotic syndrome, pemphigoid, pemphigus, polymyositis, systemic lupus erythematosus

- **Side Effects**
  Frequent
  Nausea, vomiting, anorexia (particularly during early treatment and with large doses)
  Occasional
  Rash
  Rare
  Severe nausea and vomiting with diarrhea, abdominal pain, hypersensitivity reaction

- **Serious Reactions**
  - Azathioprine use increases the risk of developing neoplasia (new abnormal-growth tumors).
  - Significant leukopenia and thrombocytopenia may occur, particularly in those undergoing kidney transplant rejection.
  - Hepatotoxicity occurs rarely.

- Severe leukopenia and/or thrombocytopenia may occur as well as macrocytic anemia and bone marrow depression; fungal, viral, bacterial, and protozoal infections may be fatal; may increase the patient's risk of neoplasia via mutagenic and carcinogenic properties (skin cancer and reticulum cell or lymphomatous tumors); temporary depression in spermatogenesis

■ **Patient/Family Education**
- The drug's therapeutic response may take up to 12 wk to appear
- Notify the physician if abdominal pain, fever, mouth sores, sore throat, or unusual bleeding occurs

■ **Monitoring Parameters**
- Hgb, WBC, monthly
- D/C if leukocytes are less than 3000/mm^3
- Therapeutic response may take 3-4 mo in rheumatoid arthritis
- CBC (especially platelet count) and serum hepatic enzyme levels weekly during the 1st month of therapy, twice monthly during the 2nd and 3rd months of treatment, and monthly thereafter

■ **Geriatric side effects at a glance:**
❑ CNS ❑ Bowel Dysfunction ❑ Bladder Dysfunction ❑ Falls

■ **U.S. Regulatory Considerations**
☑ FDA Black Box
Chronic immunosuppression may increase the risk of neoplasia.
❑ OBRA regulated in U.S. Long Term Care

azelastine

(a-zel'-as-teen)

■ **Brand Name(s):** Astelin (nasal), Optivar (ophthalmic)
Chemical Class: Phthalazinone derivative

■ **Clinical Pharmacology:**
Mechanism of Action: An antihistamine that competes with histamine for histamine receptor sites on cells in the blood vessels, GI tract, and respiratory tract. **Therapeutic Effect:** Relieves symptoms associated with seasonal allergic rhinitis, such as increased mucus production and sneezing and symptoms associated with allergic conjunctivitis, such as redness, itching, and excessive tearing.
Pharmacokinetics:

Route	Onset	Peak	Duration
Nasal spray	0.5-1 hr	2-3 hr	12 hr
Ophthalmic	N/A	3 min	8 hr

Well absorbed through nasal mucosa. Primarily excreted in feces. **Half-life:** 22 hr.

■ **Available Forms:**
  - Nasal Spray (Astelin): 137 mcg/spray.
  - Ophthalmic Solution (Optivar): 0.05%.

■ **Indications and Dosages:**
  Allergic rhinitis: Nasal 2 sprays in each nostril twice a day.
  Allergic conjunctivitis: Ophthalmic 1 drop into affected eye twice a day.

■ **Contraindications:** None known.

■ **Side Effects**
  Frequent (20%–15%)
  Headache, bitter taste
  Rare
  Nasal burning, paroxysmal sneezing, somnolence
  Ophthalmic: Transient eye burning or stinging, bitter taste, headache

■ **Serious Reactions**
  - Epistaxis occurs rarely.

Special Considerations
  - Low sedating antihistamine nasal spray with first-dose activity; note: onset of action not as fast as decongestant nasal sprays, but appropriate for prn use

■ **Patient/Family Education**
  - Advise caution with use concomitant with activities that require concentration or while operating machinery; may cause drowsiness
  - Preservative in ophth sol, benzlkonium chloride, may be absorbed by soft contact lenses; wait at least 10 min after instilling ophth sol before inserting soft contacts
  - Clear nasal passages before using azelastine
  - Prime the pump with 4 sprays or until a fine mist appears before using the nasal spray the first time. After the first use and if the pump hasn't been used for 3 or more days, prime the pump with 2 sprays or until a fine mist appears
  - Wipe the applicator tip with a clean, damp tissue and replace the cap immediately after use
  - Avoid spraying the nasal drug into the eyes
  - Avoid drinking alcoholic beverages during azelastine therapy

■ **Monitoring Parameters**
  - Therapeutic response to medication

■ **Geriatric side effects at a glance:**
  ☑ CNS ☑ Bowel Dysfunction ☑ Bladder Dysfunction ☐ Falls
  Other: Headache, alteration in taste

■ **Use with caution in older patients with:** Narrow-angle glaucoma, overflow incontinence, psychosis.

■ **U.S. Regulatory Considerations**
  ☐ FDA Black Box ☐ OBRA regulated in U.S. Long Term Care

■ **Other Uses in Geriatric Patient:** None

■ **Side Effects:**
Of particular importance in the geriatric patient: Alteration in taste may decrease food intake with possible malnutrition.

■ **Geriatric Considerations - Summary:** Azelastine is a potent H₁ receptor antagonist with minimal anticholinergic effects. It is used primarily as a nasal spray or ophthalmic solution but is well absorbed and can produce systemic effects such as headache and somnolence.

■ **References:**
1. Tinkelman DG, Bucholtz GA, Kemp JP, et al: Evaluation of the safety and efficacy of multiple doses of azelastine to adult patients with bronchial asthma over time. Am Rev Respir Dis 1990;141:569-574.
2. McTavish D, Sorkin EM: Azelastine. A review of its pharmacodynamic and pharmacokinetic properties, and therapeutic potential. Drugs 1989;38:778-800.

azithromycin

(ay-zi-thro-mye'-sin)

■ **Brand Name(s):** Zithromax, Zithromax TRI-PAK, Zithromax Z-PAK, Zmax
Chemical Class: Macrolide derivative

■ **Clinical Pharmacology:**
Mechanism of Action: A macrolide antibacterial that binds to ribosomal receptor sites of susceptible organisms, inhibiting RNA-dependent protein synthesis. **Therapeutic Effect:** Bacteriostatic or bactericidal, depending on the drug dosage.
Pharmacokinetics: Rapidly absorbed from the GI tract. Protein binding: 7%-50%. Widely distributed. Eliminated primarily unchanged by biliary excretion. **Half-life:** 68 hr.

■ **Available Forms:**
• *Tablets:* 250 mg, 500 mg, 600 mg (Zithromax). Tri-Pak: 3x500 mg (Zithromax TRI-PAK). Z-Pak: 6x250 mg (Zithromax Z-PAK).
• *Powder for Injection (Zithromax):* 500 mg.
• *Powder for Reconstitution (Zithromax):* 1 g.

■ **Indications and Dosages:**
Acute exacerbations of chronic obstructive pulmonary disease **(COPD):** PO 500 mg/day for 3 days or 500 mg on day 1, then 250 mg/day on days 2-5.
Acute bacterial sinusitis: PO (Zmax) 2 g as a single dose. PO 500 mg/day for 3 days.
Cervicitis: PO 1-2 g as single dose.
Chancroid: PO 1 g as single dose.
Mycobacterium avium complex **(MAC) prevention:** PO 1200 mg once weekly.
MAC treatment: PO 600 mg/day with ethambutol 15 mg/kg/day.
Pharyngitis, tonsillitis: PO 500 mg on day 1, then 250 mg on days 2-5.
Pneumonia, community-acquired: PO (Zmax) 2 g as a single dose. PO 500 mg on day 1, then 250 mg on days 2-5 or 500 mg/day IV for 2 days, then 500 mg/day PO to complete course of therapy.

Skin/skin-structure infections: PO 500 mg on day 1, then 250 mg on days 2-5.

- **Unlabeled Uses:** Chlamydial infections, gonococcal pharyngitis, uncomplicated gonococcal infections of the cervix, urethra, and rectum

- **Contraindications:** Hypersensitivity to other macrolide antibacterials

- **Side Effects**
  Occasional
  Nausea, vomiting, diarrhea, abdominal pain
  Rare
  Headache, dizziness, allergic reaction

- **Serious Reactions**
  - Antibiotic-associated colitis and other superinfections may result from altered bacterial balance.
  - Acute interstitial nephritis and hepatotoxicity occur rarely.

Special Considerations
  - Individualize treatment based on local susceptibility patterns.

- **Patient/Family Education**
  - Tablet may be taken without regard to food. Suspension and capsule should be taken on an empty stomach
  - Space doses evenly around the clock and continue taking azithromycin for the full course of treatment
  - If the patient must take an antacid containing aluminum or magnesium, take the drug 1 hr before or 2 hr after the antacid

- **Monitoring Parameters**
  - Evaluate the patient for signs and symptoms of superinfection, including genital or anal pruritus, sore mouth or tongue, and moderate to severe diarrhea

- **Geriatric side effects at a glance:**
  ❑ CNS ☑ Bowel Dysfunction ❑ Bladder Dysfunction ❑ Falls

- **U.S. Regulatory Considerations**
  ❑ FDA Black Box ❑ OBRA regulated in U.S. Long Term Care

aztreonam

(az'-tree-oh-nam)

- **Brand Name(s):** Azactam
  Chemical Class: Monobactam

■ Clinical Pharmacology:
Mechanism of Action: A monobactam antibacterial that inhibits bacterial cell wall synthesis. **Therapeutic Effect:** Bactericidal.
Pharmacokinetics: Completely absorbed after IM administration. Protein binding: 56%-60%. Partially metabolized by hydrolysis. Primarily excreted unchanged in urine. Removed by hemodialysis. **Half-life:** 1.4-2.2 hr (increased in impaired renal or hepatic function).

■ Available Forms:
* *Injection Powder for Reconstitution:* 500 mg, 1 g, 2 g.

■ Indications and Dosages:
UTIs: IV, IM 500 mg-1 g q8-12h.
Moderate to severe systemic infections: IV, IM 1-2 g q8-12h.
Severe or life-threatening infections: IV 2 g q6-8h.
Dosage in renal impairment: Dosage and frequency are modified based on creatinine clearance and the severity of the infection:

Creatinine Clearance	Dosage
10-30 ml/min	1-2 g initially, then ½ usual dose at usual intervals
less than 10 ml/min	1-2 g initially; then ¼ usual dose at usual intervals

■ Unlabeled Uses: Treatment of bone and joint infections

■ Contraindications: None known.

■ Side Effects
Occasional (less than 3%)
Discomfort and swelling at IM injection site, nausea, vomiting, diarrhea, rash
Rare (less than 1%)
Phlebitis or thrombophlebitis at IV injection site, abdominal cramps, headache, hypotension

■ Serious Reactions
* Antibiotic-associated colitis and other superinfections may result from altered bacterial balance.
* Severe hypersensitivity reactions, including anaphylaxis, occur rarely.

Special Considerations
* Minimal cross-reactivity between aztreonam and penicillins and cephalosporins; aztreonam and aminoglycosides have been shown to be synergistic in vitro against most strains of P. *aeruginosa*, many strains of Enterobacteriaceae, and other gram-negative aerobic bacilli
* Individualize treatment based on local susceptibility patterns.

■ Monitoring Parameters
* Signs and symptoms of superinfections, including anal or genital pruritus, black hairy tongue, vomiting, diarrhea, fever, sore throat, and ulceration or changes of oral mucosa

■ Geriatric side effects at a glance:
❑ CNS   ❑ Bowel Dysfunction   ❑ Bladder Dysfunction   ❑ Falls

bacitracin

(bass-i-tray'-sin)

■ **Brand Name(s):** AK-Tracin, Baci-IM, Baci-Rx, Ocu-Tracin, Ziba-Rx

Combinations
Rx: with neomycin, polymixin, and hydrocortisone (Cortisporin)
OTC: with neomycin and polymixin (Neosporin); with polymixin (Polysporin)
Chemical Class: *Bacillus subtilis* derivative

■ **Clinical Pharmacology:**
Mechanism of Action: An antibiotic that interferes with plasma membrane permeability and inhibits bacterial cell wall synthesis in susceptible bacteria. **Therapeutic Effect:** Bacteriostatic.
Pharmacokinetics: Not significantly absorbed following topical or ophthalmic administration.

■ **Available Forms:**
• *Powder for Irrigation*: 50,000 units.
• *Ophthalmic Ointment* (AK-Tracin): 500 units/g.
• *Topical Ointment* (Ocu-Tracin): 500 units/g.

■ **Indications and Dosages:**
Superficial ocular infections: Ophthalmic ½-inch ribbon in conjunctival sac q3-4h.
Skin abrasions, superficial skin infections: Topical Apply to affected area 1-5 times a day.
Surgical treatment and prophylaxis: Irrigation 50,000-150,000 units, as needed.

■ **Contraindications:** None known.

■ **Side Effects**
Rare
Ophthalmic: Burning, itching, redness, swelling, pain
Topical: Hypersensitivity reaction (allergic contact dermatitis, burning, inflammation, pruritus)

■ **Serious Reactions**
• None known.

■ **Patient/Family Education**
• Administer at even intervals
• Report burning, itching, increased irritation, or rash

■ **Monitoring Parameters**
  • Using the topical ointment, be alert for signs and symptoms of hypersensitivity, such as burning, inflammation, and pruritus

■ **Geriatric side effects at a glance:**
  ❏ CNS   ❏ Bowel Dysfunction   ❏ Bladder Dysfunction   ❏ Falls

■ **U.S. Regulatory Considerations**
  ❏ FDA Black Box   ❏ OBRA regulated in U.S. Long Term Care

baclofen

(bak'-loe-fen)

■ **Brand Name(s):** Lioresal, Lioresal Intrathecal
  Chemical Class: GABA chlorophenyl derivative

■ **Clinical Pharmacology:**
  Mechanism of Action: A direct-acting skeletal muscle relaxant that inhibits transmission of reflexes at the spinal cord level. **Therapeutic Effect:** Relieves muscle spasticity. **Pharmacokinetics:** Well absorbed from the GI tract. Protein binding: 30%. Partially metabolized in the liver. Primarily excreted in urine. **Half-life:** 2.5-4 hr; intrathecal: 1.5 hr.

■ **Available Forms:**
  • *Tablets:* 10 mg, 20 mg.
  • *Intrathecal Injection:* 50 mcg/ml, 500 mcg/ml, 2000 mcg/ml.

■ **Indications and Dosages:**
  Spasticity: PO Initially, 5 mg 2-3 times a day. May increase by 15 mg/day at 3-day intervals. Range: 40-80 mg/day. Maximum: 80 mg/day.
  Usual intrathecal dosage: Intrathecal 300-800 mcg/day.

■ **Unlabeled Uses:** Treatment of bladder spasms, cerebral palsy, intractable hiccups or pain, Huntington's chorea, trigeminal neuralgia

■ **Contraindications:** Skeletal muscle spasm due to cerebral palsy, Parkinson disease, rheumatic disorders, CVA, cough, intractable hiccups, neuropathic pain

■ **Side Effects**
  Frequent (greater than 10%)
  Transient somnolence, asthenia, dizziness, light-headedness, nausea, vomiting
  Occasional (10%–2%)
  Headache, paresthesia, constipation, anorexia, hypotension, confusion, nasal congestion
  Rare (less than 1%)
  Paradoxical CNS excitement or restlessness, slurred speech, tremor, dry mouth, diarrhea, nocturia, impotence

■ Serious Reactions
- Abrupt discontinuation of baclofen may produce hallucinations and seizures.
- Overdose results in blurred vision, seizures, myosis, mydriasis, severe muscle weakness, strabismus, respiratory depression, and vomiting.

Special Considerations
- Abrupt discontinuation may lead to hallucinations, spasticity, tachycardia; drug should be tapered off over 1-2 wk

■ Patient/Family Education
- Do not abruptly discontinue after long-term therapy
- Avoid hazardous activities if dizziness, drowsiness, light-headedness are present
- Avoid alcohol and CNS depressants during therapy

■ Monitoring Parameters
- CBC, liver and renal function

■ Geriatric side effects at a glance:
☑ CNS ☐ Bowel Dysfunction ☐ Bladder Dysfunction ☑ Falls

■ U.S. Regulatory Considerations
☑ FDA Black Box

Intrathecal use: Abrupt discontinuation has resulted in high fever, altered mental status, exaggerated rebound spasticity, and muscle rigidity that in rare cases advances to rhabdomyolysis, multiple organ system failure, and death.

☐ OBRA regulated in U.S. Long Term Care

balsalazide disodium

(bal-sal'-a-zide dye-soe'-dee-um)

■ Brand Name(s): Colazal
Chemical Class: 5-Amino derivative of salicylic acid

■ Clinical Pharmacology:
Mechanism of Action: A 5-aminosalicylic acid derivative that changes intestinal microflora, altering prostaglandin production and inhibiting function of natural killer cells, mast cells, neutrophils, and macrophages. **Therapeutic Effect:** Diminishes inflammatory effect in colon.

Pharmacokinetics: Low and variable absorption following PO administration. Protein binding: greater than 99%. Extensively metabolized in colon. Minimal elimination in urine and feces. **Half-life:** Unknown.

■ Available Forms:
- *Capsules:* 750 mg.

- **Indications and Dosages:**
  Ulcerative colitis: PO Three 750-mg capsules 3 times a day for 8 wk.

- **Contraindications:** Hypersensitivity to salicylates

- **Side Effects**
  Frequent (8%–6%)
  Headache, abdominal pain, nausea, diarrhea
  Occasional (4%–2%)
  Vomiting, arthralgia, rhinitis, insomnia, fatigue, flatulence, coughing, dyspepsia

- **Serious Reactions**
  - Liver toxicity occurs rarely.

Special Considerations

  - The recommended dose of 6.75 g/day provides approximately 2.4 g of free mesalamine to the colon

- **Patient/Family Education**
  - Take as directed
  - Do not chew or open balsalazide capsules
  - Notify the physician if abdominal pain, severe headache or chest pain, or unresolved diarrhea occurs

- **Monitoring Parameters**
  - Liver function test
  - Pattern of daily bowel activity and stool consistency

- **Geriatric side effects at a glance:**
  ❏ CNS ❏ Bowel Dysfunction ❏ Bladder Dysfunction ❏ Falls

- **U.S. Regulatory Considerations**
  ❏ FDA Black Box ❏ OBRA regulated in U.S. Long Term Care

becaplermin

(be-kap'-ler-min)

- **Brand Name(s):** Regranex
  Chemical Class: Recombinant human platelet-derived growth factor (rhPDGF-BB)

- **Clinical Pharmacology:**
  Mechanism of Action: A platelet-derived growth factor that heals open wounds. **Therapeutic Effect:** Stimulates body to grow new tissue.
  Pharmacokinetics: None reported.

- **Available Forms:**
  - *Gel*: 0.01% (Regranex).

- **Indications and Dosages:**
  Ulcers: Topical Apply once daily (spread evenly; cover with saline-moistened gauze dressing). After 12 hr, rinse ulcer, re-cover with saline gauze.

- **Contraindications:** Neoplasms at site of application, hypersensitivity to becaplermin or any component of the formulation

- **Side Effects**
  Occasional
  Local rash near ulcer

- **Serious Reactions**
  - None reported.

- **Patient/Family Education**
  - Refrigerate
  - Wash hands before applying

- **Monitoring Parameters**
  - If the ulcer does not decrease in size by approximately 30% after 10 wk of treatment or complete healing has not occurred in 20 wk, continued treatment should be re-assessed
  - Dose requires recalculation weekly or bi-weekly, depending on rate of change in the width and length of ulcer

- **Geriatric side effects at a glance:**
  ☐ CNS ☐ Bowel Dysfunction ☐ Bladder Dysfunction ☐ Falls

- **U.S. Regulatory Considerations**
  ☐ FDA Black Box ☐ OBRA regulated in U.S. Long Term Care

beclomethasone dipropionate

(be-kloe-meth'-a-sone)

- **Brand Name(s):** Beclovent, Beconase, Beconase AQ, Qvar, Vancenase, Vancenase AQ, Vancenase AQ DS, Vanceril, Vanceril DS
  Chemical Class: Glucocorticoid, synthetic

■ **Clinical Pharmacology:**
Mechanism of Action: An adrenocorticosteroid that prevents or controls inflammation by controlling the rate of protein synthesis; decreasing migration of polymorphonuclear leukocytes and fibroblasts; and reversing capillary permeability. **Therapeutic Effect:** Inhalation: Inhibits bronchoconstriction, produces smooth muscle relaxation, decreases mucus secretion. Intranasal: Decreases response to seasonal and perennial rhinitis.
Pharmacokinetics: Rapidly absorbed from pulmonary, nasal, and GI tissue. Undergoes extensive first-pass metabolism in the liver. Protein binding: 87%. Primarily eliminated in feces. **Half-life:** 15 hr.

■ **Available Forms:**
- *Oral Inhalation (Qvar)*. 40 mcg per inhalation, 80 mcg/inhalation.
- *Nasal Spray (Beconase AQ)*. 42 mcg/ inhalation.

■ **Indications and Dosages:**
Long-term control of bronchial asthma, reduces need for oral corticosteriod therapy for asthma : Oral Inhalation 40-160 mcg twice a day. Maximum: 320 mcg twice a day.
Rhinitis, prevention of recurrence of nasal polyps: Nasal Inhalation 1 spray in each nostril 2-4 times a day or 2 sprays twice a day. Maintenance: 1 spray 3 times a day.

■ **Unlabeled Uses:** Prevention of seasonal rhinitis (nasal form)

■ **Contraindications:** Hypersensitivity to beclomethasone, acute exacerbation of asthma, status asthmaticus

■ **Side Effects**
Frequent
Inhalation (14%-4%): Throat irritation, dry mouth, hoarseness, cough
Intranasal: Nasal burning, mucosal dryness
Occasional
Inhalation (3%-2%): Localized fungal infection (thrush)
Intranasal: Nasal-crusting epistaxis, sore throat, ulceration of nasal mucosa
Rare
Inhalation: Transient bronchospasm, esophageal candidiasis
Intranasal: Nasal and pharyngeal candidiasis, eye pain

■ **Serious Reactions**
- An acute hypersensitivity reaction, as evidenced by urticaria, angioedema, and severe bronchospasm, occurs rarely.
- A transfer from systemic to local steroid therapy may unmask previously suppressed bronchial asthma condition.

■ **Patient/Family Education**
- Rinse mouth with water following INH to decrease possibility of fungal infections, dysphonia
- Review proper MDI administration technique regularly
- Systemic corticosteroid effects from inhaled and nasal steroids inadequate to prevent adrenal insufficiency in patients withdrawn from corticosteroids abruptly
- Response to nasal steroids seen in 3 days-2 wk; discontinue if no improvement in 3 wk
- For prophylactic use, no role in acute treatment of asthma/allergy

- Taper dosage gradually; do not change dosage schedule or stop taking the drug abruptly

■ **Monitoring Parameters**
- Relief of symptoms, such as wheezing, congestion, and dyspnea

■ **Geriatric side effects at a glance:**
❑ CNS ❑ Bowel Dysfunction ❑ Bladder Dysfunction ❑ Falls

■ **U.S. Regulatory Considerations**
❑ FDA Black Box ☑ OBRA regulated in U.S. Long Term Care

belladonna alkaloids

(bell-a-don'-a al-kuh-loydz)

■ **Brand Name(s):** Antispas, Antispasmodic, Barbidonna, Barophen, Bellalphen, Bellatal, Bellergal, Bellergal-S, Bellergal-R, Chardonna-2, Donnapine, D-Tal, Haponal, Spacol, Spasmolin, Spasquid

Combinations
Rx: with butalbital (Butibel); with ergotamine and phenobarbital (Bellergal-S, Phenerbel-S); with phenobarbital (Donnatal, Donnatal Extentabs)
Chemical Class: Belladonna alkaloid

■ **Clinical Pharmacology:**
Mechanism of Action: Competitive inhibitors of the muscarinic actions of acetylcholine, acting at receptors located in exocrine glands, smooth and cardiac muscle, and intramural neurons. Composed of 3 main constituents: atropine, scopolamine, and hyoscyamine. Scopolamine exerts greater effects on the CNS, eye, and secretory glands than the constituents atropine and hyoscyamine. Atropine exerts more activity on the heart, intestine, and bronchial muscle and exhibits a more prolonged duration of action compared to scopolamine. Hyoscyamine exerts similar actions to atropine but has more potent central and peripheral nervous system effects. *Therapeutic Effect:* Peripheral anticholinergic and antispasmodic action, mild sedation.
Pharmacokinetics: None known.

■ **Available Forms:**
- *Tablet:* 40 mg phenobarbital, 0.6 mg ergotamine tartrate, 0.2 mg levorotatory alkaloids of belladonna (Bellergal, Bellergal-S, Bellergal-R, Spasmolin, Bellalphen, Antispas, Spacol, Chardonna-2, Barbidonna)
- *Tablet, Extended Release:* 0.0582 mg-0.0582 mg-48.6 mg-0.0195 mg (Donnatal Extendtabs)
- *Elixir:* 0.0194 mg-0.1037 mg-16.2 mg-0.0065 mg/5 ml (Barophen, Donnapine, Antispasmodic, Spacol, Donnatal, D-Tal, Spasquid)

■ **Indications and Dosages:**
Irritable bowel syndrome, acute enterocolitis: PO 1-2 tablets or capsules 3-4 times daily or 1-2 teaspoonfuls of elixir 3-4 times daily according to conditions and severity of symptoms.

121

■ **Contraindications:** Glaucoma, obstructive uropathy, obstructive disease of GI-anti-cholinergic tract, paralytic ileus, intestinal atony of the elderly or debilitated patient, unstable cardiovascular status in acute hemorrhage, severe ulcerative colitis especially if complicated by toxic megacolon, myasthenia gravis, hiatal hernia associated with reflux esophagitis, hypersensitivity to any component of the formulation, acute intermittent porphyria.

■ **Side Effects**

Frequent

Dry mouth, urinary retention, flushing, pupillary dilation, constipation, confusion, redness of the skin, flushing, dry skin, allergic contact dermatitis, headache, excitement, agitation, dizziness, light-headedness, drowsiness, unsteadiness, confusion, slurred speech, sedation, hyperreflexia, convulsions, vertigo, coma, mydriasis, photophobia, blurred vision, dilation of pupils

Rare

Hallucinations, acute psychosis, Stevens-Johnson syndrome, photosensitivity

■ **Serious Reactions**
- Signs and symptoms of overdose include headache, nausea, vomiting, blurred vision, dilated pupils; hot and dry skin, dizziness, dryness of the mouth, difficulty in swallowing and CNS stimulation.
- Treatment should consist of gastric lavage, emetics, and activated charcoal. If indicated, parenteral cholinergic agents such as physostigmine or bethanechol chloride should be added.

Special Considerations
- Product contains hyoscyamine, atropine, and scopolamine

■ **Patient/Family Education**
- Avoid hot environments, heat stroke may occur
- Use sunglasses when outside to prevent photophobia
- Change positions slowly to avoid light-headedness
- Avoid alcohol, CNS depressants, and tasks that require mental alertness
- Constipation, difficulty urinating, decreased sweating, drowsiness, dry mouth, increased heart rate, headache, orthostatic hypotension may occur

■ **Geriatric side effects at a glance:**
  ☑ CNS ☑ Bowel Dysfunction ☑ Bladder Dysfunction ❏ Falls
  Other: Dry mouth, blurred vision, confusion, psychosis

■ **Use with caution in older patients with:** Narrow-angle glaucoma, overflow incontinence, preexisting psychotic symptoms

■ **U.S. Regulatory Considerations**
  ❏ FDA Black Box ☑ OBRA regulated in U.S. Long Term Care

■ **Other Uses in Geriatric Patient:** Use to decrease salivation

■ **Side Effects:**
  Of *particular importance in the geriatric patient*: Delirium, possible antagonism of cholinergic drug therapy in the treatment of Alzheimer's disease.

- **Geriatric Considerations - Summary:** Alkaloids from the belladonna plant contain 3 potent anticholinergics and offer no advantage over other available drugs. Belladonna alkaloids possess potent anticholinergic effects and can cause dry mouth, blurred vision, delirium, confusion, psychosis, and increased risk of falls. This compound has no role in treating the older adult.

- **References:**
  1. Vangala V, Tueth M. Chronic anticholinergic toxicity: identification and management in older patients. Geriatrics 2003;58:36-37.
  2. Tune LE. Anticholinergic effects of medication in elderly patients. J Clin Psychiatry 2001;62(suppl 21):11-14.
  3. Ziskind AA: Transdermal scopolamine-induced pyschosis. Postgrad Med 1988;84:73-76.

belladonna and opium

(bell-a-don'-a)

- **Brand Name(s):** B & O Supprettes 15A, B & O Supprettes 16A
  Chemical Class: Belladonna alkaloid; opiate

  DEA Class: Schedule II

- **Clinical Pharmacology:**
  Mechanism of Action: Anticholinergic alkaloids that inhibit the action of acetylcholine at postganglionic (muscarinic) receptor sites. Morphine (10% of opium) depresses cerebral cortex, hypothalamus, and medullary centers. **Therapeutic Effect:** Decreases digestive secretions, increases GI muscle tone, reduces GI force, alters pain perception and emotional response to pain.
  Pharmacokinetics: Onset of action occurs within 30 min. Absorption is dependent on body hydration. Metabolized in liver to form glucuronide metabolites.

- **Available Forms:**
  - Suppository: 16.2 mg belladonna extract/30 mg opium (B & O Supprettes 15A), 16.2 mg belladonna extract/60 mg opium (B & O Supprettes 16A).

- **Indications and Dosages:**
  Analgesic, antispasmodic: Rectal 1 suppository 1-2 times/day. Maximum: 4 doses/day.

- **Unlabeled Uses:** Glaucoma, severe renal or hepatic disease, bronchial asthma, respiratory depression, convulsive disorders, acute alcoholism, hypersensitivity to belladonna or opium or its components

- **Contraindications:** None known.

- **Side Effects**
  Frequent
  Dry mouth, nose, skin and throat, decreased sweating, constipation, irritation at site of administration, drowsiness, urinary retention, dizziness

Occasional
Blurred vision, decreased flow of breast milk, bloated feeling, drowsiness, headache, intolerance to light, nervousness, flushing
Rare
Dizziness, faintness, pruritus, urticaria

■ **Serious Reactions**
  • Respiratory depression, increased intraocular pain, loss of memory, orthostatic hypotension, tachycardia, and ventricular fibrillation rarely occur.
  • Tolerance to the drug's analgesic effect and physical dependence may occur with repeated use.

■ **Patient/Family Education**
  • Moisten finger and suppository with water before inserting
  • May cause drowsiness, dry mouth, and blurred vision
  • Store at room temperature; DO NOT refrigerate

■ **Monitoring Parameters**
  • Bowel activity

■ **Geriatric side effects at a glance:**
  ☑ CNS   ☑ Bowel Dysfunction   ☑ Bladder Dysfunction   ☑ Falls
  Other: Dry mouth, blurred vision, confusion, psychosis

■ **Use with caution in older patients with:** Narrow-angle glaucoma, overflow incontinence, preexisting psychotic symptoms

■ **U.S. Regulatory Considerations**
  ❏ FDA Black Box   ☑ OBRA regulated in U.S. Long Term Care

■ **Other Uses in Geriatric Patient:** Use to decrease salivation

■ **Side Effects:**
  Of particular importance in the geriatric patient: Anticholinergic effects

■ **Geriatric Considerations - Summary:** Belladonna possesses potent anticholinergic effects and can cause dry mouth, blurred vision, delirium, confusion, psychosis, and increased risk of falls. Opium is a narcotic and when discontinued, physical dependence and withdrawal symptoms can occur. Adverse GI effects include constipation and abdominal pain. This compound has no role in treating the older adult.

■ **References:**
  1. Vangala V, Tueth M. Chronic anticholinergic toxicity: identification and management in older patients. Geriatrics 2003;58:36-37.
  2. Tune LE. Anticholinergic effects of medication in elderly patients. J Clin Psychiatry 2001;62(suppl 21):11-14.

benazepril

(ben-ay'-ze-pril)

■ **Brand Name(s):** Lotensin

Combinations
Rx: with hydrochlorothiazide (Lotensin HCT)
Rx: with amlodipine (Lotrel)
Chemical Class: Angiotensin-converting enzyme (ACE) inhibitor, nonsulfhydryl

■ **Clinical Pharmacology:**
Mechanism of Action: An ACE inhibitor that decreases the rate of conversion of angiotensin I to angiotensin II, a potent vasoconstrictor. Reduces peripheral arterial resistance. **Therapeutic Effect:** Lowers BP.
Pharmacokinetics:

Route	Onset	Peak	Duration
PO	1 hr	2-4 hr	24 hr

Partially absorbed from the GI tract. Protein binding: 97%. Metabolized in the liver to active metabolite. Primarily excreted in urine. Minimal removal by hemodialysis. **Half-life:** 35 min; metabolite 10-11 hr.

■ **Available Forms:**
• *Tablets*: 5 mg, 10 mg, 20 mg, 40 mg.

■ **Indications and Dosages:**
Hypertension (monotherapy): PO Initially, 5-10 mg/day. Range: 20-40 mg/day.
Hypertension (combination therapy): PO Discontinue diuretic 2-3 days prior to initiating benazepril, then dose as noted above. If unable to discontinue diuretic, begin benazepril at 5 mg/day.
Dosage in renal impairment: For adult patients with creatinine clearance less than 30 ml/min, initially, 5 mg/day titrated up to maximum of 40 mg/day.

■ **Unlabeled Uses:** Treatment of CHF

■ **Contraindications:** History of angioedema from previous treatment with ACE inhibitors

■ **Side Effects**
Frequent (6%–3%)
Cough, headache, dizziness
Occasional (2%)
Fatigue, somnolence or drowsiness, nausea
Rare (less than 1%)
Rash, fever, myalgia, diarrhea, loss of taste

■ **Serious Reactions**
• Excessive hypotension ("first-dose syncope") may occur in patients with CHF and in those who are severely salt or volume depleted.
• Angioedema (swelling of the face and lips) and hyperkalemia occur rarely.

- Agranulocytosis and neutropenia may be noted in those with collagen vascular disease, including scleroderma and systemic lupus erythematosus, and impaired renal function.
- Nephrotic syndrome may be noted in patients with history of renal disease.
- Hypoglycemia may occur in patients with diabetes using glucose-lowering drugs.

■ **Patient/Family Education**
- Caution with salt substitutes containing potassium chloride
- Rise slowly to sitting/standing position to minimize orthostatic hypotension
- Dizziness, fainting, light-headedness may occur during 1st few days of therapy
- May cause altered taste perception or cough; persistent dry cough usually does not subside unless medication is stopped
- Full therapeutic effect of benazepril may take 2-4 wk to appear
- Noncompliance with drug therapy or skipping drug doses may produce severe, rebound hypertension

■ **Monitoring Parameters**
- BUN, creatinine, potassium within 2 wk after initiation of therapy (increased levels may indicate acute renal failure)
- Blood pressure, CBC, urine protein levels

■ **Geriatric side effects at a glance:**
❏ CNS   ❏ Bowel Dysfunction   ❏ Bladder Dysfunction   ❏ Falls

■ **U.S. Regulatory Considerations**
☑ FDA Black Box
Although not relevant for geriatric patients, teratogenicity is associated with the use of ACE inhibitors.
❏ OBRA regulated in U.S. Long Term Care

bentoquatam

(ben'-toe-kwa-tam)

■ **Brand Name(s):** Ivy Block
Chemical Class: Organoclay compound

■ **Clinical Pharmacology:**
Mechanism of Action: An organoclay substance that absorbs and binds to urushiol, the active principle in poison oak, ivy, and sumac. **Therapeutic Effect:** Blocks urushiol skin contact and absorption.
Pharmacokinetics: None reported.

■ **Available Forms:**
- *Lotion:* 5% (Ivy Block).

- ■ **Indications and Dosages:**
  Contact dermatitis prophylaxis caused by poison oak, ivy, or sumac: Topical Apply thin film over skin at least 15 min before potential exposure. Re-apply q4h or sooner if needed.

- ■ **Contraindications:** Hypersensitivity to bentoquatam or any of its components such as methylparabens

- ■ **Side Effects**
  Occasional
  Erythema

- ■ **Serious Reactions**
  - None reported.

- ■ **Patient/Family Education**
  - To be used prior to exposure only
  - Avoid using near eyes
  - Re-apply every 4 hr, as needed

- ■ **Monitoring Parameters**
  - Therapeutic response

- ■ **Geriatric side effects at a glance:**
  ❑ CNS ❑ Bowel Dysfunction ❑ Bladder Dysfunction ❑ Falls

- ■ **U.S. Regulatory Considerations**
  ❑ FDA Black Box ❑ OBRA regulated in U.S. Long Term Care

benzocaine

(ben'-zoe-kane)

- ■ **Brand Name(s):**
  OTC: Americaine Anesthetic Lubricant, Americaine Otic, Anbesol, Anbesol Maximum Strength, Benzodent, Cepacol, Cetacaine, Chiggerex, Chiggertox, Cylex, Dermoplast, Detaine, Foille, Foille Medicated First Aid, Foille Plus, HDA Toothache, Hurricaine, Lanacane, Mycinettes, Omedia, Orabase-B, Orajel, Orajel Maximum Strength, Orasol, Otocain, Otricaine, Retre-Gel, Solarcaine, Trocaine, Zilactin-B

  Combinations
  Rx: with antipyrine (Allergen, Auralgan, Auroto); with benzethonium chloride (Americaine, Otocain); with phenylephrine (Tympagesic)
  Chemical Class: Benzoic acid derivative

- ■ **Clinical Pharmacology:**
  Mechanism of Action: A local anesthetic that blocks nerve conduction in the autonomic, sensory, and motor nerve fibers. Competes with calcium ions for membrane

binding. Reduces permeability of resting nerves to potassium and sodium ions. **Therapeutic Effect:** Produces local analgesic effect.

Pharmacokinetics: Poorly absorbed by topical administration. Well absorbed from mucous membranes and traumatized skin. Metabolized in liver and by hydrolysis with cholinesterase. Minimal excretion in urine.

■ Available Forms:

- *Cream*: 5%, 20% (Lanacane).
- *Lozenge*: 10 mg (Cepacol, Trocaine), 15 mg (Cylex, Mycinettes).
- *Oral Aerosol*: 14% (Cetacaine), 20% (Hurricaine).
- *Oral Gel*: 6.3% (Anbesol), 6.5% (HDA Toothache), 7.5% (Detaine), 10% (Orajel, Zilactin-B), 20% (Anbesol Maximum Strength, Hurricaine).
- *Oral Liquid*: 6.3% (Anbesol), 10% (Orajel), 20% (Anbesol Maximum Strength, Hurricane).
- *Oral Ointment*: 20% (Benzodent).
- *Otic Solution*: 20% (Americaine Otic, Omedia, Otocain, Otricaine).
- *Paste*: 20% (Orabase-B).
- *Topical Aerosol*: 5% (Foille, Foille Plus), 20% (Dermoplast, Solarcaine).
- *Topical Gel*: 5% (Retre-Gel), 20% (Americaine Anesthetic Lubricant).
- *Topical Liquid*: 2% (Chiggertox).
- *Topical Ointment*: 2% (Chiggerex), 5% (Foille Medicated First Aid).

■ Indications and Dosages:

Canker sores: Topical Apply gel, liquid, or ointment to affected area. Maximum: 4 times/day.

Denture irritation: Topical Apply thin layer of gel to affected area up to 4 times/day or until pain is relieved.

General lubrication: Topical Apply gel to exterior of tube or instrument prior to use.

Otitis externa, otitis media: Otic Instill 4-5 drops into external ear canal of affected ears. Repeat q1-2h as needed.

Pain and itching associated with sunburn, insect bites, minor cuts, scrapes, minor burns, minor skin irritations: Topical Apply to affected area 3-4 times/day.

Pharyngitis: PO 1 lozenge q2h. Maximum 8 lozenges/day.

Toothache: Topical Apply gel, liquid, or ointment to affected areas. Maximum: 4 times/day.

Anesthesia: Topical Apply aerosol, gel, ointment, liquid q4-12h as needed.

■ Contraindications: Hypersensitivity to benzocaine or ester-type local anesthetics, perforated tympanic membrane or ear discharge (otic preparations)

■ Side Effects

Occasional

Burning, stinging, angioedema, contact dermatitis, taste disorders

■ Serious Reactions

- None known.

■ Patient/Family Education

- Protect the solution from light and heat, do not use if it is brown or contains a precipitate
- Discard this product 6 mo after dropper is first placed in the drug solution
- Avoid contact with eyes

- Clean hands with soap and water before using benzocaine
- Do not eat for 1 hr after oral application

■ **Geriatric side effects at a glance:**
❑ CNS   ❑ Bowel Dysfunction   ❑ Bladder Dysfunction   ❑ Falls

■ **U.S. Regulatory Considerations**
❑ FDA Black Box   ❑ OBRA regulated in U.S. Long Term Care

benzonatate

(ben-zoe'-na-tate)

■ **Brand Name(s):** Tessalon, Tessalon Perles
Chemical Class: Tetracaine derivative

■ **Clinical Pharmacology:**
Mechanism of Action: A non-narcotic antitussive that anesthetizes stretch receptors in respiratory passages, lungs, and pleura. **Therapeutic Effect:** Reduces cough production.
Pharmacokinetics:

Onset	Duration
15-20 min	Up to 8 hr

■ **Available Forms:**
- *Capsules* (*Tessalon*): 100 mg, 200 mg.

■ **Indications and Dosages:**
Antitussive: PO 100 mg 3 times a day or q4h up to 600 mg/day.

■ **Contraindications:** None known.

■ **Side Effects**
Occasional
Mild somnolence, mild dizziness, constipation, GI upset, skin eruptions, nasal congestion

■ **Serious Reactions**
- A paradoxical reaction, including restlessness, insomnia, euphoria, nervousness, and tremor, has been noted.

■ **Patient/Family Education**
- Avoid driving, other hazardous activities until stabilized on this medication
- Do not chew or break capsules, will anesthetize mouth

■ **Monitoring Parameters**
  • Clinical improvement, onset of cough relief

■ **Geriatric side effects at a glance:**
  ☑ CNS ❏ Bowel Dysfunction ❏ Bladder Dysfunction ❏ Falls

■ **U.S. Regulatory Considerations**
  ❏ FDA Black Box ❏ OBRA regulated in U.S. Long Term Care

benztropine mesylate

(benz'-troe-peen mes'-sil-ate)

■ **Brand Name(s):** Cogentin
  Chemical Class: Tertiary amine

■ **Clinical Pharmacology:**
  Mechanism of Action: An antiparkinson agent that selectively blocks central cholinergic receptors, helping to balance cholinergic and dopaminergic activity. **Therapeutic Effect:** Reduces the incidence and severity of akinesia, rigidity, and tremor.
  Pharmacokinetics: Well absorbed following oral and IM administration. Oral onset of action: 1-2 hr, IM onset of action: minutes. The pharmacologic effects may not be apparent until 2-3 days after initiation of therapy and may persist for up to 24 hr after discontinuation of the drug. **Half-life:** Extended.

■ **Available Forms:**
  • *Tablets*: 0.5 mg, 1 mg, 2 mg.
  • *Injection*: 1 mg/ml.

■ **Indications and Dosages:**
  Parkinsonism: PO Initially, 0.5 mg once or twice a day. Titrate by 0.5 mg at 5- to 6-day intervals. Maximum: 4 mg/day.
  Drug-induced extrapyramidal symptoms: PO, IM 1-4 mg once or twice a day.
  Acute dystonic reactions: IV, IM Initially, 1-2 mg; then 1-2 mg PO twice a day to prevent recurrence.

■ **Contraindications:** Angle-closure glaucoma, benign prostatic hyperplasia, GI obstruction, intestinal atony, megacolon, myasthenia gravis, paralytic ileus, severe ulcerative colitis

■ **Side Effects**
  Frequent
  Somnolence, dry mouth, blurred vision, constipation, decreased sweating or urination, GI upset, photosensitivity
  Occasional
  Headache, memory loss, muscle cramps, anxiety, peripheral paresthesia, orthostatic hypotension, abdominal cramps

Rare
Rash, confusion, eye pain

■ **Serious Reactions**
- Overdose may produce severe anticholinergic effects, such as unsteadiness, somnolence, tachycardia, dyspnea, skin flushing, and severe dryness of the mouth, nose, or throat.
- Severe paradoxical reactions, marked by hallucinations, tremor, seizures, and toxic psychosis, may occur.

■ **Patient/Family Education**
- Do not discontinue abruptly
- Administer with or after meals to prevent GI upset
- Drug may increase susceptibility to heat stroke
- Dizziness, drowsiness, and dry mouth are expected responses to the drug
- Avoid tasks that require mental alertness or motor skills until response to the drug has been established

■ **Monitoring Parameters**
- Relief of symptoms, such as an improvement of masklike facial expression, muscular rigidity, shuffling gait, and resting tremors of the hands and head

■ **Geriatric side effects at a glance:**
☑ CNS ☑ Bowel Dysfunction ☑ Bladder Dysfunction ☑ Falls
Other: Dry mouth, blurred vision, somonlence, confusion, psychoses

■ **Use with caution in older patients with:** Narrow-angle glaucoma, overflow incontinence, psychosis

■ **U.S. Regulatory Considerations**
❏ FDA Black Box ☑ OBRA regulated in U.S. Long Term Care

■ **Other Uses in Geriatric Patient:** Treatment of antipsychotic-induced adverse effects

■ **Side Effects:**
Of particular importance in the geriatric patient: Anticholinergic effects

■ **Geriatric Considerations - Summary:** Benztropine and related anticholinergics present significant risk to older adults. These drugs possess potent anticholinergic effects and can cause cognitive impairment, delirium, dry mouth, blurred vision, and increased risk of falls. The use of this drug and related compounds should be limited and when used, patients should be closely monitored.

■ **References:**
1. Vangala V, Tueth M. Chronic anticholinergic toxicity: Identification and management in older patients. Geriatrics 2003;58:36-37.
2. Tune LE. Anticholinergic effects of medication in elderly patients. J Clin Psychiatry 2001;62(suppl 21):11-14.

benzylpenicilloyl polylysine

(ben'-zil-pen-i-sil' oyl pol-i-lie'-seen)

- **Brand Name(s):** Pre-Pen
  Chemical Class: Penicillin derivative

- **Clinical Pharmacology:**
  Mechanism of Action: A diagnostic agent that invokes immunoglobulin E which produces type I accelerated urticarial reactions to penicillins. **Therapeutic Effect:** A positive reaction will suggest penicillin sensitivity.
  Pharmacokinetics: Not known.

- **Available Forms:**
  - *Solution*: 0.25 ml (Pre-Pen).

- **Indications and Dosages:**
  Penicillin sensitivity: Intradermal Use a tuberculin syringe with a 26- to 30-gauge, short bevel needle. A dose of 0.01 to 0.02 ml is injected intradermally. A control of 0.9% sodium chloride should be injected about 1½ inches from the test site. Skin response usually occurs within 5-15 min. Scratch test Use a 20-gauge needle to make 3- to 5-mm nonbleeding scratch of the epidermis. Apply a small drop of solution to scratch and rub gently with applicator or toothpick. A positive reaction consists of a pale wheal surrounding the scratch site that develops within 10 min and ranges from 5-15 mm in diameter.

- **Contraindications:** Systemic or marked local reaction to its previous administration or hypersensitivity to penicillin

- **Side Effects**
  Frequent
  Skin rash
  Occasional
  Nausea

- **Serious Reactions**
  - None significant.

Special Considerations

- Does not identify those patients who react to a minor antigenic determinant (i.e., anaphylaxis); does not reliably predict the occurrence of late reactions; patients with a negative skin test may still have allergic reactions to therapeutic penicillin
- (-) Negative response: No increase in size of original bleb and/or no greater reaction than the control site
- (±) Ambiguous response: Wheal being only slightly larger than initial injection bleb, with or without accompanying erythematous flare and larger than the control site
- (+) Positive response: Itching and marked increase in size of original bleb. Wheal may exceed 20 mm in diameter and exhibit pseudopods

Patient/Family Education
- Contact the physician if pain or discomfort is severe or continues for more than 5 hr

Geriatric side effects at a glance:
☐ CNS   ☐ Bowel Dysfunction   ☐ Bladder Dysfunction   ☐ Falls

U.S. Regulatory Considerations
☐ FDA Black Box   ☐ OBRA regulated in U.S. Long Term Care

bepridil hydrochloride

(be'-pri-dil hye-droe-klor'-ide)

Brand Name(s): Vascor
Chemical Class: Diarylaminopropylamine ether

Clinical Pharmacology:
Mechanism of Action: An antihypertensive that inhibits calcium ion entry across cell membranes of cardiac and vascular smooth muscle; decreases heart rate, myocardial contractility, slows SA and AV conduction. **Therapeutic Effect:** Dilates coronary arteries, peripheral arteries/arterioles.
Pharmacokinetics: Rapidly, completely absorbed from GI tract. Undergoes first-pass metabolism in liver to active metabolite. Primarily excreted in urine. Not removed by hemodialysis. **Half-life:** less than 24 hr.

Available Forms:
- *Tablets*: 200 mg, 300 mg (Vascor).

Indications and Dosages:
Chronic stable angina: PO Initially, 200 mg/day; after 10 days, dosage may be adjusted. Maintenance: 200-400 mg/day.

Contraindications: Sick sinus syndrome/second- or third-degree AV block (except in presence of pacemaker), severe hypotension (less than 90 mm Hg, systolic), history of serious ventricular arrhythmias, uncompensated cardiac insufficiency, congenital QT interval prolongation, use with other drugs prolonging QT interval

Side Effects
Frequent
Dizziness, light-headedness, nervousness, headache, asthenia (loss of strength), hand tremor, nausea, diarrhea
Occasional
Drowsiness, insomnia, tinnitus, abdominal discomfort, palpitations, dry mouth, shortness of breath, wheezing, anorexia, constipation
Rare
Peripheral edema, anxiety, flatulence, nasal congestion, paresthesia.

133

Serious Reactions
- CHF, second- and third-degree AV block occur rarely.
- Serious arrhythmias can be induced.
- Overdosage produces nausea, drowsiness, confusion, slurred speech, profound bradycardia.

Patient/Family Education
- ECGs will be necessary during initiation of therapy and after dosage changes
- Notify provider immediately for irregular heartbeat, shortness of breath, pronounced dizziness, constipation, or hypotension
- May be taken with food or meals
- Rise slowly from lying to sitting position to avoid hypotensive effect

Monitoring Parameters
- BP, pulse, respiration, ECG intervals (PR, QRS, QT) at initiation of therapy and again after dosage increases; prolongation of QT interval by greater than 0.52 sec predisposes to proarrythmia
- Serum potassium (normalize before initiation)

Geriatric side effects at a glance:
❑ CNS   ❑ Bowel Dysfunction   ❑ Bladder Dysfunction   ❑ Falls

U.S. Regulatory Considerations
❑ FDA Black Box   ❑ OBRA regulated in U.S. Long Term Care

betamethasone

(bay-ta-meth'-a-sone)

Brand Name(s):
Abdeon, Alphatrex, Beta-Phos/AC, Betatrex, Beta-Val, Celestone, Celestone Phosphate, Celestone Soluspan, Diprolene, Luxiq, Maxivate

Combinations
Rx: with clotrimazole (Lotrisone)
Chemical Class: Glucocorticoid, synthetic

Clinical Pharmacology:
Mechanism of Action: An adrenocortical steroid that controls the rate of protein synthesis, depresses the migration of polymorphonuclear leukocytes and fibroblasts, reduces capillary permeability, and prevents or controls inflammation. *Therapeutic Effect:* Decreases tissue response to inflammatory process.
Pharmacokinetics: Rapidly and almost completely absorbed following PO administration. After topical application, limited absorption systemically. Metabolized in liver. Excreted in urine. *Half-life:* 36-54 hr.

Available Forms:
- *Tablets (Celestone)*: 0.6 mg.
- *Cream*: 0.05% (Alphatrex, Diprolene, Maxivate), 0.1% (Betatrex, Beta-Val).
- *Foam (Luxiq)*: 0.12%.
- *Gel (Diprolene)*: 0.05%.
- *Lotion*: 0.05% (Alphatrex, Diprolene, Maxivate), 0.1% (Betatrex, Beta-Val).
- *Ointment*: 0.05% (Alphatrex, Diprolene, Maxivate), 0.1% (Betatrex).
- *Syrup (Celestone)*: 0.6 mg/5 ml.
- *Injection Solution (Abdeon, Celestone Phosphate)*: 4 mg/ml.
- *Injection Suspension (Beta-Phos/AC, Celestone Soluspan)*: 3 mg acetate/3 mg betamethasone sodium phosphate.

Indications and Dosages:
Anti-inflammation, immunosuppression, corticosteroid replacement therapy: PO 0.6-7.2 mg/day. IM 0.5-9 mg/day in 2 divided doses.
Relief of inflamed and pruritic dermatoses: Topical 1-3 times a day. Foam: Apply twice a day.

Contraindications: Hypersensitivity to betamethasone, systemic fungal infections

Side Effects
Frequent
Systemic: Increased appetite, abdominal distention, nervousness, insomnia, false sense of well-being
Topical: Burning, stinging, pruritus
Occasional
Systemic: Dizziness, facial flushing, diaphoresis, decreased or blurred vision, mood swings
Topical: Allergic contact dermatitis, purpura or blood-containing blisters, thinning of skin with easy bruising, telangiectases or raised dark red spots on skin

Serious Reactions
- Prolonged use may cause HPA axis suppression.

Special Considerations
- Recommend single daily doses in AM
- Signs of adrenal insufficiency include fatigue, anorexia, nausea, vomiting, diarrhea, weight loss, weakness, dizziness, and low blood sugar; drug-induced secondary adrenocorticoid insufficiency may be minimized by gradual systemic dosage reduction; relative insufficiency may exist for up to 1 yr after discontinuation of therapy; be prepared to supplement in situations of stress
- May mask infections
- Do not give live virus vaccines to patients on prolonged therapy
- Patients on chronic steroid therapy should wear Medic Alert bracelet
- Do not use topical products on weeping, denuded, or infected areas

Patient/Family Education
- Take oral betamethasone in the morning with food or milk
- Do not abruptly discontinue drug

Monitoring Parameters
- Serum K and glucose
- Blood pressure

- Electrolytes

■ **Geriatric side effects at a glance:**
   ❑ CNS   ❑ Bowel Dysfunction   ❑ Bladder Dysfunction   ❑ Falls

■ **U.S. Regulatory Considerations**
   ❑ FDA Black Box   ❑ OBRA regulated in U.S. Long Term Care

betaxolol hydrochloride

(bay-tax'-oh-lol hye-droe-klor'-ide)

■ **Brand Name(s):** Betoptic, Betoptic S, Kerlone
   Chemical Class: β_1-Adrenergic blocker, cardioselective

■ **Clinical Pharmacology:**
   Mechanism of Action: An antihypertensive and antiglaucoma agent that blocks beta$_1$-adrenergic receptors in cardiac tissue. Reduces aqueous humor production. **Therapeutic Effect:** Slows sinus heart rate, decreases BP, and reduces intraocular pressure (IOP).
   Pharmacokinetics: Well absorbed from the GI tract. Minimal absorption after ophthalmic administration. Protein binding: 50%-60% (oral). Metabolized in liver. Primarily excreted in urine. Removed by hemodialysis. **Half-life:** 12-22 hr (half-life is increased in the elderly and patients with impaired renal function). Ophthalmic: Systemic absorption may occur.

■ **Available Forms:**
   - *Tablets (Kerlone):* 10 mg, 20 mg.
   - *Ophthalmic Solution (Betoptic):* 0.5%.
   - *Ophthalmic Suspension (Betoptic S):* 0.25%.

■ **Indications and Dosages:**
   Hypertension: PO Initially, 5 mg/day.
   Chronic open-angle glaucoma and ocular hypertension: Ophthalmic (solution) 1 drop twice a day. Ophthalmic (suspension) 1-2 drops twice a day.
   Dosage in renal impairment: For patients on dialysis, initially give 5 mg/day; increase by 5 mg/day q2wk. Maximum: 20 mg/day.

■ **Unlabeled Uses:** Treatment of angle-closure glaucoma during or after iridectomy, malignant glaucoma, secondary glaucoma; with miotics, to decrease IOP in acute and chronic angle-closure glaucoma

■ **Contraindications:** Cardiogenic shock, overt cardiac failure, second- or third-degree heart block, sinus bradycardia

■ **Side Effects**
   Betaxolol is generally well tolerated, with mild and transient side effects.

Frequent

Systemic: Hypotension manifested as dizziness, nausea, diaphoresis, headache, fatigue, constipation or diarrhea, dyspnea

Ophthalmic: Eye irritation, visual disturbances

Occasional

Systemic: Insomnia, flatulence, urinary frequency, impotence or decreased libido

Ophthalmic: Increased light sensitivity, watering of eye

Rare

Systemic: Rash, arrhythmias, arthralgia, myalgia, confusion, altered taste, increased urination

Ophthalmic: Dry eye, conjunctivitis, eye pain

■ **Serious Reactions**
- Overdose may produce profound bradycardia, hypotension, and bronchospasm.
- Abrupt withdrawal may result in diaphoresis, palpitations, headache, and tremors.
- Betaxolol administration may precipitate CHF or MI in patients with cardiac disease; thyroid storm in those with thyrotoxicosis; and peripheral ischemia in those with existing peripheral vascular disease.
- Hypoglycemia may occur in patients with previously controlled diabetes.
- Ophthalmic overdose may produce bradycardia, hypotension, bronchospasm, and acute cardiac failure.

Special Considerations
- Do not discontinue oral drug abruptly, may precipitate angina or MI
- Anaphylactic reactions may be more severe and not be as responsive to usual doses of epinephrine
- Transient stinging/discomfort is relatively common with ophthalmic preparations, notify clinician if severe
- Avoid hazardous activities if dizziness, drowsiness, light-headedness are present
- May mask the symptoms of hypoglycemia, except for sweating, in diabetic patients

■ **Monitoring Parameters**
- BP, pulse, intraocular pressure (ophth)
- Pattern of daily bowel activity and stool consistency
- Intake and output
- Weight

■ **Geriatric side effects at a glance:**
    ☑ CNS ☐ Bowel Dysfunction ☐ Bladder Dysfunction ☐ Falls
    Other: Cardiovascular and CNS effects

■ **Use with caution in older patients with:** Significant cardiovascular disease, 2nd or 3rd degree heart block, Severe sinus bradycardia, Severe respiratory disease (asthma, COPD), Diabetes, Myasthenia Gravis

■ **U.S. Regulatory Considerations**
    ☑ FDA Black Box
    In patients using <u>orally administered</u> beta-blockers, abrupt withdrawal may precipitate angina or lead to myocardial infarction or ventricular arrhythmias.
    ☐ OBRA regulated in U.S. Long Term Care

■ **Other Uses in Geriatric Patient:** None (ophthalmic)

■ **Side Effects:**
   Of particular importance in the geriatric patient: Due to systemic absorption: bradycardia, hypotension, heart failure, dizziness, fatigue, bronchospasm; due to topical
   administration: stinging, tearing, blurred vision, light sensitivity/photophobia, dryness, decreased visual acuity

■ **Geriatric Considerations - Summary:** Systemic absorption of ophthalmic drugs may
   occur and cause adverse effects in older adults. Since betaxolol is beta-selective, cardiovascular, respiratory and CNS adverse effects occur less frequently than with beta-
   nonselective topical opthalmics. These effects may still occur; therefore close monitoring for systemic side effects is warranted. Betaxolol may be less effective than the
   nonselective topical beta-blockers with an average IOP reduction of 18%-26%. Tachyphylaxis may occur after long-term therapy.

■ **References:**
   1. Marquis RE, Whitson JT. Management of glaucoma: focus on pharmacological therapy.
      Drugs & Aging 2005;22:1-22.
   2. Camras CB, Toris CB, Tamesis RR. Efficacy and adverse effects of medications used in the
      treatment of glaucoma. Drugs & Aging 1999;15:377-388.
   3. Ball S: Congestive heart failure from betaxolol (letter). Arch Ophthalmol 1987;105:320.
   4. Berry DP Jr, Van Buskirk EM, & Shields MB: Betaxolol and timolol: a comparison of efficacy
      and side effects. Arch Ophthalmol 1984; 102:42-45.

bethanechol chloride

(be-than'-e-kole klor'-ide)

■ **Brand Name(s):** Duvoid, Urecholine
   Chemical Class: Choline ester

■ **Clinical Pharmacology:**
   Mechanism of Action: A cholinergic that acts directly at cholinergic receptors in the
   smooth muscle of the urinary bladder and GI tract. Increases detrusor muscle tone.
   Therapeutic Effect: May initiate micturition and bladder emptying. Improves gastric
   and intestinal motility.
   Pharmacokinetics: Poorly absorbed following PO administration. Does not cross the
   blood-brain barrier. **Half-life:** Unknown.

■ **Available Forms:**
   • *Tablets:* 5 mg (Urecholine), 10 mg (Duvoid, Urecholine), 25 mg (Duvoid, Urecholine),
     50 mg (Duvoid, Urecholine).
   • *Subcutaneous Solution:* 5 mg/ml (Urecholine).

■ **Indications and Dosages:**
   Postoperative urine retention, atony of bladder: PO 10-50 mg 3-4 times a day. Minimum effective dose determined by giving 5-10 mg initially, then repeating same
   amount at 1-hr intervals until desired response is achieved. Subcutaneous Initially,
   2.5-5 mg. Minimum effective dose determined by giving 2.5 mg (0.5 ml), repeating
   same amount at 15- to 30-min intervals up to a maximum of 4 doses. Minimum dose
   repeated 3-4 times a day.

■ **Unlabeled Uses:** Treatment of gastroesophageal reflux, postoperative gastric atony

■ **Contraindications:** Active or latent bronchial asthma, acute inflammatory GI tract conditions, anastomosis, bladder wall instability, cardiac or coronary artery disease, epilepsy, hypertension, hyperthyroidism, hypotension, mechanical GI or urinary tract obstruction or recent GI resection, parkinsonism, peptic ulcer, pronounced bradycardia, vasomotor instability

■ **Side Effects**
Occasional
Belching, changes in vision, blurred vision, diarrhea, frequent urinary urgency
Rare
Subcutaneous: Shortness of breath, chest tightness, bronchospasm

■ **Serious Reactions**
  • Overdosage produces CNS stimulation, including insomnia, nervousness, and orthostatic hypotension, and cholinergic stimulation, such as headache, increased salivation and diaphoresis, nausea, vomiting, flushed skin, abdominal pain, and seizures.

Special Considerations
  • Recommend taking on an empty stomach to avoid nausea and vomiting

■ **Patient/Family Education**
  • Notify the physician if he or she experiences diarrhea, difficulty breathing, increased salivary secretions, irregular heartbeat, muscle weakness, nausea, severe abdominal pain, sweating, and vomiting

■ **Monitoring Parameters**
  • Fluid intake and output

■ **Geriatric side effects at a glance:**
  ❑ CNS ❑ Bowel Dysfunction ☑ Bladder Dysfunction ❑ Falls

■ **U.S. Regulatory Considerations**
  ❑ FDA Black Box ☑ OBRA regulated in U.S. Long Term Care

bimatoprost

(bi-ma'-toe-prost)

■ **Brand Name(s):** Lumigan
  Chemical Class: Prostamide analog

■ **Clinical Pharmacology:**
  Mechanism of Action: A synthetic analog of prostaglandin with ocular hypotensive activity. **Therapeutic Effect:** Reduces intraocular pressure (IOP) by increasing the outflow of aqueous humor.

Pharmacokinetics: Absorbed through the cornea and hydrolyzed to the active free acid form. Protein binding: 88%. Moderately distributed into body tissues. Metabolized in liver. Primarily excreted in urine; some elimination in feces. **Half-life:** 45 min.

- **Available Forms:**
  - *Ophthalmic Solution:* 0.03% (Lumigan).

- **Indications and Dosages:**
  Glaucoma, ocular hypertension: Ophthalmic 1 drop in affected eye(s) once daily, in the evening.

- **Contraindications:** Hypersensitivity to bimatoprost or any other component of the formulation

- **Side Effects**
  Frequent
  Conjunctival hyperemia, growth of eyelashes, and ocular pruritus
  Occasional
  Ocular dryness, visual disturbance, ocular burning, foreign body sensation, eye pain, pigmentation of the periocular skin, blepharitis, cataract, superficial punctate keratitis, eyelid erythema, ocular irritation, and eyelash darkening
  Rare
  Intraocular inflammation (iritis)

- **Serious Reactions**
  - Systemic adverse events, including infections (colds and upper respiratory tract infections), headaches, asthenia, and hirsutism, have been reported

- **Geriatric side effects at a glance:**
  ❑ CNS   ❑ Bowel Dysfunction   ❑ Bladder Dysfunction   ❑ Falls

- **U.S. Regulatory Considerations**
  ❑ FDA Black Box   ❑ OBRA regulated in U.S. Long Term Care

biperiden hydrochloride

(bye-per'-i-den hye-droe-klor'-ide)

- **Brand Name(s):** Akineton
  Chemical Class: Tertiary amine

- **Clinical Pharmacology:**
  Mechanism of Action: A weak anticholinergic that exhibits competitive antagonism of acetylcholine at cholinergic receptors in the corpus striatum, which restores balance.
  Therapeutic Effect: Antiparkinson activity.
  Pharmacokinetics: Well absorbed from GI tract. Protein binding: 23% -33%. Widely distributed. **Half-life:** 18-24 hr.

Available Forms:
- *Tablets*: 2 mg (Akineton HCl).

Indications and Dosages:
Extrapyramidal symptoms: PO 2 mg 3-4 times/day. Dosage in renal impairment.
Parkinsonism: PO 2 mg 1-3 times/day.

Unlabeled Uses: Adjunct to methadone maintenance

Contraindications: None known.

Side Effects
Frequent
Orthostatic hypotension, anorexia, headache, blurred vision, urinary retention, dry mouth or nose
Occasional
Insomnia, agitation, euphoria
Rare
Vomiting, depression, irritation or swelling of eyes, rash

Serious Reactions
- Overdosage may vary from severe anticholinergic effects, such as unsteadiness, severe drowsiness, dryness of mouth, nose, or throat, tachycardia, shortness of breath, and skin flushing.
- Also produces severe paradoxical reaction, marked by hallucinations, tremor, seizures, and toxic psychosis.

Special Considerations
- Give parenteral dose with patient recumbent to prevent postural hypotension

Patient/Family Education
- May increase susceptibility to heatstroke
- Do not discontinue drug abruptly; taper off over 1 wk
- Avoid tasks that require mental alertness or motor skills until response to the drug is established
- Dizziness, drowsiness and dry mouth are expected responses to the drug

Monitoring Parameters
- Relief of symptoms such as an improvement of masklike facial expression, muscular rigidity, shuffling gait, and resting tremors of hands and head

Geriatric side effects at a glance:
☑ CNS ☑ Bowel Dysfunction ☑ Bladder Dysfunction ☑ Falls
Other: Dry mouth, blurred vision, somonlence, confusion, psychoses

Use with caution in older patients with: Narrow-angle glaucoma, overflow incontinence, psychosis

U.S. Regulatory Considerations
❏ FDA Black Box ☑ OBRA regulated in U.S. Long Term Care

Other Uses in Geriatric Patient: Treatment of antipsychotic-induced adverse effects

■ **Side Effects:**
Of particular importance in the geriatric patient: Anticholinergic effects

■ **Geriatric Considerations - Summary:** Biperiden is a weak anticholinergic agent which still may present a risk to older adults and can cause cognitive impairment, delirium, dry mouth, blurred vision, and increased risk of falls. The use of this drug and related compounds should be limited and when used, patients should be closely monitored.

■ **References:**
1. Vangala V, Tueth M. Chronic anticholinergic toxicity: identification and management in older patients. Geriatrics 2003;58:36-37.
2. Tune LE. Anticholinergic effects of medication in elderly patients. J Clin Psychiatry 2001;62(suppl 21):11-14.
3. Fleischhacker WW, Barnas C, Gunther V, et al: Mood-altering effects of biperiden in healthy volunteers. J Affect Disord 1987; 12:153-157.

bisacodyl

(bis-a-koe'-dill)

■ **Brand Name(s):**
OTC: Alophen, Dulcolax, Fleet, Gentlax, Modane, Veracolate
Chemical Class: Diphenylmethane derivative

■ **Clinical Pharmacology:**
Mechanism of Action: A GI stimulant that has a direct effect on colonic smooth musculature by stimulating the intramural nerve plexus. *Therapeutic Effect:* Promotes fluid and ion accumulation in the colon, increasing peristalsis and producing a laxative effect.
Pharmacokinetics:

Route	Onset	Peak	Duration
PO	6-12 hr	N/A	N/A
Rectal	15-60 min	N/A	N/A

Minimal absorption following oral and rectal administration. Absorbed drug is excreted in urine; remainder is eliminated in feces.

■ **Available Forms:**
• *Tablets (Enteric-Coated [Dulcolax, Fleet]):* 5 mg.
• *Rectal Enema (Fleet):* 10 mg/1.25 oz.
• *Suppositories (Dulcolax, Fleet):* 10 mg.

■ **Indications and Dosages:**
Treatment of constipation: PO Initially, 5 mg/day. Rectal, enema One 1.25-oz bottle in a single daily dose. Rectal, suppository 5-10 mg/day.

■ **Contraindications:** Abdominal pain, appendicitis, intestinal obstruction, nausea, undiagnosed rectal bleeding, vomiting

■ **Side Effects**
Frequent
Some degree of abdominal discomfort, nausea, mild cramps, faintness

Occasional

Rectal administration: burning of rectal mucosa, mild proctitis

■ **Serious Reactions**
- Long-term use may result in laxative dependence, chronic constipation, and loss of normal bowel function.
- Prolonged use or overdose may result in electrolyte or metabolic disturbances (such as hypokalemia, hypocalcemia, and metabolic acidosis or alkalosis), as well as persistent diarrhea, vomiting, muscle weakness, malabsorption, and weight loss.

■ **Patient/Family Education**
- Do not take within 1 hr of antacids or milk
- Increasing fluid intake, exercising, and eating a high-fiber diet will promote defecation
- Notify the physician if unrelieved constipation, dizziness, muscle cramps or pain, rectal bleeding, or weakness occurs

■ **Monitoring Parameters**
- Fluid intake
- Pattern of daily bowel activity
- Electrolytes

■ **Geriatric side effects at a glance:**
❏ CNS ☑ Bowel Dysfunction ❏ Bladder Dysfunction ❏ Falls

■ **U.S. Regulatory Considerations**
❏ FDA Black Box ❏ OBRA regulated in U.S. Long Term Care

bismuth subsalicylate

(bis'-muth sub-sal-ih'-sah-late)

■ **Brand Name(s):**

OTC: Colo-Fresh, Devrom, Kaopectate, Pepto-Bismol, Pink Bismuth

Combinations
Rx: with metronidazole, tetracycline (Helidac)
Chemical Class: Salicylate derivative

■ **Clinical Pharmacology:**

Mechanism of Action: An antinauseant and antiulcer agent that absorbs water and toxins in the large intestine and forms a protective coating in the intestinal mucosa. Also possesses antisecretory and antimicrobial effects. **Therapeutic Effect:** Prevents diarrhea. Helps treat *Helicobacter pylori*–associated peptic ulcer disease.

Pharmacokinetics: Rapidly and completely absorbed following PO administration. Protein binding: greater than 90%. Primarily excreted in feces. **Terminal Half-life:** 21-72 days.

■ **Available Forms:**
  • *Caplets (Devrom)*: 200 mg.
  • *Liquid (Kaopectate, Pepto-Bismol)*: 262 mg/15 ml, 525 mg/15 ml.
  • *Tablets (Colo-Fresh)*: 324 mg.
  • *Tablets (Chewable)*: 200 mg (Devrom), 262 mg (Pepto-Bismol).

■ **Indications and Dosages:**
  Diarrhea, gastric distress: PO 2 tablets (30 ml) q30-60min. Maximum: 8 doses in 24 hr.
  H. pylori–associated duodenal ulcer, gastritis: PO 525 mg 4 times a day, with 500 mg amoxicillin and 500 mg metronidazole, 3 times a day after meals, for 7-14 days.

■ **Unlabeled Uses:** Prevention of traveler's diarrhea

■ **Contraindications:** Bleeding ulcers, gout, hemophilia, hemorrhagic states, renal impairment

■ **Side Effects**
  Frequent
  Grayish black stools
  Rare
  Constipation

■ **Serious Reactions**
  • Debilitated patients may develop impaction.

■ **Patient/Family Education**
  • Chew or dissolve in mouth; do not swallow whole
  • Shake suspension before using
  • Stop use if symptoms do not improve within 2 days or become worse, or if diarrhea is accompanied by high fever or severe abdominal pain
  • Avoid bismuth if taking aspirin or other salicylates because of the increased risk of toxicity
  • Stool may appear black or gray

■ **Monitoring Parameters**
  • Bowel sounds and daily bowel activity

■ **Geriatric side effects at a glance:**
  ❏ CNS ☑ Bowel Dysfunction ❏ Bladder Dysfunction ❏ Falls

■ **U.S. Regulatory Considerations**
  ❏ FDA Black Box ❏ OBRA regulated in U.S. Long Term Care

bisoprolol fumarate

(bis-oh'-proe-lol fyoo'-muh-rate)

■ **Brand Name(s):** Zebeta

    Combinations
    Rx: with hydrochlorothiazide (Ziac)
    Chemical Class: β_1-adrenergic blocker, cardioselective

■ **Clinical Pharmacology:**
    Mechanism of Action: An antihypertensive that blocks beta$_1$-adrenergic receptors in cardiac tissue. **Therapeutic Effect:** Slows sinus heart rate and decreases BP.
    Pharmacokinetics: Well absorbed from the GI tract. Protein binding: 26%-33%. Metabolized in the liver. Primarily excreted in urine. Not removed by hemodialysis. **Half-life:** 9-12 hr (increased in impaired renal function).

■ **Available Forms:**
    • *Tablets*: 5 mg, 10 mg.

■ **Indications and Dosages:**
    Hypertension: PO Initially, 2.5 mg/day. May increase by 2.5-5 mg/day. Maximum: 20 mg/day.
    Dosage in hepatic impairment: For patients with cirrhosis or hepatitis whose creatinine clearance is less than 40 ml/min, initially give 2.5 mg.

■ **Unlabeled Uses:** Angina pectoris, premature ventricular contractions, supraventricular arrhythmias

■ **Contraindications:** Cardiogenic shock, marked sinus bradycardia, overt cardiac failure, second- or third-degree heart block

■ **Side Effects**
    Frequent
    Hypotension manifested as dizziness, nausea, diaphoresis, headache, cold extremities, fatigue, constipation or diarrhea
    Occasional
    Insomnia, flatulence, urinary frequency, impotence or decreased libido
    Rare
    Rash, arthralgia, myalgia, confusion, altered taste

■ **Serious Reactions**
    • Overdose may produce profound bradycardia and hypotension.
    • Abrupt withdrawal may result in diaphoresis, palpitations, headache, and tremulousness.
    • Bisoprolol administration may precipitate CHF and MI in patients with heart disease, thyroid storm in those with thyrotoxicosis, and peripheral ischemia in those with existing peripheral vascular disease.
    • Hypoglycemia may occur in patients with previously controlled diabetes.
    • Thrombocytopenia, including unusual bruising and bleeding, occurs rarely.

- Property of competitive cardioselectivity yields less bronchospastic adverse effects

■ **Patient/Family Education**
- Do not abruptly discontinue bisoprolol; compliance with the therapy regimen is essential to control hypertension
- If dizziness occurs, sit or lie down immediately
- Avoid tasks that require mental alertness or motor skills until response to the drug has been established
- Do not use nasal decongestants and OTC cold preparations, especially those containing stimulants, without physician approval
- Limit alcohol and salt intake

■ **Monitoring Parameters**
- Heart rate, blood pressure
- Pattern of daily bowel activity and stool consistency
- Assess for peripheral edema

■ **Geriatric side effects at a glance:**
❑ CNS ❑ Bowel Dysfunction ❑ Bladder Dysfunction ❑ Falls

■ **U.S. Regulatory Considerations**
☑ FDA Black Box
In patients using orally administered beta-blockers, abrupt withdrawal may precipitate angina or lead to myocardial infarction or ventricular arrhythmias.
❑ OBRA regulated in U.S. Long Term Care

bitolterol mesylate

(bye-tole'-ter-ol mes'-sil-ate)

■ **Brand Name(s):** Tornalate
Chemical Class: Sympathomimetic amine; β_2-adrenergic agonist

■ **Clinical Pharmacology:**
Mechanism of Action: An antiadrenergic, sympatholytic agent that stimulates beta$_2$-adrenergic receptors in lungs. **Therapeutic Effect:** Relaxes bronchial smooth muscle, relieves bronchospasm, reduces airway resistance.
Pharmacokinetics: Onset of action is rapid with duration of 4-8 hr. Rapidly absorbed following aerosol administration. Primarily distributed to lungs. Metabolized in liver. Excreted in urine and feces. **Half-life:** 3 hr.

■ **Available Forms:**
- *Aerosol for Oral Inhalation:* 0.8% (Tornalate).
- *Solution for Oral Inhalation:* 0.2% (Tornalate).

- **Indications and Dosages:**
  Bronchospasm: Inhalation Use 2 inhalations, separated by 1- to 3-min interval. A third inhalation may be required.
  Prevention of bronchospasm: Inhalation Use 2 inhalations q8h. Do not exceed 3 inhalations q6h, or 2 inhalations q4h.

- **Unlabeled Uses:** Chronic obstructive pulmonary disease

- **Contraindications:** History of hypersensitivity to sympathomimetics, bitolterol, or any of its components.

- **Side Effects**
  Frequent
  Tremor
  Occasional
  Cough, dry or irritated mouth/throat, headache, nausea, vomiting
  Rare
  Dizziness, vertigo, palpitations, insomnia

- **Serious Reactions**
  - Although tolerance to the bronchodilating effect has not been observed, prolonged or too frequent use may lead to tolerance.
  - Severe paradoxical bronchoconstriction may occur with excessive use.

Special Considerations
  - No real clinical advantage over less expensive agents (e.g., albuterol, metaproterenol)

- **Patient/Family Education**
  - Wash inhaler in warm water and dry qd
  - If previously effective dosage regimen fails to provide usual relief, seek medical advice immediately
  - Rinse mouth with water immediately after inhalation to prevent mouth/throat dryness
  - May cause nervousness, restlessness, and insomnia; if these effects persist, notify the physician

- **Monitoring Parameters**
  - Rate, depth, rhythm, type of respiration, and quality and rate of pulse

- **Geriatric side effects at a glance:**
  ☑ CNS ☐ Bowel Dysfunction ☐ Bladder Dysfunction ☐ Falls

- **U.S. Regulatory Considerations**
  ☐ FDA Black Box ☑ OBRA regulated in U.S. Long Term Care

bivalirudin

(bye-va-leer'-u-din)

■ **Brand Name(s):** Angiomax
  Chemical Class: Hirudin derivative; thrombin inhibitor

■ **Clinical Pharmacology:**
  Mechanism of Action: An anticoagulant that specifically and reversibly inhibits thrombin by binding to its receptor sites. **Therapeutic Effect:** Decreases acute ischemic complications in patients with unstable angina pectoris.
  Pharmacokinetics:

Route	Onset	Peak	Duration
IV	Immediate	N/A	1 hr

  Primarily eliminated by kidneys. Twenty-five percent removed by hemodialysis. **Half-life:** 25 min (increased in moderate to severe renal impairment).

■ **Available Forms:**
  • Injection, Powder for Reconstitution: 250 mg.

■ **Indications and Dosages:**
  Anticoagulant in patients with unstable angina who are undergoing percutaneous transluminal coronary angioplasty (PTCA) in conjunction with aspirin: IV 0.75 mg/kg as IV bolus followed by IV infusion at rate of 1.75 mg/kg/hr for duration of procedure. After initial 4-hr infusion is completed, may give additional IV infusion at rate of 0.2 mg/kg/hr for 20 hr or less, if necessary.
  Dosage in renal impairment:

GFR	Dosage Reduced by
30-59 ml/min	20%
10-29 ml/min	60%
Dialysis	90%

■ **Contraindications:** Active major bleeding

■ **Side Effects**
  Frequent (42%)
  Back pain
  Occasional (15%-12%)
  Nausea, headache, hypotension, generalized pain
  Rare (8%-4%)
  Injection site pain, insomnia, hypertension, anxiety, vomiting, pelvic or abdominal pain, bradycardia, nervousness, dyspepsia, fever, urine retention

■ **Serious Reactions**
  • A hemorrhagic event occurs rarely and is characterized by a fall in BP or Hct.

Special Considerations
  • Safety and effectiveness have not been established in patients with unstable angina who are not undergoing PTCA or in patients with other acute coronary syndromes

- In comparative studies of PTCA in unstable angina, incidence of major bleeding lower than heparin (4% vs 9%)
- Safety and efficacy with platelet inhibitors other than aspirin (e.g., glycoprotein IIb/IIIa inhibitors) not established

■ **Patient/Family Education**
- Report blood in urine or stool
- Report discomfort or pain, especially chest pain, after treatment
- Remain on bed rest and keep the leg used during PTCA immobile, as ordered

■ **Monitoring Parameters**
- In clinical trials, the dose of bivalirudin was not titrated according to the activated clotting time (ACT)
- aPTT, Hct, BUN and serum creatinine levels, and stool or urine cultures for occult blood
- Blood pressure, pulse rate
- Assess urine for hematuria

■ **Geriatric side effects at a glance:**
❑ CNS   ❑ Bowel Dysfunction   ❑ Bladder Dysfunction   ❑ Falls

■ **U.S. Regulatory Considerations**
❑ FDA Black Box   ❑ OBRA regulated in U.S. Long Term Care

bosentan

(boe-sen'-tan)

■ **Brand Name(s):** Tracleer
  Chemical Class: Pyrimidine derivative

■ **Clinical Pharmacology:**
  Mechanism of Action: An antihypertensive that blocks endothelin-1, the neurohormone that constricts pulmonary arteries. **Therapeutic Effect:** Improves exercise ability and slows clinical worsening of pulmonary arterial hypertension (PAH).
  Pharmacokinetics: Highly bound to plasma proteins, mainly albumin. Metabolized in the liver. Eliminated by biliary excretion. **Half-life:** Approximately 5 hr.

■ **Available Forms:**
- *Tablets:* 62.5 mg, 125 mg.

■ **Indications and Dosages:**
  PAH in those with World Health Organization Class III or IV symptoms: PO 62.5 mg twice a day for 4 wk; then increase to maintenance dosage of 125 mg twice a day. When discontinuing, reduce dosage to 62.5 mg twice a day for 3-7 days to avoid clinical deterioration.
  Dosage based on transaminase elevations: Any elevation accompanied by symptoms of liver injury or serum bilirubin 2 or more times upper limit of normal, stop treatment.

AST/ALT greater than 3 or less than 6 times upper limit of normal, reduce dose or interrupt treatment. AST/ALT greater than 5 or less than 9 times upper limit of normal, stop treatment. AST/ALT greater than 8 times upper limit of normal, stop treatment.

■ **Unlabeled Uses:** CHF, pulmonary hypertension secondary to scleroderma

■ **Contraindications:** Administration with cyclosporine or glyburide

■ **Side Effects**
Occasional
Headache, nasopharyngitis, flushing
Rare
Dyspepsia (heartburn, epigastric distress), fatigue, pruritus, hypotension

■ **Serious Reactions**
• Abnormal hepatic function, lower extremity edema, and palpitations occur rarely.

Special Considerations
• Because of potential liver injury and in an effort to decrease the risk of fetal exposure, the drug may only be prescribed through the TRACLEER Access Program by calling 1-866-228-3546

■ **Monitoring Parameters**
• Hemoglobin levels at 1 and 3 mo
• Clinical symptoms of hepatic injury, including abdominal pain, fatigue, jaundice, nausea, and vomiting

■ **Geriatric side effects at a glance:**
❑ CNS   ❑ Bowel Dysfunction   ❑ Bladder Dysfunction   ❑ Falls

■ **U.S. Regulatory Considerations**
❑ FDA Black Box   ❑ OBRA regulated in U.S. Long Term Care

bretylium tosylate

(bre-til'-ee-um)

■ **Brand Name(s):** Bretylium Tosylate-Dextrose
Chemical Class: Bromobenzyl quaternary ammonium compound

■ **Clinical Pharmacology:**
Mechanism of Action: An antiarrhythmic that directly affects myocardial cell membranes. **Therapeutic Effect:** Contributes to suppression of ventricular tachycardia. **Pharmacokinetics:** Absorption is not expected to be present in peripheral blood at recommended doses. Protein binding: 1%-6%. Not metabolized. Excreted unchanged in urine. Removed by hemodialysis. **Half-life:** 6-13.5 hr.

- **Available Forms:**
  - *Injection*: 50 mg/ml (Bretylium Tosylate-Dextrose).
  - *Premix Solutions*: 500 mg/250 ml, 1000 mg/250 ml (Bretylium Tosylate-Dextrose).

- **Indications and Dosages:**

  Ventricular arrhythmias, immediate, life-threatening: IV 5 mg/kg undiluted by rapid IV injection. May increase to 10 mg/kg, repeat as needed. Maintenance: 5-10 mg/kg diluted over 8 min or longer, q6h or IV infusion at 1-2 mg/min.

  Ventricular arrhythmias, other: IM 5-10 mg/kg undiluted, may repeat at 1- to 2-hr intervals. Maintenance: 5-10 mg/kg q6-8h IV 5-10 mg/kg diluted over 8 min or longer, may repeat at 1- to 2-hr intervals. Maintenance: 5-10 mg/kg q6h or IV infusion at 1-2 mg/min.

- **Unlabeled Uses:** Treatment of cervical dystonia in patients who have developed resistance to botulinum toxin type A.

- **Contraindications:** Hypersensitivity to bretylium or any component of the formulation

- **Side Effects**

  Frequent

  Transitory hypertension followed by postural and supine hypotension in 50% of patients observed as dizziness, light-headedness, faintness, vertigo

  Occasional

  Diarrhea, loose stools, nausea, vomiting

  Rare

  Angina, bradycardia

- **Serious Reactions**
  - Respiratory depression from possible neuromuscular blockade.

- **Patient/Family Education**
  - Rise slowly from lying to sitting position and permit legs to dangle from bed for at least 5 min before standing within one hour after dose administration

- **Monitoring Parameters**
  - ECG, electrolytes, BP

- **Geriatric side effects at a glance:**
  - ❑ CNS   ❑ Bowel Dysfunction   ❑ Bladder Dysfunction   ❑ Falls

- **U.S. Regulatory Considerations**
  - ❑ FDA Black Box   ❑ OBRA regulated in U.S. Long Term Care

brimonidine tartrate

(bri-moe'-ni-deen tar'-trate)

- **Brand Name(s):** Alphagan P
  Chemical Class: α_2-Adrenergic agonist

- **Clinical Pharmacology:**
  Mechanism of Action: An ophthalmic agent that is a selective alpha$_2$-adrenergic agonist. **Therapeutic Effect:** Reduces intraocular pressure (IOP).
  Pharmacokinetics: Plasma concentrations peak within 0.5 to 2.5 hr after ocular administration. Distributed into aqueous humor. Metabolized in liver. Primarily excreted in urine. **Half-life:** 3 hr.

- **Available Forms:**
  - *Ophthalmic Solution*: 0.15% (Alphagan P) |contains Purite 0.005% as preservative|.

- **Indications and Dosages:**
  Glaucoma, ocular hypertension: Ophthalmic 1 drop in affected eye(s) 3 times/day.

- **Contraindications:** Concurrent use of monoamine oxidase (MAO) inhibitor therapy, hypersensitivity to brimonidine or any other component of the formulation

- **Side Effects**
  Occasional
  Allergic conjunctivitis, conjunctival hyperemia, eye pruritus, burning sensation, conjunctival folliculosis, oral dryness, visual disturbances

- **Serious Reactions**
  - Bradycardia, hypotension, iritis, miosis, skin reactions, including erythema, eyelid, pruritus, rash, and vasodilation, and tachycardia have been reported.

- **Geriatric side effects at a glance:**
  ❑ CNS ❑ Bowel Dysfunction ❑ Bladder Dysfunction ❑ Falls

- **U.S. Regulatory Considerations**
  ❑ FDA Black Box ❑ OBRA regulated in U.S. Long Term Care

brinzolamide

(brin-zol'-a-mide)

■ **Brand Name(s):** Azopt
   Chemical Class: Carbonic anhydrase inhibitor; sulfonamide derivative

■ **Clinical Pharmacology:**
   Mechanism of Action: An ophthalmic agent that inhibits carbonic anhydrase. Decreases aqueous humor secretion. **Therapeutic Effect:** Reduces intraocular pressure (IOP).
   Pharmacokinetics: Systemically absorbed to some degree. Protein binding: 60%. Distributed extensively in red blood cells. Sites of metabolism have not been established. Metabolized to active and inactive metabolites. Primarily excreted unchanged in urine.

■ **Available Forms:**
   • *Ophthalmic Suspension*: 1% (Azopt).

■ **Indications and Dosages:**
   Glaucoma, ocular hypertension: Ophthalmic Instill 1 drop in affected eye(s) 3 times/day.

■ **Contraindications:** Hypersensitivity to brinzolamide or any other component of the formulation

■ **Side Effects**
   Occasional
   Blurred vision, bitter taste, dry eye, ocular discharge, ocular discomfort and pain, ocular pruritus, headache, rhinitis
   Rare
   Allergic reactions, alopecia, chest pain, conjunctivitis, diarrhea, diplopia, dizziness, dry mouth, dyspnea, dyspepsia, eye fatigue, hypertonia, keratoconjunctivitis, keratopathy, kidney pain, lid margin crusting or sticky sensation, nausea, pharyngitis, tearing, urticaria

■ **Serious Reactions**
   • Electrolyte imbalance, development of an acidotic state, and possible CNS effects may occur.
   • Use with caution in patients with a history of sulfa allergy.

■ **Geriatric side effects at a glance:**
   ❏ CNS ❏ Bowel Dysfunction ❏ Bladder Dysfunction ❏ Falls

■ **U.S. Regulatory Considerations**
   ❏ FDA Black Box ❏ OBRA regulated in U.S. Long Term Care

bromfenac

(brom'-feh-nak)

- **Brand Name(s):** Xibrom

- **Clinical Pharmacology:**
  Mechanism of Action: A nonsteroidal anti-inflammatory drug (NSAID) that inhibits prostaglandin synthesis by inhibiting cyclooxygenase 1 and cyclooxygenase 2. **Therapeutic Effect:** Produces anti-inflammatory effect.
  Pharmacokinetics: The plasma concentration of bromfenac following ocular administration is unknown.

- **Available Forms:**
  - *Ophthalmic Solution*: 0.09% (Xibrom).

- **Indications and Dosages:**
  Ocular inflammation after cataract extraction: Ophthalmic Instill 1 drop into the affected eye twice daily, beginning 24 hr after surgery and continuing for 2 wk.

- **Contraindications:** Hypersensitivity to bromfenac or any component of the formulation

- **Side Effects**
  Occasional
  Abnormal sensation in eye, eye irritation, eye pain, eye pruritus, redness, headache
  Rare
  Ocular bleeding, iritis

- **Serious Reactions**
  - Keratitis occurs rarely.

- **Geriatric side effects at a glance:**
  ❏ CNS ❏ Bowel Dysfunction ❏ Bladder Dysfunction ❏ Falls

- **U.S. Regulatory Considerations**
  ❏ FDA Black Box ❏ OBRA regulated in U.S. Long Term Care

bromocriptine mesylate

(broe-moe-krip'-teen mes'-sil-ate)

■ **Brand Name(s):** Parlodel
   Chemical Class: Ergot alkaloid derivative

■ **Clinical Pharmacology:**
   Mechanism of Action: A dopamine agonist that directly stimulates dopamine receptors in the corpus striatum and inhibits prolactin secretion. Also suppresses secretion of growth hormone. **Therapeutic Effect:** Improves symptoms of parkinsonism, suppresses galactorrhea, and reduces serum growth hormone concentrations in acromegaly.
   Pharmacokinetics:

Indication	Onset	Peak	Duration
Prolactin lowering	2 hr	8 hr	24 hr
Antiparkinson	0.5-1.5 hr	2 hr	N/A
Growth hormone suppressant	1-2 hr	4-8 wk	4-8 hr

   Minimally absorbed from the GI tract. Protein binding: 90%–96%. Metabolized in the liver. Excreted in feces by biliary secretion. **Half-life:** 15 hr.

■ **Available Forms:**
   • *Capsules:* 5 mg.
   • *Tablets:* 2.5 mg.

■ **Indications and Dosages:**
   Hyperprolactinemia: PO Initially, 1.25-2.5 mg at bedtime. May increase by 2.5 mg q3-7days up to 5-7.5 mg/day in divided doses. Maintenance: 2.5 mg 2-3 times a day.
   Pituitary prolactinomas: PO Initially, 1.25 mg 2-3 times a day. May gradually increase over several weeks to 10-20 mg/day in divided doses. Maintenance: 2.5-20 mg/day in divided doses.
   Parkinsonism: PO Initially, 1.25 mg 1-2 times a day. May take single doses at bedtime. May increase by 2.5 mg/day at 14- to 28-day intervals. Maintenance: 2.5-40 mg/day in divided doses. Maximum: 100 mg/day.
   Acromegaly: PO Initially, 1.25-2.5 mg at bedtime. May increase by 1.25-2.5 mg q3-7days up to 30 mg/day in divided doses. Maintenance: 10-30 mg/day in divided doses. Maximum: 100 mg/day.

■ **Unlabeled Uses:** Treatment of cocaine addiction, hyperprolactinemia associated with pituitary adenomas, neuroleptic malignant syndrome

■ **Contraindications:** Hypersensitivity to ergot alkaloids, peripheral vascular disease, severe ischemic heart disease, uncontrolled hypertension

■ **Side Effects**
   Frequent
   Nausea (49%), headache (19%), dizziness (17%)
   Occasional (7%–3%)
   Fatigue, light-headedness, vomiting, abdominal cramps, diarrhea, constipation, nasal congestion, somnolence, dry mouth

Rare
Muscle cramps, urinary hesitancy

■ **Serious Reactions**
- Visual or auditory hallucinations have been noted in patients with Parkinson's disease.
- Long-term, high-dose therapy may produce continuing rhinorrhea, syncope, GI hemorrhage, peptic ulcer, and severe abdominal pain.

Special Considerations
- Use measures to prevent orthostatic hypotension

■ **Patient/Family Education**
- Change positions slowly and dangle the legs momentarily before standing to avoid light-headedness
- Avoid tasks that require mental alertness or motor skills until response to the drug has been established

■ **Monitoring Parameters**
- Therapeutic response

■ **Geriatric side effects at a glance:**
☑ CNS   ❑ Bowel Dysfunction   ❑ Bladder Dysfunction   ❑ Falls

■ **U.S. Regulatory Considerations**
❑ FDA Black Box   ❑ OBRA regulated in U.S. Long Term Care

brompheniramine maleate

(brome-fen-ir'-a-meen mal'-ee-ate)

■ **Brand Name(s):** BrōveX, BrōveX CT, Codimal A, Colhist, Dimetane, Dimetane Extentabs, Dimetapp, Lodrane 12 Hour, Nasahist B, ND Stat

Combinations
Rx: with pseudoephedrine, dextromethorphan (Bromadine-DM, Bromarest DX, Bromatane DX, Bromfed DM, Bromphen DX, Dimetane DX, Myphetane DX)
OTC: with pseudoephedrine (Bromfed, Drixoral)
Chemical Class: Alkylamine derivative

■ **Clinical Pharmacology:**
Mechanism of Action: An alkylamine that competes with histamine at histaminic receptor sites. Inhibits central acetylcholine. **Therapeutic Effect:** Results in anticholinergic, antipruritic, antitussive, antiemetic effects. Produces antidyskinetic, sedative effect.

Pharmacokinetics: Rapidly absorbed after PO administration. Widely distributed. Metabolized in liver. Primarily excreted in urine. **Half-life:** 25 hr.

Available Forms:
- *Tablets:* 4 mg (Dimetane).
- *Tablets, chewable (extended-release):* 12 mg (BröveX CT).
- *Tablets (extended-release):* 6 mg (Lodrane 12 Hour).
- *Tablets (timed-release):* 8 mg, 12 mg (Dimetane Extentabs).
- *Elixir:* 2 mg/5 ml (Dimetapp). Oral Suspension: 12 mg/5 ml (BröveX).

Indications and Dosages:
Allergic rhinitis, anaphylaxis, urticarial transfusion reactions, urticaria: PO 4 mg q4-6h or 8-12 mg extended/timed-release q12h.
Amelioration of allergic reactions to blood or plasma, anaphylaxis as an adjunct to epinephrine and other standard measures after the acute symptoms have been controlled, other uncomplicated allergic conditions of the immediate type when oral therapy is impossible or contraindicated: IM, IV, SC 5-20 mg/day in 2 divided doses. Maximum: 40 mg/day.

Contraindications:
Concurrent MAOI therapy, focal CNS lesions, hypersensitivity to brompheniramine or related drugs

Side Effects
Frequent
Drowsiness, dizziness, hypotension, dry mouth, nose, or throat, urinary retention, thickening of bronchial secretions
Occasional
Epigastric distress, flushing, blurred vision, tinnitus, paresthesia, sweating, chills

Serious Reactions
- Hypersensitivity reaction, such as eczema, pruritus, rash, cardiac disturbances, and photosensitivity, may occur.

Patient/Family Education
- Do not crush or chew sustained-release forms
- Use hard candy, gum, frequent rinsing of mouth for dryness
- Avoid consuming alcohol during brompheniramine therapy
- Dizziness, drowsiness, and dry mouth are expected responses to the drug
- Avoid performing tasks that require mental alertness or motor skills until response to the drug is established

Monitoring Parameters
- Blood pressure

Geriatric side effects at a glance:
☑ CNS ☑ Bowel Dysfunction ☑ Bladder Dysfunction ☐ Falls
Other: Dry mouth, blurred vision, confusion, psychoses

Use with caution in older patients with:
Narrow-angle glaucoma, overflow incontinence, psychosis.

- **U.S. Regulatory Considerations**
  - ☐ FDA Black Box ☑ OBRA regulated in U.S. Long Term Care

- **Other Uses in Geriatric Patient:** None

- **Side Effects:**
  Of particular importance in the geriatric patient: Anticholinergic effects

- **Geriatric Considerations - Summary:** Brompheniramine is a first-generation alkylamine antihistamine with potent H_1 receptor antagonism. It has anticholinergic activity and can cause somnolence. Older adults taking this drug are at risk of dizziness and hypotension.

- **References:**
  1. Klein GL, Littlejohn T, Lockhart EA, et al: Brompheniramine, terfenadine, and placebo in allergic rhinitis. Ann Allergy Asthma Immunol 1996; 77:365-370.
  2. Tune LE. Anticholinergic effects of medication in elderly patients. J Clin Psychiatry 2001;62(suppl 21):11-14.

budesonide

(byoo-des'-oh-nide)

- **Brand Name(s):** Entocort EC, Pulmicort Respules, Pulmicort Turbuhaler, Rhinocort, Rhinocort Aqua
  Chemical Class: Glucocorticoid, synthetic

- **Clinical Pharmacology:**
  Mechanism of Action: A glucocorticoid that inhibits the accumulation of inflammatory cells and decreases and prevents tissues from responding to the inflammatory process. **Therapeutic Effect:** Relieves symptoms of allergic rhinitis (inhaled) or Crohn's disease (oral).
  Pharmacokinetics: Minimally absorbed from nasal tissue; moderately absorbed from inhalation. Protein binding: 88%. Primarily metabolized in the liver. **Half-life:** 2-3 hr.

- **Available Forms:**
  - *Capsules (Entocort EC):* 3 mg.
  - *Powder for Oral Inhalation (Pulmicort Turbuhaler):* 200 mcg per inhalation.
  - *Suspension for Oral Inhalation (Pulmicort Respules):* 0.25 mg/2 ml; 0.5 mg/2 mg.
  - *Nasal Spray (Rhinocort Aqua):* 32 mcg/spray.

- **Indications and Dosages:**
  Rhinitis: Intranasal (Rhinocort Aqua) 1 spray in each nostril once a day. Maximum: 8 sprays/day.
  Bronchial asthma: Inhalation Initially, 200-400 mcg twice a day. Maximum: 800 mcg twice a day.
  Crohn's disease: PO 9 mg once a day for up to 8 wk.

- **Unlabeled Uses:** Treatment of vasomotor rhinitis

- **Contraindications:** Hypersensitivity to any corticosteroid or its components, persistently positive sputum cultures for *Candida albicans*, primary treatment of status asthmaticus, systemic fungal infections, untreated localized infection involving nasal mucosa

- **Side Effects**
  Frequent (greater than 3%)
  Nasal: Mild nasopharyngeal irritation, burning, stinging, or dryness; headache; cough
  Inhalation: Flu-like symptoms, headache, pharyngitis
  Occasional (3%-1%)
  Nasal: Dry mouth, dyspepsia, rebound congestion, rhinorrhea, loss of taste
  Inhalation: Back pain, vomiting, altered taste, voice changes, abdominal pain, nausea, dyspepsia

- **Serious Reactions**
  - An acute hypersensitivity reaction marked by urticaria, angioedema, and severe bronchospasm, occurs rarely.

Special Considerations
  - May allow discontinuation of chronic systemic corticosteroids in many patients with asthma
  - 3-7 days required for maximum benefit (nasal)

- **Patient/Family Education**
  - To be used on regular basis, not for acute symptoms
  - Use bronchodilators before oral inhaler (for patients using both)
  - Nasal vehicle may cause rhinitis
  - Notify the physician if nasal irritation occurs or if symptoms, such as sneezing, fail to improve

- **Monitoring Parameters**
  - Monitor patients switched from chronic systemic corticosteroids to avoid acute adrenal insufficiency in response to stress

- **Geriatric side effects at a glance:**
  ☑ CNS (oral)   ☑ Bowel Dysfunction (oral)   ☐ Bladder Dysfunction   ☐ Falls

- **U.S. Regulatory Considerations**
  ☑ FDA Black Box   ☑ OBRA regulated in U.S. Long Term Care

bumetanide

(byoo-met'-a-nide)

- **Brand Name(s):** Bumex
  Chemical Class: Sulfonamide derivative

- **Clinical Pharmacology:**
  Mechanism of Action: A loop diuretic that enhances excretion of sodium, chloride, and to lesser degree, potassium, by direct action at the ascending limb of the loop of Henle and in the proximal tubule. **Therapeutic Effect:** Produces diuresis.
  Pharmacokinetics:

Route	Onset	Peak	Duration
PO	30-60 min	60-120 min	4-6 hr
IV	Rapid	15-30 min	2-3 hr
IM	40 min	60-120 min	4-6 hr

  Completely absorbed from the GI tract (absorption decreased in CHF and nephrotic syndrome). Protein binding: 94%-96%. Partially metabolized in the liver. Primarily excreted in urine. Not removed by hemodialysis. **Half-life:** 1-1.5 hr.

- **Available Forms:**
  - **Tablets:** 0.5 mg, 1 mg, 2 mg.
  - **Injection:** 0.25 mg/ml.

- **Indications and Dosages:**
  Edema: PO 0.5 mg/day, increased as needed. IV, IM 0.5-2 mg/dose; may repeat in 2-3 hr. Or 0.5-1 mg/hr by continuous IV infusion.
  Hypertension: PO Initially, 0.5 mg/day. Range: 1-4 mg/day. Maximum: 5 mg/day. Larger doses may be given 2-3 doses/day.

- **Unlabeled Uses:** Treatment of hypercalcemia, hypertension

- **Contraindications:** Anuria, hepatic coma, severe electrolyte depletion

- **Side Effects**
  Expected
  Increased urinary frequency and urine volume
  Frequent
  Orthostatic hypotension, dizziness
  Occasional
  Blurred vision, diarrhea, headache, anorexia, premature ejaculation, impotence, dyspepsia
  Rare
  Rash, urticaria, pruritus, asthenia, muscle cramps, nipple tenderness

- **Serious Reactions**
  - Vigorous diuresis may lead to profound water and electrolyte depletion, resulting in hypokalemia, hyponatremia, dehydration, coma, and circulatory collapse.

- Ototoxicity—manifested as deafness, vertigo, or tinnitus—may occur, especially in patients with severe renal impairment and those taking other ototoxic drugs.
- Blood dyscrasias and acute hypotensive episodes have been reported.
- Use with caution in patients with sulfa allergy.

Special Considerations

- Cross-sensitivity with furosemide rare; may substitute bumetanide at a 1:40 ratio with furosemide in patients allergic to furosemide.
- Although allergic cross-reactivity with sulfonamide antibiotics and sulfonamide nonantibiotics has not been demonstrated, use with caution in patients with a history of severe sulfa allergies.

■ Patient/Family Education
- Take early in the day
- Rise slowly from a sitting or lying position

■ Monitoring Parameters
- *Frequent*: Electrolyte, calcium, glucose, uric acid, CO_2, BUN, creatinine during 1st months, then periodically
- *Consider*: CBC, LFTs
- Monitor for tinnitus, hearing loss (IV doses greater than 120 mg; concomitant ototoxic drugs, renal disease)

■ Geriatric side effects at a glance:
❑ CNS ❑ Bowel Dysfunction ❑ Bladder Dysfunction ❑ Falls

■ U.S. Regulatory Considerations
❑ FDA Black Box ❑ OBRA regulated in U.S. Long Term Care

buprenorphine

(byoo-pre-nor'-feen)

■ Brand Name(s): Buprenex, Subutex (sublingual)

Combinations
Rx: with naloxone (Suboxone)
Chemical Class: Opiate derivative; thebaine derivative

DEA Class: Schedule V

■ Clinical Pharmacology:
Mechanism of Action: An opioid agonist-antagonist that binds with opioid receptors in the CNS. **Therapeutic Effect:** Alters the perception of and emotional response to pain; blocks the effects of heroin and produces minimal opioid withdrawal symptoms. **Pharmacokinetics:** Rapidly absorbed following IM administration. Protein binding: Very high. Metabolized in liver. Primarily excreted in feces; minimal excretion in urine. **Half-life:** 2 hr.

■ **Available Forms:**
- *Tablets (Sublingual [Subutex])*: 2 mg, 8 mg.
- *Tablets (Sublingual [Suboxone])*: 2 mg buprenorphine/0.5 mg naloxone, 8 mg buprenorphine/2 mg naloxone.
- *Injection (Buprenex)*: 0.3 mg/ml.

■ **Indications and Dosages:**
Analgesia: IV, IM 0.15 mg q6h as needed.
Opioid dependence: Sublingual Initially, 12-16 mg/day, beginning at least 4 hr after last use of heroin or short-acting opioid. Maintenance: 16 mg/day. Range: 4-24 mg/day. Patients should be switched to buprenorphine and naloxone combination, which is preferred for maintenance treatment.

■ **Contraindications:** Hypersensitivity to buprenorphine; hypersensitivity to naloxone for those receiving the fixed combination product containing naloxone (Suboxone)

■ **Side Effects**
Frequent
Tablet: Headache, pain, insomnia, anxiety, depression, nausea, abdominal pain, constipation, back pain, weakness, rhinitis, withdrawal syndrome, infection, diaphoresis
Injection (more than 10%): Sedation
Occasional
Injection: Hypotension, respiratory depression, dizziness, headache, vomiting, nausea, vertigo

■ **Serious Reactions**
- Overdose results in cold and clammy skin, weakness, confusion, severe respiratory depression, cyanosis, pinpoint pupils, and extreme somnolence progressing to seizures, stupor, and coma.

Special Considerations
- Effective long-acting opioid agonist-antagonist; unconfirmed reported lower physical dependence; no significant advantages
- Use of SL tabs restricted to physicians licensed to treat opioid dependence
- In opioid dependence use Subutex during induction and Suboxone for unsupervised administration

■ **Patient/Family Education**
- Do not swallow SL tablets
- Change positions slowly to avoid dizziness
- Avoid tasks requiring mental alertness or motor skills until response to the drug has been established

■ **Monitoring Parameters**
- Respiration rate
- Blood pressure, pulse rate

■ **Geriatric side effects at a glance:**
❏ CNS ☑ Bowel Dysfunction ❏ Bladder Dysfunction ❏ Falls

■ **U.S. Regulatory Considerations**
❏ FDA Black Box ❏ OBRA regulated in U.S. Long Term Care

bupropion hydrochloride

(byoo-proe'-pee-on hye-droe-klor'-ide)

■ **Brand Name(s):** Wellbutrin, Wellbutrin SR, Wellbutrin XL, Zyban, Zyban SR, Zyban SR Refill
Chemical Class: Aminoketone derivative

■ **Clinical Pharmacology:**
Mechanism of Action: An aminoketone that blocks the reuptake of dopamine and norepinephrine at CNS presynaptic membranes, increasing their availability at postsynaptic receptor sites. **Therapeutic Effect:** Relieves depression and nicotine withdrawal symptoms.
Pharmacokinetics: Rapidly absorbed from the GI tract. Protein binding: 84%. Crosses the blood-brain barrier. Undergoes extensive first-pass metabolism in the liver to active metabolite. Primarily excreted in urine. **Half-life:** 14 hr.

■ **Available Forms:**
  • *Tablets (Wellbutrin):* 75 mg, 100 mg.
  • *Tablets (Extended-Release [Wellbutrin XL]):* 150 mg, 300 mg.
  • *Tablets (Sustained-Release [Wellbutrin SR]):* 100 mg, 150 mg, 200 mg.
  • *Tablets (Sustained-Release [Zyban SR, Zyban SR Refill]):* 150 mg.

■ **Indications and Dosages:**
Depression: PO (Immediate-Release) 37.5 mg twice a day. May increase by 37.5 mg q3-4 days. Maintenance: Lowest effective dosage. Maximum: 450 mg/day. PO (Sustained-Release) Initially, 50-100 mg/day. May increase by 50-100 mg/day q3-4 days. Maintenance: Lowest effective dosage. Maximum: 400 mg/day. PO (Extended-Release) 150 mg once a day. May increase to 300 mg once a day. Maximum: 450 mg a day.
Smoking cessation: PO Initially, 150 mg a day for 3 days; then 150 mg twice a day for 7-12 wk.
Dosage in liver impairment: **Mild-moderate:** use caution, reduce dosage. **Severe:** use extreme caution. Maximum dose: **Wellbutrin:** 75 mg/day **Wellbutrin SR:** 100 mg/day or 150 mg every other day **Wellbutrin XL:** 150 mg every other day **Zyban:** 150 mg every other day

■ **Unlabeled Uses:** Treatment of attention-deficit hyperactivity disorder

■ **Contraindications:** Current or prior diagnosis of anorexia nervosa or bulimia, seizure disorder, use within 14 days of MAOIs, concomitant use of other bupropion products.

■ **Side Effects**
Frequent (32%-18%)
Constipation, weight gain or loss, nausea, vomiting, anorexia, dry mouth, headache, diaphoresis, tremor, sedation, insomnia, dizziness, agitation
Occasional (10%-5%)
Diarrhea, akinesia, blurred vision, tachycardia, confusion, hostility, fatigue

■ **Serious Reactions**
  • The risk of seizures increases in patients taking more than 150 mg/dose of bupropion, in patients with a history of bulimia or seizure disorders, and in patients discontinuing drugs that may lower the seizure threshold.

- Equal efficacy as tricyclic antidepressants; advantages include minimal anticholinergic effects, lack of orthostatic hypotension, no cardiac conduction problems, absence of weight gain, no sedation
- Fewer sexual side effects than TCAs or SSRIs
- Prescribe in equally divided doses of 3 or 4 times daily to minimize risk of seizures

■ **Patient/Family Education**
- Ability to perform tasks requiring judgment or motor and cognitive skills may be impaired
- Therapeutic effects may take 2-4 wk
- Do not discontinue medication quickly after long-term use
- Take sips of tepid water or chew sugarless gum to relieve dry mouth

■ **Monitoring Parameters**
- Assess the patient's appearance, behavior, level of interest, mood, and sleep pattern to determine the drug's therapeutic effect

■ **Geriatric side effects at a glance:**
☑ CNS ☐ Bowel Dysfunction ☐ Bladder Dysfunction ☐ Falls
Other: Seizures

■ **Use with caution in older patients with:** None

■ **U.S. Regulatory Considerations**
☑ FDA Black Box
- Because there is an increased risk of suicide in children and adolescents, older adults should also be closely monitored for suicide ideation.
☐ OBRA regulated in U.S. Long Term Care

■ **Other Uses in Geriatric Patient:** Smoking cessation

■ **Side Effects:**
Of particular importance in the geriatric patient: None

■ **Geriatric Considerations - Summary:** Bupropion has several advantages as an antidepressant agent for use in older adults. It has neither the anticholinergic or cardiac toxicities of the tricyclic antidepressants, and has fewer sexual side effects than selective serotonin reuptake inhibitors. Because this drug may lower seizure threshold, it should be used with caution in older adults with increased risk of seizures (e.g., previous stroke, early-onset Alzheimer's disease).

buspirone hydrochloride

(byoo-spye'-rone hye-droe-klor'-ide)

■ **Brand Name(s):** BuSpar, BuSpar Dividose
Chemical Class: Azaspirodecanedione

■ **Clinical Pharmacology:**
Mechanism of Action: Although its exact mechanism of action is unknown, this non-barbiturate is thought to bind to serotonin and dopamine receptors in the CNS. The drug may also increase norepinephrine metabolism in the locus ceruleus. **Therapeutic Effect:** Decreased anxiety.
Pharmacokinetics: Rapidly and completely absorbed from the GI tract. Protein binding: 95%. Undergoes extensive first-pass metabolism. Metabolized in the liver to active metabolite. Primarily excreted in urine. Not removed by hemodialysis. **Half-life:** 2-3 hr.

■ **Available Forms:**
• *Tablets:* 5 mg, 7.5 mg, 10 mg (BuSpar), 15 mg (BuSpar, BuSpar Dividose), 30 mg (BuSpar Dividose).

■ **Indications and Dosages:**
Short-term management (up to 4 wk) of anxiety disorders: PO Initially, 5 mg twice a day. May increase by 5 mg/day every 2-3 days. Maximum: 60 mg/day.

■ **Unlabeled Uses:** Augmenting medication for antidepressants; management of aggression in mental retardation and secondary mental disorders, major depression, panic attack

■ **Contraindications:** Concurrent use of MAOIs, severe hepatic or renal impairment

■ **Side Effects**
Frequent (12%–6%)
Dizziness, somnolence, nausea, headache
Occasional (5%–2%)
Nervousness, fatigue, insomnia, dry mouth, light-headedness, mood swings, blurred vision, poor concentration, diarrhea, paresthesia
Rare
Muscle pain and stiffness, nightmares, chest pain, involuntary movements

■ **Serious Reactions**
• Buspirone does not appear to cause drug tolerance, psychological or physical dependence, or withdrawal syndrome.
• Overdose may produce severe nausea, vomiting, dizziness, drowsiness, abdominal distention, and excessive pupil contraction.

Special Considerations
• Advantages include less sedation (preferable in elderly), less effect on psychomotor and psychological function, minimal propensity to interact with ethanol and other CNS depressants

- Will not prevent benzodiazepine withdrawal

■ Patient/Family Education
- Optimal results may take 3-4 wk of treatment; some improvement may be seen after 7-10 days
- Drowsiness usually disappears with continued therapy
- Change positions slowly—from recumbent to sitting before standing—to avoid dizziness
- Avoid tasks that require mental alertness and motor skills until response to buspirone has been established

■ Monitoring Parameters
- Hepatic and renal function

■ Geriatric side effects at a glance:
☑ CNS ☐ Bowel Dysfunction ☐ Bladder Dysfunction ☑ Falls
Other: None

■ Use with caution in older patients with: Not recommended for use in older adults.

■ U.S. Regulatory Considerations
☐ FDA Black Box ☐ OBRA regulated in U.S. Long Term Care

■ Other Uses in Geriatric Patient: Anxiety disorders, sleep disorders, dementia-related behavior problems

■ Side Effects:
Of particular importance in the geriatric patient: Sedation

■ Geriatric Considerations - Summary: Because buspirone is less likely to cause sedation and related psychomotor problems than benzodiazepines, it may be useful in the short-term treatment of anxiety in older adults. Although it is plausible that use of buspirone would be associated with falls, this has not been well studied. Although buspirone may be helpful managing agitation in dementia, there are at least theoretical concerns that buspirone can further accelerate memory impairment in Alzheimer's disease. Because bispirone is a substrate of CYP 3A4, it should be used with caution in patients using such agents as nefazodone and amiodarone.

■ References:
1. Majercsik E, Haller J. Interactions between anxiety, social support, health status and buspirone efficacy in elderly patients. Prog Neuropsychopharmacol Biol Psychiatry 2004;28:1161-1169.
2. Cooper JP. Buspirone for anxiety and agitation in dementia. J Psychiatry Neurosci 2003;28:469.
3. Bond AJ, Wingrove J, Valerie CH, Lader MH. Treatment of generalised anxiety disorder with a short course of psychological therapy, combined with buspirone or placebo. J Affect Disord 2002;72:267-271.

butalbital compound

(byoo-tal'-bi-tal)

■ **Brand Name(s):**

Combinations

Rx: Butalbital/acetaminophen/caffeine: Amaphen, Anolor-300, Anoquan, Arcet, Butacet, Dolmar, Endolor, Esgic, Esgic-Plus, Ezol, Femcet, Fioricet, Isocet, Medigesic, Pacaps, Pharmagesic, Repan, Tencet, Triad, Two-Dyne, Zebutal

Rx: Butalbital/acetaminophen/caffeine with codeine: Ezol III, Fioricet with Codeine

Rx: Butalbital/acetaminophen: Bancap, Phrenilin, Phrenilin Forte, Sedapap-10, Triaprin

Rx: Butalbital, aspirin: Axotal

Rx: Butalbital/aspirin/caffeine: Butalgen, Fiorinal, Fiorgen, Fiormor, Fortabs, Isobutal, Isobutyl, Isolin, Isollyl, Laniroif, Lanorinal, Marnal, Tecnal, Virbutal

Rx: Butalbital/aspirin/caffeine with codeine: Ascomp with Codeine No.3, Butalbital Compound with Codeine, Butinal with Codeine No.3, Fiorinal with Codeine No.3, Idenal with Codeine, Isollyl with Codeine

Chemical Class: Barbituric acid derivative

■ **Clinical Pharmacology:**

Mechanism of Action: A barbiturate that depresses the central nervous system. **Therapeutic Effect:** Pain relief and sedation.

Pharmacokinetics: Well absorbed from the GI tract. Widely distributed to most tissues in the body. Protein binding: varies. Excreted in the urine as unchanged drug or metabolites. **Half-life:** 35 hr (butalbital).

■ **Available Forms:**
- Butalbital, acetaminophen
- *Capsules:* 50 mg butalbital and 325 mg acetaminophen (Bancap, Triaprin).
- *Capsules:* 50 mg butalbital and 650 mg acetaminophen (Bucet, Conten, Phrenilin Forte, Tencon).
- *Tablets:* 50 mg butalbital and 325 mg acetaminophen (Phrenilin).
- *Tablets:* 50 mg butalbital and 650 mg acetaminophen (Sedapap).
- Butalbital, caffeine, acetaminophen
- *Capsules:* 50 mg butalbital, 40 mg caffeine, and 325 mg acetaminophen (Amaphen, Anolor-300, Anoquan, Butacet, Dolmar, Endolor, Esgic, Ezol, Femcet, Medigesic, Pacaps, Repan, Tencet, Triad, Two-Dyne).
- *Tablets:* 50 mg butalbital, 40 mg caffeine, and 325 mg acetaminophen (Arcet, Dolmar, Esgic, Fioricet, Isocet, Pharmagesic, Repan); 50 mg butalbital, 40 mg caffeine, and 500 mg acetaminophen (Esgic-Plus, Zebutal).
- Butalbital, caffeine, acetaminophen, codeine
- *Capsules:* 50 mg butalbital, 40 mg caffeine, 325 mg acetaminophen, and 30 mg codeine phosphate (Fioricet with Codeine)
- Butalbital, aspirin
- *Tablets:* 50 mg butalbital and 650 mg aspirin (Axotal).
- Butalbital, caffeine, aspirin
- *Capsules:* 50 mg butalbital, 40 mg caffeine, and 325 mg aspirin (Butalgen, Fiorinal, Isobutal, Isollyl, Laniroif, Lanorinal, Marnal); 50 mg butalbital, 40 mg caffeine, and 330 mg aspirin (Fiorinal, Tecnal).

- *Tablets*: 50 mg butalbital, 40 mg caffeine, and 325 mg aspirin (Butalgen, Fiorgen, Fiorinal, Fiormor, Fortabs, Isobutal, Isobutyl, Isolin, Isollyl, Laniroif, Lanorinal, Marnal, Virbutal); 50 mg butalbital, 40 mg caffeine, and 330 mg aspirin (Fiorinal, Tecnal).
- Butalbital, caffeine, aspirin, codeine
- *Capsules*: 50 mg butalbital, 40 mg caffeine, 325 mg aspirin, 30 mg codeine phosphate (Ascomp with Codeine No.3, Butalbital Compound with Codeine, Butinal with Codeine No.3, Fiorinal with Codeine No.3, Idenal with Codeine, Isollyl with Codeine).

■ Indications and Dosages:
Relief of mild to moderate pain, tension headaches: PO 1-2 tablets/capsules q4h. Maximum: 6 tablets/capsules daily.

■ Contraindications:
Hypersensitivity to butalbital or any component of the formulation, porphyria

■ Side Effects
Frequent
Drowsiness, excitation, confusion, excitement, mental depression, light-headedness, dizziness, stomach upset, nausea, sleep disturbances
Rare
Rapid/irregular heartbeat, rash, itching, swelling, severe dizziness, trouble breathing, toxic epidermal necrolysis

■ Serious Reactions
- Symptoms of overdose may include vomiting, unusual drowsiness, lack of feeling alert, slow or shallow breathing, cold or clammy skin, loss of consciousness, dark urine, stomach pain, and extreme fatigue.

■ Patient/Family Education
- May cause psychological and/or physical dependence
- May cause drowsiness, use caution driving or operating machinery
- Avoid alcohol and other CNS depressants

■ Monitoring Parameters
- Liver and renal function

■ Geriatric side effects at a glance:
☑ CNS ☐ Bowel Dysfunction ☐ Bladder Dysfunction ☑ Falls
Other: Withdrawal symptoms after long-term use

■ Use with caution in older patients with:
Not recommeded for use in older adults.

■ U.S. Regulatory Considerations
☐ FDA Black Box ☑ OBRA regulated in U.S. Long Term Care

■ Other Uses in Geriatric Patient:
Anxiety disorders, sleep disorders, seizure disorders

■ Side Effects:
Of particular importance in the geriatric patient: Sedation, withdrawal symptoms when abruptly discontinued (e.g., during hospitalization) rather than tapered.

- **Geriatric Considerations - Summary:** Because barbiturates have a low therapeutic window, a wide range of drug interactions, rapid development of tolerance, and great potential for abuse and dependence, these agents are not recommended for use in older adults.

- **References:**

1. Hypnotic drugs. Med Lett Drugs Ther 2000;42:71-72.

butenafine hydrochloride

(byoo-ten'-a-feen)

- **Brand Name(s):** Mentax
  OTC: Lotrimin Ultra
  Chemical Class: Benzylamine derivative

- **Clinical Pharmacology:**
  Mechanism of Action: An antifungal agent that locks biosynthesis of ergosterol, essential for fungal cell membrane. Fungicidal. **Therapeutic Effect:** Relieves athlete's foot.
  Pharmacokinetics: Total amount absorbed into systemic circulation has not been determined. Metabolized in liver. Excreted in urine. **Half-life:** 35 hr.

- **Available Forms:**
  - **Cream:** 1% (Mentax).

- **Indications and Dosages:**
  Tinea pedis, tinea corporis, tinea cruris, tinea versicolor: Topical Apply to affected area and immediate surrounding skin daily for 4 wk.

- **Unlabeled Uses:** Onychomycosis, seborrheic dermatitis

- **Contraindications:** Hypersensitivity to butenafine or any component of the formulation

- **Side Effects**
  Occasional (2%)
  Contact dermatitis, burning/stinging, worsening of the condition
  Rare (less than 2%)
  Erythema, irritation, pruritus

- **Serious Reactions**
  - None known.

Special Considerations

- Good cutaneous absorption, prolonged skin retention, and fungicidal activity are potential advantages. Comparative trials with other agents necessary

Patient/Family Education
- Wash hands after applying medication
- Avoid contact with eyes, nose, and mouth
- Use the medication for the full length of treatment, even if symptoms have improved

Monitoring Parameters
- Skin for evidence of contact dermatitis or erythema

Geriatric side effects at a glance:
❑ CNS ❑ Bowel Dysfunction ❑ Bladder Dysfunction ❑ Falls

U.S. Regulatory Considerations
❑ FDA Black Box ❑ OBRA regulated in U.S. Long Term Care

butoconazole nitrate

(byoo-toe-ko'-na-zole ni'trāt)

Brand Name(s): Gynazole-1
OTC: Mycelex-3 2%
Chemical Class: Imidazole derivative

Clinical Pharmacology:
Mechanism of Action: An antifungal similar to imidazole derivatives that inhibits the steroid synthesis, a vital component of fungal cell formation, thereby damaging the fungal cell membrane. **Therapeutic Effect:** Fungistatic.
Pharmacokinetics: Not known.

Available Forms:
- *Cream*: 2% (Mycelex-3, OTC)
- *Cream*: 2% (Gynazole-1, prefilled applicator)

Indications and Dosages:
Treatment of candidiasis: Topical Insert 1 applicatorful intravaginally at bedtime for up to 3 or 6 days.

Contraindications: Hypersensitivity to butoconazole or any of its components

Side Effects
Occasional
Vaginal itching, burning, irritation

Serious Reactions
- Soreness, swelling, pelvic pain, or cramping rarely occurs.

- **Patient/Family Education**
  - Do not use if abdominal pain, fever, or foul-smelling discharge is present

- **Geriatric side effects at a glance:**
  - ❑ CNS   ❑ Bowel Dysfunction   ❑ Bladder Dysfunction   ❑ Falls

- **U.S. Regulatory Considerations**
  - ❑ FDA Black Box   ❑ OBRA regulated in U.S. Long Term Care

butorphanol tartrate

(byoo-tor'-fa-nole tar'-trate)

- **Brand Name(s):** Stadol, Stadol NS
  Chemical Class: Morphinian congener; opiate derivative

  DEA Class: Schedule IV

- **Clinical Pharmacology:**
  Mechanism of Action: An opioid that binds to opiate receptor sites in the CNS. Reduces intensity of pain stimuli incoming from sensory nerve endings. **Therapeutic Effect:** Alters pain perception and emotional response to pain.
  Pharmacokinetics:

Route	Onset	Peak	Duration
IM	10-30 min	30-60 min	3-4 hr
IV	less than 1 min	30 min	2-4 hr
Nasal	15 min	1-2 hr	4-5 hr

  Rapidly absorbed after IM injection. Protein binding: 80%. Extensively metabolized in the liver. Primarily excreted in urine. **Half-life:** 2.5-4 hr.

- **Available Forms:**
  - Injection (Stadol): 1 mg/ml, 2 mg/ml.
  - Nasal Spray (Stadol NS): 10 mg/ml.

- **Indications and Dosages:**
  Analgesia: IV 1 mg q4-6h as needed. IM 1 mg q4-6h as needed.
  Migraine: Nasal 1 mg or 1 spray in one nostril. May repeat in 60-90 min. May repeat 2-dose sequence q3-4h as needed. Alternatively, 2 mg or 1 spray each nostril if patient remains recumbent, may repeat in 3-4 hr.

- **Contraindications:** CNS disease that affects respirations, hypersensitivity to the preservative benzethonium chloride, physical dependence on other opioid analgesics, preexisting respiratory depression, pulmonary disease

- **Side Effects**
  Frequent
  Parenteral: Somnolence (43%), dizziness (19%)

171

Nasal: Nasal congestion (13%), insomnia (11%)

Occasional

Parenteral (3%-9%): Confusion, diaphoresis, clammy skin, lethargy, headache, nausea, vomiting, dry mouth

Nasal (3%-9%): Vasodilation, constipation, unpleasant taste, dyspnea, epistaxis, nasal irritation, upper respiratory tract infection, tinnitus

Rare

Parenteral: Hypotension, pruritus, blurred vision, sensation of heat, CNS stimulation, insomnia

Nasal: Hypertension, tremor, ear pain, paresthesia, depression, sinusitis

■ **Serious Reactions**
- Abrupt withdrawal after prolonged use may produce symptoms of narcotic withdrawal, such as abdominal cramping, rhinorrhea, lacrimation, anxiety, increased temperature, and piloerection or goose bumps.
- Overdose results in severe respiratory depression, skeletal muscle flaccidity, cyanosis, and extreme somnolence progressing to seizures, stupor, and coma.
- Tolerance to analgesic effect and physical dependence may occur with chronic use.

Special Considerations
- Chronic use can precipitate withdrawal symptoms of anxiety, agitation, mood changes, hallucinations, dysphoria, weakness, and diarrhea
- Prolonged use can result in habituation and drug-seeking behavior
- 2 mg=1 spray in each nostril

■ **Patient/Family Education**
- Change positions slowly to avoid dizziness
- Avoid tasks that require mental alertness or motor skills until response to the drug is established
- Avoid alcohol or CNS depressants during butorphanol therapy

■ **Monitoring Parameters**
- Blood pressure, heart rate, respirations

■ *Geriatric side effects at a glance:*
  ☑ CNS ☑ Bowel Dysfunction ☐ Bladder Dysfunction ☑ Falls

■ **U.S. Regulatory Considerations**
  ☐ FDA Black Box ☐ OBRA regulated in U.S. Long Term Care

cabergoline

(ca-ber'-goe-leen)

- **Brand Name(s):** Dostinex
  Chemical Class: Ergoline derivative

- **Clinical Pharmacology:**
  Mechanism of Action: Agonist at dopamine D_2 receptors suppressing prolactin secretion. **Therapeutic Effect:** Shrinks prolactinomas, restores gonadal function, improves symptoms of Parkinson's disease.
  Pharmacokinetics: Cabergoline is administered orally and undergoes significant first-pass metabolism following systemic absorption. Extensively metabolized in the liver. Elimination is primarily in the feces. **Half-life:** 80 hr.

- **Available Forms:**
  - *Tablet:* 0.5 mg

- **Indications and Dosages:**
  Hyperprolactinemia (idiopathic or primary pituitary adenomas): PO 0.25 mg 2 times per week, titrate by 0.25 mg/dose no more than every 4 wk up to 1 mg 2 times per week *Adults.* 0.5 mg 2 to 5 times per week
  Parkinson's disease: PO 0.5 mg/day and titrate to response. Mean effective dose is 3 mg/day and ranges from 0.5-6 mg/day.
  Restless legs syndrome (RLS): PO 0.5 mg once daily at bedtime, slowly titrate up until symptoms resolve or drug intolerance limits further adjustment. Mean effective dose is 2 mg/day and ranges from 1-4 mg/day.

- **Unlabeled Uses:** Parkinson's disease, RLS

- **Contraindications:** Hypersensitivity to cabergoline, ergot alkaloids or any one of its components.
  Uncontrolled hypertension.

- **Side Effects**
  ### Frequent
  Nausea, orthostatic hypotension, confusion, dyskinesia, hallucinations, peripheral edema
  ### Occasional
  Headache, vertigo, dizziness, dyspepsia, postural hypotension, constipation, asthenia, fatigue, abdominal pain, drowsiness
  ### Rare
  Vomiting, dry mouth, diarrhea, flatulence, anxiety, depression, dysmenorrhea, dyspepsia, mastalgia, paresthesias, vertigo, visual impairment, pleuropulmonary changes, pleural effusion, pulmonary fibrosis, heart failure, peptic ulcer

- **Serious Reactions**
  - Overdosage may produce nasal congestion, syncope, or hallucinations.

- More potent with longer half-life than bromocriptine or pergolide, allowing for less frequent dosing
- Initial treatment produces dramatic response; as disease progresses response duration decreases

■ Patient/Family Education
- To reduce the hypotensive effect, rise slowly from lying to sitting position and permit legs to dangle momentarily before rising

■ Monitoring Parameters
- Monitor prolactin levels monthly until prolactin levels equalize

■ Geriatric side-effects at a glance:
☑ CNS   ☐ Bowel Dysfunction   ☐ Bladder Dysfunction   ☑ Falls
Other: Orthostatic hypotension, daytime somnolence, and sudden drowsiness.

■ Use with caution in older patients with: Preexisting psychotic symptoms

■ U.S. Regulatory Considerations
☐ FDA Black Box   ☐ OBRA regulated in U.S. Long Term Care

■ Other Uses in Geriatric Patient: Restless legs syndrome

■ Side Effects:
Of particular importance in the geriatric patient: Nausea/vomiting can result in weight loss

■ Geriatric Considerations - Summary: Cabergoline is a synthetic ergot dopamine agonist that causes potent and prolonged dopamine D_2 stimulation. Cabergoline has a long elimination half-life which allows for once-daily dosing.

■ References:
1. Miyasaki JM, Martin WRW, Suchowersky O, et al. Practice parameter: initiation of treatment for Parkinson's disease: an evidence based review. Neurology 2002;58:11-17.
2. Happe S, Berger K. The association of dopamine agonists with daytime sleepiness, sleep problems and quality of life in patients with Parkinson's disease:prospective study. J Neurol 2001 248:1062-1067.
3. Hutton JT, Koller WC, Ahlskog JE, et al: Multicenter, placebo-controlled trial of cabergoline taken once daily in the treatment of Parkinson's disease. Neurology 1996; 46:1062-1065.

caffeine

(kaf'-feen)

■ **Brand Name(s):** Caffedrine, Dexitac Stay Alert Stimulant, Enerjets, Keep Alert, NoDoz, Pep-Back, Ultra Pep-Back, Quick Pep, Vivarin
Chemical Class: Xanthine derivative

■ **Clinical Pharmacology:**
Mechanism of Action: A methylxanthine and competitive inhibitor of phosphodiesterase that blocks antagonism of adenosine receptors. **Therapeutic Effect:** Stimulates respiratory center, increases minute ventilation, decreases threshold of or increases response to hypercapnia, increases skeletal muscle tone, decreases diaphragmatic fatigue, increases metabolic rate, and increases oxygen consumption.
Pharmacokinetics: Protein binding: 36%. Widely distributed through the tissues and CSF. Metabolized in liver. Excreted in urine. **Half-life:** 3-7 hr.

■ **Available Forms:**
• *Tablets*: 75 mg (Enerjets), 100 mg (Pep-Back), 150 mg (Quick Pep), 200 mg (Caffedrine Caplets, Dexitac Stay Alert Stimulant, Keep Alert, NoDoz, Ultra Pep-Back, Vivarin)

■ **Indications and Dosages:**
Drowsiness, fatigue: 200 mg no sooner than every 3-4 hr, as needed.

■ **Contraindications:** Hypersensitivity to caffeine, xanthines or any other component of the formulation

■ **Side Effects**
Occasional
Agitation, insomnia, nervousness, restlessness, GI irritation

■ **Serious Reactions**
• At high doses, caffeine can cause arrhythmias, palpitations, and tachycardia.

■ **Patient/Family Education**
• Gradual taper if used long-term to prevent withdrawal syndrome, especially headache
• Most authorities believe caffeine and other analeptics should not be used in overdose with CNS depressants and recommend other supportive therapy

■ **Monitoring Parameters**
• Blood pressure, heart rate

■ **Geriatric side effects at a glance:**
☑ CNS ☐ Bowel Dysfunction ☐ Bladder Dysfunction ☐ Falls

175

- **U.S. Regulatory Considerations**
  - ☑ FDA Black Box
  - • CNS stimulant use has a high abuse potential with the risk of dependence.
  - • Misuse may cause sudden death and serious cardiovascular adverse events.
  - ❑ OBRA regulated in U.S. Long Term Care

calcipotriene

(kal-si-poe-try'-een)

- **Brand Name(s):** Dovonex
  Chemical Class: Vitamin D analog

- **Clinical Pharmacology:**
  Mechanism of Action: A synthetic vitamin D_3 analog that regulates skin cell (keratinocyte) production and development. **Therapeutic Effect:** Preventing abnormal growth and production of psoriasis (abnormal keratinocyte growth).
  Pharmacokinetics: Minimal absorption through intact skin. Metabolized in liver.

- **Available Forms:**
  - • *Cream*: 0.005% (Dovonex).
  - • *Ointment*: 0.005% (Dovonex).
  - • *Topical Solution*: 0.005% (Dovonex).

- **Indications and Dosages:**
  Psoriasis: Topical Apply thin layer to affected skin twice daily (morning and evening); rub in gently and completely.
  Scalp psoriasis: Topical Solution Apply to lesions after combing hair.

- **Contraindications:** Hypercalcemia or evidence of vitamin D toxicity, use on face, hypersensitivity to calcipotriene or any component of the formulation

- **Side Effects**
  Frequent
  Burning, itching, skin irritation
  Occasional
  Erythema, dry skin, peeling, rash, worsening of psoriasis, dermatitis
  Rare
  Skin atrophy, hyperpigmentation, folliculitis

- **Serious Reactions**
  - • Potential for hypercalcemia may occur.

- **Patient/Family Education**
  - • Avoid contact with eyes
  - • Wash hands after application

- Report any signs of local reaction

■ **Monitoring Parameters**
- Serum calcium (if elevated discontinue therapy until normal calcium levels are restored); topical administration can yield systemic effects with excessive use
- Skin for irritation

■ **Geriatric side effects at a glance:**
❑ CNS ❑ Bowel Dysfunction ❑ Bladder Dysfunction ❑ Falls

■ **U.S. Regulatory Considerations**
❑ FDA Black Box ❑ OBRA regulated in U.S. Long Term Care

calcitonin

(kal-si-toe'-nin)

■ **Brand Name(s):** Calcimar, Cibacalcin, Fortical, Miacalcin, Miacalcin Nasal
Chemical Class: Polypeptide hormone

■ **Clinical Pharmacology:**
Mechanism of Action: A synthetic hormone that decreases osteoclast activity in bones, decreases tubular reabsorption of sodium and calcium in the kidneys, and increases absorption of calcium in the GI tract. **Therapeutic Effect:** Regulates serum calcium concentrations.
Pharmacokinetics: Injection form rapidly metabolized (primarily in kidneys); primarily excreted in urine. Nasal form rapidly absorbed. **Half-life:** 70-90 min (injection); 43 min (nasal).

■ **Available Forms:**
- *Injection (Miacalcin):* 200 international units/ml (calcitonin-salmon), 500 mg (calcitonin-human).
- *Nasal Spray (Fortical, Miacalcin Nasal):* 200 international units/activation (calcitonin-salmon).

■ **Indications and Dosages:**
Skin testing before treatment in patients with suspected sensitivity to calcitonin-salmon: Intracutaneous Prepare a 10-international units/ml dilution; withdraw 0.05 ml from a 200-international units/ml vial in a tuberculin syringe; fill up to 1 ml with 0.9% NaCl. Take 0.1 ml and inject intracutaneously on inner aspect of forearm. Observe after 15 min; a positive response is the appearance of more than mild erythema or wheal.
Paget's disease: IM, Subcutaneous Initially, 100 international units/day. Maintenance: 50 international units/day or 50-100 international units every 1-3 days. Intranasal 200-400 international units/day.
Osteoporosis imperfecta: IM, Subcutaneous 2 international units/kg 3 times a week.
Postmenopausal osteoporosis: IM, Subcutaneous 100 international units/day with adequate calcium and vitamin D intake. Intranasal 200 international units/day as a single spray, alternating nostrils daily.

Hypercalcemia: IM, Subcutaneous Initially, 4 international units/kg q12h; may increase to 8 international units/kg q12h if no response in 2 days; may further increase to 8 international units/kg q6h if no response in another 2 days.

■ **Unlabeled Uses:** Treatment of secondary osteoporosis due to drug therapy or hormone disturbance

■ **Contraindications:** Hypersensitivity to gelatin desserts or salmon protein

■ **Side Effects**
  Frequent
  IM, *Subcutaneous* (10%): Nausea (may occur 30 min after injection, usually diminishes with continued therapy), inflammation at injection site
  Nasal (12%-10%): Rhinitis, nasal irritation, redness, sores
  Occasional
  IM, *Subcutaneous* (5%-2%): Flushing of face or hands
  Nasal (5%-3%): Back pain, arthralgia, epistaxis, headache
  Rare
  IM, *Subcutaneous*: Epigastric discomfort, dry mouth, diarrhea, flatulence
  Nasal: Itching of earlobes, pedal edema, rash, diaphoresis

■ **Serious Reactions**
  • Patients with a protein allergy may develop a hypersensitivity reaction.

■ **Patient/Family Education**
  • Before 1st dose of new bottle of nasal spray, pump must be activated by holding upright and pumping nozzle 6 times until a faint spray is emitted.
  • Nausea usually decreases with continued therapy.
  • Notify the physician immediately of itching, rash, shortness of breath, or significant nasal irritation.

■ **Geriatric side effects at a glance:**
  ❑ CNS   ❑ Bowel Dysfunction   ❑ Bladder Dysfunction   ❑ Falls

■ **U.S. Regulatory Considerations**
  ❑ FDA Black Box   ❑ OBRA regulated in U.S. Long Term Care

calcitriol

(kal-si-trye'-ole)

■ **Brand Name(s):** Calcijex, Rocaltrol
  Chemical Class: ENDO-vitamin D analog

■ Clinical Pharmacology:

Mechanism of Action: A fat-soluble vitamin that is essential for absorption, utilization of calcium phosphate, and normal calcification of bone. **Therapeutic Effect:** Stimulates calcium and phosphate absorption from small intestine, promotes secretion of calcium from bone to blood, promotes renal tubule phosphate resorption, acts on bone cells to stimulate skeletal growth and on parathyroid gland to suppress hormone synthesis and secretion.

Pharmacokinetics: Rapidly absorbed from small intestine. Extensive metabolism in kidneys. Primarily excreted in feces; minimal excretion in urine. **Half-life:** 5-8 hr.

■ Available Forms:
- *Capsule:* 0.25 mcg, 0.5 mcg (Rocaltrol).
- *Injection:* 1 mcg/ml, 2 mcg/ml (Calcijex).
- *Oral Solution:* 1 mcg/ml (Rocaltrol).

■ Indications and Dosages:
Renal failure: PO 0.25 mcg/day or every other day. IV 0.5 mcg/day (0.01 mcg/kg) 3 times/wk. Dose range: 0.5-3 mcg (0.01-0.05 mcg/kg) 3 times/wk.
Hypoparathyroidism/pseudohypoparathyroidism: PO 0.5-2 mcg/day
Vitamin D-dependent rickets: PO 1 mcg once daily.
Vitamin D-resistant rickets: PO 0.015-0.02 mcg/kg once daily. Maintenance: 0.03-0.06 mcg/kg once daily. Maximum: 2 mcg once daily.

■ Contraindications:
Hypercalcemia, malabsorption syndrome, vitamin D toxicity, hypersensitivity to other vitamin D products or analogs

■ Side Effects
Occasional
Hypercalcemia, headache, irritability, constipation, metallic taste, nausea, polyuria

■ Serious Reactions
- Early signs of overdosage are manifested as weakness, headache, somnolence, nausea, vomiting, dry mouth, constipation, muscle and bone pain, and metallic taste sensation.
- Later signs of overdosage are evidenced by polyuria, polydipsia, anorexia, weight loss, nocturia, photophobia, rhinorrhea, pruritus, disorientation, hallucinations, hyperthermia, hypertension, and cardiac arrhythmias.

■ Patient/Family Education
- Adequate dietary calcium is necessary for clinical response to vitamin D therapy
- Drink plenty of liquids

■ Monitoring Parameters
- Blood Ca^{2+} and phosphate determinations must be made every week until stable, or more frequently if necessary
- Vitamin D levels also helpful, although less frequently
- BUN

■ Geriatric side effects at a glance:
❑ CNS   ❑ Bowel Dysfunction   ❑ Bladder Dysfunction   ❑ Falls

■ U.S. Regulatory Considerations
❑ FDA Black Box   ❑ OBRA regulated in U.S. Long Term Care

calcium acetate/calcium carbonate/calcium chloride/calcium citrate/calcium glubionate/calcium gluconate

■ **Brand Name(s):** Calcium acetate: PhosLo
   OTC: Calcium carbonate: Amitone, Cal-Carb Forte, Calci-Chew, Calci-Mix, Caltrate, Caltrate 600, Chooz, Dicarbosil, Florical, Maalox, Maalox Quick Dissolve, Mallamint, Mylanta, Nephro-Calci, Os-Cal 500, Oysco 500, Oyst-Cal 500, Oyster Calcium, Rolaids, Titralac, Tums, Tums Ex
   OTC: Calcium citrate: Citracal, Citracal Prenatal Rx, Cal-Citrate

■ **Brand Name(s):** Calcium glubionate: Calcione, Calciquid
   OTC: Tricalcium phosphate: Posture

   Combinations
   Rx: with cholecalciferol (Os-Cal-D)
   OTC: with sodium fluoride (Caltrate, Florical)
   Chemical Class: Divalent cation

■ **Clinical Pharmacology:**
   Mechanism of Action: An electrolyte that is essential for the function and integrity of the nervous, muscular, and skeletal systems. Calcium plays an important role in normal cardiac and renal function, respiration, blood coagulation, and cell membrane and capillary permeability. It helps regulate the release and storage of neurotransmitters and hormones, and it neutralizes or reduces gastric acid (increase pH). Calcium acetate combines with dietary phosphate to form insoluble calcium phosphate. **Therapeutic Effect:** Replaces calcium in deficiency states; controls hyperphosphatemia in end-stage renal disease.
   Pharmacokinetics: Moderately absorbed from the small intestine (absorption depends on presence of vitamin D metabolites and patient's pH). Primarily eliminated in feces.

■ **Available Forms:**
   Calcium Acetate:
   • *Gelcap (PhosLo):* 667 mg (equivalent to 169 mg elemental calcium).
   • *Tablet (PhosLo):* 667 mg (equivalent to 169 mg elemental calcium).

Calcium Carbonate:
- *Tablets*: equivalent to 500 mg elemental calcium (Os-Cal 500), equivalent to 600 mg elemental calcium (Caltrate 600).
- *Tablets* (*Chewable*): equivalent to 200 mg elemental calcium (Tums), equivalent to 500 mg elemental calcium (Os-Cal 500), 600 mg (Maalox Quick Dissolve).

Calcium Chloride:
- *Injection*: 10% (100 mg/ml) equivalent to 27.2 mg elemental calcium per ml.

Calcium Citrate:
- *Tablets*: 250 mg (equivalent to 53 mg elemental calcium) (Cal-Citrate), 950 mg (equivalent to 200 mg elemental calcium) (Citracal).

Calcium Glubionate:
- *Syrup*: 1.8 g/5 ml (equivalent to 115 mg of elemental calcium per 5 ml).

Calcium Gluconate:
- Injection: 10% (equivalent to 9 mg elemental calcium per ml).

■ Indications and Dosages:
Dietary supplement (RDA): PO 1200 mg/day. Maximum: 2.5 g/day.

Hyperphosphatemia: PO (calcium acetate) 2 tablets 3 times a day with meals. May increase gradually to bring serum phosphate level to less than 6 mg/dl as long as hypercalcemia does not develop.

Hypocalcemia: PO (calcium carbonate) 1-2 g/day in 3-4 divided doses. PO (calcium glubionate) 6-18 g/day in 4-6 divided doses. IV (calcium chloride) 0.5-1g repeated q4-6h as needed. IV (calcium gluconate) 2-15 g/24 hr.

Antacid: PO (calcium carbonate) 1-2 tabs (5-10 ml) q2h as needed.

Osteoporosis: PO (calcium carbonate) 1200 mg/day.

Cardiac arrest: IV (calcium chloride) 2-4 mg/kg. May repeat q10min.

Hypocalcemia tetany: IV (calcium chloride) 1g, may repeat in 6 hours. IV (calcium gluconate) 1-3g until therapeutic response achieved.

Supplement: PO (calcium citrate) 0.5-2g 2-4 times a day.

■ Unlabeled Uses: Treatment of hyperphosphatemia (calcium carbonate)

■ Contraindications: Calcium renal calculi, digoxin toxicity, hypercalcemia, hypercalciuria, sarcoidosis, ventricular fibrillation
Calcium acetate: Decreased renal function, hypoparathyroidism

■ Side Effects
Frequent
PO: Chalky taste

Parenteral: Hypotension; flushing; feeling of warmth; nausea; vomiting; pain, rash, redness, or burning at injection site; diaphoresis

Occasional
PO: Mild constipation, fecal impaction, peripheral edema, metabolic alkalosis (muscle pain, restlessness, slow breathing, altered taste)

Calcium carbonate: Milk-alkali syndrome (headache, decreased appetite, nausea, vomiting, unusual tiredness)

Rare
Difficult or painful urination

■ Serious Reactions
- Hypercalcemia is a serious adverse effect of calcium acetate use. Early signs include constipation, headache, dry mouth, increased thirst, irritability, decreased appetite, metallic taste, fatigue, weakness, and depression. Later signs include confusion, somnolence, hypertension, photosensitivity, arrhythmias, nausea, vomiting, and increased painful urination.

- Percentage elemental calcium content of various calcium salts: calcium acetate (25%), calcium carbonate (40%), calcium chloride (27.2%), calcium citrate (21%), calcium glubionate (6.5%), calcium gluceptate (8.2%), calcium gluconate (9.3%), calcium lactate (13%), tricalcium phosphate (39%).
- Maximum of 500 mg per dose for maximal absorption. Administer daily doses greater than 500 mg bid or tid.

■ **Patient/Family Education**
- Take tablets with a full glass of water, 30 min to 1 hr after meals
- Take calcium carbonate with food
- Separate administration of calcium from other oral drugs or fiber-containing foods by at least 2 hr
- Avoid consuming excessive amounts of alcohol, caffeine, and tobacco

■ **Monitoring Parameters**
- Serum calcium or serum ionized calcium concentrations (ionized calcium concentrations are preferable to determine free and bound calcium, especially with concurrent low serum albumin)
- Alternatively, ionized calcium can be estimated using the following rule: Total serum calcium will fall by 0.8 mg/dl for each 1.0 g/dl decrease in serum albumin concentration
- Blood pressure, ECG, serum magnesium, phosphate, and potassium levels

■ **References:**
1. Dietary Reference Intakes, www.nap.edu.

■ **Geriatric side effects at a glance:**
☐ CNS   ☑ Bowel Dysfunction   ☐ Bladder Dysfunction   ☐ Falls

■ **U.S. Regulatory Considerations**
☐ FDA Black Box   ☐ OBRA regulated in U.S. Long Term Care

candesartan cilexetil

(kan-de-sar'-tan)

■ **Brand Name(s):** Atacand
Chemical Class: Angiotensin II receptor antagonist

■ **Clinical Pharmacology:**
Mechanism of Action: An angiotensin II receptor, type AT_1, antagonist that blocks the vasoconstrictor and aldosterone-secreting effects of angiotensin II, inhibiting the binding of angiotensin II to the AT_1 receptors. **Therapeutic Effect:** Causes vasodilation, decreases peripheral resistance, and decreases BP.

Pharmacokinetics:

Route	Onset	Peak	Duration
PO	2-3 hr	6-8 hr	Greater than 24 hr

Rapidly, completely absorbed. Protein binding: greater than 99%. Undergoes minor hepatic metabolism to inactive metabolite. Excreted unchanged in urine and in the feces through the biliary system. Not removed by hemodialysis. **Half-life:** 9 hr.

■ Available Forms:
- *Tablets*: 4 mg, 8 mg, 16 mg, 32 mg.

■ Indications and Dosages:
***Hypertension alone or in combination with other* CV-antihypertensive-ARBs:** PO Initially, 16 mg once a day in those who are not volume depleted. Can be given once or twice a day with total daily doses of 8-32 mg. Give lower dosage in those treated with diuretics or with severely impaired renal function.
Heart failure: PO Initially, 4 mg once daily. May double dose at approximately 2-wk intervals up to a target dose of 32 mg/day.

■ Contraindications: Hypersensitivity to candesartan

■ Side Effects
Occasional (6%-3%)
Upper respiratory tract infection, dizziness, back and leg pain
Rare (2%-1%)
Pharyngitis, rhinitis, headache, fatigue, diarrhea, nausea, dry cough, peripheral edema

■ Serious Reactions
- Overdosage may manifest as hypotension and tachycardia. Bradycardia occurs less often. Institute supportive measures.
- Hypoglycemia may occur in patients with diabetes using glucose-lowering drugs.

Special Considerations
- Potentially as effective as or more effective than ACE inhibitors, without cough; no evidence for reduction in morbidity and mortality as first-line agents in hypertension yet; whether they provide the same cardiac and renal protection also still tentative; like ACE inhibitors, less effective in black patients

■ Patient/Family Education
- Call your clinician immediately if the following side effects are noted: wheezing; lip, throat or face swelling; hives or rash
- Avoid tasks that require mental alertness or motor skills until response to the drug has been established
- Candesartan must be taken for the rest of the patient's life to control hypertension
- Avoid exercising outside during hot weather to avoid the risks of dehydration and hypotension

■ Monitoring Parameters
- Baseline electrolytes, urinalysis, BUN and creatinine with recheck at 2-4 wk after initiation (sooner in volume-depleted patients); monitor sitting BP; watch for symptomatic hypotension, particularly in volume-depleted patients
- Maintain hydration

- **Geriatric side effects at a glance:**
  - ☐ CNS ☐ Bowel Dysfunction ☐ Bladder Dysfunction ☐ Falls

- **U.S. Regulatory Considerations**
  - ☑ FDA Black Box
  - Although not relevant for geriatric patients, teratogenicity is associated with the use of angiotensin II receptor antagonists.
  - ☐ OBRA regulated in U.S. Long Term Care

capreomycin sulfate

(kap-ree-oh-mye'-sin sul'-fate)

- **Brand Name(s):** Capastat
  Chemical Class: Polypeptide antibiotic

- **Clinical Pharmacology:**
  Mechanism of Action: A cyclic polypeptide antimicrobial but the mechanism of action is not well understood. **Therapeutic Effect:** Suppresses mycobacterial multiplication. **Pharmacokinetics:** Not well absorbed from the GI tract. Undergoes little metabolism. Primarily excreted unchanged in urine. **Half-life:** 4-6 hr (half-life is increased with impaired renal function).

- **Available Forms:**
  - Injection: 100 mg/ml (Capastat Sulfate).

- **Indications and Dosages:**
  Tuberculosis: IM 15-20 mg/kg/day for 60-120 days, followed by 1g 2-3 times/wk. Maximum: 1 g/day.

- **Unlabeled Uses:** Treatment of atypical mycobacterial infections

- **Contraindications:** Concurrent use of other ototoxic or nephrotoxic drugs, hypersensitivity to capreomycin

- **Side Effects**
  Frequent
  Ototoxicity, nephrotoxicity
  Occasional
  Eosinophilia
  Rare
  Rash, fever, urticaria, hypokalemia, thrombocytopenia, vertigo

- **Serious Reactions**
  - Renal failure, ototoxicity, and thrombocytopenia can occur.

- When used in renal insufficiency or preexisting auditory impairment, risks of additional cranial nerve VIII impairment or renal injury should be weighed against the benefits of therapy

■ **Patient/Family Education**
- Notify the physician immediately of any auditory problems

■ **Monitoring Parameters**
- Electrolytes, BUN, creatinine weekly
- Blood levels of drug
- Audiometric testing before, during, after treatment

■ **Geriatric side effects at a glance:**
☐ CNS ☐ Bowel Dysfunction ☐ Bladder Dysfunction ☐ Falls

■ **U.S. Regulatory Considerations**
☑ FDA Black Box
The use of capreomycin in patients with renal insufficiency or preexisting auditory impairment must be undertaken with great caution, and the risk of additional cranial nerve VIII impairment or renal injury should be weighed against the benefits to be derived from therapy.
☐ OBRA regulated in U.S. Long Term Care

capsaicin

(cap-say'-sin)

OTC: Zostrix, Zostrix HP
Chemical Class: Alkaloid derivative of Solanaceae plant family

■ **Clinical Pharmacology:**
Mechanism of Action: An analgesic that depletes and prevents reaccumulation of the chemomediator of pain impulses (substance P) from peripheral sensory neurons to CNS. **Therapeutic Effect:** Relieves pain.
Pharmacokinetics: None reported.

■ **Available Forms:**
- **Cream:** 0.025%, 0.075% (Zostrix).

■ **Indications and Dosages:**
Treatment of neuralgia, osteoarthritis, rheumatoid arthritis: Topical Apply directly to affected area 3-4 times/day. Continue for 14-28 days for optimal clinical response.

■ **Unlabeled Uses:** Treatment of neurogenic pain, localized pain syndromes (e.g., osteoarthritis)

■ **Contraindications:** Hypersensitivity to capsaicin or any component of the formulation

■ **Side Effects**
Frequent
Burning, stinging, erythema at site of application

■ **Serious Reactions**
- None known.

Special Considerations
- Pretreatment with topical lidocaine 5% ointment may relieve burning

■ **Patient/Family Education**
- Wash hands following use
- Transient burning may occur upon application and usually disappears after 72 hr

■ **Monitoring Parameters**
- Therapeutic response to the medication

■ **Geriatric side effects at a glance:**
❑ CNS   ❑ Bowel Dysfunction   ❑ Bladder Dysfunction   ❑ Falls

■ **U.S. Regulatory Considerations**
❑ FDA Black Box   ❑ OBRA regulated in U.S. Long Term Care

captopril

(cap'-toe-pril)

■ **Brand Name(s):** Capoten

Combinations
Rx: with hydrochlorothiazide (Capozide)
Chemical Class: Angiotensin-converting enzyme (ACE) inhibitor, nonsulfhydryl

■ **Clinical Pharmacology:**
Mechanism of Action: An ACE inhibitor that suppresses the renin-angiotensin-aldosterone system and prevents conversion of angiotensin I to angiotensin II, a potent vasoconstrictor; may also inhibit angiotensin II at local vascular and renal sites. Decreases plasma angiotensin II, increases plasma renin activity, and decreases aldosterone secretion. **Therapeutic Effect:** Reduces peripheral arterial resistance, pulmonary capillary wedge pressure; improves cardiac output and exercise tolerance.
Pharmacokinetics:

Route	Onset	Peak	Duration
PO	0.25 hr	0.5-1.5 hr	Dose related

Rapidly, well absorbed from the GI tract (absorption is decreased in the presence of food). Protein binding: 25%-30%. Metabolized in the liver. Primarily excreted in urine. Removed by hemodialysis. **Half-life:** less than 3 hr (increased in those with impaired renal function).

■ **Available Forms:**
- *Tablets:* 12.5 mg, 25 mg, 50 mg, 100 mg.

■ **Indications and Dosages:**
Hypertension: PO Initially, 12.5-25 mg 2-3 times a day. After 1-2 wk, may increase to 50 mg 2-3 times a day. Diuretic may be added if no response in additional 1-2 wk. If taken in combination with diuretic, may increase to 100-150 mg 2-3 times a day after 1-2 wk. Maintenance: 25-150 mg 2-3 times a day. Maximum: 450 mg/day.
CHF: PO Initially, 6.25-25 mg 3 times a day. Increase to 50 mg 3 times a day. After at least 2 wk, may increase to 50-100 mg 3 times a day. Maximum: 450 mg/day.
Postmyocardial infarction, impaired liver function: PO 6.25 mg a day, then 12.5 mg 3 times a day. Increase to 25 mg 3 times a day over several days up to 50 mg 3 times a day over several weeks.
Diabetic nephropathy prevention of kidney failure: PO 25 mg 3 times a day.
Dosage in renal impairment: *Creatinine clearance 10-50 ml/min.* 75% of normal dosage. *Creatinine clearance less than 10 ml/min.* 50% of normal dosage.

■ **Unlabeled Uses:** Diagnosis of anatomic renal artery stenosis, hypertensive crisis, rheumatoid arthritis

■ **Contraindications:** History of angioedema from previous treatment with ACE inhibitors

■ **Side Effects**
Frequent (7%-4%)
Rash
Occasional (4%-2%)
Pruritus, dysgeusia (altered taste)
Rare (less than 2%-0.5%)
Headache, cough, insomnia, dizziness, fatigue, paresthesia, malaise, nausea, diarrhea or constipation, dry mouth, tachycardia

■ **Serious Reactions**
- Excessive hypotension ("first-dose syncope") may occur in patients with CHF and in those who are severely salt and volume depleted.
- Angioedema (swelling of face and lips) and hyperkalemia occur rarely.
- Agranulocytosis and neutropenia may be noted in those with collagen vascular disease, including scleroderma and systemic lupus erythematosus, and impaired renal function.
- Nephrotic syndrome may be noted in those with history of renal disease.
- Hypoglycemia may occur in patients with diabetes using glucose-lowering drugs.

■ **Patient/Family Education**
- Caution with salt substitutes containing potassium chloride
- Rise slowly to sitting/standing position to minimize orthostatic hypotension
- Dizziness, fainting, light-headedness may occur during 1st few days of therapy

- May cause altered taste perception or cough; persistent dry cough usually does not subside unless medication is stopped; notify clinician if these symptoms persist
- Noncompliance with drug therapy or skipping captopril doses may cause severe, rebound hypertension

■ Monitoring Parameters
- BUN, creatinine, potassium within 2 wk after initiation of therapy (increased levels may indicate acute renal failure)
- Urinalysis for proteinuria

■ Geriatric side effects at a glance:
❑ CNS ❑ Bowel Dysfunction ❑ Bladder Dysfunction ❑ Falls

■ U.S. Regulatory Considerations
☑ FDA Black Box
Although not relevant for geriatric patients, teratogenicity is associated with the use of ACE inhibitors.
❑ OBRA regulated in U.S. Long Term Care

carbamazepine

(kar-ba-maz'-e-peen)

■ Brand Name(s): Atretol, Carbatrol, Epitol, Equetro, Tegretol, Tegretol-XR
Chemical Class: Iminostilbene derivative

■ Clinical Pharmacology:
Mechanism of Action: An iminostilbene derivative that decreases sodium and calcium ion influx into neuronal membranes, reducing post-tetanic potentiation at synapses. **Therapeutic Effect:** Reduces seizure activity.
Pharmacokinetics: Slowly and completely absorbed from the GI tract. Protein binding: 75%. Metabolized in the liver to active metabolite. Primarily excreted in urine. Not removed by hemodialysis. **Half-life:** 25-65 hr (decreased with chronic use).

■ Available Forms:
- *Capsules (Extended-Release):* 100 mg (Carbatrol, Equetro), 200 mg (Carbatrol, Equetro), 300 mg (Carbatrol, Equetro), 400 mg (Carbatrol).
- *Suspension (Tegretol):* 100 mg/5 ml.
- *Tablets (Epitol, Tegretol):* 200 mg.
- *Tablets (Chewable [Tegretol]):* 100 mg.
- *Tablets (Extended-Release [Tegretol-XR]):* 100 mg, 200 mg, 400 mg.

■ Indications and Dosages:
Seizure control: PO Initially 100 mg 1-2 times a day. May increase by 100 mg/day at weekly intervals. Usual dose 400-1000 mg/day. Maximum: 1.6-2.4 g/day.
Trigeminal neuralgia, diabetic neuropathy: PO Initially 100 mg 1-2 times a day. May increase by 100 mg/day at weekly intervals. Usual dose 400-1000 mg/day.

Bipolar disorder: PO (Equetro) Initially, 400 mg/day in 2 divided doses. May adjust dose in 200-mg increments. Maximum: 1600 mg/day in divided doses.

■ **Unlabeled Uses:** Treatment of alcohol withdrawal, diabetes insipidus, neurogenic pain, psychotic disorders

■ **Contraindications:** Concomitant use of MAOIs, history of myelosuppression, hypersensitivity to tricyclic antidepressants

■ **Side Effects**
Frequent
Drowsiness, dizziness, nausea, vomiting
Occasional
Visual abnormalities (spots before eyes, difficulty focusing, blurred vision), dry mouth or pharynx, tongue irritation, headache, fluid retention, diaphoresis, constipation or diarrhea

■ **Serious Reactions**
- Toxic reactions may include blood dyscrasias (such as aplastic anemia, agranulocytosis, thrombocytopenia, leukopenia, leukocytosis, and eosinophilia), cardiovascular disturbances (such as CHF, hypotension or hypertension, thrombophlebitis and arrhythmias), and dermatologic effects (such as rash, urticaria, pruritus, and photosensitivity).
- Abrupt withdrawal may precipitate status epilepticus.

■ **Patient/Family Education**
- Caution about driving and other activities that require alertness, at least initially
- Drug may turn urine pink to brown
- Do not take oral suspension of carbamazepine simultaneously with other liquid medicines
- Do not abruptly discontinue carbamazepine after long-term use because this may precipitate seizures

■ **Monitoring Parameters**
- CBC—aplastic anemia and agranulocytosis have been reported 5-8 times greater than in the general public
- Liver function test
- Serum drug levels (therapeutic 4-12 mcg/ml) during initial treatment

■ **Geriatric side effects at a glance:**
❑ CNS   ❑ Bowel Dysfunction   ❑ Bladder Dysfunction   ❑ Falls
Other: Hyponatremia, Osteoporosis

■ **Use with caution in older patients with:** Hepatic impairment; Patients taking diuretics, NSAIDs or with nephropathy; Sinus node dysfunction or Heart block, Osteoporosis, Unsteady gait, Urinary incontinence

■ **U.S. Regulatory Considerations**
☑ FDA Black Box
Hematologic: Aplastic anemia and agranulocytosis reported with use. Risk 5-8 times greater than in general population

❏ OBRA regulated in U.S. Long Term Care

■ **Other Uses in Geriatric Patient:** Bipolar Disorder, PTSD, Alcohol Withrawal, Neuropathic Pain

■ **Side Effects:**
Of particular importance in the geriatric patient: Delirium, confusion, cognitive impairment, drowsiness*, dizziness*, unsteadiness*, blurred vision*, diplopia*, ataxia*, anorexia, hyponatremia* (usually asymptomatic), leukopenia (usually not clinically significant), osteomalacia, rare AV block (* - adverse effects that are dose-related and often improve with dose reduction)

■ **Geriatric Considerations - Summary:** Clearance may be reduced up to 40% in older adults; therefore lower doses are generally needed to achieve therapeutic serum concentrations. Carbamazepine has mild anticholinergic actions; older adults may be more susceptible to confusion and agitation. Blurred vision and diplopia precede ataxia and serve as good monitoring parameters to prevent further toxicity. Carbamazepine may reduce bone mineral density by interfering with vitamin D catabolism. Calcium and vitamin D supplementation and monitoring of bone mineral density is recommended for older adults taking carbamazepine. In comparative studies to newer agents, carbamazepine is associated with poorer tolerability in older adults due to CNS adverse effects. In spite of the high incidence of adverse effects, carbamazepine remains first-line therapy for partial seizures and secondarily generalized seizures.

■ **References:**
1. Brodie M, Kwan P. Epilepsy in elderly people. BMJ 2005;331:1317-1322.
2. Ensrud KE, Walczak TS, Blackwell T, et al. Antiepileptic drug use increases rates of bone loss in older women: a prospective study. Neurology 2004;62:2051-2057.
3. Battino D, Croci D, Rossini A, et al. Serum carbamazepine concentrations in elderly patients: a case-matched pharmacokinetic evaluation based on therapeutic drug monitoring data. Epilepsia 2003;44:923-929.
4. Arroyo S, Kramer G. Treating epilepsy in the elderly: safety considerations. Drug Saf 2001;24:991-1015.
5. Drugs that may cause cognitive disorders in the elderly. Med Let 2000;42:111-112.
6. Faught E. Epidemiology and drug treatment of epilepsy in elderly people. Drugs Aging 1999;15:255-269.
7. Kraemer KL, Conigliaro J, Saitz R. Managing alcohol withdrawal in the elderly. Drugs Aging 1999;14:409-425.

carbamide peroxide

(kar'ba-mide per-ox'ide)

- **Brand Name(s):** Auro Ear Drops, Debrox, E-R-O Ear, Gly-Oxide, Mollifene Ear Wax Removing, Murine Ear Drops, Orajel Perioseptic, Proxigel
  OTC: (gel, solution)
  Chemical Class: Urea compound and hydrogen peroxide

- **Clinical Pharmacology:**
  Mechanism of Action: A cerumenolytic that releases oxygen on contact with moist mouth tissues to provide cleansing effects, reduce inflammation, relieve pain, and inhibit odor-forming bacteria. In the ear, oxygen is released and hydrogen peroxide is reduced to water which enables the chemical reaction. **Therapeutic Effect:** Relieves inflammation of gums and lips. Emulsifies and disperses earwax.
  Pharmacokinetics: Not known.

- **Available Forms:**
  - *Gel, Oral:* 10% (Proxigel).
  - *Solution, Oral:* 10% (Gly-Oxide), 15% (Orajel Perioseptic).
  - *Solution, Otic:* 6.5% (Auro Ear Drops, Debrox, E-R-O Ear, Mollifene Ear Wax Removing, Murine Ear Drops)

- **Indications and Dosages:**
  Earwax removal: Topical, solution Tilt head and administer 5-10 drops twice a day for up to 4 days.
  Oral lesions: Topical, gel Apply to affected area 4 times a day. Topical, solution Apply several drops undiluted on affected area 4 times a day after meals and at bedtime.

- **Unlabeled Uses:** Dental whitener

- **Contraindications:** Dizziness, ear discharge or drainage, ear injury, ear pain, irritation, or rash, hypersensitivity to carbamide peroxide or any one of its components

- **Side Effects**
  Occasional
  Oral: Gingival sensitivity

- **Serious Reactions**
  - Opportunistic infections caused by organisms like *Candida albicans* are possible with prolonged use.

- **Patient/Family Education**
  - The tip of the applicator should not enter the ear canal

- **Geriatric side effects at a glance:**
  ❑ CNS   ❑ Bowel Dysfunction   ❑ Bladder Dysfunction   ❑ Falls

- **U.S. Regulatory Considerations**
  ❑ FDA Black Box   ❑ OBRA regulated in U.S. Long Term Care

carbenicillin indanyl sodium

(kar-ben-ih-sill'-in)

- **Brand Name(s):** Geocillin
  Chemical Class: Penicillin derivative, extended-spectrum

- **Clinical Pharmacology:**
  Mechanism of Action: A penicillin that inhibits cell wall synthesis in susceptible microorganisms. **Therapeutic Effect:** Produces bactericidal effect.
  Pharmacokinetics: Moderately absorbed from the GI tract. Protein binding: 50%. Widely distributed. Partially metabolized in liver. Primarily excreted in urine. Removed by hemodialysis. **Half-life:** 1-1.5 hr (half-life increased in impaired renal function).

- **Available Forms:**
  - *Tablet*: 382 mg (Geocillin).

- **Indications and Dosages:**
  Prostatitis: PO 764 mg q6h.
  Urinary tract infection: PO 382-764 mg q6h.

- **Unlabeled Uses:** Perioperative prophylaxis

- **Contraindications:** Hypersensitivity to any penicillin

- **Side Effects**
  Frequent
  GI disturbances, including mild diarrhea, nausea, or vomiting, oral or vaginal candidiasis
  Occasional
  Generalized rash, urticaria, phlebitis, headache
  Rare
  Dizziness, seizures

- **Serious Reactions**
  - Altered bacterial balance may result in potentially fatal superinfections and antibacterial-associated colitis as evidenced by abdominal cramps, watery or severe diarrhea, and fever.
  - Severe hypersensitivity reactions, including seizures, occur rarely.

Special Considerations
NOTE: When high and rapid blood and urine levels of antibiotic are indicated, alternative parenteral therapy should be used
  - Individualize treatment based on local susceptibility patterns.

- **Patient/Family Education**
  - Take the antibiotic for the full length of treatment and evenly space doses around the clock

- Take 1 hr before or 2 hr after consuming food or beverages
- Notify the physician if diarrhea, rash, or other new symptoms occur

■ **Monitoring Parameters**
  - Intake and output, renal and hepatic function

■ **Geriatric side effects at a glance:**
  - ❑ CNS   ☑ Bowel Dysfunction   ❑ Bladder Dysfunction   ❑ Falls

■ **U.S. Regulatory Considerations**
  - ❑ FDA Black Box   ❑ OBRA regulated in U.S. Long Term Care

carbidopa; levodopa

(kar-bi-doe'-pa; lee-voe-doe'-pa)

■ **Brand Name(s):** Atamet, Parcopa, Sinemet, Sinemet CR
  Chemical Class: Catecholamine precursor

■ **Clinical Pharmacology:**
  Mechanism of Action: Levodopa is converted to dopamine in the basal ganglia thus increasing dopamine concentration in brain and inhibiting hyperactive cholinergic activity. Carbidopa prevents peripheral breakdown of levodopa, allowing more levodopa to be available for transport into the brain. **Therapeutic Effect:** Reduces tremor and other symptoms of Parkinson's disease.
  Pharmacokinetics: Carbidopa is rapidly and completely absorbed from the GI tract. Widely distributed. Excreted primarily in urine. Levodopa is converted to dopamine. Excreted primarily in urine. **Half-life:** 1-2 hr (carbidopa); 1-3 hr (levodopa).

■ **Available Forms:**
  - *Tablets (Atamet, Sinemet)*: 10 mg carbidopa/100 mg levodopa, 25 mg carbidopa/100 mg levodopa, 25 mg carbidopa/250 mg levodopa.
  - *Tablets (Oral-Disintegrating [Parcopa])*: 10 mg carbidopa/100 mg levodopa, 25 mg carbidopa/100 mg levodopa, 25 mg carbidopa/250 mg levodopa.
  - *Tablets (Extended-Release [Sinemet CR])*: 25 mg carbidopa/100 mg levodopa, 50 mg carbidopa/200 mg levodopa.

■ **Indications and Dosages:**
  Parkinsonism: PO Initially, 25 mg/100 mg twice a day. May increase as necessary. When converting a patient from Sinemet to Sinemet CR (50 mg/200 mg), dosage is based on the total daily dose of levodopa, as follows:

Sinemet	Sinemet CR
300-400 mg	1 tablet twice a day
500-600 mg	1.5 tablets twice a day or 1 tab 3 times a day
700-800 mg	4 tablets in 3 or more divided doses
900-1000 mg	5 tablets in 3 or more divided doses

Intervals between doses of Sinemet CR should be 4-8 hr while awake.

- **Contraindications:** Angle-closure glaucoma, use within 14 days of MAOIs, skin lesions (Sinemet CR), history of melanoma (Sinemet CR)

- **Side Effects**
  Frequent (90%-10%)
  Uncontrolled movements of face, tongue, arms, or upper body; nausea and vomiting (80%); anorexia (50%)
  Occasional
  Depression, anxiety, confusion, nervousness, urine retention, palpitations, dizziness, light-headedness, decreased appetite, blurred vision, constipation, dry mouth, flushed skin, headache, insomnia, diarrhea, unusual fatigue, darkening of urine and sweat
  Rare
  Hypertension, ulcer, hemolytic anemia (marked by fatigue)

- **Serious Reactions**
  - Patients on long-term therapy have a high incidence of involuntary choreiform, dystonic, and dyskinetic movements.
  - Numerous mild to severe CNS and psychiatric disturbances may occur, including reduced attention span, anxiety, nightmares, daytime somnolence, euphoria, fatigue, paranoia, psychotic episodes, depression, and hallucinations.

Special Considerations
  - If previously on levodopa, discontinue for at least 12 hr before change to carbidopa-levodopa combination

- **Patient/Family Education**
  - Limit protein taken with drug
  - Arise slowly from a reclining position
  - Wearing-off effect may occur at end of dosing interval
  - Saliva, urine, or sweat may turn dark color (red, brown, or black)
  - Delayed onset up to 1 hr with controlled-release formulation possible compared to immediate-release formulation
  - Avoid tasks that require mental alertness or motor skills until response to the drug has been established
  - Avoid alcohol
  - Notify the physician if difficulty urinating, irregular heartbeats, mental changes, severe nausea or vomiting, or uncontrolled movement of the hands, arms, legs, eyelids, face, mouth, or tongue occurs

- **Monitoring Parameters**
  - Relief of symptoms, such as improvement of masklike facial expression, muscular rigidity, shuffling gait, and resting tremors of the hands and head

- **Geriatric side effects at a glance:**
  ☐ CNS ☑ Bowel Dysfunction ☐ Bladder Dysfunction ☐ Falls
  Other: Dyskinesias

- **Use with caution in older patients with:** Psychosis

■ **U.S. Regulatory Considerations**
   ❑ FDA Black Box   ❑ OBRA regulated in U.S. Long Term Care

■ **Other Uses in Geriatric Patient:** Restless Legs Syndrome

■ **Side Effects:**
   Of particular importance in the geriatric patient: Nausea/vomiting, psychotic symptoms

■ **Geriatric Considerations - Summary:** Levodopa is a precursor to dopamine and is converted to dopamine in the CNS. Carbidopa decreases peripheral conversion and increases CNS concentrations of levodopa. While sustained-release forms may be helpful in decreasing the wearing-off of levodopa effectiveness, there may be little advantage over immediate-release preparations. This drug combination is often used as initial therapy for Parkinson's disease.

■ **References:**
   1. Miyasaki JM, Martin WRW, Suchowersky O, et al. Practice parameter: initiation of treatment for Parkinson's disease: an evidence based review. Neurology 2002;58:11-17.
   2. Fahn S, Oakes D, Shoulson I, et al. Levodopa and the progression of Parkinson's disease. N Engl J Med 2005;351:2498-2508.
   3. Koller WC, Hutton JT, Tolosa E, Capilldeo R. Immediate-release and controlled-release carbidopa/levodopa in PT: a 5-year randomized multicenter study. Neurology 1999;53:1012-1019.

carisoprodol

(kar-i-so-pro'-dol)

■ **Brand Name(s):** Soma, Vanadom

   Combinations
   Rx: with aspirin (Soma Compound); with aspirin and codeine (Soma Compound with Codeine)
   Chemical Class: Meprobamate congener

■ **Clinical Pharmacology:**
   Mechanism of Action: A centrally-acting skeletal muscle relaxant whose exact mechanism is unknown. Effects may be due to its CNS depressant actions. **Therapeutic Effect:** Relieves muscle spasms and pain.
   Pharmacokinetics: Metabolized in liver to meprobamate. Excreted in urine. **Half-life:** 8 hr.

■ **Available Forms:**
   • *Tablets (Soma, Vanadom):* 350 mg.

■ **Indications and Dosages:**
Adjunct to rest, physical therapy, analgesics, and other measures for relief of discomfort from acute, painful musculoskeletal conditions: PO 350 mg 4 times a day. Use lower initial dose and increase gradually as needed and tolerated in patients with hepatic disease.

■ **Contraindications:** Acute intermittent porphyria, sensitivity to meprobamate, mebutamate, or tybamate

■ **Side Effects**
Frequent (greater than 10%)
Somnolence
Occasional (10%-1%)
Tachycardia, facial flushing, dizziness, headache, light-headedness, dermatitis, nausea, vomiting, abdominal cramps, dyspnea

■ **Serious Reactions**
- Overdose may cause CNS and respiratory depression, shock, and coma.

Special Considerations
- Caution when used in addiction-prone individuals
- Abused on the street in conjunction with narcotics

■ **Patient/Family Education**
- Abrupt cessation may precipitate mild withdrawal symptoms such as abdominal cramps, insomnia, chills, headache, and nausea
- The drug may cause dizziness or drowsiness
- Avoid alcohol and other CNS depressants during carisoprodol therapy

■ **Monitoring Parameters**
- Relief of muscle spasm and pain

■ **Geriatric side effects at a glance:**
☑ CNS ☑ Bowel Dysfunction ☑ Bladder Dysfunction ☑ Falls
Other: Somnolence

■ **Use with caution in older patients with:** Potential for falls

■ **U.S. Regulatory Considerations**
☐ FDA Black Box ☑ OBRA regulated in U.S. Long Term Care

■ **Other Uses in Geriatric Patient:** None

■ **Geriatric Considerations - Summary:** Carisoprodol is a skeletal muscle relaxant that at higher doses can cause CNS depression. It appears to have more use with acute muscle discomfort as compared to chronic use. Carisoprodol's metabolite is meprobamate and therefore may have abuse potential and cause sedation in older adults. The risks of this drug outweigh benefits in treating older adults.

carteolol hydrochloride

(kar-tee'-oh-lole hye-droe-klor'-ide)

■ **Brand Name(s):** Cartrol, Ocupress
   Chemical Class: β-Adrenergic blocker, nonselective

■ **Clinical Pharmacology:**
   Mechanism of Action: An antihypertensive that blocks beta$_1$-adrenergic receptors at normal doses and beta$_2$-adrenergic receptors at large doses. Predominantly blocks beta$_1$-adrenergic receptors in cardiac tissue. Reduces aqueous humor production. **Therapeutic Effect:** Slows sinus heart rate, decreases cardiac output, decreases blood pressure (BP), increases airway resistance, decreases intraocular pressure (IOP). **Pharmacokinetics:** Well absorbed from the GI tract. Protein binding: unknown. Minimally metabolized in liver. Primarily excreted unchanged in urine. Not removed by hemodialysis. **Half-life:** 6 hr (increased in decreased renal function).

■ **Available Forms:**
   • *Ophthalmic Solution*: 1% (Ocupress).
   • *Tablets*: 2.5 mg, 5 mg (Cartrol).

■ **Indications and Dosages:**
   Hypertension: PO Initially, 2.5 mg/day as single dose either alone or in combination with diuretic. May increase gradually to 5-10 mg/day as a single dose. Maintenance: 2.5-5 mg/day.
   Dosage in renal impairment:

Creatinine Clearance	Dosage Interval
60 ml/min	24 hr
20-60 ml/min	48 hr
20 ml/min	72 hr

   Open-angle glaucoma, ocular hypertension: Ophthalmic 1 drop 2 times/day.

■ **Unlabeled Uses:** Combination with miotics decreases IOP in acute/chronic angle-closure glaucoma, treatment of secondary glaucoma, malignant glaucoma, angle-closure glaucoma during/after iridectomy

■ **Contraindications:** Bronchial asthma, COPD, bronchospasm, overt cardiac failure, cardiogenic shock, heart block greater than first degree, persistently severe bradycardia

■ **Side Effects**
   Frequent
   Oral: Hypotension manifested as dizziness, nausea, diaphoresis, headache, cold extremities, fatigue, constipation/diarrhea
   Ophthalmic: Redness of eye or inside of eyelids, decreased night vision
   Occasional
   Oral: Insomnia, flatulence, urinary frequency, impotence or decreased libido
   Ophthalmic: Blepharoconjunctivitis, edema, droopy eyelid, staining of cornea, blurred vision, brow ache, increased light sensitivity, burning, stinging

Rare
Rash, arthralgia, myalgia, confusion, taste disturbances

■ **Serious Reactions**
- Abrupt withdrawal (particularly in those with coronary artery disease) may produce angina or precipitate MI.
- May precipitate thyroid crisis in those with thyrotoxicosis.
- Beta-blockers may mask signs and symptoms of acute hypoglycemia (tachycardia, BP changes) in diabetic patients.

Special Considerations
- Does not alter serum cholesterol or triglycerides

■ **Patient/Family Education**
- Do not stop drug abruptly; taper over 2 wk
- Do not use OTC products containing α-adrenergic stimulants (nasal decongestants, cold remedies) unless directed by physician
- Restrict salt and alcohol intake

■ **Monitoring Parameters**
- Blood pressure, heart rate
- Daily bowel activity and stool consistency
- Intake and output

■ **Geriatric side effects at a glance:**
❑ CNS ❑ Bowel Dysfunction ❑ Bladder Dysfunction ❑ Falls
Other: Cardiovascular and CNS effects

■ **Use with caution in older patients with:** Cardiovascular disease, 2nd or 3rd degree heart block, Sinus bradycardia, Respiratory disease (asthma, COPD), Diabetes, Myasthenia Gravis

■ **U.S. Regulatory Considerations**
In patients using orally administered beta-blockers, abrupt withdrawal may precipitate angina or lead to myocardial infarction or ventricular arrhythmias.
❑ OBRA regulated in U.S. Long Term Care

■ **Other Uses in Geriatric Patient:** None (ophthalmic)

■ **Side Effects:**
Of particular importance in the geriatric patient: Due to systemic absorption: bradycardia, hypotension, dizziness, fatigue, depression, anxiety, hallucinations, bronchospasm, impotence; due to topical administration: stinging, tearing, blurred vision, light sensitivity/photophobia, dryness, decreased visual acuity

■ **Geriatric Considerations - Summary:** Carteolol decreases IOP on average 20%-32%. Systemic absorption of ophthalmic drugs may occur and cause adverse effects in older adults. Since carteolol is a nonselective beta-blocker, older adults may be more sensitive to the cardiovascular, CNS, and respiratory effects of the drug. Carteolol also possesses intrinsic sympathomimetic activity (ISA), but this does not appear to result in a lower frequency of cardiovascular adverse effects. Tachyphylaxis may occur after long-term therapy.

■ **References:**

1. Marquis RE, Whitson JT. Management of glaucoma: focus on pharmacological therapy. Drugs Aging 2005;22:1-22.
2. Camras CB, Toris CB, Tamesis RR. Efficacy and adverse effects of medications used in the treatment of glaucoma. Drugs Aging 1999;15:377-388.

carvedilol

(kar'-ve-dil-ol)

■ **Brand Name(s):** Coreg
   Chemical Class: α-Adrenergic blocker, peripheral; β-adrenergic blocker, nonselective

■ **Clinical Pharmacology:**
   Mechanism of Action: An antihypertensive that possesses nonselective beta-blocking and alpha-adrenergic blocking activity. Causes vasodilation. **Therapeutic Effect:** Reduces cardiac output, exercise-induced tachycardia, and reflex orthostatic tachycardia; reduces peripheral vascular resistance.
   Pharmacokinetics:

Route	Onset	Peak	Duration
PO	30 min	1-2 hr	24 hr

Rapidly and extensively absorbed from the GI tract. Protein binding: 98%. Metabolized in the liver. Excreted primarily via bile into feces. Minimally removed by hemodialysis. **Half-life:** 7-10 hr. Food delays rate of absorption.

■ **Available Forms:**
   • *Tablets:* 3.125 mg, 6.25 mg, 12.5 mg, 25 mg.

■ **Indications and Dosages:**
   Hypertension: PO Initially, 6.25 mg twice a day. May double at 7-to 14-day intervals to highest tolerated dosage. Maximum: 50 mg/day.
   CHF: PO Initially, 3.125 mg twice a day. May double at 2-wk intervals to highest tolerated dosage. Maximum: For patients weighing more than 85 kg, give 50 mg twice a day; for those weighing 85 kg or less, give 25 mg twice a day.
   Left ventricular dysfunction: PO Initially, 3.125-6.25 mg twice a day. May increase at intervals of 3-10 days up to 25 mg twice a day.

■ **Unlabeled Uses:** Treatment of angina pectoris, idiopathic cardiomyopathy

■ **Contraindications:** Bronchial asthma or related bronchospastic conditions, cardiogenic shock, pulmonary edema, second- or third-degree AV block, severe bradycardia

■ **Side Effects**
   Frequent (6%-4%)
   Carvedilol is generally well tolerated, with mild and transient side effects.

Fatigue, dizziness
Occasional (2%)
Diarrhea, bradycardia, rhinitis, back pain
Rare (less than 2%)
Orthostatic hypotension, somnolence, UTI, viral infection

- **Serious Reactions**
  - Overdose may produce profound bradycardia, hypotension, bronchospasm, cardiac insufficiency, cardiogenic shock, and cardiac arrest.
  - Abrupt withdrawal may result in diaphoresis, palpitations, headache, and tremors.
  - Carvedilol administration may precipitate CHF and MI in patients with heart disease; thyroid storm in those with thyrotoxicosis; and peripheral ischemia in those with existing peripheral vascular disease.
  - Hypoglycemia may occur in patients with previously controlled diabetes.

Special Considerations
  - Response less in African-Americans

- **Patient/Family Education**
  - Do not discontinue abruptly; may require taper; rapid withdrawal may produce rebound hypertension or angina
  - Careful monitoring essential when initiating therapy to detect and correct worsening symptoms of heart failure
  - If heart rate drops below 55 beats per minute, reduce dosage
  - Take with food
  - Avoid driving, hazardous tasks during initiation of therapy
  - Compliance is essential to control hypertension
  - Avoid tasks that require mental alertness or motor skills until response to the drug has been established
  - Do not take nasal decongestants and OTC cold preparations, especially those containing stimulants, without physician approval
  - Avoid alcohol and salt intake

- **Monitoring Parameters**
  - *Congestive heart failure*: Functional status, cough, dyspnea on exertion, paroxysmal nocturnal dyspnea, exercise tolerance, and ventricular function
  - *Hypertension*: Blood pressure

- **Geriatric side effects at a glance:**
  ❑ CNS   ❑ Bowel Dysfunction   ❑ Bladder Dysfunction   ❑ Falls

- **U.S. Regulatory Considerations**
  ☑ FDA Black Box
  In patients using <u>orally administered</u> beta-blockers, abrupt withdrawal may precipitate angina or lead to myocardial infarction or ventricular arrhythmias.
  ❑ OBRA regulated in U.S. Long Term Care

cascara sagrada

(cass-care-ah sah-graud'-ah)

OTC: Aromatic Cascara Fluid extract, Cascara Sagrada, Cascara Aromatic
Chemical Class: Anthraquinone derivative

■ **Clinical Pharmacology:**
Mechanism of Action: A GI stimulant that has a direct effect on colonic smooth musculature, by stimulating intramural nerve plexus. **Therapeutic Effect:** Promotes fluid and ion accumulation in the colon, increasing peristalsis and promoting a laxative effect.
Pharmacokinetics: Poorly absorbed following PO administration. Metabolized in the intestinal wall. Excreted in urine and bile. **Half life:** Unknown.

■ **Available Forms:**
 • *Liquid:* (18% alcohol) 1 g/ml.
 • *Tablets:* 150 mg, 325 mg.

■ **Indications and Dosages:**
Treatment of constipation: PO 5 ml or 1-2 tablets at bedtime.

■ **Contraindications:** Abdominal pain, appendicitis, intestinal obstruction, nausea, vomiting

■ **Side Effects**
Frequent
Pink-red, red-violet, red-brown, or yellow-brown discoloration of urine
Occasional
Some degree of abdominal discomfort, nausea, mild cramps, faintness

■ **Serious Reactions**
 • Long-term use may result in laxative dependence, chronic constipation, and loss of normal bowel function.
 • Prolonged use or overdose may result in electrolyte or metabolic disturbances (such as hypokalemia, hypocalcemia, and metabolic acidosis or alkalosis), as well as persistent diarrhea, vomiting, muscle weakness, malabsorption, and weight loss.

Special Considerations
 • Stimulant laxatives are habit forming
 • Long-term use may lead to colonic atony

■ **Patient/Family Education**
 • Urine may temporarily turn pink-red, red-violet, red-brown, or yellow-brown
 • Take measures to promote defecation, such as increasing fluid intake, exercising, and eating a high-fiber diet
 • Do not use cascara sagrada if abdominal pain, nausea, or vomiting lasting longer than 1 wk occurs
 • The liquid form contains alcohol

Monitoring Parameters
- Bowel activity and stool consistency
- Electrolytes

Geriatric side effects at a glance:
☐ CNS ☑ Bowel Dysfunction ☐ Bladder Dysfunction ☐ Falls

U.S. Regulatory Considerations
☐ FDA Black Box ☐ OBRA regulated in U.S. Long Term Care

castor oil

OTC: Emulsoil, Purge
Chemical Class: Fatty acid ester

Clinical Pharmacology:
Mechanism of Action: A laxative prepared from the bean of the castor plant but the exact mechanism of action is unknown. Acts primarily in the small intestine. May be hydrolyzed to ricinoleic acid which reduces net absorption of fluid and electrolytes and stimulates peristalsis. **Therapeutic Effect:** Increases peristalsis, promotes laxative effect.
Pharmacokinetics: Minimal absorption by the GI tract. May be metabolized like other fatty acids.

Available Forms:
- **Emulsion:** 36.4%/ml.
- **Oral Liquid:** 95% (Emulsoil, Purge).

Indications and Dosages:
Constipation: PO 15-60 ml as a single dose.

Contraindications: Abdominal pain, appendicitis, intestinal obstruction, nausea, vomiting

Side Effects
Occasional
Some degree of abdominal discomfort, nausea, mild cramps, griping, faintness

Serious Reactions
- Long-term use may result in laxative dependence, chronic constipation, and loss of normal bowel function.
- Chronic use or overdosage may result in electrolyte disturbances, such as hypokalemia, hypocalcemia, and metabolic acidosis or alkalosis, persistent diarrhea, malabsorption, and weight loss. Electrolyte disturbance may produce vomiting and muscle weakness.

Special Considerations
- Stimulant laxatives are habit forming
- Long-term use may lead to colonic atony

Patient/Family Education
- Increasing fluid intake, exercising and eating a high-fiber diet will promote defecation
- Do not take oral medications within 1 hr of taking castor oil

Monitoring Parameters
- Daily bowel activity and stool consistency
- Electrolytes

Geriatric side effects at a glance:
❑ CNS ☑ Bowel Dysfunction ❑ Bladder Dysfunction ❑ Falls

U.S. Regulatory Considerations
❑ FDA Black Box ❑ OBRA regulated in U.S. Long Term Care

cefaclor

(sef'-ah-klor)

Brand Name(s): Ceclor, Ceclor CD, Ceclor Pulvules
Chemical Class: Cephalosporin (2nd generation)

Clinical Pharmacology:
Mechanism of Action: A second-generation cephalosporin that binds to bacterial cell membranes and inhibits cell wall synthesis. **Therapeutic Effect:** Bactericidal.
Pharmacokinetics: Well absorbed from the GI tract. Protein binding: 25%. Widely distributed. Primarily excreted unchanged in urine. Moderately removed by hemodialysis. **Half-life:** 0.6-0.9 hr (increased in impaired renal function).

Available Forms:
- *Capsules (Ceclor Pulvules):* 250 mg, 500 mg.
- *Tablets (Extended-Release [Ceclor CD]):* 375 mg, 500 mg.

Indications and Dosages:
Bronchitis: PO (Extended-Release) 500 mg q12h for 7 days.
Lower respiratory tract infections: PO 250-500 mg q8h.
Pharyngitis, skin and skin-structure infections, tonsillitis: PO (Extended-Release) 375 mg q12h. PO (Regular-Release) 250-500 mg q8h.
Urinary tract infections: PO 250-500 mg q8h. PO (Extended-Release) 375-500 mg q12h.
Dosage in renal impairment: Decreased dosage may be necessary in patients with creatinine clearance less than 40 ml/min.

Contraindications: History of anaphylactic reaction to penicillins or hypersensitivity to cephalosporins

Side Effects
Frequent
Oral candidiasis, mild diarrhea, mild abdominal cramping, vaginal candidiasis

Occasional

Nausea, serum sickness–like reaction (marked by fever and joint pain; usually occurs after the second course of therapy and resolves after the drug is discontinued)

Rare

Allergic reaction (pruritus, rash, and urticaria)

■ **Serious Reactions**
- Antibiotic-associated colitis and other superinfections may result from altered bacterial balance.
- Nephrotoxicity may occur, especially in patients with preexisting renal disease.
- Patients with a history of allergies, especially to penicillin, are at increased risk for developing a severe hypersensitivity reaction, marked by severe pruritus, angioedema, bronchospasm, and anaphylaxis.

Special Considerations
- Last choice 2nd-generation cephalosporin given relative decreased activity against *Streptococcus pneumoniae* and increased side effects
- Individualize treatment based on local susceptibility patterns.

■ **Patient/Family Education**
- Administer at even intervals and continue therapy for the full course of treatment
- Administer with food or milk if the drug causes GI upset

■ **Monitoring Parameters**
- Daily bowel activity and stool consistency; although mild GI effects may be tolerable, severe symptoms may indicate the onset of antibiotic-associated colitis
- Signs and symptoms of superinfection including abdominal pain or cramping, severe mouth or tongue soreness, anal or genital pruritus or discharge, moderate to severe diarrhea, and new or increased fever

■ **Geriatric side effects at a glance:**
  ❏ CNS ❏ Bowel Dysfunction ❏ Bladder Dysfunction ❏ Falls

■ **U.S. Regulatory Considerations**
  ❏ FDA Black Box ❏ OBRA regulated in U.S. Long Term Care

cefadroxil monohydrate

(sef-ah-drox'-il mon-oh-hye'-drate)

■ **Brand Name(s):** Duricef
  Chemical Class: Cephalosporin (1st generation)

■ **Clinical Pharmacology:**
  Mechanism of Action: A first-generation cephalosporin that binds to bacterial cell membranes and inhibits cell wall synthesis. **Therapeutic Effect:** Bactericidal.

Pharmacokinetics: Well absorbed from the GI tract. Protein binding: 15%-20%. Widely distributed. Primarily excreted unchanged in urine. Removed by hemodialysis. **Half-life:** 1.2-1.5 hr (increased in impaired renal function).

- **Available Forms:**
  - *Capsules:* 500 mg.
  - *Tablets:* 1 g.

- **Indications and Dosages:**
  UTIs: PO 1-2 g/day as a single dose or in 2 divided doses.
  Skin and skin-structure infections, group A beta-hemolytic streptococcal pharyngitis, tonsillitis: PO 1-2g in 2 divided doses.
  Dosage in renal impairment: After an initial 1-g dose, dosage and frequency are modified based on creatinine clearance and the severity of the infection.

Creatinine Clearance	Dosage Interval
25-50 ml/min	500 mg q12h
10-25 ml/min	500 mg q24h
0-10 ml/min	500 mg q36h

- **Contraindications:** History of anaphylactic reaction to penicillins or hypersensitivity to cephalosporins

- **Side Effects**
  Frequent
  Oral candidiasis, mild diarrhea, mild abdominal cramping, vaginal candidiasis
  Occasional
  Nausea, unusual bruising or bleeding, serum sickness–like reaction (marked by fever and joint pain; usually occurs after the second course of therapy and resolves after the drug is discontinued)
  Rare
  Allergic reaction (rash, pruritus, urticaria), thrombophlebitis (pain, redness, swelling at injection site)

- **Serious Reactions**
  - Antibiotic-associated colitis and other superinfections may result from altered bacterial balance.
  - Nephrotoxicity may occur, especially in patients with preexisting renal disease.
  - Patients with a history of allergies, especially to penicillin, are at increased risk for developing a severe hypersensitivity reaction, marked by severe pruritus, angioedema, bronchospasm, and anaphylaxis.

Special Considerations
  - No clinical advantage over less expensive cephalexin
  - Individualize treatment based on local susceptibility patterns.

- **Patient/Family Education**
  - Administer at even intervals and continue therapy for the full course of treatment
  - Administer with food or milk if the drug causes GI upset

- **Monitoring Parameters**
  - Renal function

- Assess pattern of daily bowel activity and stool consistency; although mild GI effects may be tolerable, severe symptoms may indicate the onset of antibiotic-associated colitis
- Be alert for signs and symptoms of superinfection including abdominal pain or cramping, genital or anal pruritus or discharge, moderate to severe diarrhea, severe mouth or tongue soreness, and new or increased fever

■ **Geriatric side effects at a glance:**
❑ CNS   ❑ Bowel Dysfunction   ❑ Bladder Dysfunction   ❑ Falls

■ **U.S. Regulatory Considerations**
❑ FDA Black Box   ❑ OBRA regulated in U.S. Long Term Care

cefamandole nafate

(sef-a-man'-dole na'-fate)

■ **Brand Name(s):** Mandol
Chemical Class: Cephalosporin (2nd generation)

■ **Clinical Pharmacology:**
Mechanism of Action: A second-generation cephalosporin that binds to bacterial cell membranes. **Therapeutic Effect:** Inhibits synthesis of bacterial cell wall. Bactericidal. **Pharmacokinetics:** Well absorbed from the gastrointestinal (GI) tract. Protein binding: 56%-78%. Widely distributed. Primarily excreted unchanged in urine and high concentrations in feces. Moderately removed by hemodialysis. **Half-life:** 0.5-1 hr (half-life is increased with impaired renal function).

■ **Available Forms:**
- *Injection:* 1 g, 2 g, 10 g (Mandol).

■ **Indications and Dosages:**
Severe infections: IV, IM 500-1000 mg q4-8h. Maximum: 2g q4h.
Dosage in renal impairment:

Creatinine Clearance	Dose
25-50 ml/min	1-2g q8h
10-25 ml/min	1g q8h
10 ml/min or less	1g q12h

■ **Unlabeled Uses:** None known.

■ **Contraindications:** History of anaphylactic reaction to penicillins or hypersensitivity to cephalosporins

■ **Side Effects**
Frequent
Diarrhea, thrombophlebitis (pain, redness, swelling at injection site)

Occasional
Nausea, fever, vomiting
Rare
Allergic reaction as evidenced by pruritus, rash, and urticaria

- **Serious Reactions**
  - Antibiotic-associated colitis manifested as severe abdominal pain and tenderness, fever, and watery and severe diarrhea, and other superinfections, may result from altered bacterial balance.
  - Nephrotoxicity may occur, especially in patients with preexisting renal disease.
  - Severe hypersensitivity reaction including severe pruritus, angioedema, bronchospasm, and anaphylaxis, particularly in patients with a history of allergies, especially to penicillin, may occur.

Special Considerations
  - Individualize treatment based on local susceptibility patterns.

- **Monitoring Parameters**
  - Daily bowel activity and stool consistency; although mild GI effects may be tolerable, severe symptoms may indicate the onset of antibiotic-associated colitis
  - Be alert for signs and symptoms of superinfection including abdominal pain or cramping, anal or genital pruritus or discharge, moderate to severe diarrhea, severe mouth or tongue soreness, and new or increased fever

- **Geriatric side effects at a glance:**
  ❑ CNS   ❑ Bowel Dysfunction   ☑ Bladder Dysfunction   ❑ Falls

- **U.S. Regulatory Considerations**
  ❑ FDA Black Box   ❑ OBRA regulated in U.S. Long Term Care

cefazolin sodium

(sef-a'-zoe-lin soe'-dee-um)

- **Brand Name(s):** Ancef, Kefzol
  Chemical Class: Cephalosporin (1st generation)

- **Clinical Pharmacology:**
  Mechanism of Action: A first-generation cephalosporin that binds to bacterial cell membranes and inhibits cell wall synthesis. **Therapeutic Effect:** Bactericidal.
  Pharmacokinetics: Widely distributed. Protein binding: 85%. Primarily excreted unchanged in urine. Moderately removed by hemodialysis. **Half-life:** 1.4-1.8 hr (increased in impaired renal function).

- **Available Forms:**
  - Powder for Injection (Ancef, Kefzol): 500 mg, 1 g, 5 g, 10 g.
  - Ready-to-Hang Infusion (Ancef): 500 mg/50 ml, 1 g/50 ml.

- **Indications and Dosages:**
  Uncomplicated UTIs: IV, IM 1g q12h.
  Mild to moderate infections: IV, IM 250-500 mg q8-12h.
  Severe infections: IV, IM 0.5-1g q6-8h.
  Life-threatening infections: IV, IM 1-1.5g q6h. Maximum: 12 g/day.
  Perioperative prophylaxis: IV, IM 1g 30-60 min before surgery, 0.5-1g during surgery, and q6-8h for up to 24 hr postoperatively.
  Dosage in renal impairment: Dosing frequency is modified based on creatinine clearance.

Creatinine Clearance	Dosage Interval
10-30 ml/min	Usual dose q12h
less than 10 ml/min	Usual dose q24h

- **Contraindications:** History of anaphylactic reaction to penicillins or hypersensitivity to cephalosporins

- **Side Effects**
  Frequent
  Discomfort with IM administration, oral candidiasis, mild diarrhea, mild abdominal cramping, vaginal candidiasis
  Occasional
  Nausea, serum sickness–like reaction (marked by fever and joint pain; usually occurs after the second course of therapy and resolves after the drug is discontinued)
  Rare
  Allergic reaction (rash, pruritus, urticaria), thrombophlebitis (pain, redness, swelling at injection site)

- **Serious Reactions**
  - Antibiotic-associated colitis and other superinfections may result from altered bacterial balance.
  - Nephrotoxicity may occur, especially in patients with preexisting renal disease.
  - Patients with a history of allergies, especially to penicillin, are at increased risk for developing a severe hypersensitivity reaction, marked by severe pruritus, angioedema, bronchospasm, and anaphylaxis.

Special Considerations
  - Individualize treatment based on local susceptibility patterns.

- **Patient/Family Education**
  - IM injections may cause discomfort

- **Monitoring Parameters**
  - Signs and symptoms of superinfection

- **Geriatric side effects at a glance:**
  ☐ CNS ☑ Bowel Dysfunction ☐ Bladder Dysfunction ☐ Falls

- **U.S. Regulatory Considerations**
  ☐ FDA Black Box ☐ OBRA regulated in U.S. Long Term Care

cefdinir

(sef'-di-neer)

- **Brand Name(s):** Omnicef
  Chemical Class: Cephalosporin (3rd generation)

- **Clinical Pharmacology:**
  Mechanism of Action: A third-generation cephalosporin that binds to bacterial cell membranes and inhibits cell wall synthesis. **Therapeutic Effect:** Bactericidal.
  Pharmacokinetics: Moderately absorbed from the GI tract. Protein binding: 60%-70%. Widely distributed. Not appreciably metabolized. Primarily excreted unchanged in urine. Minimally removed by hemodialysis. **Half-life:** 1-2 hr (increased in impaired renal function).

- **Available Forms:**
  - *Capsules:* 300 mg.

- **Indications and Dosages:**
  Community-acquired pneumonia: PO 300 mg q12h for 10 days.
  Acute exacerbation of chronic bronchitis: PO 300 mg q12h for 5-10 days.
  Acute maxillary sinusitis: PO 300 mg q12h or 600 mg q24h for 10 days.
  Pharyngitis or tonsillitis: PO 300 mg q12h for 5-10 days or 600 mg q24h for 10 days.
  Uncomplicated skin or skin-structure infections: PO 300 mg q12h for 10 days.
  Dosage in renal impairment: For patients with creatinine clearance less than 30 ml/min, dosage is 300 mg/day as single daily dose. For hemodialysis patients, dosage is 300 mg or 7 mg/kg/dose every other day.

- **Contraindications:** History of anaphylactic reaction to penicillins or hypersensitivity to cephalosporins

- **Side Effects**
  Frequent
  Oral candidiasis, mild diarrhea, mild abdominal cramping, vaginal candidiasis
  Occasional
  Nausea, serum sickness–like reaction (marked by fever and joint pain; usually occurs after the second course of therapy and resolves after the drug is discontinued)
  Rare
  Allergic reaction (rash, pruritus, urticaria)

- **Serious Reactions**
  - Antibiotic-associated colitis and other superinfections may result from altered bacterial balance.
  - Nephrotoxicity may occur, especially in patients with preexisting renal disease.
  - Patients with a history of allergies, especially to penicillin, are at increased risk for developing a severe hypersensitivity reaction, marked by severe pruritus, angioedema, bronchospasm, and anaphylaxis.

Special Considerations
  - May be taken without regard to food.

- More active *in vitro* against *Staphylococcus aureus* and *Enterococcus faecalis* than cefixime, but less active against some Enterobacteriaceae.
- Individualize treatment based on local susceptibility patterns.

■ **Patient/Family Education**
- Space doses evenly around the clock and continue taking cefdinir for the full length of treatment
- Notify the physician of persistent diarrhea
- Take antacids 2 hr before or after taking cefdinir

■ **Monitoring Parameters**
- Assess pattern of daily bowel activity and stool consistency; although mild GI effects may be tolerable, severe symptoms may indicate the onset of antibiotic-associated colitis
- Be alert for signs and symptoms of superinfection including abdominal pain or cramping, anal or genital pruritus or discharge, moderate to severe diarrhea, severe mouth or tongue soreness, and new or increased fever

■ **Geriatric side effects at a glance:**
  ❑ CNS ☑ Bowel Dysfunction ❑ Bladder Dysfunction ❑ Falls

■ **U.S. Regulatory Considerations**
  ❑ FDA Black Box ❑ OBRA regulated in U.S. Long Term Care

cefditoren pivoxil

(seff-di-tore'-en pi-vox'-il)

■ **Brand Name(s):** Spectracef
  Chemical Class: Cephalosporin (3rd generation)

■ **Clinical Pharmacology:**
  Mechanism of Action: A third-generation cephalosporin that binds to bacterial cell membranes and inhibits cell wall synthesis. **Therapeutic Effect:** Bactericidal. **Pharmacokinetics:** Moderately absorbed from the GI tract. Protein binding: 88%. Not metabolized. Excreted in the urine. Minimally removed by hemodialysis. **Half-life:** 1.6 hr (half-life increased with impaired renal function).

■ **Available Forms:**
- *Tablets:* 200 mg.

■ **Indications and Dosages:**
  Pharyngitis, tonsillitis, skin infections: PO 200 mg twice a day for 10 days.
  Acute exacerbation of chronic bronchitis: PO 400 mg twice a day for 10 days.
  Community-acquired pneumonia: PO 400 mg 2 twice a day for 14 days.

Dosage in renal impairment: Dosage and frequency are modified based on creatinine clearance.

Creatinine Clearance	Dosage
50-80 ml/min	no adjustment necessary.
30-49 ml/min	200 mg twice a day
less than 30 ml/min	200 mg once a day

■ **Contraindications:** History of anaphylactic reaction to penicillins or hypersensitivity to cephalosporins

■ **Side Effects**
Occasional (11%)
Diarrhea
Rare (4%-1%)
Nausea, headache, abdominal pain, vaginal candidiasis, dyspepsia, vomiting

■ **Serious Reactions**
- Antibiotic-associated colitis and other superinfections may occur.
- Patients with a history of allergies, especially to penicillin, are at increased risk for developing a severe hypersensitivity reaction, marked by severe pruritus, angio-edema, bronchospasm, and anaphylaxis.

Special Considerations
- Older oral cephalosporins preferred; no more efficacious than 2nd-generation oral cephalosporins, no advantage over penicillin in strep pharyngitis.
- Not recommended for prolonged therapy as carnitine deficiency may result
- Individualize treatment based on local susceptibility patterns.

■ **Patient/Family Education**
- Take with meals
- Space doses evenly around the clock, do not skip doses, and continue taking cefditoren for the full course of treatment

■ **Monitoring Parameters**
- Be alert for signs and symptoms of superinfection, including abdominal pain, moderate to severe diarrhea, severe anal or genital pruritus, and stomatitis
- Assess pattern of daily bowel activity and stool consistency; severe GI effects may indicate the onset of antibiotic-associated colitis
- Monitor for carnitine deficiency, as evidenced by confusion, fatigue, hypoglycemia, and muscle damage

■ **Geriatric side effects at a glance:**
❑ CNS ☑ Bowel Dysfunction ❑ Bladder Dysfunction ❑ Falls

■ **U.S. Regulatory Considerations**
❑ FDA Black Box ❑ OBRA regulated in U.S. Long Term Care

cefepime hydrochloride

(sef'-e-pim)

■ **Brand Name(s):** Maxipime
Chemical Class: Cephalosporin (4th generation)

■ **Clinical Pharmacology:**
Mechanism of Action: A fourth-generation cephalosporin that binds to bacterial cell membranes and inhibits cell wall synthesis. **Therapeutic Effect:** Bactericidal.
Pharmacokinetics: Well absorbed after IM administration. Protein binding: 20%. Widely distributed. Primarily excreted unchanged in urine. Removed by hemodialysis. **Half-life:** 2-2.3 hr (increased in impaired renal function, and in the elderly).

■ **Available Forms:**
• *Powder for Injection:* 500 mg, 1 g, 2 g.

■ **Indications and Dosages:**
Pneumonia: IV 1-2g q12h for 7-10 days.
Intra-abdominal infections: IV 2g q12h for 10 days.
Skin and skin-structure infections: IV 2g q12h for 10 days.
UTIs: IV 0.5-2g q12h for 7-10 days.
Febrile neutropenia: IV 2g q8h.
Dosage in renal impairment: Dosage and frequency are modified based on creatinine clearance and the severity of the infection.

Creatinine Clearance	Dose Range
30-60 ml/min	0.5g q24h-2g q12h
11-29 ml/min	0.5-2g q24h
10 ml/min or less	0.25-1g q24h

■ **Contraindications:** History of anaphylactic reaction to penicillins or hypersensitivity to cephalosporins

■ **Side Effects**
Frequent
Discomfort with IM administration, oral candidiasis, mild diarrhea, mild abdominal cramping, vaginal candidiasis
Occasional
Nausea, serum sickness–like reaction (marked by fever and joint pain; usually occurs after the second course of therapy and resolves after the drug is discontinued)
Rare
Allergic reaction (rash, pruritus, urticaria), thrombophlebitis (pain, redness, swelling at injection site)

■ **Serious Reactions**
• Antibiotic-associated colitis manifested and other superinfections may result from altered bacterial balance.
• Nephrotoxicity may occur, especially in patients with preexisting renal disease.

- Patients with a history of allergies, especially to penicillin, are at increased risk for developing a severe hypersensitivity reaction, marked by severe pruritus, angio-edema, bronchospasm, and anaphylaxis.

Special Considerations
- Broad spectrum, 4th generation cephalosporin demonstrating a low potential for resistance due to lack of β-lactamase induction and low potential for selection of resistant mutant strains; as effective as ceftazidime and cefotaxime in comparative trials; twice daily dosing may add economic advantage
- Individualize treatment based on local susceptibility patterns.

■ Patient/Family Education
- IM injection may cause discomfort

■ Monitoring Parameters
- Pattern of daily bowel activity and stool consistency; although mild GI effects may be tolerable, severe symptoms may indicate the onset of antibiotic-associated coli-tis
- Intake and output and renal function test results to assess for nephrotoxicity
- Evaluate the IM injection site for induration and tenderness
- Check mouth for white patches on the mucous membranes and tongue
- Be alert for signs and symptoms of superinfection, including abdominal pain or cramping, moderate to severe diarrhea, severe anal or genital pruritus or discharge, and severe mouth or tongue soreness

■ Geriatric side effects at a glance:
❑ CNS   ☑ Bowel Dysfunction   ❑ Bladder Dysfunction   ❑ Falls

■ U.S. Regulatory Considerations
❑ FDA Black Box   ❑ OBRA regulated in U.S. Long Term Care

cefixime

(sef-ix'-eem)

■ Brand Name(s): Suprax
Chemical Class: Cephalosporin (3rd generation)

■ Clinical Pharmacology:
Mechanism of Action: A third-generation cephalosporin that binds to bacterial cell membranes and inhibits cell wall synthesis. **Therapeutic Effect:** Bactericidal.
Pharmacokinetics: Moderately absorbed from the GI tract. Protein binding: 65%-70%. Widely distributed. Primarily excreted unchanged in urine. Minimally removed by he-modialysis. **Half-life:** 3-4 hr (increased in renal impairment).

■ Available Forms:
- *Tablets*: 200 mg, 400 mg.

Indications and Dosages:

Otitis media, acute bronchitis, acute exacerbations of chronic bronchitis, pharyngitis, tonsillitis, and uncomplicated UTIs: PO 400 mg/day as a single dose or in 2 divided doses.

Uncomplicated gonorrhea: PO 400 mg as a single dose.

Dosage in renal impairment: Dosage is modified based on creatinine clearance.

Creatinine Clearance	% of Usual Dose
21-60 ml/min	75%
20 ml/min or less	50%

■ Contraindications: History of anaphylactic reaction to penicillins, hypersensitivity to cephalosporins

■ Side Effects

Frequent

Oral candidiasis, mild diarrhea, mild abdominal cramping, vaginal candidiasis

Occasional

Nausea, serum sickness–like reaction (marked by arthralgia and fever; usually occurs after 2nd course of therapy and resolves after drug is discontinued)

Rare

Allergic reaction (rash, pruritus, urticaria)

■ Serious Reactions

- Antibiotic-associated colitis and other superinfections may result from altered bacterial balance.
- Nephrotoxicity may occur, especially in patients with preexisting renal disease.
- Patients with a history of allergies, especially to penicillin, are at increased risk for developing a severe hypersensitivity reaction, marked by severe pruritus, angioedema, bronchospasm, and anaphylaxis.

Special Considerations

- No *Staphylococcus aureus* coverage
- Individualize treatment based on local susceptibility patterns.

■ Patient/Family Education

- Administer at even intervals and continue therapy for the full course of treatment
- Administer with food or milk if the drug causes GI upset

■ Monitoring Parameters

- Daily bowel activity and stool consistency; although mild GI effects may be tolerable, severe symptoms may indicate the onset of antibiotic-associated colitis
- Be alert for signs and symptoms of superinfection, including abdominal pain or cramping, anal or genital pruritus or discharge, moderate to severe diarrhea, severe mouth or tongue soreness, and new or increased fever.

■ Geriatric side effects at a glance:

❑ CNS ☑ Bowel Dysfunction ❑ Bladder Dysfunction ❑ Falls

■ U.S. Regulatory Considerations

❑ FDA Black Box ❑ OBRA regulated in U.S. Long Term Care

cefoperazone sodium

(sef-oh-per'-a-zone)

■ **Brand Name(s):** Cefobid
Chemical Class: Cephalosporin (3rd generation)

■ **Clinical Pharmacology:**
Mechanism of Action: A third-generation cephalosporin that binds to bacterial cell membranes. **Therapeutic Effect:** Inhibits synthesis of bacterial cell wall. Bactericidal. **Pharmacokinetics:** Widely distributed, including cerebrospinal fluid (CSF). Protein binding: 82%-93%. Metabolized and excreted in kidney and urine. Removed by hemodialysis. **Half-life:** 1.6-2.4 hr (half-life is increased with impaired renal function).

■ **Available Forms:**
• *Injection, premixed frozen*: 1g (Cefobid).
• *Powder for Injection*: 1 g, 2 g (Cefobid).

■ **Indications and Dosages:**
Mild to moderate infections: IM, IV 2-4 g/day in 2 divided doses q12h.
Severe or life-threatening infections: IM, IV Total daily dose and/or frequency may be increased to 6-12 g/day divided into 2, 3, or 4 equal doses of 1.5-4 g per dose.
Dosage in renal and/or hepatic impairment: Do not exceed 4 g/day in those with liver disease and/or biliary obstruction. Modification of dose usually not necessary in those with renal impairment. Dose should not exceed 1-2 g/day in those with both hepatic and substantial renal impairment.

■ **Unlabeled Uses:** Treatment of Lyme disease

■ **Contraindications:** Anaphylactic reaction to penicillins, history of hypersensitivity to cephalosporins or any one of its components.

■ **Side Effects**
Frequent
Discomfort with IM administration, oral candidiasis, mild diarrhea, mild abdominal cramping, vaginal candidiasis
Occasional
Nausea, unusual bruising/bleeding, serum sickness–like reaction
Rare
Allergic reaction, rash, pruritus, urticaria, thrombophlebitis (pain, redness, swelling at injection site)

■ **Serious Reactions**
• Antibiotic-associated colitis manifested as severe abdominal pain and tenderness, fever, and watery and severe diarrhea, and other superinfections may result from altered bacterial balance.
• Nephrotoxicity may occur, especially in patients with preexisting renal disease. Severe hypersensitivity reaction including severe pruritus, angioedema, bronchospasm, and anaphylaxis, particularly in patients with a history of allergies, especially to penicillins, may occur.

- No dose adjustment necessary in renal failure when usual doses are administered
- Individualize treatment based on local susceptibility patterns.

■ **Patient/Family Education**
- Avoid alcohol during and for 3 days after use
- Discomfort may occur with IM injection

■ **Monitoring Parameters**
- Daily bowel activity and stool consistency; although mild GI effects may be tolerable, severe symptoms may indicate the onset of antibiotic-associated colitis
- Be alert for signs and symptoms of superinfection, including abdominal pain or cramping, anal or genital pruritus or discharge, moderate to severe diarrhea, severe mouth or tongue soreness, and new or increased fever.

■ **Geriatric side effects at a glance:**
 ❑ CNS ☑ Bowel Dysfunction ❑ Bladder Dysfunction ❑ Falls

■ **U.S. Regulatory Considerations**
 ❑ FDA Black Box ❑ OBRA regulated in U.S. Long Term Care

cefotaxime sodium

(sef-oh-taks'-eem soe'-dee-um)

■ **Brand Name(s):** Claforan
 Chemical Class: Cephalosporin (3rd generation)

■ **Clinical Pharmacology:**
 Mechanism of Action: A third-generation cephalosporin that binds to bacterial cell membranes and inhibits cell wall synthesis. **Therapeutic Effect:** Bactericidal.
 Pharmacokinetics: Widely distributed, including to CSF. Protein binding: 30%-50%. Partially metabolized in the liver to active metabolite. Primarily excreted in urine. Moderately removed by hemodialysis. **Half-life:** 1 hr (increased in impaired renal function).

■ **Available Forms:**
- *Powder for Injection:* 500 mg, 1 g, 2 g, 10 g.
- *Intravenous Solution:* 1 g/50 ml, 2 g/50 ml.

■ **Indications and Dosages:**
 Uncomplicated infections: IV, IM 1g q12h.
 Mild to moderate infections: IV, IM 1-2g q8h.
 Severe infections: IV, IM 2g q6-8h.
 Life-threatening infections: IV, IM 2g q4h.
 Gonorrhea: IM (Male): 1g as a single dose. (Female): 0.5g as a single dose.
 Perioperative prophylaxis: IV, IM 1g 30-90 min before surgery.

Dosage in renal impairment: For patients with creatinine clearance less than 20 ml/min give half of dose at usual dosing intervals.

- **Unlabeled Uses:** Treatment of Lyme disease

- **Contraindications:** History of anaphylactic reaction to penicillins or hypersensitivity to cephalosporins

- **Side Effects**
  Frequent
  Discomfort with IM administration, oral candidiasis, mild diarrhea, mild abdominal cramping, vaginal candidiasis
  Occasional
  Nausea, serum sickness–like reaction (marked by fever and joint pain; usually occurs after the 2nd course of therapy and resolves after the drug is discontinued)
  Rare
  Allergic reaction (rash, pruritus, urticaria), thrombophlebitis (pain, redness, swelling at injection site)

- **Serious Reactions**
  - Antibiotic-associated colitis and other superinfections may result from altered bacterial balance.
  - Nephrotoxicity may occur, especially in patients with preexisting renal disease.
  - Patients with a history of allergies, especially to penicillin, are at increased risk for developing a severe hypersensitivity reaction, marked by severe pruritus, angioedema, bronchospasm, and anaphylaxis.

Special Considerations
  - Individualize treatment based on local susceptibility patterns.

- **Patient/Family Education**
  - IM injections may cause discomfort

- **Monitoring Parameters**
  - Daily bowel activity and stool consistency; although mild GI effects may be tolerable, severe symptoms may indicate the onset of antibiotic-associated colitis
  - Be alert for signs and symptoms of superinfection, including abdominal pain or cramping, anal or genital pruritus or itching, moderate to severe diarrhea, severe mouth or tongue soreness, and new or increased fever.

- **Geriatric side effects at a glance:**
  ❑ CNS ☑ Bowel Dysfunction ❑ Bladder Dysfunction ❑ Falls

- **U.S. Regulatory Considerations**
  ❑ FDA Black Box ❑ OBRA regulated in U.S. Long Term Care

cefotetan disodium

(sef'-oh-tee-tan dye-soe'-dee-um)

- **Brand Name(s):** Cefotan
  Chemical Class: Cephamycin

- **Clinical Pharmacology:**
  Mechanism of Action: A second-generation cephalosporin that binds to bacterial cell membranes and inhibits cell wall synthesis. **Therapeutic Effect:** Bactericidal.
  Pharmacokinetics: Protein binding: 78%-91%. Primarily excreted unchanged in urine. Minimally removed by hemodialysis. **Half-life:** 3-4.6 hr (increased in impaired renal function).

- **Available Forms:**
  - Powder for Injection: 1 g, 2 g, 10 g.
  - Intravenous Solution: 1 g/50 ml, 2 g/50 ml.

- **Indications and Dosages:**
  UTIs: IV, IM 1-2g in divided doses q12-24h.
  Mild to moderate infections: IV, IM 1-2g q12h.
  Severe infections: IV, IM 2g q12h.
  Life-threatening infections: IV, IM 3g q12h.
  Perioperative prophylaxis: IV 1-2g 30-60 min before surgery.
  Dosage in renal impairment: Dosing frequency is modified based on creatinine clearance and the severity of the infection.

Creatinine Clearance	Dosage Interval
10-30 ml/min	usual dose q24h
less than 10 ml/min	usual dose q48h

- **Contraindications:** History of anaphylactic reaction to penicillins or hypersensitivity to cephalosporins

- **Side Effects**
  Frequent
  Discomfort with IM administration, oral candidiasis, mild diarrhea, mild abdominal cramping, vaginal candidiasis
  Occasional
  Nausea, unusual bleeding or bruising, serum sickness–like reaction (marked by fever and joint pain; usually occurs after the 2nd course of therapy and resolves after the drug is discontinued)
  Rare
  Allergic reaction (rash, pruritus, urticaria), thrombophlebitis (pain, redness, swelling at injection site)

- **Serious Reactions**
  - Antibiotic-associated colitis and other superinfections may result from altered bacterial balance.
  - Nephrotoxicity may occur, especially in patients with preexisting renal disease.

218

- Patients with a history of allergies, especially to penicillin, are at increased risk for developing a severe hypersensitivity reaction, marked by severe pruritus, angioedema, bronchospasm, and anaphylaxis.

Special Considerations
- Individualize treatment based on local susceptibility patterns.

■ Patient/Family Education
- Avoid alcohol during and for 3 days after use
- IM injections may cause discomfort

■ Monitoring Parameters
- Daily bowel activity and stool consistency; although mild GI effects may be tolerable, severe symptoms may indicate the onset of antibiotic-associated colitis
- Be alert for signs and symptoms of superinfection including abdominal pain or cramping, anal or genital pruritus or discharge, moderate to severe diarrhea, severe mouth or tongue soreness, and new or increased fever.

■ Geriatric side effects at a glance:
❑ CNS ☑ Bowel Dysfunction ❑ Bladder Dysfunction ❑ Falls

■ U.S. Regulatory Considerations
❑ FDA Black Box ❑ OBRA regulated in U.S. Long Term Care

cefoxitin sodium

(se-fox'-i-tin soe'-dee-um)

■ Brand Name(s): Mefoxin
Chemical Class: Cephamycin

■ Clinical Pharmacology:
Mechanism of Action: A second-generation cephalosporin that binds to bacterial cell membranes and inhibits cell wall synthesis. Therapeutic Effect: Bactericidal.
Pharmacokinetics: Well distributed. Protein binding: 41%-75%. Primarily excreted in urine. Removed by hemodialysis. Half-life: 0.8-1 hr.

■ Available Forms:
- Powder for Injection: 1 g, 2 g, 10 g.
- Intravenous Solution: 1 g/50 ml, 2 g/50 ml.

■ Indications and Dosages:
Mild to moderate infections: IV, IM 1-2g q6-8h.
Severe infections: IV, IM 1g q4h or 2g q6-8h up to 2g q4h.
Perioperative prophylaxis: IV, IM 2g 30-60 min before surgery, then q6h for up to 24 hr after surgery.

Dosage in renal impairment: After a loading dose of 1-2 g, dosage and frequency are modified based on creatinine clearance and the severity of the infection.

Creatinine Clearance	Dosage
30-50 ml/min	1-2g q8-12h
10-29 ml/min	1-2g q12-24h
5-9 ml/min	500 mg-1g q12-24h
less than 5 ml/min	500 mg-1g q24-48h

■ **Contraindications:** History of anaphylactic reaction to penicillins or hypersensitivity to cephalosporins

■ **Side Effects**
   Frequent
   Discomfort with IM administration, oral candidiasis, mild diarrhea, mild abdominal cramping, vaginal candidiasis
   Occasional
   Nausea, serum sickness–like reaction (marked by fever and joint pain; usually occurs after the 2nd course of therapy and resolves after the drug is discontinued).
   Rare
   Allergic reaction (pruritus, rash, urticaria), thrombophlebitis (pain, redness, swelling at injection site)

■ **Serious Reactions**
   • Antibiotic-associated colitis and other superinfections may result from altered bacterial balance.
   • Nephrotoxicity may occur, especially in patients with preexisting renal disease.
   • Patients with a history of allergies, especially to penicillin, are at increased risk for developing a severe hypersensitivity reaction, marked by severe pruritus, angioedema, bronchospasm, and anaphylaxis.

Special Considerations
   • Individualize treatment based on local susceptibility patterns.

■ **Patient/Family Education**
   • IM injections may cause discomfort

■ **Monitoring Parameters**
   • Daily bowel activity and stool consistency; although mild GI effects may be tolerable, severe symptoms may indicate the onset of antibiotic-associated colitis
   • Be alert for signs and symptoms of superinfection including abdominal pain or cramping, anal or genital pruritus or discharge, moderate to severe diarrhea, severe mouth or tongue soreness, and new or increased fever.

■ **Geriatric side effects at a glance:**
   ❑ CNS ☑ Bowel Dysfunction ❑ Bladder Dysfunction ❑ Falls

■ **U.S. Regulatory Considerations**
   ❑ FDA Black Box ❑ OBRA regulated in U.S. Long Term Care

cefpodoxime proxetil

(sef-pode-ox'-eem proks'-eh-till)

- **Brand Name(s):** Vantin
  Chemical Class: Cephalosporin (2nd generation)

- **Clinical Pharmacology:**
  Mechanism of Action: A third-generation cephalosporin that binds to bacterial cell membranes and inhibits cell wall synthesis. **Therapeutic Effect:** Bactericidal.
  Pharmacokinetics: Well absorbed from the GI tract (food increases absorption). Protein binding: 21%-40%. Widely distributed. Primarily excreted unchanged in urine. Partially removed by hemodialysis. **Half-life:** 2.3 hr (increased in impaired renal function and elderly patients).

- **Available Forms:**
  - *Tablets*: 100 mg, 200 mg.

- **Indications and Dosages:**
  Chronic bronchitis, pneumonia: PO 200 mg q12h for 10-14 days.
  Gonorrhea, rectal gonococcal infection (female patients only): PO 200 mg as a single dose.
  Skin and skin-structure infections: PO 400 mg q12h for 7-14 days.
  Pharyngitis, tonsillitis: PO 100 mg q12h for 5-10 days.
  Acute maxillary sinusitis: PO 200 mg twice a day for 10 days.
  UTIs: PO 100 mg q12h for 7 days.
  Dosage in renal impairment: For patients with creatinine clearance less than 30 ml/min, usual dose is given q24h. For patients on hemodialysis, usual dose is given 3 times/wk after dialysis.

- **Contraindications:** History of anaphylactic reaction to penicillins or hypersensitivity to cephalosporins

- **Side Effects**
  Frequent
  Oral candidiasis, mild diarrhea, mild abdominal cramping, vaginal candidiasis
  Occasional
  Nausea, serum sickness–like reaction (marked by fever and joint pain; usually occurs after the 2nd course of therapy and resolves after the drug is discontinued)
  Rare
  Allergic reaction (pruritus, rash, urticaria)

- **Serious Reactions**
  - Antibiotic-associated colitis and other superinfections may result from altered bacterial balance.
  - Nephrotoxicity may occur, especially in patients with preexisting renal disease.
  - Patients with a history of allergies, especially to penicillin, are at increased risk for developing a severe hypersensitivity reaction, marked by severe pruritus, angioedema, bronchospasm, and anaphylaxis.

- Individualize treatment based on local susceptibility patterns.

■ **Monitoring Parameters**
- Pattern of daily bowel activity and stool consistency; mild GI effects may be tolerable, but severe symptoms may indicate the onset of antibiotic-associated colitis
- Assess mouth for white patches on the mucous membranes and tongue (stomatitis)
- Be alert for signs and symptoms of superinfection including abdominal pain or cramping, moderate to severe diarrhea, severe anal or genital pruritus or discharge, and severe mouth or tongue soreness

■ **Geriatric side effects at a glance:**
   ❏ CNS   ☑ Bowel Dysfunction   ❏ Bladder Dysfunction   ❏ Falls

■ **U.S. Regulatory Considerations**
   ❏ FDA Black Box   ❏ OBRA regulated in U.S. Long Term Care

cefprozil

(sef-pro'-zil)

■ **Brand Name(s):** Cefzil
   Chemical Class: Cephalosporin (2nd generation)

■ **Clinical Pharmacology:**
   Mechanism of Action: A second-generation cephalosporin that binds to bacterial cell membranes and inhibits cell wall synthesis. **Therapeutic Effect:** Bactericidal.
   Pharmacokinetics: Well absorbed from the GI tract. Protein binding: 36%-45%. Widely distributed. Primarily excreted unchanged in urine. Moderately removed by hemodialysis. **Half-life:** 1.3 hr (increased in impaired renal function).

■ **Available Forms:**
   - *Tablets*: 250 mg, 500 mg.

■ **Indications and Dosages:**
   Pharyngitis, tonsillitis: PO 500 mg q24h for 10 days.
   Acute bacterial exacerbation of chronic bronchitis, secondary bacterial infection of acute bronchitis: PO 500 mg q12h for 10 days.
   Skin and skin-structure infections: PO 250-500 mg q12h for 10 days.
   Acute sinusitis: PO 250-500 mg q12h for 10 days.
   Dosage in renal impairment: Patients with creatinine clearance less than 30 ml/min receive 50% of usual dose at usual interval.

■ **Contraindications:** History of anaphylactic reaction to penicillins or hypersensitivity to cephalosporins

Side Effects
Frequent
Oral candidiasis, mild diarrhea, mild abdominal cramping, vaginal candidiasis
Occasional
Nausea, serum sickness–like reaction (marked by fever and joint pain; usually occurs after the 2nd course of therapy and resolves after the drug is discontinued)
Rare
Allergic reaction (pruritus, rash, urticaria)

Serious Reactions
- Antibiotic-associated colitis and other superinfections may result from altered bacterial balance.
- Nephrotoxicity may occur, especially in patients with preexisting renal disease.
- Patients with a history of allergies, especially to penicillin, are at increased risk for developing a severe hypersensitivity reaction, marked by severe pruritus, angioedema, bronchospasm, and anaphylaxis.

Special Considerations
- Individualize treatment based on local susceptibility patterns.

Patient/Family Education
- Space drug doses evenly around the clock and continue cefprozil therapy for the full course of treatment
- Take with food if GI upset occurs

Monitoring Parameters
- Pattern of daily bowel activity and stool consistency; mild GI effects may be tolerable, but severe symptoms may indicate the onset of antibiotic-associated colitis
- Assess oral cavity for evidence of stomatitis
- Be alert for signs and symptoms of superinfection, including abdominal pain or cramping, moderate to severe diarrhea, severe anal or genital pruritus or discharge, and severe mouth or tongue soreness

Geriatric side effects at a glance:
❏ CNS ☑ Bowel Dysfunction ❏ Bladder Dysfunction ❏ Falls

U.S. Regulatory Considerations
❏ FDA Black Box ❏ OBRA regulated in U.S. Long Term Care

ceftazidime

(sef'-tay-zi-deem)

Brand Name(s): Ceptaz, Fortaz, Tazicef, Tazidime
Chemical Class: Cephalosporin (3rd generation)

223

■ **Clinical Pharmacology:**
Mechanism of Action: A third-generation cephalosporin that binds to bacterial cell membranes and inhibits cell wall synthesis. **Therapeutic Effect:** Bactericidal.
Pharmacokinetics: Widely distributed (including to cerebrospinal fluid [CSF]). Protein binding: 5%-17%. Primarily excreted unchanged in urine. Removed by hemodialysis. **Half-life:** 2 hr (increased in impaired renal function).

■ **Available Forms:**
- Powder for Injection (Fortaz, Tazicef, Tazidime): 500 mg, 1 g, 2 g.

■ **Indications and Dosages:**
UTIs: IV, IM 250-500 mg q12h.
Mild to moderate infections: IV, IM 1g q12h.
Uncomplicated pneumonia, skin and skin-structure infections: IV, IM 0.5-1g q12h.
Bone and joint infections: IV, IM 2g q12h.
Meningitis, serious gynecologic and intra-abdominal infections: IV, IM 2g q12h.
Dosage in renal impairment: After an initial 1-g dose, dosage and frequency are modified based on creatinine clearance and the severity of the infection.

Creatinine Clearance	Dosage
31-50 ml/min	1g q12h
16-30 ml/min	1g q24h
6-15 ml/min	500 mg q24h
less than 5 ml/min	500 mg q48h

■ **Contraindications:** History of anaphylactic reaction to penicillins or hypersensitivity to cephalosporins

■ **Side Effects**
Frequent
Discomfort with IM administration, oral candidiasis, mild diarrhea, mild abdominal cramping, vaginal candidiasis
Occasional
Nausea, serum sickness–like reaction (marked by fever and joint pain; usually occurs after the 2nd course of therapy and resolves after the drug is discontinued)
Rare
Allergic reaction (pruritus, rash, urticaria), thrombophlebitis (pain, redness, swelling at injection site)

■ **Serious Reactions**
- Antibiotic-associated colitis and other superinfections may result from altered bacterial balance.
- Nephrotoxicity may occur, especially in patients with preexisting renal disease.
- Patients with a history of allergies, especially to penicillin, are at increased risk for developing a severe hypersensitivity reaction, marked by severe pruritus, angioedema, bronchospasm, and anaphylaxis.

Special Considerations
- Especially useful for infections due to *Pseudomonas aeruginosa* (with or without an aminoglycoside)
- Individualize treatment based on local susceptibility patterns.

■ **Patient/Family Education**
- IM injections may cause discomfort

- Pattern of daily bowel activity and stool consistency; mild GI effects may be tolerable, but severe symptoms may indicate the onset of antibiotic-associated colitis
- Evaluate the IV site for phlebitis, as evidenced by heat, pain, and red streaking over the vein
- Assess the IM injection site for induration and tenderness
- Assess mouth for white patches on the mucous membranes or tongue (stomatitis)
- Be alert for signs and symptoms of superinfection, including abdominal pain or cramping, moderate to severe diarrhea, severe anal or genital pruritus or discharge, and severe mouth or tongue soreness

■ **Geriatric side effects at a glance:**
  ❑ CNS ☑ Bowel Dysfunction ❑ Bladder Dysfunction ❑ Falls

■ **U.S. Regulatory Considerations**
  ❑ FDA Black Box ❑ OBRA regulated in U.S. Long Term Care

ceftibuten

(sef-tye'-byoo-ten)

■ **Brand Name(s):** Cedax
  Chemical Class: Cephalosporin (3rd generation)

■ **Clinical Pharmacology:**
  Mechanism of Action: A third-generation cephalosporin that binds to bacterial cell membranes and inhibits cell wall synthesis. **Therapeutic Effect:** Bactericidal.
  Pharmacokinetics: Rapidly absorbed from the gastrointestinal tract. Protein binding: 65%-77%. Excreted primarily in urine. **Half-life:** 2-3 hr.

■ **Available Forms:**
- *Capsules:* 400 mg.

■ **Indications and Dosages:**
  Chronic bronchitis: PO 400 mg once a day for 10 days.
  Pharyngitis, tonsillitis: PO 400 mg once a day for 10 days.
  Dosage in renal impairment: Dosage is modified based on creatinine clearance.

Creatinine Clearance	Dosage
50 ml/min and higher	400 mg or 9 mg/kg q24h
30-49 ml/min	200 mg or 4.5 mg/kg q24h
less than 30 ml/min	100 mg or 2.25 mg/kg q24h

■ **Contraindications:** History of anaphylactic reaction to penicillins or hypersensitivity to cephalosporins

■ **Side Effects**
  Frequent
  Oral candidiasis, mild diarrhea

Occasional

Nausea, serum sickness–like reaction (marked by fever and joint pain; usually occurs after the 2nd course of therapy and resolves after the drug is discontinued)

Rare

Allergic reaction (rash, pruritus, urticaria)

■ Serious Reactions

- Antibiotic-associated colitis and other superinfections may result from altered bacterial balance.
- Nephrotoxicity may occur, especially in patients with preexisting renal disease.
- Patients with a history of allergies, especially to penicillin, are at increased risk for developing a severe hypersensitivity reaction, marked by severe pruritus, angio-edema, bronchospasm, and anaphylaxis.

Special Considerations

- Comparable to many other oral cephalosporins; may produce higher serum levels and better penetration, but unsubstantiated
- Clinical application as alternative in respiratory tract infections
- Individualize treatment based on local susceptibility patterns.

■ Patient/Family Education

- Space drug doses evenly around the clock and continue taking ceftibuten for the full course of treatment
- Take drug with food or milk if GI upset occurs

■ Monitoring Parameters

- Pattern of daily bowel activity and stool consistency; mild GI effects may be tolerable, but severe symptoms may indicate the onset of antibiotic-associated colitis
- Assess mouth for white patches on the mucous membranes and tongue (stomatitis)
- Be alert for signs and symptoms of superinfection, including abdominal pain or cramping, moderate to severe diarrhea, severe anal or genital pruritus or discharge, and severe mouth or tongue soreness

■ Geriatric side effects at a glance:

❑ CNS   ☑ Bowel Dysfunction   ❑ Bladder Dysfunction   ❑ Falls

■ U.S. Regulatory Considerations

❑ FDA Black Box   ❑ OBRA regulated in U.S. Long Term Care

ceftizoxime sodium

(sef-ti-zox'-eem)

■ **Brand Name(s):** Cefizox
   Chemical Class: Cephalosporin (3rd generation)

■ **Clinical Pharmacology:**
   Mechanism of Action: A third-generation cephalosporin that binds to bacterial cell membranes and inhibits cell wall synthesis. **Therapeutic Effect:** Bactericidal.
   Pharmacokinetics: Widely distributed (including to CSF). Protein binding: 30%. Primarily excreted unchanged in urine. Moderately removed by hemodialysis. **Half-life:** 1.7 hr (increased in impaired renal function).

■ **Available Forms:**
   • *Intravenous Solution:* 1 g/50 ml, 2 g/50 ml.
   • *Powder for Injection:* 500 mg, 1 g, 2 g, 10 g.

■ **Indications and Dosages:**
   Uncomplicated UTIs: IV, IM   500 mg q12h.
   Mild, moderate, or severe infections of the biliary, respiratory, and GU tracts; skin, bone, and intra-abdominal infections; meningitis; and septicemia: IV, IM   1-2g q8-12h.
   Life-threatening infections of the biliary, respiratory, and GU tracts; skin, bone and intra-abdominal infections; meningitis; and septicemia: IV   3-4g q8h, up to 2g q4h.
   Uncomplicated gonorrhea: IM   1g one time.
   Dosage in renal impairment: After a loading dose of 0.5-1 g, dosage and frequency are modified based on creatinine clearance and the severity of the infection.

Creatinine Clearance	Dosage
50-79 ml/min	0.5 g-1.5g q8h
5-49 ml/min	0.25 g-1g q12h
less than 5 ml/min	0.25-0.5g q24h or 0.5 g-1g q48h

■ **Contraindications:** History of anaphylactic reaction to penicillins or hypersensitivity to cephalosporins

■ **Side Effects**
   Frequent
   Discomfort with IM administration, oral candidiasis, mild diarrhea, mild abdominal cramping, vaginal candidiasis
   Occasional
   Nausea, serum sickness–like reaction (fever, joint pain; usually occurs after the 2nd course of therapy and resolves after the drug is discontinued)
   Rare
   Allergic reaction (rash, pruritus, urticaria), thrombophlebitis (pain, redness, swelling at injection site)

■ **Serious Reactions**
   • Antibiotic-associated colitis manifested and other superinfections may result from altered bacterial balance.

- Nephrotoxicity may occur, especially in patients with preexisting renal disease.
- Patients with a history of allergies, especially to penicillin, are at increased risk for developing a severe hypersensitivity reaction, marked by severe pruritus, angioedema, bronchospasm, and anaphylaxis.

Special Considerations
- Individualize treatment based on local susceptibility patterns.

■ Patient/Family Education
- IM injections may cause discomfort

■ Monitoring Parameters
- Signs and symptoms of superinfection, including abdominal pain or cramping, moderate to severe diarrhea, severe anal or genital pruritus or discharge, and severe mouth or tongue soreness
- Daily bowel activity and stool consistency; although mild GI effects may be tolerable, severe symptoms may indicate the onset of antibiotic-associated colitis

■ Geriatric side effects at a glance:
❑ CNS   ☑ Bowel Dysfunction   ❑ Bladder Dysfunction   ❑ Falls

■ U.S. Regulatory Considerations
❑ FDA Black Box   ❑ OBRA regulated in U.S. Long Term Care

ceftriaxone sodium

(sef-try-ax'-one soe'-dee-um)

■ Brand Name(s): Rocephin, Rocephin IM Convenience Kit
Chemical Class: Cephalosporin (3rd generation)

■ Clinical Pharmacology:
Mechanism of Action: A third-generation cephalosporin that binds to bacterial cell membranes and inhibits cell wall synthesis. **Therapeutic Effect:** Bactericidal.
Pharmacokinetics: Widely distributed (including to CSF). Protein binding: 83%-96%. Primarily excreted unchanged in urine. Not removed by hemodialysis. **Half-life:** 4.3-4.6 hr IV; 5.8-8.7 hr IM (increased in impaired renal function).

■ Available Forms:
- Kit (Intramuscular [Rocephin IM Convenience Kit]): 500 mg, 1 g.
- Intravenous Solution (Rocephin): 1 g/50 ml, 2 g/50 ml.
- Powder for Injection (Rocephin): 250 mg, 500 mg, 1 g, 2 g, 10 g.

■ Indications and Dosages:
Mild to moderate infections: IV, IM 1-2 g as a single dose or in 2 divided doses.
Serious infections: IV, IM Up to 4 g/day in 2 divided doses.
Lyme disease: IV 2-4 g a day for 10-14 days.

Perioperative prophylaxis: IV, IM 1g 0.5-2 hr before surgery.
Uncomplicated gonorrhea: IM 250 mg plus doxycycline one time.
Dosage in renal impairment: Dosage modification is usually unnecessary but liver and renal function test results should be monitored in those with both renal and liver impairment or severe renal impairment.

■ **Contraindications:** History of anaphylactic reaction to penicillins or hypersensitivity to cephalosporins

■ **Side Effects**
Frequent
Discomfort with IM administration, oral candidiasis, mild diarrhea, mild abdominal cramping, vaginal candidiasis
Occasional
Nausea, serum sickness–like reaction (marked by fever and joint pain; usually occurs after the 2nd course of therapy and resolves after the drug is discontinued)
Rare
Allergic reaction (rash, pruritus, urticaria), thrombophlebitis (pain, redness, swelling at injection site)

■ **Serious Reactions**
  • Antibiotic-associated colitis and other superinfections may result from altered bacterial balance.
  • Nephrotoxicity may occur, especially in patients with preexisting renal disease.
  • Patients with a history of allergies, especially to penicillin, are at increased risk for developing a severe hypersensitivity reaction, marked by severe pruritus, angioedema, bronchospasm, and anaphylaxis.

Special Considerations
  • Individualize treatment based on local susceptibility patterns.

■ **Patient/Family Education**
  • IM injections may cause discomfort

■ **Monitoring Parameters**
  • Daily bowel activity and stool consistency; although mild GI effects may be tolerable, severe symptoms may indicate the onset of antibiotic-associated colitis
  • Be alert for signs and symptoms of superinfection, including abdominal pain or cramping, anal or genital pruritus or discharge, moderate to severe diarrhea, severe mouth or tongue soreness, and new or increased fever.

■ **Geriatric side effects at a glance:**
  ❑ CNS ☑ Bowel Dysfunction ❑ Bladder Dysfunction ❑ Falls

■ **U.S. Regulatory Considerations**
  ❑ FDA Black Box ❑ OBRA regulated in U.S. Long Term Care

cefuroxime axetil/ cefuroxime sodium

(sef-yoor-ox'-eem)

■ **Brand Name(s):** Zinacef, Kefurox (as sodium), Ceftin (as axetil)
  Chemical Class: Cephalosporin (2nd generation)

■ **Clinical Pharmacology:**
  Mechanism of Action: A second-generation cephalosporin that binds to bacterial cell membranes and inhibits cell wall synthesis. **Therapeutic Effect:** Bactericidal.
  Pharmacokinetics: Rapidly absorbed from the GI tract. Protein binding: 33%-50%. Widely distributed (including to CSF). Primarily excreted unchanged in urine. Moderately removed by hemodialysis. **Half-life:** 1.3 hr (increased in impaired renal function).

■ **Available Forms:**
  • *Tablets (Ceftin):* 125 mg, 250 mg, 500 mg.
  • *Powder for Injection (Zinacef):* 750 mg, 1.5 g, 7.5 g.
  • *Powder for Injection (ADD-Vantage Vial [Zinacef]):* 750 mg, 1.5 g.
  • *Powder for Injection (Infusion Pack [Zinacef]):* 750 mg, 1.5 g.
  • *Intravenous Solution (Zinacef):* 750 mg/50 ml, 1.5 g/50 ml.

■ **Indications and Dosages:**
  Ampicillin-resistant influenza; bacterial meningitis; early Lyme disease; GU tract, gynecologic, skin, and bone infections; septicemia; gonorrhea, and other gonococcal infections:
  IV, IM 750 mg-1.5g q8h. PO 125-500 mg twice a day, depending on the infection.
  Perioperative prophylaxis: IV 1.5g 30-60 min before surgery and 750 mg q8h after surgery.
  Dosage in renal impairment: Dosage and frequency are modified based on creatinine clearance and the severity of the infection.

Creatinine Clearance	Dosage
greater than 20 ml/min	750 mg-1g q8h
10-20 ml/min	750 mg q12h
less than 10 ml/min	750 mg q24h

■ **Contraindications:** History of anaphylactic reaction to penicillins or hypersensitivity to cephalosporins

■ **Side Effects**
  Frequent
  Discomfort with IM administration, oral candidiasis, mild diarrhea, mild abdominal cramping, vaginal candidiasis
  Occasional
  Nausea, serum sickness–like reaction (marked by fever and joint pain; usually occurs after the second course of therapy and resolves after the drug is discontinued)
  Rare
  Allergic reaction (rash, pruritus, urticaria), thrombophlebitis (pain, redness, swelling at injection site)

■ Serious Reactions
- Antibiotic-associated colitis and other superinfections may result from altered bacterial balance.
- Nephrotoxicity may occur, especially in patients with preexisting renal disease.
- Patients with a history of allergies, especially to penicillin, are at increased risk for developing a severe hypersensitivity reaction, marked by severe pruritus, angioedema, bronchospasm, and anaphylaxis.

Special Considerations
- Alternative to amoxicillin or co-trimoxazole for resistant upper respiratory pathogens; expensive, but bid dosing
- Individualize treatment based on local susceptibility patterns.

■ Patient/Family Education
- Take with food
- Space doses evenly around the clock

■ Monitoring Parameters
- Assess pattern of daily bowel activity and stool consistency; although mild GI effects may be tolerable, severe symptoms may indicate the onset of antibiotic-associated colitis
- Be alert for signs and symptoms of superinfection, including abdominal pain or cramping, anal or genital pruritus or discharge, moderate to severe diarrhea, severe mouth or tongue soreness, and new or increased fever.

■ Geriatric side effects at a glance:
❑ CNS ❑ Bowel Dysfunction ❑ Bladder Dysfunction ❑ Falls

■ U.S. Regulatory Considerations
❑ FDA Black Box ❑ OBRA regulated in U.S. Long Term Care

celecoxib

(sel-eh-cox'-ib)

■ Brand Name(s): Celebrex
Chemical Class: Cyclooxygenase-2 (COX-2) inhibitor

■ Clinical Pharmacology:
Mechanism of Action: An NSAID that inhibits cyclooxygenase-2, the enzyme responsible for prostaglandin synthesis. Mechanism of action in treating familial adenomatous polyposis is unknown. **Therapeutic Effect:** Reduces inflammation and relieves pain.
Pharmacokinetics: Widely distributed. Protein binding: 97%. Metabolized in the liver. Primarily eliminated in feces. **Half-life:** 11.2 hr.

■ **Available Forms:**
- *Capsules:* 100 mg, 200 mg, 400 mg.

■ **Indications and Dosages:**
Osteoarthritis: PO 200 mg/day as a single dose or 100 mg twice a day.
Rheumatoid arthritis: PO 100-200 mg twice a day.
Acute pain: PO Initially, 400 mg with additional 200 mg on day 1, if needed. Maintenance: 200 mg twice a day as needed.
Familial adenomatous polyposis: PO 400 mg twice daily (with food).
Ankylosing spondylitis: PO 200 mg/day as a single dose or in 2 divided doses. May increase to 400 mg/day if no effect is seen after 6 wk.

■ **Contraindications:** Hypersensitivity to aspirin, NSAIDs, or sulfonamides

■ **Side Effects**
Frequent (greater than 5%)
Diarrhea, dyspepsia, headache, upper respiratory tract infection
Occasional (5%-1%)
Abdominal pain, flatulence, nausea, back pain, peripheral edema, dizziness, rash

■ **Serious Reactions**
- There is an increased risk of cardiovascular events, including MI and cerebrovascular accident, and serious, potentially life-threatening, GI bleeding.

Special Considerations
- COX-2 specific inhibition good choice for patients with inflammatory conditions who are at high risk of gastrointestinal adverse effects (e.g., older than 60 years; history of peptic ulcer disease; prolonged, high-dose NSAID therapy; concurrent use of corticosteroids or anticoagulants)

■ **Patient/Family Education**
- Take celecoxib with food if GI upset occurs
- Avoid alcohol and aspirin during celecoxib therapy because these substances increase the risk of GI bleeding

■ **Monitoring Parameters**
- Rheumatoid arthritis—Decreased acute phase reactants (ESR, C-reactive protein), pain relief, reduction in number of swollen joints, improved range of motion, less fatigue, greater functional capacity, less structural damage, maintenance of normal lifestyle
- Osteoarthritis—Decreased pain and stiffness of affected joints
- Toxicity—Initial hematocrit, fecal occult blood, then q6-12 mo; electrolytes and renal function tests q6-12 mo; LFTs q6-12 mo in high-risk patients; query patient for dyspepsia, nausea, vomiting, right upper abdominal pain, anorexia, fatigue, jaundice, edema, weight gain, decreased urine output

■ **Geriatric side effects at a glance:**
☑ CNS ☐ Bowel Dysfunction ☐ Bladder Dysfunction ☐ Falls
☑ Other: Gastropathy

■ **Use with caution in older patients with:** Renal impairment, Hepatic impairment, Cardiovascular Disease, CHF, HTN, PUD, History of GI bleeding, GERD, Bleeding and platelet disorders, History of aspirin sensitivity reaction. Also use with caution in patients taking Anticoagulants, Aspirin, and Antihypertensive agents.

- **U.S. Regulatory Considerations**
  - ☑ FDA Black Box
  - Cardiovascular risk
  - Gastrointestinal risk
  - ❑ OBRA regulated in U.S. Long Term Care

- **Other Uses in Geriatric Patient:** None

- **Side Effects:**
  Of particular importance in the geriatric patient: Confusion, cognitive impairment, delirium, hallucinations, dyspepsia, fluid retention, renal impairment

- **Geriatric Considerations - Summary:** The use of low-dose aspirin for cardioprotection negates GI protection that may be offered by celecoxib. Older adults are at higher risk for adverse GI events with a COX-2 inhibitor. Use of celecoxib does not appear to offer increased safety as compared to a nonselective NSAID plus a proton pump inhibitor. Celecoxib offers no renal protection and may exacerbate underlying renal insufficiency. Patients with CHF and HTN may experience worsening control in the presence of celecoxib due to fluid retention. Patients receiving long-term celecoxib are at increased risk for cardiovascular death, MI, and stroke; doses greater than 200 mg/day significantly elevate the risk for these outcomes.

- **References:**
  1. Savage R. Cyclo-oxygenase-2 inhibitors: when should they be used in the elderly? Drugs Aging 2005;22:185-200.
  2. NSAID alternatives. Med Lett Drugs Ther 2005;47:8.
  3. COX-2 alternatives and GI protection. Med Lett Drugs Ther 2004;46:91.
  4. What about celebrex? Med Lett Drugs Ther 2004;46:87-88.
  5. Drugs that may cause psychiatric symptoms. Med Lett Drugs Ther 2002;44:59-62.
  6. Cardiovascular safety of COX-2 inhibitors. Med Lett Drugs Ther 2001;43:99-100.
  7. Drugs that may cause cognitive disorders in the elderly. Med Let 2000;42:111-112.

cellulose sodium phosphate

(sell'u-lose so'dee-um fos'fate)

- **Brand Name(s):** Calcibind
  Chemical Class: Phosphorylated cellulose

- **Clinical Pharmacology:**
  Mechanism of Action: A nonabsorbable compound that alters urinary composition of calcium, magnesium, phosphate, and oxalate. Calcium binds to cellulose sodium phosphate, thus preventing intestinal absorption of it. **Therapeutic Effect:** Prevents the formation of kidney stones.

- **Available Forms:**
  - *Powder for Reconstitution*: 300 g (Calcibind).

■ **Indications and Dosages:**
   Hypercalciuria Type I: Acute bleeding PO Initially, 15 g/day (5g with each meal). Decrease dosage to 10 g/day when urinary calcium is less than 150 mg/day.

■ **Unlabeled Uses:** Hypercalciuria Type II

■ **Contraindications:** Primary or secondary hyperparathyroidism, including hypercalciuria (renal calcium leak), hypomagnesemic states (serum magnesium less than 1.5 mg/dl), bone disease (osteoporosis, osteomalacia, osteitis), hypocalcemic states (e.g., hypoparathyroidism, intestinal malabsorption), normal or low intestinal absorption and renal excretion of calcium, enteric hyperoxaluria, and patients with high fasting urinary calcium or hypophosphatemia.

■ **Side Effects**
   Occasional
   GI disturbance, manifested by poor taste of the drug, loose bowel movements, diarrhea, dyspepsia.

■ **Serious Reactions**
   • Hyperoxaluria and hypomagnesiuria, which negate the beneficial effect of hypocalciuria on new stone formation, magnesium depletion, and depletion of trace metals (copper, zinc, iron) may occur.

■ **Patient/Family Education**
   • Suspend each dose of cellulose sodium phosphate (CSP) powder in glass of water, soft drink, or fruit juice
   • Ingest within 30 min of a meal
   • Avoid high sodium foods, vitamin C, and dairy products
   • Reduce intake of foods high in oxalate content such as spinach, chocolate, rhubarb, and brewed tea

■ **Monitoring Parameters**
   • Serum Ca, Mg, copper, zinc, iron, parathyroid hormone, CBC every 3-6 mo
   • Serum parathyroid hormone should be obtained at least once between the 1st 2 wk to 3 mo of treatment

■ **Geriatric side effects at a glance:**
   ❑ CNS ❑ Bowel Dysfunction ❑ Bladder Dysfunction ❑ Falls

■ **U.S. Regulatory Considerations**
   ❑ FDA Black Box ❑ OBRA regulated in U.S. Long Term Care

cephalexin

(sef-a-lex'-in)

- **Brand Name(s):** Biocef, Keflex, Keftab
  Chemical Class: Cephalosporin (1st generation)

- **Clinical Pharmacology:**
  Mechanism of Action: A first-generation cephalosporin that binds to bacterial cell membranes and inhibits cell wall synthesis. **Therapeutic Effect:** Bactericidal.
  Pharmacokinetics: Rapidly absorbed from the GI tract. Protein binding: 10%-15%. Widely distributed. Primarily excreted unchanged in urine. Moderately removed by hemodialysis. **Half-life:** 0.9-1.2 hr (increased in impaired renal function).

- **Available Forms:**
  - *Capsules:* 250 mg (Keflex), 500 mg (Biocef, Keflex).
  - *Tablets:* 250 mg, 500 mg (Keftab).

- **Indications and Dosages:**
  Bone infections, prophylaxis of rheumatic fever, follow-up to parenteral therapy: PO 250-500 mg q6h up to 4 g/day.
  Streptococcal pharyngitis, skin and skin-structure infections, uncomplicated cystitis: PO 500 mg q12h.
  Dosage in renal impairment: After usual initial dose, dosing frequency is modified based on creatinine clearance and the severity of the infection.

Creatinine Clearance	Dosage Interval
10-40 ml/min	usual dose q8-12h
less than 10 ml/min	usual dose q12-24h

- **Contraindications:** History of anaphylactic reaction to penicillins or hypersensitivity to cephalosporins

- **Side Effects**
  Frequent
  Oral candidiasis, mild diarrhea, mild abdominal cramping, vaginal candidiasis
  Occasional
  Nausea, serum sickness–like reaction (marked by fever and joint pain; usually occurs after the second course of therapy and resolves after the drug is discontinued)
  Rare
  Allergic reaction (rash, pruritus, urticaria)

- **Serious Reactions**
  - Antibiotic-associated colitis and other superinfections may result from altered bacterial balance.
  - Nephrotoxicity may occur, especially in patients with preexisting renal disease.
  - Patients with a history of allergies, especially to penicillin, are at increased risk for developing a severe hypersensitivity reaction, marked by severe pruritus, angioedema, bronchospasm, and anaphylaxis.

- 1st-generation oral cephalosporin of choice
- Individualize treatment based on local susceptibility patterns.

■ **Patient/Family Education**
- Space doses evenly around the clock and continue therapy for the full course of treatment
- Take the drug with food or milk if GI upset occurs

■ **Monitoring Parameters**
- Signs and symptoms of superinfection, including abdominal pain or cramping, moderate to severe diarrhea, severe anal or genital pruritus or discharge, and severe mouth or tongue soreness
- Daily bowel activity and stool consistency; although mild GI effects may be tolerable, severe symptoms may indicate the onset of antibiotic-associated colitis

■ **Geriatric side effects at a glance:**
   ❏ CNS ☑ Bowel Dysfunction ❏ Bladder Dysfunction ❏ Falls

■ **U.S. Regulatory Considerations**
   ❏ FDA Black Box ❏ OBRA regulated in U.S. Long Term Care

cephradine

(sef'-ra-deen)

■ **Brand Name(s):** Velosef
   Chemical Class: Cephalosporin (1st generation)

■ **Clinical Pharmacology:**
   Mechanism of Action: A first-generation cephalosporin that binds to bacterial cell membranes. Inhibits synthesis of bacterial cell wall. **Therapeutic Effect:** Bactericidal. **Pharmacokinetics:** Well absorbed from the gastrointestinal (GI) tract. Protein binding: 18%-20%. Widely distributed. Primarily excreted unchanged in urine. Removed by hemodialysis. **Half-life:** 1-2 hr (half-life is increased with impaired renal function).

■ **Available Forms:**
- *Capsules*: 250 mg, 500 mg (Velosef).

■ **Indications and Dosages:**
   Mild, moderate, or severe infections of the respiratory, and genitourinary (GU) tracts; bone, joint, and skin infections; prostatitis; otitis media: PO 250-500 mg q6h. Maximum: 8 g/day.
   Dosage in renal impairment: Dosage and frequency are based on the degree of renal impairment and the severity of infection. After initial 1-g dose:

Creatinine Clearance	Dosage Interval
10-50 ml/min	250 mg q6h
0-10 ml/min	125 mg q6h

■ **Contraindications:** History of hypersensitivity to penicillins and cephalosporins

■ **Side Effects**
Frequent
Diarrhea, mild abdominal cramping, vaginal candidiasis (discharge, itching)
Occasional
Nausea, headache, unusual bruising or bleeding, serum sickness–like reaction (fever, joint pain)
Rare
Allergic reaction (rash, pruritus, urticaria)

■ **Serious Reactions**
• Antibiotic-associated colitis as evidenced by severe abdominal pain and tenderness, fever, and watery and severe diarrhea, and other superinfections may result from altered bacterial balance.
• Nephrotoxicity may occur, especially in patients with preexisting renal disease.
• Severe hypersensitivity reaction including severe pruritus, angioedema, bronchospasm, and anaphylaxis, particularly in patients with history of allergies, especially penicillin, may occur.

Special Considerations
• No advantage over cephalexin; cost should be major consideration for selection of first-generation cephalosporins
• Individualize treatment based on local susceptibility patterns.

■ **Patient/Family Education**
• Space doses evenly around the clock and continue therapy for the full length of treatment

■ **Monitoring Parameters**
• Daily bowel activity and stool consistency; although mild GI effects may be tolerable, severe symptoms may indicate the onset of antibiotic-associated colitis
• Signs and symptoms of superinfection including anal or genital pruritus, changes or ulceration of the oral mucosa, moderate to severe diarrhea, and new or increased fever

■ **Geriatric side effects at a glance:**
❑ CNS ☑ Bowel Dysfunction ❑ Bladder Dysfunction ❑ Falls

■ **U.S. Regulatory Considerations**
❑ FDA Black Box ❑ OBRA regulated in U.S. Long Term Care

cetirizine hydrochloride

(se-ti'-ra-zeen hye-droe-klor'-ide)

■ **Brand Name(s):** Zyrtec

  Combinations
  Rx: with pseudoephedrine (Zyrtec-D 12 Hour Tablets)
  Chemical Class: Piperazine derivative

■ **Clinical Pharmacology:**
  Mechanism of Action: A second-generation piperazine that competes with histamine for H_1-receptor sites on effector cells in the GI tract, blood vessels, and respiratory tract. **Therapeutic Effect:** Prevents allergic response, produces mild bronchodilation, blocks histamine-induced bronchitis.
  Pharmacokinetics:

Route	Onset	Peak	Duration
PO	less than 1 hr	4–8 hr	less than 24 hr

  Rapidly and almost completely absorbed from the GI tract (absorption not affected by food). Protein binding: 93%. Undergoes low first-pass metabolism; not extensively metabolized. Primarily excreted in urine (more than 80% as unchanged drug). **Half-life:** 6.5–10 hr.

■ **Available Forms:**
  • *Syrup*: 5 mg/5 ml.
  • *Tablets*: 5 mg, 10 mg.
  • *Tablets (Chewable)*: 5 mg, 10 mg.

■ **Indications and Dosages:**
  Allergic rhinitis, urticaria: PO Initially, 5–10 mg/day as a single or in 2 divided doses.
  Dosage in renal or hepatic impairment: For patients with renal impairment (creatinine clearance of 11–31 ml/min), those receiving hemodialysis (creatinine clearance of less than 7 ml/min), and those with hepatic impairment, dosage is decreased to 5 mg once a day.

■ **Unlabeled Uses:** Treatment of bronchial asthma

■ **Contraindications:** Hypersensitivity to cetirizine or hydroxyzine

■ **Side Effects**
  Occasional (10%–2%)
  Pharyngitis; dry mucous membranes, nose, or throat; nausea and vomiting; abdominal pain; headache; dizziness; fatigue; thickening of mucus; somnolence; photosensitivity; urine retention

■ **Serious Reactions**
  • Dizziness, sedation, and confusion may occur.

Special Considerations
  • H_1 antagonist with minimal effect on CNS; no affinity for other receptors
  • Very potent antihistamine

- Kinetics allow qd dosing and do not have cytochrome P-450 drug interactions
- Effective against itching

■ **Patient/Family Education**
- Avoid performing tasks that require alertness or motor skills until response to the drug has been established; cetirizine may cause drowsiness
- Avoid alcohol during cetirizine therapy
- Avoid prolonged exposure to sunlight

■ **Monitoring Parameters**
- Ensure that the patient with upper respiratory allergies increases fluid intake to maintain thin secretions and offset thirst
- Monitor the patient's symptoms for a therapeutic response

■ **Geriatric side effects at a glance:**
❑ CNS   ❑ Bowel Dysfunction   ❑ Bladder Dysfunction   ❑ Falls
Other: Cognitive impairment, Sedation

■ **Use with caution in older patients with:** Renal impairment, Cognitive impairment

■ **U.S. Regulatory Considerations**
❑ FDA Black Box   ❑ OBRA regulated in U.S. Long Term Care

■ **Other Uses in Geriatric Patient:** None

■ **Side Effects:**
Of *particular importance in the geriatric patient*: Impaired attention, agitation, decreased concentration, sedation, anticholinergic effects, cognitive impairment, vertigo, headache, dry mouth, urinary retention

■ **Geriatric Considerations - Summary:** Clearance and half-life are altered in older adults; therefore reduce starting dose. More sedating than fexofenadine and loratadine; consider an alternate second-generation antihistamine.

■ **References:**
1. Hansen J, Klimek L, Hormann K. Pharmacological management of allergic rhinitis in the elderly. Safety issues with oral antihistamines. Drugs Aging 2005;22:289-296.
2. Newer Antihistamines. Med Lett 2001;43.
3. Drugs that may cause cognitive disorders in the elderly. Med Lett 2000;42:111-112.
4. Mann RD, Pearce GL, Dunn N, Shakir S. Sedation with non-sedating antihistamines: four prescription-event monitoring studies in general practice. BMJ 2000;320:1184-1187.
5. Simons FER, Fraser TG, Maher J, et. al. Central nervous system effects of H1-receptor antagonists in the elderly. Ann Allergy Asthma Immunol 1999;82:157-160.

cevimeline hydrochloride

(se-vim'-e-leen hye-droe-klor'-ide)

■ **Brand Name(s):** Evoxac
Chemical Class: Oxathiolane derivative

■ **Clinical Pharmacology:**
Mechanism of Action: A cholinergic agonist that binds to muscarinic receptors of effector cells, thereby increasing secretion of exocrine glands, such as salivary glands.
Therapeutic Effect: Relieves dry mouth.
Pharmacokinetics: Rapidly absorbed following PO administration. Protein binding: less than 20%. Metabolized in liver. Primarily excreted in urine; minimal elimination in feces. **Half-life:** 5 hr.

■ **Available Forms:**
- *Capsules*: 30 mg.

■ **Indications and Dosages:**
Dry mouth: PO 30 mg 3 times a day.

■ **Contraindications:** Acute iritis, angle-closure glaucoma, uncontrolled asthma

■ **Side Effects**
Frequent (19%–11%)
Diaphoresis, headache, nausea, sinusitis, rhinitis, upper respiratory tract infection, diarrhea
Occasional (10%–3%)
Dyspepsia, abdominal pain, cough, UTI, vomiting, back pain, rash, dizziness, fatigue
Rare (2%–1%)
Skeletal pain, insomnia, hot flashes, excessive salivation, rigors, anxiety

■ **Serious Reactions**
- Cevimeline use may result in decreased visual acuity, especially at night, and impaired depth perception.

■ **Patient/Family Education**
- May cause visual disturbance, use caution driving at night or performing hazardous activities in reduced lighting
- Ensure adequate fluid intake to prevent dehydration, especially if drug causes excessive sweating

■ **Monitoring Parameters**
- Monitor patients with a cardiovascular disease for an increase in the frequency, duration, or severity of angina or changes in blood pressure or heart rate

■ **Geriatric side effects at a glance:**
  ❏ CNS ☑ Bowel Dysfunction ❏ Bladder Dysfunction ❏ Falls

■ **U.S. Regulatory Considerations**
  ❏ FDA Black Box ❏ OBRA regulated in U.S. Long Term Care

charcoal, activated

■ **Brand Name(s):** Actidose-Aqua, Actidose with Sorbitol, Aqueous CharcoAid, Charcoal Plus DS, Charcocaps, EZ-Char, Kerr Insta-Char, Liqui-Char

  Combinations
  OTC: with simethicone (Charcoal Plus, Flatulex); with sorbitol (Actidose with Sorbitol)
  Chemical Class: Carbon

■ **Clinical Pharmacology:**
  Mechanism of Action: An antidote that adsorbs (detoxifies) ingested toxic substances, irritants, intestinal gas. **Therapeutic Effect:** Inhibits gastrointestinal (GI) absorption and absorbs intestinal gas.
  Pharmacokinetics: Not orally absorbed from the GI tract. Not metabolized. Excreted in feces as charcoal. **Half-life:** Unknown.

■ **Available Forms:**
  • *Capsules, activated*: 260 mg (Charcocaps).
  • *Granules, activated*: 15g (CharcoAid-G).
  • *Liquid, activated*: 15g (Actidose-Aqua, Liqui-Char); 25g (Actidose-Aqua, Kerr Insta-Char, Liqui-Char); 50g (Actidose-Aqua, Kerr Insta-Char).
  • *Liquid, activated*: 25g (Actidose with Sorbitol, Liqui-Char, Kerr Insta-Char); 50g (Actidose with Sorbitol, Liqui-Char, Kerr Insta-Char).
  • *Pellets, activated*: 25g (EZ-Char).
  • *Powder for Suspension, activated*: 30 g, 240 g.
  • *Tablets, activated*: 250 mg (Charcol Plus DS).

■ **Indications and Dosages:**
  Acute poisoning: PO Give 30-100 g as slurry (30 g in at least 8 oz H_2O) or 12.5-50 g in aqueous or sorbitol suspension. Usually given as single dose.

■ **Contraindications:** Intestinal obstruction, GI tract not anatomically intact; patients at risk of hemorrhage or GI perforation, if use would increase risk and severity of aspiration; not effective for cyanide, mineral acids, caustic alkalis, organic solvents, iron, ethanol, methanol poisoning, lithium; do not use charcoal with sorbitol in patients with fructose intolerance, hypersensitivity to charcoal or any component of the formulation

■ **Side Effects**
  Occasional
  Diarrhea, GI discomfort, intestinal gas

Serious Reactions
- Hypernatremia, hypokalemia, and hypermagnesemia may occur with coadministration of cathartics.

Special Considerations
- Administer activated charcoal for adsorption in emergency management of poisonings as a slurry with water, a saline cathartic, or sorbitol

Patient/Family Education
- Charcoal causes stool to turn black

Monitoring Parameters
- Vital signs
- Electrolytes

Geriatric side effects at a glance:
❑ CNS ❑ Bowel Dysfunction ❑ Bladder Dysfunction ❑ Falls

U.S. Regulatory Considerations
❑ FDA Black Box ❑ OBRA regulated in U.S. Long Term Care

chloral hydrate

(klor-al hye'-drate)

Brand Name(s): Aquachloral Supprettes, Somnote
Chemical Class: Halogenated alcohol

DEA Class: Schedule IV

Clinical Pharmacology:
Mechanism of Action: A nonbarbiturate chloral derivative that produces CNS depression. *Therapeutic Effect*: Induces quiet, deep sleep, with only a slight decrease in respiratory rate and BP.
Pharmacokinetics: Readily absorbed from the GI tract following PO administration. Well absorbed following rectal administration. Protein binding: 70%-80%. Metabolized in liver and erythrocytes to the active metabolite, trichloroethanol, which may be further metabolized to inactive metabolites. Excreted in urine. *Half-life*: 7-10 hr (trichloroethanol).

Available Forms:
- *Capsules (Somnote)*: 500 mg.
- *Syrup*: 500 mg/5 ml.
- *Suppositories (Aquachloral Supprettes)*: 324 mg, 648 mg.

Indications and Dosages:
Premedication for dental or medical procedures: PO, Rectal 0.5–1 g.
Premedication for EEG: PO, Rectal 0.5–1.5 g.

■ **Contraindications:** Gastritis, marked hepatic or renal impairment, severe cardiac disease

■ **Side Effects**
Occasional
Gastric irritation (nausea, vomiting, flatulence, diarrhea), rash, sleepwalking
Rare
Headache, excitement or restlessness (particularly in patients with pain).

■ **Serious Reactions**
- Overdose may produce somnolence, confusion, slurred speech, severe incoordination, respiratory depression, and coma.
- Allergic-type reaction may occur in those with tartrazine sensitivity.

Special Considerations
- Not as effective as benzodiazepines, loses much of effectiveness for inducing and maintaining sleep after 2 wk of use

■ **Patient/Family Education**
- May cause GI upset, recommend administration with full glass of water or fruit juice; dilute syrup in a half glass of water or fruit juice

■ **Geriatric side effects at a glance:**
☑ CNS ☐ Bowel Dysfunction ☐ Bladder Dysfunction ☑ Falls
Other: Withdrawal symptoms after long-term use

■ **Use with caution in older patients with:** Not recommended for use in older adults.

■ **U.S. Regulatory Considerations**
☐ FDA Black Box ☑ OBRA regulated in U.S. Long Term Care

■ **Other Uses in Geriatric Patient:** Anxiety disorders, sleep disorders

■ **Side Effects:**
Of particular importance in the geriatric patient: Sedation, withdrawal symptoms when abruptly discontinued (e.g., during hospitalization) rather than tapered

■ **Geriatric Considerations - Summary:** Because chloral hydrate has a low therapeutic window, rapid development of tolerance, and drug interactions, it is not recommended for use in older adults.

chloramphenicol

(klor-am-fen'-i-kole)

■ **Brand Name(s):** Systemic: AK-Chlor, Chloromycetin, Chloromycetin Ophthalmic, Chloromycetin Sodium Succinate, Chloroptic, Chloroptic S.O.P., Ocu-Chlor

Combinations
Rx: Ophthalmic: Hydrocortisone acetate and polymixin B sulfate (Opthocort); hydrocortisone acetate (Chloromycetin Hydrocortisone)
Chemical Class: Dichloroacetic acid derivative

■ **Clinical Pharmacology:**
Mechanism of Action: A dichloroacetic acid derivative that inhibits bacterial protein synthesis by binding to bacterial ribosomal receptor sites. **Therapeutic Effect:** Bacteriostatic (may be bactericidal in high concentrations).
Pharmacokinetics: Rapidly and completely absorbed from the GI tract following PO administration. Well absorbed after IM administration. Some systemic absorption following ophthalmic and otic administration. Protein binding: 50%-80%. Metabolized in liver. Excreted in urine. **Half-life:** 1.5-3.5 hr.

■ **Available Forms:**
- *Powder for Injection (Chloromycetin Sodium Succinate):* 1 g.
- *Powder for Reconstitution (Ophthalmic [Chloromycetin Ophthalmic]):* 25 mg.
- *Ophthalmic Ointment (AK-Chlor, Chloroptic S.O.P., Ocu-Chlor):* 1%.
- *Ophthalmic Solution (Chloroptic, AK-Chlor, Ocu-Chlor):* 0.5%.

■ **Indications and Dosages:**
Mild to moderate infections caused by organisms resistant to other less toxic antibacterials: IV 50-100 mg/kg/day in divided doses q6h. Maximum: 4 g/day.
Usual ophthalmic dosage: 1-2 drops 4-6 times/day.

■ **Contraindications:** Hypersensitivity to chloramphenicol

■ **Side Effects**
Occasional
Systemic: Nausea, vomiting, diarrhea
Ophthalmic: Blurred vision, burning, stinging, hypersensitivity reaction
Otic: Hypersensitivity reaction
Rare
Peripheral neuritis (numbness and weakness in feet and hands), rash, shortness of breath, confusion, headache, optic neuritis (blurred vision, eye pain)

■ **Serious Reactions**
- Superinfection due to bacterial or fungal overgrowth may occur.
- There is a narrow margin between effective therapy and toxic levels producing blood dyscrasias.
- Myelosuppression, with resulting aplastic anemia, hypoplastic anemia, and pancytopenia, may occur weeks or months later.

- Because of severe adverse effects (e.g., aplastic anemia), not indicated for less serious infections; aplastic anemia reported with topical use

■ **Patient/Family Education**
- Space doses evenly around the clock
- Monitor for signs and symptoms of infection

■ **Monitoring Parameters**
- CBC with platelets and reticulocytes before and frequently during therapy (discontinue drug if bone marrow suppression occurs); serum iron and iron-binding globulin saturation may also be useful
- Serum drug level (peak 10-20 mcg/ml, trough 5-10 mcg/ml) weekly (more often in impaired hepatic, renal systems)
- Daily bowel activity and stool consistency

■ **Geriatric side effects at a glance:**
❑ CNS ❑ Bowel Dysfunction ❑ Bladder Dysfunction ❑ Falls

■ **U.S. Regulatory Considerations**
☑ FDA Black Box
Serious and fatal blood dyscrasias have occurred. Use only in serious infections.
❑ OBRA regulated in U.S. Long Term Care

chlordiazepoxide hydrochloride

(klor-dye-az-e-pox'-ide hye-droe-klor'-ide)

■ **Brand Name(s):** Libritabs, Librium, Mitran, Reposans-10

Combinations
Rx: with amitriptyline (Limbitrol DS 10-25); with clidinium (Clindex, Librax)
Chemical Class: Benzodiazepine

DEA Class: Schedule IV

■ **Clinical Pharmacology:**
Mechanism of Action: A benzodiazepine that enhances the action of the inhibitory neurotransmitter gamma-aminobutyric acid in the CNS. **Therapeutic Effect:** Produces anxiolytic effect.
Pharmacokinetics: Well absorbed from the GI tract following PO administration. Poor absorption following IM administration. Protein binding: 90%-98%. Extensively metabolized in liver. Excreted in urine. Not removed by hemodialysis. **Half-life:** 10-48 hr.

■ **Available Forms:**
- **Capsules:** 5 mg (Librium), 10 mg (Libritabs, Librium); 25 mg (Librium).
- **Injection Powder for Reconstitution (Librium):** 100 mg.

■ **Indications and Dosages:**
Alcohol withdrawal symptoms: PO 50-100 mg. May repeat q2-4h. Maximum: 300 mg/24 hr.
Anxiety: PO 5 mg 2-4 times a day. IV, IM Initially, 50-100 mg, then 25-50 mg 3-4 times a day as needed.
Preoperative anxiety: IM 50-100 mg once.

■ **Unlabeled Uses:** Treatment of panic disorder, tension headache, tremors

■ **Contraindications:** Acute alcohol intoxication, acute angle-closure glaucoma

■ **Side Effects**
Frequent
Pain at IM injection site; somnolence, ataxia, dizziness, confusion with oral dose (particularly in elderly or debilitated patients)
Occasional
Rash, peripheral edema, GI disturbances
Rare
Paradoxical CNS reactions, such as excitement or restlessness in the elderly (generally noted during first 2 wk of therapy, particularly in presence of uncontrolled pain)

■ **Serious Reactions**
- IV administration may produce pain, swelling, thrombophlebitis, and carpal tunnel syndrome.
- Abrupt or too-rapid withdrawal may result in pronounced restlessness, irritability, insomnia, hand tremors, abdominal or muscle cramps, diaphoresis, vomiting, and seizures.
- Overdose results in somnolence, confusion, diminished reflexes, and coma.

Special Considerations
- No advantage over other benzodiazepines; poor choice for elderly patients
- Do not use for everyday stress or use longer than 4 mo
- Do not discontinue medication abruptly after long-term use

■ **Patient/Family Education**
- Change positions slowly – from recumbent to sitting before standing – to prevent dizziness
- Avoid alcohol while taking this drug

■ **Geriatric side effects at a glance:**
☑ CNS ☐ Bowel Dysfunction ☐ Bladder Dysfunction ☑ Falls
Other: Withdrawal symptoms after long-term use

■ **Use with caution in older patients with:** COPD; untreated sleep apnea

■ **U.S. Regulatory Considerations**
☐ FDA Black Box ☑ OBRA regulated in U.S. Long Term Care

■ **Other Uses in Geriatric Patient:** Anxiety symptoms and related disorders, dementia-related behavioral problems, skeletal muscle strain

- **Side Effects:**
  Of particular importance in the geriatric patient: Sedation, withdrawal symptoms when abruptly discontinued (e.g., during hospitalization) rather than tapered

- **Geriatric Considerations - Summary:** Benzodiazepines are effective anxiolytic agents, and hypnotics. These drugs should be reserved for short-term use. SSRIs are preferred for long-term management of anxiety disorders in older adults, and sedating antidepressants (e.g., trazodone) or eszopiclone are preferred for long-term management of sleep problems. Long-acting benzodiazepines, including flurazepam, chlordiazepoxide, clorazepate, diazepam, clonazepam, and quazepam should generally be avoided in older adults as these agents have been associated with oversedation. On the other hand, short-acting benzodiazepines (e.g., triazolam) have been associated with a higher risk of withdrawal symptoms. When initiating therapy, benzodiazepines should be titrated carefully to avoid oversedation. In addition, many of the drugs in this class have been associated with severe withdrawal symptoms (e.g., anxiety and/or agitation, seizures) when discontinued abruptly.

- **References:**
  1. Leipzig RM, Cumming RG, Tinetti ME. Drugs and falls in older people: a systematic review and meta-analysis: I. Psychotropic drugs. J Am Geriatr Soc 1999;47:30-39.
  2. Shorr RI, Robin DW. Rational use of benzodiazepines in the elderly. Drugs Aging 1994;4:9-20.
  3. Shader RI, Greenblatt DJ. Use of benzodiazepines in anxiety disorders. N Engl J Med 1993;328:1398-1405.

chlorothiazide

(klor-oh-thye'-a-zide)

- **Brand Name(s):** Diuril, Diuril Sodium

  Combinations
  Rx: with methyldopa (Aldoclor); with reserpine (Chloroserp, Diaserp, Diupres)
  Chemical Class: Sulfonamide derivative

- **Clinical Pharmacology:**
  Mechanism of Action: A sulfonamide derivative that acts as a thiazide diuretic and antihypertensive. As a diuretic, blocks reabsorption of water and the electrolytes sodium and potassium at cortical diluting segment of distal tubule. As an antihypertensive, reduces plasma and extracellular fluid volume, decreases peripheral vascular resistance (PVR) by direct effect on blood vessels. **Therapeutic Effect:** Promotes diuresis, reduces BP.
  Pharmacokinetics: Poorly absorbed from the gastrointestinal (GI) tract. Not metabolized. Primarily excreted unchanged in urine. Not removed by hemodialysis. **Half-life:** 45-120 min.

- **Available Forms:**
  - *Powder for Injection, lyophilized:* 0.5 g.
  - *Oral Suspension:* 250 mg/5 ml (Diuril).
  - *Tablets:* 250 mg, 500 mg (Diuril).

■ **Indications and Dosages:**
  Edema, hypertension: PO 0.5-1g 1-2 times/day. May give every other day or 3-5 days/wk.
  Hypertension: IV 0.5-1g in divided doses q12-24h.

■ **Unlabeled Uses:** Treatment of diabetes insipidus, prevention of calcium-containing renal stones

■ **Contraindications:** Anuria, history of hypersensitivity to sulfonamides or thiazide diuretics, renal decompensation

■ **Side Effects**
  Expected
  Increase in urine frequency and volume
  Frequent
  Potassium depletion
  Occasional
  Postural hypotension, headache, GI disturbances, photosensitivity reaction, muscle spasms, alopecia, rash, urticaria

■ **Serious Reactions**
  • Vigorous diuresis may lead to profound water loss and electrolyte depletion, resulting in hypokalemia, hyponatremia, and dehydration.
  • Acute hypotensive episodes may occur.
  • Hyperglycemia may be noted during prolonged therapy.
  • GI upset, pancreatitis, dizziness, paresthesias, headache, blood dyscrasias, pulmonary edema, allergic pneumonitis, and dermatologic reactions occur rarely.
  • Overdosage can lead to lethargy and coma without changes in electrolytes or hydration.

Special Considerations
  • Doses above 250 mg provide no further blood pressure reduction, but are more likely to induce metabolic disturbance (hypokalemia, hyperuricemia, etc.)
  • May protect against osteoporotic hip fractures
  • Loop diuretics or metolazone more effective if CrCl less than 40-50 ml/min
  • Although allergic cross-reactivity with sulfonamide antibiotics and sulfonamide nonantibiotics has not been demonstrated, use with caution in patients with a history of severe sulfa allergies.

■ **Patient/Family Education**
  • Will increase urination temporarily (approximately 3 wk); take early in the day to prevent sleep disturbance
  • May cause sensitivity to sunlight; avoid prolonged exposure to the sun and other ultraviolet light
  • May cause gout attacks; notify clinician if sudden joint pain occurs

■ **Monitoring Parameters**
  • Weight, urine output, serum electrolytes, BUN, creatinine, CBC, uric acid, glucose, lipids

■ **Geriatric side effects at a glance:**
  ❑ CNS ❑ Bowel Dysfunction ❑ Bladder Dysfunction ❑ Falls

chloroxine

(klor-ox'-ine)

■ **Brand Name(s):** Capitrol
    Chemical Class: Hydroxyquinoline derivative

■ **Clinical Pharmacology:**
    Mechanism of Action: An antifungal that reduces scaling of the epidermis by slowing down mitotic activity. **Therapeutic Effect:** Reduces the excess scaling in patients with dandruff or seborrheic dermatitis.
    Pharmacokinetics: No studies have investigated the absorption/pharmacokinetics of chloroxine.

■ **Available Forms:**
    • *Shampoo:* 2% (Capitrol).

■ **Indications and Dosages:**
    Dandruff, seborrheic dermatitis: Shampoo affected area twice weekly.

■ **Unlabeled Uses:** None known.

■ **Contraindications:** Acutely inflamed lesions, hypersensitivity to chloroxine or any one of its components.

■ **Side Effects**
    Discoloration of light hair, skin irritation, burning

■ **Serious Reactions**
    • None known.

■ **Patient/Family Education**
    • Improvement may not occur for 14 days
    • Hair may be discolored after use
    • Avoid contact with eyes

■ **Monitoring Parameters**
    • Skin for irritation
    • Hair for discoloration

■ **Geriatric side effects at a glance:**
    ❑ CNS   ❑ Bowel Dysfunction   ❑ Bladder Dysfunction   ❑ Falls

chlorpheniramine maleate

(klor-fen-ir'-a-meen mal'-ee-ate)

OTC: Aller-Chlor, Chlor-Trimeton, Chlor-Trimeton Allergy, Chlor-Trimeton Allergy 12 Hour, Chlor-Trimeton Allergy 8 Hour, Chlorate, Chlorphen, Diabetic Tussin Allergy Relief

Combinations
Rx: with codeine (Codeprex); with hydrocodone (Tussionex); with phenylephrine and pyrilamine (Rynaton); with phenylpropanolamine (Ornade, Resaid S.R.); with pseudoephedrine (Deconamine, Fedahist)
OTC: with pseudoephedrine (Chlor-Trimeton, Dorcol Children's Cold Formula Liquid, Fedahist)
Chemical Class: Alkylamine derivative

■ **Clinical Pharmacology:**
Mechanism of Action: A propylamine derivative antihistamine that competes with histamine for histamine receptor sites on cells in the blood vessels, gastrointestinal (GI) tract, and respiratory tract. **Therapeutic Effect:** Inhibits symptoms associated with seasonal allergic rhinitis such as increased mucus production and sneezing.
Pharmacokinetics: Well absorbed after PO and parenteral administration. Food delays absorption. Widely distributed. Metabolized in liver. Primarily excreted in urine. Not removed by dialysis. **Half-life:** 20 hr.

■ **Available Forms:**
   • **Injection:** 10 mg/ml, 100 mg/ml.
   • **Syrup:** 2 mg/5 ml (Aller-Chlor, Diabetic Tussin Allergy Relief [sugar free]).
   • **Tablets:** 4 mg (Aller-Chlor, Chlor-Trimeton, Chlorate, Chlorphen).
   • **Tablets (sustained-release):** 8 mg (Chlor-Trimeton Allergy 8 Hour); 12 mg (Chlor-Trimeton Allergy 12 Hour).

■ **Indications and Dosages:**
Allergic rhinitis, common cold: PO 4 mg q6-8h or 8-12 mg (sustained-release) q8-12h. Maximum: 24 mg/day. IM, IV, SC 5-40 mg as a single dose. Maximum: 40 mg/day.

■ **Contraindications:** Hypersensitivity to chlorpheniramine or its components

■ **Side Effects**
Frequent
Drowsiness, dizziness, muscular weakness, hypotension, dry mouth, nose, throat, and lips, urinary retention, thickening of bronchial secretions
Occasional
Epigastric distress, flushing, visual or hearing disturbances, paresthesia, diaphoresis, chills

■ Serious Reactions
- Hypersensitivity reaction, such as eczema, pruritus, rash, cardiac disturbances, and photosensitivity, may occur.
- Overdosage may vary from CNS depression, including sedation, apnea, hypotension, cardiovascular collapse, or death to severe paradoxical reaction, such as hallucinations, tremor, and seizures.

Special Considerations
- More potent antihistamine than nonsedating agents (e.g., fexofenadine), good first-line choice for allergic rhinitis

■ Patient/Family Education
- Tolerance develops to sedation with chronic use
- Dizziness, drowsiness, and dry mouth are expected responses to the drug
- Avoid tasks that require mental alertness or motor skills until response to the drug is established

■ Geriatric side effects at a glance:
☑ CNS ☑ Bowel Dysfunction ☑ Bladder Dysfunction ☑ Falls
Other: Dry mouth, blurred vision, confusion, psychoses

■ Use with caution in older patients with: Narrow-angle glaucoma, overflow incontinence, psychosis.

■ U.S. Regulatory Considerations
❏ FDA Black Box ☑ OBRA regulated in U.S. Long Term Care

■ Other Uses in Geriatric Patient: None

■ Side Effects:
Of particular importance in the geriatric patient: Anticholinergic effects

■ Geriatric Considerations - Summary: Chlorpheniramine is a first-generation alkylamine antihistamine with potent H_1-receptor antagonism. It has anticholinergic activity and can cause somnolence. Older adults taking this drug are at risk of dizziness and hypotension.

■ References:
1. Bantz EW, Dolen WK, Chadwick EW, et al: Chronic chlorpheniramine therapy: subsensitivity, drug metabolism, and compliance. Ann Allergy 1987; 59:341-346.
2. Tune LE. Anticholinergic effects of medication in elderly patients. J Clin Psychiatry 2001;62(suppl 21):11-14.

chlorpromazine

(klor-proe'-ma-zeen)

- **Brand Name(s):** Thorazine
  Chemical Class: Aliphatic phenothiazine derivative

- **Clinical Pharmacology:**
  Mechanism of Action: A phenothiazine that blocks dopamine neurotransmission at postsynaptic dopamine receptor sites. Possesses strong anticholinergic, sedative, and antiemetic effects; moderate extrapyramidal effects; and slight antihistamine action. **Therapeutic Effect:** Relieves nausea and vomiting; improves psychotic conditions; controls intractable hiccups and porphyria.
  Pharmacokinetics: Rapidly absorbed after oral or IM administration. Protein binding: 92%-97%. Metabolized in the liver. Excreted in urine. **Half-life:** 6 hr.

- **Available Forms:**
  - *Oral Concentrate*: 30 mg/ml, 100 mg/ml.
  - *Syrup*: 10 mg/5 ml.
  - *Tablets*: 10 mg, 25 mg, 50 mg, 100 mg, 200 mg.
  - *Capsules (Sustained-Release)*: 30 mg, 75 mg, 150 mg.
  - *Injection*: 25 mg/ml.
  - *Suppositories*: 25 mg, 100 mg.

- **Indications and Dosages:**
  Severe nausea or vomiting: PO 10-25 mg q4-6h. IV, IM 25-50 mg q4-6h. Rectal 50-100 mg q6-8h.
  Psychotic disorders: PO 30-800 mg/day in 1-4 divided doses. IV, IM Initially, 25 mg; may repeat in 1-4 hr. May gradually increase to 400 mg q4-6h. Usual dose: 300-800 mg/day.
  Intractable hiccups: PO, IV, IM 25-50 mg 3 times a day
  Porphyria: PO 25-50 mg 3-4 times a day. IM 25 mg 3-4 times a day.

- **Unlabeled Uses:** Treatment of choreiform movement of Huntington's disease

- **Contraindications:** Comatose states, myelosuppression, severe cardiovascular disease, severe CNS depression, subcortical brain damage

- **Side Effects**
  Frequent
  Somnolence, blurred vision, hypotension, color vision or night vision disturbances, dizziness, decreased sweating, constipation, dry mouth, nasal congestion
  Occasional
  Urinary retention, photosensitivity, rash, decreased sexual function, swelling or pain in breasts, weight gain, nausea, vomiting, abdominal pain, tremors

- **Serious Reactions**
  - Extrapyramidal symptoms appear to be dose related and are divided into three categories: akathisia (including inability to sit still, tapping of feet), parkinsonian symptoms (such as mask-like face, tremors, shuffling gait, hypersalivation), and acute dystonias (including torticollis, opisthotonos, and oculogyric crisis). A dystonic reaction may also produce diaphoresis and pallor.

- Tardive dyskinesia, including tongue protrusion, puffing of the cheeks, and puckering of the mouth, is a rare reaction that may be irreversible.
- Abrupt discontinuation after long-term therapy may precipitate nausea, vomiting, gastritis, dizziness, and tremors.
- Blood dyscrasias, particularly agranulocytosis and mild leukopenia, may occur.
- Chlorpromazine may lower the seizure threshold.

■ Patient/Family Education
- Orthostasis on rising
- Avoid hot tubs, hot showers, tub baths
- Meticulous oral hygiene; frequent rinsing of mouth, sugarless gum for dry mouth
- Use a sunscreen and sunglasses
- Urine may turn pink or red
- Drowsiness generally subsides with continued therapy
- Avoid tasks that require mental alertness or motor skills until response to the drug is established
- Avoid alcohol

■ Monitoring Parameters
- Blood pressure
- CBC
- Though not used clinically, therapeutic serum level for chlorpromazine is 50-300 mcg/ml, and the toxic serum level is greater than 750 mcg/ml

■ Geriatric side effects at a glance:
☑ CNS   ☑ Bowel Dysfunction   ☑ Bladder Dysfunction   ☑ Falls

Other: Orthostatic hypotension, cardiac conduction disturbances, Torsades de Pointes, anticholinergic side effects

■ Use with caution in older patients with:
Parkinson's Disease (an atypical antipsychotic is recommended), seizure disorders, cardiovascular disease with conduction disturbance, hepatic encephalopathy, narrow-angle glaucoma, congenital prolonged Q-T syndrome or drugs which prolong Q-T interval.

■ U.S. Regulatory Considerations
❑ FDA Black Box   ☑ OBRA regulated in U.S. Long Term Care

■ Other Uses in Geriatric Patient:
Behavior disturbances in the setting of dementia

■ Side Effects:
Of *particular importance in the geriatric patient:* Tardive dyskinesia, akathisia (may appear to exacerbate behavioral disturbances), anticholinergic effects, may increase risk of sudden death

■ Geriatric Considerations - Summary:
Sink and colleagues' systematic review showed statistically significant improvements on neuropsychiatric and behavioral scales for some drugs, but improvements were small and unlikely to be clinically important. Because of documented risks and uncertain benefits, these agents should be used with caution in demented elderly persons, with frequent monitoring for side effects and a low threshold for discontinuing use.

■ **References:**
1. Leipzig RM, Cumming RG, Tinetti ME. Drugs and falls in older people: a systematic review and meta-analysis: I. Psychotropic drugs. J Am Geriatr Soc 1999;47:30-39.
2. Sink KM, Holden KF, Yaffe K. Pharmacological treatment of neuropsychiatric symptoms of dementia: a review of the evidence. JAMA 2005;293:596-608.
3. Ray WA, Meredith S, Thapa PB, et al. Antipsychotics and the risk of sudden cardiac death. Arch Gen Psychiatry 2001;58:1161-1167.

chlorpropamide

(klor-proe'-pa-mide)

■ **Brand Name(s):** Diabinese
   Chemical Class: Sulfonylurea (1st generation)

■ **Clinical Pharmacology:**
   Mechanism of Action: A first-generation sulfonylurea that promotes release of insulin from beta cells of pancreas. **Therapeutic Effect:** Lowers blood glucose concentration. **Pharmacokinetics:** Rapidly absorbed from the gastrointestinal (GI) tract. Protein binding: 60%-90%. Extensively metabolized in liver. Excreted primarily in urine. Removed by hemodialysis. **Half-life:** 30-42 hr.

■ **Available Forms:**
   • *Tablets:* 100 mg, 250 mg (Diabinese).

■ **Indications and Dosages:**
   Diabetes mellitus, combination therapy: PO Initially, 100-125 mg once a day. Maintenance: 100-250 mg once a day. Increase or decrease by 50-125 mg a day for 3- to 5-day intervals.
   Renal function impairment: Not recommended.

■ **Unlabeled Uses:** Neurogenic diabetes insipidus

■ **Contraindications:** Diabetic complications, such as ketosis, acidosis, and diabetic coma, severe liver or renal impairment, sole therapy for type 1 diabetes mellitus, or hypersensitivity to sulfonylureas

■ **Side Effects**
   Frequent
   Headache, upper respiratory tract infection
   Occasional
   Sinusitis, myalgia (muscle aches), pharyngitis, aggravated diabetes mellitus

■ **Serious Reactions**
   • Possible increased risk of cardiovascular mortality with this class of drugs.
   • Overdosage can cause severe hypoglycemia prolonged by extended half-life.

- Due to potential for prolonged hypoglycemia, other sulfonylureas should be considered before trying chlorpropamide (especially in the elderly)
- Although allergic cross-reactivity with sulfonamide antibiotics and sulfonamide nonantibiotics has not been demonstrated, use with caution in patients with a history of severe sulfa allergies.

■ Patient/Family Education

- Multiple drug interactions, including alcohol and salicylates
- Symptoms of hypoglycemia: tingling lips/tongue, nausea, confusion, fatigue, sweating, hunger, visual changes (spots)
- Carry candy, sugar packets, or other sugar supplements for immediate response to hypoglycemia
- Notify the physician if abdominal or chest pain, dark urine or light stool, hypoglycemia reactions, fever, nausea, palpitations, rash, vomiting, or yellowing of eyes or skin occurs

■ Monitoring Parameters

- Self-monitored blood glucose; glycosolated hemoglobin q3-6 mo
- Liver function

■ Geriatric side effects at a glance:

❑ CNS ❑ Bowel Dysfunction ❑ Bladder Dysfunction ❑ Falls
Other: Hypoglycemia

■ Use with caution in older patients with: Impaired hepatic function, Impaired renal function

■ U.S. Regulatory Considerations

❑ FDA Black Box ❑ OBRA regulated in U.S. Long Term Care

■ Other Uses in Geriatric Patient: Partial neurogenic diabetes insipidus

■ Side Effects:

Of *particular importance in the geriatric patient:* Hypoglycemia, dizziness, anorexia, constipation, syndrome of inappropriate antidiuretic hormone secretion (SIADH), drug-induced disulfiram-like reaction

■ Geriatric Considerations - Summary: Due to its long elimination half-life (up to 99 hr in older adults), the risk of prolonged hypoglycemia is very high. Avoid using in older adults.

■ References:

1. Drugs in the elderly. Med Lett 2006;1226:6-8.
2. Haas L. Management of diabetes mellitus medications in the nursing home. Drugs Aging 2005;22:209-218.
3. Chelliah A, Burge MR. Hypoglycemia in elderly patients with diabetes mellitus. Causes and strategies for prevention. Drugs Aging 2004;21:511-530.
4. Rosenstock J. Management of type 2 diabetes mellitus in the elderly: special considerations. Drugs Aging 2001;18:31-44.
5. Shorr RI, Ray WA, Daugherty JR, et. al. Incidence and risk factors for serious hypoglycemia in older persons using insulin or sulfonylureas. Arch Intern Med 1997;157:1681-1686.

6. Shorr RI, Ray WA, Daugherty JR, et. al. Individual sulfonylureas and serious hypoglycemia in older people. J Am Geriatr Soc 1996;44:751-755.
7. Arrigoni L, Fundak G, Horn J, et al: Chlorpropamide pharmacokinetics in young healthy adults and older diabetic patients. Clin Pharm 1987; 6:162-164.

chlorthalidone

(klor-thal'-i-doan)

■ **Brand Name(s):** Hygroton, Thalitone

Combinations
Rx: with atenolol (Tenoretic); with clonidine (Combipres, Chlorpres); with reserpine (Demi-Regroton, Regroton)
Chemical Class: Phthalimidine derivative

■ **Clinical Pharmacology:**
Mechanism of Action: A thiazide diuretic that blocks reabsorption of sodium, potassium, and water at the distal convoluted tubule; also decreases plasma and extracellular fluid volume and peripheral vascular resistance. **Therapeutic Effect:** Produces diuresis; lowers BP.
Pharmacokinetics:

Route	Onset	Peak	Duration
PO (diuretic)	2 hr	2-6 hr	Up to 36 hr

Rapidly absorbed from the GI tract. Excreted unchanged in urine. **Half-life:** 35-50 hr. Onset of antihypertensive effect: 3-4 days; optimal therapeutic effect: 3-4 wk.

■ **Available Forms:**
• *Tablets (Hygroton, Thalitone):* 15 mg, 25 mg, 50 mg, 100 mg.

■ **Indications and Dosages:**
Hypertension, edema: PO Initially, 12.5-25 mg/day or every other day.

■ **Contraindications:** Anuria, history of hypersensitivity to sulfonamides or thiazide diuretics, renal decompensation

■ **Side Effects**
Expected
Increase in urinary frequency and urine volume

Frequent
Potassium depletion (rarely produces symptoms)

Occasional
Anorexia, impotence, diarrhea, orthostatic hypotension, GI disturbances, photosensitivity

Rare
Rash

- **Serious Reactions**
  - Vigorous diuresis may lead to profound water and electrolyte depletion, resulting in hypokalemia, hyponatremia, and dehydration.
  - Acute hypotensive episodes may occur.
  - Hyperglycemia may occur during prolonged therapy.
  - Overdose can lead to lethargy and coma without changes in electrolytes or hydration.

Special Considerations
  - Doses above 25 mg provide no further blood pressure reduction, but are more likely to induce metabolic disturbance (hypokalemia, hyperuricemia, etc.)
  - May protect against osteoporotic hip fractures
  - Loop diuretics or metolazone more effective if CrCl less than 40-50 ml/min
  - Although allergic cross-reactivity with sulfonamide antibiotics and sulfonamide nonantibiotics has not been demonstrated, use with caution in patients with a history of severe sulfa allergies.

- **Patient/Family Education**
  - Will increase urination temporarily (approximately 3 wk); take early in the day to prevent sleep disturbance
  - May cause sensitivity to sunlight; avoid prolonged exposure to the sun and other ultraviolet light
  - May cause gout attacks; notify clinician if sudden joint pain occurs
  - Take chlorthalidone with food to avoid GI distress, preferably early in the morning to avoid nighttime urination
  - Change positions slowly to reduce the drug's hypotensive effect

- **Monitoring Parameters**
  - Weight, urine output, serum electrolytes, BUN, creatinine, CBC, uric acid, glucose, lipids

- **Geriatric side effects at a glance:**
  - ❑ CNS ❑ Bowel Dysfunction ❑ Bladder Dysfunction ❑ Falls

- **U.S. Regulatory Considerations**
  - ❑ FDA Black Box ❑ OBRA regulated in U.S. Long Term Care

chlorzoxazone

(klor-zox'-a-zone)

- **Brand Name(s):** (Parafon Forte DSC, Remular, Remular-S)
  Chemical Class: Benzoxazole derivative

- **Clinical Pharmacology:**
  Mechanism of Action: A skeletal muscle relaxant that inhibits transmission of reflexes at the spinal cord level. **Therapeutic Effect:** Relieves muscle spasticity.

Pharmacokinetics: Readily absorbed from the GI tract. Metabolized in liver. Primarily excreted in urine. **Half-life:** 1.1 hr.

■ **Available Forms:**
- *Caplets:* 500 mg (Parafon Forte DSC).
- *Tablets:* 250 mg.

■ **Indications and Dosages:**
Musculoskeletal pain: PO 250-500 mg 3-4 times/day. Maximum: 750 mg 3-4 times/ day.

■ **Contraindications:** Hypersensitivity to chlorzoxazone or any one of its components.

■ **Side Effects**
Frequent
Drowsiness, fever, headache
Occasional
Nausea, vomiting, stomach cramps, rash

■ **Serious Reactions**
- Overdosage results in nausea, vomiting, diarrhea, and hypotension.

■ **Patient/Family Education**
- Potential for psychological dependency
- Drowsiness usually diminishes with continued therapy

■ **Monitoring Parameters**
- CBC
- Liver and renal function

■ **Geriatric side effects at a glance:**
☑ CNS   ☑ Bowel Dysfunction   ☑ Bladder Dysfunction   ☑ Falls
Other: Decreased mental alertness

■ **Use with caution in older patients with:** Potential for falls

■ **U.S. Regulatory Considerations**
☐ FDA Black Box   ☑ OBRA regulated in U.S. Long Term Care

■ **Other Uses in Geriatric Patient:** None

■ **Side Effects:**
Of particular importance in the geriatric patient: None

■ **Geriatric Considerations - Summary:** Chlorzoxazone is a centrally acting skeletal muscle relaxant that at higher doses can cause CNS depression. It appears to have modest clinical benefits and is most often used for acute muscle discomfort as compared to chronic muscle pain. It is often taken in combination with acetaminophen. Transient CNS depressant effects place the older adult at risk for falls and related accidents when taking this drug.

cholestyramine resin

(koe-less-tir'-a-meen)

- **Brand Name(s):** Questran, Questran Light, LoCHOLEST, LoCHOLEST Light, Prevalite
  Chemical Class: CV-Lipid-bile acid sequestrant

- **Clinical Pharmacology:**
  Mechanism of Action: An antihyperlipoproteinemic that binds with bile acids in the intestine, forming an insoluble complex. Binding results in partial removal of bile acid from enterohepatic circulation. **Therapeutic Effect:** Removes LDL cholesterol from plasma.
  Pharmacokinetics: Not absorbed from the GI tract. Decreases in serum LDL apparent in 5-7 days and in serum cholesterol in 1 mo. Serum cholesterol returns to baseline levels about 1 mo after drug is discontinued.

- **Available Forms:**
  - *Powder for Oral Suspension:* 4 g/5 g (Questran Light), 4 g/9 g (Prevalite, Questran).

- **Indications and Dosages:**
  Hypercholesterolemia: PO Initially, 4g 1-2 times a day. Maintenance: 8-16 g/day in divided doses. Maximum: 24 g/day.
  Pruritus: PO Initially, 4g 1-2 times a day. Maintenance: 8-16 g/day in divided doses. Maximum: 24 g/day.

- **Unlabeled Uses:** Treatment of diarrhea (due to bile acids), hyperoxaluria

- **Contraindications:** Complete biliary obstruction, hypersensitivity to cholestyramine or tartrazine (frequently seen in aspirin hypersensitivity)

- **Side Effects**
  Frequent
  Constipation (may lead to fecal impaction), nausea, vomiting, abdominal pain, indigestion
  Occasional
  Diarrhea, belching, bloating, headache, dizziness
  Rare
  Gallstones, peptic ulcer disease, malabsorption syndrome

- **Serious Reactions**
  - GI tract obstruction, hyperchloremic acidosis, and osteoporosis secondary to calcium excretion may occur.
  - High dosage may interfere with fat absorption, resulting in steatorrhea.

Special Considerations
  - Avoid use in patients with elevated triglycerides

- **Patient/Family Education**
  - Give all other medications 1 hr before or 4 hr after cholestyramine to avoid poor absorption

- Mix drug with applesauce or noncarbonated beverage (2-6 oz), let stand for 2 min; do not take dry
- Take cholestyramine before meals and drink several glasses of water between meals

■ **Monitoring Parameters**
- Daily bowel activity and stool consistency

■ **Geriatric side effects at a glance:**
☐ CNS   ☑ Bowel Dysfunction   ☐ Bladder Dysfunction   ☐ Falls

■ **U.S. Regulatory Considerations**
☐ FDA Black Box   ☐ OBRA regulated in U.S. Long Term Care

choline magnesium trisalicylate

(koe'-leen mag-nees'-ee-um trye-sal'-eh-si-late)

■ **Brand Name(s):** Tricosal, Trilisate
Chemical Class: Salicylate derivative

■ **Clinical Pharmacology:**
Mechanism of Action: A nonsteroidal salicylate that inhibits prostaglandin synthesis and acts on the hypothalamus heat-regulating center. **Therapeutic Effect:** Reduces inflammatory response and intensity of pain stimulus reaching sensory nerve endings. **Pharmacokinetics:** Rapidly absorbed from GI tract. Oral route onset 1 hr, peak 2 hr, and duration 9-17 hr. Protein binding: High. Widely distributed. Excreted in urine. **Half-life:** 2-3 hr.

■ **Available Forms:**
- **Tablets:** 500 mg, 750 mg, 1000 mg (Tricosal, Trilisate).
- **Liquid:** 500 mg/5ml (Trilisate).

■ **Indications and Dosages:**
Analgesic, acute painful shoulder, anti-inflammatory, antipyretic: PO Initially, 500 mg-1500 mg q8-12h, then 1-4.5 g/day.

■ **Contraindications:** Allergy to tartrazine dye, bleeding disorders, GI bleeding or ulceration, history of hypersensitivity to choline magnesium trisalicylate, aspirin, or NSAIDs.

■ **Side Effects**
Side effects appear less frequently with short-term treatment.
Occasional
Nausea, dyspepsia (heartburn, indigestion, epigastric pain), tinnitus

Rare

Anorexia, headache, vomiting, flatulence, dizziness, somnolence, insomnia, fatigue, hearing impairment

- **Serious Reactions**
  - High doses may produce GI bleeding.
  - Overdosage may be characterized by ringing in ears, generalized pruritus (may be severe), headache, dizziness, flushing, tachycardia, hyperventilation, sweating, and thirst.

Special Considerations

- Consider for patients with GI intolerance to aspirin or patients in whom interference with normal platelet function by aspirin or other NSAIDs is undesirable

- **Patient/Family Education**
  - Solution may be mixed with fruit juice just before administration; do not mix with antacid
  - Report any ringing in the ears or persistent GI pain

- **Monitoring Parameters**
  - Liver and renal function studies, stool for occult blood and Hct if long-term therapy

- **Geriatric side effects at a glance:**
  - ☐ CNS   ☐ Bowel Dysfunction   ☐ Bladder Dysfunction   ☐ Falls
  - ☑ Other: Gastropathy

- **Use with caution in older patients with:** Renal impairment, Hepatic impairment, CHF, HTN, PUD, History of GI bleeding, GERD, Gout, History of aspirin sensitivity reaction. Also use with caution in patients taking Anticoagulants, Aspirin, and Antihypertensive agents.

- **U.S. Regulatory Considerations**
  - ☐ FDA Black Box   ☐ OBRA regulated in U.S. Long Term Care

- **Other Uses in Geriatric Patient:** None

- **Side Effects:**
  Of particular importance in the geriatric patient: Confusion, cognitive impairment, delirium, dizziness, dyspepsia, fluid retention, renal impairment

- **Geriatric Considerations - Summary:** As a nonacetylated salicylate, choline magnesium salicylate does not adversely affect platelet function and is associated with fewer adverse GI and renal effects. A preferred analgesic and anti-inflammatory agent for use in older adults. Use of NSAIDs in older adults increases the risk of GI complications including gastric ulceration, bleeding, and perforation. These complications are not necessarily preceded by less severe GI symptoms. Concomitant use of a proton pump inhibitor or misoprostol reduces the risk for gastric ulceration and bleeding, but may not prevent long-term GI toxicity.

- **References:**
  1. COX-2 alternatives and GI protection. Med Lett Drugs Ther 2004;46:91.
  2. Drugs that may cause cognitive disorders in the elderly. Med Lett Drugs Ther 2000;42:111-112.

ciclopirox

(sye-kloe-peer'-ox)

■ **Brand Name(s):** Loprox, Penlac
   Chemical Class: N-Hydroxypyridinone derivative

■ **Clinical Pharmacology:**
   Mechanism of Action: An antifungal that inhibits the transport of essential elements in the fungal cell, thereby interfering with biosynthesis in fungi. **Therapeutic Effect:** Results in fungal cell death.
   Pharmacokinetics: Absorbed through intact skin. Distributed to epidermis, dermis, including hair, hair follicles, and sebaceous glands. Protein binding: 98%. Primarily excreted in urine and to a lesser extent in feces. **Half-life:** 1.7 hr.

■ **Available Forms:**
   - *Cream*: 0.77% (Loprox).
   - *Gel*: 0.77% (Loprox).
   - *Lotion*: 0.77% (Loprox TS).
   - *Shampoo*: 0.77% (Loprox).
   - *Topical Solution, nail lacquer*: 8% (Penlac).

■ **Indications and Dosages:**
   Tinea pedis: Topical Apply 2 times a day until signs and symptoms significantly improve.
   Tinea cruris, Tinea corporis: Topical Apply 2 times a day until signs and symptoms significantly improve.
   Onychomycosis: Topical (solution) Apply to the affected area (nails) daily. Remove with alcohol every 7 days.
   Seborrheic dermatitis: Shampoo Apply to affected scalp areas 2 times a day, in the morning and evening for 4 wk.

■ **Contraindications:** Hypersensitivity to ciclopirox or any one of its components

■ **Side Effects**
   Rare
   Topical: Irritation, burning, redness, pain at the site of application

■ **Serious Reactions**
   - None known.

Special Considerations
   - Use of nail lacquer requires monthly removal of the unattached, infected nails by a health care professional; in clinical trials less than 12% of patients achieved a clear or almost clear nail

■ **Patient/Family Education**
   Cream/gel/lotion:
   - Continue medication for several days after condition clears

- Consult prescriber if no improvement after 4 wk of treatment
- Avoid contact with eyes and mouth

Nail lacquer:
- 48 wk of daily applications considered full treatment, may take 6 mo before seeing improvement

■ **Geriatric side effects at a glance:**
  ❑ CNS ❑ Bowel Dysfunction ❑ Bladder Dysfunction ❑ Falls

■ **U.S. Regulatory Considerations**
  ❑ FDA Black Box ❑ OBRA regulated in U.S. Long Term Care

cidofovir

(si-dof'-o-veer)

■ **Brand Name(s):** Vistide
  Chemical Class: Acyclic purine nucleoside analog

■ **Clinical Pharmacology:**
  Mechanism of Action: An anti-infective that inhibits viral DNA synthesis by incorporating itself into the growing viral DNA chain. **Therapeutic Effect:** Suppresses replication of cytomegalovirus (CMV).
  Pharmacokinetics: Protein binding: less than 6%. Excreted primarily unchanged in urine. Effect of hemodialysis unknown. **Elimination half-life:** 1.4-3.8 hr.

■ **Available Forms:**
  - *Injection:* 75 mg/ml (5-ml ampule).

■ **Indications and Dosages:**
  CMV *retinitis in patients with* AIDS (*in combination with probenecid*): IV infusion Induction: Usual dosage, 5 mg/kg at constant rate over 1 hr once weekly for 2 consecutive wk. Give 2g of PO probenecid 3 hr before cidofovir dose, and then give 1g 2 hr and 8 hr after completion of the 1-hr cidofovir infusion (total of 4 g). In addition, give 1 L of 0.9% NaCl over 1-2 hr immediately before the cidofovir infusion. If tolerated, a second liter may be infused over 1-3 hr at the start of the infusion or immediately afterward. Maintenance: 5 mg/kg cidofovir at constant rate over 1 hr once every 2 wk.
  Dosage in renal impairment: Changes during therapy. If creatinine increases by 0.3-0.4 mg/dl, reduce dose to 3 mg/kg; if creatinine increases by 0.5 mg/dl or greater or development of 3+ or greater proteinuria, discontinue therapy. Preexisting renal impairment. Do not use with serum creatinine greater than 1.5 mg/dl, creatinine clearance less than 55 ml/min, or urine protein 100 mg/dl or greater (2+ or greater proteinuria).

■ **Unlabeled Uses:** Treatment of acyclovir-resistant herpes simplex virus, adenovirus, foscarnet-resistant CMV, ganciclovir-resistant CMV, varicella-zoster virus

■ **Contraindications:** Direct intraocular injection, history of clinically severe hypersensitivity to probenecid or other sulfa-containing drugs, renal function impairment (serum creatinine level greater than 1.5 mg/dl, creatinine clearance of 55 ml/min or less, or urine protein level greater than 100 mg/dl)

■ **Side Effects**
Frequent
Nausea, vomiting (65%), fever (57%), asthenia (46%), rash (30%), diarrhea (27%), headache (27%), alopecia (25%), chills (24%), anorexia (22%), dyspnea (22%), abdominal pain (17%)

■ **Serious Reactions**
- Serious adverse reactions may include proteinuria (80%), nephrotoxicity (53%), neutropenia (31%), elevated serum creatinine levels (29%), infection (24%), anemia (20%), ocular hypotony (a decrease in intraocular pressure 12%), and pneumonia (9%).
- Concurrent use of probenecid may produce a hypersensitivity reaction characterized by a rash, fever, chills, and anaphylaxis.
- Acute renal failure occurs rarely.

Special Considerations
- Concurrent high-dose PO probenecid plus saline hydration reduces nephrotoxicity; procedure: probenecid 2g 3 hr prior to INF, then 1g at 2 and 8 hr after INF; normal saline 1000 ml over 1 hr immediately prior to INF

■ **Patient/Family Education**
- Complete the full course of probenecid with each dose of cidofovir
- Male patients should practice barrier contraceptive methods during and for 3 mo after treatment
- It is important to have regular follow-up ophthalmologic exams

■ **Monitoring Parameters**
- Renal function, urinalysis (especially serum creatinine and urine protein prior to each dose), and blood chemistry (to include serum uric acid, phosphate, and bicarbonate), white counts with differential during intravenous therapy
- Periodically evaluate the patient's visual acuity and check for ocular symptoms

■ **Geriatric side effects at a glance:**
❑ CNS   ❑ Bowel Dysfunction   ❑ Bladder Dysfunction   ❑ Falls

■ **U.S. Regulatory Considerations**
☑ FDA Black Box
Risk of nephrotoxicity and neutropenia. Reduce risk for nephrotoxicity with IV prehydration (normal saline) and administration of probenecid.
❑ OBRA regulated in U.S. Long Term Care

cilostazol

(sil-oh'-sta-zol)

- **Brand Name(s):** Pletal
  Chemical Class: Quinolinone derivative

- **Clinical Pharmacology:**
  Mechanism of Action: A phosphodiesterase III inhibitor that inhibits platelet aggregation. Dilates vascular beds with greatest dilation in femoral beds. **Therapeutic Effect:** Improves walking distance in patients with intermittent claudication.
  Pharmacokinetics: Moderately absorbed from the GI tract. Protein binding: 95%–98%. Extensively metabolized in the liver. Excreted primarily in the urine and, to a lesser extent, in the feces. Not removed by hemodialysis. **Half-life:** 11–13 hr. Therapeutic effect is usually noted in 2–4 wk but may take as long as 12 wk.

- **Available Forms:**
  - *Tablets*: 50 mg, 100 mg.

- **Indications and Dosages:**
  Intermittent claudication: PO 100 mg twice a day at least 30 min before or 2 hr after meals. 50 mg twice a day during concurrent therapy with clarithromycin, diltiazem, erythromycin, fluconazole, fluoxetine, omeprazole, or sertraline.

- **Contraindications:** CHF of any severity (see FDA Black Box); hemostatic disorders or active pathologic bleeding, such as bleeding peptic ulcer and intracranial bleeding

- **Side Effects**
  Frequent (34%–10%)
  Headache, diarrhea, palpitations, dizziness, pharyngitis
  Occasional (7%–3%)
  Nausea, rhinitis, back pain, peripheral edema, dyspepsia, abdominal pain, tachycardia, cough, flatulence, myalgia
  Rare (2%–1%)
  Leg cramps, paresthesia, rash, vomiting

- **Serious Reactions**
  - Signs and symptoms of overdose are noted by severe headache, diarrhea, hypotension, and cardiac arrhythmias.

Special Considerations
  - Cilostazol has been shown, in a multicenter, randomized, double-blind study (DP-PARA 2), to be superior to pentoxifylline for treatment of claudication symptoms

- **Patient/Family Education**
  - Take ½ hr before meal or 2 hr after meal
  - Avoid taking cilostazol with grapefruit juice because it may increase the drug's blood concentration and risk of toxicity

- **Monitoring Parameters**
  - Beneficial effects usually seen in 2–4 wk, may take up to 12 wk
  - Assess for relief of cramping in the feet, calf muscles, thighs, and buttocks during exercise

- **Geriatric side effects at a glance:**
  - ☐ CNS ☐ Bowel Dysfunction ☐ Bladder Dysfunction ☐ Falls

- **U.S. Regulatory Considerations**
  - ☑ FDA Black Box
  - Contraindicated in CHF of any severity
  - ☐ OBRA regulated in U.S. Long Term Care

cimetidine

(sye-met'-i-deen)

- **Brand Name(s):** Tagamet
  OTC: Tagamet HB
  Chemical Class: Imidazole derivative

- **Clinical Pharmacology:**
  Mechanism of Action: A GI H_2-blocker and gastric acid secretion inhibitor that inhibits histamine action at H_2-receptor sites of parietal cells. **Therapeutic Effect:** Inhibits gastric acid secretion during fasting, at night, or when stimulated by food, caffeine, or insulin.
  Pharmacokinetics: Well absorbed from the GI tract. Protein binding: 15%–20%. Widely distributed. Metabolized in the liver. Primarily excreted in urine. Not removed by hemodialysis. **Half-life:** 2 hr; increased with impaired renal function.

- **Available Forms:**
  - *Tablets* (Tagamet HB): 100 mg, 200 mg.
  - *Tablets* (Tagamet): 200 mg, 300 mg, 400 mg, 800 mg.
  - *Liquid* (Tagamet): 300 mg/5 ml.
  - *Liquid* (Tagamet HB): 200 mg/20 ml.
  - *Injection* (Tagamet): 150 mg/ml.

- **Indications and Dosages:**
  Active ulcer: PO 300 mg 4 times a day or 400 mg twice a day or 800 mg at bedtime. IV, IM 300 mg q6h or 150 mg as single dose followed by 37.5 mg/hr continuous infusion.
  Prevention of duodenal ulcer: PO 400-800 mg at bedtime.
  Gastric hypersecretory secretions: PO, IV, IM 300-600 mg q6h. Maximum: 2400 mg/day.
  Gastrointestinal reflux disease: PO 800 mg twice a day or 400 mg 4 times a day for 12 wk.
  OTC use: PO 100 mg up to 30 min before meals. Maximum: 2 doses/day.
  Prevention of upper GI bleeding: IV Infusion 50 mg/hr.

Dosage in renal impairment: Dosage is based on a 300-mg dose. Dosage interval is modified based on creatinine clearance.

Creatinine Clearance	Dosage Interval
greater than 40 ml/min	q6h
20–40 ml/min	q8h or decrease dose by 25%
less than 20 ml/min	q12h or decrease dose by 50%

Give after hemodialysis and q12h between dialysis sessions.

■ **Unlabeled Uses:** Prevention of aspiration pneumonia; treatment of acute urticaria, chronic warts, upper GI bleeding

■ **Contraindications:** Hypersensitivity to other H_2-antagonists

■ **Side Effects**
  Occasional (4%–2%)
  Headache
  Severely ill patients, patients with impaired renal function: Confusion, agitation, psychosis, depression, anxiety, disorientation, hallucinations. Effects reverse 3-4 days after discontinuance.
  Rare (less than 2%)
  Diarrhea, dizziness, somnolence, nausea, vomiting, gynecomastia, rash, impotence

■ **Serious Reactions**
  • Rapid IV administration may produce cardiac arrhythmias and hypotension.

Special Considerations
  • Generic formulations offer less costly alternative for patients not at risk for drug interactions

■ **Patient/Family Education**
  • Stagger doses of cimetidine and antacids
  • IM injection may produce transient discomfort at injection site. Avoid tasks that require mental alertness or motor skills until response to the drug is established
  • Avoid smoking
  • Notify the physician if blood in vomitus or stool, or dark, tarry stool occurs

■ **Monitoring Parameters**
  • Blood pressure for hypotension during IV infusion
  • Blood in stool
  • Mental status, especially in those with impaired renal function

■ **Geriatric side effects at a glance:**
  ☑ CNS ❑ Bowel Dysfunction ❑ Bladder Dysfunction ❑ Falls
  Other: Cognitive impairment, delirium

■ **Use with caution in older patients with:** Impaired renal function, Cognitive impairment

■ **U.S. Regulatory Considerations**
  ❑ FDA Black Box ❑ OBRA regulated in U.S. Long Term Care

■ **Other Uses in Geriatric Patient:** Acute allergic reactions, urticaria (in addition to antihistamine therapy)

■ **Side Effects:**
Of *particular importance in the geriatric patient*: Anticholinergic effects, delirium, confusion, drowsiness, agitation, headaches, diarrhea, gynecomastia

■ **Geriatric Considerations - Summary:** Adjust dose based on creatinine clearance. Many drug interactions due to inhibitory effect on cytochromes 3A4, 2D6, and 1A2. Not effective in preventing NSAID-induced gastric ulceration and bleeding; proton-pump inhibitors should be used for this indication instead. Due to greater potential for CNS adverse effects and drug interactions as compared to other H$_2$-blockers, consider an alternate H$_2$-blocker when this drug class is indicated for treatment.

■ **References:**
1. Gawrich S, Shaker R. Medical management of nocturnal symptoms of gastro-oesophageal reflux disease in the elderly. Drugs Aging 2003;20:509-516.
2. Tune LE. Anticholinergic effects of medication in elderly patients. J Clin Psychiatry 2001;62(suppl 21):11-14.
3. Thomson ABR. Gastro-oesophageal reflux in the elderly. Role of drug therapy in management. Drugs Aging 2001;18:409-414.
4. Drugs that may cause cognitive disorders in the elderly. Med Lett 2000;42:111-112.

cinacalcet hydrochloride

(sin-a-cal'-set hye-droe-klor'-ide)

■ **Brand Name(s):** Sensipar
Chemical Class: Calcimimetic agent

■ **Clinical Pharmacology:**
Mechanism of Action: A calcium receptor agonist that increases the sensitivity of the calcium-sensing receptor on the parathyroid gland to extracellular calcium, thus lowering the parathyroid hormone (PTH) levels. **Therapeutic Effect:** Decreases serum calcium and PTH levels.
Pharmacokinetics: Extensively distributed after PO administration. Protein binding: 93%-97%. Rapidly and extensively metabolized by multiple enzymes. Primarily eliminated in urine with a lesser amount excreted in feces. **Half-life:** 30-40 hr.

■ **Available Forms:**
• *Tablets*: 30 mg, 60 mg, 90 mg.

■ **Indications and Dosages:**
Hypercalcemia in parathyroid carcinoma: PO Initially, 30 mg twice a day. Titrate dosage sequentially (60 mg twice a day, 90 mg twice a day, and 90 mg 3-4 times a day) every 2-4 wk as needed to normalize serum calcium levels.
Secondary hyperparathyroidism in patients on dialysis: PO Initially, 30 mg once a day. Titrate dosage sequentially (60, 90, 120, and 180 mg once a day) every 2-4 wk.

■ **Unlabeled Uses:** Primary hyperthyroidism

■ **Contraindications:** None known.

- **Side Effects**
    Frequent (31%-21%)
    Nausea, vomiting, diarrhea
    Occasional (15%-10%)
    Myalgia, dizziness
    Rare (7%-5%)
    Asthenia, hypertension, anorexia, noncardiac chest pain

- **Serious Reactions**
    - Overdose may lead to hypocalcemia.

Special Considerations
    - Can be used alone or in combination with vitamin D sterols and/or phosphate binders

- **Patient/Family Education**
    - Take with food or shortly after a meal. Do not divide tablets
    - Notify the health care provider immediately if diarrhea or vomiting occurs.

- **Monitoring Parameters**
    - Serum calcium and phosphorus within 1 wk
    - iPTH 1-4 wk after initiation or dose adjustment
    - Once maintenance dose established, serum calcium and phosphorus qmo, iPTH q1-3 mo to target of 150-300 pg/ml
    - Pattern of daily bowel activity and stool consistency

- **Geriatric side effects at a glance:**
    ❑ CNS ❑ Bowel Dysfunction ❑ Bladder Dysfunction ❑ Falls

- **U.S. Regulatory Considerations**
    ❑ FDA Black Box ❑ OBRA regulated in U.S. Long Term Care

ciprofloxacin hydrochloride

(sip-ro-floks'-a-sin hye-droe-klor'-ide)

- **Brand Name(s):** Ciloxan (ophthalmic), Cipro, Cipro I.V., Cipro XR
    Chemical Class: Fluoroquinolone derivative

- **Clinical Pharmacology:**
    Mechanism of Action: A fluoroquinolone that inhibits the enzyme DNA gyrase in susceptible bacteria, interfering with bacterial cell replication. **Therapeutic Effect:** Bactericidal.
    Pharmacokinetics: Well absorbed from the GI tract (food delays absorption). Protein binding: 20%-40%. Widely distributed (including to CSF). Metabolized in the liver to active metabolite. Primarily excreted in urine. Minimal removal by hemodialysis.
    Half-life: 4-6 hr (increased in impaired renal function and the elderly).

Available Forms:
- *Tablets (Cipro)*: 100 mg, 250 mg, 500 mg, 750 mg.
- *Tablets (Extended-Release [Cipro XR])*: 500 mg, 1000 mg.
- *Infusion (Cipro I.V.)*: 200 mg/100 ml, 400 mg/200 ml.
- *Intravenous Solution (Cipro I.V.)*: 10 mg/ml.
- *Ophthalmic Ointment (Ciloxan)*: 0.3%.
- *Ophthalmic Suspension (Ciloxan)*: 0.3%.
- *Oral Suspension, Powder for Reconstitution (Cipro)*: 250 mg/5 ml, 500 mg/5 ml.

Indications and Dosages:
Bone, joint infections: IV 400 mg q12h for 4-6 wk. PO 500 mg q12h for 4-6 wk.
Conjunctivitis: Ophthalmic 1-2 drops q2h for 2 days, then 2 drops q4h for next 5 days.
Corneal ulcer: Ophthalmic 2 drops q15min for 6 hr, then 2 drops q30min for the remainder of first day, 2 drops q1h on second day, and 2 drops q4h on days 3-14.
Febrile neutropenia: IV 400 mg q8h for 7-14 days (in combination).
Gonorrhea: PO 250 mg as a single dose.
Infectious diarrhea: PO 500 mg q12h for 5-7 days.
Intra-abdominal infections (with metronidazole): IV 400 mg q12h for 7-14 days. PO 500 mg q12h for 7-14 days.
Lower respiratory tract infections: IV 400 mg q12h for 7-14 days. PO 500 mg q12h for 7-14 days (750 mg q12h for 7-14 days for severe or complicated infections).
Nosocomial pneumonia: IV 400 mg q8h for 10-14 days.
Prostatitis: IV 400 mg q12h for 28 days. PO 500 mg q12h for 28 days.
Sinusitis: IV 400 mg q12h for 10 days. PO 500 mg q12h for 10 days.
Skin and skin-structure infections: IV 400 mg q12h for 7-14 days. PO 500 mg q12h for 7-14 days (750 mg q12h for severe or complicated infections).
Susceptible infections: IV 400 mg q8-12h. PO 500-750 mg q12h.
UTIs: IV 200 mg q12h for 7-14 days (400 mg q12h for severe or complicated infections). PO 100-250 mg q12h for 3 days for acute uncomplicated infections; 250 mg q12h for 7-14 days for mild to moderate infections; 500 mg q12h for 7-14 days for severe or complicated infections.
Dosage in renal impairment: Dosage and frequency are modified based on creatinine clearance and the severity of the infection.

Creatinine Clearance	Dosage Interval
less than 30 ml/min	usual dose q18-24h

Hemodialysis: 250-500 mg q24h (after dialysis).
Peritoneal Dialysis: 250-500 mg q24h (after dialysis).

Unlabeled Uses: Treatment of chancroid

Contraindications: Hypersensitivity to ciprofloxacin or other quinolones; for ophthalmic administration: vaccinia, varicella, epithelial herpes simplex, keratitis, mycobacterial infection, fungal disease of ocular structure, use after uncomplicated removal of a foreign body

Side Effects
Frequent (5%-2%)
Nausea, diarrhea, dyspepsia, vomiting, constipation, flatulence, confusion, crystalluria
Ophthalmic: Burning, crusting in corner of eye
Occasional (less than 2%)
Abdominal pain or discomfort, headache, rash
Ophthalmic: Bad taste, sensation of something in eye, eyelid redness or itching

Rare (less than 1%)
Dizziness, confusion, tremors, hallucinations, hypersensitivity reaction, insomnia, dry mouth, paresthesia

■ **Serious Reactions**
- Superinfection (especially enterococcal or fungal), nephropathy, cardiopulmonary arrest, chest pain, and cerebral thrombosis may occur.
- Hypersensitivity reactions, including photosensitivity (as evidenced by rash, pruritus, blisters, edema, and burning skin), have occurred in patients receiving fluoroquinolones.
- Sensitization to the ophthalmic form of the drug may contraindicate later systemic use of ciprofloxacin.
- Tendon effects, including ruptures of shoulder, hand, Achilles tendon or other tendons, may occur. Risk increases with concomitant corticosteroid use, especially in the elderly.

Special Considerations
- Reserve use for UTI to documented pseudomonal infection or complicated UTI
- Individualize treatment based on local susceptibility patterns.

■ **Patient/Family Education**
- Do not skip drug doses; take for the full course of therapy
- Take with meals and an 8-oz glass of water
- Do not take antacids within 2 hr of taking ciprofloxacin
- Your tendons may be more easily injured while taking this medication. Monitor for pain or swelling in your knee, ankle, shoulder, elbow, or wrist.
- Your skin may be more sensitive to sunlight while taking this medication. Wear sunscreen when outdoors. Avoid sunlamps and tanning beds.
- This medication may make you dizzy or drowsy. Avoid driving or other activities requiring you to be alert.

■ **Monitoring Parameters**
- Therapeutic response to medication
- Daily bowel activity and stool consistency. Although mild GI effects may be tolerable, severe symptoms may indicate the onset of antibiotic-associated colitis.
- Signs and symptoms of superinfection include abdominal pain or cramping, anal or genital pruritus or discharge, moderate to severe diarrhea, severe mouth or tongue soreness, and new or increased fever.

■ **Geriatric side effects at a glance:**
☑ CNS ☐ Bowel Dysfunction ☐ Bladder Dysfunction ☐ Falls

■ **U.S. Regulatory Considerations**
☐ FDA Black Box ☐ OBRA regulated in U.S. Long Term Care

citalopram hydrobromide

(sye-tal'-oh-pram hye-droe-broe'-mide)

■ **Brand Name(s):** Celexa
Chemical Class: Bicyclic phthalane derivative

■ **Clinical Pharmacology:**
Mechanism of Action: A selective serotonin reuptake inhibitor that blocks the uptake of the neurotransmitter serotonin at CNS presynaptic neuronal membranes, increasing its availability at postsynaptic receptor sites. **Therapeutic Effect:** Relieves depression.
Pharmacokinetics: Well absorbed after PO administration. Protein binding: 80%. Primarily metabolized in the liver. Primarily excreted in feces with a lesser amount eliminated in urine. **Half-life:** 35 hr.

■ **Available Forms:**
  • *Oral Solution*: 10 mg/5 ml.
  • *Tablets*: 10 mg, 20 mg, 40 mg.

■ **Indications and Dosages:**
Depression: PO 20 mg/day. May titrate to 40 mg/day only for nonresponding patients.

■ **Unlabeled Uses:** Treatment of alcohol abuse, dementia, diabetic neuropathy, obsessive-compulsive disorder, panic disorder, smoking cessation

■ **Contraindications:** Sensitivity to citalopram, use within 14 days of MAOIs

■ **Side Effects**
Frequent (21%–11%)
Nausea, dry mouth, somnolence, insomnia, diaphoresis
Occasional (8%–4%)
Tremor, diarrhea, abnormal ejaculation, dyspepsia, fatigue, anxiety, vomiting, anorexia
Rare (3%–2%)
Sinusitis, sexual dysfunction, abdominal pain, agitation, decreased libido

■ **Serious Reactions**
  • Overdose is manifested as dizziness, drowsiness, tachycardia, somnolence, confusion, and seizures.

Special Considerations
  • No clinical advantage over other SSRIs

■ **Patient/Family Education**
  • Therapeutic response may take 5-6 wk; most commonly taken once daily in the afternoon or evening
  • Do not discontinue citalopram abruptly or increase the dosage
  • Avoid alcohol while taking citalopram

- Avoid tasks that require mental alertness or motor skills until response to the drug has been established
- Take sips of tepid water and chew sugarless gum to help relieve dry mouth

■ **Monitoring Parameters**
- Closely supervise the suicidal patient during early therapy; as depression lessens, the patient's energy level improves, increasing the risk of suicide
- Assess the patient's appearance, behavior, level of interest, mood, and sleep pattern to determine the drug's therapeutic effect

■ **Geriatric side effects at a glance:**
❏ CNS ☑ Bowel Dysfunction ❏ Bladder Dysfunction ☑ Falls
Other: Hyponatremia, weight gain (long term)

■ **Use with caution in older patients with:** None

■ **U.S. Regulatory Considerations**
☑ FDA Black Box
- There is an increased risk of suicide in children and adolescents.
- Older adults should be closely monitored for suicidal ideation.
☑ OBRA regulated in U.S. Long Term Care

■ **Other Uses in Geriatric Patient:** Anxiety symptoms and related disorders

■ **Side Effects:**
Of particular importance in the geriatric patient: Hyponatremia, withdrawal symptoms when abruptly discontinued (e.g., during hospitalization) rather than tapered

■ **Geriatric Considerations - Summary:** These agents are now considered by many the first-line therapy for treatment of depression in older adults. They are also effective in the management of symptoms of anxiety. Although these agents appear to have a more favorable side-effect profile than tricyclic antidepressants for most older adults, it is important to note that some of these agents have the potential significant drug interactions, have been associated with falls, and require careful attention to electrolyte status. In addition, many of the drugs in this class have been associated with severe withdrawal symptoms (e.g., nausea and/or vomiting, dizziness, headaches, lethargy or light-headedness, anxiety and/or agitation) when discontinued abruptly.

■ **References:**
1. Cadieux RJ. Antidepressant drug interactions in the elderly. Understanding the P-450 system is half the battle in reducing risks. Postgrad Med 1999;106:231-240, 245.
2. Roose SP, Laghrissi-Thode F, Kennedy JS, et al. Comparison of paroxetine and nortriptyline in depressed patients with ischemic heart disease. JAMA 1998;279:287-291.
3. Thapa PB, Gideon P, Cost TW, et al. Antidepressants and the risk of falls among nursing home residents. N Engl J Med 1998;339:875-882.
4. Bouman WP, Pinner G, Johnson H. Incidence of selective serotonin reuptake inhibitor (SSRI) induced hyponatraemia due to the syndrome of inappropriate antidiuretic hormone (SIADH) secretion in the elderly. Int J Geriatr Psychiatry 1998;13:12-15.

clarithromycin

(clare-i-thro-mye'-sin)

■ **Brand Name(s):** Biaxin, Biaxin XL, Biaxin XL-Pak
  Chemical Class: Macrolide derivative

■ **Clinical Pharmacology:**
  Mechanism of Action: A macrolide that binds to ribosomal receptor sites of susceptible organisms, inhibiting protein synthesis of the bacterial cell wall. **Therapeutic Effect:** Bacteriostatic; may be bactericidal with high dosages or very susceptible microorganisms.
  Pharmacokinetics: Well absorbed from the GI tract. Protein binding: 65%-75%. Widely distributed. Metabolized in the liver to active metabolite. Primarily excreted in urine. Not removed by hemodialysis. **Half-life:** 3-7 hr; metabolite 5-7 hr (increased in impaired renal function).

■ **Available Forms:**
  - *Oral Suspension* (Biaxin): 125 mg/5 ml, 250 mg/5 ml.
  - *Tablets* (Biaxin): 250 mg, 500 mg.
  - *Tablets* (Extended-Release [Biaxin XL, Biaxin XL Pak]): 500 mg.

■ **Indications and Dosages:**
  Bronchitis: PO 250-500 mg q12h for 7-14 days. PO (Extended-Release) 1g once daily for 7 days.
  Skin, soft tissue infections: PO 250 mg q12h for 7-14 days.
  Mycobacterium avium complex (MAC) prophylaxis: PO 500 mg twice a day.
  MAC treatment: PO 500 mg twice a day in combination.
  Pharyngitis, tonsillitis: PO 250 mg q12h for 10 days.
  Pneumonia: PO 250 mg q12h for 7-14 days. PO (Extended-Release) 1 g/day.
  Maxillary sinusitis: PO 500 mg q12h or 1000 mg (2×500 mg extended-release) once daily for 14 days.
  Helicobacter pylori: PO 500 mg q8-12h for 10-14 days in combination.
  Dosage in renal impairment: For patients with creatinine clearance less than 30 ml/min, reduce dose by 50% and administer once or twice a day.

■ **Contraindications:** Hypersensitivity to other macrolide antibacterials

■ **Side Effects**
  Occasional (6%-3%)
  Diarrhea, nausea, altered taste, abdominal pain
  Rare (2%-1%)
  Headache, dyspepsia

■ **Serious Reactions**
  - Antibiotic-associated colitis and other superinfections may result from altered bacterial balance.
  - Hepatotoxicity and thrombocytopenia occur rarely.

• Individualize treatment based on local susceptibility patterns.

■ Patient/Family Education
• Take extended-release tablet with food, immediate-release tablets and granules without regard to food
• Do NOT refrigerate suspension
• Take clarithromycin tablets with 8 oz of water; the tablets and oral suspension may be taken with or without food
• Space doses evenly around the clock and continue taking clarithromycin for the full course of treatment

■ Monitoring Parameters
• Pattern of daily bowel activity and stool consistency; mild GI effects may be tolerable, but severe symptoms may indicate the onset of antibiotic-associated colitis
• Be alert for signs and symptoms of superinfection, including abdominal pain, anal or genital pruritus, moderate to severe diarrhea, and mouth soreness

■ Geriatric side effects at a glance:
☑ CNS ☑ Bowel Dysfunction ☐ Bladder Dysfunction ☐ Falls

■ U.S. Regulatory Considerations
☐ FDA Black Box ☐ OBRA regulated in U.S. Long Term Care

clemastine fumarate

(klem'-as-teen)

■ Brand Name(s): Contac 12 Hour Allergy, Dayhistol Allergy, Tavist Allergy

Combinations
OTC: with pseudoephedrine and acetaminophen (Tavist Allergy/Sinus/Headache Tablets)
Chemical Class: Ethanolamine derivative

■ Clinical Pharmacology:
Mechanism of Action: An ethanolamine that competes with histamine on effector cells in the GI tract, blood vessels, and respiratory tract. *Therapeutic Effect:* Relieves allergy symptoms, including urticaria, rhinitis, and pruritus.
Pharmacokinetics:

Route	Onset	Peak	Duration
PO	15-60 min	5-7 hr	10-12 hr

Well absorbed from the GI tract. Metabolized in the liver. Excreted primarily in urine.
Half-life: 21 hr.

■ Available Forms:
• *Syrup* (Tavist): 0.67 mg/5 ml.
• *Tablets*: 1.34 mg (Contac 12 Hour Allergy), 2.68 mg (Tavist).

■ **Indications and Dosages:**
  Allergic rhinitis, urticaria: PO 1.34 mg 1-2 times a day.

■ **Contraindications:** Angle-closure glaucoma, hypersensitivity to clemastine, use within 14 days of MAOIs

■ **Side Effects**
  Frequent
  Somnolence, dizziness, hypotension, urine retention, thickening of bronchial secretions, dry mouth, nose, or throat
  Occasional
  Epigastric distress, flushing, blurred vision, tinnitus, paresthesia, diaphoresis, chills

■ **Serious Reactions**
  • A hypersensitivity reaction, marked by eczema, pruritus, rash, cardiac disturbances, angioedema, and photosensitivity, may occur.
  • Overdose symptoms may vary from CNS depression, including sedation, apnea, cardiovascular collapse, and death to severe paradoxical reaction, such as hallucinations, tremor, and seizures.

Special Considerations

  • No advantage over loratadine or cetirizine; lower doses associated with less sedation and efficacy

■ **Patient/Family Education**
  • Dizziness, drowsiness, and dry mouth are expected side effects of clemastine
  • Avoid performing tasks that require mental alertness or motor skills until response to the drug has been established
  • Avoid alcohol during clemastine therapy

■ **Geriatric side effects at a glance:**
  ☑ CNS ☑ Bowel Dysfunction ☑ Bladder Dysfunction ☐ Falls
  Other: Dry mouth, blurred vision, confusion, psychoses

■ **Use with caution in older patients with:** Narrow-angle glaucoma, overflow incontinence, psychosis.

■ **U.S. Regulatory Considerations**
  ☐ FDA Black Box ☑ OBRA regulated in U.S. Long Term Care

■ **Other Uses in Geriatric Patient:** Sedation, motion sickness

■ **Side Effects:**
  Of particular importance in the geriatric patient: Anticholinergic effects

■ **Geriatric Considerations - Summary:** Clemastine is a first-generation ethanolamine antihistamine with potent H_1-receptor antagonism. It also has significant anticholinergic activity and causes somnolence at normal doses. Older adults taking this drug are at risk of dizziness and hypotension and clemastine would not be considered a drug of choice for this population. Federal guidelines discourage the use of ethanolamines as sedatives in older adults.

- **References:**
    1. Hagermark O, Levander S, Stahle M: A comparison of antihistaminic and sedative effects of some H_1-receptor antagonists. Acta Derm Venereol 1985;114:155-156.
    2. Tune LE. Anticholinergic effects of medication in elderly patients. J Clin Psychiatry 2001;62(suppl 21):11-14.
    3. Gengo F, Gabos C, Miller JK: The pharmacodynamics of diphenhydramine-induced drowsiness and changes in mental performance. Clin Pharmacol Ther 1989;45:15-21.

clindamycin

(klin-da-mye'-sin)

- **Brand Name(s):** Cleocin HCl, Cleocin Ovules, Cleocin Phosphate, Cleocin T, Cleocin Vaginal, Clinda-Derm, Clindagel, Clindamax, Clindesse, Clindets Pledget
  Chemical Class: Lincomycin derivative

- **Clinical Pharmacology:**
  Mechanism of Action: A lincosamide antibacterial that inhibits protein synthesis of the bacterial cell wall by binding to bacterial ribosomal receptor sites. Topically, it decreases fatty acid concentration on the skin. **Therapeutic Effect:** Bacteriostatic. Prevents outbreaks of acne vulgaris.
  Pharmacokinetics: Rapidly absorbed from the GI tract. Protein binding: 92%-94%. Widely distributed. Metabolized in the liver to some active metabolites. Primarily excreted in urine. Not removed by hemodialysis. **Half-life:** 2.4-3 hr (increased in impaired renal function and premature infants).

- **Available Forms:**
  - *Capsules (Cleocin HCl)*: 75 mg, 150 mg, 300 mg.
  - *Intravenous Solution (Cleocin Phosphate)*: 150 mg/ml, 300 mg-5%/50 ml, 600 mg-5%/50 ml, 900 mg-5%/50 ml.
  - *Topical Gel (Cleocin T, Clindagel, Clindamax)*: 1%.
  - *Topical Lotion (Cleocin T)*: 1%.
  - *Topical Solution (Cleocin T, Clinda-Derm)*: 1%.
  - *Topical Swab (Cleocin T, Clindets Pledget)*: 1%.
  - *Vaginal Cream (Cleocin Vaginal)*: 2%.
  - *Vaginal Suppository (Cleocin Ovules)*: 100 mg.

- **Indications and Dosages:**
  Susceptible infections: IV, IM 600-2700 mg/day in 2-4 divided doses. PO 150-450 mg q6h.
  Bacterial vaginosis: PO 300 mg twice a day for 7 days. Intravaginal One applicatorful at bedtime for 3-7 days or 1 suppository at bedtime for 3 days. Intravaginal (Clindesse cream) One applicatorful once at any time of the day.
  Acne vulgaris: Topical Apply thin layer to affected area twice a day.

- **Unlabeled Uses:** Treatment of actinomycosis, babesiosis, erysipelas, malaria, otitis media, *Pneumocystis carinii* pneumonia, sinusitis, toxoplasmosis

- **Contraindications:** History of antibacterial-associated colitis, regional enteritis, or ulcerative colitis; hypersensitivity to clindamycin or lincomycin; known allergy to tartrazine dye

- **Side Effects**
  Frequent
  Systemic: Abdominal pain, nausea, vomiting, diarrhea
  Topical: Dry scaly skin
  Vaginal: Vaginitis, pruritus
  Occasional
  Systemic: Phlebitis or thrombophlebitis with IV administration, pain and induration at IM injection site, allergic reaction, urticaria, pruritus
  Topical: Contact dermatitis, abdominal pain, mild diarrhea, burning or stinging
  Vaginal: Headache, dizziness, nausea, vomiting, abdominal pain
  Rare
  Vaginal: Hypersensitivity reaction

- **Serious Reactions**
  - Antibiotic-associated colitis and other superinfections may occur during and several weeks after clindamycin therapy (including the topical form).
  - Blood dyscrasias (leukopenia, thrombocytopenia) and nephrotoxicity (proteinuria, azotemia, oliguria) occur rarely.

Special Considerations
  - Most active antibiotic against anaerobes
  - Preferred topical antiacne antibiotic
  - Individualize treatment based on local susceptibility patterns.

- **Patient/Family Education**
  - Avoid intercourse and use of vaginal products (tampons, douches) when using the vag cream or suppositories
  - Vaginal cream contains mineral oil and vaginal suppositories contain an oleaginous base which may weaken rubber or latex products such as condoms, avoid use within 72 hr following treatment with vaginal cream or suppositories
  - Space doses evenly around the clock and continue taking clindamycin for the full course of treatment
  - Do not apply topical preparations near the eyes

- **Monitoring Parameters**
  - Daily bowel activity and stool consistency
  - Skin for dryness, irritation and rash with topical application
  - Signs and symptoms of superinfection, such as anal or genital pruritus, a change in oral mucosa, increased fever, and severe diarrhea

- **Geriatric side effects at a glance:**
  ☐ CNS ☑ Bowel Dysfunction ☐ Bladder Dysfunction ☐ Falls

- **U.S. Regulatory Considerations**
  ☑ FDA Black Box
  IV, IM, and oral administration: Risk for pseudomembranous colitis that may range from mild to severe or life-threatening. Reserve for use in serious infections only.
  ☐ OBRA regulated in U.S. Long Term Care

clioquinol; hydrocortisone

(kly-oh-kwin'-ole)

OTC: Ala-Quin, Dek-Quin, Vioform-Hydrocortisone Cream, Vioform-Hydrocortisone Mild Cream, Vioform-Hydrocortisone Mild Ointment, Vioform-Hydrocortisone Ointment
Chemical Class: Hydroxyquinoline derivative

■ Clinical Pharmacology:
Mechanism of Action: Clioquinol is a broad-spectrum antibacterial agent but the mechanism of action is unknown. Hydrocortisone is a corticosteroid that diffuses across cell membranes, forms complexes with specific receptors and further binds to DNA and stimulates transcription of mRNA (messenger RNA) and subsequent protein synthesis of various enzymes thought to be ultimately responsible for the anti-inflammatory effects of corticosteroids applied topically to the skin. **Therapeutic Effect:** Alters membrane function and produces antibacterial activity.
Pharmacokinetics: Clioquinol may be absorbed through the skin in sufficient amounts.

■ Available Forms:
- *Cream:* 3% clioquinol and 0.5% hydrocortisone (Ala-Quin, Vioform-Hydrocortisone Mild Cream); 3% clioquinol and 1% hydrocortisone (Vioform-Hydrocortisone Cream, Dek-Quin).
- *Ointment:* 3% clioquinol and 1% hydrocortisone (Vioform-Hydrocortisone Mild Ointment).

■ Indications and Dosages:
Antibacterial, antifungal skin conditions: Topical Apply to skin 3-4 times/day.

■ Contraindications: Lesions of the eye, tuberculosis of skin, diaper rash, hypersensitivity to clioquinol or hydrocortisone or any other component of the formulation

■ Side Effects
Occasional
Blistering, burning, itching, peeling, skin rash, redness, swelling

■ Serious Reactions
- Thinning of skin with easy bruising may occur with prolonged use.

Special Considerations
- Potential neurotoxicity with absorption (with occlusion); since other agents without this toxicity exist, questionable utility

■ Patient/Family Education
- Avoid contact with eyes
- Rub the topical form well into affected areas
- Medication may stain fabrics, skin, hair, and nails yellow

Monitoring Parameters
- Skin for irritation
- Therapeutic response

Geriatric side effects at a glance:
☐ CNS   ☐ Bowel Dysfunction   ☐ Bladder Dysfunction   ☐ Falls

U.S. Regulatory Considerations
☐ FDA Black Box   ☐ OBRA regulated in U.S. Long Term Care

clobetasol propionate

(klo-bet'-a-sol proe'-pi-on-ate)

- **Brand Name(s):** Cormax, Olux, Temovate
  Chemical Class: Corticosteroid, synthetic

- **Clinical Pharmacology:**
  Mechanism of Action: A corticosteroid that inhibits accumulation of inflammatory cells at inflammation sites, phagocytosis, lysosomal enzyme release, and synthesis or release of mediators of inflammation. **Therapeutic Effect:** Decreases or prevents tissue response to inflammatory process.
  Pharmacokinetics: May be absorbed from intact skin. Metabolized in liver. Excreted in the urine.

- **Available Forms:**
  - *Cream:* 0.05% (Cormax, Temovate).
  - *Cream, in emollient base:* 0.05% (Temovate).
  - *Foam:* 0.05% (Olux).
  - *Gel:* 0.05% (Temovate).
  - *Ointment:* 0.05% (Cormax, Temovate).
  - *Topical Solution:* 0.05% (Cormax, Temovate).

- **Indications and Dosages:**
  Anti-inflammatory, corticosteroid replacement therapy: Topical Apply 2 times/day for 2 wk. Foam Apply 2 times/day for 2 wk.

- **Contraindications:** Hypersensitivity to clobetasol or other corticosteroids.

- **Side Effects**
  Frequent
  Local irritation, dry skin, itching, redness
  Occasional
  Allergic contact dermatitis
  Rare
  Cushing's syndrome, numbness of fingers, skin atrophy

Serious Reactions
- Overdosage can occur from topically applied clobetasol propionate absorbed in sufficient amounts to produce systemic effects producing reversible adrenal suppression, manifestations of Cushing's syndrome, hyperglycemia, and glucosuria in some patients.

Special Considerations
- No demonstrated superiority over other high-potency agents; cost should govern use

Patient/Family Education
- Apply sparingly only to affected area
- Avoid contact with the eyes
- Do not put bandages or dressings over treated area unless directed by clinician
- Do not use on weeping, denuded, or infected areas
- Discontinue drug, notify clinician if local irritation or fever develops

Monitoring Parameters
- Therapeutic response to medication

Geriatric side effects at a glance:
❏ CNS   ❏ Bowel Dysfunction   ❏ Bladder Dysfunction   ❏ Falls

U.S. Regulatory Considerations
❏ FDA Black Box   ❏ OBRA regulated in U.S. Long Term Care

clocortolone pivalate

(kloe-kor'-toe-lone piv'-a-late)

Brand Name(s): Cloderm
Chemical Class: Corticosteroid, synthetic

Clinical Pharmacology:
Mechanism of Action: A topical corticosteroid that inhibits accumulation of inflammatory cells at inflammation sites, suppresses mitotic activity, and causes vasoconstriction. **Therapeutic Effect:** Decreases or prevents tissue response to inflammatory process.
Pharmacokinetics: Absorption is variable and dependent upon many factors including integrity of skin, dose, vehicle used, and use of occlusive dressings. Small amounts may be absorbed from the skin. Metabolized in liver. Excreted in the urine and feces.

Available Forms:
- *Cream*: 0.1%.

Indications and Dosages:
Dermatoses: Topical Apply 1-4 times/day.

- **Contraindications:** Hypersensitivity to clocortolone pivalate or other corticosteroids; viral, fungal, or tubercular skin lesions

- **Side Effects**
  Occasional
  Local irritation, burning, itching, redness, allergic contact dermatitis
  Rare
  Hypertrichosis, hypopigmentation, maceration of skin, miliaria, perioral dermatitis, skin atrophy, striae

- **Serious Reactions**
  - Overdosage can occur from topically applied clocortolone pivalate absorbed in sufficient amounts to produce systemic effects in some patients.

Special Considerations
  - No demonstrated superiority over other low-potency agents; cost should govern use

- **Patient/Family Education**
  - Apply sparingly only to affected area
  - Avoid contact with the eyes
  - Do not put bandages or dressings over treated area unless directed by clinician
  - Discontinue drug, notify clinician if local irritation or fever develops
  - Do not use on weeping, denuded, or infected areas

- **Monitoring Parameters**
  - Therapeutic response to medication

- **Geriatric side effects at a glance:**
  ❑ CNS   ❑ Bowel Dysfunction   ❑ Bladder Dysfunction   ❑ Falls

- **U.S. Regulatory Considerations**
  ❑ FDA Black Box   ❑ OBRA regulated in U.S. Long Term Care

clofazimine

(kloe-faz'-i-meen)

- **Brand Name(s):** Lamprene
  Chemical Class: Iminophenazine dye

- **Clinical Pharmacology:**
  Mechanism of Action: An antibiotic that binds to mycobacterial DNA. **Therapeutic Effect:** Inhibits mycobacterial growth and produces anti-inflammatory action.

Pharmacokinetics: Variable absorption following PO administration. Due to its high lipophilicity, clofazimine is deposited primarily in fatty tissue. Metabolized in liver. Primarily excreted in feces and minimal elimination in urine. **Half-life**: 70 days (following long-term therapy).

■ **Available Forms:**
- *Capsules*: 50 mg.

■ **Indications and Dosages:**
Leprosy: PO 100 mg/day in combination with dapsone and rifampin for 3 yr, then 100 mg/day as monotherapy.
Erythema nodosum: PO 100-200 mg/day for up to 3 mo, then 100 mg/day.

■ **Contraindications:** None known.

■ **Side Effects**
Frequent (greater than 10%)
Dry skin, abdominal pain, nausea, vomiting, diarrhea, skin discoloration (pink to brownish-black)
Occasional (10%-1%)
Rash; pruritus; eye irritation; discoloration of sputum, sweat, and urine

■ **Serious Reactions**
- Severe abdominal pain and bleeding have been reported.

Special Considerations
- Use in conjunction with other antileprosy agents to prevent development of resistance

■ **Patient/Family Education**
- May discolor skin from pink to brownish-black, as well as discoloring the conjunctivae, lacrimal fluid, sweat, sputum, urine, and feces; skin discoloration may take several months or years to disappear after discontinuation of therapy
- Take with meals to decrease GI discomfort

■ **Geriatric side effects at a glance:**
❏ CNS   ❏ Bowel Dysfunction   ❏ Bladder Dysfunction   ❏ Falls

■ **U.S. Regulatory Considerations**
❏ FDA Black Box   ❏ OBRA regulated in U.S. Long Term Care

clomipramine hydrochloride

(kloe-mi'-pra-meen hye-droe-klor'-ide)

- **Brand Name(s):** Anafranil
  Chemical Class: Dibenzocycloheptene derivative; tertiary amine

- **Clinical Pharmacology:**
  Mechanism of Action: A tricyclic antidepressant that blocks the reuptake of neurotransmitters, such as norepinephrine and serotonin, at CNS presynaptic membranes, increasing their availability at postsynaptic receptor sites. **Therapeutic Effect:** Reduces obsessive-compulsive behavior.
  Pharmacokinetics: Well absorbed from GI tract. Protein binding: 97%. Principally bound to albumin. Distributed into cerebrospinal fluid. Metabolized in the liver. Undergoes extensive first-pass effect. Excreted in urine and feces. Half-life: 19-37 hr.

- **Available Forms:**
  - *Capsules*: 25 mg, 50 mg, 75 mg.

- **Indications and Dosages:**
  Obsessive-compulsive disorder: PO Initially, 25 mg/day. May gradually increase to 100 mg/day in the first 2 wk. Maximum: 250 mg/day.

- **Unlabeled Uses:** Treatment of bulimia nervosa, cataplexy associated with narcolepsy, depression, neurogenic pain, panic disorder, ejaculatory disorders, pervasive developmental disorder

- **Contraindications:** Acute recovery period after MI, use within 14 days of MAOIs

- **Side Effects**
  Frequent
  Somnolence, fatigue, dry mouth, blurred vision, constipation, sexual dysfunction (42%), ejaculatory failure (20%), impotence, weight gain (18%), delayed micturition, orthostatic hypotension, diaphoresis, impaired concentration, increased appetite, urine retention
  Occasional
  GI disturbances (such as nausea, GI distress, and metallic taste), asthenia, aggressiveness, muscle weakness
  Rare
  Paradoxical reactions (agitation, restlessness, nightmares, insomnia), extrapyramidal symptoms (particularly fine hand tremor), laryngitis, seizures

- **Serious Reactions**
  - Overdose may produce seizures; cardiovascular effects, such as severe orthostatic hypotension, dizziness, tachycardia, palpitations, and arrhythmias; and altered temperature regulation, including hyperpyrexia or hypothermia.
  - Abrupt discontinuation after prolonged therapy may produce headache, malaise, nausea, vomiting, and vivid dreams.
  - Anemia and agranulocytosis have been noted.

■ **Patient/Family Education**
- Beneficial effects may take 2-3 wk
- Use caution while driving or during other activities requiring alertness; may cause drowsiness
- Avoid alcohol and other CNS depressants
- Do not discontinue abruptly
- Tolerance to postural hypotension, sedative, and anticholinergic effects usually develops during early therapy

■ **Monitoring Parameters**
- Supervise suicidal-risk patient closely during early therapy (as depression lessens, energy level improves, increasing suicidal potential)
- Assess appearance, behavior, speech pattern, level of interest, and mood

■ **Geriatric side effects at a glance:**
☑ CNS   ☑ Bowel Dysfunction   ☑ Bladder Dysfunction   ☑ Falls
Other: Orthostatic hypotension, cardiac conduction disturbances, anticholinergic side effects

■ **Use with caution in older patients with:** Cardiovascular disease, prostatic hyptertrophy or other conditions which increase the risk of urinary retention

■ **U.S. Regulatory Considerations**
☑ FDA Black Box
- Because there is an increased risk of suicide in children and adolescents, older adults should also be closely monitored for suicide ideation.
☑ OBRA regulated in U.S. Long Term Care

■ **Other Uses in Geriatric Patient:** Neuropathic pain, urge urinary incontinence

■ **Side Effects:**
Of particular importance in the geriatric patient: Anticholinergic effects, extrapyramidal symptoms, high doses (greater than 100 mg) may increase risk of sudden death

■ **Geriatric Considerations - Summary:** Although tricyclic antidepressants are effective in the treatment of major depression in older adults, the side-effect profile and low toxic-to-therapeutic ratio relegate them to second-line agents (after serotonin reuptake inhibitors) for most older patients. These agents are effective in the treatment of urge urinary incontinence and neuropathic pain, but must be monitored closely. Of the tricyclic antidepressants, imipramine and amitryptyline have the highest anticholinergic activity and may be useful for management of incontinence, but should otherwise be avoided.

■ **References:**
1. Leipzig RM, Cumming RG, Tinetti ME. Drugs and falls in older people: a systematic review and meta-analysis: I. Psychotropic drugs. J Am Geriatr Soc 1999;47:30-39.
2. Cadieux RJ. Antidepressant drug interactions in the elderly. Understanding the P-450 system is half the battle in reducing risks. Postgrad Med 1999;106:231-240, 245.
3. Ray WA, Meredith S, Thapa PB, et al. Cyclic antidepressants and the risk of sudden cardiac death. Clin Pharmacol Ther 2004;75:234-241.

4. Roose SP, Laghrissi-Thode F, Kennedy JS, et al. Comparison of paroxetine and nortriptyline in depressed patients with ischemic heart disease. JAMA 1998;279:287-291.

clonazepam

(kloe-na'-zi-pam)

- **Brand Name(s):** Klonopin, Klonopin Wafer
  Chemical Class: Benzodiazepine

  DEA Class: Schedule IV

- **Clinical Pharmacology:**
  Mechanism of Action: A benzodiazepine that depresses all levels of the CNS; inhibits nerve impulse transmission in the motor cortex and suppresses abnormal discharge in petit mal seizures. **Therapeutic Effect:** Produces anxiolytic and anticonvulsant effects.
  Pharmacokinetics: Well absorbed from the GI tract. Protein binding: 85%. Metabolized in the liver. Excreted in urine. Not removed by hemodialysis. **Half-life:** 18-50 hr.

- **Available Forms:**
  - *Tablets (Klonopin):* 0.5 mg, 1 mg, 2 mg.
  - *Tablets (Disintegrating [Klonopin Wafer]):* 0.125 mg, 0.25 mg, 0.5 mg, 1 mg, 2 mg.

- **Indications and Dosages:**
  Adjunctive treatment of Lennox-Gastaut syndrome (petit mal variant) and akinetic, myoclonic, and absence (petit mal) seizures: PO 1.5 mg/day; may be increased in 0.5- to 1-mg increments every 3 days until seizures are controlled. Don't exceed maintenance dosage of 20 mg/day.
  Panic disorder: PO Initially, 0.25 mg twice a day; increased in increments of 0.125-0.25 mg twice a day every 3 days. Maximum: 4 mg/day.

- **Unlabeled Uses:** Adjunctive treatment of seizures; treatment of simple, complex partial, and tonic-clonic seizures

- **Contraindications:** Narrow-angle glaucoma, significant hepatic disease, hypersensitivity to benzodiazepines

- **Side Effects**
  Frequent
  Mild, transient drowsiness; ataxia; behavioral disturbances (aggression, irritability, agitation)
  Occasional
  Rash, ankle or facial edema, nocturia, dysuria, change in appetite or weight, dry mouth, sore gums, nausea, blurred vision
  Rare
  Paradoxical CNS reactions, including excitement or restlessness (particularly in the presence of uncontrolled pain).

■ **Serious Reactions**
  • Abrupt withdrawal may result in pronounced restlessness, irritability, insomnia, hand tremors, abdominal or muscle cramps, diaphoresis, vomiting, and status epilepticus.
  • Overdose results in somnolence, confusion, diminished reflexes, and coma.

Special Considerations
  • Up to 30% of patients have shown a loss of anticonvulsant activity, often within 3 mo of administration; dosage adjustment may reestablish efficacy

■ **Patient/Family Education**
  • Do not take more than prescribed amount, may be habit-forming
  • Avoid driving, activities that require alertness; drowsiness may occur
  • Avoid alcohol ingestion or other CNS depressants
  • Do not discontinue medication abruptly after long-term use

■ **Monitoring Parameters**
  • Although relationship between serum concentrations and seizure control is not well established and not used clinically, proposed therapeutic concentrations are 20-80 ng/ml; potentially toxic concentrations greater than 80 ng/ml
  • Close attention to seizure frequency is important in order to detect the emergence of tolerance
  • CBC and blood chemistry tests periodically to assess hepatic and renal function for patients on long-term therapy

■ **Geriatric side effects at a glance:**
  ☑ CNS   ☐ Bowel Dysfunction   ☐ Bladder Dysfunction   ☑ Falls
  Other: Withdrawal symptoms after long-term use

■ **Use with caution in older patients with:** COPD; untreated sleep apnea

■ **U.S. Regulatory Considerations**
  ☐ FDA Black Box   ☑ OBRA regulated in U.S. Long Term Care

■ **Other Uses in Geriatric Patient:** Anxiety symptoms and related disorders, dementia-related behavioral problems, neuropathic pain, restless legs syndrome

■ **Side Effects:**
  Of particular importance in the geriatric patient: Sedation, withdrawal symptoms when abruptly discontinued (e.g., during hospitalization) rather than tapered

■ **Geriatric Considerations - Summary:** Benzodiazepines are effective anxiolytic agents, and hypnotics. These drugs should be reserved for short-term use. SSRIs are preferred for long-term management of anxiety disorders in older adults, and sedating antidepressants (e.g., trazodone) or eszopiclone are preferred for long-term management of sleep problems. Long-acting benzodiazepines, including flurazepam, chlordiazepoxide, clorazepate, diazepam, clonazepam, and quazepam, should generally be avoided in older adults as these agents have been associated with oversedation. On the other hand, short-acting benzodiazepines (e.g., triazolam) have been associated with a higher risk of withdrawal symptoms. When initiating therapy, benzodiazepines should be titrated carefully to avoid oversedation. In addition, many of the drugs in this class have been associated with severe withdrawal symptoms (e.g., anxiety and/or agitation, seizures) when discontinued abruptly.

■ **References:**
1. Leipzig RM, Cumming RG, Tinetti ME. Drugs and falls in older people: a systematic review and meta-analysis: I. Psychotropic drugs. J Am Geriatr Soc 1999;47:30-39.
2. Shorr RI, Robin DW. Rational use of benzodiazepines in the elderly. Drugs Aging 1994;4:9-20.
3. Shader RI, Greenblatt DJ. Use of benzodiazepines in anxiety disorders. N Engl J Med 1993;328:1398-1405.

clonidine

(kloe'-ni-deen)

■ **Brand Name(s):** Catapres, Catapres-TTS-1, Catapres-TTS-2, Catapres-TTS-3, Clonidine TTS-1, Clonidine TTS-2, Clonidine TTS-3, Duraclon

Combinations
Rx: with chlorthalidone (Chlorpres, Combipress)
Chemical Class: Imidazoline derivative

■ **Clinical Pharmacology:**
Mechanism of Action: An antiadrenergic, sympatholytic agent that prevents pain signal transmission to the brain and produces analgesia at pre- and post-alpha-adrenergic receptors in the spinal cord. **Therapeutic Effect:** Reduces peripheral resistance; decreases BP and heart rate.
Pharmacokinetics:

Route	Onset	Peak	Duration
PO	0.5-1 hr	2-4 hr	Up to 8 hr

Well absorbed from the GI tract. Transdermal best absorbed from the chest and upper arm; least absorbed from the thigh. Protein binding: 20%–40%. Metabolized in the liver. Primarily excreted in urine. Minimally removed by hemodialysis. **Half-life:** 12–16 hr (increased with impaired renal function).

■ **Available Forms:**
- *Tablets (Catapres):* 0.1 mg, 0.2 mg, 0.3 mg.
- *Transdermal Patch:* 2.5 mg (release at 0.1 mg/24 hr) (Catapres-TTS-1, Clonidine TTS-1); 5 mg (release at 0.2 mg/24 hr)(Catapres-TTS-2, Clonidine TTS-2); 7.5 mg (release at 0.3 mg/24 hr)(Catapres-TTS-3, Clonidine TTS-3).
- *Injection (Duraclon):* 100 mcg/ml, 500 mcg/ml.

■ **Indications and Dosages:**
Hypertension: PO Initially, 0.1 mg at bedtime. May increase gradually. Transdermal System delivering 0.1 mg/24 hr up to 0.6 mg/24 hr q7 days.
Severe pain: Epidural 30–40 mcg/hr.

■ **Unlabeled Uses:** Diagnosis of pheochromocytoma, opioid withdrawal, prevention of migraine headaches, treatment of diarrhea in diabetes mellitus, menopausal flushing

■ **Contraindications:** Epidural contraindicated in those patients with bleeding diathesis or infection at the injection site, those receiving anticoagulation therapy

■ Side Effects
Frequent
Dry mouth (40%), somnolence (33%), dizziness (16%), sedation, constipation (10%)
Occasional (5%–1%)
Tablets, injection: Depression, swelling of feet, loss of appetite, decreased sexual ability, itching eyes, dizziness, nausea, vomiting, nervousness
Transdermal: Itching, reddening or darkening of skin
Rare (less than 1%)
Nightmares, vivid dreams, cold feeling in fingers and toes

■ Serious Reactions
- Overdose produces profound hypotension, irritability, bradycardia, respiratory depression, hypothermia, miosis (pupillary constriction), arrhythmias, and apnea.
- Abrupt withdrawal may result in rebound hypertension associated with nervousness, agitation, anxiety, insomnia, hand tingling, tremor, flushing, and diaphoresis.

■ Patient/Family Education
- Avoid hazardous activities, since drug may cause drowsiness
- Do not discontinue oral drug abruptly or withdrawal symptoms may occur (anxiety, increased BP, headache, insomnia, increased pulse, tremors, nausea, sweating)
- Response may take 2-3 days if drug is given transdermally
- Do not use OTC (cough, cold, or allergy) products unless directed by clinician
- Rise slowly to sitting or standing position to minimize orthostatic hypotension
- Dizziness, fainting, light-headedness may occur during 1st few days of therapy
- May cause dry mouth; use hard candy, saliva product, or frequent rinsing of mouth

■ Monitoring Parameters
- Blood pressure (posturally), blood glucose in patients with diabetes mellitus, confusion, mental depression
- Daily bowel activity and stool consistency

■ Geriatric side effects at a glance:
☑ CNS ☐ Bowel Dysfunction ☐ Bladder Dysfunction ☐ Falls

■ Use with caution in older patients with: Renal impairment

■ U.S. Regulatory Considerations
☑ FDA Black Box
Although not relevent in geriatric patients, epidural administration of clonidine is not recommended.
☐ OBRA regulated in U.S. Long Term Care

■ Other Uses in Geriatric Patient: Menopausal vasomotor symptoms, Alcohol withdrawal, PTSD, Excessive salivation or drug-induced sialorrhea

■ Side Effects:
Of particular importance in the geriatric patient: Case reports of confusion associated with somnolence, dementia, sedation, dizziness, orthostasis, dry mouth, constipation

- **Geriatric Considerations - Summary:** Discontinuation of clonidine is likely to require a slow taper. If the patient is receiving a concomitant beta-blocker, the beta-blocker must be tapered and discontinued before discontinuing clonidine. Clonidine discontinuation in the presence of a beta-blocker can lead to severe hypertension and cardiovascular events due to unopposed alpha-receptor stimulation. CNS effects often preclude its use in older adults. A higher clonidine dose (0.4 mg/day) is generally needed to control peri- or postmenopausal vasomotor symptoms; however, adverse effects often make it difficult to achieve effective doses.

- **References:**
  1. Drugs that may cause cognitive disorders in the elderly. Med Lett 2000;42:111-112.
  2. Barton D, Loprinzi C, Wahner-Roedler D. Hot flashes: aetiology and management. Drugs Aging 2001;8:591-606.
  3. Nagamani M, Kelver ME, Smith ER. Treatment of menopausal hot flashes with transdermal administration of clonidine. Am J Obstet Gynecol 1987;156:561-565.

clopidogrel bisulfate

(kloh-pid'-oh-grel bye-sul'-fate)

- **Brand Name(s):** Plavix
  Chemical Class: Thienopyridine derivative

- **Clinical Pharmacology:**
  Mechanism of Action: A thienopyridine derivative that inhibits binding of the enzyme adenosine phosphate (ADP) to its platelet receptor and subsequent ADP-mediated activation of a glycoprotein complex. **Therapeutic Effect:** Inhibits platelet aggregation.
  Pharmacokinetics:

Route	Onset	Peak	Duration
PO	1 hr	2 hr	N/A

  Rapidly absorbed. Protein binding: 98%. Extensively metabolized by the liver. Eliminated equally in the urine and feces. **Half-life:** 8 hr.

- **Available Forms:**
  - *Tablets:* 75 mg.

- **Indications and Dosages:**
  MI, *stroke reduction*: PO 75 mg once a day.
  ***Acute coronary syndrome*:** PO Initially, 300 mg loading dose, then 75 mg once a day (in combination with aspirin).

- **Unlabeled Uses:** Graft patency (saphenous vein), mitral regurgitation, mitral stenosis, noncardioembolic stroke, percutaneous coronary intervention

- **Contraindications:** Active bleeding, coagulation disorders, severe hepatic disease

- **Side Effects**
  Frequent (15%)
  Skin disorders

Occasional (8%–6%)
Upper respiratory tract infection, chest pain, flu-like symptoms, headache, dizziness, arthralgia
Rare (5%–3%)
Fatigue, edema, hypertension, abdominal pain, dyspepsia, diarrhea, nausea, epistaxis, dyspnea, rhinitis

■ Serious Reactions

- Agranulocytosis, aplastic anemia/pancytopenia, and thrombotic thrombocytopenic purpura (TTP) occur rarely.
- Cases of bleeding with fatal outcome (especially intracranial, GI, and retroperitoneal hemorrhage) have been reported.
- Hepatitis, hypersensitivity reactions, anaphylactoid reactions, and angioedema have also been reported.

Special Considerations

- Comparative studies indicate that the drug is at least as effective as aspirin; comparisons with ticlopidine lacking, however; no frequent CBC monitoring necessary
- Should probably replace ticlopidine as an aspirin alternative
- 28 × the cost of an equivalent supply of aspirin

■ Patient/Family Education

- Inform clinician of signs and symptoms of bleeding prior to surgery, dental work; inform clinician of sore throat, fever, etc. (consider neutropenia)
- Notify the dentist and other physicians of clopidogrel therapy before surgery is scheduled or new drugs are prescribed

■ Monitoring Parameters

- Platelet count for thrombocytopenia
- Hgb, WBC count, and BUN, serum bilirubin, creatinine, AST and ALT levels
- Evaluate for signs and symptoms of hepatic insufficiency during clopidogrel therapy

■ Geriatric side effects at a glance:
  ❏ CNS ❏ Bowel Dysfunction ❏ Bladder Dysfunction ❏ Falls

■ U.S. Regulatory Considerations
  ❏ FDA Black Box ☑ OBRA regulated in U.S. Long Term Care

clorazepate dipotassium

(klor-az'-e-pate)

- **Brand Name(s):** Gen-Xene, Tranxene, Tranxene-SD
  Chemical Class: Benzodiazepine

  DEA Class: Schedule IV

- **Clinical Pharmacology:**
  Mechanism of Action: A benzodiazepine that depresses all levels of the CNS, including limbic and reticular formation, by binding to benzodiazepine receptor sites on the gamma-aminobutyric acid (GABA) receptor complex. Modulates GABA, a major inhibitory neurotransmitter in the brain. **Therapeutic Effect:** Produces anxiolytic effect, suppresses seizure activity.

- **Available Forms:**
  - *Tablets (Tranxene T-Tab):* 3.75 mg, 7.5 mg, 15 mg.
  - *Tablets (Sustained-Release):* 11.25 mg (Tranxene SD Half-Strength); 22.5 mg (Tranxene-SD).

- **Indications and Dosages:**
  Anxiety: PO (Regular-Release) 7.5-15 mg 2-4 times a day. PO (Sustained-Release) 11.25 mg or 22.5 mg once a day at bedtime.
  Anticonvulsant: PO Initially, 7.5 mg 2-3 times a day. May increase by 7.5 mg at weekly intervals. Maximum: 90 mg/day.
  Alcohol withdrawal: PO Initially, 30 mg, then 15 mg 2-4 times a day on first day. Gradually decrease dosage over subsequent days. Maximum: 90 mg/day.

- **Contraindications:** Acute narrow-angle glaucoma

- **Side Effects**
  Frequent
  Somnolence
  Occasional
  Dizziness, GI disturbances, nervousness, blurred vision, dry mouth, headache, confusion, ataxia, rash, irritability, slurred speech
  Rare
  Paradoxical CNS reactions, such as excitement or restlessness in the elderly or debilitated (generally noted during first 2 weeks of therapy, particularly in presence of uncontrolled pain)

- **Serious Reactions**
  - Abrupt or too-rapid withdrawal may result in pronounced restlessness, irritability, insomnia, hand tremors, abdominal or muscle cramps, diaphoresis, vomiting, and seizures.
  - Overdose results in somnolence, confusion, diminished reflexes, and coma.

Special Considerations
  - Do not use for everyday stress or for longer than 4 mo
  - No advantage over diazepam

- **Patient/Family Education**
  - Do not discontinue medication abruptly after long-term use
  - Avoid tasks that require mental alertness or motor skills until response to the drug has been established
  - Change positions slowly—from recumbent to sitting before standing—to prevent dizziness
  - Avoid smoking and consuming alcoholic beverages during therapy

- **Monitoring Parameters**
  - Therapeutic response, characterized by a calm facial expression and decreased restlessness in anxious patients and a decrease in intensity or frequency of seizures in patients with seizure disorder

- **Geriatric side effects at a glance:**
  ☑ CNS   ☐ Bowel Dysfunction   ☐ Bladder Dysfunction   ☑ Falls
  Other: Withdrawal symptoms after long-term use

- **Use with caution in older patients with:** COPD; untreated sleep apnea

- **U.S. Regulatory Considerations**
  ☐ FDA Black Box   ☑ OBRA regulated in U.S. Long Term Care

- **Other Uses in Geriatric Patient:** Anxiety symptoms and related disorders, dementia-related behavioral problems

- **Side Effects:**
  Of particular importance in the geriatric patient: Sedation, withdrawal symptoms when abruptly discontinued (e.g., during hospitalization) rather than tapered

- **Geriatric Considerations - Summary:** Benzodiazepines are effective anxiolytic agents, and hypnotics. These drugs should be reserved for short-term use. SSRIs are preferred for long-term management of anxiety disorders in older adults, and sedating antidepressants (e.g., trazodone) or eszopiclone are preferred for long-term management of sleep problems. Long-acting benzodiazepines, including flurazepam, chlordiazepoxide, clorazepate, diazepam, clonazepam, and quazepam, should generally be avoided in older adults as these agents have been associated with oversedation. On the other hand, short-acting benzodiazepines (e.g., triazolam) have been associated with a higher risk of withdrawal symptoms. When initiating therapy, benzodiazepines should be titrated carefully to avoid oversedation. In addition, many of the drugs in this class have been associated with severe withdrawal symptoms (e.g., anxiety and/or agitation, seizures) when discontinued abruptly.

- **References:**
  1. Leipzig RM, Cumming RG, Tinetti ME. Drugs and falls in older people: a systematic review. and meta-analysis: I. Psychotropic drugs. J Am Geriatr Soc 1999;47:30-39.
  2. Shorr RI, Robin DW. Rational use of benzodiazepines in the elderly. Drugs Aging 1994;4:9-20.
  3. Shader RI, Greenblatt DJ. Use of benzodiazepines in anxiety disorders. N Engl J Med 1993;328:1398-1405.

clotrimazole

(kloe-trim'-a-zole)

■ **Brand Name(s):**
OTC: Mycelex, Mycelex OTC, Lotrimin, Gyne-Lotrimin, Trivagizole 3

Combinations
Rx: with betamethasone dipropionate (Lotrisone)
Chemical Class: Imidazole derivative

■ **Clinical Pharmacology:**
Mechanism of Action: An antifungal that binds with phospholipids in fungal cell membrane. The altered cell membrane permeability. **Therapeutic Effect:** Inhibits yeast growth.
Pharmacokinetics: Poorly, erratically absorbed from GI tract. Bound to oral mucosa. Absorbed portion metabolized in liver. Eliminated in feces. Topical: Minimal systemic absorption (highest concentration in stratum corneum). Intravaginal: Small amount systemically absorbed. **Half-life:** 3.5-5 hr.

■ **Available Forms:**
- *Combination Pack*: Vaginal tablet 100 mg and vaginal cream 1% (Mycelex-7).
- *Lotion*: 1% (Lotrimin).
- *Topical Cream*: 1% (Lotrimin, Lotrimin AF, Mycelex, Mycelex OTC).
- *Topical Solution*: 1% (Lotrimin, Lotrimin AF, Mycelex, Mycelex OTC).
- *Troches*: 10 mg (Mycelex).
- *Vaginal Cream*: 1% (Gyne-Lotrimin, Mycelex-7), 2% (Gyne-Lotrimin 3, Mycelex-3, Trivagizole 3).
- *Vaginal Tablets*: 100 mg, 500 mg (Gyne-Lotrimin, Mycelex-7).

■ **Indications and Dosages:**
Oropharyngeal candidiasis treatment: PO 10 mg 5 times/day for 14 days.
Oropharyngeal candidiasis prophylaxis: PO 10 mg 3 times/day.
Dermatophytosis, cutaneous candidiasis: Topical 2 times/day. Therapeutic effect may take up to 8 wk.
Vulvovaginal candidiasis: Vaginal (Tablets) 1 tablet (100 mg) at bedtime for 7 days; 2 tablets (200 mg) at bedtime for 3 days; or 500-mg tablet one time. Vaginal (Cream) 1 applicatorful at bedtime for 7-14 days.

■ **Unlabeled Uses:** *Topical*: Treatment of paronychia, tinea barbae, tinea capitis.

■ **Contraindications:** Hypersensitivity to clotrimazole or any component of the formulation

■ **Side Effects**
Frequent
Oral: Nausea, vomiting, diarrhea, abdominal pain
Occasional
Topical: Itching, burning, stinging, erythema, urticaria
Vaginal: Mild burning (tablets/cream); irritation, cystitis (cream)
Rare
Vaginal: Itching, rash, lower abdominal cramping, headache

Serious Reactions

- None reported.

Patient/Family Education

- Continue for the full length of therapy
- Avoid contact with eyes
- Refrain from sexual intercourse or advise partner to use a condom during therapy

Monitoring Parameters

- Skin for blistering or urticaria
- With vaginal therapy, evaluate for vulvovaginal irritation, abdominal cramping, urinary frequency, and discomfort

Geriatric side effects at a glance:

☐ CNS ☐ Bowel Dysfunction ☐ Bladder Dysfunction ☐ Falls

U.S. Regulatory Considerations

☐ FDA Black Box ☐ OBRA regulated in U.S. Long Term Care

clozapine

(klo'-za-peen)

■ **Brand Name(s):** Clozaril, FazaClo
   Chemical Class: Dibenzodiazepine derivative

■ **Clinical Pharmacology:**
   Mechanism of Action: A dibenzodiazepine derivative that interferes with the binding of dopamine at dopamine receptor sites; binds primarily at nondopamine receptor sites. **Therapeutic Effect:** Diminishes schizophrenic behavior.
   Pharmacokinetics: Absorbed rapidly and almost completely. Distributed rapidly and extensively. Crosses the blood-brain barrier. Protein binding: 95%. Metabolized in the liver. Excreted in urine and feces. **Half-life:** 8 hr.

■ **Available Forms:**
   - *Tablets (Clozaril)*: 12.5 mg, 25 mg, 100 mg.
   - *Tablets (Oral-Disintegrating[FazaClo])*: 25 mg, 100 mg.

■ **Indications and Dosages:**
   Schizophrenic disorders, reduce suicidal behavior: PO Initially, 25 mg/day. May increase by 25 mg/day. Maximum: 450 mg/day.

■ **Contraindications:** Coma, concurrent use of other drugs that may suppress bone marrow function, history of clozapine-induced agranulocytosis or severe granulocytopenia, myeloproliferative disorders, severe CNS depression

Side Effects

Frequent

Somnolence (39%), salivation (31%), tachycardia (25%), dizziness (19%), constipation (14%)

Occasional

Hypotension (9%); headache (7%); tremor, syncope, diaphoresis, dry mouth (6%); nausea, visual disturbances (5%); nightmares, restlessness, akinesia, agitation, hypertension, abdominal discomfort or heartburn, weight gain (4%)

Rare

Rigidity, confusion, fatigue, insomnia, diarrhea, rash

Serious Reactions

- **Alert**: Blood dyscrasias, particularly agranulocytosis and mild leukopenia, may occur.
- Seizures occur in about 3% of patients.
- Overdose produces CNS depression (including sedation, coma, and delirium), respiratory depression, and hypersalivation.

Special Considerations

- The risk of agranulocytosis and seizures limits use to patients who have failed to respond or were unable to tolerate treatment with appropriate courses of standard antipsychotics.
- Advise patients to report immediately the appearance of lethargy, weakness, fever, sore throat, malaise, mucous membrane ulceration, or other possible signs of infection.
- Patients cannot be reinitiated on clozapine if WBC counts fall below 2000/mm^3 or ANC falls below 1000/mm^3 during clozapine therapy.

Patient/Family Education

- Do not abruptly withdraw from long-term drug therapy.
- Drowsiness generally subsides during continued therapy.
- Avoid tasks that require mental alertness or motor skills until response to the drug is established.
- Avoid alcohol.

Monitoring Parameters

- WBC at baseline and then qwk for first 6 mo, every other week thereafter if WBC counts maintained (WBC ≥3000/mm^3, ANC ≥1500/mm^3); WBC counts qwk for at least 4 wk after discontinuation.
- Blood pressure, LFTs
- Pulse for tachycardia
- Assess for therapeutic response (interest in surroundings, improvement in self-care, increased ability to concentrate, relaxed facial expression)

Geriatric side effects at a glance:

☑ CNS ☑ Bowel Dysfunction ☑ Bladder Dysfunction ☑ Falls

Other: Agranulocytosis, cardiovascular collapse, seizures, weight gain, glucose intolerance, diabetes, orthostatic hypotension, extrapyramidal symptoms

Use with caution in older patients with: Diabetes, glucose intolerance, cardiovascular disease

■ U.S. Regulatory Considerations
☑ FDA Black Box

There is an increased risk of death in older patients with dementia. Although the causes of death were varied, most of the deaths appeared to be either cardiovascular (e.g., heart failure, sudden death) or infectious (e.g., pneumonia) in nature. This drug is not approved for treatment of patients with dementia-related psychosis.

☑ OBRA regulated in U.S. Long Term Care

■ Other Uses in Geriatric Patient: Behavior disturbances in the setting of dementia

■ Side Effects:
Of particular importance in the geriatric patient: Weight gain, glucose intolerance, diabetes, increased risk of death

■ Geriatric Considerations - Summary: Direct comparisons between older and newer antipsychotic drugs in demented elderly persons are scarce. Newer agents have the theoretical advantage of a lower incidence of tardive dyskinesia but may cause weight gain, impaired glycemic control, and increased risk for cardiovascular events. These agents should be used with caution in demented elderly persons, with frequent monitoring for side effects and a low threshold for discontinuing use. Indeed, the Food and Drug Administration has recently released an advisory about these medications outlining the risk for increased mortality. Because of the special toxicities associated with clozapine, above and beyond class-related effects, this drug is not recommended for first-line use in older adults.

■ References:
1. Sink KM, Holden KF, Yaffe K. Pharmacological treatment of neuropsychiatric symptoms of dementia: a review of the evidence. JAMA 2005;293:596-608.
2. Alexopoulos GS, Streim J, Carpenter D, Docherty JP. Using antipsychotic agents in older patients. J Clin Psychiatry 2004;65 (suppl 2):5-99.
3. Deaths with antipsychotics in elderly patients with behavioral disturbances. Available at: www.fda.gov/cder/drug/advisory/antipsychotics.htm.
4. Herst L, Powell G. Is clozapine safe in the elderly? Aust N Z J Psychiatry 1997;31:411-417.

co-trimoxazole (sulfamethoxazole and trimethoprim)

(koe-trye-mox'a-zole; sul-fa-meth-ox'-a-zole; trye-meth'-oh-prim)

■ Brand Name(s): Bactrim, Bactrim DS, Bactrim Pediatric, Bethaprim, Septra, Septra DS, Sulfatrim Suspension, Uroplus, Uroplus DS
Chemical Class: Dihydrofolate reductase inhibitor (trimethoprim); sulfonamide derivative (sulfamethoxazole)

■ **Clinical Pharmacology:**
Mechanism of Action: A sulfonamide and folate antagonist that blocks bacterial synthesis of essential nucleic acids. **Therapeutic Effect:** Bactericidal in susceptible microorganisms.
Pharmacokinetics: Rapidly and well absorbed from the GI tract. Protein binding: 45%-60%. Widely distributed. Metabolized in the liver. Excreted in urine. Minimally removed by hemodialysis. **Half-life:** sulfamethoxazole 6-12 hr, trimethoprim 8-10 hr (increased in impaired renal function).

■ **Available Forms:**
- Alert All dosage forms have same 5:1 ratio of sulfamethoxazole (SMX) to trimethoprim (TMP).
- *Tablets* (Bactrim, Septra, Uroplus): SMX 400 mg and TMP 80 mg.
- *Tablets* (Double Strength [Bactrim DS, Septra DS, Uroplus DS]): SMX 800 mg and TMP 160 mg.
- *Injection:* SMX 80 mg and TMP 16 mg per ml.

■ **Indications and Dosages:**
Chronic bronchitis: PO 1 double-strength or 2 single-strength tablets or 20-ml suspension q12h for 14 days.
Pneumocystis carinii pneumonia (PCP) prophylaxis: PO 1 double-strength tablet daily or 3 times a week or 1 single-strength tablet daily.
PCP Treatment: PO, IV 15-20 mg/kg as trimethoprim a day in 4 divided doses for 14-21 days.
Shigellosis: PO 1 double-strength tablet or 2 single-strength tablets or 20-ml suspension q12h for 5 days.
UTIs: PO 1 double-strength or 2 single-strength tablets or 20-ml suspension q12h for 10-14 days.
Traveler's diarrhea: PO 1 double-strength or 2 single-strength tablets or 20-ml suspension q12h for 5 days.
Dosage in renal impairment: Dosage and frequency are modified based on creatinine clearance, the severity of the infection, and the serum concentration of the drug. For those with creatinine clearance of 15-30 ml/min, a 50% dosage reduction is recommended.

■ **Unlabeled Uses:** Treatment of bacterial endocarditis; gonorrhea; meningitis; septicemia; sinusitis; and biliary tract, bone, joint, chancroid, chlamydial, intra-abdominal, skin, and soft tissue infections

■ **Contraindications:** Hypersensitivity to trimethoprim or any sulfonamides, megaloblastic anemia due to folate deficiency.

■ **Side Effects**
Frequent
Anorexia, nausea, vomiting, rash (generally 7-14 days after therapy begins), urticaria
Occasional
Diarrhea, abdominal pain, pain or irritation at the IV infusion site
Rare
Headache, vertigo, insomnia, seizures, hallucinations, depression

■ **Serious Reactions**
- Rash, fever, sore throat, pallor, purpura, cough, and shortness of breath may be early signs of serious adverse reactions.

- Fatalities have occasionally occurred after Stevens-Johnson syndrome, toxic epidermal necrolysis, fulminant hepatic necrosis, agranulocytosis, aplastic anemia, and other blood dyscrasias in patients taking sulfonamides.
- Myelosuppression, decreased platelet count, and severe dermatologic reactions may occur.

Special Considerations

- Pay special attention to complaints of skin rash, especially those involving mucous membranes (could signify early Stevens-Johnson syndrome), sore throat, mouth sores, fever, or unusual bruising or bleeding
- Individualize treatment based on local susceptibility patterns.

■ Patient/Family Education

- Take oral doses with 8 oz of water and drink several extra glasses of water each day
- Space drug doses evenly around the clock and continue taking for the full course of treatment
- Notify the physician immediately if any new symptom, especially bleeding, bruising, fever, sore throat, and a rash or other skin changes, occurs
- Your skin may be more sensitive to sunlight while taking this medication. Wear sunscreen outdoors. Avoid sunlamps and tanning beds.

■ Monitoring Parameters

- Baseline and periodic CBC for patients on long-term or high-dose therapy
- Intake and output
- Skin for pallor, purpura, and rash
- Renal and liver function
- Vital signs
- Daily bowel activity and stool consistency. Although mild GI effects may be tolerable, severe symptoms may indicate the onset of antibiotic-associated colitis.
- Signs and symptoms of superinfection include abdominal pain or cramping, anal or genital pruritus or discharge, moderate to severe diarrhea, severe mouth or tongue soreness, and new or increased fever.

■ Geriatric side effects at a glance:
❏ CNS ❏ Bowel Dysfunction ❏ Bladder Dysfunction ❏ Falls

■ U.S. Regulatory Considerations
❏ FDA Black Box ❏ OBRA regulated in U.S. Long Term Care

codeine phosphate/codeine sulfate

(koe'-deen foss'-fate/koe'-deen sul'-fate)

■ **Brand Name(s):** Codeine Phosphate, Codeine Sulfate

Combinations
Rx: with acetaminophen (Tylenol No. 2, Tylenol No. 3, Tylenol No. 4); with aspirin (Empirin No. 3, Empirin No. 4); with chlorpheniramine (Codeprex); with guaifenesin (Robitussin AC); with APAP (Capital, Aceta); with APAP, butalbital, caffeine (Fioricet, Phenaphen); with aspirin (Fiorinal)
Chemical Class: Natural opium alkaloid; phenanthrene derivative

DEA Class: Schedule II

■ Clinical Pharmacology:
Mechanism of Action: An opioid agonist that binds to opioid receptors at many sites in the CNS, particularly in the medulla. This action inhibits the ascending pain pathways. **Therapeutic Effect:** Alters the perception of and emotional response to pain, suppresses cough reflex.
Pharmacokinetics: Well absorbed following PO administration. Protein binding: Very low. Metabolized in liver. Excreted in urine. **Half-life:** 2.5-3.5 hr.

■ Available Forms:
- *Tablets (phosphate):* 30 mg, 60 mg.
- *Tablets (sulfate):* 15 mg, 30 mg, 60 mg.
- *Oral Solution:* 15 mg/5 ml.
- *Injection:* 15 mg/ml, 30 mg/ml, 60 mg/ml.

■ Indications and Dosages:
Analgesia: PO, IM, Subcutaneous 30 mg q4–6h. Range: 15–60 mg.
Cough: PO 10–20 mg q4–6h.
Dosage in renal impairment: Dosage is modified based on creatinine clearance.

Creatinine Clearance	Dosage
10-50 ml/min	75% of usual dose
less than 10 ml/min	50% of usual dose

■ Unlabeled Uses: Treatment of diarrhea

■ Contraindications: None known.

■ Side Effects
Frequent
Constipation, somnolence, nausea, vomiting
Occasional
Paradoxical excitement, confusion, palpitations, facial flushing, decreased urination, blurred vision, dizziness, dry mouth, headache, hypotension (including orthostatic hypotension), decreased appetite, injection site redness, burning, or pain
Rare
Hallucinations, depression, abdominal pain, insomnia

■ Serious Reactions
- Too-frequent use may result in paralytic ileus.
- Overdose may produce cold and clammy skin, confusion, seizures, decreased BP, restlessness, pinpoint pupils, bradycardia, respiratory depression, decreased LOC, and severe weakness.
- The patient who uses codeine repeatedly may develop a tolerance to the drug's analgesic effect as well as physical dependence.

■ **Patient/Family Education**
- Minimize nausea by administering with food and remain lying down following dose
- Do not administer agonist/antagonist analgesics (i.e., pentazocine, nalbuphine, butorphanol, dezocine, buprenorphine) to patient who has received a prolonged course of codeine (a pure agonist). In opioid-dependent patients, mixed agonist/antagonist analgesics may precipitate withdrawal symptoms
- Change positions slowly to avoid orthostatic hypotension
- Avoid tasks that require mental alertness or motor skills until his or her response to the drug has been established
- Avoid alcohol during codeine therapy

■ **Monitoring Parameters**
- Clinical improvement and onset of pain or cough relief
- Bowel activity and stool consistency

■ **Geriatric side effects at a glance:**
☑ CNS   ☑ Bowel Dysfunction   ☑ Bladder Dysfunction   ☑ Falls

■ **U.S. Regulatory Considerations**
☐ FDA Black Box   ☑ OBRA regulated in U.S. Long Term Care

colchicine

(kol'-chi-seen)

■ **Brand Name(s):** Colchicine

> Combinations
> **Rx:** with probenicid (Proben-C, Colbenemid)
> **Chemical Class:** *Colchicum autumnale* alkaloid

■ **Clinical Pharmacology:**
Mechanism of Action: An alkaloid that decreases leukocyte motility, phagocytosis, and lactic acid production. **Therapeutic Effect:** Decreases urate crystal deposits and reduces inflammatory process.
Pharmacokinetics: Rapidly absorbed from the GI tract. Highest concentration is in the liver, spleen, and kidney. Protein binding: 30%–50%. Reenters the intestinal tract by biliary secretion and is reabsorbed from the intestines. Partially metabolized in the liver. Eliminated primarily in feces.

■ **Available Forms:**
- *Tablets:* 0.5 mg, 0.6 mg.
- *Injection:* 0.5 mg/ml.

■ **Indications and Dosages:**
Acute gouty arthritis: PO Initially, 0.6-1.2 mg; then 0.6 mg q1-2h until pain is relieved or nausea, vomiting, or diarrhea occurs. Total dose: 6 mg. IV Initially, 1-2 mg; then 0.5 mg q6h until satisfactory response. Maximum: 4 mg/wk or 4 mg/one course of treatment. If pain recurs, may give 1-2 mg/day for several days but no sooner than 7 days after a full course of IV therapy (total of 4 mg).
Chronic gouty arthritis: PO 0.6 mg every other day up to 3 times a day.

■ **Unlabeled Uses:** To reduce frequency of recurrence of familial Mediterranean fever; treatment of acute calcium pyrophosphate deposition, amyloidosis, biliary cirrhosis, recurrent pericarditis, sarcoid arthritis

■ **Contraindications:** Blood dyscrasias; severe cardiac, GI, hepatic, or renal disorders

■ **Side Effects**
Frequent
PO: Nausea, vomiting, abdominal discomfort
Occasional
PO: Anorexia
Rare
Hypersensitivity reaction, including angioedema
Parenteral: Nausea, vomiting, diarrhea, abdominal discomfort, pain or redness at injection site, neuritis in injected arm

■ **Serious Reactions**
- Bone marrow depression, including aplastic anemia, agranulocytosis, and thrombocytopenia, may occur with long-term therapy.
- Overdose initially causes a burning feeling in the skin or throat, severe diarrhea, and abdominal pain. The patient then experiences fever, seizures, delirium, and renal impairment, marked by hematuria and oliguria. The third stage of overdose causes hair loss, leukocytosis, and stomatitis.

■ **Patient/Family Education**
- Limit intake of high purine foods, such as fish and organ meats, and drink 8-10 eight-oz glasses of fluid daily while taking colchicine
- Notify the physician if fever, numbness, skin rash, sore throat, fatigue, unusual bleeding or bruising, or weakness occurs
- Discontinue colchicine as soon as gout pain is relieved, or at the first appearance of diarrhea, nausea, or vomiting

■ **Monitoring Parameters**
- CBC, platelets, reticulocytes before and during therapy (q3mo)
- Fluid intake and output
- Serum uric acid level
- Therapeutic response, including improved joint range of motion and reduced joint tenderness, redness, and swelling

■ **Geriatric side effects at a glance:**
❑ CNS   ☑ Bowel Dysfunction   ❑ Bladder Dysfunction   ❑ Falls

■ **U.S. Regulatory Considerations**
❑ FDA Black Box   ❑ OBRA regulated in U.S. Long Term Care

colesevelam

(koh-le-sev'-e-lam)

■ **Brand Name(s):** Welchol
  Chemical Class: Hydrophilic nonabsorbed polymer

■ **Clinical Pharmacology:**
  Mechanism of Action: A lipid-bile acid sequestrant and nonsystemic polymer that binds with bile acids in the intestines, preventing their reabsorption and removing them from the body. **Therapeutic Effect:** Decreases LDL cholesterol.
  Pharmacokinetics: Not absorbed. Primarily eliminated in feces.

■ **Available Forms:**
  • *Tablets*: 625 mg.

■ **Indications and Dosages:**
  To decrease LDL cholesterol level in primary hypercholesterolemia (Fredrickson type IIa): PO 3 tablets with meals twice a day or 6 tablets once a day with a meal. May increase daily dose to 7 tablets a day.

■ **Contraindications:** Complete biliary obstruction

■ **Side Effects**
  Frequent (12%–8%)
  Flatulence, constipation, infection, dyspepsia (heartburn, epigastric distress)

■ **Serious Reactions**
  • GI tract obstruction may occur.

Special Considerations
  • Combination colesevelam and an HMG-CoA reductase inhibitor is effective in further lowering serum total cholesterol and LDL-cholesterol levels beyond that achieved by either agent alone

■ **Patient/Family Education**
  • Tablets should be taken with a liquid, and with a meal
  • Follow the prescribed diet
  • Periodic laboratory tests are an essential part of therapy
  • Do not take any medications, including OTC drugs, without physician approval

■ **Monitoring Parameters**
  • Plasma lipids
  • Pattern of daily bowel activity and stool consistency

■ **Geriatric side effects at a glance:**
  ❑ CNS ❑ Bowel Dysfunction ❑ Bladder Dysfunction ❑ Falls

colestipol hydrochloride

(koe-les'-ti-pole hye-droe-klor'-ide)

■ **Brand Name(s):** Colestid
Chemical Class: CV-Lipid-bile acid sequestrant

■ **Clinical Pharmacology:**
Mechanism of Action: An antihyperlipoproteinemic that binds with bile acids in the intestine, forming an insoluble complex. Binding results in partial removal of bile acid from enterohepatic circulation. **Therapeutic Effect:** Removes low-density lipoproteins (LDL) and cholesterol from plasma.
Pharmacokinetics: Not absorbed from the gastrointestinal (GI) tract. Excreted in the feces.

■ **Available Forms:**
- *Granules*: 5-g packet (Colestid).
- *Tablet*: 1g (Colestid).

■ **Indications and Dosages:**
Primary hypercholesterolemia: PO, granules Initially, 5g 1-2 times/day. Range: 5-30 g/day once or in divided doses. PO, tablets Initially, 2g 1-2 times/day. Range: 2-16 g/day.

■ **Unlabeled Uses:** Treatment of diarrhea (due to bile acids); hyperoxaluria

■ **Contraindications:** Complete biliary obstruction, hypersensitivity to bile acid sequestering resins

■ **Side Effects**
Frequent
Constipation (may lead to fecal impaction), nausea, vomiting, stomach pain, indigestion
Occasional
Diarrhea, belching, bloating, headache, dizziness
Rare
Gallstones, peptic ulcer, malabsorption syndrome

■ **Serious Reactions**
- GI tract obstruction, hyperchloremic acidosis, and osteoporosis secondary to calcium excretion may occur.
- High dosage may interfere with fat absorption, resulting in steatorrhea.

- Bile acid sequestrant choice should be based on cost and patient acceptability
- Give all other medications 1 hr before colestipol or 4 hr after colestipol to avoid poor absorption

■ Patient/Family Education
- Mix the powder with 3 to 6 oz fruit juice, milk, soup, or water; place the powder on the surface of a liquid for 1 to 2 min to prevent lumping and then mix the powder into liquid; never take colestipol in its dry form
- Take colestipol before meals and drink several glasses of water between meals
- Eat high-fiber foods such as fruits, whole grain cereals, and vegetables to reduce the risk of constipation

■ Monitoring Parameters
- Daily bowel activity and stool consistency
- Blood chemistry test

■ Geriatric side effects at a glance:
❏ CNS ☑ Bowel Dysfunction ❏ Bladder Dysfunction ❏ Falls

■ U.S. Regulatory Considerations
❏ FDA Black Box ❏ OBRA regulated in U.S. Long Term Care

cortisone acetate

(kor'-ti-sone)

■ Brand Name(s): Cortone
Chemical Class: Glucocorticoid

■ Clinical Pharmacology:
Mechanism of Action: An adrenocortical steroid that inhibits the accumulation of inflammatory cells at inflammation sites, phagocytosis, lysosomal enzyme release and synthesis, and release of mediators of inflammation. **Therapeutic Effect:** Prevents or suppresses cell-mediated immune reactions. Decreases or prevents tissue response to inflammatory process.
Pharmacokinetics: Rapidly and almost completely absorbed after PO administration. Protein binding: 90%. Metabolized in liver. Excreted in urine. **Half-life:** Unknown.

■ Available Forms:
- *Tablets:* 5 mg, 10 mg, 25 mg.
- *Injectable Suspension:* 25 mg/ml, 50 mg/ml.

■ Indications and Dosages:
Adrenocortical insufficiency: PO 12-15 mg/m^2 divided as two-thirds in the morning and one-third in the afternoon.
Inflammatory conditions: PO 25-300 mg/day. IM 25-300 mg/day.

■ **Contraindications:** Hypersensitivity to corticosteroids, administration of live virus vaccine, peptic ulcers (except in life-threatening situations), systemic fungal infection

■ **Side Effects**
Frequent
Insomnia, heartburn, anxiety, abdominal distention, increased diaphoresis, acne, mood swings, increased appetite, facial flushing, delayed wound healing, increased susceptibility to infection, diarrhea or constipation
Occasional
Headache, edema, change in skin color, frequent urination
Rare
Tachycardia, allergic reaction (such as rash and hives), psychological changes, hallucinations, depression

■ **Serious Reactions**
• Long-term therapy may cause hypocalcemia, hypokalemia, muscle wasting in arms and legs, osteoporosis, spontaneous fractures, amenorrhea, cataracts, glaucoma, peptic ulcer disease, and CHF.
• Abrupt withdrawal following long-term therapy may cause anorexia, nausea, fever, headache, joint pain, rebound inflammation, fatigue, weakness, lethargy, dizziness, and orthostatic hypotension.

Special Considerations
• Increased dose of rapidly acting corticosteroids may be necessary in patient subjected to unusual stress
• May mask infections
• Do not give live virus vaccines to patients on prolonged therapy
• Patients on chronic steroid therapy should wear medical bracelet
• Drug-induced adrenocorticoid insufficiency may be minimized by gradual systemic dosage reduction; relative insufficiency may exist for up to 1 yr after discontinuation
• Symptoms of adrenal insufficiency include: nausea, fatigue, anorexia, hypotension, hypoglycemia, fever

■ **Patient/Family Education**
• Report fever, muscle aches, sore throat, and sudden weight gain or swelling

■ **Monitoring Parameters**
• Serum K and glucose
• Edema, blood pressure, CHF, mental status, weight
• For patients on long-term therapy, signs and symptoms of hypocalcemia (such as muscle twitching, cramps, and positive Chvostek's or Trousseau's signs), or hypokalemia (such as ECG changes, nausea and vomiting, irritability, weakness and muscle cramps, and numbness or tingling, especially in the lower extremities)

■ **Geriatric side effects at a glance:**
☑ CNS ❑ Bowel Dysfunction ❑ Bladder Dysfunction ❑ Falls

■ **U.S. Regulatory Considerations**
❑ FDA Black Box ☑ OBRA regulated in U.S. Long Term Care

cosyntropin

(kos-syn-troe'-pin)

- **Brand Name(s):** Cortrosyn
  Chemical Class: ACTH derivative

- **Clinical Pharmacology:**
  Mechanism of Action: A glucocorticoid that stimulates initial reaction in synthesis of adrenal steroids from cholesterol. **Therapeutic Effect:** Increases endogenous corticoid synthesis.
  Pharmacokinetics: None reported.

- **Available Forms:**
  - *Powder for Reconstitution:* 0.25 mg (Cortrosyn).

- **Indications and Dosages:**
  Screening test for adrenal function: IM 0.25-0.75 mg one time. IV infusion 0.25 mg in D_5W or 0.9% NaCl infused at rate of 0.04 mg/hr.

- **Contraindications:** Hypersensitivity to cosyntropin or corticotropin

- **Side Effects**
  Occasional
  Nausea, vomiting
  Rare
  Hypersensitivity reaction (fever, pruritus)

- **Serious Reactions**
  - None reported.

- **Patient/Family Education**
  - Explain procedure and purpose of test to the patient

- **Monitoring Parameters**
  - Check plasma cortisol levels at baseline and 30-60 min after drug is administered; normal adrenal function indicated by an increase of at least 70 mcg/l or a measured level of 20 mcg

- **Geriatric side effects at a glance:**
  ☑ CNS ❏ Bowel Dysfunction ❏ Bladder Dysfunction ❏ Falls

- **U.S. Regulatory Considerations**
  ❏ FDA Black Box ☑ OBRA regulated in U.S. Long Term Care

cromolyn sodium

(kroe'-moe-lin)

■ **Brand Name(s):** *Inhalation:* Intal

■ **Brand Name(s):** *Ophthalmic:* Crolom, Opticrom

■ **Brand Name(s):** *Oral:* Gastrocrom

■ **Brand Name(s):** *Nasal:* Nasalcrom
   Chemical Class: Mast cell stabilizer

■ **Clinical Pharmacology:**
   Mechanism of Action: An antiasthmatic and antiallergic agent that prevents mast cell release of histamine, leukotrienes, and slow-reacting substances of anaphylaxis by inhibiting degranulation after contact with antigens. **Therapeutic Effect:** Helps prevent symptoms of asthma, allergic rhinitis, mastocytosis, and exercise-induced bronchospasm.
   Pharmacokinetics: Minimal absorption after PO, inhalation, or nasal administration. Absorbed portion excreted in urine or by biliary system. **Half-life:** 80–90 min.

■ **Available Forms:**
   • *Oral Concentrate (Gastrocrom):* 100 mg/5ml.
   • *Oral Capsules (Gastrocrom):* 100 mg.
   • *Nasal Spray (Nasalcrom):* 40 mg/ml.
   • *Solution for Nebulization (Intal):* 10 mg/ml.
   • *Solution for Oral Inhalation (Intal):* 800 mcg/inhalation.
   • *Ophthalmic Solution (Crolom, Opticrom):* 4%.

■ **Indications and Dosages:**
   Asthma: Inhalation (nebulization) 20 mg 3-4 times a day. Aerosol Spray Initially, 2 sprays 4 times a day. Maintenance: 2-4 sprays 3-4 times a day.
   Prevention of bronchospasm: Inhalation (nebulization) 20 mg within 1 hr before exercise or exposure to allergens. Aerosol Spray 2 sprays within 1 hr before exercise or exposure to allergens
   Food allergy, inflammatory bowel disease: PO 200-400 mg 4 times a day.
   Allergic rhinitis: Intranasal 1 spray each nostril 3-4 times a day. May increase up to 6 times a day.
   Systemic mastocytosis: PO 200 mg 4 times a day.
   Conjunctivitis: Ophthalmic 1-2 drops in both eyes 4-6 times a day.

■ **Contraindications:** Status asthmaticus

■ **Side Effects**
   Frequent
   PO: Headache, diarrhea
   Inhalation: Cough, dry mouth and throat, stuffy nose, throat irritation, unpleasant taste
   Nasal: Nasal burning, stinging, or irritation; increased sneezing
   Ophthalmic: Eye burning or stinging

Occasional

PO: Rash, abdominal pain, arthralgia, nausea, insomnia

Inhalation: Bronchospasm, hoarseness, lacrimation

Nasal: Cough, headache, unpleasant taste, postnasal drip

Ophthalmic: Lacrimation and itching of eye

Rare

Inhalation: Dizziness, painful urination, arthralgia, myalgia, rash

Nasal: Epistaxis, rash

Ophthalmic: Chemosis or edema of conjunctiva, eye irritation

■ Serious Reactions

- Anaphylaxis occurs rarely when cromolyn is given by the inhalation, nasal, or oral route.

■ Patient/Family Education

- Therapeutic effect in asthma may take up to 4 wk
- Administer cromolyn at regular intervals
- Explain to the patient how to use a Spinhaler if he or she is to receive cromolyn by nebulization or inhalation capsules
- Rinse mouth with water immediately after inhalation to prevent mouth and throat dryness
- Drink plenty of fluids to decrease the thickness of lung secretions

■ Monitoring Parameters

- Pulse rate and quality and respiratory rate, depth, rhythm, and type
- Observe the patient for cyanosis manifested as lips and fingernails with a blue or dusky color in light-skinned patients; a gray color in dark-skinned patients
- Auscultate the patient's breath sounds for crackles, rhonchi, and wheezing

■ Geriatric side effects at a glance:

❏ CNS   ❏ Bowel Dysfunction   ❏ Bladder Dysfunction   ❏ Falls

■ U.S. Regulatory Considerations

❏ FDA Black Box   ❏ OBRA regulated in U.S. Long Term Care

crotamiton

(kroe-tam'-i-ton)

■ Brand Name(s): Eurax

Chemical Class: Chloroformate salt

■ Clinical Pharmacology:

Mechanism of Action: A scabicidal agent whose exact mechanism is unknown. **Therapeutic Effect:** Scabicidal activity against **Sarcoptes scabiei**.

Pharmacokinetics: Not known.

■ **Available Forms:**
- *Cream*: 10% (Eurax).
- *Lotion*: 10% (Eurax).

■ **Indications and Dosages:**
Treatment of scabies: Topical Wash and scrub away loose scales and towel dry. Apply a thin layer and massage into skin over the entire body with special attention to skin folds, creases, and interdigital spaces. Repeat application in 24 hr. Take a cleansing bath 48 hr after the final application. Treatment may be repeated after 7-10 days if live mites are still present.
Pruritus: Topical Massage into affected areas until medication is completely absorbed. Repeat as needed.

■ **Unlabeled Uses:** Folliculitis, pediculosis

■ **Contraindications:** Hypersensitivity to crotamiton or any one of its components

■ **Side Effects**
Occasional
Itching, burning, irritation, warm sensation, contact dermatitis

■ **Serious Reactions**
- None known.

■ **Patient/Family Education**
- 60 g is sufficient for 2 applications
- Reapply locally during 48-hr treatment period after handwashing, etc.
- A cleansing bath should be taken 48 hr after the last application
- After treatment, use topical corticosteroids to decrease contact dermatitis, antihistamines for pruritus; pruritus may continue for 4-6 wk
- Wash all contaminated clothing and bed linens to avoid reinfestation
- It is important to massage into the skin, especially to skin folds, digits, and creases

■ **Monitoring Parameters**
- Check the skin for local burning, itching, and irritation

■ **Geriatric side effects at a glance:**
❑ CNS ❑ Bowel Dysfunction ❑ Bladder Dysfunction ❑ Falls

■ **U.S. Regulatory Considerations**
❑ FDA Black Box ❑ OBRA regulated in U.S. Long Term Care

cyanocobalamin

(sye-an-oh-koe-bal'-a-min)

■ **Brand Name(s):** Cobal-1000, Cobolin-M, Crystal B-12, Cyomin, Depo-Cobalin, LA-12, Liver, Nascobal, Neuroforte-R, Vita #12, Vitabee 12, Vitamin B-12
Chemical Class: NUTR-vitamin B complex

■ **Clinical Pharmacology:**
Mechanism of Action: Acts as a coenzyme for various metabolic functions, including fat and carbohydrate metabolism and protein synthesis. **Therapeutic Effect:** Necessary for cell growth and replication, hematopoiesis, and myelin synthesis.
Pharmacokinetics: In the presence of calcium, absorbed systemically in lower half of ileum. Initially, bound to intrinsic factor; this complex passes down intestine, binding to receptor sites on ileal mucosa. Protein binding: High. Metabolized in the liver. Primarily eliminated unchanged in urine. **Half-life:** 6 days.

■ **Available Forms:**
- *Tablets*: 50 mcg, 100 mcg, 250 mcg, 500 mcg, 1000 mcg, 5000 mcg.
- *Tablets* (*Extended-Release*): 1500 mcg.
- *Injection*: 1000 mcg/ml.
- *Nasal Gel* (*Nascobal*): 500 mcg/0.1 ml.

■ **Indications and Dosages:**
Dietary supplement (RDA): PO 2.4 mcg/day.
Pernicious anemia: IM, Subcutaneous 100 mcg/day for 7 days, then every other day for 7 days, then every 3-4 days for 2-3 weeks. Maintenance: 100 mcg/mo (oral 1000-2000 mcg/day). Intranasal 500 mcg once a week.
Uncomplicated NUTR-vitamin B$_{12}$ deficiency: PO 1000-2000 mcg/day IM, Subcutaneous 100 mcg/day for 5-10 days, followed by 100-200 mcg/mo.
Complicated vitamin B$_{12}$ deficiency: IM, Subcutaneous 1000 mcg (with IM or IV folic acid 15 mg) as a single dose, then 1000 mcg/day plus oral folic acid 5 mg/day for 7 days.

■ **Contraindications:** Folic acid deficiency anemia, hereditary optic nerve atrophy, history of allergy to cobalamins

■ **Side Effects**
Occasional
Diarrhea, pruritus

■ **Serious Reactions**
- Impurities in preparation may cause a rare allergic reaction.
- Peripheral vascular thrombosis, pulmonary edema, hypokalemia, and CHF may occur.

Special Considerations
- Nutritional sources: egg yolks, fish, organ meats, dairy products, clams, oysters

311

Patient/Family Education
- Lifetime treatment may be necessary with pernicious anemia
- Report symptoms of infection
- Eat foods rich in vitamin B_{12} including clams, dairy products, egg yolks, fermented cheese, herring, muscle and organ meats, oysters, and red snapper

Monitoring Parameters
- CBC with reticulocyte count after 1st wk of therapy
- Serum potassium level, which normally ranges from 3.5-5 mEq/L, and serum cyanocobalamin level, which normally ranges from 200-800 mcg/ml
- Evaluate the patient for reversal of deficiency symptoms (anorexia, ataxia, fatigue, hyporeflexia, insomnia, irritability, loss of positional sense, pallor, and palpitations on exertion); a therapeutic response to treatment usually occurs within 48 hr

Geriatric side effects at a glance:
❑ CNS   ❑ Bowel Dysfunction   ❑ Bladder Dysfunction   ❑ Falls

U.S. Regulatory Considerations
❑ FDA Black Box   ❑ OBRA regulated in U.S. Long Term Care

Reference:
1. Dietary Reference Intakes, www.nap.edu

cyclobenzaprine hydrochloride

(sye-kloe-ben'-za-preen)

Brand Name(s): Flexeril
Chemical Class: Tricyclic amine

Clinical Pharmacology:
Mechanism of Action: A centrally acting skeletal muscle relaxant that reduces tonic somatic muscle activity at the level of the brainstem. **Therapeutic Effect:** Relieves local skeletal muscle spasm.
Pharmacokinetics:

Route	Onset	Peak	Duration
PO	1 hr	3-4 hr	12-24 hr

Well but slowly absorbed from the GI tract. Protein binding: 93%. Metabolized in the GI tract and the liver. Primarily excreted in urine. **Half-life:** 1-3 days.

Available Forms:
- **Tablets:** 5 mg, 10 mg.

Indications and Dosages:
Acute, painful musculoskeletal conditions: PO 5 mg 3 times a day.

Dosage in hepatic impairment: *Mild:* 5 mg 3 times a day. *Moderate and severe:* Not recommended.

■ **Unlabeled Uses:** Treatment of fibromyalgia

■ **Contraindications:** Acute recovery phase of MI, arrhythmias, CHF, heart block, conduction disturbances, hyperthyroidism, use within 14 days of MAOIs

■ **Side Effects**
  Frequent
  Somnolence (39%), dry mouth (27%), dizziness (11%)
  Rare (3%–1%)
  Fatigue, asthenia, blurred vision, headache, nervousness, confusion, nausea, constipation, dyspepsia, unpleasant taste

■ **Serious Reactions**
  • Overdose may result in visual hallucinations, hyperactive reflexes, muscle rigidity, vomiting, and hyperpyrexia.

Special Considerations
  • Avoid use in elderly due to anticholinergic side effects

■ **Patient/Family Education**
  • Use caution with alcohol, other CNS depressants
  • Avoid with hazardous activities if drowsiness or dizziness occur
  • Drowsiness usually diminishes with continued therapy
  • Change positions slowly to help avoid the drug's hypotensive effects
  • Sip tepid water and chew sugarless gum to relieve dry mouth

■ **Monitoring Parameters**
  • Evidence of a therapeutic response, such as decreased skeletal muscle pain, stiffness, and tenderness and improved mobility

■ **Geriatric side effects at a glance:**
  ☑ CNS   ☑ Bowel Dysfunction   ☑ Bladder Dysfunction   ☑ Falls
  Other: Dry mouth, blurred vision, confusion, psychoses

■ **Use with caution in older patients with:** Narrow-angle glaucoma, overflow incontinence, psychosis.

■ **U.S. Regulatory Considerations**
  ☐ FDA Black Box   ☑ OBRA regulated in U.S. Long Term Care

■ **Other Uses in Geriatric Patient:** None

■ **Side Effects:**
  Of particular importance in the geriatric patient: Delirium, possible antagonism of cholinergic drug therapy in the treatment of Alzheimer's disease; sedation

■ **Geriatric Considerations - Summary:** Cyclobenzaprine is a skeletal muscle relaxant which is structurally related to the tricyclic antidepressants with anticholinergic properties and it is very sedating. It is used for acute muscle pain and should not be used chronically. Its usefulness in the older adult is limited by its potential to cause adverse effects.

■ **References:**
1. Katz WA, Dube J: Cyclobenzaprine in the treatment of acute muscle spasm: review of a decade of clinical experience. Clin Ther 1988;10:216-229.

cyclophosphamide

(sye-kloe-fos'-fa-mide)

■ **Brand Name(s):** Cytoxan, Cytoxan Lyophilized, Neosar
Chemical Class: Nitrogen mustard, synthetic

■ **Clinical Pharmacology:**
Mechanism of Action: An alkylating agent that inhibits DNA and RNA protein synthesis by cross-linking with DNA and RNA strands, preventing cell growth. Cell cycle–phase nonspecific. **Therapeutic Effect:** Potent immunosuppressant.
Pharmacokinetics: Well absorbed from the GI tract. Protein binding: low. Crosses the blood-brain barrier. Metabolized in the liver to active metabolites. Primarily excreted in urine. Removed by hemodialysis. **Half-life:** 3-12 hr.

■ **Available Forms:**
- *Tablets (Cytoxan):* 25 mg, 50 mg.
- *Powder for Injection (Neosar):* 100 mg, 200 mg, 500 mg, 1 g, 2 g.
- *Powder for Injection (Lyophilized [Cytoxan Lyophilized]):* 100 mg, 200 mg, 500 mg, 1 g, 2 g.

■ **Indications and Dosages:**
Ovarian adenocarcinoma, breast carcinoma, Hodgkin's disease, non-Hodgkin's lymphoma, multiple myeloma, leukemia (acute lymphoblastic, acute myelogenous, acute monocytic, chronic granulocytic, chronic lymphocytic), mycosis fungoides, disseminated neuroblastoma, retinoblastoma: PO 1-5 mg/kg/day. IV 40-50 mg/kg in divided doses over 2-5 days; or 10-15 mg/kg every 7-10 days or 3-5 mg/kg twice a week.
Biopsy-proven minimal-change nephrotic syndrome: PO 2.5-3 mg/kg/day for 60-90 days.

■ **Unlabeled Uses:** Adrenocortical, bladder, cervical, endometrial, prostatic, testicular carcinomas; Ewing's sarcoma; multiple sclerosis; non-small cell, small cell lung cancer; organ transplant rejection; osteosarcoma; ovarian germ cell, primary brain, trophoblastic tumors; rheumatoid arthritis; soft tissue sarcomas; systemic dermatomyositis; systemic lupus erythematosus; Wilms' tumor

■ **Contraindications:** Severe bone marrow suppression

■ **Side Effects**
Expected
Marked leukopenia 8-15 days after initial therapy
Frequent
Nausea, vomiting (beginning about 6 hr after administration and lasting about 4 hr); alopecia (33%)

Occasional
Diarrhea, darkening of skin and fingernails, stomatitis, headache, diaphoresis
Rare
Pain or redness at injection site

■ Serious Reactions
- Cyclophosphamide's major toxic effect is myelosuppression resulting in blood dyscrasias, such as leukopenia, anemia, thrombocytopenia, and hypoprothrombinemia.
- Expect leukopenia to resolve in 17-28 days. Anemia generally occurs after large doses or prolonged therapy. Thrombocytopenia may occur 10-15 days after drug initiation.
- Hemorrhagic cystitis occurs commonly in long-term therapy.
- Pulmonary fibrosis and cardiotoxicity have been noted with high doses.
- Amenorrhea, azoospermia, and hyperkalemia may also occur.

■ Patient/Family Education
- Drink plenty of fluids before, during, and after therapy and void frequently to prevent cystitis
- Avoid receiving vaccinations without the physician's approval and avoid contact with anyone who has recently received a live-virus vaccine because cyclophosphamide lowers the body's resistance
- Report easy bruising, fever, signs of local infection, sore throat, or unusual bleeding from any site
- Hair loss is reversible, but new hair may have a different color or texture

■ Monitoring Parameters
- CBC, differential, platelet count qwk; withhold drug if WBC is less than 4000/mm^3 or platelet count is less than 75,000/mm^3
- Renal function studies: BUN, UA, serum uric acid; urine CrCl before, during therapy
- Intake and output; report fall in urine output 30 ml/hr or lower

■ Geriatric side effects at a glance:
❑ CNS   ❑ Bowel Dysfunction   ❑ Bladder Dysfunction   ❑ Falls

■ U.S. Regulatory Considerations
❑ FDA Black Box   ❑ OBRA regulated in U.S. Long Term Care

cycloserine

(sye-kloe-ser'-een)

■ **Brand Name(s):** Seromycin
Chemical Class: *Streptomyces orchidaceus* product

■ **Clinical Pharmacology:**
Mechanism of Action: An antitubercular that inhibits cell wall synthesis by competing with the amino acid, D-alanine, for incorporation into the bacterial cell wall. **Therapeutic Effect:** Causes disruption of bacterial cell wall. Bactericidal or bacteriostatic.
Pharmacokinetics: Readily absorbed from the gastrointestinal (GI) tract. No protein binding. Widely distributed (including cerebrospinal fluid [CSF]). Metabolized in liver. Primarily excreted in urine. Removed by hemodialysis. **Half-life:** 10 hr.

■ **Available Forms:**
  • *Capsules*: 250 mg (Seromycin).

■ **Indications and Dosages:**
Tuberculosis: 250 mg q12h for 14 days, then 500 mg-1g/day in 2 divided doses for 18-24 mo. Maximum: 1g as a single daily dose.
Dosage in renal impairment:

Creatinine Clearance	Dosage Interval
10-50 ml/min	q24h
less than 10 ml/min	q36-48h

■ **Unlabeled Uses:** Gaucher's disease, acute urinary tract infections

■ **Contraindications:** Epilepsy, depression, severe anxiety, psychosis, severe renal insufficiency, excessive concurrent use of alcohol, history of hypersensitivity reactions with previous cycloserine therapy

■ **Side Effects**
Occasional
Drowsiness, headache, dizziness, vertigo, seizures, confusion, psychosis, paresis, tremor, vitamin B_{12} deficiency, folate deficiency, cardiac arrhythmias, increased liver enzymes

■ **Serious Reactions**
  • Neurotoxicity, as evidenced by confusion, agitation, CNS depression, psychosis, coma, and seizures, occurs rarely.
  • Neurotoxic effects of cycloserine may be treated and prevented with the administration of 200-300 mg of pyridoxine daily.

Special Considerations
  • L-enantiomer (1-cycloserine) in Gaucher's disease (Orphan Drug)
  • Pyridoxine may prevent neurotoxicity (200-300 mg/day)

- Avoid concurrent alcohol
- Cycloserine may cause drowsiness, mental confusion, dizziness, or tremors
- Do not skip doses

■ **Monitoring Parameters**
- Mental status closely and liver function tests qwk
- Monitor cycloserine concentrations; toxicity is greatly increased at levels more than 30 mcg/ml

■ **Geriatric side effects at a glance:**
   ❏ CNS   ❏ Bowel Dysfunction   ❏ Bladder Dysfunction   ❏ Falls

■ **U.S. Regulatory Considerations**
   ❏ FDA Black Box   ❏ OBRA regulated in U.S. Long Term Care

cyclosporine

(sye-kloe-spor'-in)

■ **Brand Name(s):** Gengraf, Neoral, Restasis, Sandimmune
Chemical Class: Cyclic peptide

■ **Clinical Pharmacology:**
Mechanism of Action: A cyclic polypeptide that inhibits both cellular and humoral immune responses by inhibiting interleukin-2, a proliferative factor needed for T-cell activity. **Therapeutic Effect:** Prevents organ rejection and relieves symptoms of psoriasis and arthritis.
Pharmacokinetics: Variably absorbed from the GI tract. Protein binding: 90%. Widely distributed. Metabolized in the liver. Eliminated primarily by biliary or fecal excretion. Not removed by hemodialysis. **Half-life:** Adults, 10-27 hr; children, 7-19 hr.

■ **Available Forms:**
- Capsules (Softgel [Gengraf, Neoral, Sandimmune]): 25 mg, 100 mg.
- Oral Solution (Sandimmune): 50-ml bottle with calibrated liquid measuring device.
- Injection (Sandimmune): 50 mg/ml.
- Ophthalmic Emulsion (Restasis): 0.05%.

■ **Indications and Dosages:**
Transplantation, prevention of organ rejection: PO 10-18 mg/kg/dose given 4-12 hr prior to organ transplantation. Maintenance: 5-15 mg/kg/day in divided doses then tapered to 3-10 mg/kg/day. IV Initially, 5-6 mg/kg/dose given 4-12 hr prior to organ transplantation. Maintenance: 2-10 mg/kg/day in divided doses.
Rheumatoid arthritis: PO Initially, 2.5 mg/kg a day in 2 divided doses. May increase by 0.5-0.75 mg/kg/day. Maximum: 4 mg/kg/day.
Psoriasis: PO Initially, 2.5 mg/kg/day in 2 divided doses. May increase by 0.5 mg/kg/day. Maximum: 4 mg/kg/day.
Dry eye: Ophthalmic Instill 1 drop in each affected eye q12h.

- **Unlabeled Uses:** Treatment of alopecia areata, aplastic anemia, atopic dermatitis, Behçet's disease, biliary cirrhosis, prevention of corneal transplant rejection

- **Contraindications:** History of hypersensitivity to cyclosporine or polyoxyethylated castor oil

- **Side Effects**
  Frequent
  Mild to moderate hypertension (26%), hirsutism (21%), tremor (12%)
  Occasional (4%–2%)
  Acne, leg cramps, gingival hyperplasia (marked by red, bleeding, and tender gums), paresthesia, diarrhea, nausea, vomiting, headache
  Rare (less than 1%)
  Hypersensitivity reaction, abdominal discomfort, gynecomastia, sinusitis

- **Serious Reactions**
  - Mild nephrotoxicity occurs in 25% of renal transplant patients, 38% of cardiac transplant patients, and 37% of liver transplant patients, generally 2-3 mo after transplantation (more severe toxicity generally occurs soon after transplantation). Hepatotoxicity occurs in 4% of renal transplant patients, 7% of cardiac transplant patients, and 4% of liver transplant patients, generally within the first mo after transplantation. Both toxicities usually respond to dosage reduction.
  - Severe hyperkalemia and hyperuricemia occur occasionally.

Special Considerations
  - Neoral has increased bioavailability compared to Sandimmune (do NOT use interchangeably)

- **Patient/Family Education**
  - Oral sol may be mixed with milk, chocolate milk, or orange juice to improve palatability. Do not mix with grapefruit juice (increased cyclosporine levels).
  - Ophth product may be used with artificial tears—allow 15-min interval between products
  - Essential to repeat blood testing on a routine basis while receiving medication
  - Headache and tremor may occur as a response to medication

- **Monitoring Parameters**
  - Renal function studies: BUN, creatinine qmo during treatment, 3 mo after treatment
  - Liver function studies and serum levels during treatment
  - Blood level monitoring: maintenance of 24-hr trough levels of 250-800 ng/ml (whole blood, RIA) or 50-300 ng/ml (plasma, RIA) should minimize side effects and rejection events
  - Potassium level for evidence of hyperkalemia
  - Blood pressure

- **Geriatric side effects at a glance:**
  ☐ CNS ☐ Bowel Dysfunction ☐ Bladder Dysfunction ☐ Falls

- **U.S. Regulatory Considerations**
  ☑ FDA Black Box
  - Prescribed by experienced physicians
  - Increased susceptibility to infection

- Increased risk of neoplasia
- Nephrotoxicity and hypertension
- ❏ OBRA regulated in U.S. Long Term Care

cyproheptadine hydrochloride

(si-proe-hep'-ta-deen hye-droe-klor'-ide)

■ **Brand Name(s):** Periactin
Chemical Class: Piperidine derivative

■ **Clinical Pharmacology:**
Mechanism of Action: An antihistamine that competes with histamine at histaminic receptor sites. Anticholinergic effects cause drying of nasal mucosa. **Therapeutic Effect:** Relieves allergic conditions (urticaria, pruritus).
Pharmacokinetics: Well absorbed from GI tract. Metabolized in liver. Primarily eliminated in feces. **Half-life:** 16 hr.

■ **Available Forms:**
- *Syrup*: 2 mg/5 ml (Periactin).
- *Tablets*: 4 mg (Periactin).

■ **Indications and Dosages:**
Allergic condition: PO 4 mg 2 times/day. May increase dose but do not exceed 0.5 mg/kg/day.

■ **Contraindications:** Acute asthmatic attack, patients receiving MAO inhibitors, history of hypersensitivity to antihistamines

■ **Side Effects**
Frequent
Drowsiness, dizziness, muscular weakness, dry mouth/nose/throat/lips, urinary retention, thickening of bronchial secretions
Occasional
Sedation, dizziness, hypotension
Rare
Epigastric distress, flushing, visual disturbances, hearing disturbances, paresthesia, sweating, chills

■ **Serious Reactions**
- Hypersensitivity reaction (eczema, pruritus, rash, cardiac disturbances, angioedema, photosensitivity) may occur.
- Overdosage may vary from CNS depression (sedation, apnea, cardiovascular collapse, death) to severe paradoxical reaction (hallucinations, tremor, seizures).

■ **Patient/Family Education**
  - Dry mouth, drowsiness, and dizziness are expected responses to the drug
  - Avoid tasks that require mental alertness or motor skills until response to the drug is established

■ **Monitoring Parameters**
  - Blood pressure

■ **Geriatric side effects at a glance:**
  ☑ CNS ☑ Bowel Dysfunction ☑ Bladder Dysfunction ❑ Falls
  Other: Dry mouth, somnolence, restlessness, confusion, psychoses

■ **Use with caution in older patients with:** Narrow-angle glaucoma, overflow incontinence, orthostatic hypotension, taking drugs that increase serotonin activity.

■ **U.S. Regulatory Considerations**
  ❑ FDA Black Box ☑ OBRA regulated in U.S. Long Term Care

■ **Other Uses in Geriatric Patient:** Appetite stimulation, pruritus

■ **Side Effects:**
  Of particular importance in the geriatric patient: Anticholinergic effects

■ **Geriatric Considerations - Summary:** Cyproheptadine is a first-generation piperidine antihistamine with potent H_1-receptor antagonism and significant anticholinergic activity. This drug also has the unique property of being a serotonin antagonist. It has CNS depressant effects, causing drowsiness and confusion. Older adults taking this drug are at risk of dizziness and hypotension. Cyproheptadine's antiserotonin activity can result in decreased efficacy of antidepressants that potentiate serotonin.

■ **References:**
  1. Tune LE. Anticholinergic effects of medication in elderly patients. J Clin Psychiatry 2001;62(suppl 21):11-14.
  2. McDaniel WW: Serotonin syndrome: early management with cyproheptadine. Ann Pharmacother 2001; 35:870-873.

dalteparin sodium

(dal-te-pa'-rin soe'-dee-um)

■ **Brand Name(s):** Fragmin
  Chemical Class: Heparin derivative, depolymerized; low-molecular-weight heparin

■ **Clinical Pharmacology:**
  Mechanism of Action: An antithrombin that inhibits factor Xa and thrombin in the presence of low-molecular-weight heparin. Only slightly influences platelet aggregation, PT, and aPTT. *Therapeutic Effect:* Produces anticoagulation.

Route	Onset	Peak	Duration
Subcutaneous	N/A	4 hr	N/A

Protein binding: less than 10%. **Half-life**: 3-5 hr.

■ Available Forms:

- *Syringe*: 2500 international units/0.2 ml, 5000 international units/0.2 ml, 7500 international units/0.3 ml, 10,000 international units/ml.
- *Vial*: 10,000 international units/ml, 25,000 international units/ml.

■ Indications and Dosages:

Low- to moderate-risk abdominal surgery: Subcutaneous 2500 international units 1-2 hr before surgery, then daily for 5-10 days.

High-risk abdominal surgery: Subcutaneous 5000 international units 1-2 hr before surgery, then daily for 5-10 days.

Total hip surgery: Subcutaneous 2500 international units 1-2 hr before surgery, then 2500 units 6 hr after surgery, then 5000 units/day for 7-10 days.

Unstable angina, non–Q-wave MI: Subcutaneous 120 international units/kg q12h (maximum: 10,000 international units/dose) given with aspirin until clinically stable.

Prevention of deep vein thrombosis (DVT) or pulmonary edema in the acutely ill patient: Subcutaneous 5000 international units once a day.

■ Contraindications:
Active major bleeding; concurrent heparin therapy; hypersensitivity to dalteparin, heparin, or pork products; thrombocytopenia associated with positive in vitro test for antiplatelet antibody

■ Side Effects

Occasional (7%–3%)

Hematoma at injection site

Rare (less than 1%)

Hypersensitivity reaction (chills, fever, pruritus, urticaria, asthma, rhinitis, lacrimation, headache); mild, local skin irritation

■ Serious Reactions

- Overdose may lead to bleeding complications ranging from local ecchymoses to major hemorrhage.
- Thrombocytopenia occurs rarely.

Special Considerations

- Cannot be used interchangeably (unit for unit) with unfractionated heparin or other low-molecular-weight heparins

■ Patient/Family Education

- Usual length of dalteparin therapy is 5-10 days
- Notify the physician of signs of bleeding, breathing difficulty, bruising, dizziness, fever, itching, light-headedness, rash, and swelling
- Rotate injection sites daily
- Perform an ice massage at the injection site shortly before injection, to prevent excessive bruising

■ Monitoring Parameters

- CBC with platelets, stool occult blood, urinalysis
- Monitoring aPTT is NOT required

- Assess for signs of bleeding, including bleeding at surgical or injection sites or from gums, hematuria, blood in stool, bruising, and petechiae

■ **Geriatric side effects at a glance:**
❏ CNS ❏ Bowel Dysfunction ❏ Bladder Dysfunction ❏ Falls

■ **U.S. Regulatory Considerations**
☑ FDA Black Box
Increased risk of spinal/epidural hematomas with neuraxial anesthesia or spinal puncture. Risk is further increased by use of indwelling spinal catheters, repeated/traumatic epidural/spinal puncture, or use of drugs affecting hemostasis (NSAIDs, anticoagulants, platelet inhibitors).
❏ OBRA regulated in U.S. Long Term Care

danazol

(da'-na-zole)

■ **Brand Name(s):** Danocrine
Chemical Class: ENDO-androgen; ethisterone derivative

■ **Clinical Pharmacology:**
Mechanism of Action: A testosterone derivative that suppresses the pituitary-ovarian axis by inhibiting the output of pituitary gonadotropins. Causes atrophy of both normal and ectopic endometrial tissue in endometriosis. Follicle-stimulating hormone (FSH) and luteinizing hormone (LH) are depressed in fibrocystic breast disease. Inhibits steroid synthesis and binding of steroids to their receptors in breast tissues. Increases serum levels of esterase inhibitor. **Therapeutic Effect:** Produces anovulation and amenorrhea, reduces the production of estrogen, corrects biochemical deficiency as seen in hereditary angioedema.
Pharmacokinetics: Well absorbed from gastrointestinal (GI) tract. Metabolized in liver, primarily to 2-hydroxymethylethisterone. Excreted in urine. **Half-life:** 4.5 hr.

■ **Available Forms:**
- *Capsules*: 50 mg, 100 mg, 200 mg (Danocrine).

■ **Indications and Dosages:**
Fibrocystic breast disease: PO 100-400 mg/day in 2 divided doses.
Hereditary angioedema: PO Initially, 200 mg 2-3 times/day. Decrease dose by 50% or less at 1-3 mo intervals. If attack occurs, increase dose by up to 200 mg/day.

■ **Unlabeled Uses:** Treatment of gynecomastia, menorrhagia

■ **Contraindications:** Cardiac impairment, hypercalcemia, prostatic or breast cancer in males, severe liver or renal disease

■ **Side Effects**
Frequent
Females: Decreased breast size, increased weight

Occasional

Males/females: Edema, rhabdomyolysis (muscle cramps, unusual fatigue), virilism (acne, oily skin), flushed skin, altered moods

Rare

Males/females: Hematuria, gingivitis, carpal tunnel syndrome, cataracts, severe headache, vomiting, rash, photosensitivity

Females: Enlarged clitoris, hoarseness, deepening voice, hair growth, monilial vaginitis

Males: Decreased testicle size.

■ **Serious Reactions**
- Jaundice may occur in those receiving 400 mg/day or more.
- Liver dysfunction, eosinophilia, thrombocytopenia, and pancreatitis occur rarely.

Special Considerations
- Drug of choice for treating all types of hereditary angioedema in the elderly
- Breast pain should be treated conservatively (analgesics, supportive bra). Hormonal therapy is not innocuous. Symptoms usually return after discontinuation
- Ovarian function usually returns within 60-90 days after discontinuation

■ **Patient/Family Education**
- Essential to repeat blood testing on a routine basis while receiving medication
- Notify physician promptly of masculinizing effects (may not be reversible), weight gain, muscle cramps, or fatigue

■ **Monitoring Parameters**
- Potassium, blood sugar, urine glucose during long-term therapy
- Weight 2-3 times/week; report more than 5 lb/week gain or swelling of fingers or feet
- Blood pressure
- Check for jaundice

■ **Geriatric side effects at a glance:**
    ❑ CNS   ❑ Bowel Dysfunction   ❑ Bladder Dysfunction   ❑ Falls

■ **U.S. Regulatory Considerations**
    ❑ FDA Black Box   ❑ OBRA regulated in U.S. Long Term Care

dantrolene sodium

(dan'-troe-leen)

■ **Brand Name(s):** Dantrium
    Chemical Class: Hydantoin derivative

■ **Clinical Pharmacology:**

Mechanism of Action: A skeletal muscle relaxant that reduces muscle contraction by interfering with release of calcium ion. Reduces calcium ion concentration. **Therapeutic Effect:** Dissociates excitation-contraction coupling. Interferes with catabolic process associated with malignant hyperthermic crisis.

Pharmacokinetics: Poorly absorbed from the GI tract. Protein binding: High. Metabolized in the liver. Primarily excreted in urine. **Half-life:** IV: 4-8 hr; PO: 8.7 hr.

■ **Available Forms:**
- *Capsules (Dantrium)*: 25 mg, 50 mg, 100 mg.
- *Powder for Injection (Dantrium Intravenous)*: 20-mg vial.

■ **Indications and Dosages:**

Spasticity: PO Initially, 25 mg/day. Increase to 25 mg 2-4 times a day, then by 25-mg increments up to 100 mg 2-4 times a day.

Prevention of malignant hyperthermic crisis: PO 4-8 mg/kg/day in 3-4 divided doses 1-2 days before surgery; give last dose 3-4 hr before surgery. IV 2.5 mg/kg about 1.25 hr before surgery.

Management of malignant hyperthermic crisis: IV Initially a minimum of 1 mg/kg rapid IV; may repeat up to total cumulative dose of 10 mg/kg. May follow with 4-8 mg/kg/day PO in 4 divided doses up to 3 days after crisis.

■ **Unlabeled Uses:** Relief of exercise-induced pain in patients with muscular dystrophy, treatment of flexor spasms and neuroleptic malignant syndrome

■ **Contraindications:** Active hepatic disease

■ **Side Effects**

Frequent
Drowsiness, dizziness, weakness, general malaise, diarrhea (mild)

Occasional
Confusion, diarrhea (may be severe), headache, insomnia, constipation, urinary frequency

Rare
Paradoxical CNS excitement or restlessness, paresthesia, tinnitus, slurred speech, tremor, blurred vision, dry mouth, nocturia, impotence, rash, pruritus

■ **Serious Reactions**
- There is a risk of hepatotoxicity, most notably in females, and those taking other medications concurrently.
- Overt hepatitis noted most frequently between 3rd and 12th mo of therapy.
- Overdosage results in vomiting, muscular hypotonia, muscle twitching, respiratory depression, and seizures.

Special Considerations
- Use carefully where spasticity is utilized to sustain upright posture and balance in locomotion or to obtain or maintain increased function
- Discontinue after 6 wk if improvement does not occur
- Use lowest dose possible (hepatotoxicity dose-related)

■ **Patient/Family Education**
- IV therapy may decrease grip strength and increase weakness of leg muscles, especially walking down stairs
- Caution driving or operating hazardous machinery

- Avoid tasks that require mental alertness or motor skills until response to the drug is established
- Notify the physician if bloody or tarry stools, continued weakness, diarrhea, fatigue, itching, nausea, or skin rash occurs

■ **Monitoring Parameters**
- Baseline and periodic LFTs (AST, ALT, alk phosphatase, total bilirubin)

■ **Geriatric side effects at a glance:**
❑ CNS   ❑ Bowel Dysfunction   ☑ Bladder Dysfunction   ☑ Falls

■ **U.S. Regulatory Considerations**
☑ FDA Black Box
Hepatotoxicity
☑ OBRA regulated in U.S. Long Term Care

dapsone

(dap'-sone)

■ **Brand Name(s):** Dapsone
Chemical Class: Sulfone

■ **Clinical Pharmacology:**
Mechanism of Action: An antibiotic that is a competitive antagonist of para-aminobenzoic acid (PABA); it prevents normal bacterial utilization of PABA for synthesis of folic acid. **Therapeutic Effect:** Inhibits bacterial growth.
Pharmacokinetics: Slowly absorbed from the GI tract. Protein binding: 70%-90%. Metabolized in liver. Excreted in urine. **Half-life:** 10-50 hr.

■ **Available Forms:**
- **Tablets:** 25 mg, 100 mg.

■ **Indications and Dosages:**
Leprosy: PO 50-100 mg/day for 3-10 yr.
Dermatitis herpetiformis: PO Initially, 50 mg/day. May increase up to 300 mg/day.
Pneumocystis carinii pneumonia (PCP): PO 100 mg/day in combination with trimethoprim for 21 days.
Prevention of PCP: PO 100 mg/day.

■ **Unlabeled Uses:** Treatment of inflammatory bowel disorders, malaria

■ **Contraindications:** None known.

■ **Side Effects**
Frequent (greater than 10%)
Hemolytic anemia, methemoglobinemia, rash

Occasional (10%-1%)
Hemolysis, photosensitivity reaction

■ **Serious Reactions**
  • Agranulocytosis and blood dyscrasias may occur.

Special Considerations
  • Use in conjunction with either rifampin or clofazimine to prevent development of drug resistance and reduce infectiousness of patient with leprosy more quickly

■ **Patient/Family Education**
  • Full therapeutic effects on leprosy may not occur for several mo; compliance with dosage schedule, duration is necessary
  • Frequent blood tests are necessary, especially during early dapsone therapy
  • Notify the physician and discontinue if a rash occurs
  • Report persistent fatigue, fever, or sore throat
  • Avoid overexposure to sun or ultraviolet light

■ **Monitoring Parameters**
  • CBC weekly for the 1st mo, qmo for 6 mo, and semiannually thereafter
  • Periodic LFTs
  • Skin for a dermatologic reaction
  • Signs and symptoms of hemolysis, such as jaundice

■ **Geriatric side effects at a glance:**
  ❏ CNS   ❏ Bowel Dysfunction   ❏ Bladder Dysfunction   ❏ Falls

■ **U.S. Regulatory Considerations**
  ❏ FDA Black Box   ❏ OBRA regulated in U.S. Long Term Care

daptomycin

(dap'-toe-mye-sin)

■ **Brand Name(s):** Cubicin
  Chemical Class: Lipopeptide, cyclic

■ **Clinical Pharmacology:**
  Mechanism of Action: A lipopeptide antibacterial agent that binds to bacterial membranes and causes a rapid depolarization of the membrane potential. The loss of membrane potential leads to inhibition of protein, DNA, and RNA synthesis. **Therapeutic Effect:** Bactericidal.
  Pharmacokinetics: Widely distributed. Protein binding: 90%. Primarily excreted unchanged in urine. Moderately removed by hemodialysis. **Half-life:** 7-8 hr (increased in impaired renal function).

- **Available Forms:**
  - *Powder for Injection*: 250 mg/vial, 500 mg/vial.

- **Indications and Dosages:**
  Complicated skin and skin-structure infections: IV 4 mg/kg every 24 hr for 7-14 days.
  Dosage in renal impairment: For patients with creatinine clearance of less than 30 ml/min, dosage is 4 mg/kg q48h for 7-14 days.

- **Contraindications:** None known.

- **Side Effects**
  Frequent (6%-5%)
  Constipation, nausea, peripheral injection site reactions, headache, diarrhea
  Occasional (4%-3%)
  Insomnia, rash, vomiting
  Rare (less than 3%)
  Pruritus, dizziness, hypotension

- **Serious Reactions**
  - Skeletal muscle myopathy, characterized by muscle pain and weakness, particularly of the distal extremities, occurs rarely.
  - Antibiotic-associated colitis and other superinfections may result from altered bacterial balance.

Special Considerations
  - Experience with coadministration of HMG-CoA reductase inhibitors and daptomycin is limited; consider holding HMG-CoA reductase inhibitors in patients receiving daptomycin
  - Not effective for pneumonia even due to susceptible organisms

- **Patient/Family Education**
  - Notify the physician if headache, nausea, rash, severe diarrhea, new muscle weakness, or any other new symptoms occur

- **Monitoring Parameters**
  - CPK (weekly; discontinue in symptomatic patients with CPK elevation greater than 1000 U/L (5× ULN), or in asymptomatic patients with CPK greater than 10× ULN
  - Check for white patches on the mucous membranes and tongue
  - Pattern of daily bowel activity and stool consistency; mild GI effects may be tolerable, but severe symptoms may indicate the onset of antibiotic-associated colitis
  - Be alert for signs and symptoms of superinfection, including abdominal pain, moderate to severe diarrhea, severe anal or genital pruritus, and severe mouth soreness

- **Geriatric side effects at a glance:**
  ❑ CNS ❑ Bowel Dysfunction ❑ Bladder Dysfunction ❑ Falls

- **U.S. Regulatory Considerations**
  ❑ FDA Black Box ❑ OBRA regulated in U.S. Long Term Care

darbepoetin alfa

(dar-be-poe'-e-tin al'-fa)

- **Brand Name(s):** Aranesp
  Chemical Class: Amino acid glycoprotein

- **Clinical Pharmacology:**
  Mechanism of Action: A glycoprotein that stimulates formation of RBCs in bone marrow; increases serum half-life of epoetin. **Therapeutic Effect:** Induces erythropoiesis and release of reticulocytes from bone marrow.
  Pharmacokinetics: Well absorbed after subcutaneous administration. **Half-life:** 48.5 hr.

- **Available Forms:**
  - *Injection:* 25 mcg/ml, 40 mcg/ml, 60 mcg/ml, 100 mcg/ml, 150 mcg/ml, 200 mcg/ml, 300 mcg/ml.
  - *Prefilled Syringe:* 25 mcg/0.42 ml, 40 mcg/0.4 ml, 60 mcg/0.3 ml, 100 mcg/0.5 ml, 200 mcg/0.4 ml, 300 mcg/0.6 ml, 500 mcg/ml.

- **Indications and Dosages:**
  Anemia in chronic renal failure: IV Bolus, Subcutaneous Initially, 0.45 mcg/kg once weekly. Adjust dosage to achieve and maintain a target Hgb not to exceed 12 g/dl. Do not increase dosage more frequently than once monthly. Limit increases in Hgb by less than 1 g/dl over any 2-wk period.
  Anemia associated with chemotherapy: IV, Subcutaneous 2.25 mcg/kg/dose once a week. May increase up to 4.5 mcg/kg/dose once a week.

- **Contraindications:** History of sensitivity to mammalian cell-derived products or human albumin, uncontrolled hypertension

- **Side Effects**
  Frequent
  Myalgia, hypertension or hypotension, headache, diarrhea
  Occasional
  Fatigue, edema, vomiting, reaction at administration site, asthenia, dizziness

- **Serious Reactions**
  - Vascular access thrombosis, CHF, sepsis, arrhythmias, and anaphylactic reaction occur rarely.

Special Considerations
  - Two formulations available, one containing polysorbate 80, the other containing human albumin; a theoretical risk for Creutzfeldt-Jakob disease exists with the albumin formulation but is considered extremely remote
  - Advantage over erythropoietin is decreased frequency of dosing

- **Patient/Family Education**
  - Educate about blood pressure monitoring
  - Proper instruction for home administration if deemed appropriate

- Report severe headache
- Avoid tasks that require mental alertness or motor skills until response to the drug is established

■ Monitoring Parameters
- Hematocrit/hemoglobin weekly for 4 wk or until stable; if Hb increases >1.0 g/dL in any 2-wk period, decrease dose (possible increased seizure risk); target Hb level to not exceed 12 g/L
- Serum ferritin, transferrin saturation; supplemental iron recommended if ferritin <100 mcg/L or transferrin saturation <20%
- If lack of response or failure to maintain response occurs, check for causative factors (e.g., folate or vitamin B_{12} deficiency, occult blood loss, malignancy)
- Blood pressure aggressively for an increase because 25% of patients taking darbepoetin alfa require antihypertensive therapy and dietary restrictions

■ Geriatric side effects at a glance:
❑ CNS   ❑ Bowel Dysfunction   ❑ Bladder Dysfunction   ❑ Falls

■ U.S. Regulatory Considerations
❑ FDA Black Box   ❑ OBRA regulated in U.S. Long Term Care

darifenacin

(dare-ih-fen'-ah-sin)

■ Brand Name(s): Enablex

■ Clinical Pharmacology:
Mechanism of Action: A urinary antispasmodic agent that acts as a direct antagonist at muscarinic receptor sites in cholinergically innervated organs. Blockade of the receptors limits bladder contractions. **Therapeutic Effect:** Reduces symptoms of bladder irritability and overactivity; improves bladder capacity.
Pharmacokinetics: Well absorbed after PO administration. Protein binding: 98%. Extensively metabolized in the liver. Primarily excreted in urine with a lesser amount eliminated in feces. **Half-life:** 13-19 hr.

■ Available Forms:
- *Tablets* (*Extended-Release*): 7.5 mg, 15 mg.

■ Indications and Dosages:
Overactive bladder: PO Initially, 7.5 mg once daily. If response is not adequate after at least 2 wk, dosage may be increased to 15 mg once daily.
Dosage in hepatic impairment: For patients with moderate hepatic impairment, maximum dosage is 7.5 mg once daily.

■ Contraindications: GI or GU obstruction, paralytic ileus, severe hepatic impairment, uncontrolled angle-closure glaucoma, urine retention

■ **Side Effects**
   Frequent (35%-21%)
   Dry mouth, constipation
   Occasional (8%-4%)
   Dyspepsia, headache, nausea, abdominal pain
   Rare (3%-2%)
   Asthenia, diarrhea, dizziness, dry eyes

■ **Serious Reactions**
   • UTI occurs occasionally.

■ **Geriatric side effects at a glance:**
   ☑ CNS   ☑ Bowel Dysfunction   ☑ Bladder Dysfunction   ☑ Falls
   Other: Dry mouth, blurred vision, dizziness, somnolence

■ **Use with caution in older patients with:** Tachyarrythmias, overflow incontinence.

■ **U.S. Regulatory Considerations**
   ❑ FDA Black Box   ❑ OBRA regulated in U.S. Long Term Care

■ **Other Uses in Geriatric Patient:** None

■ **Side Effects:**
   Of particular importance in the geriatric patient: Delirium, possible antagonism of cholinergic drug therapy in the treatment of Alzheimer's disease.

■ **Geriatric Considerations - Summary:** Darifenacin and other newer anticholinergic drugs are moderately effective in the treatment of urge urinary incontinence and offer the potential benefit of selective antagonism of muscarinic receptors with less potential for CNS adverse effects. The relative safety and efficacy of these agents, which are significantly more expensive, has not been well studied to determine if they are superior to longer-acting anticholinergic formulations. These newer drugs can produce anticholinergic adverse effects including cognitive impairment, dry mouth, blurred vision, and increased risk of falls.

■ **References:**
   1. Hay-Smith J, Herbison P, Ellis G, Moore K. Anticholinergic drugs versus placebo for overactive bladder syndrome in adults. Cochrane Database of Systematic Reviews 2003;3.
   2. Lipton RB. Assessment of cognitive function of the elderly population: effects of darifenacin. J Urol 2005;173:493.
   3. Tune LE. Anticholinergic effects of medication in elderly patients. J Clin Psychiatry 2001;62(suppl 21):11-14.
   4. Ouslander JG. Management of overactive bladder. N Engl J Med 2004;350:786-799.

deferoxamine mesylate

(de-fer-ox'-a-meen mes'-sil-ate)

- **Brand Name(s):** Desferal
  Chemical Class: Siderochrome

- **Clinical Pharmacology:**
  Mechanism of Action: An antidote that binds with iron to form complex. **Therapeutic Effect:** Promotes urine excretion of acute iron poisoning.
  Pharmacokinetics: Well absorbed after IM, SC administration. Widely distributed. Rapidly metabolized in tissues, plasma. Excreted in urine, eliminated in feces via biliary excretion. Removed by hemodialysis. **Half-life:** 6 hr.

- **Available Forms:**
  - *Injection*: 500 mg (Desferal Mesylate).

- **Indications and Dosages:**
  Acute iron intoxication: IM Initially, 90 mg/kg, then 45 mg/kg up to 1g q4-12h. Maximum: 6 g/day. IV 15 mg/kg/hr up to 90 mg/kg q8hr. Maximum: 6 g/day.
  Chronic iron overload: Subcutaneous 1-2 g/day (20-40 mg/kg) over 8-24 hr. IM 0.5-1 g/day. In addition to IM, 2g infused at rate not to exceed 15 mg/kg/hr.

- **Contraindications:** Severe renal disease, anuria, primary hemochromatosis, hypersensitivity to deferoxamine mesylate or any component of the formulation

- **Side Effects**
  Frequent
  Pain, induration at injection site, urine color change (to orange-rose)
  Occasional
  Abdominal discomfort, diarrhea, leg cramps, impaired vision

- **Serious Reactions**
  - Neurotoxicity, including high-frequency hearing loss, has been reported.

Special Considerations

  - Acute iron intoxication
  - Deferoxamine indicated if:
    - Free serum iron present
    - Patient symptomatic
    - Serum iron greater than 350 mcg/dL

- **Patient/Family Education**
  - May turn urine red
  - Discomfort may occur at site of injection

- **Monitoring Parameters**
  - Visual acuity tests, slit-lamp examinations, funduscopy, and audiometry are recommended periodically in patients treated for prolonged periods of time

- BUN, creatinine, CrCl
- Serum iron levels

■ **Geriatric side effects at a glance:**
  ❏ CNS ❏ Bowel Dysfunction ❏ Bladder Dysfunction ❏ Falls

■ **U.S. Regulatory Considerations**
  ❏ FDA Black Box ❏ OBRA regulated in U.S. Long Term Care

delavirdine mesylate

(de-la-vir'-deen mes'-sil-ate)

■ **Brand Name(s):** Rescriptor
  Chemical Class: Arylpiperazine derivative; non-nucleoside reverse transcriptase inhibitor

■ **Clinical Pharmacology:**
  Mechanism of Action: A non-nucleoside reverse transcriptase inhibitor that binds directly to HIV-1 reverse transcriptase and blocks RNA- and DNA-dependent DNA polymerase activities. **Therapeutic Effect:** Interrupts HIV replication, slowing the progression of HIV infection.
  Pharmacokinetics: Rapidly absorbed after PO administration. Protein binding: 98%. Primarily distributed in plasma. Metabolized in the liver. Eliminated in feces and urine. **Half-life:** 2-11 hr.

■ **Available Forms:**
  - *Tablets:* 100 mg, 200 mg.

■ **Indications and Dosages:**
  HIV infection (in combination with other ID-antiretrovirals): PO 400 mg 3 times a day.

■ **Contraindications:** None known.

■ **Side Effects**
  Frequent (18%)
  Rash, pruritus
  Occasional (greater than 2%)
  Headache, nausea, diarrhea, fatigue, anorexia

■ **Serious Reactions**
  - Hepatic failure, severe rash, hemolytic anemia, rhabdomyolysis, erythema multiforme, Stevens-Johnson syndrome, and acute kidney failure have been reported.

Special Considerations
  - Always check updated treatment guidelines before initiating or changing antiretroviral therapy. (http://AIDSinfo.nih.gov)

- ■ **Patient/Family Education**
  - May take without regard to food; patients with achlorhydria should take with acidic beverage (orange or cranberry juice); may cause alcohol intolerance
  - Do not take any other medications, including OTC drugs, without notifying the physician
  - Delavirdine is not a cure for HIV infection, nor does it reduce the risk of transmitting HIV to others

- ■ **Monitoring Parameters**
  - CBC, hepatic, and renal function
  - Skin for rash
  - Daily pattern of bowel activity and stool consistency
  - Assess eating pattern, and monitor for nausea and weight loss

- ■ **Geriatric side effects at a glance:**
  - ❑ CNS ❑ Bowel Dysfunction ❑ Bladder Dysfunction ❑ Falls

- ■ **U.S. Regulatory Considerations**
  - ❑ FDA Black Box ❑ OBRA regulated in U.S. Long Term Care

demeclocycline hydrochloride

(dem-e-kloe-sye'-kleen hye-droe-klor'-ide)

- ■ **Brand Name(s):** Declomycin
  Chemical Class: Tetracycline derivative

- ■ **Clinical Pharmacology:**
  Mechanism of Action: A tetracycline antibacterial that inhibits bacterial protein synthesis by binding to ribosomal receptor sites; also inhibits ADH-induced water reabsorption. **Therapeutic Effect:** Bacteriostatic; also produces water diuresis.
  Pharmacokinetics: Food and dairy products interfere with absorption. Protein binding: 41%-91%. Metabolized in liver. Excreted in urine. Removed by hemodialysis. **Half-life:** 10-15 hr.

- ■ **Available Forms:**
  - *Tablets*: 150 mg, 300 mg.

- ■ **Indications and Dosages:**
  Mild to moderate infections, including acne, pertussis, chronic bronchitis, and UTIs: PO 150 mg 4 times a day or 300 mg 2 times a day.
  Uncomplicated gonorrhea: PO Initially, 600 mg, then 300 mg q12h for 4 days for total of 3 g.
  Syndrome of inappropriate ADH secretion (SIADH): PO Initially, 900-1200 mg/day in 3-4 divided doses, then decrease dose to 600-900 mg/day in divided doses.

333

■ **Contraindications:** None known.

■ **Side Effects**
Frequent
Anorexia, nausea, vomiting, diarrhea, dysphagia, possibly severe photosensitivity, (with moderate to high demeclocycline dosage).
Occasional
Urticaria, rash; diabetes insipidus syndrome, marked by polydipsia, polyuria, and weakness (with long-term therapy).

■ **Serious Reactions**
• Superinfection (especially fungal), anaphylaxis, and benign intracranial hypertension occur rarely.

Special Considerations
• No advantages over other tetracyclines as anti-infective; higher incidence of phototoxicity; active against water intoxication and SIADH
• Individualize treatment based on local susceptibility patterns

■ **Patient/Family Education**
• Sunscreen does not seem to decrease photosensitivity
• Avoid milk products; take with full glass of water on an empty stomach 1 hr before meals or 2 hr after meals
• Space drug doses evenly around the clock and continue taking demeclocycline for the full course of treatment

■ **Monitoring Parameters**
• LFTs during prolonged administration
• Skin for rash
• Daily bowel activity and stool consistency. Although mild GI effects may be tolerable, severe symptoms may indicate the onset of antibiotic-associated colitis.
• Signs and symptoms of superinfection include abdominal pain or cramping, anal or genital pruritus or discharge, moderate to severe diarrhea, severe mouth or tongue soreness, and new or increased fever.

■ **Geriatric side effects at a glance:**
❏ CNS   ☑ Bowel Dysfunction   ❏ Bladder Dysfunction   ❏ Falls

■ **U.S. Regulatory Considerations**
❏ FDA Black Box   ❏ OBRA regulated in U.S. Long Term Care

desipramine hydrochloride

(dess-ip'-ra-meen)

- **Brand Name(s):** Norpramin
  Chemical Class: Dibenzazepine derivative; secondary amine

- **Clinical Pharmacology:**
  Mechanism of Action: A tricyclic antidepressant that blocks the reuptake of neurotransmitters, such as norepinephrine and serotonin, at presynaptic membranes, increasing their availability at postsynaptic receptor sites. Also has anticholinergic activity. **Therapeutic Effect:** Relieves depression.
  Pharmacokinetics: Rapidly and well absorbed from the GI tract. Protein binding: 90%. Metabolized in the liver. Primarily excreted in urine. Minimally removed by hemodialysis. **Half-life:** 12-27 hr.

- **Available Forms:**
  - *Tablets*: 10 mg, 25 mg, 50 mg, 75 mg, 100 mg, 150 mg.

- **Indications and Dosages:**
  Depression: PO Initially, 10-25 mg/day. May gradually increase to 75-100 mg/day. Maximum: 300 mg/day.

- **Unlabeled Uses:** Treatment of cataplexy associated with narcolepsy, cocaine withdrawal, neurogenic pain, panic disorder

- **Contraindications:** Angle-closure glaucoma, use within 14 days of MAOIs

- **Side Effects**
  Frequent
  Somnolence, fatigue, dry mouth, blurred vision, constipation, delayed micturition, orthostatic hypotension, diaphoresis, impaired concentration, increased appetite, urine retention
  Occasional
  GI disturbances (such as nausea, GI distress, metallic taste)
  Rare
  Paradoxical reactions (agitation, restlessness, nightmares, insomnia), extrapyramidal symptoms (particularly fine hand tremor)

- **Serious Reactions**
  - Overdose may produce confusion, seizures, somnolence, arrhythmias, fever, hallucinations, dyspnea, vomiting, and unusual fatigue or weakness.
  - Abrupt discontinuation after prolonged therapy may produce severe headache, malaise, nausea, vomiting, and vivid dreams.

Special Considerations

- Equally effective as other tricyclic antidepressants for depression; fewer anticholinergic effects than tertiary amines, less orthostasis, and mild stimulatory property

Patient/Family Education
- Therapeutic effects may take 4-6 wk
- Use caution in driving or other activities requiring alertness
- Avoid alcohol and other CNS depressants
- Do not discontinue abruptly after long-term use
- Change positions slowly to avoid hypotensive effect

Monitoring Parameters
- Determination of desipramine plasma concentrations is not routinely recommended but may be useful in identifying toxicity, drug interactions, or noncompliance (adjustments in dosage should be made according to clinical response, not plasma concentrations); therapeutic level is 50-200 ng/ml
- Supervise suicidal-risk patient closely during early therapy (as depression lessens, energy level improves, increasing suicide potential)
- Assess appearance, behavior, speech pattern, level of interest, mood

Geriatric side effects at a glance:
☑ CNS ☑ Bowel Dysfunction ☑ Bladder Dysfunction ☑ Falls
Other: Orthostatic hypotension, cardiac conduction disturbances, anticholinergic side effects

Use with caution in older patients with: Cardiovascular disease, prostatic hyptertrophy or other conditions which increase the risk of urinary retention

U.S. Regulatory Considerations
☑ FDA Black Box
- Because there is an increased risk of suicide in children and adolescents, older adults should also be closely monitored for suicide ideation.
☑ OBRA regulated in U.S. Long Term Care

Other Uses in Geriatric Patient: Neuropathic pain, urge urinary incontinence

Side Effects:
Of particular importance in the geriatric patient: Anticholinergic effects, extrapyramidal symptoms, high doses (>100 mg) may increase risk of sudden death

Geriatric Considerations - Summary: Although tricyclic antidepressants are effective in the treatment of major depression in older adults, the side-effect profile and low toxic-to-therapeutic ratio relegate them to second-line agents (after serotonin reuptake inhibitors) for most older patients. These agents are effective in the treatment of urge urinary incontinence and neuropathic pain, but must be monitored closely. Of the tricyclic antidepressants, imipramine and amitryptyline have the highest anticholinergic activity and may be best choice in this class for management of incontinence, but should otherwise be avoided.

References:
1. Leipzig RM, Cumming RG, Tinetti ME. Drugs and falls in older people: a systematic review and meta-analysis: I. Psychotropic drugs. J Am Geriatr Soc 1999;47:30-39.
2. Cadieux RJ. Antidepressant drug interactions in the elderly. Understanding the P-450 system is half the battle in reducing risks. Postgrad Med 1999;106:231-240, 245.
3. Ray WA, Meredith S, Thapa PB, et al. Cyclic antidepressants and the risk of sudden cardiac death. Clin Pharmacol Ther 2004;75:234-241.
4. Roose SP, Laghrissi-Thode F, Kennedy JS, et al. Comparison of paroxetine and nortriptyline in depressed patients with ischemic heart disease. JAMA 1998;279:287-291.

desirudin

(deh-seer'-ew-din)

■ **Brand Name(s):** Iprivask
   Chemical Class: Hirudin derivative; thrombin inhibitor

■ **Clinical Pharmacology:**
   Mechanism of Action: An anticoagulant that binds specifically and directly to thrombin, inhibiting free circulating and clot-bound thrombin. **Therapeutic Effect:** Prolongs the clotting time of human plasma.
   Pharmacokinetics: Completely absorbed. Distributed in extracellular space. Metabolized and eliminated by the kidney. **Half-life:** 2–3 hr.

■ **Available Forms:**
   • *Powder for Injection*: 15-mg vial with diluent (diluent includes 0.6 ml mannitol (3%) in water for injection).

■ **Indications and Dosages:**
   Prevention of deep vein thrombosis (DVT) in patients undergoing hip replacement surgery: Subcutaneous Initially, 15 mg q12h given 5–15 min before surgery but following induction of regional block anesthesia, if used. May administer up to 12 days post surgery.
   Moderate renal impairment (creatinine clearance 31–60 ml/min or higher): Subcutaneous 5 mg q12h.
   Severe renal impairment (creatinine clearance less than 31 ml/min): Subcutaneous 1.7 mg q12h.

■ **Contraindications:** Hypersensitivity to natural or recombinant hirudins (anticoagulation factors), active bleeding, irreversible coagulation disorders

■ **Side Effects**
   Frequent (6%)
   Hematoma
   Occasional (4%–2%)
   Injection site mass, wound secretion, nausea, hypersensitivity reaction

■ **Serious Reactions**
   • *Alert* When neuraxial anesthesia (epidural/spinal anesthesia) or spinal puncture is employed, patients anticoagulated or scheduled to be anticoagulated with selective inhibitors of thrombin such as desirudin may be at risk of developing an epidural or spinal hematoma which can result in long-term or permanent paralysis.
   • Serious or major hemorrhage and anaphylactic reaction occur rarely.

■ **Patient/Family Education**
   • Use an electric razor and soft toothbrush to prevent bleeding during therapy
   • Do not take other medications, including OTC drugs (especially aspirin), without physician approval

- Report black or red stool, coffee-ground vomitus, dark or red urine, or red-speckled mucus from cough

■ **Monitoring Parameters**
- If CrCl less than 60 ml/min, monitor aPTT and serum Cr at least daily; if aPTT exceeds 2× control, interrupt therapy until the value returns to less than 2× control and then resume therapy at a reduced dose guided by the initial degree of aPTT abnormality
- Assess for abdominal or back pain, a decrease in blood pressure and Hct, an increase in pulse rate, and severe headache because these signs may indicate hemorrhage
- Assess the patient's gums for erythema and gingival bleeding, skin for bruises, and urine for hematuria
- Examine the patient for excessive bleeding from minor cuts and scratches

■ **Geriatric side effects at a glance:**
  ❑ CNS ❑ Bowel Dysfunction ❑ Bladder Dysfunction ❑ Falls

■ **U.S. Regulatory Considerations**
  ☑ FDA Black Box
  Increased risk of spinal/epidural hematomas with neuraxial anesthesia or spinal puncture. Risk is further increased by use of indwelling spinal catheters, repeated/traumatic epidural/spinal puncture, or use of drugs affecting hemostasis (NSAIDs, anticoagulants, platelet inhibitors).
  ❑ OBRA regulated in U.S. Long Term Care

desloratadine

(des-lor-at'-a-deen)

■ **Brand Name(s):** Clarinex, Clarinex RediTabs
  Chemical Class: Piperidine derivative

■ **Clinical Pharmacology:**
  Mechanism of Action: A nonsedating antihistamine that exhibits selective peripheral histamine H_1-receptor blocking action. Competes with histamine at receptor sites.
  Therapeutic Effect: Prevents allergic responses mediated by histamine, such as rhinitis and urticaria.
  Pharmacokinetics: Rapidly and almost completely absorbed from the GI tract. Distributed mainly in liver, lungs, GI tract, and bile. Metabolized in the liver to active metabolite and undergoes extensive first-pass metabolism. Eliminated in urine and feces. **Half-life:** 27 hr (increased in the elderly and in renal or hepatic impairment).

■ **Available Forms:**
- *Tablets (Clarinex):* 5 mg.
- *Tablets (Orally-Disintegrating [Clarinex RediTabs]):* 2.5 mg, 5 mg.
- *Syrup (Clarinex):* 2.5 mg/5 ml.

■ Indications and Dosages:
Allergic rhinitis, urticaria: PO 5 mg once a day.
Dosage in hepatic or renal impairment: Dosage is decreased to 5 mg every other day.

■ Contraindications: None known.

■ Side Effects
Frequent (12%)
Headache
Occasional (3%)
Dry mouth, somnolence
Rare (less than 3%)
Fatigue, dizziness, diarrhea, nausea

■ Serious Reactions
- None known.

Special Considerations
- No advantage over loratadine (parent compound), which is available OTC
- Intranasal corticosteroids are preferred therapy unless allergy symptoms are mild and infrequent
- Reserve for patients unable to tolerate sedating antihistamines like chlorpheniramine

■ Patient/Family Education
- May be taken without regard to meals
- Take orally-disintegrating tabs immediately after opening the blister packet
- Desloratadine does not cause drowsiness
- Avoid alcohol during therapy

■ Monitoring Parameters
- Therapeutic response

■ Geriatric side effects at a glance:
❑ CNS   ❑ Bowel Dysfunction   ❑ Bladder Dysfunction   ❑ Falls
Other: Cognitive impairment, Sedation

■ Use with caution in older patients with: Hepatic impairment, Renal impairment, Cognitive impairment

■ U.S. Regulatory Considerations
❑ FDA Black Box   ❑ OBRA regulated in U.S. Long Term Care

■ Other Uses in Geriatric Patient: None

■ Side Effects:
Of particular importance in the geriatric patient: Impaired attention, decreased concentration, sedation, potential for anticholinergic effects, cognitive impairment, headaches, dry mouth

■ Geriatric Considerations - Summary: A preferred agent for older adults when an antihistamine is indicated.

■ **References:**
1. Hansen J, Klimek L, Hormann K. Pharmacological management of allergic rhinitis in the elderly. Safety issues with oral antihistamines. Drugs Aging 2005;22:289-296.
2. Affrime M, Gupta S, Banfield C, Cohen A. A pharmacokinetic profile of desloratadine in healthy adults, including elderly. Clin Pharmacokin 2002;41(Suppl 1):13-19.
3. Newer antihistamines. Med Lett 2001;43.
4. Drugs that may cause cognitive disorders in the elderly. Med Lett 2000;42:111-112.

desmopressin

(des-moe-press'-in)

■ **Brand Name(s):** DDAVP, DDAVP Nasal, DDAVP Rhinal Tube, Minirin, Stimate
Chemical Class: Arginine vasopressin analog

■ **Clinical Pharmacology:**
Mechanism of Action: A synthetic pituitary hormone that increases reabsorption of water by increasing permeability of collecting ducts of the kidneys. Also serves as a plasminogen activator. **Therapeutic Effect:** Increases plasma factor VIII (antihemophilic factor). Decreases urinary output.
Pharmacokinetics:

Route	Onset	Peak	Duration
PO	1 hr	2-7 hr	6-8 hr
IV	15-30 min	1.5-3 hr	N/A
Intranasal	15 min-1 hr	1-5 hr	5-21 hr

Poorly absorbed after oral or nasal administration. Metabolism: Unknown. **Half-life:** Oral: 1.5-2.5 hr. Intranasal: 3.3-3.5 hr. IV: 0.4-4 hr.

■ **Available Forms:**
• *Tablets* (DDAVP): 0.1 mg, 0.2 mg.
• *Injection* (DDAVP): 4 mcg/ml.
• *Nasal Solution* (DDAVP): 0.01%.
• *Nasal Spray*: 0.01 mg/inhalation (DDAVP Nasal), 0.15 mg/inhalation (Stimate).

■ **Indications and Dosages:**
Central cranial diabetes insipidus: PO Initially, 0.05 mg twice a day. Range: 0.1-1.2 mg/day in 2-3 divided doses. IV, Subcutaneous 2-4 mcg/day in 2 divided doses or 1/10 of maintenance intranasal dose. Intranasal (use 100 mcg/ml concentration) 5-40 mcg (0.05-0.4 ml) in 1-3 doses/day.
Hemophilia A, von Willebrand's Disease (Type I): IV Infusion 0.3 mcg/kg diluted in 50 ml 0.9% NaCl. Intranasal (use 1.5 mg/ml concentration providing 150 mcg/spray) *Weight more than 50 kg.* 300 mcg; use 1 spray in each nostril. *Weight 50 kg or less.* 150 mcg as a single spray.

■ **Unlabeled Uses:** Prophylaxis and treatment of central diabetes insipidus, treatment of hemophilia A, von Willebrand's disease

■ **Contraindications:** Hemophilia A with factor VIII levels less than 5%; hemophilia B; severe type I, type IIB, or platelet-type von Willebrand's disease

Side Effects
Occasional
IV: Pain, redness, or swelling at injection site; headache; abdominal cramps; vulval pain; flushed skin; mild BP elevation; nausea with high dosages
Nasal: Rhinorrhea, nasal congestion, slight BP elevation

Serious Reactions
- Water intoxication or hyponatremia, marked by headache, somnolence, confusion, decreased urination, rapid weight gain, seizures, and coma, may occur in overhydration.

Patient/Family Education
- Nasal tube delivery system is supplied with a flexible calibrated plastic tube (rhinyle); draw sol into the rhinyle, insert 1 end of tube into nostril, blow on the other end to deposit sol deep into nasal cavity
- Ingest only enough water to satisfy thirst
- Report abdominal cramps, headache, heartburn, nausea, or shortness of breath

Monitoring Parameters
- Diabetes insipidus: Urine volume and osmolality, plasma osmolality
- Hemophilia A: Determine factor VIII coagulant activity before injecting desmopressin for hemostasis; if activity is <5% of normal, do not rely on desmopressin
- Von Willebrand's disease: Assess levels of factor VIII coagulant, factor VIII antigen, and ristocetin cofactor; skin bleeding time may also be helpful

Geriatric side effects at a glance:
❑ CNS ❑ Bowel Dysfunction ❑ Bladder Dysfunction ❑ Falls

U.S. Regulatory Considerations
❑ FDA Black Box ❑ OBRA regulated in U.S. Long Term Care

desonide

(dess'-oh-nide)

Brand Name(s): Delonide, DesOwen, Tridesilon
Chemical Class: Corticosteroid, synthetic

Clinical Pharmacology:
Mechanism of Action: A topical corticosteroid that has anti-inflammatory, antipruritic, and vasoconstrictive properties. The exact mechanism of the anti-inflammatory process is unclear. **Therapeutic Effect:** Reduces or prevents tissue response to the inflammatory process.
Pharmacokinetics: Large variation in absorption determined by many factors. Metabolized in the liver. Primarily excreted by the kidneys and small amounts in the bile.

341

■ **Available Forms:**
- *Lotion*: 0.05% (DesOwen).
- *Cream*: 0.05% (DesOwen).
- *Ointment*: 0.05% (DesOwen, Tridesilon).

■ **Indications and Dosages:**
Dermatoses: Topical Apply sparingly 2-3 times/day.
Otitis externa: Aural Instill 3 to 4 drops into the ear 3-4 times/day.

■ **Contraindications:** Perforated eardrum, history of hypersensitivity to desonide or other corticosteroids

■ **Side Effects**
Occasional
Burning and stinging at site of application, dryness, skin peeling, contact dermatitis

■ **Serious Reactions**
- The serious reactions of long-term therapy (greater than 2 wk) and the addition of occlusive dressings are reversible hypothalamic-pituitary-adrenal (HPA) axis suppression, manifestations of Cushing's syndrome, hyperglycemia, and glucosuria.

■ **Patient/Family Education**
- Apply sparingly only to affected area
- Avoid contact with the eyes
- Do not put bandages or dressings over treated area unless directed by clinician
- Discontinue drug and notify clinician if local irritation or fever develops
- Do not use on weeping, denuded, or infected areas

■ **Monitoring Parameters**
- Skin for rash

■ **Geriatric side effects at a glance:**
❑ CNS ❑ Bowel Dysfunction ❑ Bladder Dysfunction ❑ Falls

■ **U.S. Regulatory Considerations**
❑ FDA Black Box ❑ OBRA regulated in U.S. Long Term Care

desoximetasone

(des-ox-i-met'-a-sone)

- **Brand Name(s):** Topicort, Topicort LP
  Chemical Class: Corticosteroid, synthetic

- **Clinical Pharmacology:**
  Mechanism of Action: A high-potency, fluoronated topical corticosteroid that has anti-inflammatory, antipruritic, and vasoconstrictive properties. The exact mechanism of the anti-inflammatory process is unclear. **Therapeutic Effect:** Reduces tissue response to the inflammatory process.
  Pharmacokinetics: Large variation in absorption among sites. Protein binding in varying degrees. Metabolized in liver. Primarily excreted in urine.

- **Available Forms:**
  - *Cream*: 0.25% (Topicort), 0.05% (Topicort LP).
  - *Gel*: 0.05% (Topicort).
  - *Ointment*: 0.25% (Topicort).

- **Indications and Dosages:**
  Dermatoses: Topical Apply sparingly 2 times/day.

- **Unlabeled Uses:** Eczema, psoriasis vulgaris

- **Contraindications:** History of hypersensitivity to desoximetasone or other corticosteroids

- **Side Effects**
  Frequent
  Itching, redness, irritation, burning at site of application
  Occasional
  Dryness, folliculitis, hypertrichosis, acneiform eruptions, hypopigmentation, perioral dermatitis
  Rare
  Allergic contact dermatitis, adrenal suppression, atrophy, striae, miliaria, photosensitivity

- **Serious Reactions**
  - Serious reactions of long-term therapy (greater than 2 weeks) and addition of occlusive dressings are reversible hypothalamic-pituitary-adrenal (HPA) axis suppression, manifestations of Cushing's syndrome, hyperglycemia, and glucosuria.
  - Abruptly withdrawing the drug after long-term therapy may require supplemental systemic corticosteroids.

Special Considerations
  - Potent, fluorinated topical corticosteroid with comparable efficacy to fluocinonide, diflorasone, amcinonide, betamethasone, dipropionate, and halcinonide; cost should govern use

■ Patient/Family Education
- Apply sparingly only to affected area
- Avoid contact with the eyes
- Do not put bandages or dressings over treated area unless directed by clinician
- Discontinue drug, notify clinician if local irritation or fever develops
- Do not use on weeping, denuded, or infected areas

■ Monitoring Parameters
- Be alert for signs and symptoms of infection such as fever and sore throat that indicate reduced immune response

■ Geriatric side effects at a glance:
❏ CNS ❏ Bowel Dysfunction ❏ Bladder Dysfunction ❏ Falls

■ U.S. Regulatory Considerations
❏ FDA Black Box ❏ OBRA regulated in U.S. Long Term Care

dexamethasone

(dex-a-meth'-a-sone)

■ Brand Name(s): Adrenocot, Cortastat, Cortastat 10, Cortastat LA, Dalalone, Dalalone D.P., Dalalone L.A., Decadron, Decadron 5-12 Pak, Decadron Phosphate Injectable, Decaject, De-Sone LA, Dexacen-4, Dexamethasone Intensol, Dexasone, Dexasone LA, Dexpak Taperpak, Hexadrol, Hexadrol Phosphate, Maxidex, Solurex, Solurex LA

Combinations
Rx: with neomycin, (NeoDecadron, Ak-Neo-Dex); with neomycin and polymixin B (Dexacidin, Maxitrol, Dexasporin); with tobramycin (Tobradex); with lidocaine (Decadron with Xylocaine)
Chemical Class: Glucocorticoid, synthetic

■ Clinical Pharmacology:
Mechanism of Action: A long-acting glucocorticoid that inhibits accumulation of inflammatory cells at inflammation sites, phagocytosis, lysosomal enzyme release and synthesis, and release of mediators of inflammation. **Therapeutic Effect:** Prevents and suppresses cell and tissue immune reactions and inflammatory process.
Pharmacokinetics: Rapidly, completely absorbed from the GI tract after oral administration. Widely distributed. Protein binding: High. Metabolized in the liver. Primarily excreted in urine. Minimally removed by hemodialysis. **Half-life:** 3-4.5 hr.

■ Available Forms:
- *Nasal Aerosol:* 100 mcg.
- *Ophthalmic Ointment (Decadron, Maxidex):* 0.05% .
- *Ophthalmic Solution (Decadron):* 0.1%.
- *Ophthalmic Suspension (Maxidex):* 0.1%.
- *Oral Concentrate (Dexamethasone Intensol):* 1 mg/ml.
- *Oral Solution:* 0.5 mg/5 ml, 1 mg/ml.

344

- **Tablets:** 0.25 mg, 0.5 mg (Decadron), 0.75 mg (Decadron, Decadron 5-12 Pak), 1 mg, 1.5 mg (Dexpak Taperpak), 2 mg, 4 mg (Decadron, Hexadrol), 6 mg.
- **Topical Aerosol:** 0.01%, 0.04%.
- **Topical Cream (Decadron):** 0.1%,
- **Topical Gel:** 0.1%.
- **Injectable Solution:** 4 mg/ml (Adrenocot, Cortastat, Dalalone, Decadron Phosphate Injectable, Decaject, Dexacen-4, Dexasone, Hexadrol Phosphate, Solurex), 10 mg/ml (Cortastat 10, Dexasone, Hexadrol Phosphate).
- **Injectable Suspension:** 8 mg/ml (Cortastat LA, Dalalone L.A., De-Sone LA, Dexasone LA, Solurex LA), 16 mg/ml (Dalalone D.P.).

■ Indications and Dosages:
Anti-inflammatory: PO, IV, IM 0.75-9 mg/day in divided doses q6-12h.
Cerebral edema: IV Initially, 10 mg, then 4 mg (IV or IM) q6h.
Nausea and vomiting in chemotherapy patients: IV 8-20 mg once, then 4 mg (PO) q4–6h or 8 mg q8h.
Usual topical dosage: Topical Apply to affected area 3-4 times a day.
Usual ophthalmic dosage, ocular inflammatory conditions: Ointment Thin coating 3-4 times/day. Suspension Initially, 2 drops q1h while awake and q2h at night for 1 day, then reduce to 3-4 times/day.

■ Unlabeled Uses: Antiemetic, croup

■ Contraindications: Active untreated infections, fungal, tuberculosis, or viral diseases of the eye

■ Side Effects
Frequent
Inhalation: Cough, dry mouth, hoarseness, throat irritation
Intranasal: Burning, mucosal dryness
Ophthalmic: Blurred vision
Systemic: Insomnia, facial swelling or cushingoid appearance, moderate abdominal distention, indigestion, increased appetite, nervousness, facial flushing, diaphoresis
Occasional
Inhalation: Localized fungal infection, such as thrush
Intranasal: Crusting inside nose, nosebleed, sore throat, ulceration of nasal mucosa
Ophthalmic: Decreased vision, watering of eyes, eye pain, burning, stinging, redness of eyes, nausea, vomiting
Systemic: Dizziness, decreased or blurred vision
Topical: Allergic contact dermatitis, purpura or blood-containing blisters, thinning of skin with easy bruising, telangiectasis or raised dark red spots on skin
Rare
Inhalation: Increased bronchospasm, esophageal candidiasis
Intranasal: Nasal and pharyngeal candidiasis, eye pain
Systemic: General allergic reaction (such as rash and hives); pain, redness, or swelling at injection site; psychological changes; false sense of well-being; hallucinations; depression

■ Serious Reactions
- Long-term therapy may cause muscle wasting (especially in the arms and legs), osteoporosis, spontaneous fractures, cataracts, glaucoma, peptic ulcer disease, and CHF.
- The ophthalmic form may cause glaucoma, ocular hypertension, and cataracts.

- Abrupt withdrawal following long-term therapy may cause severe joint pain, severe headache, anorexia, nausea, fever, rebound inflammation, fatigue, weakness, lethargy, dizziness, and orthostatic hypotension.

Special Considerations
- Signs of adrenal insufficiency include fatigue, anorexia, nausea, vomiting, diarrhea, weight loss, weakness, dizziness, and low blood sugar; drug-induced secondary adrenocorticoid insufficiency and low blood sugar; drug-induced adrenocorticoid insufficiency may be minimized by gradual systemic dosage reduction; relative insufficiency may exist for up to 1 yr after discontinuation; therefore, be prepared to supplement in situations of stress
- May mask infections
- Do not give live virus vaccines to patients on prolonged therapy
- Patients on chronic steroid therapy should wear medical alert bracelet

■ Monitoring Parameters
- Potassium and blood sugar during long-term therapy
- Check lens and intraocular pressure frequently during prolonged use of ophthalmic preparations

■ Patient/Family Education
- Do not abruptly discontinue the drug or change the dosage or schedule; the drug must be withdrawn gradually under medical supervision
- Report fever, muscle aches, sore throat, and sudden weight gain or swelling.
- Severe stress, including serious infection, surgery, or trauma, may require an increase in dexamethasone dosage
- Inform the dentist and other physicians if he or she is taking dexamethasone or has taken it within the past 12 mo
- Use the topical form after a bath or shower for best absorption
- Steroids often cause mood swings, ranging from euphoria to depression

■ Geriatric side effects at a glance:
☑ CNS   ☐ Bowel Dysfunction   ☐ Bladder Dysfunction   ☐ Falls

■ U.S. Regulatory Considerations
☐ FDA Black Box   ☑ OBRA regulated in U.S. Long Term Care

dexchlorpheniramine maleate

(dex'-klor-fen-eer'-a-meen mal'-ee-ate)

■ Brand Name(s): Polaramine, Polaramine Repetabs

Combinations
Rx: with guaifenesin, pseudoephedrine (Polaramine Expectorant)
Chemical Class: Alkylamine derivative

■ **Clinical Pharmacology:**
Mechanism of Action: A propylamine derivative that competes with histamine for H_1-receptor sites on effector cells in the gastrointestinal (GI) tract, blood vessels, and respiratory tract. Dexchlorpheniramine is the dextro-isomer of chlorpheniramine and is approximately two times more active. **Therapeutic Effect:** Prevents allergic response, produces mild bronchodilation, blocks histamine-induced bronchitis.
Pharmacokinetics:

Route	Onset	Peak	Duration
PO	0.5 hr	1-2 hr	3-6 hr

Well absorbed from the GI tract. Protein binding: 70%. Widely distributed. Metabolized in liver to active metabolite, undergoes extensive first-pass metabolism. Excreted primarily in urine. Not removed by hemodialysis. **Half-life:** 20 hr.

■ **Available Forms:**
- *Tablets:* 2 mg (Polaramine [DSC]).
- *Extended-Release Tablets:* 4 mg, 6 mg (Polaramine Repetabs).
- *Syrup:* 2 mg/ 5 ml (Polaramine).

■ **Indications and Dosages:**
Allergic rhinitis, common cold: PO 2 mg q4-6h or 4-6 mg timed-release at bedtime or q8-10h.

■ **Unlabeled Uses:** Asthma, chemotherapy-induced stomatitis, dermographia, familial immunodeficiency disease, malaria, mastocytosis, Meniere's disease, nausea, neurocysticercosis, otitis media, psoriasis, radiocontrast media reactions, urticaria

■ **Contraindications:** History of hypersensitivity to antihistamines

■ **Side Effects**
Frequent
Drowsiness, dizziness, headache, dry mouth, nose, or throat, urinary retention, thickening of bronchial secretions, sedation, hypotension
Occasional
Epigastric distress, flushing, blurred vision, tinnitus, paresthesia, sweating, chills

■ **Serious Reactions**
- Hypersensitivity reaction, such as eczema, pruritus, rash, cardiac disturbances, and photosensitivity, may occur.
- Overdosage may vary from CNS depression, including sedation, apnea, hypotension, cardiovascular collapse, or death to severe paradoxical reaction, such as hallucinations, tremor, and seizures.

Special Considerations
- Active dextro-isomer of chlorpheniramine

■ **Patient/Family Education**
- The patient may develop tolerance to the drug's sedative effect
- Avoid performing tasks that require mental alertness or motor skills until response to the drug is established

- Notify the physician if he or she experiences visual disturbances
- Dizziness, drowsiness, and dry mouth are expected side effects of dexchlorpheniramine
- Avoid alcohol

■ **Geriatric side effects at a glance:**
☑ CNS   ☑ Bowel Dysfunction   ☑ Bladder Dysfunction   ❑ Falls
Other: Dry mouth, blurred vision, confusion, psychoses

■ **Use with caution in older patients with:** Narrow-angle glaucoma, overflow incontinence, psychosis.

■ **U.S. Regulatory Considerations**
❑ FDA Black Box   ❑ OBRA regulated in U.S. Long Term Care

■ **Other Uses in Geriatric Patient:** None

■ **Side Effects:**
Of particular importance in the geriatric patient: Anticholinergic effects

■ **Geriatric Considerations - Summary:** Dexchlorpheniramine is a first-generation alkylamine antihistamine with potent H_1-receptor antagonism. It has anticholinergic properties and can cause somnolence. Older adults taking this drug are at risk of dizziness and hypotension.

■ **References:**
1. Bantz EW, Dolen WK, Chadwick EW, et al. Chronic chlorpheniramine therapy: subsensitivity, drug metabolism, and compliance. Ann Allergy 1987; 59:341-346.
2. Tune LE. Anticholinergic effects of medication in elderly patients. J Clin Psychiatry 2001;62(suppl 21):11-14.

dexmethylphenidate hydrochloride

(dex-meth-ill-fen'-i-date hye-droe-klor'-ide)

■ **Brand Name(s):** Focalin, Focalin XR
Chemical Class: Piperidine derivative of amphetamine

■ **Clinical Pharmacology:**
Mechanism of Action: A CNS stimulant that blocks the reuptake of norepinephrine and dopamine into presynaptic neurons, increasing the release of these neurotransmitters into the synaptic cleft. **Therapeutic Effect:** Decreases motor restlessness and fatigue; increases motor activity, mental alertness, and attention span; elevates mood.

Pharmacokinetics:

Route	Onset	Peak	Duration
PO	N/A	N/A	4-5 hr

Readily absorbed from the GI tract. Plasma concentrations increase rapidly. Metabolized in the liver. Excreted unchanged in urine. **Half-life:** 2.2 hr.

■ Available Forms:

- *Tablets (Focalin):* 2.5 mg, 5 mg, 10 mg.
- *Capsules (Extended-Release [Focalin XR]):* 5 mg, 10 mg, 20 mg.

■ Indications and Dosages:

Attention-deficit hyperactivity disorder (ADHD): PO (Patients new to dexmethylphenidate or methylphenidate) 2.5 mg twice a day (5 mg/day). May adjust dosage in 2.5- to 5-mg increments. Maximum: 20 mg/day. PO (Patients currently taking methylphenidate) Half the methylphenidate dosage. Maximum: 20 mg/day. PO [Exended-Release (Patients new to dexmethylphenidate or methylphenidate)] Initially, 10 mg/day. PO [Extended-Release (Patients currently taking methylphenidate)] Half the methylphenidate dosage. Maximum: 20 mg/day. Patients using Focalin may be switched to the same daily dose for Focalin XR.

■ Contraindications: Diagnosis or family history of Tourette's syndrome; glaucoma; history of marked agitation, anxiety, or tension; motor tics; use within 14 days of MAOIs

■ Side Effects

Frequent

Abdominal pain, nausea, anorexia, fever

Occasional

Tachycardia, arrhythmias, palpitations, insomnia, twitching

Rare

Blurred vision, rash, arthralgia

■ Serious Reactions

- Withdrawal after prolonged therapy may unmask symptoms of the underlying disorder.
- Dexmethylphenidate may lower the seizure threshold in those with a history of seizures.
- Overdose produces excessive sympathomimetic effects, including vomiting, tremor, hyperreflexia, seizures, confusion, hallucinations, and diaphoresis.
- Neuroleptic malignant syndrome occurs rarely.

Special Considerations

- No clinical data to support use of this agent over racemic methylphenidate

■ Patient/Family Education

- Take last dose late afternoon or early evening to prevent insomnia
- Reinforce habit-forming potential of medication; caution against taking more than required dose
- Avoid tasks that require mental alertness or motor skills until response to the drug has been established

- **Monitoring Parameters**
  - Improvement of clinical symptoms, lack of adverse effects; periodic complete blood count with differential, routine blood chemistry; growth determinations (body weight and height), blood pressure, pulse rate

- **Geriatric side effects at a glance:**
  ☑ CNS ☐ Bowel Dysfunction ☐ Bladder Dysfunction ☐ Falls

- **U.S. Regulatory Considerations**
  ☑ FDA Black Box
  - CNS stimulant use has a high abuse potential with the risk of dependence.
  - Misuse may cause sudden death and serious cardiovascular adverse events.
  - Reports of psychotic episodes.
  - Use caution when withdrawing drug.
  ☐ OBRA regulated in U.S. Long Term Care

dextroamphetamine sulfate

(dex-troe-am-fet'-a-meen sul'-fate)

- **Brand Name(s):** Dexedrine, Dexedrine Spansule, Dextrostat
  Chemical Class: D-β-phenyl-isopropylamine

  DEA Class: Schedule II

- **Clinical Pharmacology:**
  Mechanism of Action: An amphetamine that enhances the action of dopamine and norepinephrine by blocking their reuptake from synapses; also inhibits monoamine oxidase and facilitates the release of catecholamines. **Therapeutic Effect:** Increases motor activity and mental alertness; decreases motor restlessness, drowsiness, and fatigue; suppresses appetite.
  Pharmacokinetics: Well absorbed following PO administration. Metabolized in liver. Excreted in urine. Removed by hemodialysis. **Half-life:** 7-34 hr.

- **Available Forms:**
  - *Capsules (Sustained-Release [Dexedrine Spansule]):* 5 mg, 10 mg, 15 mg.
  - *Tablets:* 5 mg (Dexedrine), 10 mg (Dexedrine, Dextrostat).

- **Indications and Dosages:**
  Narcolepsy: PO Initially, 10 mg/day. Increase by 10 mg/day at weekly intervals until therapeutic response is achieved.
  Appetite suppressant: PO 5-30 mg daily in divided doses of 5-10 mg each, given 30-60 min before meals; or 1 extended-release capsule in the morning.

- **Contraindications:** Advanced arteriosclerosis, agitated states, glaucoma, history of drug abuse, hypersensitivity to sympathomimetic amines, hyperthyroidism, moderate to severe hypertension, symptomatic cardiovascular disease, use within 14 days of MAOIs

Side Effects

Frequent

Irregular pulse, increased motor activity, talkativeness, nervousness, mild euphoria, insomnia

Occasional

Headache, chills, dry mouth, GI distress, worsening depression in patients who are clinically depressed, tachycardia, palpitations, chest pain, dizziness, decreased appetite

Serious Reactions

- Overdose may produce skin pallor or flushing, arrhythmias, and psychosis.
- Abrupt withdrawal after prolonged use of high doses may produce lethargy lasting for weeks.

Special Considerations

- Use for obesity should be reserved for patients failing to respond to alternative therapy; weigh the limited benefit against the substantial risk of addiction and dependence

Patient/Family Education

- Tolerance or dependency is common
- Avoid OTC preparations unless approved by clinician
- Do not crush or chew sustained-release dosage forms
- Take dextroamphetamine early in the day
- Avoid performing tasks that require mental alertness or motor skills until response to the drug has been established
- Notify the physician if decreased appetite, dizziness, dry mouth, or pronounced nervousness occurs

Monitoring Parameters

- Blood pressure
- Weight
- CNS for overstimulation

Geriatric side effects at a glance:

☑ CNS   ❑ Bowel Dysfunction   ❑ Bladder Dysfunction   ❑ Falls

U.S. Regulatory Considerations

☑ FDA Black Box
- CNS stimulant use has a high abuse potential with the risk of dependence.
- Misuse may cause sudden death and serious cardiovascular adverse events.

❑ OBRA regulated in U.S. Long Term Care

dextromethorphan hydrobromide

(dex-troe-meth-or'-fan hye-droe-broe'-mide)

- **Brand Name(s):** Benylin Adult, Creomulsion Cough, Creo-Terpin, Delsym, Dexalone, ElixSure Cough, Hold DM, Scot-Tussin DM Cough Chasers, Silphen DM, Simply Cough
  OTC: Robitussin CoughGels, Robitussin Honey Cough, Robitussin Maximum Strength Cough, Vicks 44 Cough Relief

  Combinations
  OTC: with benzocaine (Spec T, Vicks Formula 44 cough control discs, Vicks cough silencers); with guaifenesin (Robitussin DM)
  Chemical Class: Levorphanol derivative

- **Clinical Pharmacology:**
  Mechanism of Action: A chemical relative of morphine without the narcotic properties that acts on the cough center in the medulla oblongata by elevating the threshold for coughing. **Therapeutic Effect:** Suppresses cough.
  Pharmacokinetics: Rapidly absorbed from the gastrointestinal (GI) tract. Distributed into cerebrospinal fluid (CSF). Extensively and poorly metabolized in liver to dextrorphan (active metabolite). Excreted unchanged in urine. **Half-life:** 1.4-3.9 hr (parent compound), 3.4-5.6 hr (dextrorphan).

- **Available Forms:**
  - *Gelcap:* 15 mg (Robitussin CoughGels), 30 mg (Dexalone).
  - *Liquid:* 5 mg/5ml (Simply Cough), 10 mg/5 ml (Vicks 44 Cough Relief), 10 mg/15 ml (Creo-Terpin).
  - *Lozenges:* 5 mg (Hold DM, Scot-Tussin DM Cough Chasers).
  - *Suspension (Extended-Release):* 30 mg/5 ml (Delsym).
  - *Syrup:* 7.5 mg/5 ml (ElixSure Cough), 10 mg/5 ml (Robitussin Honey Cough, Silphen DM), 15 mg/5 ml (Benylin Adult, Robitussin Maximum Strength Cough), 20 mg/15 ml (Creomulsion Cough).

- **Indications and Dosages:**
  Cough: PO 10-20 mg q4h. Maximum: 120 mg/day.

- **Unlabeled Uses:** N-methyl-D-aspartate (NMDA) antagonist in cerebral injury

- **Contraindications:** Coadministration with monoamine oxidase inhibitors (MAOIs), hypersensitivity to dextromethorphan or its components

- **Side Effects**
  Rare
  Abdominal discomfort, constipation, dizziness, drowsiness, GI upset, nausea

- **Serious Reactions**
  - Overdosage may result in muscle spasticity, increase or decrease in blood pressure, blurred vision, blue fingernails and lips, nausea, vomiting, hallucinations, and respiratory depression.

- **Patient/Family Education**
  - Avoid performing tasks that require mental alertness or motor skills until response to the drug is established
  - Do not take dextromethorphan for chronic cough
  - Maintain adequate hydration by drinking plenty of fluids
  - Notify the physician if cough persists or if fever, rash, headache, or sore throat is present with cough

- **Monitoring Parameters**
  - Clinical improvement and onset of relief of cough

- **Geriatric side effects at a glance:**
  - ❑ CNS ❑ Bowel Dysfunction ❑ Bladder Dysfunction ❑ Falls

- **U.S. Regulatory Considerations**
  - ❑ FDA Black Box ❑ OBRA regulated in U.S. Long Term Care

diazepam

(dye-az'-e-pam)

- **Brand Name(s):** Diastat, Diazepam Intensol, Dizac, Valium
  Chemical Class: Benzodiazepine

  DEA Class: Schedule IV

- **Clinical Pharmacology:**
  Mechanism of Action: A benzodiazepine that depresses all levels of the CNS by enhancing the action of gamma-aminobutyric acid, a major inhibitory neurotransmitter in the brain. **Therapeutic Effect:** Produces anxiolytic effect, elevates the seizure threshold, produces skeletal muscle relaxation.
  Pharmacokinetics:

Route	Onset	Peak	Duration
PO	30 min	1-2 hr	2-3 hr
IV	1-5 min	15 min	15-60 min
IM	15 min	30-90 min	30-90 min

Well absorbed from the GI tract. Widely distributed. Protein binding: 98%. Metabolized in the liver to active metabolite. Excreted in urine. Minimally removed by hemodialysis. **Half-life:** 20-70 hr (increased in hepatic dysfunction and the elderly).

- **Available Forms:**
  - *Oral Concentrate* (Diazepam Intensol): 5 mg/ml.
  - *Oral Solution*: 5 mg/5 ml.
  - *Tablets* (Valium): 2 mg, 5 mg, 10 mg.
  - *Injection*: 5 mg/ml.

- *Rectal Gel (Diastat)*: 5 mg/ml.

■ Indications and Dosages:
Anxiety, skeletal muscle relaxation: PO 2-5 mg 2-4 times a day. IV, IM 2-10 mg repeated in 3-4 hr.
Preanesthesia: IV 5-15 mg 5-10 min before procedure.
Alcohol withdrawal: PO 10 mg 3-4 times during first 24 hr, then reduced to 5-10 mg 3-4 times a day as needed IV, IM Initially, 10 mg, followed by 5-10 mg q3-4h.
Status epilepticus: IV 5-10 mg q10-15min up to 30 mg/8 hr.
Control of increased seizure activity in patients with refractory epilepsy who are on stable regimens of anticonvulsants: Rectal Gel 0.2 mg/kg; may be repeated in 4-12 hr.

■ Unlabeled Uses: Treatment of panic disorder, tension headache, tremors

■ Contraindications: Angle-closure glaucoma, coma, preexisting CNS depression, respiratory depression, severe and uncontrolled pain

■ Side Effects
Frequent
Pain with IM injection, somnolence, fatigue, ataxia
Occasional
Slurred speech, orthostatic hypotension, headache, hypoactivity, constipation, nausea, blurred vision
Rare
Paradoxical CNS reactions, such as excitement or restlessness in the elderly or debilitated (generally noted during first 2 wk of therapy, particularly in presence of uncontrolled pain)

■ Serious Reactions
- IV administration may produce pain, swelling, thrombophlebitis, and carpal tunnel syndrome.
- Abrupt or too-rapid withdrawal may result in pronounced restlessness, irritability, insomnia, hand tremor, abdominal or muscle cramps, diaphoresis, vomiting, and seizures.
- Abrupt withdrawal in patients with epilepsy may produce an increase in the frequency or severity of seizures.
- Overdose results in somnolence, confusion, diminished reflexes, and coma.

Special Considerations
- Flumazenil (Mazicon), a benzodiazepine receptor antagonist, is indicated for complete or partial reversal of the sedative effects of benzodiazepines

■ Patient/Family Education
- Avoid driving, activities that require alertness; drowsiness may occur
- Avoid alcohol, other psychotropic medications unless prescribed by clinician
- Do not take the rectal form of the drug more than once every 5 days or more than 5 times a month

■ Monitoring Parameters
- Blood pressure, heart rate, respiratory rate; therapeutic response in patients with seizure disorder, a decrease in the frequency or intensity of seizures; in patients with anxiety, a calm facial expression and decreased restlessness; in patients with musculoskeletal spasm, decreased intensity of skeletal muscle pain

- Though not used to monitor treatment, the therapeutic serum level for diazepam is 0.5 to 2 mcg/ml, and the toxic serum level is greater than 3 mcg/ml

■ **Geriatric side effects at a glance:**
☑ CNS ☐ Bowel Dysfunction ☐ Bladder Dysfunction ☑ Falls
Other: Withdrawal symptoms after long-term use

■ **Use with caution in older patients with:** Concurrent treatment with potent CYP 3A4 inhibitors (e.g., nefazodone) leads to increased plasma concentrations of diazepam; COPD; untreated sleep apnea

■ **U.S. Regulatory Considerations**
☐ FDA Black Box ☑ OBRA regulated in U.S. Long Term Care

■ **Other Uses in Geriatric Patient:** Anxiety symptoms and related disorders, dementia-related behavioral problems

■ **Side Effects:**
Of particular importance in the geriatric patient: Sedation, withdrawal symptoms when abruptly discontinued (e.g., during hospitalization) rather than tapered

■ **Geriatric Considerations - Summary:** Benzodiazepines are effective anxiolytic agents, and hypnotics. These drugs should be reserved for short-term use. SSRIs are preferred for long-term management of anxiety disorders in older adults, and sedating antidepressants (e.g., trazodone) or eszopiclone are preferred for long-term management of sleep problems. Long-acting benzodiazepines, including flurazepam, chlordiazepoxide, clorazepate, diazepam, clonazepam, and quazepam should generally be avoided in older adults as these agents have been associated with oversedation. On the other hand, short-acting benzodiazepines (e.g., triazolam) have been associated with a higher risk of withdrawal symptoms. When initiating therapy, benzodiazepines should be titrated carefully to avoid oversedation. In addition, many of the drugs in this class have been associated with severe withdrawal symptoms (e.g., anxiety and/or agitation, seizures) when discontinued abruptly.

■ **References:**

1. Leipzig RM, Cumming RG, Tinetti ME. Drugs and falls in older people: a systematic review and meta-analysis: I. Psychotropic drugs. J Am Geriatr Soc 1999;47:30-39.
2. Shorr RI, Robin DW. Rational use of benzodiazepines in the elderly. Drugs Ageing 1994;4:9-20.
3. Shader RI, Greenblatt DJ. Use of benzodiazepines in anxiety disorders. N Engl J Med 1993;328:1398-1405.

diclofenac

(dye-kloe'-fen-ak)

■ **Brand Name(s):** Cataflam, Solaraze, Voltaren, Voltaren Ophthalmic, Voltaren XR

Combinations
Rx: with misoprostol (Arthotec)
Chemical Class: Phenylacetic acid derivative

■ **Clinical Pharmacology:**
Mechanism of Action: An NSAID that inhibits prostaglandin synthesis, reducing the intensity of pain. Also constricts the iris sphincter. May inhibit angiogenesis (the formation of blood vessels) by inhibiting substance P or blocking the angiogenic effects of prostaglandin E. **Therapeutic Effect:** Produces analgesic and anti-inflammatory effects. Prevents miosis during cataract surgery. May reduce angiogenesis in inflamed tissue.
Pharmacokinetics:

Route	Onset	Peak	Duration
PO	30 min	2-3 hr	Up to 8 hr

Completely absorbed from the GI tract; penetrates cornea after ophthalmic administration (may be systemically absorbed). Protein binding: greater than 99%. Widely distributed. Metabolized in the liver. Primarily excreted in urine. Minimally removed by hemodialysis. **Half-life:** 1.2-2 hr.

■ **Available Forms:**
- *Topical Gel (Solaraze):* 3%.
- *Tablets (Immediate-Release [Cataflam]):* 50 mg.
- *Tablets (Delayed-Release [Voltaren]):* 25 mg, 50 mg, 75 mg.
- *Tablets (Extended-Release [Voltaren XR]):* 100 mg.
- *Ophthalmic Solution (Voltaren Ophthalmic):* 0.1%.

■ **Indications and Dosages:**
Osteoarthritis: PO (Cataflam, Voltaren) 50 mg 2-3 times a day. PO (Voltaren XR) 100-200 mg/day as a single dose.
Rheumatoid arthritis: PO (Cataflam, Voltaren) 50 mg 2-4 times a day. Maximum: 225 mg/day. PO (Voltaren XR) 100 mg once a day. Maximum: 100 mg twice a day.
Ankylosing spondylitis: PO (Voltaren) 100-125 mg/day in 4-5 divided doses.
Actinic keratoses: Topical Apply twice a day to lesion for 60-90 days.
Cataract surgery: Ophthalmic Apply 1 drop to eye 4 times a day commencing 24 hr after cataract surgery. Continue for 2 wk afterward.
Pain, relief of photophobia in patients undergoing corneal refractive surgery: Ophthalmic Apply 1-2 drops to affected eye 1 hr before surgery, within 15 min after surgery, then 4 times a day for up to 3 days.

■ **Unlabeled Uses:** Treatment of vascular headaches (oral); to reduce the occurrence and severity of cystoid macular edema after cataract surgery (ophthalmic form)

■ **Contraindications:** Hypersensitivity to aspirin, diclofenac, and other NSAIDs; porphyria

- **Side Effects**
  Frequent (9%–4%)
  PO: Headache, abdominal cramps, constipation, diarrhea, nausea, dyspepsia
  Ophthalmic: Burning or stinging on instillation, ocular discomfort
  Occasional (3%–1%)
  PO: Flatulence, dizziness, epigastric pain
  Ophthalmic: Ocular itching or tearing
  Rare (less than 1%)
  PO: Rash, peripheral edema or fluid retention, visual disturbances, vomiting, drowsiness

- **Serious Reactions**
  - Overdose may result in acute renal failure.
  - Rare reactions with long-term use include peptic ulcer disease, GI bleeding, gastritis, a severe hepatic reaction (jaundice), nephrotoxicity (hematuria, dysuria, proteinuria), and a severe hypersensitivity reaction (bronchospasm or angioedema).

Special Considerations
  - No significant advantage over other NSAIDs; cost should govern use

- **Patient/Family Education**
  - Swallow diclofenac tablets whole and do not crush or chew them
  - Take diclofenac with food or milk if GI upset occurs
  - Avoid alcohol and aspirin during diclofenac therapy because these substances increase the risk of GI bleeding
  - Notify the physician if a persistent headache, black stools, changes in vision, pruritus, rash, or weight gain occurs
  - Do not use hydrogel soft contact lenses during ophthalmic diclofenac therapy
  - Notify the physician if rash occurs while using topical diclofenac

- **Monitoring Parameters**
  - Initial hematocrit and fecal occult blood test within 3 mo of starting regular chronic therapy; repeat every 6-12 mo (more frequently in high-risk patients (>65 years, peptic ulcer disease, concurrent steroids or anticoagulants); electrolytes, creatinine, and BUN within 3 mo of starting regular chronic therapy; repeat every 6-12 mo
  - Complete healing of actinic keratoses may not be evident for up to 30 days post cessation of therapy
  - Daily bowel activity and stool consistency
  - Therapeutic response, such as improved grip strength, increased joint mobility, and decreased joint pain, tenderness, stiffness, and swelling

- **Geriatric side effects at a glance:**
  ☑ CNS ☐ Bowel Dysfunction ☐ Bladder Dysfunction ☐ Falls
  ☑ Other: Gastropathy

- **Use with caution in older patients with:** Renal impairment, Hepatic impairment, CHF, HTN, PUD, History of GI bleeding, GERD, Bleeding and platelet disorders, History of aspirin sensitivity reaction. Also use with caution in patients taking Anticoagulants, Aspirin, and Antihypertensive agents.

- **U.S. Regulatory Considerations**
  ☑ FDA Black Box
  - Cardiovascular risk

- Gastrointestinal risk
- [ ] OBRA regulated in U.S. Long Term Care

■ **Other Uses in Geriatric Patient:** Acute Gout

■ **Side Effects:**
Of particular importance in the geriatric patient: Confusion, cognitive impairment, delirium, dizziness, dyspepsia, fluid retention, renal impairment

■ **Geriatric Considerations - Summary:** Use of NSAIDs in older adults increases the risk of GI complications including gastric ulceration, bleeding, and perforation. These complications are not necessarily preceded by less severe GI symptoms. Concomitant use of a proton pump inhibitor or misoprostol reduces the risk for gastric ulceration and bleeding, but may not prevent long-term GI toxicity. No clinical data exist to support reduced GI toxicity with the use of diclofenac.

■ **References:**
1. COX-2 alternatives and GI protection. Med Lett Drugs Ther 2004;46:91.
2. Drugs that may cause cognitive disorders in the elderly. Med Lett Drugs Ther 2000;42:111-112.

dicloxacillin sodium

(dye-klox'-a-sill-in soe'-dee-um)

■ **Brand Name(s):** Dycil, Pathocil
Chemical Class: Penicillin derivative, penicillinase-resistant

■ **Clinical Pharmacology:**
Mechanism of Action: A penicillin that acts as a bactericidal in susceptible microorganisms. **Therapeutic Effect:** Inhibits bacterial cell wall synthesis.
Pharmacokinetics: Well absorbed from gastrointestinal (GI) tract. Rate and extent reduced by food. Distributed throughout body including CSF. Protein binding: 96%. Partially metabolized in liver. Primarily excreted in feces and urine. Not removed by hemodialysis. **Half-life:** 0.7 hr.

■ **Available Forms:**
- *Capsules:* 250 mg, 500 mg (Dycil, Pathocil).

■ **Indications and Dosages:**
Respiratory tract infection, staphylococcal and streptococcal infections: PO 125-250 mg q6h.

■ **Contraindications:** Hypersensitivity to any penicillin

■ **Side Effects**
Frequent
GI disturbances (mild diarrhea, nausea, or vomiting), headache

Occasional
Generalized rash, urticaria

- **Serious Reactions**
  - Altered bacterial balance may result in potentially fatal superinfections and anti-bacterial-associated colitis as evidenced by abdominal cramps, watery or severe diarrhea, and fever.
  - Severe hypersensitivity reactions, including anaphylaxis and acute interstitial nephritis occur rarely.

- **Patient/Family Education**
  - Should be taken with water 1 hr before or 2 hr after meals on an empty stomach
  - Continue dicloxacillin for the full length of treatment
  - Notify the physician if diarrhea, rash, or other new symptoms occur
  - Individualize treatment based on local susceptibility patterns.

- **Monitoring Parameters**
  - CBC
  - Renal function
  - Urinalysis
  - Daily bowel activity and stool consistency. Although mild GI effects may be tolerable, severe symptoms may indicate the onset of antibiotic-associated colitis.
  - Signs and symptoms of superinfection include abdominal pain or cramping, anal or genital pruritus or discharge, moderate to severe diarrhea, severe mouth or tongue soreness, and new or increased fever.

- **Geriatric side effects at a glance:**
  ☐ CNS ☑ Bowel Dysfunction ☐ Bladder Dysfunction ☐ Falls

- **U.S. Regulatory Considerations**
  ☐ FDA Black Box ☐ OBRA regulated in U.S. Long Term Care

dicyclomine hydrochloride

(dye-sye'-kloe-meen hye-droe-klor'-ide)

- **Brand Name(s):** Bentyl, Dicyclocot
  Chemical Class: Tertiary amine

- **Clinical Pharmacology:**
  Mechanism of Action: A GI antispasmodic and anticholinergic agent that directly acts as a relaxant on smooth muscle. **Therapeutic Effect:** Reduces tone and motility of GI tract.

Pharmacokinetics:

Route	Onset	Peak	Duration
PO	1-2 hr	N/A	4 hr

Readily absorbed from the GI tract. Widely distributed. Metabolized in the liver. **Half-life:** 9-10 hr.

■ **Available Forms:**
- *Capsules (Bentyl)*: 10 mg.
- *Tablets (Bentyl)*: 20 mg.
- *Syrup (Bentyl)*: 10 mg/5 ml.
- *Injection (Bentyl, Dicyclocot)*: 10 mg/ml.

■ **Indications and Dosages:**
Functional disturbances of GI motility: PO 10–20 mg 4 times a day. May increase up to 160 mg/day. IM 20 mg q4–6h.

■ **Contraindications:** Bladder neck obstruction due to prostatic hyperplasia, coronary vasospasm, intestinal atony, myasthenia gravis in patients not treated with neostigmine, narrow-angle glaucoma, obstructive disease of the GI tract, paralytic ileus, severe ulcerative colitis, tachycardia secondary to cardiac insufficiency or thyrotoxicosis, toxic megacolon, unstable cardiovascular status in acute hemorrhage

■ **Side Effects**
Frequent
Dry mouth (sometimes severe), constipation, diminished sweating ability
Occasional
Blurred vision; photophobia; urinary hesitancy; somnolence (with high dosage); agitation, excitement, confusion, or somnolence noted (even with low dosages); transient light-headedness (with IM route), irritation at injection site (with IM route)
Rare
Confusion, hypersensitivity reaction, increased IOP, nausea, vomiting, unusual fatigue

■ **Serious Reactions**
- Overdose may produce temporary paralysis of ciliary muscle; pupillary dilation; tachycardia; palpitations; hot, dry, or flushed skin; absence of bowel sounds; hyperthermia; increased respiratory rate; ECG abnormalities; nausea; vomiting; rash over face or upper trunk; CNS stimulation; and psychosis (marked by agitation, restlessness, rambling speech, visual hallucinations, paranoid behavior, and delusions, followed by depression).

Special Considerations
- Not for intravenous use

■ **Patient/Family Education**
- Avoid becoming overheated while exercising in hot weather because this may cause heatstroke
- Avoid hot baths and saunas
- Avoid tasks that require mental alertness or motor skills until response to the drug has been established
- Do not take antacids or antidiarrheals within 1 hr of taking dicyclomine because these drugs decrease dicyclomine's effectiveness

■ **Monitoring Parameters**
  • Evaluate the patient for urine retention
  • Blood pressure, body temperature
  • Bowel sounds for peristalsis, and mucous membranes and skin turgor for hydration status
  • Daily bowel activity and stool consistency

■ **Geriatric side effects at a glance:**
  ☑ CNS ☑ Bowel Dysfunction ☑ Bladder Dysfunction ☐ Falls
  Other: Dry mouth, blurred vision, somnolence

■ **Use with caution in older patients with:** Prostate hypertrophy, dementia

■ **U.S. Regulatory Considerations**
  ☐ FDA Black Box ☑ OBRA regulated in U.S. Long Term Care

■ **Other Uses in Geriatric Patient:** Urinary incontinence

■ **Side Effects:**
  Of particular importance in the geriatric patient: Anticholinergic effects

■ **Geriatric Considerations - Summary:** Dicyclomine is a weak anticholinergic but has the potential to cause adverse effects in the older adult, including urinary retention, hypotension, and confusion. The potential for adverse effects limits the usefulness of this drug for older adults.

didanosine

(dye-dan'-o-seen)

■ **Brand Name(s):** Videx, Videx-EC
  Chemical Class: Nucleoside analog

■ **Clinical Pharmacology:**
  Mechanism of Action: A purine nucleoside analog that is intracellularly converted into a triphosphate, which interferes with RNA-directed DNA polymerase (reverse transcriptase). **Therapeutic Effect:** Inhibits replication of retroviruses, including HIV.
  Pharmacokinetics: Variably absorbed from the GI tract. Protein binding: less than 5%. Rapidly metabolized intracellularly to active form. Primarily excreted in urine. Partially (20%) removed by hemodialysis. **Half-life:** 1.5 hr; metabolite: 8-24 hr.

■ **Available Forms:**
  • *Capsules (Delayed-Release)*: 125 mg (Videx), 200 mg (Videx-EC), 250 mg (Videx-EC), 400 mg (Videx-EC).
  • *Powder for Oral Solution (Videx)*: 100 mg, 167 mg, 250 mg.
  • *Tablets (Chewable [Videx])*: 25 mg, 50 mg, 100 mg, 150 mg, 200 mg.

■ Indications and Dosages:

HIV infection (in combination with other ID-antiretrovirals): PO (Chewable Tablets) *Weight 60 kg and more.* 200 mg q12h or 400 mg once a day. *Weight less than 60 kg.* 125 mg q12h or 250 mg once a day. PO (Delayed-Release Capsules) *Weight 60 kg and more.* 400 mg once a day. *Weight less than 60 kg.* 250 mg once a day. PO (Oral Solution) *Weight 60 kg and more.* 250 mg q12h. *Weight less than 60 kg.* 167 mg q12h.

Dosage in renal impairment: Patients weighing less than 60 kg:

CrCl	Tablets	Oral Solution	Delayed- Release Capsules
30-59 ml/min	75 mg twice a day	100 mg twice a day	125 mg once a day
10-29 ml/min	100 mg once a day	100 mg once a day	125 mg once a day
less than 10 ml/min	75 mg once a day	100 mg once a day	N/A

CrCl = creatinine clearance

Patients weighing 60 kg or more:

CrCl	Tablets	Oral Solution	Delayed- Release Capsules
30-59 ml/ min	100 mg twice a day	100 mg twice a day	200 mg once a day
10-29 ml/ min	150 mg once a day	167 mg once a day	125 mg once a day
less than 10 ml/ min	100 mg once a day	100 mg once a day	125 mg once a day

CrCl = creatinine clearance

■ Contraindications: Hypersensitivity to didanosine or any of its components

■ Side Effects

Frequent (greater than 10%)
Diarrhea, neuropathy, chills and fever

Occasional (9%-2%)
Rash, pruritus, headache, abdominal pain, nausea, vomiting, pneumonia, myopathy, decreased appetite, dry mouth, dyspnea

■ Serious Reactions

- Pneumonia and opportunistic infections occur occasionally.
- Peripheral neuropathy, potentially fatal pancreatitis, retinal changes, and optic neuritis are the major toxic effects.

Special Considerations

- Always check updated treatment guidelines before initiating or changing antiretroviral therapy. (http://AIDSinfo.nih.gov)

■ Patient/Family Education

- Administer on empty stomach
- Shake the oral suspension well before using it, keep it refrigerated, and discard the solution after 30 days and obtain a new supply
- Avoid consuming alcohol
- Notify the physician if nausea or vomiting, numbness, or persistent, severe abdominal pain occurs
- Didanosine is not a cure for HIV infection, nor does it reduce the risk of transmitting HIV to others

■ Monitoring Parameters

- Amylase, lipase, ophthalmologic examinations
- Suspend use until pancreatitis excluded if patient develops nausea, abdominal pain
- Tablets contain 264.5 mg sodium, packets 1380 mg sodium
- Weight
- Pattern of daily bowel activity and stool consistency

- Signs and symptoms of peripheral neuropathy, including burning feet, restless legs syndrome (inability to find a comfortable position for legs and feet), and lack of co-ordination
- Skin for eruptions and a rash
- Signs and symptoms of opportunistic infections, including cough or other respiratory symptoms, fever, and oral mucosa changes

■ **Geriatric side effects at a glance:**
  ❑ CNS ❑ Bowel Dysfunction ❑ Bladder Dysfunction ❑ Falls

■ **U.S. Regulatory Considerations**
  ☑ FDA Black Box
  Pancreatitis, hepatotoxicity with steatosis, lactic acidosis.
  ❑ OBRA regulated in U.S. Long Term Care

diethylpropion hydrochloride

(die-ethyl-prop'-ion hye-droe-klor'-ide)

■ **Brand Name(s):** Tenuate, Tenuate Dospan
  Chemical Class: Phenethylamine derivative

  DEA Class: Schedule IV

■ **Clinical Pharmacology:**
  Mechanism of Action: A sympathomimetic amine that stimulates the release of norepinephrine and dopamine. **Therapeutic Effect:** Decreases appetite.
  Pharmacokinetics: Rapidly absorbed from the gastrointestinal (GI) tract. Widely distributed. Metabolized in liver to active metabolite and undergoes extensive first-pass metabolism. Excreted in urine. Unknown if removed by hemodialysis. **Half-life:** 4-6 hr.

■ **Available Forms:**
  • *Tablets*: 25 mg (Tenuate).
  • *Tablets* (*Extended-Release*): 75 mg (Tenuate Dospan).

■ **Indications and Dosages:**
  Obesity: PO 25 mg 3 times/day before meals. (Extended-Release) 75 mg at midmorning.

■ **Unlabeled Uses:** Migraines

■ **Contraindications:** Agitated states, use of MAOIs within 14 days, glaucoma, history of drug abuse, hyperthyroidism, advanced arteriosclerosis or severe cardiovascular disease, severe hypertension, and hypersensitivity to sympathomimetic amines

Side Effects

Frequent

Elevated blood pressure, nervousness, insomnia

Occasional

Dizziness, drowsiness, tremor, headache, nausea, stomach pain, fever, rash

Rare

Agranulocytosis, leukopenia, blurred vision, psychosis, CVA, seizure

Serious Reactions

- Overdose may produce agitation, tachycardia, palpitations, cardiac irregularities, chest pain, psychotic episode, seizures, and coma.
- Hypersensitivity reactions and blood dyscrasias occur rarely.

Special Considerations

- Tolerance to anorectic effects may develop within weeks; cross-tolerance is almost universal
- Measure the limited usefulness against the inherent risks (habituation) of this agent
- Most patients will eventually regain weight lost during use of this product

Patient/Family Education

- Notify the physician if any increase in seizures, fever, nervousness, palpitations, skin rash, or vomiting occurs
- Avoid alcohol
- Take the last dose of diethylpropion in the early morning to avoid insomnia
- Avoid consuming caffeine during diethylpropion therapy
- Do not abruptly discontinue the drug after prolonged use

Monitoring Parameters

- Blood pressure
- CBC

Geriatric side effects at a glance:

❑ CNS ❑ Bowel Dysfunction ❑ Bladder Dysfunction ❑ Falls

U.S. Regulatory Considerations

❑ FDA Black Box ❑ OBRA regulated in U.S. Long Term Care

diflorasone diacetate

(die-floor'-a-sone dye-as'-uh-tate)

- **Brand Name(s):** Maxiflor, Psorcon, Psorcon E
  Chemical Class: Corticosteroid, synthetic

■ **Clinical Pharmacology:**
Mechanism of Action: A high-potency, fluorinated corticosteroid that decreases inflammation by suppression of migration of polymorphonuclar leukocytes and reversal of increased capillary permeability. The exact mechanism of the anti-inflammatory process is unclear. **Therapeutic Effect:** Decreases or prevents tissue response to the inflammatory process.
Pharmacokinetics: Poor absorption; occlusive dressings increase absorption. Metabolized in liver. Primarily excreted in urine.

■ **Available Forms:**
- *Cream*: 0.05% (Maxiflor, Psorcon).
- *Ointment*: 0.05% (Maxiflor, Psorcon).
- *Ointment, Emollient*: 0.05% (Psorcon E).

■ **Indications and Dosages:**
Dermatoses : Topical (Cream) Apply sparingly 2- 4 times/day. (Ointment) Apply sparingly 1- 3 times/day.

■ **Unlabeled Uses:** Psoriasis

■ **Contraindications:** History of hypersensitivity to diflorasone or other corticosteroids

■ **Side Effects**
Rare
Itching, redness, dryness, irritation, burning at site of application, arthralgia, folliculitis, maceration, muscle atrophy, secondary infection

■ **Serious Reactions**
- Overdosage symptoms include moon face, central obesity, hypertension, diabetes, hyperlipidemia, peptic ulcer, increased susceptibility to infection, electrolyte and fluid imbalance, psychosis, and hallucinations.
- The serious reactions of long-term therapy (greater than 2 wk) and the addition of occlusive dressings are reversible hypothalamic-pituitary-adrenal (HPA) axis suppression, manifestations of Cushing's syndrome, hyperglycemia, and glucosuria.

Special Considerations
- No demonstrated superiority over other high-potency agents; cost should govern use

■ **Patient/Family Education**
- Apply sparingly only to affected area
- Avoid contact with the eyes
- Do not put bandages or dressings over treated area unless directed by clinician
- Discontinue drug, notify clinician if local irritation or fever develops
- Do not use on weeping, denuded, or infected areas
- Notify the physician if fever or rash occurs
- Avoid exposure to sunlight

■ **Monitoring Parameters**
- Skin for rash
- Discontinue the use of diflorasone if no improvement is seen; reassess diagnosis

- **Geriatric side effects at a glance:**
  - ☐ CNS ☐ Bowel Dysfunction ☐ Bladder Dysfunction ☐ Falls

- **U.S. Regulatory Considerations**
  - ☐ FDA Black Box ☐ OBRA regulated in U.S. Long Term Care

diflunisal

(dye-floo'-ni-sal)

- **Brand Name(s):** Dolobid
  Chemical Class: Salicylate derivative

- **Clinical Pharmacology:**
  Mechanism of Action: A nonsteroidal anti-inflammatory that inhibits prostaglandin synthesis, reducing inflammatory response and intensity of pain stimulus reaching sensory nerve endings. **Therapeutic Effect:** Produces analgesic and anti-inflammatory effect.
  Pharmacokinetics:

Route	Onset	Peak	Duration
PO	1 hr	2-3 hr	8-12 hr

  Completely absorbed from the GI tract. Widely distributed. Protein binding: greater than 99%. Metabolized in liver. Primarily excreted in urine. Not removed by hemodialysis. **Half-life:** 8-12 hr.

- **Available Forms:**
  - *Tablets:* 250 mg, 500 mg.

- **Indications and Dosages:**
  Mild to moderate pain: PO Initially, 0.5-1 g, then 250-500 mg q8-12h. Maximum: 1.5 g/day.
  Osteoarthritis: PO 500-750 mg/day in divided doses.
  Rheumatoid arthritis: PO 0.5-1 g/day in 2 divided doses. Maximum: 1.5 g/day.

- **Unlabeled Uses:** Treatment of psoriatic arthritis, vascular headache

- **Contraindications:** Active GI bleeding, factor VII or factor IX deficiencies, hypersensitivity to aspirin or NSAIDs

- **Side Effects**
  Side effects are less common with short-term treatment.
  Occasional (9%-3%)
  Nausea, dyspepsia (heartburn, indigestion, epigastric pain), diarrhea, headache, rash
  Rare (3%-1%)
  Vomiting, constipation, flatulence, dizziness, somnolence, insomnia, fatigue, tinnitus

■ **Serious Reactions**
- Overdosage may produce drowsiness, vomiting, nausea, diarrhea, hyperventilation, tachycardia, diaphoresis, stupor, and coma.
- Peptic ulcer, GI bleeding, gastritis, and severe hepatic reaction, including cholestasis, jaundice occur rarely.
- Nephrotoxicity, including dysuria, hematuria, proteinuria, and nephrotic syndrome, and severe hypersensitivity reaction, marked by bronchospasm and angioedema, occur rarely.

Special Considerations
- No significant advantage over other NSAIDs; cost should govern use

■ **Patient/Family Education**
- Swallow tablets whole; do not chew or crush
- Take diflunisal with food or milk if GI upset occurs
- Notify the physician if GI distress, headache, or rash occurs

■ **Monitoring Parameters**
- Initial hematocrit and fecal occult blood test within 3 mo of starting regular chronic therapy; repeat every 6-12 mo (more frequently in high-risk patients ($>$ 65 years, peptic ulcer disease, concurrent steroids or anticoagulants); electrolytes, creatinine, and BUN within 3 mo of starting regular chronic therapy; repeat every 6-12 mo
- Skin for rash
- Daily bowel activity and stool consistency
- Therapeutic response for improved grip strength, increased joint mobility, reduced joint tenderness, and relief of pain, stiffness, and swelling

■ **Geriatric side effects at a glance:**
☑ CNS   ☐ Bowel Dysfunction   ☐ Bladder Dysfunction   ☐ Falls
☑ Other: Gastropathy

■ **Use with caution in older patients with:** Renal impairment, Hepatic impairment, CHF, HTN, PUD, History of GI bleeding, GERD, Bleeding and platelet disorders, History of aspirin sensitivity reaction. Also use with caution in patients taking Anticoagulants, Aspirin, and Antihypertensive agents.

■ **U.S. Regulatory Considerations**
☑ FDA Black Box
- Cardiovascular risk
- Gastrointestinal risk
☐ OBRA regulated in U.S. Long Term Care

■ **Other Uses in Geriatric Patient:** Acute Gout

■ **Side Effects:**
   Of particular importance in the geriatric patient: Confusion, cognitive impairment, delirium, dizziness, dyspepsia, fluid retention, renal impairment

■ **Geriatric Considerations - Summary:** Use of NSAIDs in older adults increases the risk of GI complications including gastric ulceration, bleeding, and perforation. These complications are not necessarily preceded by less severe GI symptoms. Concomitant use of a proton pump inhibitor or misoprostol reduces the risk for gastric ulceration and bleeding, but may not prevent long-term GI toxicity.

■ **References:**
1. COX-2 alternatives and GI protection. Med Lett Drugs Ther 2004;46:91.
2. Drugs that may cause cognitive disorders in the elderly. Med Lett Drugs Ther 2000;42:111-112.

digoxin

(di-jox'-in)

■ **Brand Name(s):** Digitek, Lanoxicaps, Lanoxin
Chemical Class: Digitalis glycoside

■ **Clinical Pharmacology:**
Mechanism of Action: A cardiac inotropic agent that increases the influx of calcium from extracellular to intracellular cytoplasm. **Therapeutic Effect:** Potentiates the activity of the contractile cardiac muscle fibers and increases the force of myocardial contraction. Slows the heart rate by decreasing conduction through the SA and AV nodes.
Pharmacokinetics:

Route	Onset	Peak	Duration
PO	0.5-2 hr	28 hr	3-4 days
IV	5-30 min	1-4 hr	3-4 days

Readily absorbed from the GI tract. Widely distributed. Protein binding: 30%. Partially metabolized in the liver. Primarily excreted in urine. Minimally removed by hemodialysis. **Half-life:** 36–48 hr (increased with impaired renal function and in the elderly).

■ **Available Forms:**
- *Capsules (Lanoxicaps):* 50 mcg, 100 mcg, 200 mcg.
- *Elixir (Lanoxin):* 50 mcg/ml.
- *Tablets (Digitek, Lanoxin):* 125 mcg, 250 mcg.
- *Injection (Lanoxin):* 100 mcg/ml, 250 mcg/ml.

■ **Indications and Dosages:**
Rapid loading dose for the management and treatment of CHF; control of ventricular rate in patients with atrial fibrillation; treatment and prevention of recurrent paroxysmal atrial tachycardia: PO Initially, 0.5-0.75 mg, additional doses of 0.125-0.375 mg at 6- to 8-hr intervals. Range: 0.75-1.25 mg. IV 0.6-1 mg.
Maintenance dosage for CHF; control of ventricular rate in patients with atrial fibrillation; treatment and prevention of recurrent paroxysmal atrial tachycardia: PO, IV 0.125-0.375 mg/day.
Dosage in renal impairment: Dosage adjustment is based on creatinine clearance. Total digitalizing dose: decrease by 50% in end-stage renal disease.

Creatinine Clearance	Dosage
10-50 ml/min	25%-75% usual
less than 10 ml/min	10%-25% usual

■ **Contraindications:** Ventricular fibrillation, ventricular tachycardia unrelated to CHF

Side Effects

None known. However, there is a very narrow margin of safety between a therapeutic and toxic result. Long-term therapy may produce mammary gland enlargement in women but is reversible when drug is withdrawn.

Serious Reactions

- The most common early manifestations of digoxin toxicity are GI disturbances (anorexia, nausea, vomiting) and neurologic abnormalities (fatigue, headache, depression, weakness, drowsiness, confusion, nightmares).
- Facial pain, personality change, and ocular disturbances (photophobia, light flashes, halos around bright objects, yellow or green color perception) may be noted.

Special Considerations

- Preferred digitalis glycoside
- Rule out digitalis toxicity if nausea, vomiting, arrhythmias develop
- Listed adverse effects are mostly signs of toxicity

Patient/Family Education

- Take apical pulse and notify the physician of a pulse rate of 60 beats/minute or less or a rate less than that indicated by the physician
- Carry or wear identification that he or she is receiving digoxin and to inform dentists and other physicians about digoxin therapy
- Do not take OTC medications without physician approval
- Notify the physician if decreased appetite, diarrhea, nausea, visual changes, or vomiting occurs

Monitoring Parameters

- Heart rate and rhythm, periodic ECGs
- Serum potassium, magnesium, calcium, creatinine
- Serum digoxin levels when compliance, effectiveness, or systemic availability is questioned or toxicity suspected
- Obtain serum drug concentrations at least 8-12 hr after a dose (preferably prior to next scheduled dose); therapeutic range 0.5-2.0 ng/ml

Geriatric side effects at a glance:

☑ CNS   ☑ Bowel Dysfunction   ☐ Bladder Dysfunction   ☐ Falls

Side effects of particular importance   May cause anorexia

U.S. Regulatory Considerations

☐ FDA Black Box   ☐ OBRA regulated in U.S. Long Term Care

digoxin immune FAB

(di-jox'-in)

■ **Brand Name(s):** Digibind, DigiFab
   Chemical Class: Antibody fragment

■ **Clinical Pharmacology:**
   Mechanism of Action: An antidote that binds molecularly to digoxin in the extracellular space. **Therapeutic Effect:** Makes digoxin unavailable for binding at its site of action on cells in the body.
   Pharmacokinetics:

Route	Onset	Peak	Duration
IV	30 min	N/A	3-4 days

   Widely distributed into extracellular space. Excreted in urine. **Half-life:** 15-20 hr.

■ **Available Forms:**
   • *Powder for Injection*: 38-mg vial (Digibind), 40-mg vial (DigiFab).

■ **Indications and Dosages:**
   Potentially life-threatening digoxin overdose: IV Dosage varies according to amount of digoxin to be neutralized. Refer to manufacturer's dosing guidelines.

■ **Contraindications:** None known.

■ **Side Effects**
   Rare
   Allergic reaction

■ **Serious Reactions**
   • Hyperkalemia may occur as a result of digitalis toxicity. Signs and symptoms of hyperkalemia include diarrhea, paresthesia of extremities, heaviness of legs, decreased BP, cold skin, grayish pallor, hypotension, mental confusion, irritability, flaccid paralysis, tented T waves, widening QRS interval, and ST depression.
   • Hypokalemia may develop rapidly when the effect of digitalis is reversed. Signs and symptoms of hypokalemia include muscle cramping, nausea, vomiting, hypoactive bowel sounds, abdominal distention, difficulty breathing, and orthostatic hypotension.
   • Low cardiac output and CHF may occur rarely.

■ **Patient/Family Education**
   • Before discharge, review the digoxin dosages carefully with the patient, and make sure he or she knows how to take the drug as prescribed
   • Follow-up care, including monitoring serum digoxin level, is important to maintain
   • Notify the physician if anorexia, nausea, vomiting, or visual changes occurs

Monitoring Parameters
- Potassium, serum digoxin level prior to therapy
- Continuous ECG monitoring
- Blood pressure
- Signs and symptoms of an arrhythmia (such as palpitations), or heart failure (such as dyspnea and edema) if the digoxin level falls below the therapeutic level

Geriatric side effects at a glance:
❑ CNS ❑ Bowel Dysfunction ❑ Bladder Dysfunction ❑ Falls

U.S. Regulatory Considerations
❑ FDA Black Box ❑ OBRA regulated in U.S. Long Term Care

dihydroergotamine mesylate

(dye-hye-droe-er-got'-a-meen mes'-sil-ate)

■ **Brand Name(s):** D.H.E.45, Migranal
Chemical Class: Ergot alkaloid

■ **Clinical Pharmacology:**
Mechanism of Action: An ergotamine derivative, alpha-adrenergic blocker that directly stimulates vascular smooth muscle. May also have antagonist effects on serotonin. **Therapeutic Effect:** Peripheral and cerebral vasoconstriction.
Pharmacokinetics: Slow, incomplete absorption from the gastrointestinal (GI) tract; rate of absorption of intranasal route varies. Protein binding: greater than 90%. Undergoes extensive first-pass metabolism in liver. Metabolized to active metabolite. Eliminated in feces via biliary system. **Half-life:** 7-9 hr.

■ **Available Forms:**
- *Injection:* 1 mg/ml (D.H.E.45).
- *Nasal Spray:* 4 mg/ml [0.5mg/spray] (Migranal).

■ **Indications and Dosages:**
Migraine headaches, cluster headaches: IM, Subcutaneous 1 mg at onset of headache; repeat hourly. Maximum: 3 mg/day; 6 mg/wk. IV 1 mg at onset of headache; repeat hourly. Maximum: 2 mg/day; 6 mg/wk. Intranasal 1 spray (0.5 mg) into each nostril; repeat in 15 min. Maximum: 4 sprays/day; 8 sprays/wk.

■ **Contraindications:** Coronary artery disease, hypertension, impaired liver or renal function, malnutrition, peripheral vascular diseases, such as thromboangiitis obliterans, syphilitic arteritis, severe arteriosclerosis, thrombophlebitis, Raynaud's disease, sepsis, severe pruritus

■ **Side Effects**
Occasional
Cough, dizziness, rhinitis, altered taste, throat and nose irritation

Rare

Muscle pain, fatigue, diarrhea, upper respiratory tract infection, dyspepsia

■ **Serious Reactions**
- Prolonged administration or excessive dosage may produce ergotamine poisoning manifested as nausea, vomiting, weakness of legs, pain in limb muscles, numbness and tingling of fingers or toes, precordial pain, tachycardia or bradycardia, and hypertension or hypotension.
- Localized edema and itching due to vasoconstriction of peripheral arteries and arterioles may occur.
- Feet or hands will become cold, pale, and numb.
- Muscle pain will occur when walking and later, even at rest.
- Gangrene may occur.
- Occasionally confusion, depression, drowsiness, and seizures appear.

Special Considerations
- Considered alternative abortive acute migraine agent; nasal spray less effective than triptans

■ **Patient/Family Education**
- Initiate therapy at first sign of attack
- Prolonged use may lead to withdrawal headaches
- Notify the physician if the dihydroergotamine dosage does not relieve vascular headaches, or if irregular heartbeat, nausea, numbness or tingling of the fingers and toes, pain or weakness of the extremities, or vomiting occurs

■ **Monitoring Parameters**
- Therapeutic response to medication

■ **Geriatric side effects at a glance:**
   ❑ CNS   ❑ Bowel Dysfunction   ❑ Bladder Dysfunction   ❑ Falls

■ **U.S. Regulatory Considerations**
   ☑ FDA Black Box
- Can result in serious peripheral edema
- Concurrent use with CYP3A4 inhibitors contraindicated
   ❑ OBRA regulated in U.S. Long Term Care

dihydrotachysterol

(dye-hye-droe-tak-iss'-ter-ole)

■ **Brand Name(s):** DHT, DHT Intensol, Hytakerol
   Chemical Class: Sterol derivative

■ **Clinical Pharmacology:**
Mechanism of Action: A fat-soluble vitamin that is essential for absorption, utilization of calcium phosphate, and normal calcification of bone. **Therapeutic Effect:** Stimulates calcium and phosphate absorption from small intestine, promotes secretion of calcium from bone to blood, promotes renal tubule phosphate resorption, acts on bone cells to stimulate skeletal growth and on parathyroid gland to suppress hormone synthesis and secretion.
Pharmacokinetics: Well absorbed from small intestine. Metabolized in liver. Eliminated via biliary system; excreted in urine. **Half-life:** Unknown.

■ **Available Forms:**
- *Oral Solution*: 0.2 mg/ml (DHT Intensol).
- *Capsule*: 0.125 mg (Hytakerol).
- *Tablets*: 0.125 mg, 0.2 mg, 0.4 mg (DHT).

■ **Indications and Dosages:**
Hypoparathyroidism: PO Initially, 0.8-2.4 mg/day for several days. Maintenance: 0.2-1 mg/day.
Nutritional rickets: PO 0.5 mg as a single dose or 13-50 mcg/day until healing occurs.
Renal osteodystrophy: PO 0.25-0.6 mg/24 hr adjusted as necessary to achieve normal serum calcium levels and promote bone healing.

■ **Contraindications:** Hypercalcemia, malabsorption syndrome, vitamin D toxicity, hypersensitivity to vitamin D products or analogs

■ **Side Effects**
Occasional
Nausea, vomiting

■ **Serious Reactions**
- Early signs of overdosage are manifested as weakness, headache, somnolence, nausea, vomiting, dry mouth, constipation, muscle and bone pain, and metallic taste sensation.
- Later signs of overdosage are evidenced by polyuria, polydipsia, anorexia, weight loss, nocturia, photophobia, rhinorrhea, pruritus, disorientation, hallucinations, hyperthermia, hypertension, and cardiac arrhythmias.

Special Considerations
- Vitamin D analog of choice for prevention and treatment of renal osteodystrophy; less expensive than calcitriol

■ **Patient/Family Education**
- Compliance with dosage instructions, diet (evaluate vitamin D ingested in fortified foods, maintain adequate calcium intake) is essential
- Drink plenty of fluids

■ **Monitoring Parameters**
- Serum Ca^{2+} and phosphate
- If adverse reactions occur, rule out hypercalcemia, worsening renal function
- BUN, serum alkaline phosphatase, serum creatinine
- Fluid intake

■ **Geriatric side effects at a glance:**
❏ CNS ❏ Bowel Dysfunction ❏ Bladder Dysfunction ❏ Falls

diltiazem hydrochloride

(dil-tye'-a-zem hye-droe-klor'-ide)

■ **Brand Name(s):** Cardizem, Cardizem CD, Cardizem LA, Cardizem SR, Cartia, Dilacor XR, Diltia XT, Taztia XT, Tiazac

Combinations
Rx: with enalapril (Teczem)
Chemical Class: Benzothiazepine

■ **Clinical Pharmacology:**
Mechanism of Action: An antianginal, antihypertensive, and antiarrhythmic agent that inhibits calcium movement across cardiac and vascular smooth-muscle cell membranes. This action causes the dilation of coronary arteries, peripheral arteries, and arterioles. **Therapeutic Effect:** Decreases heart rate and myocardial contractility, slows SA and AV conduction, and decreases total peripheral vascular resistance by vasodilation.
Pharmacokinetics:

Route	Onset	Peak	Duration
PO	0.5-1 hr	N/A	N/A
PO (extended-release)	2-3 hr	N/A	N/A
IV	3 min	N/A	N/A

Well absorbed from the GI tract. Protein binding: 70%-80%. Undergoes first-pass metabolism in the liver to active metabolite. Primarily excreted in urine. Not removed by hemodialysis. **Half-life:** 3-8 hr.

■ **Available Forms:**
- *Capsules (Sustained-Release [Cardizem SR]):* 60 mg, 90 mg, 120 mg.
- *Capsules (Extended-Release [Cardizem CD]):* 120 mg (Cardizem CD, Cartia XT, Dilacor XR, Diltia XT, Taztia XT, Tiazac), 180 mg (Cardizem CD, Cartia XT, Dilacor XR, Diltia XT, Taztia XT, Tiazac), 240 mg (Cardizem CD, Cartia XT, Dilacor XR, Diltia XT, Taztia XT, Tiazac), 300 mg (Cardizem CD, Cartia XT, Taztia XT, Tiazac), 360 mg (Cardizem CD, Taztia XT, Tiazac), 420 mg (Tiazac).
- *Tablets (Cardizem):* 30 mg, 60 mg, 90 mg, 120 mg.
- *Tablets (Extended-Release [Cardizem LA]):* 120 mg, 180 mg, 240 mg, 300 mg, 360 mg, 420 mg.
- *Injection (Ready-to-Hang Infusion):* 1 mg/ml.

■ **Indications and Dosages:**
Angina: PO (Cardizem) Initially, 30 mg 4 times a day. Range: 180-360 mg/day. PO (Cardizem CD, Cartia XT, Dilacor XR, Diltia XT, Tiazac) Initially, 120-180 mg/day. Maximum: 480 mg/day. PO (Cardizem LA) Initially, 180 mg/day. May increase at 7-14-day intervals. Maximum: 360 mg/day.

Hypertension: PO (Cardizem CD, Cartia XT, Dilacor XR, Diltia XT, Tiazac) Initially, 180-240 mg/day. Range: 180-420 mg/day, Tiazac: 120-540 mg/day. PO (Cardizem SR) Initially, 60-120 mg twice a day. May increase at 14-day intervals. Maintenance: 240-360 mg/day. PO (Cardizem LA) Initially, 180-240 mg/day. May increase at 14-day intervals. Range: 120-540 mg/day.

Temporary control of rapid ventricular rate in atrial fibrillation or flutter, rapid conversion of paroxysmal supraventricular tachycardia to normal sinus rhythm: IV push Initially, 0.25 mg/kg actual body weight over 2 min. May repeat in 15 min at dose of 0.35 mg/kg actual body weight. Subsequent doses individualized. IV Infusion After initial bolus injection, may begin infusion at 5-10 mg/hr; may increase by 5 mg/hr up to a maximum of 15 mg/hr. Infusion duration should not exceed 24 hr.

■ **Contraindications:** Acute MI, pulmonary congestion, hypersensitivity to diltiazem or other antihypertensives, second- or third-degree AV block (except in the presence of a pacemaker), severe hypotension (less than 90 mm Hg, systolic), sick sinus syndrome

■ **Side Effects**

Frequent (10%–5%)

Peripheral edema, dizziness, light-headedness, headache, bradycardia, asthenia (loss of strength, weakness)

Occasional (5%–2%)

Nausea, constipation, flushing, ECG changes

Rare (less than 2%)

Rash, micturition disorder (polyuria, nocturia, dysuria, frequency of urination), abdominal discomfort, somnolence

■ **Serious Reactions**

• Abrupt withdrawal may increase frequency or duration of angina.
• CHF and second- and third-degree AV block occur rarely.
• Overdose produces nausea, somnolence, confusion, slurred speech, and profound bradycardia.

■ **Patient/Family Education**

• Do not abruptly discontinue diltiazem
• Rise slowly from a lying position to a sitting position and wait momentarily before standing to avoid diltiazem's hypotensive effect
• Avoid tasks that require mental alertness or motor skills until response to the drug has been established
• Notify the physician if constipation, irregular heartbeat, nausea, pronounced dizziness, or shortness of breath occurs

■ **Monitoring Parameters**

• Blood pressure
• ECG
• Liver and renal function
• Assess the patient for peripheral edema behind the medial malleolus in ambulatory patients or in the sacral area in bedridden patients

■ **Geriatric side effects at a glance:**

❑ CNS ❑ Bowel Dysfunction ❑ Bladder Dysfunction ❑ Falls

dimenhydrinate

(dye-men-hye'-dri-nate)

■ **Brand Name(s):** Dramamine, Motion-Aid
Chemical Class: Ethanolamine derivative

■ **Clinical Pharmacology:**
Mechanism of Action: An antihistamine and anticholinergic that competes for H_1-receptor sites on effector cells of the GI tract, blood vessels, and respiratory tract. The anticholinergic action diminishes vestibular stimulation and depresses labyrinthine function. **Therapeutic Effect:** Prevents symptoms of motion sickness.
Pharmacokinetics: Well absorbed following PO administration. Metabolized in liver. Excreted in urine. **Half-life:** Unknown.

■ **Available Forms:**
- *Tablets* (*Chewable* [*Dramamine*]): 50 mg.
- *Tablets* (*Dramamine*): 50 mg.
- *Injectable Solution* (*Motion-Aid*): 50 mg/ml.

■ **Indications and Dosages:**
Motion sickness: PO 50-100 mg q4-6h. Maximum: 400 mg/day. IM 50-100 mg q4-6h as needed. IV 50 mg over 2 min.

■ **Contraindications:** Hypersensitivity to diphenhydramine

■ **Side Effects**
Frequent
Dry mouth
Occasional
Hypotension, palpitations, tachycardia, headache, somnolence, dizziness, anorexia, constipation, dysuria, blurred vision, tinnitus, wheezing, chest tightness
Rare
Photosensitivity, rash, urticaria

■ **Serious Reactions**
- None significant.

■ **Patient/Family Education**
- For prevention of motion sickness administer at least 30 min before exposure to motion
- May cause drowsiness, dizziness, and dry mouth

- Avoid tasks requiring mental alertness or motor skills until response to the drug has been established
- Avoid prolonged sun exposure

■ **Monitoring Parameters**
- Blood pressure
- Signs and symptoms of motion sickness

■ **Geriatric side effects at a glance:**
☑ CNS ☑ Bowel Dysfunction ☑ Bladder Dysfunction ❑ Falls
Other: Dry mouth, blurred vision, confusion, psychoses

■ **Use with caution in older patients with:** Narrow-angle glaucoma, overflow incontinence, psychosis.

■ **U.S. Regulatory Considerations**
❑ FDA Black Box ❑ OBRA regulated in U.S. Long Term Care

■ **Other Uses in Geriatric Patient:** Sedation, antihistamine

■ **Side Effects:**
Of particular importance in the geriatric patient: Anticholinergic effects

■ **Geriatric Considerations - Summary:** Dimenhydrinate is a first-generation ethanolamine antihistamine with potent H_1-receptor antagonism. It also has significant anticholinergic properties and causes somnolence at normal doses. Older adults taking this drug are at risk of dizziness and hypotension and dimenhydrinate would not be considered a drug of choice for this population.

■ **References:**
1. Hagermark O, Levander S, Stahle M: A comparison of antihistaminic and sedative effects of some H_1-receptor antagonists. Acta Derm Venereol 1985; 114:155-156.
2. Tune LE. Anticholinergic effects of medication in elderly patients. J Clin Psychiatry 2001;62(suppl 21):11-14.

dimercaprol

(dye-mer-kap'-role)

■ **Brand Name(s):** BAL in Oil
Chemical Class: Dithiol derivative

■ **Clinical Pharmacology:**
Mechanism of Action: A chelating agent that contains two sulfhydryl groups that form a stable, nontoxic chelate 5-membered heterocyclic ring with heavy metals. **Therapeutic Effect:** Prevents the metal from combining with sulfhydryl groups on physiologic proteins and keeps them inactive until they can be excreted.

Pharmacokinetics: Time to peak after IM administration occurs in 30-60 min. Widely distributed to all tissues including the brain and, mainly, intracellular space. Rapidly metabolized by the liver to inactive metabolites. Excreted in the urine and bile. Removed by hemodialysis. **Half-life:** 4 hr.

■ **Available Forms:**
- *Injection, Oil:* 100 mg/ml (BAL in Oil).

■ **Indications and Dosages:**
Poisoning, arsenic (mild): IM   2.5 mg/kg 4 times/day for 2 days, 2 times on day 3, then once daily for 10 days or recovery.
Poisoning, arsenic (severe): IM   3 mg/kg q4h for 2 days, 4 times on day 3, then twice daily for 10 days or recovery.
Poisoning, gold (mild): IM   2.5 mg/kg 4 times/day for 2 days, 2 times on day 3, then once daily for 10 days or recovery.
Poisoning, gold (severe): IM   3 mg/kg q4h for 2 days, 4 times on day 3, then twice daily for 10 days or until recovery.
Poisoning, lead (mild): IM   Initially, 4 mg/kg, then 3 mg/kg q4h for 2-7 days in combination with edetate calcium disodium injection at different injection sites.
Poisoning, lead (severe): IM   4 mg/kg q4h for 2-7 days in combination with edetate calcium disodium injection at different injection sites.
Poisoning, mercury: IM   5 mg/kg for 1 day, followed by 2.5 mg/kg 1 or 2 times/day for 10 days.
Dosage in renal impairment: 2 mg/kg q12h during dialysis.

■ **Unlabeled Uses:** Antimony poisoning, bismuth poisoning, selenium poisoning, silver poisoning, vanadium poisoning

■ **Contraindications:** Acute renal impairment, organic (short-chain alkyl) mercury poisoning, G6PD deficiency (unless a life-threatening situation exists), hepatic insufficiency (unless due to arsenic poisoning), use of iron, cadmium or selenium poisoning, hypersensitivity to dimercaprol or any component of the formulations

■ **Side Effects**
Frequent
Hypertension, dose-related tachycardia, headache
Occasional
Nausea, vomiting
Rare
Burning eyes, lips, mouth, throat and penis, nervousness, pain at injection site, salivation, fever, dysuria

■ **Serious Reactions**
- Abscess formation at injection site, blepharospasm, convulsions, thrombocytopenia, and transient neutropenia occur rarely.

Special Considerations
- Administer by deep IM injection only

■ **Patient/Family Education**
- Frequent blood and urine tests are required

■ **Monitoring Parameters**
- Blood pressure, pulse
- BUN, Cr, urine pH (alkaline urinary pH decreases renal damage)

- Specific heavy metal levels

■ **Geriatric side effects at a glance:**
❏ CNS ❏ Bowel Dysfunction ❏ Bladder Dysfunction ❏ Falls

■ **U.S. Regulatory Considerations**
❏ FDA Black Box ❏ OBRA regulated in U.S. Long Term Care

diphenhydramine hydrochloride

(dye-fen-hye'-dra-meen hye-droe-klor'-ide)

■ **Brand Name(s):** Banaril, Benadryl, Diphedryl, Diphen, Diphenhist, Nytol
OTC: Allermax, Banophen, Banophen Caplets, Belix, Benadryl 25, Benylin Cough, Bydramine Cough, Diphen Cough, Dormarex 2, Genahist, Gen-D-phen, Hydramine Cough, Nidryl, Nordryl Cough, Phendry, Uni-Bent Cough

Combinations
OTC: with acetaminophen (Excedrin PM, Extra Strength Tylenol PM, Sominex Pain Relief, Unisom with Pain Relief); with calamine (Caladryl)
Chemical Class: Ethanolamine derivative

■ **Clinical Pharmacology:**
Mechanism of Action: An ethanolamine that competitively blocks the effects of histamine at peripheral H_1-receptor sites. **Therapeutic Effect:** Produces anticholinergic, antipruritic, antitussive, antiemetic, antidyskinetic, and sedative effects.
Pharmacokinetics:

Route	Onset	Peak	Duration
PO	15-30 min	1-4 hr	4-6 hr
IV, IM	less than 15 min	1-4 hr	4-6 hr

Well absorbed after PO or parenteral administration. Protein binding: 98%-99%. Widely distributed. Metabolized in the liver. Primarily excreted in urine. **Half-life:** 1-4 hr.

■ **Available Forms:**
- *Capsules:* 25 mg (Banophen, Diphen, Genahist), 50 mg (Nytol).
- *Syrup (Diphen, Diphenhist):* 12.5 mg/5 ml.
- *Tablets (Banophen, Benadryl, Genahist, Nytol):* 25 mg, 50 mg.
- *Injection (Benadryl):* 50 mg/ml.
- *Cream (Benadryl):* 1%, 2%.
- *Spray (Benadryl):* 1%, 2%.

■ **Indications and Dosages:**
Moderate to severe allergic reaction: PO, IV, IM 25-50 mg q4h. Maximum: 400 mg/day.
Motion sickness: PO 25-50 mg q4-6h. Maximum: 300 mg/day.

Parkinson's disease: PO 25-50 mg 3-4 times a day.
Antitussive: PO 5 mg q4h. Maximum: 150 mg/day.
Nighttime sleep aid: PO 50 mg at bedtime.
Pruritus: Topical Apply 1% or 2% cream or spray 3–4 times a day.

■ **Contraindications:** Acute exacerbation of asthma, use within 14 days of MAOIs

■ **Side Effects**
Frequent
Somnolence, dizziness, muscle weakness, hypotension, urine retention, thickening of bronchial secretions, dry mouth, nose, throat, or lips
Occasional
Epigastric distress, flushing, visual or hearing disturbances, paresthesia, diaphoresis, chills

■ **Serious Reactions**
- Hypersensitivity reactions, such as eczema, pruritus, rash, cardiac disturbances, and photosensitivity, may occur.
- Overdose symptoms may vary from CNS depression, including sedation, apnea, hypotension, cardiovascular collapse, and death, to severe paradoxical reactions, such as hallucinations, tremor, and seizures.

■ **Patient/Family Education**
- Dizziness, drowsiness, and dry mouth are expected side effects of diphenhydramine, but the patient may develop a tolerance to the drug's sedative effects
- Avoid performing tasks that require mental alertness or motor skills until response to the drug has been established
- Avoid alcohol

■ **Monitoring Parameters**
- Blood pressure

■ **Geriatric side effects at a glance:**
☑ CNS ☑ Bowel Dysfunction ☑ Bladder Dysfunction ☑ Falls
Other: Dry mouth, blurred vision, confusion, psychoses

■ **Use with caution in older patients with:** Narrow-angle glaucoma, overflow incontinence, psychosis.

■ **U.S. Regulatory Considerations**
☐ FDA Black Box ☑ OBRA regulated in U.S. Long Term Care

■ **Other Uses in Geriatric Patient:** Sedation, motion sickness, topical anesthetic

■ **Side Effects:**
Of particular importance in the geriatric patient: Anticholinergic effects

■ **Geriatric Considerations - Summary:** Diphenhydramine is a first-generation ethanolamine antihistamine with potent H_1-receptor antagonism. It also has significant anticholinergric properties and causes somnolence at normal doses. Older adults taking this drug are at risk of dizziness and hypotension and diphenhydramine would not be considered a drug of choice for this population. Federal guidelines discourage the use of ethanolamines as sedatives in older adults.

■ **References:**
1. Agostini JV, Leo-Summers LS, Inouye SK. Cognitive and other adverse effects of diphenhydramine use in hospitalized older patients. Arch Intern Med 2001; 161:2091-2097.
2. Tune LE. Anticholinergic effects of medication in elderly patients. J Clin Psychiatry 2001;62(suppl 21):11-14.
3. Gengo F, Gabos C, Miller JK. The pharmacodynamics of diphenhydramine-induced drowsiness and changes in mental performance. Clin Pharmacol Ther 1989; 45:15-21.

dipivefrin hydrochloride

(dye-pi'-ve-frin hye-droe-klor'-ide)

■ **Brand Name(s):** Propine
Chemical Class: Diesterified epinephrine derivative

■ **Clinical Pharmacology:**
Mechanism of Action: A prodrug of epinephrine that penetrates into anterior chamber of the eye through its lipophilic character. **Therapeutic Effect:** Reduces intraocular pressure.
Pharmacokinetics: Onset of action occurs within 30 min and peak effect in 1 hr. Dipivefrin is more lipophilic than epinephrine. Distributed to cornea. Dipivefrin is converted to epinephrine inside the eye by enzyme hydrolysis.

■ **Available Forms:**
• *Ophthalmic Solution*: 1 mg/ml (Propine).

■ **Indications and Dosages:**
Glaucoma, open-angle: Ophthalmic, Topical Instill 1 drop of 0.1% solution in affected eye(s) q12h.

■ **Contraindications:** Narrow-angle glaucoma, hypersensitivity to dipivefrin or any component of the formulation

■ **Side Effects**
Occasional
Blurred vision, burning or stinging of eye, mydriasis, headache
Rare
Follicular conjunctivitis

■ **Serious Reactions**
• Signs of systemic absorption include hypertension, arrhythmias, and tachycardia.
• Follicular conjunctivitis has been reported.

■ **Geriatric side effects at a glance:**
❑ CNS ❑ Bowel Dysfunction ❑ Bladder Dysfunction ❑ Falls

381

dipyridamole

(dye-peer-id'-a-mole)

■ **Brand Name(s):** Persantine

Combinations
Rx: with aspirin (Aggrenox)
Chemical Class: Pyrimidine derivative

■ **Clinical Pharmacology:**
Mechanism of Action: A blood modifier and platelet aggregation inhibitor that inhibits the activity of adenosine deaminase and phosphodiesterase, enzymes causing accumulation of adenosine and cyclic adenosine monophosphate. **Therapeutic Effect:** Inhibits platelet aggregation; may cause coronary vasodilation.
Pharmacokinetics: Slowly, variably absorbed from the GI tract. Widely distributed. Protein binding: 91%-99%. Metabolized in the liver. Primarily eliminated via biliary excretion. **Half-life:** 10-15 hr.

■ **Available Forms:**
  • **Tablets:** 25 mg, 50 mg, 75 mg.
  • **Injection:** 5 mg/ml.

■ **Indications and Dosages:**
Prevention of thromboembolic disorders: PO 75-100 mg 4 times a day in combination with other medications.
Diagnostic aid: IV **Based on weight.** 0.142 mg/kg/min infused over 4 min; although a maximum hasn't been determined, doses greater than 60 mg have been determined to be unnecessary for any patient.

■ **Unlabeled Uses:** Reduces risk of reinfarction in patients recovering from MI, treatment of transient ischemic attacks (TIAs)

■ **Contraindications:** None known.

■ **Side Effects**
  Frequent (14%)
  Dizziness
  Occasional (6%–2%)
  Abdominal distress, headache, rash
  Rare (less than 2%)
  Diarrhea, vomiting, flushing, pruritus

■ **Serious Reactions**
  • Overdose produces peripheral vasodilation, resulting in hypotension.

■ Patient/Family Education
- Avoid alcohol; drinking three or more alcoholic beverages a day increases the risk of stomach bleeding and dizziness, possibly resulting in a fall
- Try dry toast or unsalted crackers to relieve nausea
- Therapeutic response may not be achieved before 2 to 3 mo of continuous therapy
- Use caution when rising suddenly from lying or sitting position

■ Monitoring Parameters
- Blood pressure for hypotension
- Skin for rash

■ Geriatric side effects at a glance:
❑ CNS ❑ Bowel Dysfunction ❑ Bladder Dysfunction ❑ Falls

■ U.S. Regulatory Considerations
❑ FDA Black Box ❑ OBRA regulated in U.S. Long Term Care

dirithromycin

(dye-rith-roe-mye′-sin)

■ Brand Name(s): Dynabac, Dynabac D5-Pak
Chemical Class: Macrolide derivative

■ Clinical Pharmacology:
Mechanism of Action: A macrolide that binds to ribosomal receptor sites of susceptible organisms, inhibiting bacterial protein synthesis. **Therapeutic Effect:** Bactericidal or bacteriostatic, depending on drug dosage.
Pharmacokinetics: Rapidly absorbed from the GI tract. Protein binding: 15%-30%. Widely distributed into tissues and within cells. Eliminated primarily unchanged by biliary excretion. Not removed by hemodialysis. **Half-life:** 30-44 hr.

■ Available Forms:
- *Tablets* (*Enteric-Coated* [*Dynabac, Dynabac D5-Pak*]): 250 mg.

■ Indications and Dosages:
Pharyngitis, tonsillitis: PO 500 mg once a day for 10 days.
Acute or chronic bronchitis, skin and skin-structure infections: PO 500 mg once a day for 7 days.
Community-acquired pneumonia: PO 500 mg once a day for 14 days.

■ Contraindications: Hypersensitivity to other macrolide antibacterials

383

■ **Side Effects**
   Frequent (10%-8%)
   Abdominal pain, headache, nausea, diarrhea
   Occasional (3%-2%)
   Vomiting, dyspepsia, dizziness, nonspecific pain, asthenia
   Rare (less than 2%)
   Increased cough, flatulence, rash, dyspnea, pruritus and urticaria, insomnia

■ **Serious Reactions**
   • Antibiotic-associated colitis and other superinfections may result from altered bacterial balance.

Special Considerations

   • Long $t_{1/2}$ and higher tissue concentrations allow qd dosing; however, the improved antimicrobial activity against *Haemophilus influenzae* and lower incidence of GI adverse effects have not been realized with this agent; azithromycin probably best choice pending further comparisons
   • Individualize treatment based on local susceptibility patterns.

■ **Patient/Family Education**
   • Take with food or within 1 hr of having eaten
   • Continue therapy for the full length of treatment
   • If the patient must take an antacid containing aluminum or magnesium, take the drug 1 hr before or 2 hr after the antacid

■ **Monitoring Parameters**
   • WBC count to determine if the infection is improving
   • Evaluate for diarrhea, GI discomfort, headache, and nausea
   • Daily bowel activity and stool consistency. Although mild GI effects may be tolerable, severe symptoms may indicate the onset of antibiotic-associated colitis.
   • Signs and symptoms of superinfection include abdominal pain or cramping, anal or genital pruritus or discharge, moderate to severe diarrhea, severe mouth or tongue soreness, and new or increased fever.

■ **Geriatric side effects at a glance:**
   ❑ CNS ☑ Bowel Dysfunction ❑ Bladder Dysfunction ❑ Falls

■ **U.S. Regulatory Considerations**
   ❑ FDA Black Box ❑ OBRA regulated in U.S. Long Term Care

disopyramide phosphate

(dye-soe-peer'-a-mide foss'-fate)

- **Brand Name(s):** Norpace, Norpace CR
  Chemical Class: Pyramide derivative

- **Clinical Pharmacology:**
  Mechanism of Action: An antiarrhythmic that prolongs the refractory period of the cardiac cell by direct effect, decreasing myocardial excitability and conduction velocity. **Therapeutic Effect:** Depresses myocardial contractility. Has anticholinergic and negative inotropic effects.
  Pharmacokinetics: Rapidly and almost completely absorbed from the GI tract. Protein binding: 50%-65%. Metabolized in liver. Excreted in urine. Removed by hemodialysis. **Half-life:** 4-10 hr.

- **Available Forms:**
  - *Capsules (Norpace)* : 100 mg, 150 mg.
  - *Capsules (Extended-Release [Norpace CR])*: 100 mg, 150 mg.

- **Indications and Dosages:**
  Suppression and prevention of ventricular ectopy, unifocal or multifocal premature ventricular contractions, paired ventricular contractions (couplets), and episodes of ventricular tachycardia: PO *Weight 50 kg and more.* 150 mg q6h (300 mg q12h with extended-release). *Weight less than 50 kg.* 100 mg q6h (200 mg q12h with extended-release).
  Dosage in renal impairment: With or without loading dose of 150 mg:

Creatinine Clearance	Dosage
40 ml/min and higher	100 mg q6h (extended-release 200 mg q12h)
30-39 ml/min	100 mg q8h
15-29 ml/min	100 mg q12h
less than 15 ml/min	100 mg q24h

  Dosage in liver impairment: 100 mg q6h (200 mg q12h with extended-release).
  Dosage in cardiomyopathy, cardiac decompensation: No loading dose; 100 mg q6-8h with gradual dosage adjustments.

- **Unlabeled Uses:** Prophylaxis and treatment of supraventricular tachycardia

- **Contraindications:** Cardiogenic shock, congenital QT prolongation, narrow-angle glaucoma (unless patient is undergoing cholinergic therapy), preexisting second- or third-degree AV block, preexisting urinary retention

- **Side Effects**
  Frequent (greater than 9%)
  Dry mouth (32%), urinary hesitancy, constipation
  Occasional (9%–3%)
  Blurred vision, dry eyes, nose, or throat, urinary retention, headache, dizziness, fatigue, nausea
  Rare (less than 1%)
  Impotence, hypotension, edema, weight gain, shortness of breath, syncope, chest pain, nervousness, diarrhea, vomiting, decreased appetite, rash, itching

■ Serious Reactions
- May produce or aggravate CHF.
- May produce severe hypotension, shortness of breath, chest pain, syncope (especially in patients with primary cardiomyopathy or CHF).
- Hepatotoxicity occurs rarely.

Special Considerations
- Due to potential for prodysrhythmic effects, use for asymptomatic PVCs or lesser dysrhythmias should be avoided

■ Patient/Family Education
- Notify the physician if productive cough or shortness of breath occurs
- Do not take nasal decongestants or OTC cold preparations, especially those containing stimulants, without consulting the physician for approval
- Limit alcohol and salt consumption

■ Monitoring Parameters
- Monitor ECG closely; if PR, QRS, or QT interval increase by 25%, stop drug
- Therapeutic plasma levels are 2-4 mcg/ml
- Blood glucose, liver enzymes, and serum alkaline phosphatase, bilirubin, and potassium, AST (SGOT), and ALT (SGPT) levels
- Intake and output
- Signs and symptoms of CHF including cough, dyspnea (particularly on exertion), fatigue, and rales at the base of the lungs

■ Geriatric side effects at a glance:
❑ CNS   ☑ Bowel Dysfunction   ❑ Bladder Dysfunction   ❑ Falls

■ U.S. Regulatory Considerations
☑ FDA Black Box   ❑ OBRA regulated in U.S. Long Term Care
- Proarrhythmic effects

dobutamine hydrochloride

(doe-byoo'-ta-meen hye-droe-klor'-ide)

Chemical Class: Catecholamine, synthetic

■ Clinical Pharmacology:
Mechanism of Action: A direct-acting inotropic agent acting primarily on beta$_1$-adrenergic receptors. **Therapeutic Effect:** Decreases preload and afterload, and enhances myocardial contractility, stroke volume, and cardiac output. Improves renal blood flow and urine output.

Pharmacokinetics:

Route	Onset	Peak	Duration
IV	1-2 min	10 min	length of infusion

Metabolized in the liver. Primarily excreted in urine. Not removed by hemodialysis.
Half-life: 2 min.

■ **Available Forms:**
- *Infusion (Ready-to-use)*: 1 mg/ml, 2 mg/ml, 4 mg/ml.
- *Injection*: 12.5-mg/ml vial.

■ **Indications and Dosages:**
Short-term management of cardiac decompensation: IV Infusion 2.5-20 mcg/kg/min. Rarely, drug can be infused at a rate of up to 40 mcg/kg/min to increase cardiac output.

■ **Contraindications:** Hypovolemia patients, idiopathic hypertrophic subaortic stenosis, sulfite sensitivity

■ **Side Effects**
Frequent (greater than 5%)
Increased heart rate, increased BP
Occasional (5%–3%)
Pain at injection site
Rare (3%–1%)
Nausea, headache, anginal pain, shortness of breath, fever

■ **Serious Reactions**
- Overdose may produce a marked increase in heart rate (by 30 beats/min or higher), marked increase in BP (by 50 mm Hg or higher), anginal pain, and premature ventricular contractions (PVCs).

■ **Patient/Family Education**
- Report chest pain or palpitations during the infusion or pain or burning at the IV site

■ **Monitoring Parameters**
- Continuously monitor ECG, BP, and PCWP
- Signs and symptoms of infiltration of the IV solution, which can cause local inflammatory changes and possible dermal necrosis
- Intake and output
- Serum potassium levels
- Dobutamine plasma levels; dobutamine's therapeutic range is 40-190 ng/ml

■ **Geriatric side effects at a glance:**
❑ CNS ❑ Bowel Dysfunction ❑ Bladder Dysfunction ❑ Falls

■ **U.S. Regulatory Considerations**
❑ FDA Black Box ❑ OBRA regulated in U.S. Long Term Care

docusate

(dok'-yoo-sate)

OTC: *Docusate Sodium*: Colace, Dioeze, Diocto, DOK, DOSS DSS, Ducosoft-S, Modane Soft, Regulax SS
OTC: *Docusate Calcium*: Sulfolax, Surfak Stool Softener

Combinations
OTC: with senna concentrate (Senokot-S); with phenolphthalein (Doxidan); with casanthranol (Peri-Colace); with cascara sagrada (Nature's Remedy)
Chemical Class: Anionic surfactant

■ Clinical Pharmacology:
Mechanism of Action: A bulk-producing laxative that decreases surface film tension by mixing liquid and bowel contents. **Therapeutic Effect:** Increases infiltration of liquid to form a softer stool.
Pharmacokinetics: Minimal absorption from the GI tract. Acts in small and large intestines. Results usually occur 1-2 days after first dose, but may take 3-5 days.

■ Available Forms:
- *Capsules*: 50 mg (Colace), 100 mg (Colace, Ducosoft-S), 240 mg (Surfak).
- *Liquid (Colace)*: 50 mg/5 ml (sodium).
- *Syrup (Colace, Diocto)*: 60 mg/15 ml.

■ Indications and Dosages:
Stool softener: PO 50-500 mg/day in 1-4 divided doses.

■ Contraindications: Acute abdominal pain, concomitant use of mineral oil, intestinal obstruction, nausea, vomiting

■ Side Effects
Occasional
Mild GI cramping, throat irritation (with liquid preparation)
Rare
Rash

■ Serious Reactions
- None known.

■ Patient/Family Education
- Drink plenty of water during administration
- Institute measures to promote defecation, such as increasing fluid intake, exercising, and eating a high-fiber diet
- Notify the physician if unrelieved constipation, dizziness, muscle cramps or pain, rectal bleeding, or weakness occurs
- Notify the physician of sudden changes in bowel habits or over 2 wk duration

- **Monitoring Parameters**
  - Daily bowel activity and stool consistency
  - Bowel sounds for peristalsis

- **Geriatric side effects at a glance:**
  ☐ CNS ☑ Bowel Dysfunction ☐ Bladder Dysfunction ☐ Falls

- **U.S. Regulatory Considerations**
  ☐ FDA Black Box ☐ OBRA regulated in U.S. Long Term Care

dofetilide

(doe-fet'-il-ide)

- **Brand Name(s):** Tikosyn
  Chemical Class: Methanesulfonanilide derivative

- **Clinical Pharmacology:**
  Mechanism of Action: A selective potassium channel blocker that prolongs repolarization without affecting conduction velocity by blocking one or more time-dependent potassium currents. Dofetilide has no effect on sodium channels or adrenergic alpha or beta receptors. **Therapeutic Effect:** Terminates reentrant tachyarrhythmias, preventing reinduction.
  Pharmacokinetics: Well absorbed from the GI tract. Protein binding: 60%-70%. Metabolized in liver. Primarily excreted in urine; minimal elimination in feces. **Half-life:** 7.5-10 hr.

- **Available Forms:**
  - *Capsules:* 125 mcg, 250 mcg, 500 mcg.

- **Indications and Dosages:**
  Maintain normal sinus rhythm after conversion from atrial fibrillation or flutter: PO Individualized using a seven-step dosing algorithm dependent upon calculated creatinine clearance and QT interval measurements.

- **Contraindications:** Concurrent use of drugs that prolong the QT interval; concurrent use of amiodarone, megestrol, prochlorperazine, or verapamil; congenital or acquired prolonged QT syndrome; paroxysmal atrial fibrillation; severe renal impairment

- **Side Effects**
  Occasional (less than 5%)
  Headache, chest pain, dizziness, dyspnea, nausea, insomnia, back and abdominal pain, diarrhea, rash

- **Serious Reactions**
  - Angioedema, bradycardia, cerebral ischemia, facial paralysis, and serious ventricular arrhythmias or various forms of heart block may be noted.

389

Patient/Family Education
- Take without regard to food
- Dofetilide therapy compliance is essential and dosing instructions must be followed diligently
- Notify the physician if dizziness, severe diarrhea, or other adverse effects occur

Monitoring Parameters
- ECG, QTc intervals, renal function

Geriatric side effects at a glance:
❑ CNS ❑ Bowel Dysfunction ❑ Bladder Dysfunction ❑ Falls

U.S. Regulatory Considerations
☑ FDA Black Box ❑ OBRA regulated in U.S. Long Term Care

dolasetron mesylate

(dol-a'-se-tron mes'-sil-ate)

Brand Name(s): Anzemat
Chemical Class: Nonbenzamide

Clinical Pharmacology:
Mechanism of Action: A 5-HT$_3$-receptor antagonist that acts centrally in the chemoreceptor trigger zone and peripherally at the vagal nerve terminals. **Therapeutic Effect:** Prevents nausea and vomiting.
Pharmacokinetics: Readily absorbed from the GI tract after PO administration. Protein binding: 69%-77%. Metabolized in the liver. Primarily excreted in urine. Unknown if removed by hemodialysis. **Half-life:** 5-10 hr.

Available Forms:
- *Tablets*: 50 mg, 100 mg.
- *Injection*: 20 mg/ml in single-use 0.625-ml amps, 0.625-ml fill in 2-ml Carpuject, and 5-ml vials.

Indications and Dosages:
Prevention of chemotherapy-induced nausea and vomiting: PO 100 mg within 1 hr of chemotherapy. IV 1.8 mg/kg as a single dose 30 min before chemotherapy. Maximum: 100 mg.
Treatment or prevention of postoperative nausea or vomiting: PO 100 mg within 2 hr of surgery. IV 12.5 mg 15 min before cessation of anesthesia or as soon as nausea occurs.

Unlabeled Uses: Radiation therapy–induced nausea and vomiting

- **Contraindications:** None known.

- **Side Effects**
  Frequent (10%-5%)
  Headache, diarrhea, fatigue
  Occasional (5%-1%)
  Fever, dizziness, tachycardia, dyspepsia

- **Serious Reactions**
  - Overdose may produce a combination of CNS stimulant and depressant effects.

Special Considerations
  - No obvious advantage over other agents in this class (ondansetron, granisetron)

- **Patient/Family Education**
  - Do not cut, break, or chew film-coated tablets
  - The postoperative patient should report nausea as soon as it occurs because prompt administration of the drug increases its effectiveness
  - The patient should try other methods of reducing nausea, such as lying quietly and avoiding strong odors

- **Monitoring Parameters**
  - Relief of nausea and vomiting
  - ECG

- **Geriatric side effects at a glance:**
  ❏ CNS   ❏ Bowel Dysfunction   ❏ Bladder Dysfunction   ❏ Falls

- **U.S. Regulatory Considerations**
  ❏ FDA Black Box   ❏ OBRA regulated in U.S. Long Term Care

donepezil hydrochloride

(doe-nep'-e-zil hye-droe-klor'-ide)

- **Brand Name(s):** Aricept, Aricept ODT
  Chemical Class: Cholinesterase inhibitor; piperidine derivative

- **Clinical Pharmacology:**
  Mechanism of Action: A cholinesterase inhibitor that inhibits the enzyme acetylcholinesterase, thus increasing the concentration of acetylcholine at cholinergic synapses and enhancing cholinergic function in the CNS. **Therapeutic Effect:** Slows the progression of Alzheimer's disease.
  Pharmacokinetics: Well absorbed after PO administration. Protein binding: 96%. Extensively metabolized. Eliminated in urine and feces. **Half-life:** 70 hr.

■ **Available Forms:**
   • *Tablets (Aricept)*: 5 mg, 10 mg.
   • *Tablets (Orally-Disintegrating [Aricept ODT])*: 5 mg, 10 mg.

■ **Indications and Dosages:**
   Alzheimer's disease: PO Initially, 5 mg/day at bedtime. May increase at 4- to 6-wk interval to 10 mg/day at bedtime.

■ **Unlabeled Uses:** Treatment of attention-deficit hyperactivity disorder, autism, behavioral syndromes in dementia

■ **Contraindications:** History of hypersensitivity to piperidine derivatives

■ **Side Effects**
   Frequent (11%-8%)
   Nausea, diarrhea, headache, insomnia, nonspecific pain, dizziness
   Occasional (6%-3%)
   Mild muscle cramps, fatigue, vomiting, anorexia, ecchymosis
   Rare (3%-2%)
   Depression, abnormal dreams, weight loss, arthritis, somnolence, syncope, frequent urination

■ **Serious Reactions**
   • Overdose may result in cholinergic crisis, characterized by severe nausea, increased salivation, diaphoresis, bradycardia, hypotension, flushed skin, abdominal pain, respiratory depression, seizures, and cardiorespiratory collapse. Increasing muscle weakness may result in death if respiratory muscles are involved. The antidote is 1-2 mg IV atropine sulfate with subsequent doses based on therapeutic response.

Special Considerations
   • Advantages over the cholinesterase inhibitors include qd dosing and apparent lack of liver toxicity

■ **Patient/Family Education**
   • May be taken with or without food
   • Notify the physician if abdominal pain, diarrhea, excessive sweating or salivation, dizziness, or nausea and vomiting occur
   • Donepezil is not a cure for Alzheimer's disease but may slow the progression of its symptoms

■ **Monitoring Parameters**
   • Close monitoring for clinical improvement and periodic reassessment of need for continued therapy
   • Monitor the patient's behavioral, cognitive, and functional status
   • Monitor the patient for cholinergic reactions, such as diaphoresis, dizziness, excessive salivation, facial warmth, abdominal cramps or discomfort, lacrimation, pallor, and urinary urgency
   • Monitor the patient for diarrhea, headache, insomnia, and nausea

■ **Geriatric side effects at a glance:**
   ❑ CNS ☑ Bowel Dysfunction ❑ Bladder Dysfunction ❑ Falls
   Other: Anorexia, weight loss, bradycardia

- **Use with caution in older patients with:** None

- **U.S. Regulatory Considerations**
  ❑ FDA Black Box   ❑ OBRA regulated in U.S. Long Term Care

- **Other Uses in Geriatric Patient:** None

- **Side Effects:**
  Of particular importance in the geriatric patient: None

- **Geriatric Considerations - Summary:** Donepezil is modestly effective for treatment of cognitive decline associated with Alzheimer's disease. Compared to placebo, persons using donepezil have less decline in performance on cognitive tests, but many patients derive no clinical benefit, and there is no evidence the drug delays disability or institutionalization. Donepezil is expensive, and not cost-effective for this indication. Persons using drugs to treat Alzheimer's disease should be monitored closely, and prescribers should have a low threshold for discontinuing these agents if no clinical benefit is observed.

- **References:**
  1. Courtney C, Farrell D, Gray R, et al. Long-term donepezil treatment in 565 patients with Alzheimer's disease (AD2000): randomised double-blind trial. Lancet 2004;363:2105-2115.
  2. Cummings JL. Alzheimer's disease. N Engl J Med 2004;351:56-67.
  3. Kaduszkiewicz H, Zimmermann T, Beck-Bornholdt HP, et al. Cholinesterase inhibitors for patients with Alzheimer's disease: systematic review of randomised clinical trials. BMJ 2005;331:321-327.

dopamine hydrochloride

(doe'-pa-meen)

Chemical Class: Catecholamine, synthetic

- **Clinical Pharmacology:**
  Mechanism of Action: A sympathomimetic (adrenergic agonist) that stimulates adrenergic receptors. Effects are dose dependent. Low dosages (less than 5 mcg/kg/min) stimulate dopaminergic receptors, causing renal vasodilation. Low to moderate dosages (10 mcg/kg/min or less) have a positive inotropic effect by direct action and release of norepinephrine. High dosages (greater than 10 mcg/kg/min) stimulate alpha-receptors. **Therapeutic Effect:** With low dosages, increases renal blood flow, urine flow, and sodium excretion. With low to moderate dosages, increases myocardial contractility, stroke volume, and cardiac output. With high dosages, increases peripheral resistance, renal vasoconstriction, and systolic and diastolic BP.
  Pharmacokinetics:

Route	Onset	Peak	Duration
IV	1-2 min	N/A	less than 10 min

Widely distributed. Does not cross blood-brain barrier. Metabolized in the liver, kidney, and plasma. Primarily excreted in urine. Not removed by hemodialysis. **Half-life:** 2 min.

■ **Available Forms:**
  • *Injection*: 40 mg/ml, 80 mg/ml, 160 mg/ml.
  • *Injection (Premix with dextrose)*: 80 mg/100 ml, 160 mg/100 ml, 320 mg/100 ml.

■ **Indications and Dosages:**
  Treatment and prevention of acute hypotension; shock (associated with cardiac decompensation, MI, open heart surgery, renal failure, or trauma), treatment of low cardiac output, treatment of CHF: IV 1 mcg/kg/min up to 50 mcg/kg/min titrated to desired response.

■ **Contraindications:** Pheochromocytoma, sulfite sensitivity, uncorrected tachyarrhythmias, ventricular fibrillation

■ **Side Effects**
  Frequent
  Headache, ectopic beats, tachycardia, anginal pain, palpitations, vasoconstriction, hypotension, nausea, vomiting, dyspnea
  Occasional
  Piloerection or goose bumps, bradycardia, widening of QRS complex

■ **Serious Reactions**
  • High doses may produce ventricular arrhythmias.
  • Patients with occlusive vascular disease are at high risk for further compromise of circulation to the extremities, which may result in gangrene.
  • Tissue necrosis with sloughing may occur with extravasation of IV solution.

Special Considerations
  • *Dilute before use if not prediluted;* antidote for extravasation: infiltrate area as soon as possible with 10-15 ml NS containing 5-10 mg phentolamine

■ **Patient/Family Education**
  • Report chest pain or palpitations during the infusion or pain or burning at the IV site

■ **Monitoring Parameters**
  • Urine flow, cardiac output, blood pressure, pulmonary wedge pressure
  • Immediately notify the physician if the patient experiences arrhythmias, decreased peripheral circulation (marked by cold, pale, or mottled extremities), decreased urine output, or significant changes in BP or heart rate. Also notify the physician if the patient fails to respond to increase or decrease in infusion rate
  • Taper the dopamine dosage before discontinuing the drug because abrupt cessation of dopamine therapy may result in marked hypotension
  • Be alert to excessive vasoconstriction as evidenced by decreased urine output, disproportionate increase in diastolic BP, and increased arrhythmias or heart rate. Slow or temporarily stop the dopamine infusion and notify the physician if excessive vasoconstriction occurs

■ **Geriatric side effects at a glance:**
  ❑ CNS   ❑ Bowel Dysfunction   ❑ Bladder Dysfunction   ❑ Falls

■ **U.S. Regulatory Considerations**
  ❑ FDA Black Box   ❑ OBRA regulated in U.S. Long Term Care

dorzolamide hydrochloride; timolol maleate

(door-zol'-a-mide hye-droe-klor'-ide; tim'-oh-lol mal'-ee-ate)

- **Brand Name(s):** Cosopt

- **Clinical Pharmacology:**
  Mechanism of Action: A combination ophthalmic agent that inhibits carbonic anhydrase and blocks beta-adrenergic receptors. Reduces aqueous humor production.
  Therapeutic Effect: Reduces intraocular pressure (IOP).
  Pharmacokinetics: None reported.

- **Available Forms:**
  - *Ophthalmic Solution*: 2% dorzolamide hydrochloride and 0.5% timolol maleate (Cosopt).

- **Indications and Dosages:**
  Glaucoma, ocular hypertension: Ophthalmic 1 drop in affected eye(s) twice daily.

- **Contraindications:** Bronchial asthma or chronic obstructive pulomonary disease, cardiogenic shock, overt cardiac failure, second and third degree AV block, severe sinus bradycardia, hypersensitivity to dorzolamide, timolol, or any other component of the formulation

- **Side Effects**
  Frequent
  Conjunctival hyperemia, growth of eyelashes, ocular pruritus, taste perversion
  Occasional
  Ocular dryness and itching, visual disturbance, ocular burning, foreign body sensation, eye pain, pigmentation of the periocular skin, blepharitis, cataract, superficial punctate keratitis, eyelid erythema, ocular irritation, eyelash darkening
  Rare
  Intraocular inflammation (iritis), hypotension, depression, dizziness, dry mouth, nausea, vomiting, tearing

- **Serious Reactions**
  - Systemic adverse events, including infections (colds and upper respiratory tract infections), headaches, asthenia, and hirsutism, have been reported.
  - Bronchospasm and myocardial infarction have also been reported.
  - Use with caution in patients with a history of sulfa allergy.

- **Geriatric side effects at a glance:**
  ❑ CNS ❑ Bowel Dysfunction ❑ Bladder Dysfunction ❑ Falls

- **U.S. Regulatory Considerations**
  ❑ FDA Black Box ❑ OBRA regulated in U.S. Long Term Care

doxapram hydrochloride

(dox'-a-pram)

- **Brand Name(s):** Dopram
  Chemical Class: Pyrrolidinone derivative

- **Clinical Pharmacology:**
  Mechanism of Action: A central nervous system stimulant that directly stimulates the respiratory center in the medulla or indirectly by effects on the carotid. **Therapeutic Effect:** Increases pulmonary ventilation by increasing resting minute ventilation, tidal volume, respiratory frequency, and inspiratory neuromuscular drive, and enhances the ventilatory response to carbon dioxide.
  Pharmacokinetics: IV onset 20-40 sec, peak 1-2 min, duration 5-12 min. Metabolized in the liver to metabolites, ketodoxapram (active) and desethyldoxapram (inactive). Partially excreted in the urine. Not removed by hemodialysis. **Half-life:** 2.4-9.9 hr.

- **Available Forms:**
  - *Injection*: 20 mg/ml (Dopram).

- **Indications and Dosages:**
  Chronic obstructive pulmonary disease (COPD): IV Infusion Initially, 1-2 mg/min. Maximum: 3 g/day for no more than 2 hr.
  Drug-induced CNS depression: IV Injection Initially, 1-2 mg/kg, repeat after 5 min. May repeat at 1-2 hour intervals, until sustained consciousness. Maximum: 3 g/day. IV Infusion Initially, bolus dose of 2 mg/kg, repeat after 5 min. If no response, wait 1-2 hr and repeat. If stimulation is noted, initiate infusion at 1-3 mg/min. Infusion should not be continued for more than 2 hr. Maximum: 3 g/day.
  Respiratory depression: IV Injection Initially, 0.5-1 mg/kg. May repeat at 5-min intervals in patients who demonstrate initial response. Maximum: 2 mg/kg. IV Infusion Initially, 5 mg/min until adequate response or adverse effects are seen. Decrease to 1-3 mg/min. Maximum: 4 mg/kg.

- **Unlabeled Uses:** Sleep apnea, congenital central hypoventilation syndrome, obesity-hypoventilation syndrome, postanesthetic respiratory depression, shivering

- **Contraindications:** Convulsive disorders, cardiovascular impairment, head injury or cerebral vascular accident, severe hypertension, mechanical ventilation disorders, hypersensitivity to doxapram.

- **Side Effects**
  Occasional
  Flushing, sweating, pruritus, disorientation, headache, dizziness, hyperactivity, convulsions, dyspnea, cough, tachypnea, hiccough, rebound hypoventilation, phlebitis, variations in heart rate, arrhythmias, chest pain, nausea, vomiting, diarrhea, stimulation of urinary bladder with spontaneous voiding.

- **Serious Reactions**
  - Overdosage may produce extensions of the pharmacologic effects of the drug. Excessive pressor effect, skeletal muscle hyperactivity, tachycardia, and enhanced deep tendon reflexes may be early signs of overdosage.

- **Patient/Family Education**
  - Notify the nurse on duty immediately of trouble breathing

- **Monitoring Parameters**
  - Baseline ABG then q30 min (for use in COPD)
  - Blood pressure, heart rate, deep tendon reflexes

- **Geriatric side effects at a glance:**
  - ❑ CNS ❑ Bowel Dysfunction ❑ Bladder Dysfunction ❑ Falls

- **U.S. Regulatory Considerations**
  - ❑ FDA Black Box ❑ OBRA regulated in U.S. Long Term Care

doxazosin mesylate

(dox-ay'-zoe-sin mes'-sil-ate)

- **Brand Name(s):** Cardura, Cardura XL
  Chemical Class: Quinazoline derivative

- **Clinical Pharmacology:**
  Mechanism of Action: An antihypertensive that selectively blocks alpha$_1$-adrenergic receptors, decreasing peripheral vascular resistance. **Therapeutic Effect:** Causes peripheral vasodilation and lowers BP. Also relaxes smooth muscle of bladder and prostate.
  Pharmacokinetics:

Route	Onset	Peak	Duration
PO	N/A	2-6 hr	24 hr

  Well absorbed from the GI tract. Protein binding: 98%–99%. Metabolized in the liver. Primarily eliminated in feces. Not removed by hemodialysis. **Half-life:** 19–22 hr.

- **Available Forms:**
  - *Tablets*: 1 mg, 2 mg, 4 mg, 8 mg.

- **Indications and Dosages:**
  Mild to moderate hypertension: PO Initially, 1 mg once a day. May increase to a maximum of 16 mg/day.
  Benign prostatic hyperplasia: PO Initially, 1 mg/day. May increase q1–2 wk. Maximum: 8 mg/day.

- **Contraindications:** Hypersensitivity to other quinazolines

- **Side Effects**
  Frequent (20%–10%)
  Dizziness, asthenia, headache, edema

397

Occasional (9%–3%)
Nausea, pharyngitis, rhinitis, pain in extremities, somnolence
Rare (3%–1%)
Palpitations, diarrhea, constipation, dyspnea, myalgia, altered vision, dizziness, nervousness

■ **Serious Reactions**
- First-dose syncope (hypotension with sudden loss of consciousness) may occur 30 to 90 min following initial dose of 2 mg or greater, a too-rapid increase in dosage, or addition of another antihypertensive agent to therapy. First-dose syncope may be preceded by tachycardia (pulse rate of 120-160 beats/minute).

Special Considerations
- The doxazosin arm of the ALLHAT study was stopped early; the doxazosin group had a 25% greater risk of combined cardiovascular disease events which was primarily accounted for by a doubled risk of CHF vs the chlorthalidone group; doxazosin was also found to be less effective at controlling systolic BP an average of 3 mm Hg; may want to consider primary antihypertensives in addition to alpha-blockers for BPH symptoms
- Use as a single antihypertensive agent limited by tendency to cause sodium and water retention and increased plasma volume

■ **Patient/Family Education**
- Alert patient to the possibility of syncopal and orthostatic symptoms, especially with first dose ("1st-dose syncope")
- Initial dose should be administered at bedtime in the smallest possible dose
- Full therapeutic effect may not appear for 3-4 wk
- Avoid performing tasks that require mental alertness or motor skills until response to doxazosin has been established

■ **Monitoring Parameters**
- Blood pressure
- Pulse
- Assess for edema and headache

■ **Geriatric side effects at a glance:**
☑ CNS   ☐ Bowel Dysfunction   ☐ Bladder Dysfunction   ☑ Falls
Other: Orthostatic Hypotension, Worsening of urge or mixed urinary incontinence

■ **Use with caution in older patients with:** Congestive heart failure, patients taking medications for impotence (e.g., vardenafil, sildenafil, or tadalafil).

■ **U.S. Regulatory Considerations**
☐ FDA Black Box   ☐ OBRA regulated in U.S. Long Term Care

■ **Side Effects:**
Of particular importance in the geriatric patient: Orthostatic Hypotension, Worsening of urge or mixed urinary incontinence

■ **Geriatric Considerations - Summary:** Alpha-adrenergic blockers are modestly effective alone, and in combination with 5-alpha reductase inhibitors (e.g., finasteride) in the treatment of urinary obstructive symptoms related to benign prostatic hyperplasia. The main side effect of these agents is orthostatic hypotension, and in hypertensive patients, these agents may increase the risk of congestive heart failure as reported in the ALLHAT study.

■ **References:**
1. Lepor H, Williford WO, Barry MJ, et al. The efficacy of terazosin, finasteride, or both in benign prostatic hyperplasia. Veterans Affairs Cooperative Studies Benign Prostatic Hyperplasia Study Group. N Engl J Med 1996;335:533-539.
2. McConnell JD, Roehrborn CG, Bautista OM, et al. The long-term effect of doxazosin, finasteride, and combination therapy on the clinical progression of benign prostatic hyperplasia. N Engl J Med 2003;349:2387-2398.
3. Major cardiovascular events in hypertensive patients randomized to doxazosin vs chlorthalidone: the antihypertensive and lipid-lowering treatment to prevent heart attack trial (ALLHAT). ALLHAT Collaborative Research Group. JAMA 2000;283:1967-1975.

doxepin hydrochloride

(dox'-eh-pin hye-droe-klor'-ide)

■ **Brand Name(s):** Prudoxin, Sinequan, Zonalon
  Chemical Class: Dibenzoxepin derivative; tertiary amine

■ **Clinical Pharmacology:**
  Mechanism of Action: A tricyclic antidepressant, antianxiety agent, antineuralgic agent, antipruritic, and antiulcer agent that increases synaptic concentrations of norepinephrine and serotonin. **Therapeutic Effect:** Produces antidepressant and anxiolytic effects.
  Pharmacokinetics: Rapidly and well absorbed from the GI tract. Protein binding: 80%-85%. Metabolized in the liver to active metabolite. Primarily excreted in urine. Not removed by hemodialysis. **Half-life:** 6-8 hr. Topical: Absorbed through the skin. Distributed to body tissues. Metabolized to active metabolite. Excreted in urine.

■ **Available Forms:**
  • *Capsules (Sinequan):* 10 mg, 25 mg, 50 mg, 75 mg, 100 mg, 150 mg.
  • *Oral Concentrate (Sinequan):* 10 mg/ml.
  • *Cream (Prudoxin, Zonalon):* 5%.

■ **Indications and Dosages:**
  Depression, anxiety: PO Initially, 10-25 mg at bedtime. May increase by 10-25 mg/day every 3-7 days. Maximum: 75 mg/day.
  Pruritus associated with eczema: Topical Apply thin film 4 times a day.

■ **Unlabeled Uses:** Treatment of neurogenic pain, panic disorder; prevention of vascular headache, pruritus in idiopathic urticaria

■ **Contraindications:** Angle-closure glaucoma, hypersensitivity to other tricyclic antidepressants, urine retention

■ **Side Effects**
  Frequent
  Oral: Orthostatic hypotension, somnolence, dry mouth, headache, increased appetite, weight gain, nausea, unusual fatigue, unpleasant taste

Topical: Edema; increased pruritus and eczema; burning, tingling, or stinging at application site; altered taste; dizziness; drowsiness; dry skin; dry mouth; fatigue; headache; thirst

Occasional

Oral: Blurred vision, confusion, constipation, hallucinations, difficult urination, eye pain, irregular heartbeat, fine muscle tremors, nervousness, impaired sexual function, diarrhea, diaphoresis, heartburn, insomnia

Topical: Anxiety, skin irritation or cracking, nausea

Rare

Oral: Allergic reaction, alopecia, tinnitus, breast enlargement

Topical: Fever, photosensitivity

■ **Serious Reactions**
- Abrupt or too-rapid withdrawal may result in headache, malaise, nausea, vomiting, and vivid dreams.
- Overdose may produce seizures, dizziness, and cardiovascular effects, such as severe orthostatic hypotension, tachycardia, palpitations, and arrhythmias.

Special Considerations
- Equally effective as other tricyclic antidepressants for depression; distinguishing characteristics include sedative, anxiolytic, antihistaminic properties

■ **Patient/Family Education**
- Therapeutic effects may take 4-6 wk
- Do not discontinue abruptly after long-term use
- If drowsiness occurs with top application, decrease surface area being treated or number of daily applications
- Change positions slowly to avoid hypotensive effect
- Tolerance to postural hypotension, sedative and anticholinergic effects usually develops during early therapy
- Avoid tasks that require mental alertness or motor skills until response to the drug has been established

■ **Monitoring Parameters**
- CBC; ECG; mental status: mood, sensorium, affect, suicidal tendencies
- Supervise the suicidal-risk patient closely during early therapy (as depression lessens, energy level improves, increasing suicidal potential)
- Assess appearance, behavior, speech pattern, level of interest, and mood

■ **Geriatric side effects at a glance:**
  ☑ CNS ☑ Bowel Dysfunction ☑ Bladder Dysfunction ☑ Falls
  Other: Orthostatic hypotension, cardiac conduction disturbances, anticholinergic side effects

■ **Use with caution in older patients with:** Cardiovascular disease, prostatic hyptertrophy or other conditions which increase the risk of urinary retention

■ **U.S. Regulatory Considerations**
  ☑ FDA Black Box
- Because there is an increased risk of suicide in children and adolescents, older adults should also be closely monitored for suicide ideation.
  ☑ OBRA regulated in U.S. Long Term Care

- **Other Uses in Geriatric Patient:** Neuropathic pain, urge urinary incontinence
- **Side Effects:**
  Of particular importance in the geriatric patient: Anticholinergic effects, extrapyramidal symptoms, high doses may increase risk of sudden death

- **Geriatric Considerations - Summary:** Although tricyclic antidepressants are effective in the treatment of major depression in older adults, the side-effect profile and low toxic-to-therapeutic ratio relegate them to second-line agents (after serotonin reuptake inhibitors) for most older patients. These agents are effective in the treatment of urge urinary incontinence and neuropathic pain, but must be monitored closely. Of the tricyclic antidepressants, imipramine and amitryptyline have the highest anticholinergic activity and may be best choice in this class for management of incontinence, but should otherwise be avoided.

- **References:**
  1. Leipzig RM, Cumming RG, Tinetti ME. Drugs and falls in older people: a systematic review and meta-analysis: I. Psychotropic drugs. J Am Geriatr Soc 1999;47:30-39.
  2. Cadieux RJ. Antidepressant drug interactions in the elderly. Understanding the P-450 system is half the battle in reducing risks. Postgrad Med 1999;106:231-240, 245.
  3. Ray WA, Meredith S, Thapa PB, et al. Cyclic antidepressants and the risk of sudden cardiac death. Clin Pharmacol Ther 2004;75:234-241.
  4. Roose SP, Laghrissi-Thode F, Kennedy JS, et al. Comparison of paroxetine and nortriptyline in depressed patients with ischemic heart disease. JAMA 1998;279:287-291.

doxercalciferol

(docks-er-kal-sif'-e-role)

- **Brand Name(s):** Hectorol
  Chemical Class: Vitamin D analog

- **Clinical Pharmacology:**
  Mechanism of Action: A fat-soluble vitamin that is essential for absorption, utilization of calcium phosphate, and normal calcification of bone. **Therapeutic Effect:** Stimulates calcium and phosphate absorption from small intestine, promotes secretion of calcium from bone to blood, promotes renal tubule phosphate resorption, acts on bone cells to stimulate skeletal growth and on parathyroid gland to suppress hormone synthesis and secretion.
  Pharmacokinetics: Readily absorbed from small intestine. Metabolized in liver. Partially eliminated in urine. Not removed by hemodialysis. **Half-life:** up to 96 hr.

- **Available Forms:**
  - *Capsule:* 2.5 mcg (Hectorol).
  - *Injection:* 2 mcg/ml (Hectorol).

- **Indications and Dosages:**
  Secondary hyperparathyroidism, dialysis patients: IV Titrate dose to lower iPTH to 150-300 pg/ml. Adjust dose at 8-wk intervals to a maximum dose of 18 mcg/wk. Initially, if iPTH level is more than 400 pg/ml, give 4 mcg 3 times/wk after dialysis, ad-

ministered as a bolus dose. Dose Titration iPTH level decreased by 50% and more than 300 pg/ml: Dose may be increased by 1-2 mcg at 8-wk intervals as needed. iPTH level 150-300 pg/ml: Maintain the current dose. iPTH level <100 pg/ml: Suspend drug for 1 week and resume at a reduced dose of at least 1 mcg lower. PO Dialysis patients: Titrate dose to lower iPTH to 150-300 pg/ml. Adjust dose at 8-week intervals to a maximum dose of 20 mcg 3 times/week. Initially, if iPTH is more than 400 pg/ml, give 10 mcg 3 times/week at dialysis. Dose titration iPTH level decreased by 50% and more than 300 pg/ml: Increase dose to 12.5 mcg 3 times/week for 8 more weeks. This titration process may continue at 8-wk intervals. Each increase should be by 2.5 mcg/dose. iPTH level 150-300 pg/ml: Maintain current dose. iPTH level less than 100 pg/ml: Suspend drug for 1 week and resume at a reduced dose. Decrease each dose by at least 2.5 mcg. **Secondary hyperparathyroidism, predialysis patients:** PO Titrate dose to lower iPTH to 35-70 pg/ml with stage 3 disease or to 70-110 pg/ml with stage 4 disease. Dose may be adjusted at 2-week intervals with a maximum dose of 3.5 mcg/day. Begin with 1 mcg/day. Dose titration iPTH level more than 70 pg/ml with stage 3 disease or more than 110 pg/ml with stage 4 disease: Increase dose by 0.5 mcg every 2 weeks as needed. iPTH level 35-70 pg/ml with stage 3 disease or 70-110 pg/ml with stage 4 disease: Maintain current dose. iPTH level less than 35 pg/ml with stage 3 disease or less than 70 pg/ml with stage 4 disease: Suspend drug for 1 week, then resume at a reduced dose of at least 0.5 mcg lower.

■ **Contraindications:** Hypercalcemia, malabsorption syndrome, vitamin D toxicity, hypersensitivity to doxercalciferol or other vitamin D analogs

■ **Side Effects**
Occasional
Edema, headache, malaise, dizziness, nausea, vomiting, dyspnea
Rare
Bradycardia, sleep disorder, pruritus, anorexia, constipation

■ **Serious Reactions**
• Early signs of overdosage are manifested as weakness, headache, somnolence, nausea, vomiting, dry mouth, constipation, muscle and bone pain, and metallic taste sensation.
• Later signs of overdosage are evidenced by polyuria, polydipsia, anorexia, weight loss, nocturia, photophobia, rhinorrhea, pruritus, disorientation, hallucinations, hyperthermia, hypertension, and cardiac arrhythmias.

Special Considerations
• Do not take Ca supplements, vitamin D, or Mg-containing antacids

■ **Patient/Family Education**
• Avoid magnesium-containing antacids
• Notify the physician if weakness, loss of appetite, nausea, vomiting, excessive thirst, dry mouth, or muscle or bone pain occurs

■ **Monitoring Parameters**
• iPTH, serum Ca and serum phosphate qwk during titration
• D/C drug if hypercalcemia, hyperphosphatemia, or serum Ca × serum phosphate product >70, resume when parameters decreased, at a dose 2.5 mcg or less
• Urinary Ca, alkaline phosphatase, renal function tests

■ **Geriatric side effects at a glance:**
❑ CNS   ❑ Bowel Dysfunction   ❑ Bladder Dysfunction   ❑ Falls

doxycycline

(dox-i-sye'-kleen)

■ **Brand Name(s):** Adoxa, Atridox, Doryx, Doxy-100, Doxy Caps, Doxychel Hyclate, Mono-dox, Periostat, Vibramycin, Vibra-Tabs
Chemical Class: Tetracycline derivative

■ **Clinical Pharmacology:**
Mechanism of Action: A tetracycline antibacterial that inhibits bacterial protein synthesis by binding to ribosomes. **Therapeutic Effect:** Bacteriostatic.
Pharmacokinetics: Rapidly and almost completely absorbed after PO administration. Protein binding: greater than 90%. Metabolized in liver. Partially excreted in urine; partially eliminated in bile. **Half-life:** 15-24 hr.

■ **Available Forms:**
- *Capsules:* 50 mg (Monodox), 75 mg (Doryx), 100 mg (Doryx, Monodox, Vibramycin).
- *Oral Suspension* (*Vibramycin*): 25 mg/5 ml.
- *Syrup* (*Vibramycin*): 50 mg/5 ml.
- *Tablets:* 20 mg (Periostat), 50 mg (Adoxa), 75 mg (Adoxa), 100 mg (Adoxa, Vibra-Tabs).
- *Injection, Powder for Reconstitution* (*Doxy-100*): 100 mg.

■ **Indications and Dosages:**
Respiratory, skin, and soft-tissue infections; UTIs; pelvic inflammatory disease* (PID); *brucellosis; trachoma; Rocky Mountain spotted fever; typhus; Q fever; rickettsia; severe acne* (Adoxa); *smallpox; psittacosis; ornithosis; granuloma inguinale; lymphogranuloma venereum; intestinal amebiasis* (adjunctive treatment); *prevention of rheumatic fever:
PO Initially, 100 mg q12h, then 100 mg/day as single dose or 50 mg q12h for severe infections. IV Initially, 200 mg as 1-2 infusions; then 100-200 mg/day in 1-2 divided doses.
Acute gonococcal infections: PO Initially, 200 mg, then 100 mg at bedtime on first day; then 100 mg twice a day for 14 days.
Syphilis: PO, IV 200 mg/day in divided doses for 14-28 days.
Traveler's diarrhea: PO 100 mg/day during a period of risk (up to 14 days) and for 2 days after returning home.
Periodontitis: PO 20 mg twice a day.

■ **Unlabeled Uses:** Treatment of atypical mycobacterial infections, gonorrhea, malaria, rheumatoid arthritis; prevention of Lyme disease; prevention or treatment of traveler's diarrhea.

■ **Contraindications:** Hypersensitivity to tetracyclines or sulfites, severe hepatic dysfunction

403

Side Effects

Frequent

Anorexia, nausea, vomiting, diarrhea, dysphagia, possibly severe photosensitivity

Occasional

Rash, urticaria

Serious Reactions

- Superinfection (especially fungal) and benign intracranial hypertension (headache, visual changes) may occur.
- Hepatoxicity, fatty degeneration of the liver, and pancreatitis occur rarely.

Special Considerations

- Tetracycline of choice due to broad spectrum, long t½, superior tissue penetration, and excellent oral absorption
- Individualize treatment based on local susceptibility patterns.

Patient/Family Education

- Do not take with antacids, iron products
- Take with food
- Continue taking doxycycline for the full course of therapy
- Avoid overexposure to sun or ultraviolet light to prevent photosensitivity reactions

Monitoring Parameters

- Skin for rash
- Monitor the patient's LOC because of the potential for benign intracranial hypertension
- Daily bowel activity and stool consistency. Although mild GI effects may be tolerable, severe symptoms may indicate the onset of antibiotic-associated colitis.
- Signs and symptoms of superinfection include abdominal pain or cramping, anal or genital pruritus or discharge, moderate to severe diarrhea, severe mouth or tongue soreness, and new or increased fever.

Geriatric side effects at a glance:

❑ CNS   ☑ Bowel Dysfunction   ❑ Bladder Dysfunction   ❑ Falls

U.S. Regulatory Considerations

❑ FDA Black Box   ❑ OBRA regulated in U.S. Long Term Care

dronabinol

(droe-nab'-i-nol)

Brand Name(s): Marinol
Chemical Class: Cannabinoid derivative

■ **Clinical Pharmacology:**
Mechanism of Action: An antiemetic and GI-appetite stimulant that may act by inhibiting vomiting control mechanisms in the medulla oblongata. **Therapeutic Effect:** Inhibits vomiting and stimulates appetite.
Pharmacokinetics: Well absorbed after PO administration. Protein binding: 97%. Undergoes first-pass metabolism. Is highly lipid soluble. Primarily excreted in feces.
Half-life: 4 hr.

■ **Available Forms:**
- *Capsules (Gelatin [Marinol]):* 2.5 mg, 5 mg, 10 mg.

■ **Indications and Dosages:**
Prevention of chemotherapy-induced nausea and vomiting: PO Initially, 5 mg/m^2 1-3 hr before chemotherapy, then q2-4h after chemotherapy for total of 4-6 doses a day. May increase by 2.5 mg/m^2 up to 15 mg/m^2 per dose.
Appetite stimulant: PO Initially, 2.5 mg twice a day (before lunch and dinner). Range: 2.5-20 mg/day.

■ **Unlabeled Uses:** Postoperative nausea and vomiting

■ **Contraindications:** Treatment of nausea and vomiting not caused by chemotherapy, hypersensitivity to sesame oil or tetrahydrocannabinol products

■ **Side Effects**
Frequent (24%-3%)
Euphoria, dizziness, paranoid reaction, somnolence
Occasional (3%-1%)
Asthenia, ataxia, confusion, abnormal thinking, depersonalization
Rare (less than 1%)
Diarrhea, depression, nightmares, speech difficulties, headache, anxiety, tinnitus, flushed skin

■ **Serious Reactions**
- Mild intoxication may produce increased sensory awareness (including taste, smell, and sound), altered time perception, reddened conjunctiva, dry mouth, and tachycardia.
- Moderate intoxication may produce memory impairment and urine retention.
- Severe intoxication may produce lethargy, decreased motor coordination, slurred speech, and orthostatic hypotension.

Special Considerations
- May have additive sedative or behavioral effects with CNS depressants
- Use caution escalating the dose because of increased frequency of adverse reactions at higher doses

■ **Patient/Family Education**
- Drowsiness usually disappears with continued therapy
- Change positions slowly—from recumbent, to sitting, before standing—to prevent dizziness
- Avoid tasks that require mental alertness or motor skills until response to the drug has been established

- Do not use other medications, including OTC drugs, without consulting the physician
- Avoid alcohol

■ Monitoring Parameters
- Monitor patients with history of psychiatric illness

■ Geriatric side effects at a glance:
☑ CNS ☐ Bowel Dysfunction ☐ Bladder Dysfunction ☐ Falls

■ U.S. Regulatory Considerations
☐ FDA Black Box ☐ OBRA regulated in U.S. Long Term Care

droperidol

(droe-per'-i-dole)

■ Brand Name(s): Inapsine

Combinations
Rx: with fentanyl (Innovar)
Chemical Class: Butyrophenone derivative

■ Clinical Pharmacology:
Mechanism of Action: A general anesthetic and antiemetic agent that antagonizes dopamine neurotransmission at synapses by blocking postsynaptic dopamine receptor sites; partially blocks adrenergic receptor binding sites. *Therapeutic Effect:* Produces tranquilization, antiemetic effect.
Pharmacokinetics: Onset of action occurs within 30 min. Well absorbed. Metabolized in liver. Excreted in urine and feces. *Half-life:* 2.3 hr.

■ Available Forms:
- *Injection:* 2.5 mg/ml (Inapsine).

■ Indications and Dosages:
Preoperative: IM, IV 2.5-10 mg 30-60 min before induction of general anesthesia.
Adjunct for induction of general anesthesia: IV 0.22-0.275 mg/kg.
Adjunct for maintenance of general anesthesia: IV 1.25-2.5 mg.
Diagnostic procedures w/o general anesthesia: IM 2.5-10 mg 30-60 min before procedure. If needed, may give additional doses of 1.25-2.5 mg (usually by IV injection).

■ Contraindications: Known or suspected QT prolongation, hypersensitivity to droperidol or any component of the formulation

■ Side Effects
Frequent
Mild to moderate hypotension

406

Occasional

Tachycardia, postop drowsiness, dizziness, chills, shivering

Rare

Postop nightmares, facial sweating, bronchospasm

- **Serious Reactions**
  - Extrapyramidal symptoms may appear as akathisia (motor restlessness) and dystonias: torticollis (neck muscle spasm), opisthotonos (rigidity of back muscles), and oculogyric crisis (rolling back of eyes).
  - Overdosage includes symptoms of hypotension, tachycardia, hallucinations, and extrapyramidal symptoms.
  - Prolonged QT interval, seizures, and arrhythmias have been reported.

- **Patient/Family Education**
  - Change positions slowly to avoid orthostatic hypotension
  - Avoid tasks that require mental alertness or motor skills until response to the drug is established

- **Monitoring Parameters**
  - QT prolongation has occurred in patients with no known CV disease and with doses at or below recommended doses; reserve use for patients who fail to show response to other adequate treatments
  - Baseline ECG, blood pressure, heart rate, respiratory rate; if QT >440 msec for males or >450 msec for females, do not use droperidol
  - Therapeutic response from anxiety
  - Monitor for extrapyramidal symptoms

- **Geriatric side effects at a glance:**
  ☑ CNS ☑ Bowel Dysfunction ☐ Bladder Dysfunction ☑ Falls
  Other: Orthostatic hypotension, cardiac conduction disturbances, anticholinergic side effects.

- **Use with caution in older patients with:** Parkinson's disease (an atypical antipsychotic is recommended), seizure disorders, cardiovascular disease with conduction disturbance, hepatic encephalopathy, narrow-angle glaucoma, congenital prolonged Q-T syndrome or drugs which prolong Q-T interval, drugs which inhibit or utilize 26D substrate of cytochrome P450.

- **U.S. Regulatory Considerations**
  ☑ FDA Black Box
  - QT prolongation/torsades de pointes at usual doses
  - For refractory disease only
  ☑ OBRA regulated in U.S. Long Term Care

- **Other Uses in Geriatric Patient:** Management of agitation secondary to delirium, antiemetic

- **Side Effects:**
  Of particular importance in the geriatric patient: Tardive dyskinesia, akathisia (may appear to exacerbate behavioral disturbances), anticholinergic effects, may increase risk of sudden death

- **Geriatric Considerations - Summary:** Droperidol may be useful in the management of severly agitated older adults. It may be faster acting than haloperidol, and may cause less respiratory depression than some benzodiazepines, but is associated with a higher risk of hypotension. Because this agent has been associated (in high doses) with torsades de pointes, we recommend checking an ECG (for QT interval) prior to administration of droperidol.

- **References:**
  1. Knott JC, Taylor DM, Castle DJ. Randomized clinical trial comparing intravenous midazolam and droperidol for sedation of the acutely agitated patient in the emergency department. Ann Emerg Med 2006;47:61-67.
  2. Martel M, Sterzinger A, Miner J, et al. Management of acute undifferentiated agitation in the emergency department: a randomized double-blind trial of droperidol, ziprasidone, and midazolam. Acad Emerg Med 2005;12:1167-1172.

drotrecogin alfa

(droe-tre-koe'-jin al'-fa)

- **Brand Name(s):** Xigris
  Chemical Class: Glycoprotein

- **Clinical Pharmacology:**
  Mechanism of Action: A recombinant form of human-activated protein C that exerts an antithrombotic effect by inhibiting Factors Va and VIIIa and may exert an indirect profibrinolytic effect by inhibiting plasminogen activator inhibitor-1 and limiting the generation of activated thrombin-activatable-fibrinolysis-inhibitor. The drug may also exert an anti-inflammatory effect by inhibiting tumor necrosis factor (TNF) production by monocytes, by blocking leukocyte adhesion to selectins, and by limiting thrombin-induced inflammatory responses. **Therapeutic Effect:** Produces anti-inflammatory, antithrombotic, and profibrinolytic effects.
  Pharmacokinetics: Inactivated by endogenous plasma protease inhibitors. Clearance occurs within 2 hr of initiating infusion. **Half-life:** 1.6 hr.

- **Available Forms:**
  - *Powder for Infusion*: 5 mg, 20 mg.

- **Indications and Dosages:**
  Severe sepsis: IV Infusion 24 mcg/kg/hr for 96 hr. Immediately stop infusion if clinically significant bleeding is identified

- **Contraindications:** Active internal bleeding, evidence of cerebral herniation, intracranial neoplasm or mass lesion, presence of an epidural catheter, recent (within the past 3 mo) hemorrhagic stroke, recent (within the past 2 mo) intracranial or intraspinal surgery or severe head trauma, trauma with an increased risk of life-threatening bleeding

- **Side Effects**
  None known.

- **Serious Reactions**
  - Bleeding (intrathoracic, retroperitoneal, GI, GU, intra-abdominal, intracranial) occurs in about 2% of patients.

Special Considerations

- The efficacy of drotrecogin alfa was studied in an international, multicenter, randomized, double-blind, placebo-controlled trial (PROWESS) of 1690 patients with severe sepsis (Bernard GR, et al. Efficacy and safety of recombinant human activated protein C for severe sepsis. N Engl J Med. 2001;344:699-709); entry criteria included a systemic inflammatory response presumed due to infection and at least one associated acute organ dysfunction; acute organ dysfunction was defined as one of the following: cardiovascular dysfunction (shock, hypotension, or the need for vasopressor support despite adequate fluid resuscitation); respiratory dysfunction [relative hypoxemia (PaO_2/FiO_2 ratio <250); renal dysfunction (oliguria despite adequate fluid resuscitation); thrombocytopenia (platelet count <80,000/mm^3 or 50% decrease from the highest value the previous 3 days); or metabolic acidosis with elevated lactic acid concentrations
- The primary efficacy endpoint was all-cause mortality assessed 28 days after the start of study drug administration; prospectively defined subsets for mortality analyses included groups defined by APACHE II score (a score designed to assess risk of mortality based on acute physiology and chronic health evaluation, see http://www.sfar.org/scores2/scores2.html); the APACHE II score was calculated from physiologic and laboratory data obtained within the 24-hr period immediately preceding the start of study drug administration irrespective of the preceding length of stay in the intensive care unit; the study was terminated after a planned interim analysis due to significantly decreased mortality in patients on drotrecogin alfa than in patients on placebo (210/850, 25% vs 259/840, 31% p=0.005); the observed mortality difference between drotrecogin alfa and placebo was limited to the half of patients with higher risk of death, i.e., APACHE II score >25, the third and fourth quartile APACHE II scores (mortality 31% with treatment, 44% with placebo); the efficacy of drotrecogin alfa has not been established in patients with lower risk of death, e.g., APACHE II score <25

- **Patient/Family Education**
  - Inform the patient that bleeding may occur for up to 28 days after treatment; warn the patient to immediately notify the physician if signs or symptoms of unusual bleeding occur

- **Monitoring Parameters**
  - CBC with platelets, INR
  - Monitor the patient closely for hemorrhagic complications

- **Geriatric side effects at a glance:**
  - ❑ CNS   ❑ Bowel Dysfunction   ❑ Bladder Dysfunction   ❑ Falls

- **U.S. Regulatory Considerations**
  - ❑ FDA Black Box   ❑ OBRA regulated in U.S. Long Term Care

duloxetine hydrochloride

(du-lox'-uh-teen hye-droe-klor'-ide)

■ **Brand Name(s):** Cymbalta
  Chemical Class: Aryloxypropylamine

■ **Clinical Pharmacology:**
  Mechanism of Action: An antidepressant that appears to inhibit serotonin and nor-epinephrine reuptake at CNS neuronal presynaptic membranes; is a less potent inhibitor of dopamine reuptake. **Therapeutic Effect:** Relieves depression.
  Pharmacokinetics: Well absorbed from the GI tract. Protein binding: greater than 90%. Extensively metabolized to active metabolites. Excreted primarily in urine and, to a lesser extent, in feces. **Half-life:** 8-17 hr.

■ **Available Forms:**
  • *Capsules:* 20 mg, 30 mg, 60 mg.

■ **Indications and Dosages:**
  Major depressive disorder: PO 20 mg twice a day, increased up to 60 mg/day as a single dose or in 2 divided doses.
  Diabetic neuropathy pain: PO 60 mg once a day.

■ **Unlabeled Uses:** Treatment of chronic pain syndromes, fibromyalgia, stress incontinence, urinary incontinence

■ **Contraindications:** End-stage renal disease (creatinine clearance less than 30 ml/min), severe hepatic impairment, uncontrolled angle-closure glaucoma, use within 14 days of MAOIs

■ **Side Effects**
  Frequent (20%-11%)
  Nausea, dry mouth, constipation, insomnia
  Occasional (9%-5%)
  Dizziness, fatigue, diarrhea, somnolence, anorexia, diaphoresis, vomiting
  Rare (4%-2%)
  Blurred vision, erectile dysfunction, delayed or failed ejaculation, anorgasmia, anxiety, decreased libido, hot flashes

■ **Serious Reactions**
  • Duloxetine use may slightly increase the patient's heart rate.
  • Colitis, dysphagia, gastritis, and irritable bowel syndrome occur rarely.

Special Considerations
  • Place in therapy: Similar to venlafaxine, with less risk of increased blood pressure; alternative in major depression in poor responders to other agents; at least as effective as tricyclics, but with lower toxicity; more efficacious than SSRIs

■ **Patient/Family Education**
  • Therapeutic response may take 4-6 wk; be alert for emergence of anxiety, agitation, panic, mania, or worsening of depressive state

- Do not abruptly discontinue duloxetine
- Avoid tasks that require mental alertness or motor skills until response to the drug has been established
- Do not consume large amounts of alcohol to prevent liver damage

■ Monitoring Parameters
- *Efficacy*: resolution/improvement in symptoms of depression
- *Toxicity*: blood pressure and pulse in patients prior to initiating treatment and periodically thereafter; Signs of toxicity: somnolence, sleep disturbances, persistent GI symptoms
- Liver function test results for patients on long-term duloxetine therapy

■ Geriatric side effects at a glance:
☐ CNS   ☑ Bowel Dysfunction   ☐ Bladder Dysfunction   ☑ Falls

■ Use with caution in older patients with: Narrow-angle glaucoma, patients prone to urinary retention (e.g., prostatic hypertrophy)

■ U.S. Regulatory Considerations
☑ FDA Black Box
- Because there is an increased risk of suicide in children and adolescents, older adults should also be closely monitored for suicide ideation.
☐ OBRA regulated in U.S. Long Term Care

■ Other Uses in Geriatric Patient: Anxiety symptoms and related disorders, stress urinary incontinence

■ Side Effects:
Of particular importance in the geriatric patient: Although not well docuemented, other agents with serotonergic activity have been associated with hyponatremia and withdrawal symptoms when abruptly discontinued (e.g., during hospitalization) rather than tapered.

■ Geriatric Considerations - Summary: Compared to placebo, duloxetine is effective for the treatent of depression and painful diabetic neuropathy. Few head-to-head studies are available comparing duloxetine to other agents in the treatment of depression or painful neuropathy. Because this agent may increase urethral sphincter activity, it is now being assessed as an agent for the treatment of stress urinary incontinence. This same property may increase the risk of urinary retention, although this has not been well documented. Duloxetine has not been well studied with respect to falls.

■ References:
1. Kirwin JL, Goren JL. Duloxetine: a dual serotonin-norepinephrine reuptake inhibitor for treatment of major depressive disorder. Pharmacotherapy 2005;25:396-410.
2. Schuessler B, Baessler K. Pharmacologic treatment of stress urinary incontinence: expectations for outcome. Urology 2003;62:31-38.
3. Goldstein DJ, Lu Y, Detke MJ, et al. Duloxetine vs. placebo in patients with painful diabetic neuropathy. Pain 2005;116:109-118.

dyphylline

(dye'-fi-lin)

■ **Brand Name(s):** Dilor, Lufyllin

Combinations
Rx: with guaifenesin (Dilex-G, Dilor-G, Lufyllin-GG); with ephedrine, guaifenesin, phenobarbital (Lufyllin-EPG)
Chemical Class: Xanthine derivative

■ **Clinical Pharmacology:**
Mechanism of Action: A xanthine derivative that acts as a bronchodilator by directly relaxing smooth muscle of the bronchial airway and pulmonary blood vessels similar to theophylline. ***Therapeutic Effect:*** Relieves bronchospasm, increases vital capacity, produces cardiac, and skeletal muscle stimulation.
Pharmacokinetics: Rapid absorption after PO administration. Excreted in urine. ***Half-life:*** 2 hr.

■ **Available Forms:**
- *Elixir:* 100 mg/15 ml (Lufyllin).
- *Injection:* 250 mg/ml (Dilor).
- *Tablet:* 200 mg, 400 mg (Dilor, Lufyllin).

■ **Indications and Dosages:**
Chronic bronchospasm, asthma: PO 15 mg/kg 4 times/day. IM 250-500 mg. Maximum: 15 mg/kg q6h.
Dosage in renal impairment:

Creatinine Clearance	Dosage Percent
50-80 ml/min	Administer 75% of dose
10-50 ml/min	Administer 50% of dose
<10 ml/min	Administer 25% of dose

■ **Contraindications:** Uncontrolled arrhythmias, hyperthyroidism, history of hypersensitivity to dyphylline, related xanthine derivatives, or any component of the formulation

■ **Side Effects**
Frequent
Tachycardia, nervousness, restlessness
Occasional
Heartburn, vomiting, headache, mild diuresis, insomnia, nausea

■ **Serious Reactions**
- Ventricular arrhythmias, hypotension, circulatory failure, seizures, hyperglycemia, and syndrome of inappropriate antidiuretic hormone (SIADH) have been reported.

Special Considerations
- Though better tolerated, significantly less bronchodilating activity vs theophylline. Serious dosing errors possible if dyphylline monitored with theophylline serum assays

Monitoring Parameters
- Minimal effective serum concentration 12 mcg/ml
- Signs of clinical improvement such as cessation of clavicular retractions, quieter and slower respirations, and a relaxed facial expression
- Examine the patient's lips and fingernails for evidence of oxygen depletion such as blue or gray lips, blue or dusky colored fingernails in light-skinned patients, and gray fingernails in dark-skinned patients

Geriatric side effects at a glance:
☑ CNS   ☐ Bowel Dysfunction   ☐ Bladder Dysfunction   ☐ Falls

U.S. Regulatory Considerations
☐ FDA Black Box   ☑ OBRA regulated in U.S. Long Term Care

econazole nitrate

(e-kone'-a-zole nye'-trate)

Brand Name(s): Spectazole
Chemical Class: Imidazole derivative

Clinical Pharmacology:
Mechanism of Action: An imidazole derivative that changes the permeability of the fungal cell wall. **Therapeutic Effect:** Inhibits fungal biosynthesis of triglycerides, phospholipids. Fungistatic.
Pharmacokinetics: Low systemic absorption. Protein binding: 98%. Metabolized in liver to more than 20 metabolites. Primarily excreted in urine; minimal excretion in feces. Not removed by hemodialysis.

Available Forms:
- *Cream*: 1% (Spectazole).

Indications and Dosages:
Treatment of tinea pedis, tinea cruris, tinea corporis, tinea versicolor: Topical Apply once daily to affected area for 2-4 wk.

Unlabeled Uses: Cutaneous candidiasis, otomycosis

Contraindications: Hypersensitivity to econazole

Side Effects
Occasional (10%-1%)
Vulvar/vaginal burning
Rare (less than 1%)
Itching and burning of sexual partner, polyuria, vulvar itching, soreness, edema, discharge

413

Serious Reactions
- None known.

Patient/Family Education
- For external use only; avoid contact with eyes; cleanse skin with soap and water and dry thoroughly prior to application
- Use medication for full treatment time outlined by clinician, even though symptoms may have improved
- Notify clinician if no improvement after 2 wk (jock itch, ringworm) or 4 wk (athlete's foot)

Monitoring Parameters
- Evaluate the patient's skin for itching, irritation, or rash

Geriatric side effects at a glance:
❑ CNS   ❑ Bowel Dysfunction   ❑ Bladder Dysfunction   ❑ Falls

U.S. Regulatory Considerations
❑ FDA Black Box   ❑ OBRA regulated in U.S. Long Term Care

edetate calcium disodium (calcium EDTA)

(ed'-eh-tate kal'-see-um dye-soe'-dee-um)

■ **Brand Name(s):** Calcium Disodium Versenate
Chemical Class: Chelating agent

■ **Clinical Pharmacology:**
Mechanism of Action: A chelating agent that reduces blood concentration of heavy metals, especially lead, forming stable complexes. **Therapeutic Effect:** Allows heavy metal excretion in urine.
Pharmacokinetics: Well absorbed after parenteral administration; poorly absorbed from the gastrointestinal (GI) tract. Penetrates to extracellular fluid and slowly diffuses into cerebrospinal fluid (CSF). No metabolism occurs. Excreted in the urine either unchanged or as the metal chelates. **Half-life:** 20-60 min (IV), 1.5 hr (IM).

■ **Available Forms:**
- *Injection*: 200 mg/ml (Calcium Disodium Versenate).

■ **Indications and Dosages:**
Diagnosis of lead poisoning: IM, IV 500 mg/m². Maximum: 1 g/m²/day divided in equal doses 8-12 hr apart for 5 days, skip 2-4 days and repeat course if needed.

Lead poisoning (without encephalopathy): IM/IV 1-1.5 g/m² daily for 3-5 days (if blood lead concentration >100 mcg/dl, calcium edetate usually given with dimercaprol.) Allow at least 2-4 days, up to 2-3 wk between courses of therapy. Patients should not be given more than 2 courses of therapy.

Lead poisoning (with encephalopathy): IM Initially, dimercaprol 4 mg/kg; then give dimercaprol 4 mg/kg and calcium EDTA 250 mg/m²; then 4 hr later and q4h for 5 days.

■ **Contraindications:** Anuria, severe renal disease, hypersensitivity to EDTA or any component of the formulation

■ **Side Effects**
Frequent
Chills, fever, anorexia, headache, histamine-like reaction (sneezing, stuffy nose, watery eyes), decreased BP, nausea, vomiting, thrombophlebitis
Rare
Frequent urination, secondary gout (severe pain in feet, knees, elbows).

■ **Serious Reactions**
• Drug may produce same signs of renal damage as severe acute lead poisoning (proteinuria, microscopic hematuria). Transient anemia/bone marrow depression, hypercalcemia (constipation, drowsiness, dry mouth, metallic taste) occurs occasionally.

■ **Patient/Family Education**
• Notify clinician immediately if no urine output in a 12-hr period

■ **Monitoring Parameters**
• Urinalysis and urine sediment daily during therapy to detect signs of progressive renal tubular damage
• Renal function tests, liver function tests, and serum electrolytes before and periodically during therapy
• ECG during IV therapy
• BUN

■ **Geriatric side effects at a glance:**
❑ CNS   ❑ Bowel Dysfunction   ❑ Bladder Dysfunction   ❑ Falls

■ **U.S. Regulatory Considerations**
☑ FDA Black Box
Increased intracranial pressure when administered intravenously
❑ OBRA regulated in U.S. Long Term Care

edetate disodium

(ed'-eh-tate dye-soe'-dee-um)

- **Brand Name(s):** Disotate, Endrate
  Chemical Class: Chelating agent

- **Clinical Pharmacology:**
  Mechanism of Action: A chelating agent that forms a soluble chelate with calcium, resulting in rapid decrease in plasma calcium concentrations. **Therapeutic Effect:** Allows calcium to be excreted in urine.
  Pharmacokinetics: Distributed in extracellular fluid and does not appear in red blood cells. No metabolism occurs. Rapidly excreted in the urine. **Half-life:** 1.4-3 hr.

- **Available Forms:**
  - Injection: 150 mg/ml (Disotate, Endrate).

- **Indications and Dosages:**
  Digitalis toxicity, hypercalcemia: IV 500 mg/kg/day over 3 hr or more, daily for 5 days, skip 2 days, repeat as needed up to 15 doses. Maximum: 3 g/day.

- **Contraindications:** Anuria, renal impairment, hypersensitivity to EDTA or any component of the formulation

- **Side Effects**
  Frequent
  Abdominal cramps or pain, diarrhea, nausea, vomiting, circumoral paresthesia, headache, numbness, postural hypotension
  Rare
  Exfoliative dermatitis, toxic skin and mucous membrane reactions, thrombophlebitis (at injection site)

- **Serious Reactions**
  - Nephrotoxicity may occur with excessive dosages.
  - Hypomagnesemia may occur with prolonged use.

Special Considerations
  - Have patient remain supine for a short time after INF due to the possibility of orthostatic hypotension
  - Additives may be incompatible with the reconstituted (diluted) solution required for IV infusion

- **Monitoring Parameters**
  - ECG, blood pressure during INF
  - Renal function before and during therapy
  - Serum calcium, magnesium, potassium levels
  - BUN

- **Geriatric side effects at a glance:**
  - ❏ CNS   ❏ Bowel Dysfunction   ❏ Bladder Dysfunction   ❏ Falls

- **U.S. Regulatory Considerations**
  - ☑ FDA Black Box
  - Increased intracranial pressure when administered intravenously
  - ❏ OBRA regulated in U.S. Long Term Care

edrophonium chloride

(ed-roe-foe'-nee-um klor'-ide)

- **Brand Name(s):** Enlon, Reversol, Tensilon

  Combinations
  Rx: with atropine (Enlon-Plus)
  Chemical Class: Cholinesterase inhibitor; quaternary ammonium derivative

- **Clinical Pharmacology:**
  Mechanism of Action: A parasympathetic, anticholinesterase agent that inhibits destruction of acetylcholine by acetylcholinesterase, thus causing accumulation of acetylcholine at cholinergic synapses. Results in an increase in cholinergic responses such as miosis, increased tonus of intestinal and skeletal muscles, bronchial and ureteral constriction, bradycardia, and increased salivary and sweat gland secretions.
  Therapeutic Effect: Diagnosis of myasthenia gravis.
  Pharmacokinetics: Onset of action occurs within 30-60 sec and has duration of 10 min. Rapid absorption after IV administration. Exact method of metabolism is unknown. Rapidly excreted in urine. **Half-life:** 1.8 hr.

- **Available Forms:**
  - Injection: 10 mg/ml (Enlon, Reversol, Tensilon).

- **Indications and Dosages:**
  Diagnosis of myasthenia gravis: IV 2-mg test dose over 15-30 sec. If no reaction in 45 sec, give additional dose of 8 mg. Test dose may be repeated after 30 min. IM/SC Initially, 10 mg as a single dose. If no cholinergic reaction occurs, give 2 mg 30 minutes later to rule out false-negative reaction.
  Neuromuscular blockade antagonism: IV 10 mg over 30-45 sec. May be repeated as needed until a cholinergic response is detected. Maximum: 40 mg.
  Dosage in renal impairment: Dose may need to be reduced in patients with chronic renal failure.

- **Contraindications:** Gastrointestinal (GI) or genitourinary (GU) obstruction, hypersensitivity to edrophonium, sulfites, or any component of the formulation

- **Side Effects**
  Frequent
  Increase salivation, intestinal secretions, lacrimation, urinary urgency, hyperperistalsis, sweating

Occasional
Bradycardia, hypotension, convulsions, dysphagia, nausea, vomiting, diarrhea
Rare
Bronchoconstriction, cardiac arrest, central respiratory paralysis

- **Serious Reactions**
  - Overdosage causes symptoms of cholinergic crisis such as muscle weakness, nausea, vomiting, miosis, bronchospasm, and respiratory paralysis.

Special Considerations

  - Since symptoms of anticholinesterase overdose (cholinergic crisis) may mimic underdosage (myasthenic weakness), their condition may be worsened by the use of this drug

- **Patient/Family Education**
  - Notify the physician or health care advisor of difficulty breathing, dizziness, muscle cramps and spasms, or vomiting
  - Side effects of the drug should not last long because the effects of the drug are short-lived

- **Monitoring Parameters**
  - Preinjection and postinjection strength
  - Heart rate, respiratory rate, blood pressure

- **Geriatric side effects at a glance:**
  ☐ CNS ☐ Bowel Dysfunction ☐ Bladder Dysfunction ☐ Falls

- **U.S. Regulatory Considerations**
  ☐ FDA Black Box ☐ OBRA regulated in U.S. Long Term Care

efalizumab

(e-fa-li-zoo'-mab)

- **Brand Name(s):** Raptiva
  Chemical Class: Monoclonal antibody

- **Clinical Pharmacology:**
  Mechanism of Action: A monoclonal antibody that interferes with lymphocyte activation by binding to the lymphocyte antigen, inhibiting the adhesion of leukocytes to other cell types. **Therapeutic Effect:** Prevents the release of cytokines and the growth and migration of circulating total lymphocytes, predominant in psoriatic lesions.
  Pharmacokinetics: Clearance is affected by body weight, not by gender or race, after subcutaneous injection. Serum concentration reaches steady state at 4 wk. Mean time to elimination: 25 days.

■ Available Forms:
- *Powder for Injection*: 150 mg, designed to deliver 125 mg/1.25 ml.

■ Indications and Dosages:
Psoriasis: Subcutaneous Initially, 0.7 mg/kg followed by weekly doses of 1 mg/kg. Maximum: 200 mg (single dose).

■ Contraindications: Concurrent use of immunosuppressive agents, hypersensitivity to any murine or humanized monoclonal antibody preparation

■ Side Effects
Frequent (32%–10%)
Headache, chills, nausea, injection site pain
Occasional (8%–7%)
Myalgia, flu-like symptoms, fever
Rare (4%)
Back pain, acne

■ Serious Reactions
- Hypersensitivity reaction, malignancies, serious infections (abscess, cellulitis, postoperative wound infection, pneumonia), thrombocytopenia, and worsening of psoriasis occur rarely.

Special Considerations
- Evaluate for latent tuberculosis infection with a tuberculin skin test before initiation of therapy

■ Patient/Family Education
- Intended for use under the guidance and supervision of clinician; patients may self-inject if appropriate and with medical follow-up, after proper training in injection technique, including proper syringe and needle disposal
- Efalizumab treatment increases the risk of developing an infection
- Notify the health care provider if bleeding from the gums, bruising or petechiae of the skin, or signs of infection occur
- Do not undergo phototherapy treatments

■ Monitoring Parameters
- **Efficacy:** Improvement of clinical signs/symptoms of psoriasis (e.g., itching, redness, scaling, psoriatic body surface area coverage); PASI scores are based on plaque thickness, scaling, and redness, adjusted for percentage of affected body surface area; quality of life assessments
- **Toxicity:** CBC with differential periodically, particularly platelets; vital signs in patients with a history of hypersensitivity to any medication (first injection); temperature periodically (infection)

■ Geriatric side effects at a glance:
❑ CNS   ❑ Bowel Dysfunction   ❑ Bladder Dysfunction   ❑ Falls

■ U.S. Regulatory Considerations
❑ FDA Black Box   ❑ OBRA regulated in U.S. Long Term Care

efavirenz

(e-fa-veer'-ens)

- **Brand Name(s):** Sustiva
  Chemical Class: Benzoxazinone, substituted; non-nucleoside reverse transcriptase inhibitor

- **Clinical Pharmacology:**
  Mechanism of Action: A non-nucleoside reverse transcriptase inhibitor that inhibits the activity of HIV reverse transcriptase of HIV-1 and the transcription of HIV-1 RNA to DNA. **Therapeutic Effect:** Interrupts HIV replication, slowing the progression of HIV infection.
  Pharmacokinetics: Rapidly absorbed after PO administration. Protein binding: 99%. Metabolized to major isoenzymes in the liver. Eliminated in urine and feces. **Half-life:** 40-55 hr.

- **Available Forms:**
  - *Capsules:* 50 mg, 100 mg, 200 mg.
  - *Tablets:* 600 mg.

- **Indications and Dosages:**
  HIV infection (in combination with other ID-antiretrovirals): PO 600 mg once a day at bedtime.

- **Contraindications:** Concurrent use with ergot derivatives, midazolam, or triazolam; efavirenz as monotherapy

- **Side Effects**
  Frequent (52%)
  Mild to severe: Dizziness, vivid dreams, insomnia, confusion, impaired concentration, amnesia, agitation, depersonalization, hallucinations, euphoria, somnolence (mild symptoms don't interfere with daily activities; severe symptoms interrupt daily activities)
  Occasional
  Mild to moderate: Maculopapular rash (27%); nausea, fatigue, headache, diarrhea, fever, cough (less than 26%) (moderate symptoms may interfere with daily activities)

- **Serious Reactions**
  - Serious psychiatric adverse experiences (aggressive reactions, agitation, delusions, emotional lability, mania, neurosis, paranoia, psychosis, suicide) have been reported.

Special Considerations
  - Always check updated treatment guidelines before initiating or changing antiretroviral therapy. (http://AIDSinfo.nih.gov)

- **Patient/Family Education**
  - May be taken without regard for meals; absorption increased by a high-fat meal, which should be avoided

- Take at bedtime for first 2-4 wk of therapy; may continue at bedtime if desired
- Use caution in driving or other activities requiring alertness
- Avoid alcohol ingestion
- CNS and psychological side effects, such as delusions, depression, dizziness, and impaired concentration, occur in more than half of patients taking this drug; notify the physician if these symptoms continue or become problematic

■ Monitoring Parameters
- ALT, AST, CBC, cholesterol, triglycerides
- Monitor the patient for adverse CNS and psychological effects, such as abnormal dreams, dizziness, impaired concentration, insomnia, severe acute depression (including suicidal ideation or attempts), and somnolence. Be aware that insomnia may begin during the first or second day of therapy and generally resolves in 2-4 wk
- Assess skin for rash

■ Geriatric side effects at a glance:
❑ CNS ❑ Bowel Dysfunction ❑ Bladder Dysfunction ❑ Falls

■ U.S. Regulatory Considerations
❑ FDA Black Box ❑ OBRA regulated in U.S. Long Term Care

eflornithine

(ee-flor'-ni-theen)

■ Brand Name(s): Vaniqa
Chemical Class: Ornithine decarboxylase inhibitor

■ Clinical Pharmacology:
Mechanism of Action: A topical antiprotozoal that inhibits ornithine decarboxylase cell division and synthetic function in the skin. **Therapeutic Effect:** Reduces rate of hair growth.
Pharmacokinetics: Absorption is less than 1% from intact skin. Not metabolized. Primarily excreted as unchanged drug in urine. **Half life:** 8 hr.

■ Available Forms:
- Cream: 13.9% (Vaniqa).

■ Indications and Dosages:
For reduction of unwanted facial hair in women: Topical Apply thin layer to affected area of face and adjacent involved areas under chin; rub in thoroughly. Use twice daily at least 8 hr apart. Do not wash area for at least 4 hr.

■ Contraindications: Hypersensitivity to eflornithine or any component of the formulation

Side Effects

Frequent

Acne

Occasional

Headache, stinging/burning skin, dry skin, pruritus, erythema

Rare

Tingling skin, rash, dyspepsia (heartburn, GI distress)

Serious Reactions

- Bleeding skin, cheilitis, contact dermatitis, herpes simplex, lip swelling, nausea, numbness, rosacea, and weakness have been reported.

Special Considerations

- The most frequent, serious, toxic effect of eflornithine is myelosuppression, which may be unavoidable if successful treatment is to be completed; decisions to modify dosage or to interrupt or cease treatment depend on the severity of the observed adverse event(s) and the availability of support facilities

Patient/Family Education

- Take for the full length of treatment
- Notify the physician of rash, skin irritation, or intolerance

Monitoring Parameters

- Serial audiograms if feasible
- CBC with platelets before and twice weekly during therapy and qwk after completion of therapy until hematologic values return to baseline levels
- Follow-up for at least 24 mo is advised to ensure further therapy should relapses occur

Geriatric side effects at a glance:

❑ CNS   ❑ Bowel Dysfunction   ❑ Bladder Dysfunction   ❑ Falls

U.S. Regulatory Considerations

❑ FDA Black Box   ❑ OBRA regulated in U.S. Long Term Care

eletriptan

(el-ih-trip'-tan)

Brand Name(s): Relpax

Chemical Class: Serotonin derivative

Clinical Pharmacology:

Mechanism of Action: A serotonin receptor agonist that binds selectively to vascular receptors, producing a vasoconstrictive effect on cranial blood vessels. **Therapeutic Effect:** Relieves migraine headache.

Pharmacokinetics: Well absorbed after PO administration. Metabolized by the liver to inactive metabolite. Eliminated in urine. **Half-life:** 4.4 hr (increased in hepatic impairment and the elderly (older than 65 yr).

■ **Available Forms:**
  • *Tablets*: 20 mg, 40 mg.

■ **Indications and Dosages:**
  Acute migraine headache: PO 20-40 mg. If headache improves but then returns, dose may be repeated after 2 hr. Maximum: 80 mg/day.

■ **Contraindications:** Arrhythmias associated with conduction disorders, cerebrovascular syndrome including strokes and transient ischemic attacks (TIAs), coronary artery disease, hemiplegic or basilar migraine, ischemic heart disease, peripheral vascular disease including ischemic bowel disease, severe hepatic impairment, uncontrolled hypertension, use within 24 hr of treatment with another 5-HT$_1$ agonist, an ergotamine-containing or ergot-type medication such as dihydroergotamine (DHE) or methysergide

■ **Side Effects**
  Occasional (6%-5%)
  Dizziness, somnolence, asthenia, nausea
  Rare (3%-2%)
  Paresthesia, headache, dry mouth, warm or hot sensation, dyspepsia, dysphagia

■ **Serious Reactions**
  • Cardiac reactions (including ischemia, coronary artery vasospasm, and MI) and noncardiac vasospasm-related reactions (such as hemorrhage and cerebrovascular accident [CVA]) occur rarely, particularly in patients with hypertension, diabetes, or a strong family history of coronary artery disease; obese patients; smokers.

Special Considerations
  • First dose should be administered under medical supervision, particularly in patients with risk factors for coronary artery disease

■ **Patient/Family Education**
  • Use for treatment of migraines, not prophylaxis
  • Swallow the tablets whole, do not crush or break them
  • Take a single dose of eletriptan as soon as migraine symptoms appear
  • Avoid tasks that require mental alertness or motor skills until response to the drug has been established
  • Notify the physician immediately if palpitations, pain or tightness in the chest or throat, pain or weakness in the extremities, or sudden or severe abdominal pain occurs
  • Lie down in a dark, quiet room for additional benefit after taking eletriptan

■ **Monitoring Parameters**
  • *Efficacy*: Headache response 1-4 hr after a dose (reduction from moderate or severe pain to minimal or no pain); headache recurrence within 24 hr
  • *Toxicity*: Vital signs (pulse, blood pressure), electrocardiogram, particularly in patient with coronary artery disease risk factors

- **Geriatric side effects at a glance:**
  - ☐ CNS   ☐ Bowel Dysfunction   ☐ Bladder Dysfunction   ☐ Falls

- **U.S. Regulatory Considerations**
  - ☐ FDA Black Box   ☐ OBRA regulated in U.S. Long Term Care

emtricitabine

(em-tri-sit'-uh-bean)

- **Brand Name(s):** Emtriva

  Combinations
  Rx: with tenofovir (Truvada)
  Chemical Class: Nucleoside analog

- **Clinical Pharmacology:**
  Mechanism of Action: An antiretroviral that inhibits HIV-1 reverse transcriptase by incorporating itself into viral DNA, resulting in chain termination. **Therapeutic Effect:** Interrupts HIV replication, slowing the progression of HIV infection.
  Pharmacokinetics: Rapidly and extensively absorbed from the GI tract. Excreted primarily in urine (86%) and, to a lesser extent, in feces (14%); 30% removed by hemodialysis. Unknown if removed by peritoneal dialysis. **Half-life:** 10 hr.

- **Available Forms:**
  - *Capsules*: 200 mg.

- **Indications and Dosages:**
  HIV infection (in combination with other antiretrovirals): PO 200 mg once a day.
  Dosage in renal impairment: Dosage and frequency are modified based on creatinine clearance.

Creatinine Clearance	Dosage
30-49 ml/min	200 mg q48h
15-29 ml/min	200 mg q72h
less than 15 ml/min, hemodialysis patients	200 mg q96h

- **Contraindications:** None known.

- **Side Effects**
  Frequent (23%-13%)
  Headache, rhinitis, rash, diarrhea, nausea
  Occasional (14%-4%)
  Cough, vomiting, abdominal pain, insomnia, depression, paresthesia, dizziness, peripheral neuropathy, dyspepsia, myalgia
  Rare (3%-2%)
  Arthralgia, abnormal dreams

424

- **Serious Reactions**
  - Lactic acidosis and hepatomegaly with steatosis occur rarely and may be severe.

Special Considerations

- Current treatment guidelines use emtricitabine as an alternative to lamivudine in the nucleoside reverse transcriptase "backbone" that is part of combination antiretroviral therapy; it has no known advantages over lamivudine
- Reduced susceptibility to emtricitabine is associated with HIV reverse transcriptase gene mutation M184V/I
- Always check updated treatment guidelines before initiating or changing antiretroviral therapy (http://AIDSinfo.nih.gov)

- **Patient/Family Education**
  - Success of an antiretroviral regimen requires >95% adherence to dosing schedule
  - Emtricitabine use may cause a redistribution of body fat
  - Continue taking the drug for the full course of treatment
  - Emtricitabine is not a cure for HIV infection, nor does it reduce the risk of transmitting HIV to others

- **Monitoring Parameters**
  - CBC, renal function, ALT, AST, triglycerides, HIV RNA, CD4 count
  - Daily pattern of bowel activity and stool consistency
  - Skin for rash and urticaria

- **Geriatric side effects at a glance:**
  ☐ CNS ☑ Bowel Dysfunction ☐ Bladder Dysfunction ☐ Falls

- **U.S. Regulatory Considerations**
  ☑ FDA Black Box
  Lactic acidosis and severe hepatomegaly with steatosis
  ☐ OBRA regulated in U.S. Long Term Care

enalapril maleate

(e-nal'-a-pril mal'-ee-ate)

- **Brand Name(s):** Enalaprilat, Enalaprit Novaplus, Vasotec

  Combinations
  Rx: with diltiazem (Teczem); with felodipine (Lexxel); with hydrochlorothiazide (Vaseretic)
  Chemical Class: Angiotensin-converting enzyme (ACE) inhibitor, nonsulfhydryl

- **Clinical Pharmacology:**
  Mechanism of Action: This ACE inhibitor suppresses the renin-angiotensin-aldosterone system, and prevents conversion of angiotensin I to angiotensin II, a potent vasoconstrictor; may inhibit angiotensin II at local vascular, renal sites. Decreases plasma

angiotensin II, increases plasma renin activity, decreases aldosterone secretion. **Therapeutic Effect:** In hypertension, reduces peripheral arterial resistance. In congestive heart failure (CHF), increases cardiac output; decreases peripheral vascular resistance, BP, pulmonary capillary wedge pressure, heart size.
Pharmacokinetics:

Route	Onset	Peak	Duration
PO	1 hr	4-6 hr	24 hr
IV	15 min	1-4 hr	6 hr

Readily absorbed from the GI tract (not affected by food). Protein binding: 50%-60%. Converted to active metabolite. Primarily excreted in urine. Removed by hemodialysis. **Half-life:** 11 hr (half-life is increased in those with impaired renal function).

■ **Available Forms:**
  • *Tablets*: 2.5 mg, 5 mg, 10 mg, 20 mg.
  • *Injection*: 1.25 mg/ml.

■ **Indications and Dosages:**
  Hypertension alone or in combination with other CV-antihypertensive-ACEs: PO Initially, 2.5-5 mg/day. May increase at 1-2 wk intervals. Range: 10-40 mg/day in 1-2 divided doses. IV 0.625-1.25 mg q6h up to 5 mg q6h.
  Adjunctive therapy for CHF: PO Initially, 2.5-5 mg/day. Range: 5-20 mg/day in 2 divided doses.
  Dosage in renal impairment: Dosage is modified based on creatinine clearance.

Creatinine Clearance	% Usual Dose
10-50 ml/min	75-100
less than 10 ml/min	50

■ **Unlabeled Uses:** Diabetic nephropathy, hypertension due to scleroderma renal crisis, hypertensive crisis, idiopathic edema, renal artery stenosis, rheumatoid arthritis, post MI for prevention of ventricular failure

■ **Contraindications:** History of angioedema from previous treatment with ACE inhibitors

■ **Side Effects**
  Frequent (7%-5%)
  Headache, dizziness
  Occasional (3%-2%)
  Orthostatic hypotension, fatigue, diarrhea, cough, syncope
  Rare (less than 2%)
  Angina, abdominal pain, vomiting, nausea, rash, asthenia (loss of strength, energy), syncope

■ **Serious Reactions**
  • Excessive hypotension ("first-dose syncope") may occur in patients with CHF and in those who are severely salt or volume depleted.
  • Angioedema (swelling of face, lips) and hyperkalemia occur rarely.
  • Agranulocytosis and neutropenia may be noted in patients with collagen vascular diseases, including scleroderma and systemic lupus erythematosus, and impaired renal function.
  • Nephrotic syndrome may be noted in those with history of renal disease.
  • Hypoglycemia may occur in patients with diabetes using glucose-lowering drugs.

■ Patient/Family Education
- Caution with salt substitutes containing potassium chloride
- Rise slowly to sitting/standing position to minimize orthostatic hypotension
- Dizziness, fainting, light-headedness may occur during first few days of therapy
- May cause altered taste perception or cough; persistent dry cough usually does not subside unless medication is stopped; notify clinician if these symptoms persist
- Noncompliance with drug therapy or skipping drug doses may produce severe, rebound hypertension
- Notify the physician if diarrhea, difficulty breathing, excessive perspiration, vomiting, or swelling of the face, lips, or tongue occurs

■ Monitoring Parameters
- BUN, creatinine, potassium within 2 wk after initiation of therapy (increased levels may indicate acute renal failure)
- Blood pressure
- Daily bowel activity and stool consistency

■ Geriatric side effects at a glance:
❏ CNS ❏ Bowel Dysfunction ❏ Bladder Dysfunction ❏ Falls

■ U.S. Regulatory Considerations
☑ FDA Black Box

Although not relevant for geriatric patients, teratogenicity is associated with the use of ACE inhibitors.

❏ OBRA regulated in U.S. Long Term Care

enfuvirtide

(en-fyoo'-vir-tide)

■ Brand Name(s): Fuzeon
Chemical Class: Fusion inhibitor, HIV; polypeptide, synthetic

■ Clinical Pharmacology:
Mechanism of Action: A fusion inhibitor that interferes with the entry of HIV-1 into CD4+ cells by inhibiting the fusion of viral and cellular membranes. **Therapeutic Effect:** Impairs HIV replication, slowing the progression of HIV infection.
Pharmacokinetics: Comparable absorption when injected into subcutaneous tissue of abdomen, arm, or thigh. Protein binding: 92%. Undergoes catabolism to amino acids. **Half-life:** 3.8 hr.

■ Available Forms:
- *Powder for Injection*: 108-mg (approximately 90 mg/ml when reconstituted) vials.

- **Indications and Dosages:**
  HIV *infection (in combination with other antiretrovirals)*: Subcutaneous 90 mg (1 ml) twice a day.

- **Contraindications:** None known.

- **Side Effects**
  Expected (98%)
  Local injection site reactions (pain, discomfort, induration, erythema, nodules, cysts, pruritus, ecchymosis)
  Frequent (26%-16%)
  Diarrhea, nausea, fatigue
  Occasional (11%-4%)
  Insomnia, peripheral neuropathy, depression, cough, decreased appetite or weight loss, sinusitis, anxiety, asthenia, myalgia, cold sores
  Rare (3%-2%)
  Constipation, influenza, upper abdominal pain, anorexia, conjunctivitis

- **Serious Reactions**
  - Enfuvirtide use may potentiate bacterial pneumonia.
  - Hypersensitivity (rash, fever, chills, rigors, hypotension), thrombocytopenia, neutropenia, and renal insufficiency or failure may occur rarely.

Special Considerations
- Not active against HIV-2
- In heavily pretreated patients, randomized to receiving an "optimized" backbone regimen (based on treatment history and resistance testing) versus an optimized backbone regimen plus enfuvirtide, changes in HIV RNA at 24 wk were -0.73 $\log_{10}$ copies/ml and -1.52 $\log_{10}$ copies/ml, respectively; CD4 cell count changes from baseline were 35 and 71 cells/mm^3, respectively; clinical outcomes were not improved by enfuvirtide during this study
- Always check updated treatment guidelines before initiating or changing antiretroviral therapy. (http://AIDSinfo.nih.gov)

- **Patient/Family Education**
  - Injection site reactions occur commonly
  - Hypersensitivity reactions have included individually and in combination: rash, fever, nausea and vomiting, chills, rigors, hypotension
  - Increased rate of bacterial pneumonia was observed in subjects treated with enfuvirtide in clinical trials (4.68 pneumonia events per 100 patient-years in the treatment group versus 0.61 events per 100 patient-years in the control group)
  - More information is available for patients at www.FUZEON.com, or 877-438-9366
  - Take for the full course of treatment
  - Enfuvirtide is not a cure for HIV infection, nor does it reduce the risk of transmitting HIV to others; continue practices to prevent transmission of HIV

- **Monitoring Parameters**
  - CBC with differential (eosinophilia), ALT, AST, triglycerides
  - Skin for a hypersensitivity reaction and local injection site reactions
  - Observe for evidence of fatigue or nausea
  - Signs and symptoms of depression

■ **Geriatric side effects at a glance:**
  ❏ CNS ☑ Bowel Dysfunction ❏ Bladder Dysfunction ❏ Falls

■ **U.S. Regulatory Considerations**
  ❏ FDA Black Box ❏ OBRA regulated in U.S. Long Term Care

enoxaparin sodium

(ee-nox-a-pa'-rin soe'-dee-um)

■ **Brand Name(s):** Lovenox
  Chemical Class: Heparin derivative, depolymerized; low-molecular-weight heparin

■ **Clinical Pharmacology:**
  Mechanism of Action: A low-molecular-weight heparin that potentiates the action of antithrombin III and inactivates coagulation factor Xa. **Therapeutic Effect:** Produces anticoagulation. Does not significantly influence bleeding time, PT, or aPTT.
  Pharmacokinetics:

Route	Onset	Peak	Duration
Subcutaneous	N/A	3-5 hr	12 hr

  Well absorbed after subcutaneous administration. Eliminated primarily in urine. Not removed by hemodialysis. **Half-life:** 4.5 hr.

■ **Available Forms:**
  • *Injection*: 30 mg/0.3 ml, 40 mg/0.4 ml, 60 mg/0.6 ml, 80 mg/0.8 ml, 100 mg/ml, 120 mg/0.8 ml, 150 mg/ml in prefilled syringes.

■ **Indications and Dosages:**
  Prevention of deep vein thrombosis (DVT) after hip and knee surgery: Subcutaneous 30 mg twice a day, generally for 7-10 days.
  Prevention of DVT after abdominal surgery: Subcutaneous 40 mg a day for 7-10 days.
  Prevention of long-term DVT in nonsurgical acute illness: Subcutaneous 40 mg once a day for 3 wk.
  Prevention of ischemic complications of unstable angina and non-Q-wave MI (with oral aspirin therapy): Subcutaneous 1 mg/kg q12h.
  Acute DVT: Subcutaneous 1 mg/kg q12h or 1.5 mg/kg once daily.
  Dosage in renal impairment: Clearance of enoxaparin is decreased when creatinine clearance is less than 30 ml/min. Monitor patient and adjust dosage as necessary. When enoxaparin is used in abdominal, hip, or knee surgery or acute illness, the dosage in renal impairment is 30 mg once a day. When enoxaparin is used to treat DVT, angina, or MI the dosage in renal impairment is 1 mg/kg once a day.

■ **Unlabeled Uses:** Prevention of DVT following general surgical procedures

■ **Contraindications:** Active major bleeding, concurrent heparin therapy, hypersensitivity to heparin or pork products, thrombocytopenia associated with positive in vitro test for antiplatelet antibodies

■ **Side Effects**
   Occasional (4%–1%)
   Injection site hematoma, nausea, peripheral edema

■ **Serious Reactions**
   • Overdose may lead to bleeding complications ranging from local ecchymoses to major hemorrhage. Antidote: Protamine sulfate (1% solution) equal to the dose of enoxaparin injected. One mg protamine sulfate neutralizes 1 mg enoxaparin. A second dose of 0.5 mg protamine sulfate per 1 mg enoxaparin may be given if aPTT tested 2-4 hr after first injection remains prolonged.

Special Considerations
   • Cannot be used interchangeably with unfractionated heparin or other low-molecular-weight heparins
   • 1.5 mg/kg qd dosing should not be used in patients with cancer or obese patients

■ **Patient/Family Education**
   • Administer by deep SC inj into abdominal wall; alternate inj sites
   • Report any unusual bruising or bleeding to clinician
   • The usual length of therapy is 7-10 days
   • Use an electric razor and soft toothbrush to prevent bleeding during therapy
   • Do not take other medications, including OTC drugs (especially aspirin), without physician approval

■ **Monitoring Parameters**
   • CBC with platelets, stool occult blood, urinalysis
   • Monitoring aPTT is NOT required
   • Assess for signs of bleeding, including bleeding at injection or surgical sites or from gums, blood in stool, bruising, hematuria, and petechiae

■ **Geriatric side effects at a glance:**
   ❑ CNS   ❑ Bowel Dysfunction   ❑ Bladder Dysfunction   ❑ Falls

■ **U.S. Regulatory Considerations**
   ☑ FDA Black Box
   Increased risk of spinal/epidural hematomas with neuraxial anesthesia or spinal puncture. Risk is further increased by use of indwelling spinal catheters, repeated/traumatic epidural/spinal puncture, or use of drugs affecting hemostasis (NSAIDs, anticoagulants, platelet inhibitors).
   ❑ OBRA regulated in U.S. Long Term Care

entacapone

(en-ta'-ka-pone)

- **Brand Name(s):** Comtan
  Chemical Class: Catechol-O-methyltransferase (COMT) inhibitor; nitrocatechol

- **Clinical Pharmacology:**
  Mechanism of Action: An antiparkinson agent that inhibits the enzyme, catechol-O-methyltransferase (COMT), potentiating dopamine activity and increasing the duration of action of levodopa. **Therapeutic Effect:** Decreases signs and symptoms of Parkinson's disease.
  Pharmacokinetics: Rapidly absorbed after PO administration. Protein binding: 98%. Metabolized in the liver. Primarily eliminated by biliary excretion. Not removed by hemodialysis. **Half-life:** 2.4 hr.

- **Available Forms:**
  - *Tablets*: 200 mg.

- **Indications and Dosages:**
  Adjunctive treatment of Parkinson's disease: PO 200 mg concomitantly with each dose of carbidopa and levodopa up to a maximum of 8 times a day (1600 mg).

- **Contraindications:** Hypersensitivity, use within 14 days of MAOIs

- **Side Effects**
  Frequent (greater than 10%)
  Dyskinesia, nausea, dark yellow or orange urine and sweat, diarrhea
  Occasional (9%-3%)
  Abdominal pain, vomiting, constipation, dry mouth, fatigue, back pain
  Rare (less than 2%)
  Anxiety, somnolence, agitation, dyspepsia, flatulence, diaphoresis, asthenia, dyspnea

- **Serious Reactions**
  - Hallucinations have been reported.

- **Patient/Family Education**
  - Take entacapone with carbidopa and levodopa for best results
  - Avoid tasks that require mental alertness or motor skills until response to the drug has been established
  - Entacapone may cause sweat or urine to turn dark yellow or orange
  - Notify the physician if uncontrolled movement of the hands, arms, legs, eyelids, face, mouth, or tongue occurs

- **Monitoring Parameters**
  - Blood pressure
  - Monitor for dyskinesia, diarrhea, and orthostatic hypotension
  - Assess for relief of symptoms, including improvement of masklike facial expression, muscular rigidity, shuffling gait, and resting tremors of the hands and head

■ **Geriatric side effects at a glance:**
  ❏ CNS   ❏ Bowel Dysfunction   ❏ Bladder Dysfunction   ❏ Falls
  Other: Gastrointestinal discomfort, urine discoloration

■ **Use with caution in older patients with:** Psychotic symptoms, orthostatic hypotension

■ **U.S. Regulatory Considerations**
  ❏ FDA Black Box   ❏ OBRA regulated in U.S. Long Term Care

■ **Other Uses in Geriatric Patient:** Restless Legs Syndrome

■ **Side Effects:**
  Of particular importance in the geriatric patient: Dyskinesias, hallucinations

■ **Geriatric Considerations - Summary:** Entacapone inhibits peripheral COMT and increases levodopa's effects. Its primary role is as adjunctive therapy to prolong the beneficial effects of levodopa and to decrease end-of-dose fluctuations in response to treatment. Concurrent use of levodopa is necessary for entacapone to be effective and unlike tolcapone, hepatic monitoring is not required.

■ **References:**
  1. Kieburtz K, et al. Entacapone improves motor fluctuations in levodopa-treated Parkinson's disease patients. Ann Neurol 1997;52:747-755.
  2. Rine UK, Larsen JP, Siden A, et al. Entacapone enhances the response to levodopa in parkinsonian patients with motor fluctuations. Neurology 1998;51:278-285.
  3. Kaakkola S. Clinical pharmacology, therapeutic use and potential of COMT inhibitors in Parkinson's disease. Drugs 2000; 59:1233-1250.

entecavir

(en-te'-ka-veer)

■ **Brand Name(s):** Baraclude

■ **Clinical Pharmacology:**
  Mechanism of Action: A guanosine nucleoside analog that inhibits hepatitis B viral polymerase, which blocks reverse transcriptase activity. **Therapeutic Effect:** Interferes with viral DNA synthesis.
  Pharmacokinetics: Poorly absorbed from the gastrointestinal (GI) tract. Protein binding: 13%. Widely distributed. Partially metabolized in liver. Excreted primarily in urine.
  Half-life: 128-149 hr (longer in renal impairment).

■ **Available Forms:**
  • *Tablets:* 0.5 mg, 1 mg.
  • *Oral Solution:* 0.05 mg/ml.

- **Indications and Dosages:**
  Chronic hepatitis B: PO 0.5 mg once a day.
  Dosage in renal impairment:

Creatinine Clearance	Dosage
greater than 50 ml/min	0.5 mg once a day
30-49 ml/min	0.25 mg once a day
10-29 ml/min	0.15 mg once a day
less than 10 ml/min	0.05 mg once a day

- **Contraindications:** Hypersensitivity to entecavir or any component of the formulation

- **Side Effects**
  Occasional
  Headache, fatigue, dizziness, nausea
  Rare
  Diarrhea, dyspepsia, vomiting

- **Serious Reactions**
  - *Alert* Lactic acidosis and severe hepatomegaly may occur.

Special Considerations

  - Always check updated treatment guidelines before initiating or changing antiretroviral therapy. (http://AIDSinfo.nih.gov)

- **Geriatric side effects at a glance:**
  ☐ CNS   ☐ Bowel Dysfunction   ☐ Bladder Dysfunction   ☐ Falls

- **U.S. Regulatory Considerations**
  ☐ FDA Black Box   ☐ OBRA regulated in U.S. Long Term Care

ephedrine

(eh-fed'-rin)

OTC: Pretz-D, Kondon's Nasal

Combinations
Rx: with potassium iodide, phenobarbital, theophylline (Quadrinal), with hydroxyzine, theophylline (Hydrophed DF, Marax-DF); with guaifenesin (Broncholate, Ephex SR)
Chemical Class: Catecholamine

- **Clinical Pharmacology:**
  Mechanism of Action: An adrenergic agonist that stimulates alpha-adrenergic receptors causing vasoconstriction and pressor effects, $beta_1$-adrenergic receptors, resulting in cardiac stimulation, and $beta_2$-adrenergic receptors, resulting in bronchial dilation and vasodilation. **Therapeutic Effect:** Increases BP and pulse rate.

433

Pharmacokinetics: Well absorbed after nasal and parenteral absorption. Metabolized in liver. Excreted in urine. **Half-life:** 3-6 hr.

■ **Available Forms:**
- *Capsules:* 25 mg.
- *Injection:* 50 mg/ml.
- *Intranasal spray:* 0.25% (Pretz-D).

■ **Indications and Dosages:**
Asthma: PO 25-50 mg q3-4h as needed.
Hypotension: IM 25-50 mg as a single dose. Maximum 150 mg/day. IV 5 mg/dose slow IVP as prevention. 10-25 mg/dose slow IVP repeated q5-10min as treatment. Maximum: 150 mg/day. SC 25-50 q4-6h. Maximum 150 mg/day.
Nasal congestion: PO 25-50 mg q6h as needed. Nasal 2-3 sprays into each nostril q4h

■ **Unlabeled Uses:** Obesity, propofol-induced pain, radiocontrast media reactions

■ **Contraindications:** Anesthesia with cyclopropane or halothane, diabetes (ephedrine injection), hypersensitivity to ephedrine or other sympathomimetic amines, hypertension or other cardiovascular disorders, thyrotoxicosis

■ **Side Effects**
Frequent
Systemic: Hypertension, anxiety
Occasional
Systemic: Nausea, vomiting, palpitations, tremor
Nasal: Burning, stinging, runny nose, dryness of mucosa. Prolonged use may result in rebound congestion.
Rare
Psychosis, decreased urination, necrosis at injection site from repeated injections

■ **Serious Reactions**
- Excessive doses may cause hypertension, intracranial hemorrhage, anginal pain, and fatal arrhythmias.
- Prolonged or excessive use may result in metabolic acidosis due to increased serum lactic acid concentrations.
- Observe for disorientation, weakness, hyperventilation, headache, nausea, vomiting, and diarrhea.

Special Considerations
- Found in many OTC weight-loss products containing MaHuang; use should be avoided
- Manage rebound congestion by stopping ephedrine; one nostril at a time, substitute systemic decongestant and/or nasal steroid

■ **Patient/Family Education**
- May cause wakefulness or nervousness; take last dose 4-6 hr prior to bedtime
- Do not use nasal products for more than 3-5 days to prevent rebound congestion
- Avoid consuming an excessive amount of caffeine derivatives such as chocolate, cocoa, coffee, cola, or tea
- Report any unusual side effects including headaches, dizziness, and fast heartbeat

■ **Monitoring Parameters**
- Heart rate, ECG, blood pressure (when using for vasopressor effect)
- Urine output
- Mental status changes

■ **Geriatric side effects at a glance:**
☑ CNS   ☐ Bowel Dysfunction   ☑ Bladder Dysfunction   ☐ Falls

■ **U.S. Regulatory Considerations**
☐ FDA Black Box   ☐ OBRA regulated in U.S. Long Term Care

epinephrine

(ep-i-nef'-rin)

■ **Brand Name(s):** Adrenalin, Adrenalin Topical, Epifrin, EpiPen, EpiPen 2-Pak, EpiPen Auto Injector, Sus-Phrine Injection
OTC: Adrenalin, AsthmaHaler Mist, Asthma-Nefrin, microNefrin, Nephron, Primatene Mist, S-2

Combinations
Rx: with etidocaine (Duranest with Epinephrine); with prilocaine (Citanest Forte); with lidocaine (Xylocaine with Epinephrine); with pilocarpine (E-Pilo Ophthalmic)
Chemical Class: Catecholamine

■ **Clinical Pharmacology:**
Mechanism of Action: A sympathomimetic, adrenergic agonist that stimulates alpha-adrenergic receptors causing vasoconstriction and pressor effects, beta$_1$-adrenergic receptors, resulting in cardiac stimulation, and beta$_2$-adrenergic receptors, resulting in bronchial dilation and vasodilation. With ophthalmic form, increases outflow of aqueous humor from anterior eye chamber. **Therapeutic Effect:** Relaxes smooth muscle of the bronchial tree, produces cardiac stimulation, and dilates skeletal muscle vasculature. The ophthalmic form dilates pupils and constricts conjunctival blood vessels.

Pharmacokinetics:

Route	Onset	Peak	Duration
IM	5-10 min	20 min	1-4 hr
Subcutaneous	5-10 min	20 min	1-4 hr
Inhalation	3-5 min	20 min	1-3 hr
Ophthalmic	1 hr	4-8 hr	12-24 hr

Well absorbed after parenteral administration; minimally absorbed after inhalation. Metabolized in the liver, other tissues, and sympathetic nerve endings. Excreted in urine. The ophthalmic form may be systemically absorbed as a result of drainage into nasal pharyngeal passages. Mydriasis occurs within several min and persists several hr; vasoconstriction occurs within 5 min, and lasts less than 1 hr.

■ **Available Forms:**
- *Injection* (*Adrenalin*): 0.1 mg/ml, 1 mg/ml.
- *Injection*: 0.3 mg/0.3 ml (EpiPen Auto Injector), 0.15 mg/0.3 ml (EpiPen 2-Pak).

- *Inhalation (Aerosol [Primatene Mist])*: 0.2 mg/inhalation.
- *Inhalation Solution*: 1%, 2.25%.
- *Ophthalmic Solution (Epifrin)*: 0.5%, 1%, 2%.
- *Subcutaneous Suspension (Sus-Phrine Injection)*: 5 mg/ml.
- *Topical Solution (Adrenalin, Topical)*: 1:100.

■ Indications and Dosages:
Anaphylaxis: IM 0.3 mg (0.3 ml of 1:1000 solution). May repeat if anaphylaxis persists.
Asthma: Subcutaneous 0.2-0.5 mg (0.2-0.5 ml of 1:1000 solution) q2h as needed. In severe attacks, may repeat q20min times 3 doses. Inhalation 1 inhalation, wait at least 1 min. May repeat once. Do not use again for at least 3 hr.
Cardiac arrest: IV Initially, 1 mg. May repeat q3-5min as needed.
Hypersensitivity reaction: IM, Subcutaneous 0.3-0.5 mg q15-20min Inhalation 1 inhalation, may repeat in at least 1 min. Give subsequent doses no sooner than 3 hr. Nebulizer 1-3 deep inhalations. Give subsequent doses no sooner than 3 hr.
Glaucoma: Ophthalmic 1-2 drops 1-2 times a day.

■ Unlabeled Uses:
Systemic: Treatment of gingival or pulpal hemorrhage, priapism
Ophthalmic: Treatment of conjunctival congestion during surgery, secondary glaucoma

■ Contraindications:
Cardiac arrhythmias, cerebrovascular insufficiency, hypertension, hyperthyroidism, ischemic heart disease, narrow-angle glaucoma, shock

■ Side Effects
Frequent
Systemic: Tachycardia, palpitations, nervousness
Ophthalmic: Headache, eye irritation, watering of eyes
Occasional
Systemic: Dizziness, light-headedness, facial flushing, headache, diaphoresis, increased BP, nausea, trembling, insomnia, vomiting, fatigue
Ophthalmic: Blurred or decreased vision, eye pain
Rare
Systemic: Chest discomfort or pain, arrhythmias, bronchospasm, dry mouth or throat

■ Serious Reactions
- Excessive doses may cause acute hypertension or arrhythmias.
- Prolonged or excessive use may result in metabolic acidosis due to increased serum lactic acid concentrations. Metabolic acidosis may cause disorientation, fatigue, hyperventilation, headache, nausea, vomiting, and diarrhea.

■ Patient/Family Education
- Do not exceed recommended doses
- Wait at least 3-5 min between inhalations with MDI
- Notify clinician of dizziness or chest pain
- Do not use nasal preparations for >3-5 days to prevent rebound congestion
- To avoid contamination of ophth preparations, do not touch tip of container to any surface
- Do not use ophth preparations while wearing soft contact lenses
- Transitory stinging may occur on instillation of ophth preparations
- Report any decrease in visual acuity immediately

- Use of OTC asthma preparations containing epinephrine should be discouraged
- Avoid consuming excessive amounts of caffeine derivatives such as chocolate, cocoa, coffee, cola, and tea

■ **Monitoring Parameters**
  - Blood pressure, heart rate
  - Intraocular pressure
  - Breath sounds for crackles, rhonchi, and wheezing
  - ECG and patient's condition, especially in the patient with cardiac arrest

■ **Geriatric side effects at a glance:**
  ☑ CNS ☐ Bowel Dysfunction ☑ Bladder Dysfunction ☐ Falls

■ **U.S. Regulatory Considerations**
  ☐ FDA Black Box ☐ OBRA regulated in U.S. Long Term Care

eplerenone

(e-pler'-en-one)

■ **Brand Name(s):** Inspra
  Chemical Class: Pregnene methyl ester

■ **Clinical Pharmacology:**
  Mechanism of Action: An aldosterone receptor antagonist that binds to the mineralocorticoid receptors in the kidney, heart, blood vessels, and brain, blocking the binding of aldosterone. **Therapeutic Effect:** Reduces BP.
  Pharmacokinetics: Absorption unaffected by food. Protein binding: 50%. No active metabolites. Excreted in the urine with a lesser amount eliminated in the feces. Not removed by hemodialysis. **Half-life:** 4-6 hr.

■ **Available Forms:**
  - *Tablets*: 25 mg, 50 mg.

■ **Indications and Dosages:**
  Hypertension: PO 50 mg once a day. If 50 mg once a day produces an inadequate BP response, may increase dosage to 50 mg twice a day. If patient is concurrently receiving erythromycin, saquinavir, verapamil, or fluconazole, reduce initial dose to 25 mg once a day.
  CHF *following* MI: PO Initially, 25 mg once a day. If tolerated, titrate up to 50 mg once a day within 4 wk.

■ **Contraindications:** Concurrent use of potassium supplements or potassium-sparing diuretics (such as amiloride, spironolactone, and triamterene), or strong inhibitors of the cytochrome P450 3A4 enzyme system (including ketoconazole and itraconazole), creatinine clearance less than 50 ml/min, serum creatinine level greater than 2 mg/dl in males or 1.8 mg/dl in females, serum potassium level greater than 5.5 mEq/L, type 2 diabetes mellitus with microalbuminuria

- **Side Effects**
  Rare (3%–1%)
  Dizziness, diarrhea, cough, fatigue, flu-like symptoms, abdominal pain

- **Serious Reactions**
  - Hyperkalemia may occur, particularly in patients with type 2 diabetes mellitus and microalbuminuria.

Special Considerations

- Primary advantage of eplerenone over spironolactone is a potentially decreased incidence of endocrine-related adverse effects, such as gynecomastia or sexual dysfunction

- **Patient/Family Education**
  - Avoid tasks that require mental alertness or motor skills until response to the drug has been established
  - Do not break, crush, or chew film-coated tablets
  - Avoid exercising outside during hot weather because of the risks of dehydration and hypotension

- **Monitoring Parameters**
  - *Efficacy*: Blood pressure, heart rate, ECG, urine output, cardiac output, improvement in symptoms of heart failure
  - *Toxicity*: Serum electrolytes (especially potassium), renal function tests, BP, ECG (hyperkalemia), signs and symptoms of toxicity

- **Geriatric side effects at a glance:**
  ❑ CNS ❑ Bowel Dysfunction ❑ Bladder Dysfunction ❑ Falls

- **U.S. Regulatory Considerations**
  ❑ FDA Black Box ❑ OBRA regulated in U.S. Long Term Care

epoetin alfa

(eh-poh'-ee-tin al'-fa)

- **Brand Name(s):** Epogen, Procrit
  Chemical Class: Amino acid glycoprotein

- **Clinical Pharmacology:**
  Mechanism of Action: A glycoprotein that stimulates division and differentiation of erythroid progenitor cells in bone marrow. **Therapeutic Effect:** Induces erythropoiesis and releases reticulocytes from bone marrow.
  Pharmacokinetics: Well absorbed after subcutaneous administration. Following administration, an increase in reticulocyte count occurs within 10 days, and increases in Hgb, Hct, and RBC count are seen within 2-6 wk. **Half-life:** 4-13 hr.

- **Available Forms:**
  - Injection (*Epogen, Procrit*): 2000 units/ml, 3000 units/ml, 4000 units/ml, 10,000 units/ml, 20,000 units/ml, 40,000 units/ml.

- **Indications and Dosages:**

  Treatment of anemia in chemotherapy patients: IV, Subcutaneous 150 units/kg/dose 3 times a wk. Maximum: 1200 units/kg/wk.

  Reduction of allogenic blood transfusions in elective surgery: Subcutaneous 300 units/kg/day 10 days before day of, and 4 days after, surgery.

  Chronic renal failure: IV Bolus, Subcutaneous Initially, 50-100 units/kg 3 times a wk. Target Hct range: 30%-36%. Adjust dosage no earlier than 1-mo intervals unless prescribed. Decrease dosage if Hct is increasing and approaching 36%. Plan to temporarily withhold doses if Hct continues to rise and to reinstate lower dosage when Hct begins to decrease. If Hct increases by more than 4 points in 2 wk, monitor Hct twice a wk for 2-6 wk. Increase dose if Hct does not increase 5-6 points after 8 wk (with adequate iron stores) and if Hct is below target range. Maintenance: *For patients on dialysis:* 75 units/kg 3 times a wk. Range: 12.5-525 units/kg. *For patients not on dialysis:* 75–150 units/kg/wk.

  HIV infection in patients treated with AZT: IV, Subcutaneous Initially, 100 units/kg 3 times a wk for 8 wk; may increase by 50-100 units/kg 3 times a wk. Evaluate response q4-8wk thereafter. Adjust dosage by 50-100 units/kg 3 times a wk. If dosages larger than 300 units/kg 3 times a wk are not eliciting response, it is unlikely patient will respond. Maintenance: Titrate to maintain desired Hct.

- **Unlabeled Uses:** Anemia associated with frequent blood donations, anemia in critically ill patients, malignancy, management of hepatitis C, myelodysplastic syndromes

- **Contraindications:** History of sensitivity to mammalian cell-derived products or human albumin, uncontrolled hypertension

- **Side Effects**

  Patients receiving chemotherapy

  Frequent (20%–17%)

  Fever, diarrhea, nausea, vomiting, edema

  Occasional (13%–11%)

  Asthenia, shortness of breath, paresthesia

  Rare (5%–3%)

  Dizziness, trunk pain

  Patients with chronic renal failure

  Frequent (24%–11%)

  Hypertension, headache, nausea, arthralgia

  Occasional (9%–7%)

  Fatigue, edema, diarrhea, vomiting, chest pain, skin reactions at administration site, asthenia, dizziness

  Patients with HIV infection treated with AZT

  Frequent (38%–15%)

  Fever, fatigue, headache, cough, diarrhea, rash, nausea

  Occasional (14%–9%)

  Shortness of breath, asthenia, skin reaction at injection site, dizziness

- **Serious Reactions**
  - Hypertensive encephalopathy, thrombosis, cerebrovascular accident, MI, and seizures have occurred rarely.

- Hyperkalemia occurs occasionally in patients with chronic renal failure, usually in those who do not conform to medication regimen, dietary guidelines, and frequency of dialysis regimen.

Special Considerations

- Iron supplementation should be given during therapy to provide for increased requirements during expansion of red cell mass secondary to marrow stimulation by erythropoietin
- Use prior to elective surgery should be limited to patients with presurgery hemoglobin of >10 but ≤13 g/dl undergoing noncardiac, nonvascular procedures

■ Patient/Family Education

- Do not shake vials as this may denature the glycoprotein rendering the drug inactive
- Notify clinician if severe headache develops
- Frequent blood tests required to determine optimal dose
- Avoid potentially hazardous activities during the first 90 days of therapy; there is an increased risk of seizure development in patients with chronic renal failure during the first 90 days of therapy

■ Monitoring Parameters

- Hct (target range 30%-33%, max 36%), serum iron, ferritin (keep >100 ng/dl)
- Baseline erythropoietin level (treatment of patients with erythropoietin levels >200 mU/ml is not recommended)
- Blood pressure
- BUN, uric acid, creatinine, phosphorus, potassium on a regular basis
- Body temperature, especially in patients receiving chemotherapy and in patients with HIV infection treated with zidovudine

■ Geriatric side effects at a glance:
❑ CNS   ❑ Bowel Dysfunction   ❑ Bladder Dysfunction   ❑ Falls

■ U.S. Regulatory Considerations
❑ FDA Black Box   ❑ OBRA regulated in U.S. Long Term Care

epoprostenol sodium, prostacyclin

(e-poe-pros'-ten-ol soe'-dee-um, pros-tuh-sahy-klin)

■ Brand Name(s): Flolan
Chemical Class: Prostaglandin I_2

■ Clinical Pharmacology:
Mechanism of Action: An antihypertensive that directly dilates pulmonary and systemic arterial vascular beds and inhibits platelet aggregation. **Therapeutic Effect:** Reduces right and left ventricular afterload; increases cardiac output and stroke volume.

Pharmacokinetics: Extensively metabolized by rapid hydrolysis at neutral pH in blood and by enzymatic degradation. The metabolites are excreted in urine. **Half-life:** 3-5 min.

■ Available Forms:
- Injection, Powder for Reconstitution: 0.5 mg, 1.5 mg.

■ Indications and Dosages:
Long-term treatment of New York Heart Association Class III and IV primary pulmonary hypertension: IV Infusion Procedure to determine dose range: Initially, 2 ng/kg/min, increased in increments of 2 ng/kg/min q15min until dose-limiting adverse effects occur. Chronic Infusion: Start at 4 ng/kg/min less than the maximum dose rate tolerated during acute dose ranging (or one half of the maximum rate if rate was less than 5 ng/kg/min).

■ Unlabeled Uses:
Cardiopulmonary bypass surgery; hemodialysis; pulmonary hypertension associated with acute respiratory distress syndrome, systemic lupus erythematosus, or congenital heart disease; refractory CHF; severe community-acquired pneumonia

■ Contraindications:
Long-term use in patients with CHF (severe ventricular systolic dysfunction)

■ Side Effects
Frequent
Acute phase: Flushing (58%), headache (49%), nausea (32%), vomiting (32%), hypotension (16%), anxiety (11%), chest pain (11%), dizziness (8%)
Chronic phase: (greater than 20%): Dyspnea, asthenia, dizziness, headache, chest pain, nausea, vomiting, palpitations, edema, jaw pain, tachycardia, flushing, myalgia, nonspecific muscle pain, paresthesia, diarrhea, anxiety, chills, fever, or flu-like symptoms
Occasional
Acute phase (5%-2%): Bradycardia, abdominal pain, muscle pain, dyspnea, back pain
Chronic phase (20%-10%): Rash, depression, hypotension, pallor, syncope, bradycardia, ascites
Rare
Acute phase: Paresthesia
Chronic phase (less than 2%): Diaphoresis, dyspepsia, tachycardia

■ Serious Reactions
- Overdose may cause hyperglycemia or ketoacidosis manifested as increased urination, thirst, and fruitlike breath odor.
- Angina, MI, and thrombocytopenia occur rarely.
- Abrupt withdrawal, including a large reduction in dosage or interruption in drug delivery, may produce rebound pulmonary hypertension as evidenced by dyspnea, dizziness, and asthenia.

Special Considerations
- Clinically shown to improve exercise capacity, dyspnea, and fatigue as early as 1st week of therapy
- Drug is administered chronically on an ambulatory basis with a portable infusion pump through a permanent central venous catheter; peripheral IV infusions may be used temporarily until central venous access obtained
- Patients must be taught sterile technique, drug reconstitution, and care of catheter

- Do not interrupt infusion or decrease rate abruptly, may cause rebound symptoms (dyspnea, dizziness, asthenia, death)
- Unless contraindicated, patients should be anticoagulated to reduce risk of pulmonary thromboembolism or systemic embolism through a patent foramen ovale

■ Patient/Family Education
- Therapy will be necessary for a prolonged period, possibly years
- Brief interruptions in drug delivery may result in rapidly worsening symptoms

■ Monitoring Parameters
- Postural BP and heart rate for several hr following dosage adjustments
- Assess for a therapeutic response as evidenced by decreased chest pain, dyspnea on exertion, fatigue, pulmonary arterial pressure, pulmonary vascular resistance, and syncope, and improved pulmonary function

■ Geriatric side effects at a glance:
❑ CNS ❑ Bowel Dysfunction ❑ Bladder Dysfunction ❑ Falls

■ U.S. Regulatory Considerations
❑ FDA Black Box ❑ OBRA regulated in U.S. Long Term Care

eprosartan mesylate

(ep-roe-sar'-tan mes'-sil-ate)

■ Brand Name(s): Teveten
Chemical Class: Angiotensin II receptor antagonist

■ Clinical Pharmacology:
Mechanism of Action: An angiotensin II receptor antagonist that blocks the vasoconstrictor and aldosterone-secreting effects of angiotensin II, inhibiting the binding of angiotensin II to the AT_1 receptors. *Therapeutic Effect:* Causes vasodilation, decreases peripheral resistance, and decreases BP.
Pharmacokinetics: Rapidly absorbed after PO administration. Protein binding: 98%. Undergoes first-pass metabolism in the liver to active metabolites. Excreted in urine and biliary system. Minimally removed by hemodialysis. *Half-life:* 5–9 hr.

■ Available Forms:
- *Tablets:* 400 mg, 600 mg.

■ Indications and Dosages:
Hypertension: PO Initially, 600 mg/day. Range: 400–800 mg/day.

■ Contraindications: Bilateral renal artery stenosis, hyperaldosteronism

■ Side Effects
Occasional (5%–2%)
Headache, cough, dizziness

442

Rare (less than 2%)

Muscle pain, fatigue, diarrhea, upper respiratory tract infection, dyspepsia

■ Serious Reactions

- Overdosage may manifest as hypotension and tachycardia. Bradycardia occurs less often.
- Hypoglycemia may occur in patients with diabetes using glucose-lowering drugs.

Special Considerations

- Potentially as effective as or more effective than angiotensin-converting enzyme inhibitors, without cough; no evidence yet for reduction in morbidity and mortality as first-line agents in hypertension; whether they provide the same cardiac and renal protection also still tentative; like ACE inhibitors, less effective in black patients

■ Patient/Family Education

- Call your clinician immediately if note following side effects: wheezing; lip, throat, or face swelling; hives or rash
- Avoid tasks that require mental alertness or motor skills until response to the drug has been established
- Restrict alcohol and sodium consumption while taking eprosartan, adhere to the provided diet, and control weight
- Do not exercise outside during hot weather because of the risks of dehydration and hypotension

■ Monitoring Parameters

- Baseline electrolytes, urinalysis, BUN, and creatinine with recheck at 2-4 wk after initiation (sooner in volume-depleted patients); monitor sitting blood pressure; watch for symptomatic hypotension, particularly in volume-depleted patients

■ Geriatric side effects at a glance:

❑ CNS   ❑ Bowel Dysfunction   ❑ Bladder Dysfunction   ❑ Falls

■ U.S. Regulatory Considerations

☑ FDA Black Box

Although not relevant for geriatric patients, teratogenicity is associated with the use of angiotensin II receptor antagonists.

❑ OBRA regulated in U.S. Long Term Care

eptifibatide

(ep-tih-fib'-ah-tide)

■ **Brand Name(s):** Integrilin
  Chemical Class: Glycoprotein (GP) IIb/IIIa inhibitor

■ **Clinical Pharmacology:**
  Mechanism of Action: A glycoprotein IIb/IIIa inhibitor that rapidly inhibits platelet aggregation by preventing binding of fibrinogen to receptor sites on platelets. **Therapeutic Effect:** Prevents closure of treated coronary arteries. Also prevents acute cardiac ischemic complications.
  Pharmacokinetics: Protein binding: 25%. Excreted in urine. **Half-life:** 2.5 hr.

■ **Available Forms:**
  • *Injection Solution:* 0.75 mg/ml, 2 mg/ml.

■ **Indications and Dosages:**
  Adjunct to percutaneous coronary intervention (PCI): IV Bolus, IV Infusion 180 mcg/kg before PCI initiation; then continuous drip of 2 mcg/kg/min and a second 180 mcg/kg bolus 10 min after the first. Maximum: 15 mg/h. Continue until hospital discharge or for up to 18-24 hr. Minimum 12 hr is recommended. Concurrent aspirin and heparin therapy is recommended.
  Acute coronary syndrome: IV Bolus, IV Infusion 180 mcg/kg bolus then 2 mcg/kg/min until discharge or coronary artery bypass graft, up to 72 hr. Maximum: 15 mg/h. Concurrent aspirin and heparin therapy is recommended.
  Dosage in renal impairment: Creatinine clearance less than 50 ml/min. Use 180 mcg/kg bolus (maximum 22.6 mg) and 1 mcg/kg/min infusion (maximum: 7.5 mg/h).

■ **Contraindications:** Active internal bleeding, AV malformation or aneurysm, history of cerebrovascular accident (CVA) within 2 yr or CVA with residual neurologic defect, history of vasculitis, intracranial neoplasm, oral anticoagulant use within last 7 days unless PT is less than 1.22 times the control, recent (6 wk or less) GI or GU bleeding, recent (6 wk or less) surgery or trauma, prior IV dextran use before or during percutaneous transluminal coronary angioplasty (PTCA), severe uncontrolled hypertension, thrombocytopenia (less than 100,000 cells/μl)

■ **Side Effects**
  Occasional (7%)
  Hypotension

■ **Serious Reactions**
  • Minor to major bleeding complications may occur, most commonly at arterial access site for cardiac catheterization.

Special Considerations
  • When bleeding cannot be controlled with pressure, discontinue INF
  • Most major bleeding occurs at arterial access site for cardiac catheterization; prior to pulling femoral artery sheath, discontinue heparin for 3-4 hr and document activated clotting time (ACT) <150 sec or aPTT <45 sec; achieve sheath hemostasis 2-4 hr before discharge

- In patients who undergo CABG, discontinue eptifibatide INF prior to surgery
- Eptifibatide, tirofiban, and abciximab can all decrease the incidence of cardiac events associated with acute coronary syndromes; direct comparisons are needed to establish which, if any, is superior; for angioplasty, until more data become available, abciximab appears to be the drug of choice

■ Patient/Family Education
- Report bleeding from surgical site, chest pain, or dyspnea
- Use an electric razor and soft toothbrush, to prevent bleeding during eptifibatide therapy
- Do not take other medications, including OTC drugs (especially aspirin), without physician approval
- Report black or red stool, coffee-ground emesis, dark or red urine, or red-speckled mucus from cough

■ Monitoring Parameters
- Platelet count, hemoglobin, hematocrit, PT/aPTT (baseline, within 6 hr following bolus dose, then daily thereafter)
- In patients undergoing PCI, also measure ACT; maintain aPTT between 50 and 70 sec unless PCI is to be performed; during PCI, maintain ACT between 300 and 350 sec

■ Geriatric side effects at a glance:
❑ CNS   ❑ Bowel Dysfunction   ❑ Bladder Dysfunction   ❑ Falls

■ U.S. Regulatory Considerations
❑ FDA Black Box   ❑ OBRA regulated in U.S. Long Term Care

ergoloid mesylates

(er'-goe-loid mess'-i-lates)

■ Brand Name(s): Gerimal, Hydergine
Chemical Class: Ergot alkaloid

■ Clinical Pharmacology:
Mechanism of Action: An ergot alkaloid that centrally acts and decreases vascular tone, slows heart rate. Peripheral action blocks alpha-adrenergic receptors. **Therapeutic Effect:** Improved O_2 uptake and improves cerebral metabolism.
Pharmacokinetics: Rapidly, incompletely absorbed from GI tract. Metabolized in liver. Eliminated primarily in feces. **Half-life:** 2-5 hr.

■ Available Forms:
- *Capsules:* 1 mg (Hydergine).
- *Oral Solution:* 1 mg/ml (Hydergine).
- *Tablets:* 1 mg (Gerimal, Hydergine).
- *Tablets, sublingual:* 1 mg (Gerimal, Hydergine).

- **Indications and Dosages:**
  Age-related decline in mental capacity: PO Initially, 1 mg 3 times/day. Range: 1.5-12 mg/day.

- **Contraindications:** Acute or chronic psychosis (regardless or etiology), hypersensitivity to ergoloid mesylates or any component of the formulation

- **Side Effects**
  Occasional
  GI distress, transient nausea, sublingual irritation

- **Serious Reactions**
  - Overdose may produce blurred vision, dizziness, syncope, headache, flushed face, nausea, vomiting, decreased appetite, stomach cramps, and stuffy nose.

- **Patient/Family Education**
  - Results may not be observed for 3-4 wk
  - May cause transient GI disturbances; allow sublingual tablets to completely dissolve under tongue; do not chew or crush sublingual tablets

- **Monitoring Parameters**
  - Before prescribing, exclude the possibility that the patient's signs and symptoms arise from a potentially reversible and treatable condition
  - Periodically reassess the diagnosis and the benefit of current therapy to the patient; discontinue if no benefit
  - Pulse
  - Therapeutic response and improvement

- **Geriatric side effects at a glance:**
  ☑ CNS ❑ Bowel Dysfunction ❑ Bladder Dysfunction ❑ Falls

- **Use with caution in older patients with:** Liver disease

- **U.S. Regulatory Considerations**
  ❑ FDA Black Box ❑ OBRA regulated in U.S. Long Term Care

- **Other Uses in Geriatric Patient:** Attempt to improve or delay cognitive decline associated with Alzheimer's disease or vascular dementia.

- **Side Effects:**
  Of particular importance in the geriatric patient: Orthostatic hypotension

- **Geriatric Considerations - Summary:** Once popular for the treatment of cognitive impairment assciated with Alzheimer's disease or vascular dementia. There is no evidence that ergoloid mesylates are effective for either of these conditions. Unless an individual patient has experienced an observable improvement using ergoloid mesylates, these agents should be avoided.

References:
1. Olin J, Schneider L, Novit A, Luczak S. Hydergine for dementia. Cochrane Database Syst Rev 2001;CD000359
2. Schneider LS, Olin JT. Overview of clinical trials of hydergine in dementia. Arch Neurol 1994;51:787-798.
3. Thompson TL, Filley CM, Mitchell WD, et al. Lack of efficacy of hydergine in patients with Alzheimer's disease. N Engl J Med 1990;323:445-448.

ergotamine tartrate/ dihydroergotamine

(er-got'-a-meen tar'-trate dye-hye-droe-er-got'-a-meen, -min)

■ **Brand Name(s):** Ergomar, DHE 45, Migranal

Combinations
Rx: with caffeine (Cafergot, Ercaf, Wigraine); with belladonna alkaloids, phenobarbital (Bellergal-S), DHE 45, Ergomar, Migranal
Chemical Class: Ergot alkaloid

■ **Clinical Pharmacology:**
Mechanism of Action: An ergotamine derivative and alpha-adrenergic blocker that directly stimulates vascular smooth muscle, resulting in peripheral and cerebral vasoconstriction. May also have antagonist effects on serotonin. **Therapeutic Effect:** Suppresses vascular headaches.
Pharmacokinetics: Slowly and incompletely absorbed from the GI tract; rapidly and extensively absorbed after rectal administration. Protein binding: greater than 90%. Undergoes extensive first-pass metabolism in the liver to active metabolite. Eliminated in feces by the biliary system. **Half-life:** 21 hr.

■ **Available Forms:**
- *Tablets (Sublingual [Ergomar]):* 2 mg.
- *Injection (DHE 45):* 1 mg/ml.
- *Nasal Spray (Migranal):* 0.5 mg/spray.
- *Suppositories (ergotamine and caffeine):* 2 mg, with 100 mg caffeine.

■ **Indications and Dosages:**
Vascular headaches: PO (Cafergot [fixed-combination of ergotamine and caffeine]) 2 mg at onset of headache, then 1-2 mg q30min. Maximum: 6 mg/episode; 10 mg/wk. IV 1 mg at onset of headache; may repeat hourly. Maximum: 2 mg/day; 6 mg/wk. Sublingual 1 tablet at onset of headache, then 1 tablet q30min. Maximum: 3 tablets/24 hr; 5 tablets/wk. IM, Subcutaneous (dihydroergotamine) 1 mg at onset of headache; may repeat hourly. Maximum: 3 mg/day; 6 mg/wk. Intranasal 1 spray (0.5 mg) into each nostril; may repeat in 15 min. Maximum: 4 sprays/day; 8 sprays/wk. Rectal 1 suppository at onset of headache; may repeat dose in 1 hr. Maximum: 2 suppositories/episode; 5 suppositories/wk.

■ **Unlabeled Uses:** Prevention of deep venous thrombosis, prevention and treatment of orthostatic hypotension, pulmonary thromboembolism

447

- **Contraindications:** Coronary artery disease, hypertension, impaired hepatic or renal function, malnutrition, peripheral vascular diseases (such as thromboangiitis obliterans, syphilitic arteritis, severe arteriosclerosis, thrombophlebitis, and Raynaud's disease), sepsis, severe pruritus

- **Side Effects**
  Occasional (5%-2%)
  Cough, dizziness
  Rare (less than 2%)
  Myalgia, fatigue, diarrhea, upper respiratory tract infection, dyspepsia

- **Serious Reactions**
  - Prolonged administration or excessive dosage may produce ergotamine poisoning, manifested as nausea and vomiting; paresthesia, muscle pain or weakness; precordial pain; tachycardia or bradycardia; and hypertension or hypotension. Vasoconstriction of peripheral arteries and arterioles may result in localized edema and pruritus. Muscle pain will occur when walking and later, even at rest. Other rare effects include confusion, depression, drowsiness, seizures, and gangrene.

- **Patient/Family Education**
  - Initiate therapy at first sign of attack
  - DO NOT exceed recommended dosage
  - Notify clinician of irregular heartbeat, nausea, vomiting, numbness or tingling of fingers or toes, pain or weakness of extremities
  - Regular use may lead to withdrawal headaches

- **Monitoring Parameters**
  - Monitor the patient closely for evidence of ergotamine overdose from prolonged administration or excessive dosage

- **Geriatric side effects at a glance:**
  ☐ CNS ☑ Bowel Dysfunction ☐ Bladder Dysfunction ☐ Falls

- **U.S. Regulatory Considerations**
  ☑ FDA Black Box
  - Concurrent use with CYP3A4 inhibitors is contraindicated.
  - Can result in serious peripheral ischemia.
  ☑ OBRA regulated in U.S. Long Term Care

erlotinib

(er-loe'-tye-nib)

■ **Brand Name(s):** Tarceva

■ **Clinical Pharmacology:**
Mechanism of Action: A human epidermal growth factor that inhibits tyrosine kinases (TK) associated with transmembrane cell surface receptors found on both normal and cancer cells. One such receptor is epidermal growth factor receptor (EGFR). **Therapeutic Effect:** TK activity appears to be vitally important to cell proliferation and survival. **Pharmacokinetics:** About 60% is absorbed after PO administration; bioavailability is increased by food to almost 100%. Protein binding: 93%. Extensively metabolized in liver. Primarily eliminated in feces; minimal excretion in urine. **Half-life:** 36 hr.

■ **Available Forms:**
  • *Tablets:* 25 mg, 100 mg, 150 mg.

■ **Indications and Dosages:**
Overactive bladder: PO Initially, 7.5 mg once a day. If response is not adequate after a minimum of 2 wk, dosage may be increased to 15 mg once daily. Do not exceed 7.5 mg once a day in patients with moderate hepatic impairment.

■ **Contraindications:** None known.

■ **Side Effects**
Frequent (35%-21%)
Dry mouth, constipation
Occasional (8%-4%)
Dyspepsia, headache, nausea, abdominal pain
Rare (3%-2%)
Asthenia, diarrhea, dizziness, ocular dryness

■ **Serious Reactions**
  • Urinary tract infection occurs occasionally.
  • GI bleeding and increased hepatic enzymes have been reported.

■ **Geriatric side effects at a glance:**
  ❑ CNS ☑ Bowel Dysfunction ❑ Bladder Dysfunction ❑ Falls

■ **U.S. Regulatory Considerations**
  ❑ FDA Black Box ❑ OBRA regulated in U.S. Long Term Care

ertapenem

(er-ta-pen'-em)

- **Brand Name(s):** Invanz
  Chemical Class: Carbapenem

- **Clinical Pharmacology:**
  Mechanism of Action: A carbapenem that penetrates the bacterial cell wall of microorganisms and binds to penicillin-binding proteins, inhibiting cell wall synthesis. **Therapeutic Effect:** Produces bacterial cell death.
  Pharmacokinetics: Almost completely absorbed after IM administration. Protein binding: 85%-95%. Widely distributed. Primarily excreted in urine with smaller amount eliminated in feces. Removed by hemodialysis. **Half-life:** 4 hr.

- **Available Forms:**
  - Injection Powder for Reconstitution: 1-g.

- **Indications and Dosages:**
  Intra-abdominal infection: IV, IM 1 g/day for 5-14 days.
  Skin and skin-structure infection: IV, IM 1 g/day for 7-14 days.
  Pneumonia, UTI: IV, IM 1 g/day for 10-14 days.
  Pelvic infection: IV, IM 1 g/day for 3-10 days.
  Dosage in renal impairment: For adults and elderly patients with creatinine clearance less than 30 ml/min, dosage is 500 mg once a day.

- **Contraindications:** History of hypersensitivity to beta-lactams (imipenem and cilastin, meropenem), hypersensitivity to amide-type local anesthetics (IM)

- **Side Effects**
  Frequent (10%-6%)
  Diarrhea, nausea, headache
  Occasional (5%-2%)
  Altered mental status, insomnia, rash, abdominal pain, constipation, vomiting, edema, fever
  Rare (less than 2%)
  Dizziness, cough, oral candidiasis, anxiety, tachycardia, phlebitis at IV site

- **Serious Reactions**
  - Antibiotic-associated colitis and other superinfections may occur.
  - Anaphylactic reactions have been reported.
  - Seizures may occur in those with CNS disorders (including patients with brain lesions or a history of seizures), bacterial meningitis, or severe renal impairment.

Special Considerations
  - Daily dosing is advantage over imipenem or meropenem
  - Individualize treatment based on local susceptibility patterns.

- **Patient/Family Education**
  - Notify the physician if diarrhea, a rash, seizures, tremors, or any other new symptoms occur

- **Monitoring Parameters**
  - Skin for rash
  - Hydration status, check for nausea and vomiting
  - IV injection site for inflammation
  - Mental status, and watch for seizures and tremors
  - Sleep pattern for evidence of insomnia
  - Daily bowel activity and stool consistency. Although mild GI effects may be tolerable, severe symptoms may indicate the onset of antibiotic-associated colitis.
  - Signs and symptoms of superinfection include abdominal pain or cramping, anal or genital pruritus or discharge, moderate to severe diarrhea, severe mouth or tongue soreness, and new or increased fever.

- **Geriatric side effects at a glance:**
  - ☑ CNS   ☑ Bowel Dysfunction   ☐ Bladder Dysfunction   ☐ Falls

- **U.S. Regulatory Considerations**
  - ☐ FDA Black Box   ☐ OBRA regulated in U.S. Long Term Care

erythromycin

(er-ith-roe-mye'-sin)

- **Brand Name(s):** (A/T/S, Akne-Mycin, EES, Emgel, E-Mycin, Eryc, Erycette, EryDerm, Erygel, Erymax, EryPed, Ery-Tab, Erythra-Derm, Erythrocin, PCE Dispertab, Romycin, Roymicin, Staticin, Theramycin, Theramycin Z, T-Stat)

  Combinations
  Rx: with benzoyl peroxide (Benzamycin)
  Chemical Class: Macrolide derivative

- **Clinical Pharmacology:**
  Mechanism of Action: A macrolide that reversibly binds to bacterial ribosomes, inhibiting bacterial protein synthesis. **Therapeutic Effect:** Bacteriostatic.
  Pharmacokinetics: Variably absorbed from the GI tract (depending on dosage form used). Protein binding: 70%-90%. Widely distributed. Metabolized in the liver. Primarily eliminated in feces by bile. Not removed by hemodialysis. **Half-life:** 1.4-2 hr (increased in impaired renal function).

- **Available Forms:**
  - *Topical Gel (A/T/S, Emgel, Erygel):* 2%.
  - *Injection Powder for Reconstitution (Erythrocin):* 500 mg, 1 g.
  - *Ophthalmic Ointment (Roymicin):* 0.5%.
  - *Topical Ointment (Akne-Mycin):* 2%.

451

- *Topical Solution*: 1.5% (Staticin), 2% (A/T/S, Erymax, EryDerm, Erythra-Derm, Romycin, Theramycin Z, T-Stat).
- *Topical Swab (Erycette*, T-Stat) : 2%.
- *Tablets (Chewable [EryPed])*: 200 mg.
- *Tablets*: 250 mg (E-Mycin, Ery-Tab, Erythrocin), 333 mg (Ery-Tab, E-Mycin, PCE Dispertab), 400 mg (EES), 500 mg (E-Mycin, Ery-Tab, Erythrocin, PCE Dispertab).
- *Capsules (Enteric-Coated [Eryc])*: 250 mg.

■ Indications and Dosages:

Mild to moderate infections of the upper and lower respiratory tract, pharyngitis, skin infections: PO 250 mg q6h, 500 mg q12h, or 333 mg q8h. Maximum: 4 g/day. IV 15-20 mg/kg/day in divided doses. Maximum: 4 g/day.

Preoperative intestinal antisepsis: PO 1g at 1 pm, 2 pm, and 11 pm on day before surgery (with neomycin).

Acne vulgaris: Topical Apply thin layer to affected area twice a day.

■ Unlabeled Uses: Systemic: Treatment of acne vulgaris, chancroid, *Campylobacter* enteritis, gastroparesis, Lyme disease, diabetic gastroparesis

Topical: Treatment of minor bacterial skin infections
Ophthalmic: Treatment of blepharitis, conjunctivitis, keratitis, chlamydial trachoma

■ Contraindications: History of hepatitis due to macrolides; hypersensitivity to macrolides; preexisting hepatic disease.

■ Side Effects

Frequent
IV: Abdominal cramping or discomfort, phlebitis or thrombophlebitis
Topical: Dry skin (50%)

Occasional
Nausea, vomiting, diarrhea, rash, urticaria

Rare
Ophthalmic: Sensitivity reaction with increased irritation, burning, itching, and inflammation
Topical: Urticaria

■ Serious Reactions

- Antibiotic-associated colitis and other superinfections may occur.
- High dosages in patients with renal impairment may lead to reversible hearing loss.
- Anaphylaxis and hepatotoxicity occur rarely.
- Ventricular arrhythmias and prolonged QT interval occur rarely with the IV drug form.

Special Considerations

- Individualize treatment based on local susceptibility patterns.

■ Patient/Family Education

- Take with food to minimize GI discomfort
- Take each dose with 180-240 ml of water
- Wash, rinse, and dry affected area prior to top application
- Keep top preparations away from eyes, nose, and mouth
- Ophth ointments may cause temporary blurring of vision following administration
- Space doses evenly around the clock and continue erythromycin therapy for the full course of treatment

- Wait at least 1 hr before using other topical acne preparations containing abrasive or peeling agents, such as medicated soaps, and cosmetics or aftershave containing alcohol

■ Monitoring Parameters
- LFTs if hepatotoxicity suspected
- Check daily for vein irritation and phlebitis in patients receiving IV forms
- Skin for rash
- Signs of hearing loss because high dosages can cause hearing loss in patients with hepatic or renal dysfunction
- Daily bowel activity and stool consistency. Although mild GI effects may be tolerable, severe symptoms may indicate the onset of antibiotic-associated colitis.
- Signs and symptoms of superinfection include abdominal pain or cramping, anal or genital pruritus or discharge, moderate to severe diarrhea, severe mouth or tongue soreness, and new or increased fever.

■ Geriatric side effects at a glance:
❑ CNS   ☑ Bowel Dysfunction   ❑ Bladder Dysfunction   ❑ Falls

■ U.S. Regulatory Considerations
❑ FDA Black Box   ❑ OBRA regulated in U.S. Long Term Care

escitalopram oxalate

(es-sye-tal'-oh-pram ok'-sal-ate)

■ Brand Name(s): Lexapro
Chemical Class: Bicyclic phthalane derivative

■ Clinical Pharmacology:
Mechanism of Action: A selective serotonin reuptake inhibitor that blocks the uptake of the neurotransmitter serotonin at neuronal presynaptic membranes, increasing its availability at postsynaptic receptor sites. **Therapeutic Effect:** Relieves depression. **Pharmacokinetics:** Well absorbed after PO administration. Primarily metabolized in the liver. Primarily excreted in feces with a lesser amount eliminated in urine. **Half-life:** 35 hr.

■ Available Forms:
- *Oral Solution*: 5 mg/5 ml.
- *Tablets*: 5 mg, 10 mg, 20 mg.

■ Indications and Dosages:
Depression, generalized anxiety disorder (GAD): PO 10 mg/day.

■ Unlabeled Uses: Mixed anxiety and depressive disorder

■ Contraindications: Use within 14 days of MAOIs

Side Effects

Frequent (21%-11%)
Nausea, dry mouth, somnolence, insomnia, diaphoresis

Occasional (8%-4%)
Tremor, diarrhea, abnormal ejaculation, dyspepsia, fatigue, anxiety, vomiting, anorexia

Rare (3%-2%)
Sinusitis, sexual dysfunction, menstrual disorder, abdominal pain, agitation, decreased libido

Serious Reactions
- Overdose is manifested as dizziness, drowsiness, tachycardia, somnolence, confusion, and seizures.

Special Considerations
- Patent extension for a useful agent; not different from citalopram

Patient/Family Education
- Do not discontinue escitalopram or increase the dosage
- Avoid alcohol while taking escitalopram
- Avoid tasks that require mental alertness or motor skills until response to the drug has been established

Monitoring Parameters
- Improvement of symptoms of depression or anxiety/depression, suicidal ideation, signs of toxicity (e.g., somnolence, sleep disturbances, persistent GI symptoms)

Geriatric side effects at a glance:
☐ CNS   ☑ Bowel Dysfunction   ☐ Bladder Dysfunction   ☑ Falls
Other: Hyponatremia, weight gain (long term)

Use with caution in older patients with: None

U.S. Regulatory Considerations
☑ FDA Black Box
- Because there is an increased risk of suicide in children and adolescents, older adults should also be closely monitored for suicide ideation.
☑ OBRA regulated in U.S. Long Term Care

Other Uses in Geriatric Patient: Anxiety symptoms and related disorders

Side Effects:
Of particular importance in the geriatric patient: Hyponatremia, withdrawal symptoms when abruptly discontinued (e.g., during hospitalization) rather than tapered

Geriatric Considerations - Summary: These agents are now considered by many the first-line therapy for treatment of depression in older adults. They are also effective in the management of symptoms of anxiety. Although these agents appear to have a more favorable side-effect profile than tricyclic antidepressants for most older adults, it is important to note that some of these agents have potential significant drug interactions, have been associated with falls, and require careful attention to elec-

trolyte status. In addition, many of the drugs in this class have been associated with severe withdrawal symptoms (e.g., nausea and/or vomiting, dizziness, headaches, lethargy or light-headedness, anxiety and/or agitation) when discontinued abruptly.

■ **References:**

1. Cadieux RJ. Antidepressant drug interactions in the elderly. Understanding the P-450 system is half the battle in reducing risks. Postgrad Med 1999;106:231-240, 245.
2. Roose SP, Laghrissi-Thode F, Kennedy JS, et al. Comparison of paroxetine and nortriptyline in depressed patients with ischemic heart disease. JAMA 1998;279:287-291.
3. Thapa PB, Gideon P, Cost TW, et al. Antidepressants and the risk of falls among nursing home residents. N Engl J Med 1998;339:875-882.
4. Bouman WP, Pinner G, Johnson H. Incidence of selective serotonin reuptake inhibitor (SSRI) induced hyponatraemia due to the syndrome of inappropriate antidiuretic hormone (SIADH) secretion in the elderly. Int J Geriatr Psychiatry 1998;13:12-15.

esmolol hydrochloride

(ess'-moe-lol hye-droe-klor'-ide)

■ **Brand Name(s):** Brevibloc
  Chemical Class: β_1-adrenergic blocker, cardioselective

■ **Clinical Pharmacology:**
  Mechanism of Action: An antiarrhythmic that selectively blocks beta$_1$-adrenergic receptors. **Therapeutic Effect:** Slows sinus heart rate, decreases cardiac output, reducing BP.
  Pharmacokinetics: Rapidly metabolized primarily by esterase in the cytosol of red blood cells. Protein binding: 55%. Less than 1%-2% excreted in urine. **Half-life:** 9 min.

■ **Available Forms:**
  • *Injection:* 10 mg/ml, 20 mg/ml, 250 mg/ml.

■ **Indications and Dosages:**
  Arrhythmias: IV Initially, loading dose of 500 mcg/kg/min for 1 min, followed by 50 mcg/kg/min for 4 min. If optimum response is not attained in 5 min, give second loading dose of 500 mcg/kg/min for 1 min, followed by infusion of 100 mcg/kg/min for 4 min. Additional loading doses can be given and infusion increased by 50 mcg/kg/min, up to 200 mcg/kg/min, for 4 min. Once desired response is attained, cease loading dose and increase infusion by no more than 25 mcg/kg/min. Interval between doses may be increased to 10 min. Infusion usually administered over 24-48 hr in most patients. Range: 50-200 mcg/kg/min, with average dose of 100 mcg/kg/min.
  Intraoperative tachycardia or hypertension (immediate control): IV Initially, 80 mg over 30 sec, then 150 mcg/kg/min infusion up to 300 mcg/kg/min.

■ **Contraindications:** Cardiogenic shock, overt cardiac failure, second- and third-degree heart block, sinus bradycardia

■ **Side Effects**
  Frequent
  Esmolol is generally well tolerated, with transient and mild side effects.

Hypotension (systolic BP less than 90 mm Hg) manifested as dizziness, nausea, diaphoresis, headache, cold extremities, fatigue
Occasional
Anxiety, drowsiness, flushed skin, vomiting, confusion, inflammation at injection site, fever

■ **Serious Reactions**
- Overdose may produce profound hypotension, bradycardia, dizziness, syncope, drowsiness, breathing difficulty, bluish fingernails or palms of hands, and seizures.
- Esmolol administration may potentiate insulin-induced hypoglycemia in diabetic patients.

Special Considerations
- Transfer to alternative agent (e.g., propranolol, digoxin, verapamil): ½ hr after first dose of alternative agent, reduce esmolol INF rate by 50%; following second dose of alternative agent, monitor patient's response and, if satisfactory control is maintained for the first hr, discontinue esmolol INF
- Do not discontinue abruptly; may require taper; rapid withdrawal may produce rebound hypertension or angina

■ **Patient/Family Education**
- Blood pressure and heart rate should be continuously monitored during esmolol therapy
- Report cold extremities, dizziness, faintness, or nausea

■ **Monitoring Parameters**
- *Angina*: Reduction in nitroglycerin usage; frequency, severity, onset, and duration of angina pain; heart rate
- *Arrhythmias*: Heart rate
- *Hypertension*: Blood pressure
- *Postmyocardial infarction*: Left ventricular function, lower resting heart rate
- *Toxicity*: Blood glucose, bronchospasm, hypotension, bradycardia, depression, confusion, hallucination, sexual dysfunction

■ **Geriatric side effects at a glance:**
❑ CNS ❑ Bowel Dysfunction ❑ Bladder Dysfunction ❑ Falls

■ **U.S. Regulatory Considerations**
☑ FDA Black Box
In patients using orally administered beta-blockers, abrupt withdrawal may precipitate angina or lead to myocardial infarction or ventricular arrhythmias.
❑ OBRA regulated in U.S. Long Term Care

esomeprazole

(es-om-eh-pray'-zole)

■ **Brand Name(s):** Nexium, Nexium IV
  Chemical Class: Benzimidazole derivative

■ **Clinical Pharmacology:**
  Mechanism of Action: A proton pump inhibitor that is converted to active metabolites that irreversibly bind to and inhibit hydrogen-potassium adenosine triphosphates, an enzyme on the surface of gastric parietal cells. Inhibits hydrogen ion transport into gastric lumen. **Therapeutic Effect:** Increases gastric pH, reducing gastric acid production.
  Pharmacokinetics: Well absorbed after oral administration. Protein binding: 97%. Extensively metabolized by the liver. Primarily excreted in urine. **Half-life:** 1-1.5 hr.

■ **Available Forms:**
  • *Capsules (Delayed-Release, Magnesium [Nexium]):* 20 mg, 40 mg.
  • *Powder for Solution (Sodium [Nexium IV]):* 20 mg, 40 mg.

■ **Indications and Dosages:**
  Erosive esophagitis: PO 20-40 mg once daily for 4-8 wk. IV 20 or 40 mg once daily by IV injection over at least 3 min or IV infusion over 10-30 minutes.
  To maintain healing of erosive esophagitis: PO 20 mg/day.
  Gastroesophageal reflux disease, to reduce the risk of NSAID-induced gastric ulcer: PO 20 mg once a day for 4 wk.
  Duodenal ulcer caused by Helicobacter pylori: PO 40 mg (esomeprazole) once a day, with amoxicillin 1000 mg and clarithromycin 500 mg twice a day for 10 days.

■ **Contraindications:** Hypersensitivity to benzimidazoles

■ **Side Effects**
  Frequent (7%)
  Headache
  Occasional (3%–2%)
  Diarrhea, abdominal pain, nausea
  Rare (less than 2%)
  Dizziness, asthenia or loss of strength, vomiting, constipation, rash, cough

■ **Serious Reactions**
  • None known.

Special Considerations
  • S-isomer of omeprazole (racemate)
  • No advantage over other proton pump inhibitors; cost should govern choice
  • Notify the physician if headache occurs during therapy

■ **Patient/Family Education**
  • Take at least 1 hr before meals

- Capsules may be opened, mixed with cold applesauce and swallowed immediately without chewing for patients who cannot swallow capsules whole

■ **Monitoring Parameters**
- Therapeutic response (relief of GI symptoms)

■ **Geriatric side effects at a glance:**
❑ CNS ❑ Bowel Dysfunction ❑ Bladder Dysfunction ❑ Falls

■ **U.S. Regulatory Considerations**
❑ FDA Black Box ❑ OBRA regulated in U.S. Long Term Care

estazolam

(es-ta'-zoe-lam)

■ **Brand Name(s):** ProSom
Chemical Class: Benzodiazepine

DEA Class: Schedule IV

■ **Clinical Pharmacology:**
Mechanism of Action: A benzodiazepine that enhances action of gamma-aminobutyric acid (GABA) neurotransmission in the central nervous system (CNS). **Therapeutic Effect:** Produces depressant effect at all levels of CNS.
Pharmacokinetics: Rapidly absorbed from gastrointestinal (GI) tract. Protein binding: 93%. Metabolized in liver. Primarily excreted in urine, minimal in feces. **Half-life:** 10-24 hr.

■ **Available Forms:**
- *Tablets*: 1 mg, 2 mg (ProSom).

■ **Indications and Dosages:**
Insomnia: PO 0.5-1 mg at bedtime.

■ **Contraindications:** Hypersensitivity to other benzodiazepines

■ **Side Effects**
Frequent
Drowsiness, sedation, rebound insomnia (may occur for 1-2 nights after drug is discontinued), dizziness, confusion, euphoria
Occasional
Weakness, anorexia, diarrhea
Rare
Paradoxical CNS excitement, restlessness

■ **Serious Reactions**
- Overdosage results in somnolence, confusion, diminished reflexes, and coma.

- **Patient/Family Education**
  - Do not discontinue abruptly after prolonged therapy
  - May experience disturbed sleep for the first or second night after discontinuing the drug
  - Avoid alcohol
  - Smoking decreases the drug's effectiveness

- **Monitoring Parameters**
  - Therapeutic response—decrease in number of nocturnal awakenings, increase in length of sleep

- **Geriatric side effects at a glance:**
  ☑ CNS   ☐ Bowel Dysfunction   ☐ Bladder Dysfunction   ☑ Falls
  Other: Withdrawal symptoms after long-term use

- **Use with caution in older patients with:** COPD; untreated sleep apnea

- **U.S. Regulatory Considerations**
  ☐ FDA Black Box   ☑ OBRA regulated in U.S. Long Term Care

- **Other Uses in Geriatric Patient:** Anxiety symptoms and related disorders, dementia-related behavioral problems

- **Side Effects:**
  Of particular importance in the geriatric patient: Sedation, withdrawal symptoms when abruptly discontinued (e.g., during hospitalization) rather than tapered.

- **Geriatric Considerations - Summary:** Benzodiazepines are effective anxiolytic agents, and hypnotics. These drugs should be reserved for short-term use. SSRIs are preferred for long-term management of anxiety disorders in older adults, and sedating antidepressants (e.g., trazodone) or eszopiclone are preferred for long-term management of sleep problems. Long-acting benzodiazepines, including flurazepam, chlordiazepoxide, clorazepate, diazepam, clonazepam, and quazepam should generally be avoided in older adults as these agents have been associated with oversedation. On the other hand, short-acting benzodiazepines (e.g., triazolam) have been associated with a higher risk of withdrawal symptoms. When initiating therapy, benzodiazepines should be titrated carefully to avoid oversedation. In addition, many of the drugs in this class have been associated with severe withdrawal symptoms (e.g., anxiety and/or agitation, seizures) when discontinued abruptly.

- **References:**
  1. Leipzig RM, Cumming RG, Tinetti ME. Drugs and falls in older people: a systematic review and meta-analysis: I. Psychotropic drugs. J Am Geriatr Soc 1999;47:30-39.
  2. Shorr RI, Robin DW. Rational use of benzodiazepines in the elderly. Drugs Aging 1994;4:9-20.
  3. Shader RI, Greenblatt DJ. Use of benzodiazepines in anxiety disorders. N Engl J Med 1993;328:1398-1405.

estradiol

(ess-tra-dye'-ole)

■ **Brand Name(s):** Alora, Climara, Del-estrogen, Depo-Estradiol, Esclim, Estrace, Estraderm, Estrasorb, Estring, EstroGel, Femring, Menostar, Vagifem,Vivelle, Vivelle-Dot
Chemical Class: ENDO-estrogen derivative

■ **Clinical Pharmacology:**
Mechanism of Action: An estrogen that increases synthesis of DNA, RNA, and proteins in target tissues; reduces release of gonadotropin-releasing hormone from the hypothalamus; and reduces follicle-stimulating hormone and luteinizing hormone (LH) release from the pituitary. **Therapeutic Effect:** Promotes normal growth, promotes development of female sex organs, and maintains GU function and vasomotor stability. Prevents accelerated bone loss by inhibiting bone resorption, restoring balance of bone resorption and formation. Inhibits LH and decreases serum testosterone concentration.
Pharmacokinetics: Well absorbed from the GI tract. Widely distributed. Protein binding: 50%-80%. Metabolized in the liver. Primarily excreted in urine. **Half-life:** Unknown.

■ **Available Forms:**
- *Tablets (Estrace):* 0.5 mg, 1 mg, 2 mg.
- *Emulsion (Topical [Estrasorb]):* 2.5 mg/g.
- *Injection (Cypionate [Depo-Estradiol]):* 5 mg/ml.
- *Injection (Valerate [Del-estrogen]):* 10 mg/ml.
- *Topical Gel (EstroGel):* 1.25 g.
- *Transdermal System (Alora):* twice weekly: 0.025 mg, 0.05 mg, 0.075 mg, 0.1 mg.
- *Transdermal System (Climara):* once weekly: 0.025 mg, 0.0375 mg, 0.05 mg, 0.06 mg, 0.075 mg, 0.1 mg.
- *Transdermal System (Esclim):* twice weekly: 0.025 mg, 0.0375 mg, 0.05 mg, 0.075 mg, 0.1 mg.
- *Transdermal System (Estraderm):* twice weekly: 0.05 mg, 0.1 mg.
- *Transdermal System (Menostar):* once a week: 1 mg.
- *Transdermal System (Vivelle):* twice weekly: 0.025 mg, 0.0375 mg, 0.05 mg, 0.075 mg, 0.1 mg.
- *Transdermal System (Vivelle-Dot):* twice weekly: 0.0375 mg, 0.05 mg, 0.075 mg, 0.1 mg.
- *Vaginal Cream (Estrace):* 0.1 mg/g.
- *Vaginal Ring (Estring):* 2 mg.
- *Vaginal Ring (Femring):* 0.05 mg.
- *Vaginal Tablet (Vagifem):* 25 mcg.

■ **Indications and Dosages:**
Prostate cancer: IM (estradiol valerate) 30 mg or more q1-2 wk. PO 10 mg 3 times a day for at least 3 mo.
Breast cancer: PO 10 mg 3 times a day for at least 3 mo.
Osteoporosis prophylaxis in postmenopausal females: PO 0.5 mg/day cyclically (3 weeks on, 1 week off). Transdermal (Climara) Initially, 0.025 mg weekly, adjust dose as needed. Transdermal (Alora, Vivelle, Vivelle-Dot) Initially, 0.025 mg patch twice weekly, adjust dose as needed. Transdermal (Estraderm) 0.05 mg twice weekly. Transdermal (Menostar) 1 mg weekly.

Female hypoestrogenism: PO 1-2 mg/day, adjust dose as needed. IM (cypionate) 1.5-2 mg monthly. IM (estradiol valerate) 10-20 mg q4wk.

Vasomotor symptoms associated with menopause: PO 1-2 mg/day cyclically (3 weeks on, 1 week off), adjust dose as needed. IM (estradiol cypionate) 1-5 mg q3-4wk. IM (estradiol valerate) 10-20 mg q4wk. Topical emulsion (Estrasorb) 3.84g once a day in the morning. Topical Gel (Estrogel) 1.25 g/day. Transdermal (Climara) 0.025 mg weekly. Adjust dose as needed. Transdermal (Alora, Esclim, Estraderm, Vivelle-Dot) 0.05 mg twice a week. Transdermal (Vivelle) 0.0375 mg twice a week. Vaginal Ring (Femring) 0.05 mg. May increase to 0.1 mg if needed.

Vaginal atrophy: Vaginal Ring (Estring) 2 mg.

Atrophic vaginitis: Vaginal Tablet (Vagifem) Initially, 1 tablet/day for 2 weeks. Maintenance: 1 tablet twice a week.

■ **Unlabeled Uses:** Treatment of Turner's syndrome

■ **Contraindications:** Abnormal vaginal bleeding, active arterial thrombosis, blood dyscrasias, estrogen-dependent cancer, known or suspected breast cancer, thrombophlebitis or thromboembolic disorders, thyroid dysfunction

■ **Side Effects**

Frequent

Anorexia, nausea, swelling of breasts, peripheral edema marked by swollen ankles and feet

Transdermal: Skin irritation, redness

Occasional

Vomiting, especially with high doses; headache that may be severe; intolerance to contact lenses; hypertension; glucose intolerance; brown spots on exposed skin

Vaginal: Local irritation, vaginal discharge

Rare

Chorea or involuntary movements, hirsutism or abnormal hairiness, loss of scalp hair, depression

■ **Serious Reactions**

- Estrogen therapy may increase the risk of developing coronary heart disease, hypercalcemia, gallbladder disease, cerebrovascular disease, and breast cancer.
- Prolonged administration increases the risk of gallbladder disease, thromboembolic disease, and breast, cervical, vaginal, endometrial, and hepatic carcinoma.
- Cholestatic jaundice occurs rarely.

Special Considerations

- Progestins recommended in nonhysterectomized women. Estring may have minimal systemic absorption

■ **Patient/Family Education**

- Limit alcohol and caffeine intake
- Stop smoking tobacco
- Report calf or chest pain, depression, numbness or weakness of an extremity, severe abdominal pain, shortness of breath, speech or vision disturbance, sudden headache, unusual bleeding, or vomiting

■ **Monitoring Parameters**

- Blood pressure, weight, blood glucose, liver function, and serum calcium levels

■ **U.S. Regulatory Considerations**
   ☑ FDA Black Box
   There is an increased risk of cardiovascular disease, endometrial cancer, thromboembolic disease, and worsening dementia.
   ❑ OBRA regulated in U.S. Long Term Care

■ **Geriatric Considerations - Summary:** Estrogens should be avoided in patients with cognitive impairment.

estrogens, conjugated

(ess'-troe-jens, kon'-joo-gay-ted)

■ **Brand Name(s):** Cenestin, Enjuvia, Premarin, Premarin Intravenous, Premarin Vaginal

Combinations
Rx: with medroxyprogesterone (Prempro [daily product], Premphase [cycled product]); with meprobamate (PMB); with methyltestosterone (Premarin with methyltestosterone)
Chemical Class: ENDO-estrogen derivative

■ **Clinical Pharmacology:**
Mechanism of Action: An estrogen that increases synthesis of DNA, RNA, and various proteins in target tissues; reduces release of gonadotropin-releasing hormone from the hypothalamus; and reduces follicle-stimulating hormone (FSH) and luteinizing hormone (LH) release from the pituitary gland. ***Therapeutic Effect:*** Promotes normal growth, promotes development of femal sex organs, and maintains GU function and vasomotor stability. Prevents accelerated bone loss by inhibiting bone resorption, restoring balance of bone resorption and formation. Inhibits LH and decreases serum concentration of testosterone.
Pharmacokinetics: Well absorbed from the GI tract. Widely distributed. Protein binding: 50%-80%. Metabolized in the liver. Primarily excreted in urine.

■ **Available Forms:**
   • *Tablets:* 0.3 mg (Cenestin, Premarin), 0.45 mg (Cenestin, Premarin), 0.625 mg (Cenestin, Enjuvia, Premarin), 0.9 mg (Cenestin, Premarin), 1.25 mg (Cenestin, Enjuvia, Premarin), 2.5 mg (Cenestin, Premarin).
   • *Injection (Premarin Intravenous):* 25 mg.
   • *Vaginal Cream (Premarin Vaginal):* 0.625 mg/g.

■ **Indications and Dosages:**
Vasomotor symptoms associated with menopause, atrophic vaginitis, kraurosis vulvae:
PO 0.3-0.625 mg/day cyclically (21 days on, 7 days off) or continuously. Intravaginal 0.5-2 g/day cyclically, such as 21 days on and 7 days off.

Female hypogonadism: PO 0.3-0.625 mg/day in divided doses for 20 days; then a rest period of 10 days.

Female castration, primary ovarian failure: PO Initially, 1.25 mg/day cyclically. Adjust dosage, upward or downward, according to severity of symptoms and patient response. For Maintenance, adjust dosage to lowest level that will provide effective control.

Osteoporosis: PO 0.3-0.625 mg/day, cyclically, such as 25 days on and 5 days off.

Breast cancer: PO 10 mg 3 times a day for at least 3 mo.

Prostate cancer: PO 1.25-2.5 mg 3 times a day.

Abnormal uterine bleeding: PO 1.25 mg q4h for 24 hr, then 1.25 mg/day for 7-10 days. IV, IM 25 mg; may repeat once in 6-12 hr.

■ **Unlabeled Uses:** Prevention of estrogen deficiency–induced premenopausal osteoporosis

Cream: Prevention of nosebleeds

■ **Contraindications:** Breast cancer with some exceptions, hepatic disease, thrombophlebitis, undiagnosed vaginal bleeding

■ **Side Effects**

Frequent

Vaginal bleeding, breast pain or tenderness; gynecomastia

Occasional

Headache, hypertension, intolerance to contact lenses

High-doses: Anorexia, nausea

Rare

Loss of scalp hair, depression

■ **Serious Reactions**

• Prolonged administration may increase the risk of breast, cervical, endometrial, hepatic, and vaginal carcinoma; cerebrovascular disease, coronary heart disease, gallbladder disease, and hypercalcemia.

Special Considerations

• Progestins recommended in nonhysterectomized women
• Premarin is derived from pregnant mare's urine; Cenestin from yams and soy. Although probably therapeutically equivalent, they are not substitutable by the pharmacist
• Consider topical products if treatment is solely for vulvar or vaginal atrophy
• Currently recommended that use of hormone replacement therapy be limited to treating symptomatic women, preferably for 5 yr or less. Risk felt to outweigh benefit in asymptomatic women using only for prophylaxis of other conditions

■ **Patient/Family Education**

• Avoid smoking because of the increased risk of blood clot formation and MI
• Diet and exercise are important when conjugated estrogens are taken to retard osteoporosis
• Report abnormal vaginal bleeding, depression, or signs and symptoms of blood clots
• Perform breast self-examination monthly
• Report weekly weight gain of more than 5 lb

Monitoring Parameters
- Blood pressure periodically
- Weight
- Signs and symptoms of thromboembolic or thrombotic disorders, including loss of coordination, numbness or weakness of an extremity, shortness of breath, speech or vision disturbance, sudden severe headache, and pain in the chest, leg, or groin

Geriatric side effects at a glance:
☐ CNS   ☐ Bowel Dysfunction   ☐ Bladder Dysfunction   ☐ Falls

U.S. Regulatory Considerations
☑ FDA Black Box
There is an increased risk of cardiovascular disease, endometrial cancer, thromboembolic disease, and worsening dementia.
☐ OBRA regulated in U.S. Long Term Care

Geriatric Considerations - Summary: Estrogens should be avoided in patients with cognitive impairment.

estrogens, esterified

(ess'-troe-jens, ess'-ter-i-fyed)

Brand Name(s): Estratab, Menest

Combinations
Rx: with methyltestosterone (Estratest, Menogen)
Chemical Class: ENDO-estrogen derivative

Clinical Pharmacology:
Mechanism of Action: A combination of sodium salts of sulfate esters of estrogenic substances (principal component is estrone) that increases synthesis of DNA, RNA, and various proteins in responsive tissues. Reduces release of gonadotropin-releasing hormone, reducing follicle-stimulating hormone (FSH) and luteinizing hormone (LH). **Therapeutic Effect:** Promotes vasomotor stability, maintains genitourinary (GU) function, normal growth, development of female sex organs. Prevents accelerated bone loss by inhibiting bone resorption, restoring balance of bone resorption and formation.
Pharmacokinetics: Readily absorbed from the gastrointestinal (GI) tract. Widely distributed. Protein binding: 50%-80%. Rapidly metabolized in liver and GI tract to estrone sulfate and conjugated and unconjugated metabolites. Excreted in urine and bile. **Half-life:** Unknown.

Available Forms:
- *Tablets:* 0. 3 mg (Menest), 0. 625 mg (Estratab).

Indications and Dosages:
Vasomotor symptoms associated with menopause, atrophic vaginitis, kraurosis vulvae:
PO 0.3-1.25 mg/day.

Female hypogonadism: PO 2.5-7.5 mg/day in divided doses for 20 days; rest 10 days.
Female castration, primary ovarian failure: PO Initially, 1. 25 mg/day cyclically.
Breast cancer: PO 10 mg 3 times/day for at least 3 mo.
Prostate cancer: PO 1.25-2. 5 mg 3 times/day.

■ **Contraindications:** Breast cancer with some exceptions, liver disease, thrombophlebitis, undiagnosed vaginal bleeding

■ **Side Effects**
Frequent
Breast pain or tenderness, gynecomastia
Occasional
Headache, increased blood pressure (BP), intolerance to contact lenses, nausea
Rare
Loss of scalp hair, clinical depression

■ **Serious Reactions**
• Prolonged administration may increase risk of gallbladder, thromboembolic disease, breast, cervical, vaginal, endometrial, and liver carcinoma.

Special Considerations
• Progestins recommended in nonhysterectomized women

■ **Patient/Family Education**
• Avoid smoking because of the increased risk of blood clot formation and MI
• Report abnormal vaginal bleeding, depression, or signs and symptoms of blood clots
• Perform breast self-examination monthly
• Report weekly weight gain of more than 5 lb

■ **Monitoring Parameters**
• Blood pressure periodically
• Weight
• Signs and symptoms of thromboembolic or thrombotic disorders, including loss of coordination, numbness or weakness of an extremity, shortness of breath, speech or vision disturbance, sudden severe headache, and pain in the chest, leg, or groin

■ **Geriatric side effects at a glance:**
❑ CNS ❑ Bowel Dysfunction ❑ Bladder Dysfunction ❑ Falls

■ **U.S. Regulatory Considerations**
☑ FDA Black Box
There is an increased risk of cardiovascular disease, endometrial cancer, thromboembolic disease, and worsening dementia.
❑ OBRA regulated in U.S. Long Term Care

■ **Geriatric Considerations - Summary:** Estrogens should be avoided in patients with cognitive impairment.

estrone

(ess'-trone)

■ **Brand Name(s):** Estragyn 5, Estro-A, Estrogenic, Estrogens, Kestrone 5
  Chemical Class: ENDO-estrogen derivative

■ **Clinical Pharmacology:**
  Mechanism of Action: An estrogen that increases synthesis of DNA, RNA, proteins in target tissues; reduces release of gonadotropin-releasing hormone from hypothalamus; reduces follicle-stimulating hormone (FSH) and luteinizing hormone (LH) release from the pituitary. **Therapeutic Effect:** Promotes normal growth, development of female sex organs, maintaining genitourinary (GU) function, vasomotor stability. Prevents accelerated bone loss by inhibiting bone resorption, restoring balance of bone resorption and formation. Inhibits LH, decreases serum concentration of testosterone.
  Pharmacokinetics: Well absorbed from the gastrointestinal (GI) tract. Widely distributed. Protein binding: 50%-80%. Metabolized in liver as well as a certain proportion excreted into the bile and reabsorbed from the intestine. Primarily excreted in urine. **Half-life:** Unknown.

■ **Available Forms:**
  • Injection: 2 mg/ml (Estro-A, Estrogenic, Estrogens), 5 mg/ml (Estragyn 5, Kestrone 5).

■ **Indications and Dosages:**
  Atrophic vaginitis, female castration, female hypogonadism, kraurosis vulvae, menopausal symptoms, primary ovarian failure, prostatic carcinoma: IM Initially, 0.1 or 0.5 mg 2-3 times weekly cyclically (21 days on; 7 days off or continuously). When progestin is given concomitantly, begin progestin after 10-13 days of each estrogen cycle.

■ **Contraindications:** Abnormal vaginal bleeding, active arterial thrombosis, blood dyscrasias, estrogen-dependent cancer, known or suspected breast cancer, thrombophlebitis or thromboembolic disorders, hypersensitivity to estrone or any of its components.

■ **Side Effects**
  Occasional
  Edema, weight change, breast tenderness, nervousness, insomnia, fatigue, dizziness
  Rare
  Alopecia, mental depression, dermatologic changes, headache, fever, nausea

■ **Serious Reactions**
  • Thrombophlebitis, pulmonary or cerebral embolism, and retinal thrombosis occur rarely.

Special Considerations
  • Progestins recommended in nonhysterectomized women
  • Consider topical products if treatment is solely for vulvar or vaginal atrophy

- Currently recommended that use of hormone replacement therapy be limited to treating symptomatic women, preferably for 5 yr or less. Risk felt to outweigh benefit in asymptomatic women using only for prophylaxis of other conditions

■ **Patient/Family Education**
- Avoid smoking because of the increased risk of blood clot formation and MI
- Report abnormal vaginal bleeding, depression, or signs and symptoms of blood clots
- Perform breast self-examination monthly
- Report weekly weight gain of more than 5 lb

■ **Monitoring Parameters**
- Blood pressure periodically
- Blood glucose levels, hepatic enzymes, serum calcium levels
- Weight
- Signs and symptoms of thromboembolic or thrombotic disorders, including loss of coordination, numbness or weakness of an extremity, shortness of breath, speech or vision disturbance, sudden severe headache, and pain in the chest, leg, or groin

■ **Geriatric side effects at a glance:**
❑ CNS ❑ Bowel Dysfunction ❑ Bladder Dysfunction ❑ Falls

■ **U.S. Regulatory Considerations**
☑ FDA Black Box
There is an increased risk of cardiovascular disease, endometrial cancer, thromboembolic disease, and worsening dementia.
❑ OBRA regulated in U.S. Long Term Care

■ **Geriatric Considerations - Summary:** Estrogens should be avoided in patients with cognitive impairment.

estropipate

(es-troe-pih'-pate)

■ **Brand Name(s):** Ogen, Ortho-Est
  Chemical Class: ENDO-estrogen derivative

■ **Clinical Pharmacology:**
  Mechanism of Action: An estrogen that increases synthesis of DNA, RNA, and proteins in target tissues; reduces release of gonadotropin-releasing hormone from the hypothalamus; and reduces follicle-stimulating hormone (FSH) and luteinizing hormone (LH) from the pituitary. **Therapeutic Effect:** Promotes normal growth, promotes development of female sex organs, and maintains GU function and vasomotor stability. Prevents accelerated bone loss by inhibiting bone resorption, restoring balance of bone resorption and formation. Inhibits LH and decreases serum testosterone concentration.

Pharmacokinetics: Readily absorbed through the skin, mucous membranes, and GI tract. Widely distributed. Protein binding: 50%-80%. Metabolized in the liver. Primarily excreted in urine. **Half-life**: 12-20 hr.

■ **Available Forms:**
  • *Tablets (Ogen, Ortho-Est)*: 0.625 mg (0.75 mg estropipate), 1.25 mg (1.5 mg estropipate), 2.5 mg (3 mg estropipate).
  • *Vaginal Cream (Ogen)*: 1.5 mg/g.

■ **Indications and Dosages:**
  Vasomotor symptoms, atrophic vaginitis, kraurosis vulvae: PO 0.625-5 mg/day cyclically.
  Atrophic vaginitis, kraurosis vulvae: Intravaginal 2-4 g/day cyclically.
  Female hypogonadism, castration, primary ovarian failure: PO 1.25-7.5 mg/day for 21 days; then off for 8-10 days. Repeat if bleeding does not occur by end of off cycle.
  Prevention of osteoporosis: PO 0.625 mg/day (25 days of 31-day cycle/mo).

■ **Contraindications:** Abnormal vaginal bleeding, active arterial thrombosis, blood dyscrasias, estrogen-dependent cancer, known or suspected breast cancer, thrombophlebitis or thromboembolic disorders, thyroid dysfunction

■ **Side Effects**
  Frequent
  Anorexia, nausea, swelling of breasts, peripheral edema marked by swollen ankles and feet
  Occasional
  Vomiting, especially with high doses; headache that may be severe; intolerance to contact lenses; hypertension; glucose intolerance; brown spots on exposed skin
  Vaginal: Local irritation, vaginal discharge
  Rare
  Chorea or involuntary movements, hirsutism or abnormal hairiness, loss of scalp hair, depression

■ **Serious Reactions**
  • Prolonged administration may increase the risk of breast, cervical, endometrial, hepatic, and vaginal carcinoma; cerebrovascular disease, coronary heart disease, gallbladder disease, and hypercalcemia.
  • Cholestatic jaundice occurs rarely.

Special Considerations
  • Unopposed estrogen increases risk of endometrial cancer; recommended administration of concurrent progestational agents for nonhysterectomized women

■ **Patient/Family Education**
  • Avoid smoking because of the increased risk of blood clot formation and MI
  • Remain recumbent for at least 30 minutes after vaginal application and do not use tampons during estropipate therapy
  • Report depression or abnormal vaginal bleeding

■ **Monitoring Parameters**
  • Signs and symptoms of thromboembolic or thrombotic disorders, including loss of coordination, numbness or weakness of an extremity, shortness of breath, speech or vision disturbance, sudden severe headache, and pain in the chest, leg, or groin

- **Geriatric side effects at a glance:**
  - ❑ CNS ❑ Bowel Dysfunction ❑ Bladder Dysfunction ❑ Falls

- **U.S. Regulatory Considerations**
  - ☑ FDA Black Box

  There is an increased risk of cardiovascular disease, endometrial cancer, thromboembolic disease, and worsening dementia.
  - ❑ OBRA regulated in U.S. Long Term Care

- **Geriatric Considerations - Summary:** Estrogens should be avoided in patients with cognitive impairment.

eszopiclone

(es-zoe'-pi-clone)

- **Brand Name(s):** Lunesta

- **Clinical Pharmacology:**

  Mechanism of Action: A nonbenzodiazepine that may interact with GABA-receptor complexes at binding domains located close to or allosterically coupled to benzodiazepine receptors. **Therapeutic Effect:** Induces sleep and helps maintain sleep at night.

  Pharmacokinetics: Rapidly absorbed after PO administration. Weakly bound to plasma proteins. Metabolized in the liver. Excreted in urine. **Half-life:** 5-6 hr.

- **Available Forms:**
  - *Tablets* (*Film-Coated*): 1 mg, 2 mg, 3 mg.

- **Indications and Dosages:**

  Insomnia: PO Initially, 1 mg before bedtime. Maximum: 2 mg.

  Difficulty maintaining sleep: PO 2 mg before bedtime.

- **Contraindications:** None known.

- **Side Effects**

  Frequent (34%-21%)

  Unpleasant taste, headache

  Occasional (10%-4%)

  Somnolence, dry mouth, dyspepsia, dizziness, nervousness, nausea, rash, pruritus, depression, diarrhea

  Rare (3%-2%)

  Hallucinations, anxiety, confusion, abnormal dreams, decreased libido, neuralgia.

- **Serious Reactions**
  - Chest pain and peripheral edema occur occasionally.

- **Geriatric side effects at a glance:**
  ☑ CNS ❑ Bowel Dysfunction ❑ Bladder Dysfunction ☑ Falls
  Other: Unpleasant taste

- **Use with caution in older patients with:** Concurrent treatment with potent CYP 3A4 inhibitors (e.g., nefazodone); COPD; untreated sleep apnea

- **U.S. Regulatory Considerations**
  ❑ FDA Black Box ❑ OBRA regulated in U.S. Long Term Care

- **Other Uses in Geriatric Patient:** Hypnotic

- **Side Effects:**
  Of particular importance in the geriatric patient: Sedation

- **Geriatric Considerations - Summary:** Eszopiclone is the only hypnotic which has been shown to maintain efficacy over long-term use (6 months) and may have a role in the management of chronic sleep problems in older adults. Because eszopiclone is a substrate of CYP C3A, and 2E1, it should be used with caution, especially with drugs such as nefazodone, clarithromycin, and amiodarone. This agent has been newly approved for use in the US and has not been well studied in terms of falls or other geriatric side effects.

- **References:**
  1. McCall WV. Diagnosis and management of insomnia in older people. J Am Geriatr Soc 2005;53:S272-S277
  2. Eszopiclone (Lunesta), a new hypnotic. Med Lett Drugs Ther 2005;47:17-19.

etanercept

(eh-tan'-er-sept)

- **Brand Name(s):** Enbrel
  Chemical Class: Recombinant human fusion protein

- **Clinical Pharmacology:**
  Mechanism of Action: A protein that binds to tumor necrosis factor (TNF), blocking its interaction with cell surface receptors. Elevated levels of TNF, which is involved in inflammatory and immune responses, are found in the synovial fluid of rheumatoid arthritis patients. *Therapeutic Effect:* Relieves symptoms of rheumatoid arthritis. *Pharmacokinetics:* Well absorbed after subcutaneous administration. *Half-life:* 115 hr.

- **Available Forms:**
  - *Powder for Injection:* 25 mg.
  - *Prefilled Syringe:* 50 mg.

■ **Indications and Dosages:**
Rheumatoid arthritis, psoriatic arthritis, ankylosing spondylitis: Subcutaneous 25 mg twice weekly given 72-96 hr apart. Alternative weekly dosing: 0.8 mg/kg/dose once a week. Maximum: 50 mg/week. Maximum: 25 mg/dose.
Plaque psoriasis: Subcutaneous 50 mg twice a week (give 3-4 days apart) for 3 mo. Maintenance: 50 mg once a week.

■ **Unlabeled Uses:** Treatment of Crohn's disease, reactive arthritis

■ **Contraindications:** Serious active infection or sepsis

■ **Side Effects**
Frequent (37%)
Injection site erythema, pruritus, pain, and swelling; abdominal pain, vomiting
Occasional (16%-4%)
Headache, rhinitis, dizziness, pharyngitis, cough, asthenia, abdominal pain, dyspepsia
Rare (less than 3%)
Sinusitis, allergic reaction

■ **Serious Reactions**
- Infections (such as pyelonephritis, cellulitis, osteomyelitis, wound infection, leg ulcer, septic arthritis, diarrhea, bronchitis, and pneumonia) occur in 38%-29% of patients.
- Rare adverse effects include heart failure, hypertension, hypotension, pancreatitis, GI hemorrhage, and dyspnea. The patient also may develop autoimmune antibodies.

Special Considerations
- Immunizations should be up to date prior to starting therapy

■ **Patient/Family Education**
- Review injection techniques to ensure safe self-administration
- Avoid receiving live-virus vaccines during treatment
- Notify the physician if bleeding, bruising, pallor, or persistent fever occurs
- Reassure the patient that injection site reactions generally occur in the first month of treatment and decrease in frequency with continued etanercept therapy

■ **Monitoring Parameters**
- Efficacy: ESR, C-reactive protein, rheumatoid factor, improvement in tender/painful swollen joints, quality of life
- Temporarily discontinue therapy and expect to treat the patient with varicella-zoster immune globulin, as prescribed, if the patient experiences significant exposure to varicella virus during treatment

■ **Geriatric side effects at a glance:**
❑ CNS ❑ Bowel Dysfunction ❑ Bladder Dysfunction ❑ Falls

■ **U.S. Regulatory Considerations**
❑ FDA Black Box ❑ OBRA regulated in U.S. Long Term Care

ethambutol hydrochloride

(e-tham'-byoo-tole hye-droe-klor'-ide)

■ **Brand Name(s):** Myambutol
Chemical Class: Diisopropylethylene diamide derivative

■ **Clinical Pharmacology:**
Mechanism of Action: An isonicotinic acid derivative that interferes with RNA synthesis. **Therapeutic Effect:** Suppresses the multiplication of mycobacteria.
Pharmacokinetics: Rapidly and well absorbed from the GI tract. Protein binding: 20%-30%. Widely distributed. Metabolized in the liver. Primarily excreted in urine. Removed by hemodialysis. **Half-life:** 3-4 hr (increased in impaired renal function).

■ **Available Forms:**
• *Tablets:* 100 mg, 400 mg.

■ **Indications and Dosages:**
Tuberculosis, other myobacterial diseases: PO 15-25 mg/kg/day. Maximum: 1.6 g/dose.
Dosage in renal impairment: Dosage interval is modified based on creatinine clearance.

Creatinine Clearance	Dosage Interval
10-50 ml/min	q24-36h
less than 10 ml/min	q48h

■ **Unlabeled Uses:** Treatment of atypical mycobacterial infections such as *Mycobacterium avium* complex (MAC)

■ **Contraindications:** Optic neuritis

■ **Side Effects**
Occasional
Acute gouty arthritis (chills, pain, swelling of joints with hot skin), confusion, abdominal pain, nausea, vomiting, anorexia, headache
Rare
Rash, fever, blurred vision, eye pain, red-green color blindness

■ **Serious Reactions**
• Optic neuritis (more common with high-dosage or long-term ethambutol therapy), peripheral neuritis, thrombocytopenia, and an anaphylactoid reaction occur rarely.

Special Considerations
• Initial therapy in tuberculosis should include 4 drugs: isoniazid, rifampin, pyrazinamide, and ethambutol, until drug susceptibility results available

■ **Patient/Family Education**
• Administer with meals to decrease GI symptoms
• Do not skip drug doses and take ethambutol for the full course of therapy, which may be months or years

- Notify the physician immediately of any visual problems; effects are generally reversible after ethambutol is discontinued, but in rare cases they may take up to a year to resolve or may become permanent
- Promptly report burning, numbness, or tingling of the feet or hands, as well as pain and swelling of joints

■ Monitoring Parameters
- Perform visual acuity testing before beginning therapy and periodically during drug administration (qmo if dose >15 mg/kg/day)
- Serum uric acid levels; assess the patient for signs and symptoms of gout, including hot, painful, or swollen joints, especially in the ankle, big toe, or knee
- Signs and symptoms of peripheral neuritis, as evidenced by burning, numbness, or tingling of the extremities

■ Geriatric side effects at a glance:
❏ CNS ❏ Bowel Dysfunction ❏ Bladder Dysfunction ❏ Falls

■ U.S. Regulatory Considerations
❏ FDA Black Box ❏ OBRA regulated in U.S. Long Term Care

ethinyl estradiol

(eth'-in-il es-tra-dye'-ole)

■ Brand Name(s): Estinyl
Chemical Class: ENDO-estrogen derivative

■ Clinical Pharmacology:
Mechanism of Action: A synthetic derivative of estradiol that increases synthesis of DNA, RNA, proteins in target tissues; reduces release of gonadotropin-releasing hormone from hypothalamus; reduces follicle-stimulating hormone (FSH) and luteinizing hormone (LH) release from the pituitary. **Therapeutic Effect:** Promotes normal growth, development of female sex organs, maintaining genitourinary (GU) function, vasomotor stability. Prevents accelerated bone loss by inhibiting bone resorption, restoring balance of bone resorption and formation. Inhibits LH, decreases serum concentration of testosterone.

Pharmacokinetics: Well absorbed from the gastrointestinal (GI) tract. Widely distributed. Protein binding: 50%-80%. Rapidly metabolized in liver to estrone and estriol. Excreted in urine and feces. **Half-life:** 8-25 hr.

■ Available Forms:
- *Tablets:* 0.02 mg, 0.05 mg, 0.5 mg (Estinyl).

■ Indications and Dosages:
Female hypogonadism: PO 0.05 mg 1-3 times/day during the first 2 wk of menstrual cycle, followed by progesterone during the last half of cycle for 3-6 mo.
Menopausal symptoms: PO 0.02- 0.05 mg/day cyclically (3 wk on, 1 wk off).
Breast cancer: PO 1 mg 3 times/day for at least 3 mo.

Prostate cancer: PO 0.15-2 mg/day.

■ **Contraindications:** Abnormal vaginal bleeding, active arterial thrombosis, blood dyscrasias, estrogen-dependent cancer, known or suspected breast cancer, thrombophlebitis or thromboembolic disorders, thyroid dysfunction, hypersensitivity to estrongens

■ **Side Effects**
Frequent
Anorexia, nausea, swelling of breasts, peripheral edema, evidenced by swollen ankles, feet
Occasional
Vomiting, especially with high dosages, headache that may be severe, intolerance to contact lenses, increased blood pressure (BP), glucose intolerance, brown spots on exposed skin
Rare
Chorea or involuntary movements, hirsutism or abnormal hairiness, loss of scalp hair, depression

■ **Serious Reactions**
• Prolonged administration increases risk of gallbladder disease, thromboembolic disease, and breast, cervical, vaginal, endometrial, and liver carcinoma.
• Cholestatic jaundice occurs rarely.

Special Considerations
• Unopposed estrogen increases risk of endometrial cancer; recommended administration of concurrent progestational agents for nonhysterectomized women

■ **Patient/Family Education**
• Limit alcohol and caffeine intake
• Stop smoking tobacco
• Report calf or chest pain, depression, numbness or weakness of an extremity, severe abdominal pain, shortness of breath, speech or vision disturbance, sudden headache, unusual bleeding, or vomiting

■ **Monitoring Parameters**
• Blood pressure periodically
• Weight
• Signs and symptoms of thromboembolic or thrombotic disorders, including loss of coordination, numbness or weakness of an extremity, shortness of breath, speech or vision disturbance, sudden severe headache, and pain in the chest, leg, or groin

■ **Geriatric side effects at a glance:**
❏ CNS ❏ Bowel Dysfunction ❏ Bladder Dysfunction ❏ Falls

■ **U.S. Regulatory Considerations**
☑ FDA Black Box
There is an increased risk of cardiovascular disease, endometrial cancer, thromboembolic disease, and worsening dementia.
❏ OBRA regulated in U.S. Long Term Care

■ **Geriatric Considerations - Summary:** Estrogens should be avoided in patients with cognitive impairment.

ethionamide

(e-thye-on'-am-ide)

■ **Brand Name(s):** Trecator-SC
Chemical Class: Thiomine derivative

■ **Clinical Pharmacology:**
Mechanism of Action: An antitubercular agent that inhibits peptide synthesis. **Therapeutic Effect:** Suppresses mycobacterial multiplication. Bactericidal.
Pharmacokinetics: Rapidly absorbed from the gastrointestinal (GI) tract. Widely distributed. Protein binding: 10%. Metabolized in liver. Primarily excreted in urine. Removed by hemodialysis. **Half-life:** 2-3 hr (half-life is increased with impaired renal function).

■ **Available Forms:**
• *Tablets:* 250 mg (Trecator).

■ **Indications and Dosages:**
Tuberculosis: PO 500-1000 mg/day as a single to 3 divided doses.
Dosage in renal impairment: Creatinine clearance less than 50 ml/min, reduce dose by 50%.

■ **Unlabeled Uses:** Treatment of atypical mycobacterial infections

■ **Contraindications:** Severe hepatic impairment, hypersensitivity to ethionamide

■ **Side Effects**
Occasional
Abdominal pain, nausea, vomiting, weakness, postural hypotension, psychiatric disturbances, drowsiness, dizziness, headache, confusion, anorexia, headache, metallic taste, anorexia, diarrhea, stomatitis, peripheral neuritis
Rare
Rash, fever, blurred vision, optic neuritis, seizures, hypothyroidism, hypoglycemia, gynecomastia, thrombocytopenia, jaundice

■ **Serious Reactions**
• Peripheral neuropathy, anorexia, and joint pain rarely occur.

Special Considerations
• Use only with at least 1 other effective antituberculous agent

■ **Monitoring Parameters**
• Serum transaminases (AST, ALT) biweekly during therapy

■ **Geriatric side effects at a glance:**
☑ CNS ❑ Bowel Dysfunction ❑ Bladder Dysfunction ❑ Falls

ethosuximide

(eth-oh-sux'-i-mide)

■ **Brand Name(s):** Zarontin
  Chemical Class: Succinimide derivative

■ **Clinical Pharmacology:**
  Mechanism of Action: An anticonvulsant that increases the seizure threshold and suppresses paroxysmal spike-and-wave pattern in absence seizures; depresses nerve transmission in the motor cortex. **Therapeutic Effect:** Produces anticonvulsant activity.
  Pharmacokinetics: Well absorbed from the GI tract. Metabolized in liver. Excreted in urine. Removed by hemodialysis. **Half-life:** 50-60 hr (in adults); 30 hr (in children).

■ **Available Forms:**
  • **Capsule:** 100 mg, 150 mg, 200 mg, 250 mg (Zarontin).
  • **Syrup:** 250 mg/5 ml (Zarontin).

■ **Indications and Dosages:**
  Absence seizures : PO Initially, 250 mg/day or 15 mg/kg/day in 2 divided doses. Maintenance: 15-40 mg/kg/day in 2 divided doses. Use with caution in patients with renal impairment.

■ **Unlabeled Uses:** None known.

■ **Contraindications:** Hypersensitivity to succinimides

■ **Side Effects**
  Occasional
  Dizziness, drowsiness, double vision, headache, ataxia, nausea, diarrhea, vomiting, somnolence, urticaria
  Rare
  Arganulocytosis, gum hypertrophy, leukopenia, myopia, swelling of the tongue, systemic lupus erythematosus, vaginal bleeding

■ **Serious Reactions**
  • Abrupt withdrawal may increase seizure frequency.
  • Overdosage results in nausea, vomiting, and CNS depression including coma with respiratory depression.

■ **Patient/Family Education**
  • Take doses at regularly spaced intervals
  • OK with food or milk

- Avoid alcohol and tasks that require mental alertness or motor skills until response to the drug is established
- Notify the physician if fever, rash, or swelling of glands occurs

■ **Monitoring Parameters**
- Blood counts, renal function tests, liver function tests, urinalysis periodically
- Therapeutic serum concentrations 40-100 mcg/ml
- Evidence of toxicity such as bruising, fever, joint pain, mouth ulcerations, sore throat, and unusual bleeding

■ **Geriatric side effects at a glance:**
  ❏ CNS ❏ Bowel Dysfunction ❏ Bladder Dysfunction ❏ Falls

■ **U.S. Regulatory Considerations**
  ❏ FDA Black Box ❏ OBRA regulated in U.S. Long Term Care

etidronate disodium

(ee-tid'-roe-nate dye-soe'-dee-um)

■ **Brand Name(s):** Didronel
Chemical Class: Pyrophosphate analog

■ **Clinical Pharmacology:**
Mechanism of Action: A bisphosphonate that decreases mineral release and matrix in bone and inhibits osteocytic osteolysis. **Therapeutic Effect:** Decreases bone resorption.
Pharmacokinetics: Variable absorption following PO administration. Not metabolized. Approximately 50% of drug is excreted in urine. Unabsorbed drug is excreted intact in feces. **Half-life:** 1-6 hr (oral); 6 hr (IV).

■ **Available Forms:**
- *Tablets* (Didronel): 200 mg, 400 mg.
- *Injection* (Didronel I.V.): 300-mg ampule (50 mg/ml).

■ **Indications and Dosages:**
Paget's disease: PO Initially, 5-10 mg/kg/day not to exceed 6 mo, or 11-20 mg/kg/day not to exceed 3 mo. Repeat only after drug-free period of at least 90 days.
Heterotopic ossification caused by spinal cord injury: PO 20 mg/kg/day for 2 wk; then 10 mg/kg/day for 10 wk.
Heterotopic ossification complicating total hip replacement: PO 20 mg/kg/day for 1 mo before surgery; then 20 mg/kg/day for 3 mo after surgery.
Hypercalcemia associated with malignancy: IV 7.5 mg/kg/day for 3 days. For retreatment, allow 7 days between treatment courses. Follow with oral therapy on day after last infusion. Begin with 20 mg/kg/day for 30 days; may extend up to 90 days.

■ **Contraindications:** Clinically overt osteomalacia

■ Side Effects
Frequent
Nausea; diarrhea; continuing or more frequent bone pain in patients with Paget's disease
Occasional
Bone fractures, especially of the femur
Parenteral: Metallic, altered taste
Rare
Hypersensitivity reaction, osteonecrosis of the jaw

■ Serious Reactions
- Nephrotoxicity, including hematuria, dysuria, and proteinuria, has occurred with parenteral route.

Special Considerations
- A dental examination with appropriate preventive dentistry should be considered prior to treatment with bisphosphonates in patients with concomitant risk factors (e.g., cancer, chemotherapy, corticosteroid use, poor oral hygiene). While on bisphosphonate treatment, patients with concomitant risk factors should avoid invasive dental procedures if possible. For patients who develop osteonecrosis of the jaw while on bisphosphonate therapy, dental surgery may exacerbate the condition. For patients requiring dental procedures, there are no data available to suggest whether discontinuation of bisphosphonate treatment reduces the risk of osteonecrosis of the jaw.

■ Patient/Family Education
- Administer on empty stomach with H_2O, 2 hr ac
- Exceeding the 2-wk treatment periods for osteoporosis may lead to bone demineralization and osteomalacia
- It may take up to 3 mo for a noticeable therapeutic response
- Consume calcium-rich foods, such as dairy products and milk
- Inform your dentist if you are taking this drug.
- If you develop jaw pain, loose teeth, or signs of oral infection, immediately inform your doctor.

■ Monitoring Parameters
- Electrolytes, BUN, fluid intake and output in patients with impaired renal function
- Assess the patient for diarrhea

■ Geriatric side effects at a glance:
❑ CNS   ❑ Bowel Dysfunction   ❑ Bladder Dysfunction   ❑ Falls

■ U.S. Regulatory Considerations
❑ FDA Black Box   ❑ OBRA regulated in U.S. Long Term Care

etodolac

(e-toe'-doe-lak)

- **Brand Name(s):** Lodine, Lodine XL
  Chemical Class: Acetic acid derivative

- **Clinical Pharmacology:**
  Mechanism of Action: An NSAID that produces analgesic and anti-inflammatory effects by inhibiting prostaglandin synthesis. **Therapeutic Effect:** Reduces the inflammatory response and intensity of pain.
  Pharmacokinetics:

Route	Onset	Peak	Duration
PO (analgesic)	30 min	N/A	4-12 hr

Completely absorbed from the GI tract. Protein binding: greater than 99%. Widely distributed. Metabolized in the liver. Primarily excreted in urine. Not removed by hemodialysis. **Half-life:** 6-7 hr.

- **Available Forms:**
  - *Capsules (Lodine):* 200 mg, 300 mg.
  - *Tablets (Lodine):* 400 mg, 500 mg.
  - *Tablets (Extended-Release [Lodine XL]):* 400 mg, 500 mg, 600 mg.

- **Indications and Dosages:**
  Osteoarthritis, rheumatoid arthritis: PO (Immediate-Release) Initially, 300 mg 2-3 times a day or 400-500 mg twice a day. Maintenance: 600-1000 mg/day in 2-4 divided doses. PO (Extended-Release) 400-1000 mg once daily. Maximum: 1200 mg/day.
  Analgesia: PO 200-400 mg q6-8h as needed. Maximum: 1200 mg/day.

- **Unlabeled Uses:** Treatment of acute gouty arthritis, vascular headache

- **Contraindications:** Active peptic ulcer disease, chronic inflammation of GI tract, GI bleeding or ulceration, history of hypersensitivity to aspirin or NSAIDs

- **Side Effects**
  Occasional (9%–4%)
  Dizziness, headache, abdominal pain or cramps, bloated feeling, diarrhea, nausea, indigestion
  Rare (3%–1%)
  Constipation, rash, pruritus, visual disturbances, tinnitus

- **Serious Reactions**
  - Overdose may result in acute renal failure.
  - There is an increased risk of cardiovascular events (including MI and CVA) and serious and potentially life-threatening GI bleeding.
  - Rare reactions with long-term use include peptic ulcer disease, GI bleeding, gastritis, severe hepatic reactions (jaundice), nephrotoxicity (hematuria, dysuria, proteinuria), and a severe hypersensitivity reaction (bronchospasm, angioedema).

- **Patient/Family Education**
  - Swallow etodolac capsules whole and do not open, chew, or crush them
  - Take etodolac with food, milk, or antacids if GI distress occurs
  - Notify the physician if edema, GI distress, headache, rash, signs of bleeding or visual disturbances occur
  - Avoid alcohol and aspirin during etodolac therapy because these substances increase the risk of GI bleeding
  - Avoid performing tasks that require mental alertness or motor skills until response to the drug has been established

- **Monitoring Parameters**
  - Initial hematocrit and fecal occult blood test within 3 mo of starting regular chronic therapy; repeat every 6-12 mo (more frequently in high-risk patients [>65 years, peptic ulcer disease, concurrent steroids or anticoagulants]); electrolytes, creatinine, and BUN within 3 mo of starting regular chronic therapy; repeat every 6-12 mo
  - Therapeutic response, such as improved grip strength, increased joint mobility, and decreased pain, tenderness, stiffness, and swelling

- **Geriatric side effects at a glance:**
  - ☑ CNS ☐ Bowel Dysfunction ☐ Bladder Dysfunction ☐ Falls
  - ☑ Other: Gastropathy

- **Use with caution in older patients with:** Renal impairment, Hepatic impairment, CHF, HTN, PUD, History of GI bleeding, GERD, Bleeding and platelet disorders, History of aspirin sensitivity reaction. Also use with caution in patients taking Anticoagulants, Aspirin, and Antihypertensive agents.

- **U.S. Regulatory Considerations**
  - ☑ FDA Black Box
  - Cardiovascular risk
  - Gastrointestinal risk
  - ☐ OBRA regulated in U.S. Long Term Care

- **Other Uses in Geriatric Patient:** Acute Gout

- **Side Effects:**
  Of particular importance in the geriatric patient: Confusion, cognitive impairment, delirium, dizziness, dyspepsia, fluid retention, renal impairment

- **Geriatric Considerations - Summary:** A preferred agent in older adults due to its association with fewer GI adverse effects. Use of NSAIDs in older adults increases the risk of GI complications including gastric ulceration, bleeding, and perforation. These complications are not necessarily preceded by less severe GI symptoms. Concomitant use of a proton pump inhibitor or misoprostol reduces the risk for gastric ulceration and bleeding, but may not prevent long-term GI toxicity. No clinical data exist to support reduced GI toxicity with the use of etodolac.

- **References:**
  1. COX-2 alternatives and GI protection. Med Lett Drugs Ther 2004;46:91.
  2. Drugs that may cause cognitive disorders in the elderly. Med Lett Drugs Ther 2000;42:111-112.

exenatide

(ex-en'-a-tide)

■ **Brand Name(s):** Byetta

■ **Clinical Pharmacology:**
Mechanism of Action: An incretin mimetic agent that mimics the enhancement of glucose-dependent insulin secretion and several other antihyperglycemic actions of incretins. Incretins, such as glucagon-like peptide-1 (GLP-1), enhance glucose-dependent insulin secretion and exhibit other antihyperglycemic actions following release into circulation from the gut. **Therapeutic Effect:** Controls glucose levels in diabetic patients.
Pharmacokinetics: Following subcutaneous administration, exenatide reaches median peak plasma concentrations in 2.1 hr. Excreted in the kidney predominantly by glomerular filtration with subsequent proteolytic degradation. **Half-life:** 2.4 hr.

■ **Available Forms:**
  • *Solution for Subcutaneous Injection* (**Byetta**): 250 mcg/ml.

■ **Indications and Dosages:**
Type 2 diabetes mellitus, as an adjunct in patients taking metformin, a sulfonylurea, or a combination of metformin and a sulfonylurea but have not achieved adequate glycemic control: Subcutaneous Initially, 5 mcg administered twice daily 60 min before the morning and evening meals. The dose may be increased to 10 mcg twice daily after 1 mo of therapy.

■ **Contraindications:** Hypersensitivity to exenatide or any component of the formulation

■ **Side Effects**
  Frequent
  Nausea, vomiting, diarrhea, jittery feeling, dizziness, headache, dyspepsia
  Occasional
  Jittery feeling, dizziness, headache, dyspepsia
  Rare
  Weakness, decreased appetite, gastroesophageal reflux disease, hyperhidrosis

■ **Serious Reactions**
  • Jittery feeling, dizziness, headache, dyspepsia

■ **Geriatric side effects at a glance:**
  ❑ CNS ❑ Bowel Dysfunction ❑ Bladder Dysfunction ❑ Falls

■ **U.S. Regulatory Considerations**
  ❑ FDA Black Box ❑ OBRA regulated in U.S. Long Term Care

ezetimibe

(ez-et'-i-mibe)

■ **Brand Name(s):** Zetia

Combinations
Rx: with simvastatin (Vytorin)
Chemical Class: Substituted azetidinone

■ **Clinical Pharmacology:**
Mechanism of Action: An antihyperlipidemic that inhibits cholesterol absorption in the small intestine, leading to a decrease in the delivery of intestinal cholesterol to the liver. **Therapeutic Effect:** Reduces total serum cholesterol, LDL cholesterol, and triglyceride levels; and increases HDL cholesterol concentration.
Pharmacokinetics: Well absorbed following oral administration. Protein binding: greater than 90%. Metabolized in the small intestine and liver. Excreted by the kidneys and bile. **Half-life:** 22 hr.

■ **Available Forms:**
  • *Tablets:* 10 mg.

■ **Indications and Dosages:**
Hypercholesterolemia: PO Initially, 10 mg once a day, given with or without food. If the patient is also receiving a bile acid sequestrant, give ezetimibe at least 2 hr before or at least 4 hr after the bile acid sequestrant.
Sitosterolemia: PO 10 mg/day.

■ **Contraindications:** Concurrent use of a hydroxymethylglutaryl-CoA (HMG-CoA) reductase inhibitor (atorvastatin, fluvastatin, lovastatin, pravastatin, or simvastatin) in patients with active hepatic disease or unexplained persistent elevations in serum transaminase levels, moderate or severe hepatic insufficiency

■ **Side Effects**
Occasional (4%–3%)
Back pain, diarrhea, arthralgia, sinusitis, abdominal pain
Rare (2%)
Cough, pharyngitis, fatigue

■ **Serious Reactions**
  • Hepatitis, hypersensitivity reactions, myopathy, and rhabdomyolysis occur rarely.

Special Considerations
  • Modest cholesterol reductions as monotherapy (15%); primary use in combination with statins to achieve and sustain LDL goals

■ **Patient/Family Education**
  • Periodic laboratory tests are an essential part of therapy
  • Do not discontinue ezetimibe without physician approval

■ Monitoring Parameters
- Lipid profile, LFTs, serum CPK, electrolytes, blood glucose, signs and symptoms of toxicity (GI symptoms, headache, rash); pattern of daily bowel activity and stool consistency

■ Geriatric side effects at a glance:
❑ CNS ☑ Bowel Dysfunction ❑ Bladder Dysfunction ❑ Falls

■ U.S. Regulatory Considerations
❑ FDA Black Box ❑ OBRA regulated in U.S. Long Term Care

famciclovir

(fam-sye'-kloe-veer)

■ Brand Name(s): Famvir
Chemical Class: Acyclic purine nucleoside analog

■ Clinical Pharmacology:
Mechanism of Action: A synthetic nucleoside that inhibits viral DNA synthesis. **Therapeutic Effect:** Suppresses replication of herpes simplex virus and varicella-zoster virus.

Pharmacokinetics: Rapidly and extensively absorbed after PO administration. Protein binding: 20%-25%. Rapidly metabolized to penciclovir by enzymes in the GI wall, liver, and plasma. Eliminated unchanged in urine. Removed by hemodialysis. **Half-life:** 2 hr.

■ Available Forms:
- *Tablets*: 125 mg, 250 mg, 500 mg.

■ Indications and Dosages:
Herpes zoster: PO 500 mg q8h for 7 days.
Genital herpes, first episode: PO 250 mg 3 times a day for 7-10 days.
Recurrent genital herpes: PO 125 mg twice a day for 5 days.
Suppression of recurrent genital herpes: PO 250 mg twice a day for up to 1 yr.
Recurrent herpes simplex: PO 500 mg twice a day for 7 days.
Dosage in renal impairment: Dosage and frequency are modified based on creatinine clearance.

Creatinine Clearance	Herpes Zoster	Genital Herpes
40-59 ml/min	500 mg q12h	125 mg q12h
20-39 ml/min	500 mg q24h	125 mg q24h
less than 20 ml/min	250 mg q24h	125 mg q24h

Dosage in hemodialysis patients: For adults with herpes zoster, give 250 mg after each dialysis treatment; for adults with genital herpes, give 125 mg after each dialysis treatment.

■ Contraindications: Hypersensitivity to penciclovir cream

■ **Side Effects**
Frequent
Headache (23%), nausea (12%)
Occasional (10%-2%)
Dizziness, somnolence, numbness of feet, diarrhea, vomiting, constipation, decreased appetite, fatigue, fever, pharyngitis, sinusitis, pruritus
Rare (less than 2%)
Insomnia, abdominal pain, dyspepsia, flatulence, back pain, arthralgia

■ **Serious Reactions**
- Urticaria, hallucinations, and confusion (including delirium, disorientation, confusional state, occurring predominantly in the elderly) have been reported.

Special Considerations
- Reserve chronic suppressive therapy for patients without prodromal symptoms who have frequent recurrences

■ **Patient/Family Education**
- Drink adequate fluids
- Keep fingernails short and hands clean
- Do not touch the lesions for the duration of an outbreak to prevent cross-contamination and spreading the infection to new sites
- Space doses evenly around the clock and take famciclovir for the full course of treatment
- Notify the physician if the lesions fail to improve or if they recur

■ **Monitoring Parameters**
- Assess for signs and symptoms of neurologic effects, including dizziness and headache

■ **Geriatric side effects at a glance:**
❑ CNS ❑ Bowel Dysfunction ❑ Bladder Dysfunction ❑ Falls

■ **U.S. Regulatory Considerations**
❑ FDA Black Box ❑ OBRA regulated in U.S. Long Term Care

famotidine

(fa-moe'-ti-deen)

■ **Brand Name(s):** Pepcid, Pepcid RPD
OTC: Mylanta AR, Pepcid AC

Combinations
OTC: with calcium carbonate and magnesium hydroxide (Pepcid Complete)
Chemical Class: Thiazole derivative

Clinical Pharmacology:

Mechanism of Action: A GI H_2-blocker and gastric acid secretion inhibitor that inhibits histamine action at histamine 2 receptors of parietal cells. **Therapeutic Effect:** Inhibits gastric acid secretion when fasting, at night, or when stimulated by food, caffeine, or insulin.

Pharmacokinetics:

Route	Onset	Peak	Duration
PO	1 hr	1-4 hr	10-12 hr
IV	1 hr	0.5-3 hr	10-12 hr

Rapidly, incompletely absorbed from the GI tract. Protein binding: 15%-20%. Partially metabolized in the liver. Primarily excreted in urine. Not removed by hemodialysis. **Half-life:** 2.5-3.5 hr (increased with impaired renal function).

Available Forms:
- *Oral Suspension* (**Pepcid**): 40 mg/5 ml.
- *Tablets*: 10 mg (**Pepcid AC**), 20 mg (**Pepcid, Pepcid AC**), 40 mg (**Pepcid**).
- *Tablets (Chewable* [**Pepcid AC**]): 10 mg.
- *Capsules* (**Pepcid AC**): 10 mg.
- *Injection* (**Pepcid**): 10 mg/ml.

Indications and Dosages:
Acute treatment of duodenal and gastric ulcers: PO 40 mg/day at bedtime.
Duodenal ulcer maintenance: PO 20 mg/day at bedtime.
Gastroesophageal reflux disease: PO 20 mg twice a day.
Esophagitis: PO 2-40 mg twice a day.
Hypersecretory conditions: PO Initially, 20 mg q6h. May increase up to 160 mg q6h.
Acid indigestion, heartburn (over-the-counter): PO 10-20 mg 15-60 min before eating. Maximum: 2 doses per day.
Usual parenteral dosage: IV 20 mg q12h.
Dosage in renal impairment: Dosing frequency is modified based on creatinine clearance.

Creatinine Clearance	Dosing Frequency
10-50 ml/min	q24h
less than 10 ml/min	q36-48h

Unlabeled Uses:
Autism, prevention of aspiration pneumonitis, *Helicobacter pylori* eradication

Contraindications:
None known.

Side Effects
Occasional (5%)
Headache
Rare (2% or less)
Constipation, diarrhea, dizziness

Serious Reactions
- None known.

Special Considerations
- No advantage over other agents in this class, base selection on cost

Patient/Family Education
- Stagger doses of famotidine and antacids

- May take famotidine without regard to meals but that it's best taken after meals or at bedtime
- Notify the physician if headache occurs
- Avoid alcohol, aspirin, and coffee, all of which may cause GI distress, during famotidine therapy
- Contact the physician if persistent acid indigestion, heartburn, or sour stomach persists despite the medication

■ **Monitoring Parameters**
  - Pattern of bowel activity and stool consistency

■ **Geriatric side effects at a glance:**
  ☑ CNS ☐ Bowel Dysfunction ☐ Bladder Dysfunction ☐ Falls
  Other: Cognitive impairment

■ **Use with caution in older patients with:** Renal impairment, Cognitive impairment

■ **U.S. Regulatory Considerations**
  ☐ FDA Black Box ☐ OBRA regulated in U.S. Long Term Care

■ **Other Uses in Geriatric Patient:** Acute allergic reactions, urticaria (in addition to antihistamine therapy)

■ **Side Effects:**
  Of particular importance in the geriatric patient: Delirium, confusion, dizziness, headache, constipation, diarrhea

■ **Geriatric Considerations - Summary:** Adjust dose based on creatinine clearance. Not effective in preventing NSAID-induced gastric ulceration and bleeding; proton pump inhibitors should be used for this indication instead.

■ **References:**
  1. Gawrich S, Shaker R. Medical management of nocturnal symptoms of gastro-oesophageal reflux disease in the elderly. Drugs Aging 2003;20:509-516.
  2. Thomson ABR. Gastro-oesophageal reflux in the elderly. Role of drug therapy in management. Drugs Aging 2001;18:409-414.
  3. Drugs that may cause cognitive disorders in the elderly. Med Lett 2000;42:111-112.

felodipine

(fell-o'-da-peen)

■ **Brand Name(s):** Plendil

  Combinations
  Rx: with enalapril (Lexxel)
  Chemical Class: Dihydropyridine

■ Clinical Pharmacology:

Mechanism of Action: An antihypertensive and antianginal agent that inhibits calcium movement across cardiac and vascular smooth-muscle cell membranes. Potent peripheral vasodilator (does not depress SA or AV nodes). **Therapeutic Effect:** Increases myocardial contractility, heart rate, and cardiac output; decreases peripheral vascular resistance and BP.

Pharmacokinetics:

Route	Onset	Peak	Duration
PO	2-5 hr	N/A	N/A

Rapidly, completely absorbed from the GI tract. Protein binding: greater than 99%. Undergoes first-pass metabolism in the liver. Primarily excreted in urine. Not removed by hemodialysis. **Half-life:** 11–16 hr.

■ Available Forms:

- *Tablets* (*Extended-Release*): 2.5 mg, 5 mg, 10 mg.

■ Indications and Dosages:

Hypertension: PO Initially, 2.5 mg/day. Adjust dosage at no less than 2-wk intervals. Maintenance: 2.5-10 mg/day. Range: 2.5-20 mg/day. *Patients with impaired hepatic function.* Initially, 2.5 mg/day. Adjust dosage at no less than 2-wk intervals. Maintenance: 2.5-10 mg/day. Range: 2.5-20 mg/day.

■ Unlabeled Uses: Treatment of CHF, chronic angina pectoris, Raynaud's phenomenon

■ Contraindications: None known.

■ Side Effects

Frequent (22%-18%)
Headache, peripheral edema
Occasional (6%-4%)
Flushing, respiratory infection, dizziness, light-headedness, asthenia (loss of strength, weakness)
Rare (less than 3%)
Paresthesia, abdominal discomfort, nervousness, muscle cramping, cough, diarrhea, constipation

■ Serious Reactions

- Overdose produces nausea, somnolence, confusion, slurred speech, hypotension, and bradycardia.

Special Considerations

- Results of V-HeFT III indicate felodipine may be used safely in patients with left ventricular dysfunction

■ Patient/Family Education

- Administer as whole tablet (do not crush or chew)
- Avoid grapefruit juice (see drug interactions)
- Do not abruptly discontinue felodipine; compliance with the therapy regimen is essential to control hypertension
- Rise slowly from a lying to a sitting position and wait momentarily before standing to avoid felodipine's hypotensive effect
- Avoid tasks that require mental alertness or motor skills until response to the drug has been established

- Notify the physician if an irregular heartbeat, nausea, prolonged dizziness, or shortness of breath occurs

■ **Monitoring Parameters**
- Liver function
- Pulse for bradycardia
- Skin for flushing

■ **Geriatric side effects at a glance:**
☐ CNS ☐ Bowel Dysfunction ☐ Bladder Dysfunction ☐ Falls

■ **U.S. Regulatory Considerations**
☐ FDA Black Box ☐ OBRA regulated in U.S. Long Term Care

fenofibrate

(fen-oh-fye'-brate)

■ **Brand Name(s):** Antara, Lipidil Supra, Lofibra, Tricor, Triglide
Chemical Class: Fibric acid derivative

■ **Clinical Pharmacology:**
Mechanism of Action: An antihyperlipidemic that enhances synthesis of lipoprotein lipase and reduces triglyceride-rich lipoproteins and VLDLs. **Therapeutic Effect:** Increases VLDL catabolism and reduces total plasma triglyceride levels.
Pharmacokinetics: Well absorbed from the GI tract. Absorption increased when given with food. Protein binding: 99%. Rapidly metabolized in the liver to active metabolite. Excreted primarily in urine; lesser amount in feces. Not removed by hemodialysis. **Half-life:** 20 hr.

■ **Available Forms:**
- **Capsules:** 43 mg (Antara), 67 mg (Lofibra), 87 mg (Antara), 130 mg (Antara), 134 mg (Lofibra), 200 mg (Lipidil Supra, Lofibra).
- **Tablets:** 48 mg (Tricor), 50 mg (Triglide), 145 mg (Tricor), 160 mg (Triglide).

■ **Indications and Dosages:**
Hypertriglyceridemia: PO (Antara) 43-130 mg/day. PO (Lofibra) 67-200 mg/day with meals. PO (Tricor) 48-145 mg/day. PO (Triglide) 50-160 mg/day.
Hypercholesterolemia: PO (Antara) 130 mg/day. PO (Lofibra) 200 mg/day with meals. PO (Tricor) 145 mg/day. PO (Triglide) 160 mg/day.

■ **Contraindications:** Gallbladder disease, severe renal or hepatic dysfunction (including primary biliary cirrhosis, unexplained persistent liver function abnormality)

■ **Side Effects**
Frequent (8%-4%)
Pain, rash, headache, asthenia or fatigue, flu symptoms, dyspepsia, nausea or vomiting, rhinitis

Occasional (3%-2%)
Diarrhea, abdominal pain, constipation, flatulence, arthralgia, decreased libido, dizziness, pruritus
Rare (less than 2%)
Increased appetite, insomnia, polyuria, cough, blurred vision, eye floaters, earache

■ **Serious Reactions**
- Fenofibrate may increase excretion of cholesterol into bile, leading to cholelithiasis.
- Pancreatitis, hepatitis, thrombocytopenia, and agranulocytosis occur rarely.

Special Considerations
- Plasma concentrations of fenofibric acid after administration of 54-mg and 160-mg tablets are equivalent to 67-mg and 200-mg capsules

■ **Patient/Family Education**
- Signs, symptoms, and resources for management of myositis
- Take with food
- Notify the physician if constipation, diarrhea, or nausea becomes severe
- Notify the physician if dizziness, insomnia, muscle pain, rash, or skin irritation occurs

■ **Monitoring Parameters**
- Serum cholesterol, triglycerides, LDL-cholesterol, HDL-cholesterol, LFTs (serum transaminases), periodic CBC, serum CK

■ **Geriatric side effects at a glance:**
  ❏ CNS ❏ Bowel Dysfunction ❏ Bladder Dysfunction ❏ Falls

■ **U.S. Regulatory Considerations**
  ❏ FDA Black Box ❏ OBRA regulated in U.S. Long Term Care

fenoldopam mesylate

(fhe-knowl'-doh-pam mes'-sil-ate)

■ **Brand Name(s):** Corlopam
  Chemical Class: Benzazepine derivative

■ **Clinical Pharmacology:**
  Mechanism of Action: A rapid-acting vasodilator. An agonist for D_1-like dopamine receptors; also produces vasodilation in coronary, renal, mesenteric, and peripheral arteries. **Therapeutic Effect:** Reduces systolic and diastolic BP and increases heart rate. **Pharmacokinetics:** After IV administration, metabolized in the liver. Primarily excreted in urine. Unknown if removed by hemodialysis. **Half-life:** Approximately 5 min.

■ Available Forms:
- *Injection*: 10 mg/ml.

■ Indications and Dosages:
Short-term management of severe hypertension when rapid, but quickly reversible emergency reduction of BP is clinically indicated, including malignant hypertension with deteriorating end-organ function: IV Infusion (continuous) Initially, 0.1 mcg/kg/min. May increase in increments of 0.05-0.1 mcg/kg/min until target BP is achieved. Usual length of treatment is 1-6 hr with tapering of dose q15-30min. Average rate: 0.25-0.5 mcg/kg/min. Maximum rate: 1.6 mcg/kg/min.

■ Unlabeled Uses: Prevention of contrast media-induced nephrotoxicity

■ Contraindications: Sensitivity to sulfites

■ Side Effects
Expected
Beta-blockers may cause unforeseen hypotension.
Occasional
Headache (7%), flushing (3%), nausea (4%), hypotension (2%)
Rare (2% or less)
Nervousness or anxiety, vomiting, constipation, nasal congestion, diaphoresis, back pain

■ Serious Reactions
- Excessive hypotension occurs occasionally.
- Substantial tachycardia may lead to ischemic cardiac events or worsened heart failure.
- Allergic-type reactions, including anaphylaxis and life-threatening asthmatic exacerbation, may occur in patients with sulfite sensitivity.

Special Considerations
- *Preparation of infusion solution*: Contents of ampules must be diluted prior to infusion: 1 ml of 10 mg/ml solution in 250 ml 0.9% sodium chloride or 5% dextrose yields a final concentration of 40 mcg/ml
- *Potential advantage over sodium nitroprusside in hypertensive crisis*: Induction of natriuresis, diuresis; ability to increase creatinine clearance, preserve renal function

■ Patient/Family Education
- Change positions slowly to avoid orthostasis

■ Monitoring Parameters
- Blood pressure, pulse, serum electrolytes, urine volume, urinary sodium, serum creatinine, blood urea nitrogen, electrocardiogram, hepatic function tests, infusion rate

■ Geriatric side effects at a glance:
❑ CNS ❑ Bowel Dysfunction ❑ Bladder Dysfunction ❑ Falls

■ U.S. Regulatory Considerations
❑ FDA Black Box ❑ OBRA regulated in U.S. Long Term Care

fenoprofen calcium

(fen-oh-proe'-fen kal'-see-um)

■ **Brand Name(s):** Nalfon
   Chemical Class: Propionic acid derivative

■ **Clinical Pharmacology:**
   Mechanism of Action: An NSAID that produces analgesic and anti-inflammatory effects by inhibiting prostaglandin synthesis. **Therapeutic Effect:** Reduces the inflammatory response and intensity of pain.
   Pharmacokinetics: Rapidly absorbed following PO administration. Protein binding: 99%. Metabolized in liver. Primarily excreted in urine; small amount excreted in feces.
   Half-life: 3 hr.

■ **Available Forms:**
   • *Capsules*: 200 mg, 300 mg.
   • *Tablets*: 600 mg.

■ **Indications and Dosages:**
   Mild to moderate pain: PO 200 mg q4-6h as needed.
   Rheumatoid arthritis, osteoarthritis: PO 300-600 mg 3-4 times a day.

■ **Unlabeled Uses:** Treatment of ankylosing spondylitis, psoriatic arthritis, vascular headaches

■ **Contraindications:** Active peptic ulcer disease, chronic inflammation of GI tract, GI bleeding or ulceration, history of hypersensitivity to aspirin or NSAIDs, significant renal impairment

■ **Side Effects**
   Frequent (9%-3%)
   Headache, somnolence, dyspepsia, nausea, vomiting, constipation
   Occasional (2%-1%)
   Dizziness, pruritus, nervousness, asthenia, diarrhea, abdominal cramps, flatulence, tinnitus, blurred vision, peripheral edema and fluid retention

■ **Serious Reactions**
   • Overdose may result in acute hypotension and tachycardia.
   • Rare reactions with long-term use include peptic ulcer disease, GI bleeding, gastritis, severe hepatic reaction (jaundice), nephrotoxicity (hematuria, dysuria, proteinuria), and a severe hypersensitivity reaction (bronchospasm, angioedema).

Special Considerations
   • No significant advantage over other NSAIDs; cost should govern use

■ **Patient/Family Education**
   • Swallow fenoprofen capsules whole and do not chew or crush them
   • Take with food or milk if GI upset occurs

- Avoid tasks that require mental alertness or motor skills until response to the drug has been established
- Avoid alcohol and aspirin during fenoprofen therapy because these substances increase the risk of GI bleeding

■ Monitoring Parameters
- Initial hematocrit and fecal occult blood test within 3 mo of starting regular chronic therapy; repeat every 6-12 mo (more frequently in high-risk patients [>65 years, peptic ulcer disease, concurrent steroids or anticoagulants]); electrolytes, creatinine, and BUN within 3 mo of starting regular chronic therapy; repeat every 6-12 mo
- Pattern of daily bowel activity and stool consistency
- Therapeutic response, such as improved grip strength, increased joint mobility, and decreased pain, stiffness, and swelling

■ Geriatric side effects at a glance:
    ☑ CNS   ☐ Bowel Dysfunction   ☐ Bladder Dysfunction   ☐ Falls
    ☑ Other: Gastropathy

■ Use with caution in older patients with:
Renal impairment, Hepatic impairment, CHF, HTN, PUD, History of GI bleeding, GERD, Bleeding and platelet disorders, History of aspirin sensitivity reaction. Also use with caution in patients taking Anticoagulants, Aspirin, and Antihypertensive agents.

■ U.S. Regulatory Considerations
    ☑ FDA Black Box
- Cardiovascular risk
- Gastrointestinal risk
    ☐ OBRA regulated in U.S. Long Term Care

■ Other Uses in Geriatric Patient: Acute Gout

■ Side Effects:
Of particular importance in the geriatric patient: Confusion, cognitive impairment, delirium, dizziness, dyspepsia, fluid retention, renal impairment

■ Geriatric Considerations - Summary:
Use with caution due to the higher risk of GI adverse events. Not a preferred NSAID in older adults. Use of NSAIDs in older adults increases the risk of GI complications including gastric ulceration, bleeding, and perforation. These complications are not necessarily preceded by less severe GI symptoms. Concomitant use of a proton pump inhibitor or misoprostol reduces the risk for gastric ulceration and bleeding, but may not prevent long-term GI toxicity.

■ References:
1. COX-2 alternatives and GI protection. Med Lett Drugs Ther 2004;46:91.
2. Drugs that may cause cognitive disorders in the elderly. Med Lett Drugs Ther 2000;42:111-112.

fentanyl citrate

(fen'-ta-nill sit'-trate)

■ **Brand Name(s):** Injection: Sublimaze

■ **Brand Name(s):** Transdermal: Duragesic

■ **Brand Name(s):** Lozenge: Actiq

> Combinations
> **Rx:** with droperidol (Innovar)
> **Chemical Class:** Opiate derivative; phenylpiperidine derivative
>
> DEA Class: Schedule II

■ **Clinical Pharmacology:**
Mechanism of Action: An opioid agonist that binds to opioid receptors in the CNS, reducing stimuli from sensory nerve endings and inhibiting ascending pain pathways.
Therapeutic Effect: Alters pain reception and increases the pain threshold.
Pharmacokinetics:

Route	Onset	Peak	Duration
IV	1-2 min	3-5 min	0.5-1 hr
IM	7-15 min	20-30 min	1-2 hr
Transdermal	6-8 hr	24 hr	72 hr
Transmucosal	5-15 min	20-30 min	1-2 hr

Well absorbed after IM or topical administration. Transmucosal form absorbed through the buccal mucosa and GI tract. Protein binding: 80%-85%. Metabolized in the liver. Primarily eliminated by biliary system. **Half-life:** 2-4 hr IV; 17 hr transdermal; 6.6 hr transmucosal.

■ **Available Forms:**
- Injection (Sublimaze): 50 mcg/ml.
- Transdermal Patch (Duragesic): 12 mcg/hr, 25 mcg/hr, 50 mcg/hr, 75 mcg/hr, 100 mcg/hr.
- Transmucosal Lozenges (Actiq): 200 mcg, 400 mcg, 600 mcg, 800 mcg, 1200 mcg, 1600 mcg.

■ **Indications and Dosages:**
Sedation in minor procedures, analgesia: IV, IM 0.5-1 mcg/kg/dose; may repeat in 30-60 min.
Preoperative sedation, postoperative pain, adjunct to regional anesthesia: IV, IM 50-100 mcg/dose.
Adjunct to general anesthesia: IV 2-50 mcg/kg.
Usual transdermal dose: Initially, 25 mcg/hr. May increase after 3 days.
Usual transmucosal dose: 200-400 mcg for breakthrough cancer pain.
Usual epidural dose: Bolus dose of 100 mcg, followed by continuous infusion of 10 mcg/ml concentration at 4-12 ml/hr.
Continuous analgesia: IV Bolus dose of 1-2 mcg/kg, followed by continuous infusion of 1 mcg/kg/hr. Range: 1-5 mcg/kg/hr.

Dosage in renal impairment: Dosage is modified based on creatinine clearance.

Creatinine Clearance	Dosage
10-50 ml/min	75% of usual dose
less than 10 ml/min	50% of usual dose

- **Contraindications:** Increased intracranial pressure, severe hepatic or renal impairment, severe respiratory depression

- **Side Effects**

  Frequent

  IV: Postoperative drowsiness, nausea, vomiting

  Transdermal **(10%-3%):** Headache, pruritus, nausea, vomiting, diaphoresis, dyspnea, confusion, dizziness, somnolence, diarrhea, constipation, decreased appetite

  Occasional

  IV: Postoperative confusion, blurred vision, chills, orthostatic hypotension, constipation, difficulty urinating

  Transdermal **(3%-1%):** Chest pain, arrhythmias, erythema, pruritus, swelling of skin, syncope, agitation, tingling or burning of skin

- **Serious Reactions**
  - Overdose or too-rapid IV administration may produce severe respiratory depression and skeletal and thoracic muscle rigidity (which may lead to apnea), laryngospasm, bronchospasm, cold and clammy skin, cyanosis, and coma.
  - The patient who uses fentanyl repeatedly may develop a tolerance to the drug's analgesic effect.

Special Considerations

- Increased skin temperature increases absorption rate of transdermal preparation
- Lozenge should be used only in a monitored anesthesia care setting
- Following removal of transdermal system, 17 hr are required for 50% decrease in serum fentanyl concentrations
- Do not administer agonist/antagonist analgesics (i.e., pentazocine, nalbuphine, butorphanol, dezocine, buprenorphine) to patient who has received a prolonged course of fentanyl (a pure agonist). In opioid-dependent patients, mixed agonist/antagonist analgesics may precipitate withdrawal symptoms

- **Patient/Family Education**
  - Use fentanyl as directed to avoid an overdosage; prolonged use of the drug may cause physical dependence
  - Discontinue fentanyl slowly after long-term use
  - Avoid alcohol during fentanyl therapy and consult the physician before taking any other drugs
  - Avoid tasks requiring mental alertness or motor skills until response to the drug has been established

- **Monitoring Parameters**
  - Blood pressure, heart rate, respiratory rate, and oxygen saturation
  - Relief of pain

- **Geriatric side effects at a glance:**

  ☑ CNS ☑ Bowel Dysfunction ☑ Bladder Dysfunction ☑ Falls

■ **U.S. Regulatory Considerations**
  ☑ FDA Black Box
  • High abuse potential and risk of respiratory depression with overdose.
  • Use in opioid-tolerant patients
  • Close monitoring with CYP3A4 inhibitors
  ☑ OBRA regulated in U.S. Long Term Care

ferrous fumarate/ferrous gluconate/ferrous sulfate

(fer'-rous fume'-ah-rate/fer'-rous glue'-kuh-nate/fer'-rous sul'-fate)

■ **Brand Name(s):** (ferrous fumarate) Femiron, Feostat, Ferro-Sequels, Nephro-Fer

■ **Brand Name(s):** (ferrous gluconate) Fergon

■ **Brand Name(s):** (ferrous sulfate) Fer-In-Sol, Fer-Iron, Slow-Fe
  Chemical Class: Iron preparation

■ **Clinical Pharmacology:**
  Mechanism of Action: An enzymatic mineral that is an essential component in the formation of Hgb, myoglobin, and enzymes. Promotes effective erythropoiesis and transport and utilization of oxygen (O_2). **Therapeutic Effect:** Prevents iron deficiency. **Pharmacokinetics:** Absorbed in the duodenum and upper jejunum. Ten percent absorbed in patients with normal iron stores; increased to 20%-30% in those with inadequate iron stores. Primarily bound to serum transferrin. Excreted in urine, sweat, and sloughing of intestinal mucosa. **Half-life:** 6 hr.

■ **Available Forms:**
  Ferrous fumarate:
  • *Tablets*: 63 mg (20 mg elemental iron) (Femiron), 350 mg (115 mg elemental iron) (Nephro-Fer).
  • *Tablets (Chewable [Feostat])*: 100 mg (33 mg elemental iron).
  • *Tablets (Time-Release [Ferro-Sequels])*: 150 mg (50 mg elemental iron).
  Ferrous gluconate:
  • *Tablets*: 240 mg (27 mg elemental iron) (Fergon), 325 mg (36 mg elemental iron).
  Ferrous sulfate:
  • *Tablets*: 325 mg (65 mg elemental iron).
  • *Tablets (Timed-Release [Slow Fe])*: 160 mg (50 mg elemental iron).
  • *Elixir*: 220 mg/5 ml (44 mg elemental iron per 5 ml).
  • *Oral Drops (Fer-In-Sol, Fer-Iron)*: 75 mg/0.6 ml.

■ **Indications and Dosages:**
  Iron deficiency anemia: PO (ferrous fumarate) 60-100 mg twice a day. PO (ferrous gluconate) 60 mg 2-4 times a day. PO (ferrous sulfate) 325 mg 2-4 times a day. Dosage is expressed in terms of milligrams of elemental iron, degree of anemia, patient

495

weight, and presence of any bleeding. Expect to use periodic hematologic determinations as guide to therapy.

***Prevention of iron deficiency*:** PO (ferrous fumarate) 60-100 mg/day. PO (ferrous gluconate) 60 mg/day. PO (ferrous sulfate) 325 mg/day.

■ **Contraindications:** Hemochromatosis, hemosiderosis, hemolytic anemias, peptic ulcer disease, regional enteritis, ulcerative colitis

■ **Side Effects**

Occasional

Nausea, abdominal or stomach pain, abdominal cramping

Rare

Heartburn, anorexia, constipation, diarrhea

■ **Serious Reactions**
- Large doses may aggravate existing GI tract disease, such as peptic ulcer disease, regional enteritis, and ulcerative colitis.
- Severe iron poisoning is manifested as vomiting, severe abdominal pain, diarrhea, and dehydration, followed by hyperventilation, pallor or cyanosis, and cardiovascular collapse.

■ **Patient/Family Education**
- Best absorbed on empty stomach, may take with food if GI upset occurs
- Drink liquid iron preparations in water or juice and through a straw to prevent tooth stains
- Do not crush tablets
- 4-6 mo of therapy generally required
- Iron changes stools black or dark green

■ **Monitoring Parameters**
- Hemoglobin, hematocrit, reticulocyte count, ferritin and serum iron levels, and total iron-binding capacity
- Pattern of daily bowel activity and stool consistency
- Clinical improvement and record relief of iron deficiency symptoms (fatigue, headache, irritability, pallor, and paresthesia of extremities)

■ **Geriatric side effects at a glance:**
❑ CNS ☑ Bowel Dysfunction ❑ Bladder Dysfunction ❑ Falls

■ **U.S. Regulatory Considerations**
❑ FDA Black Box ❑ OBRA regulated in U.S. Long Term Care

fexofenadine hydrochloride

(fex-oh-fen'-eh-deen hye-droe-klor'-ide)

- **Brand Name(s):** Allegra

  Combinations
  Rx: with pseudoephedrine (Allegra-D)
  Chemical Class: Piperidine derivative

- **Clinical Pharmacology:**
  Mechanism of Action: A piperidine that competes with histamine for H_1-receptor sites on effector cells. **Therapeutic Effect:** Relieves allergic rhinitis symptoms.
  Pharmacokinetics: Rapidly absorbed after PO administration. Protein binding: 60%-70%. Does not cross the blood-brain barrier. Minimally metabolized. Eliminated in feces and urine. Not removed by hemodialysis. **Half-life: 14.4 hr (increased in renal impairment).**

- **Available Forms:**
  - *Tablets*: 30 mg, 60 mg, 180 mg.

- **Indications and Dosages:**
  Allergic rhinitis, urticaria: PO   60 mg twice a day or 180 mg once a day.
  Dosage in renal impairment: Dosage is reduced to 60 mg once a day.

- **Contraindications:** None known.

- **Side Effects**
  Rare (less than 2%)
  Somnolence, headache, fatigue, nausea, vomiting, abdominal distress

- **Serious Reactions**
  - In rare cases, hypersensitivity reactions including rash, urticaria, pruritus, with manifestations characterized as angioedema, chest tightness, dyspnea, flushing, and systemic anaphylaxis have been reported.

Special Considerations

  - Essentially the same as terfenadine without the potential for QT prolongation; relatively weak antihistamine with minimal sedation

- **Patient/Family Education**
  - Avoid performing tasks that require mental alertness or motor skills until response to the drug has been established
  - Drinking coffee or tea may help reduce drowsiness
  - Avoid alcohol during antihistamine therapy

- **Monitoring Parameters**
  - Assess for relief of allergy symptoms including rhinorrhea, sneezing, itching, and red, watery eyes

- **Geriatric side effects at a glance:**
  - ☐ CNS   ☐ Bowel Dysfunction   ☐ Bladder Dysfunction   ☐ Falls
  - Other: Cognitive impairment, Sedation

- **Use with caution in older patients with:** Cognitive impairment

- **U.S. Regulatory Considerations**
  - ☐ FDA Black Box   ☐ OBRA regulated in U.S. Long Term Care

- **Other Uses in Geriatric Patient:** None

- **Side Effects:**
  - *Of particular importance in the geriatric patient:* Anticholinergic effects

- **Geriatric Considerations - Summary:** One of the least likely antihistamines to cause CNS effects. No dose adjustments required in older adults with decreased renal function. Slow metabolizers likely to experience increased side effects and anticholinergic effects. Increased risk of sedation at higher doses.

- **References:**
  1. Hansen J, Klimek L, Hormann K. Pharmacological management of allergic rhinitis in the elderly. Safety issues with oral antihistamines. Drugs Aging 2005;22:289-296.
  2. Newer antihistamines. Med Lett 2001;43.
  3. Drugs that may cause cognitive disorders in the elderly. Med Lett 2000;42:111-112.
  4. Mann RD, Pearce GL, Dunn N, Shakir S. Sedation with non-sedating antihistamines: four prescription-event monitoring studies in general practice. BMJ 2000;320:1184-1187.

finasteride

(fin-as'-tur-ide)

- **Brand Name(s):** Proscar, Propecia
  - **Chemical Class:** 5α-Reductase inhibitor

- **Clinical Pharmacology:**
  - **Mechanism of Action:** An androgen hormone inhibitor that inhibits 5-alpha reductase, an intracellular enzyme that converts testosterone into dihydrotestosterone (DHT) in the prostate gland, resulting in a decreased serum DHT level. **Therapeutic Effect:** Reduces size of the prostate gland.
  - **Pharmacokinetics:**

Route	Onset	Peak	Duration
PO	24 hr	1-2 days	5-7 days

  Rapidly absorbed from the GI tract. Protein binding: 90%. Widely distributed. Metabolized in the liver. **Half-life:** 6-8 hr. Onset of clinical effect: 3-6 mo of continued therapy.

- **Available Forms:**
  - • *Tablets:* 1 mg (Propecia), 5 mg (Proscar).

- **Indications and Dosages:**
  Benign prostatic hyperplasia (BPH): PO 5 mg once a day (for a minimum of 6 mo).
  Hair loss: PO 1 mg/day.

- **Unlabeled Uses:** Adjuvant monotherapy after radical prostatectomy in treatment of prostate cancer, female hirsutism

- **Contraindications:** Exposure to the patient's semen or handling of finasteride tablets by those who are or may be pregnant

- **Side Effects**
  Rare (4%-2%)
  Gynecomastia, sexual dysfunction (impotence, decreased libido, decreased volume of ejaculate)

- **Serious Reactions**
  - Hypersensitivity reactions, including rash, pruritus, urticaria, circumoral swelling, and testicular pain, have been reported.

Special Considerations
- Minimal benefit for benign prostatic hypertrophy if the prostate is not very large; response is not immediate
- Combination therapy with α-blocker may be optimal for more rapid relief of BPH symptoms
- Whether long-term treatment can reduce prostate cancer risk is unknown; decreases prostate-specific antigen (PSA)

- **Patient/Family Education**
  - Condoms should be used if the female partner is at risk of pregnancy
  - Women who are or may be pregnant should not handle finasteride tablets or be exposed to semen because of the potential risk to a fetus
  - Withdrawal of drug for hair loss leads to reversal within 12 mo
  - Finasteride may cause impotence and decrease ejaculate volume
  - Take the drug for at least 6 mo
  - It is unknown if taking this drug decreases the need for surgery

- **Monitoring Parameters**
  - 6-12 mo of therapy may be necessary in some patients to assess effectiveness (BPH), 3 or more mo for hair loss
  - Fluid intake and output

- **Geriatric side effects at a glance:**
  ❑ CNS   ❑ Bowel Dysfunction   ❑ Bladder Dysfunction   ❑ Falls

- **U.S. Regulatory Considerations**
  ❑ FDA Black Box   ❑ OBRA regulated in U.S. Long Term Care

flavoxate hydrochloride

(fla-vox'-ate hye-droe-klor'-ide)

■ **Brand Name(s):** Urispas
Chemical Class: Flavone derivative

■ **Clinical Pharmacology:**
Mechanism of Action: An anticholinergic that relaxes detrusor and other smooth muscle by cholinergic blockade, counteracting muscle spasm in the urinary tract. **Therapeutic Effect:** Produces anticholinergic, local anesthetic, and analgesic effects, relieving urinary symptoms.
Pharmacokinetics: Unknown absorption, distribution, metabolism. Protein binding: 50%-80%. Excreted in urine. **Half-life:** 10-20 hr.

■ **Available Forms:**
• *Tablets:* 100 mg.

■ **Indications and Dosages:**
To relieve symptoms of cystitis, prostatitis, urethritis, urethrocystitis, or urethrotrigonitis: PO 100-200 mg 3-4 times a day.

■ **Contraindications:** Duodenal or pyloric obstruction, GI hemorrhage or obstruction, ileus, lower urinary tract obstruction

■ **Side Effects**
Frequent
Somnolence, dry mouth and throat
Occasional
Constipation, difficult urination, blurred vision, dizziness, headache, increased light sensitivity, nausea, vomiting, abdominal pain, confusion
Rare
Hypersensitivity, increased IOP, leukopenia

■ **Serious Reactions**
• Overdose may produce anticholinergic effects, including unsteadiness, severe dizziness, somnolence, fever, facial flushing, dyspnea, nervousness, and irritability.

Special Considerations
• Urinary antispasmodic that is no more effective than propantheline or other similar agents

■ **Patient/Family Education**
• Avoid performing tasks that require mental alertness or motor skills until response to the drug has been established
• Be aware of signs and symptoms of flavoxate overdose, including unsteadiness, severe dizziness, drowsiness, fever, flushed face, shortness of breath, nervousness, and irritability

- **Monitoring Parameters**
  - Monitor for symptomatic relief
  - Observe patient for confusion

- **Geriatric side effects at a glance:**
  ☑ CNS ☑ Bowel Dysfunction ☑ Bladder Dysfunction ☐ Falls
  Other: Dry mouth, blurred vision, somnolence

- **Use with caution in older patients with:** Prostate hypertrophy, dementia

- **U.S. Regulatory Considerations**
  ☐ FDA Black Box ☑ OBRA regulated in U.S. Long Term Care

- **Other Uses in Geriatric Patient:** None

- **Side Effects:**
  Of particular importance in the geriatric patient: None

- **Geriatric Considerations - Summary:** Flavoxate has anticholinergic activity and has the potential to cause adverse effects in the older adult, including urinary retention, hypotension, and confusion. There are no well controlled studies that show efficacy over placebo in the treatment of the overactive bladder. The potential for adverse effects limits the usefulness of this drug for older adults.

- **References:**
  1. Hashim H, Abrams P. Treatment of overactive bladder. Drugs 2004; 64:1644-1654.

flecainide acetate

(fle'-kah-nide as'-eh-tate)

- **Brand Name(s):** Tambocor
  Chemical Class: Benzamide derivative

- **Clinical Pharmacology:**
  Mechanism of Action: An antiarrhythmic that slows atrial, AV, His-Purkinje, and intraventricular conduction. Decreases excitability, conduction velocity, and automaticity.
  Therapeutic Effect: Controls atrial, supraventricular, and ventricular arrhythmias.
  Pharmacokinetics: Almost completely absorbed following PO administration. Protein binding: 40%. Metabolized in liver. Excreted in urine. **Half-life:** 19-22 hr.

- **Available Forms:**
  - *Tablets:* 50 mg, 100 mg.

- **Indications and Dosages:**
  Life-threatening ventricular arrhythmias, sustained ventricular tachycardia: PO Initially, 100 mg q12h, increased by 100 mg (50 mg twice a day) every 4 days until effective dose or maximum of 400 mg/day is attained.

Paroxysmal supraventricular tachycardias (PSVT), paroxysmal atrial fibrillation (PAF):
PO Initially, 50 mg q12h, increased by 100 mg (50 mg twice a day) every 4 days until effective dose or maximum of 300 mg/day is attained.

■ **Contraindications:** Cardiogenic shock, preexisting second- or third-degree AV block, right bundle-branch block (without presence of a pacemaker)

■ **Side Effects**
  Frequent (19%-10%)
  Dizziness, dyspnea, headache
  Occasional (9%-4%)
  Nausea, fatigue, palpitations, chest pain, asthenia (loss of strength, energy), tremor, constipation

■ **Serious Reactions**
  • Flecainide may worsen existing arrhythmias or produce new ones.
  • CHF may occur or existing CHF may worsen.
  • Overdose may increase QRS duration, prolong QT interval, cause conduction disturbances, reduce myocardial contractility, and cause hypotension.

Special Considerations
  • Not first-line therapy
  • Reserve for resistant arrhythmias due to proarrhythmic effects
  • Initiate therapy in facilities capable of providing continuous ECG monitoring and managing life-threatening dysrhythmias

■ **Patient/Family Education**
  • Side effects of flecainide therapy generally disappear with continued use or decreased dosage
  • Do not abruptly discontinue the medication
  • Do not use nasal decongestants or OTC cold preparations without physician approval
  • Use caution when performing tasks that require mental alertness or motor skills
  • Notify the physician if chest pain, faintness, or palpitations occur

■ **Monitoring Parameters**
  • Monitor trough plasma levels periodically, especially in patients with moderate to severe chronic renal failure or severe hepatic disease and CHF; therapeutic range 0.2-1 mcg/ml
  • Pulse for irregular rate and quality
  • ECG for changes, particularly widening of the QRS complex or prolongation of the QT interval
  • Evidence of CHF, including weight gain, pulmonary crackles, and dyspnea
  • Intake and output; a decrease in urine output may indicate CHF

■ **Geriatric side effects at a glance:**
  ❑ CNS ❑ Bowel Dysfunction ❑ Bladder Dysfunction ❑ Falls

■ **U.S. Regulatory Considerations**
  ☑ FDA Black Box
  • An excessive mortality or nonfatal cardiac arrest rate was observed in patients with non-life-threatening ventricular arrhythmias who had a recent MI.

- Ventricular proarrhythmic effects have been observed in patients with atrial fibrillation/flutter. This drug is not recommended in patients with chronic atrial fibrillation.
- Pulmonary fibrosis, interstitial pneumonitis, fibrosing alveolitis, pulmonary edema, and pneumonitis have been reported.
- ❑ OBRA regulated in U.S. Long Term Care

fluconazole

(floo-con'-a-zole)

- ■ **Brand Name(s):** Diflucan
  Chemical Class: Triazole derivative
- ■ **Clinical Pharmacology:**
  Mechanism of Action: A fungistatic antifungal that interferes with cytochrome P-450, an enzyme necessary for ergosterol formation. **Therapeutic Effect:** Directly damages fungal membrane, altering its function.
  Pharmacokinetics: Well absorbed from GI tract. Widely distributed, including to CSF. Protein binding: 11%. Partially metabolized in liver. Excreted unchanged primarily in urine. Partially removed by hemodialysis. **Half-life:** 20-30 hr (increased in impaired renal function).

- ■ **Available Forms:**
  - *Tablets:* 50 mg, 100 mg, 150 mg, 200 mg.
  - *Powder for Oral Suspension:* 10 mg/ml, 40 mg/ml.
  - *Injection:* 2 mg/ml (in 100- or 200-ml containers).

- ■ **Indications and Dosages:**
  Oropharyngeal candidiasis: PO, IV 200 mg once, then 100 mg/day for at least 14 days.
  Esophageal candidiasis: PO, IV 200 mg once, then 100 mg/day (up to 400 mg/day) for 21 days and at least 14 days following resolution of symptoms.
  Vaginal candidiasis: PO 150 mg once.
  Prevention of candidiasis in patients undergoing bone marrow transplantation: PO 400 mg/day
  Systemic candidiasis: PO, IV 400 mg once, then 200 mg/day (up to 400 mg/day) for at least 28 days and at least 14 days following resolution of symptoms.
  Urinary candidiasis: PO, IV 50-200 mg/day.
  Cryptococcal meningitis: PO, IV 400 mg once, then 200 mg/day (up to 800 mg/day) for 10-12 wk after CSF becomes negative (200 mg/day for suppression of relapse in patients with AIDS).
  Onychomycosis: PO 150 mg/wk.
  Dosage in renal impairment: After a loading dose of 400 mg, the daily dosage is based on creatinine clearance.

Creatinine Clearance	% of Recommended Dose
greater than 50 ml/min	100
21-50 ml/min	50
11-20 ml/min	25
Dialysis	Dose after dialysis

- **Unlabeled Uses:** Treatment of coccidioidomycosis, cryptococcosis, fungal pneumonia, onychomycosis, ringworm of the hand, septicemia

- **Contraindications:** None known.

- **Side Effects**
  Occasional (4%-1%)
  Hypersensitivity reaction (including chills, fever, pruritus, and rash), dizziness, drowsiness, headache, constipation, diarrhea, nausea, vomiting, abdominal pain

- **Serious Reactions**
  - Exfoliative skin disorders, serious hepatic effects, and blood dyscrasias (such as eosinophilia, thrombocytopenia, anemia, and leukopenia) have been reported rarely.

- **Patient/Family Education**
  - Do not drive or use machinery until response to the drug is established
  - Notify the physician if dark urine, pale stool, rash with or without itching, or yellow skin or eyes develops
  - The patient with an oropharyngeal infection should maintain good oral hygiene
  - Consult the physician before taking any other medications

- **Monitoring Parameters**
  - Periodic liver function tests with prolonged therapy
  - CBC, renal function, platelet count, serum potassium levels
  - Signs and symptoms of a hypersensitivity reaction, including chills and fever
  - Take temperature daily
  - Daily pattern of bowel activity and stool consistency

- **Geriatric side effects at a glance:**
  ☑ CNS   ☐ Bowel Dysfunction   ☐ Bladder Dysfunction   ☐ Falls

- **U.S. Regulatory Considerations**
  ☐ FDA Black Box   ☐ OBRA regulated in U.S. Long Term Care

flucytosine

(floo-sye'-toe-seen)

- **Brand Name(s):** Ancobon
  Chemical Class: Pyrimidine derivative, fluorinated

- **Clinical Pharmacology:**
  Mechanism of Action: An antifungal that penetrates fungal cells and is converted to fluorouracil which competes with uracil interfering with fungal RNA and protein synthesis. **Therapeutic Effect:** Damages fungal membrane.

Pharmacokinetics: Well absorbed from gastrointestinal (GI) tract. Widely distributed, including cerebrospinal fluid (CSF). Protein binding: 2%-4%. Metabolized in liver. Partially removed by hemodialysis. **Half-life:** 3-8 hr (half-life is increased with impaired renal function).

■ Available Forms:
- *Capsule:* 250 mg, 500 mg.

■ Indications and Dosages:
Fungal infections, candidiasis, cryptococcosis: PO 50 to 150 mg/kg/day in 4 equally divided doses.

Dosage in renal function impairment: Based on creatinine clearance:

Creatinine Clearance	Dosage Interval
20-40 ml/min	q12h
10-20 ml/min	q24h
0-10 ml/min	q24-48h

■ Contraindications: Hypersensitivity to flucytosine

■ Side Effects
Occasional
Pruritus, rash, photosensitivity, dizziness, drowsiness, headache, diarrhea, nausea, vomiting, abdominal pain, increased liver enzymes, jaundice, increased BUN and creatinine, weakness, hearing loss

■ Serious Reactions
- Hepatic dysfunction and severe bone marrow suppression occur rarely.

Special Considerations
- Rarely used as monotherapy; generally used in combination with amphotericin B

■ Patient/Family Education
- Reduce or avoid GI upset by taking caps a few at a time over a 15-min period
- Continue therapy for the full length of treatment and space doses evenly around the clock
- Notify the physician if unexplained fever, sore throat, rash or hives, trouble breathing, yellow skin or eyes, persistent chest pain, or blood urine develops

■ Monitoring Parameters
- Creatinine, BUN, alk phosphatase, AST, ALT, CBC
- Serum flucytosine concentrations (therapeutic range 25-100 mcg/ml)
- Be alert to bone marrow suppressive symptoms

■ Geriatric side effects at a glance:
❏ CNS ❏ Bowel Dysfunction ❏ Bladder Dysfunction ❏ Falls

■ U.S. Regulatory Considerations
❏ FDA Black Box ❏ OBRA regulated in U.S. Long Term Care

fludrocortisone acetate

(floo-droe-kor'-tis-sone as'-e-tate)

- **Brand Name(s):** Florinef Acetate
  Chemical Class: ENDO-mineralocorticoid, synthetic

- **Clinical Pharmacology:**
  Mechanism of Action: A mineralocorticoid that acts at distal tubules. **Therapeutic Effect:** Increases potassium and hydrogen ion excretion. Replaces sodium loss and raises blood pressure (with low dosages). Inhibits endogenous adrenal cortical secretion, thymic activity, and secretion of corticotropin by pituitary gland (with higher dosages).
  Pharmacokinetics: Well absorbed from the GI tract. Protein binding: 42%. Widely distributed. Metabolized in the liver and kidney. Primarily excreted in urine. **Half-life:** 3.5 hr.

- **Available Forms:**
  - *Tablets*: 0.1 mg.

- **Indications and Dosages:**
  Addison's disease: PO 0.05–0.1 mg/day. Range: 0.1 mg 3 times a wk to 0.2 mg/day. Administration with cortisone or hydrocortisone preferred.
  Salt-losing adrenogenital syndrome: PO 0.1–0.2 mg/day.

- **Unlabeled Uses:** Treatment of acidosis in renal tubular disorders, idiopathic orthostatic hypotension

- **Contraindications:** CHF, systemic fungal infection

- **Side Effects**
  Frequent
  Increased appetite, exaggerated sense of well-being, abdominal distention, weight gain, insomnia, mood swings
  High dosages, prolonged therapy, too-rapid withdrawal, increased susceptibility to infection with masked signs and symptoms, delayed wound healing, hypokalemia, hypocalcemia, GI distress, diarrhea or constipation, hypertension
  Occasional
  Headache, dizziness, gastric ulcer development
  Rare
  Hypersensitivity reaction

- **Serious Reactions**
  - Long-term therapy may cause muscle wasting (especially in the arms and legs), osteoporosis, spontaneous fractures, amenorrhea, cataracts, glaucoma, peptic ulcer disease, and CHF.
  - Abruptly withdrawing the drug after long-term therapy may cause anorexia, nausea, fever, headache, joint pain, rebound inflammation, fatigue, weakness, lethargy, dizziness, and orthostatic hypotension.

Patient/Family Education
- Notify clinician of dizziness, severe headache, swelling of feet or lower legs, unusual weight gain
- Do not discontinue abruptly
- Maintain careful personal hygiene and avoid exposure to disease or trauma
- Severe stress, such as serious infection, surgery, or trauma may require an increase in the fludrocortisone dosage
- Steroids often cause mood swings, ranging from euphoria to depression

Monitoring Parameters
- Serum electrolytes, blood pressure, serum renin
- Taper dosage slowly if fludrocortisones is to be discontinued

Geriatric side effects at a glance:
❏ CNS ❏ Bowel Dysfunction ❏ Bladder Dysfunction ❏ Falls

U.S. Regulatory Considerations
❏ FDA Black Box ❏ OBRA regulated in U.S. Long Term Care

flumazenil

(floo-may'-zuh-nil)

Brand Name(s): Romazicon
Chemical Class: Imidazobenzodiazepine derivative

Clinical Pharmacology:
Mechanism of Action: An antidote that antagonizes the effect of benzodiazepines on the gamma-aminobutyric acid receptor complex in the CNS. **Therapeutic Effect:** Reverses sedative effect of benzodiazepines.
Pharmacokinetics:

Route	Onset	Peak	Duration
IV	1-2 min	6-10 min	less than 1 hr

Duration and degree of benzodiazepine reversal depend on dosage and plasma concentration. Protein binding: 50%. Metabolized by the liver; excreted in urine.

Available Forms:
- *Injection*: 0.1 mg/ml.

Indications and Dosages:
Reversal of conscious sedation or general anesthesia: IV Initially, 0.2 mg (2 ml) over 15 sec; may repeat dose in 45 sec; then at 60-sec intervals. Maximum: 1 mg (10-ml) total dose.

507

Benzodiazepine overdose: IV Initially, 0.2 mg (2 ml) over 30 sec; if desired level of consciousness (LOC) is not achieved after 30 sec, 0.3 mg (3 ml) may be given over 30 sec. Further doses of 0.5 mg (5 ml) may be administered over 30 sec at 60-sec intervals. Maximum: 3 mg (30 ml) total dose.

■ **Contraindications:** Anticholinergic signs (such as mydriasis, dry mucosa, and hypoperistalsis), arrhythmias, cardiovascular collapse, history of hypersensitivity to benzodiazepines, patients with signs of serious cyclic antidepressant overdose (such as motor abnormalities), patients who have been given a benzodiazepine for control of a potentially life-threatening condition (such as control of status epilepticus or increased intracranial pressure [ICP])

■ **Side Effects**
Frequent (11%-4%)
Agitation, anxiety, dry mouth, dyspnea, insomnia, palpitations, tremors, headache, blurred vision, dizziness, ataxia, nausea, vomiting, pain at injection site, diaphoresis
Occasional (3%-1%)
Fatigue, flushing, auditory disturbances, thrombophlebitis, rash
Rare (less than 1%)
Urticaria, pruritus, hallucinations

■ **Serious Reactions**
• Toxic effects, such as seizures and arrhythmias, of other drugs taken in overdose, especially tricyclic antidepressants, may emerge with reversal of sedative effect of benzodiazepines.
• Flumazenil may provoke a panic attack in those with a history of panic disorder.

■ **Patient/Family Education**
• Resedation may occur; do not engage in any activities requiring complete alertness or operate hazardous machinery or a motor vehicle until at least 18-24 hr after discharge
• Do not use any alcohol or nonprescription drugs for 18-24 hr after flumazenil administration

■ **Monitoring Parameters**
• Monitor for seizures, sedation, respiratory depression, or other residual benzodiazepine effects for an appropriate period (up to 120 min) based on dose and duration of effect of the benzodiazepine employed; pharmacokinetics of benzodiazepines are not altered in the presence of flumazenil
• Heart rate and rhythm and blood pressure
• Monitor and maintain a patent airway and prepare to assist with ventilation if flumazenil does not fully reverse the respiratory depressant effects of the benzodiazepine
• Closely monitor for return of unconsciousness or narcosis for at least 1 hr after the patient is fully alert

■ **Geriatric side effects at a glance:**
❑ CNS   ❑ Bowel Dysfunction   ❑ Bladder Dysfunction   ❑ Falls

■ **U.S. Regulatory Considerations**
❑ FDA Black Box   ❑ OBRA regulated in U.S. Long Term Care

flunisolide

(floo-niss'-oh-lide)

- **Brand Name(s):** AeroBid, AeroBid-M, Nasalide, Nasarel
  Chemical Class: Glucocorticoid, synthetic

- **Clinical Pharmacology:**
  Mechanism of Action: An adrenocorticosteroid that controls the rate of protein synthesis, depresses migration of polymorphonuclear leukocytes, reverses capillary permeability, and stabilizes lysosomal membranes. **Therapeutic Effect:** Prevents or controls inflammation.
  Pharmacokinetics: Rapidly absorbed from lungs and GI tract following inhalation. About 50% of dose is absorbed from the nasal mucosa following intranasal administration. Metabolized in liver. Partially excreted in urine and feces. **Half-life:** 1-2 hr.

- **Available Forms:**
  - *Aerosol with Adapter (AeroBid):* 250 mcg/activation.
  - *Aerosol (AeroBid-M):* 250 mcg/activation.
  - *Nasal Spray (Nasalide, Nasarel):* 25 mcg/activation.

- **Indications and Dosages:**
  Long-term control of bronchial asthma, assists in reducing or discontinuing oral corticosteroid therapy: Inhalation 2 inhalations twice a day, morning and evening. Maximum: 4 inhalations twice a day.
  Relief of symptoms of perennial and seasonal rhinitis: Intranasal Initially, 2 sprays each nostril twice a day, may increase at 4-7 day intervals to 2 sprays 3 times a day. Maximum: 8 sprays in each nostril daily.

- **Unlabeled Uses:** To prevent recurrence of nasal polyps after surgery

- **Contraindications:** Hypersensitivity to any corticosteroid, persistently positive sputum cultures for *Candida albicans,* primary treatment of status asthmaticus, systemic fungal infections

- **Side Effects**
  Frequent
  Inhalation (25%-10%): Unpleasant taste, nausea, vomiting, sore throat, diarrhea, upset stomach, cold symptoms, nasal congestion
  Occasional
  Inhalation (9%-3%): Dizziness, irritability, nervousness, tremors, abdominal pain, heartburn, oropharynx candidiasis, edema
  Nasal: Mild nasopharyngeal irritation or dryness, rebound congestion, bronchial asthma, rhinorrhea, altered taste

- **Patient/Family Education**
  - To be used on a regular basis, not for acute symptoms
  - Use bronchodilators before oral inhaler (for patients using both)

- Nasal sol may cause drying and irritation of nasal mucosa
- Clear nasal passages prior to use of nasal sol
- Maintain fastidious oral hygiene; rinse mouth with water immediately after inhalation to prevent mouth and throat dryness and a fungal infection
- Drink plenty of fluids to decrease the thickness of lung secretions
- Notify the physician if nasal irritation occurs or if symptoms, such as sneezing, fail to improve

■ Monitoring Parameters
- Monitor patients switched from chronic systemic corticosteroids to avoid acute adrenal insufficiency in response to stress
- Pulse rate and quality and respiratory rate, depth, rhythm, and type
- ABG levels
- Breath sounds for rales, rhonchi, and wheezing

■ Geriatric side effects at a glance:
❑ CNS ❑ Bowel Dysfunction ❑ Bladder Dysfunction ❑ Falls

■ U.S. Regulatory Considerations
❑ FDA Black Box ❑ OBRA regulated in U.S. Long Term Care

fluocinolone acetonide

(floo-oh-sin'-oh-lone a-seat'-oh-nide)

■ Brand Name(s): Capex, Derma-Smoothe/FS, FS Shampoo, Synalar

Combinations
Rx: with hydroquinone/tretinoin (Tri-Luma)
Chemical Class: Corticosteroid, synthetic

■ Clinical Pharmacology:
Mechanism of Action: A fluorinated topical corticosteroid that controls the rate of protein synthesis; depresses migration of polymorphonuclear leukocytes and fibroblasts; reduces capillary permeability; prevents or controls inflammation. *Therapeutic Effect:* Decreases tissue response to inflammatory process.
Pharmacokinetics: Use of occlusive dressings may increase percutaneous absorption. Protein binding: more than 90%. Excreted in urine. *Half-life:* Unknown.

■ Available Forms:
- *Cream:* 0.01%, 0.025% (Synalar).
- *Oil:* 0.01% (Derma-Smoothe/FS).
- *Ointment:* 0.025% (Synalar).
- *Shampoo:* 0.01% (Capex).
- *Solution:* 0.01% (Synalar).

■ Indications and Dosages:
Atopic dermatitis: Topical Apply 3 times/day.

Scalp psoriasis: Topical Apply to damp or wet hair and leave on overnight or for at least 4 hr. Remove by washing hair with shampoo.
Seborrheic dermatitis, scalp: Shampoo Apply once daily; allow it to remain on scalp for at least 5 min.

■ **Unlabeled Uses:** Vitiligo

■ **Contraindications:** Hypersensitivity to fluocinolone or other corticosteroids

■ **Side Effects**
Occasional
Burning, dryness, itching, stinging
Rare
Allergic contact dermatitis, purpura or blood-containing blisters, thinning of skin with easy bruising, telangiectasis or raised dark red spots on skin

■ **Serious Reactions**
• When taken in excessive quantities, HPA axis suppression may occur.

Special Considerations
• Topical oil contains refined peanut oil

■ **Patient/Family Education**
• Apply sparingly only to affected area
• Avoid contact with eyes
• Do not put bandages or dressings over treated area unless directed by clinician
• Do not use on weeping, denuded, or infected areas
• Discontinue drug, notify clinician if local irritation or fever develops

■ **Monitoring Parameters**
• Assess for improvement of skin conditions, relief of pruritus, and healing of lesions

■ **Geriatric side effects at a glance:**
❏ CNS   ❏ Bowel Dysfunction   ❏ Bladder Dysfunction   ❏ Falls

■ **U.S. Regulatory Considerations**
❏ FDA Black Box   ❏ OBRA regulated in U.S. Long Term Care

fluocinonide

(floo-oh-sin'-oh-nide)

■ **Brand Name(s):** Lidex, Lidex-E
Chemical Class: Corticosteroid, synthetic

■ **Clinical Pharmacology:**
Mechanism of Action: A topical corticosteroid that has anti-inflammatory, antipruritic, and vasoconstrictive properties. The exact mechanism of the anti-inflammatory

process is unclear. **Therapeutic Effect:** Reduces or prevents tissue response to the inflammatory process.
Pharmacokinetics: Well absorbed systemically. Large variation in absorption among sites. Protein binding: varies. Metabolized in liver. Primarily excreted in urine.

■ **Available Forms:**
- *Cream (anhydrous emollient)*: 0.05% (Lidex).
- *Cream (aqueous emollient)*: 0.05% (Lidex-E).
- *Gel*: 0.05% (Lidex).
- *Ointment*: 0.05% (Lidex).
- *Solution*: 0.05% (Lidex).

■ **Indications and Dosages:**
Dermatoses: Topical Apply sparingly 2-4 times/day.

■ **Contraindications:** History of hypersensitivity to fluocinonide or other corticosteroids

■ **Side Effects**
Occasional
Itching, redness, irritation, burning at site of application, dryness, folliculitis, acneiform eruptions, hypopigmentation
Rare
Allergic contact dermatitis, maceration of the skin, secondary infection, skin atrophy

■ **Serious Reactions**
- The serious reactions of long-term therapy and the addition of occlusive dressings are reversible hypothalamic-pituitary-adrenal (HPA) axis suppression, manifestations of Cushing's syndrome, hyperglycemia, and glucosuria.

■ **Patient/Family Education**
- Apply sparingly only to affected area
- Avoid contact with eyes
- Do not put bandages or dressings over treated area unless directed by clinician
- Do not use on weeping, denuded, or infected areas
- Discontinue drug, notify clinician if local irritation or fever develops
- Avoid exposure to sunlight

■ **Monitoring Parameters**
- Skin for rash or irritation

■ **Geriatric side effects at a glance:**
❑ CNS   ❑ Bowel Dysfunction   ❑ Bladder Dysfunction   ❑ Falls

■ **U.S. Regulatory Considerations**
❑ FDA Black Box   ❑ OBRA regulated in U.S. Long Term Care

fluoxetine hydrochloride

(floo-ox'-e-teen hye-droe-klor'-ide)

■ **Brand Name(s):** Prozac, Prozac Weekly, Rapiflux, Sarafem

Combinations
Rx: with olanzapine (Symbyax)
Chemical Class: Aryloxypropylamine

■ **Clinical Pharmacology:**
Mechanism of Action: A psychotherapeutic agent that selectively inhibits serotonin uptake in the CNS, enhancing serotonergic function. **Therapeutic Effect:** Relieves depression; reduces obsessive-compulsive and bulimic behavior.
Pharmacokinetics: Well absorbed from the GI tract. Crosses the blood-brain barrier. Protein binding: 94%. Metabolized in the liver to active metabolite. Primarily excreted in urine. Not removed by hemodialysis. **Half-life:** 2-3 days; metabolite 7-9 days.

■ **Available Forms:**
- *Capsules:* 10 mg (Prozac, Sarafem), 20 mg (Prozac, Sarafem), 40 mg (Prozac).
- *Capsules (Delayed-Release[Prozac Weekly]):* 90 mg.
- *Oral Solution (Prozac):* 20 mg/5 ml.
- *Tablets (Prozac, Rapiflux):* 10 mg, 20 mg.

■ **Indications and Dosages:**
Depression: PO *Elderly.* Initially, 10 mg/day. May increase by 10-20 mg q2wk. Maximum: 60 mg/day.
Panic disorder: PO Initially, 10 mg/day. May increase to 20 mg/day after 1 week. Maximum: 60 mg/day.
Bulimia nervosa: PO 60 mg each morning.
Obsessive-compulsive disorder (OCD): PO 40-80 mg/day.

■ **Unlabeled Uses:** Treatment of body dysmorphic disorder, fibromyalgia, hot flashes, post-traumatic stress duisorder, Raynaud's phenomena

■ **Contraindications:** Use within 14 days of MAOIs

■ **Side Effects**
Frequent (more than 10%)
Headache, asthenia, insomnia, anxiety, nervousness, somnolence, nausea, diarrhea, decreased appetite
Occasional (9%-2%)
Dizziness, tremor, fatigue, vomiting, constipation, dry mouth, abdominal pain, nasal congestion, diaphoresis, rash
Rare (less than 2%)
Flushed skin, light-headedness, impaired concentration

■ **Serious Reactions**
- Overdose may produce seizures, nausea, vomiting, agitation, and restlessness.

■ **Patient/Family Education**
  - Therapeutic response may take 4-6 wk
  - May cause insomnia, administer in AM; sedating antidepressants, in small doses (i.e., trazodone 50 mg), frequently administered hs, concurrently
  - Avoid tasks that require mental alertness or motor skills until response to the drug has been established
  - Avoid alcohol

■ **Monitoring Parameters**
  - Closely supervise suicidal patients during early therapy; as depression lessens, the patient's energy level improves, increasing the suicide potential
  - Assess the patient's appearance, behavior, level of interest, mood, and sleep pattern before and during therapy
  - Pattern of daily bowel activity and stool consistency
  - Skin for rash
  - Blood glucose level and serum alkaline phosphatase, bilirubin, sodium, AST (SGOT) and ALT (SGPT) levels

■ **Geriatric side effects at a glance:**
    ❏ CNS   ☑ Bowel Dysfunction   ❏ Bladder Dysfunction   ☑ Falls
    Other: Hyponatremia, weight gain (long term)

■ **Use with caution in older patients with:** None

■ **U.S. Regulatory Considerations**
    ☑ FDA Black Box
  - Because there is an increased risk of suicide in children and adolescents, older adults should also be closely monitored for suicide ideation.
    ☑ OBRA regulated in U.S. Long Term Care

■ **Other Uses in Geriatric Patient:** Anxiety symptoms and related disorders

■ **Side Effects:**
    Of particular importance in the geriatric patient: Hyponatremia, withdrawal symptoms when abruptly discontinued (e.g., during hospitalization) rather than tapered

■ **Geriatric Considerations - Summary:** These agents are now considered by many the first-line therapy for treatment of depression in older adults. They are also effective in the management of symptoms of anxiety. Although these agents appear to have a more favorable side-effect profile than tricyclic antidepressants for most older adults, it is important to note that some of these agents have the potential for significant drug interactions, have been associated with falls, and require careful attention to electrolyte status. In addition, many of the drugs in this class have been associated with severe withdrawal symptoms (e.g., nausea and/or vomiting, dizziness, headaches, lethargy or light-headedness, anxiety and/or agitation) when discontinued abruptly.

■ **References:**
  1. Cadieux RJ. Antidepressant drug interactions in the elderly. Understanding the P-450 system is half the battle in reducing risks. Postgrad Med 1999;106:231-240, 245.
  2. Roose SP, Laghrissi-Thode F, Kennedy JS, et al. Comparison of paroxetine and nortriptyline in depressed patients with ischemic heart disease. JAMA 1998;279:287-291.

3. Thapa PB, Gideon P, Cost TW, et al. Antidepressants and the risk of falls among nursing home residents. N Engl J Med 1998;339:875-882.
4. Bouman WP, Pinner G, Johnson H. Incidence of selective serotonin reuptake inhibitor (SSRI) induced hyponatraemia due to the syndrome of inappropriate antidiuretic hormone (SIADH) secretion in the elderly. Int J Geriatr Psychiatry 1998;13:12-15.

fluoxymesterone

(floo-ox-i-mes'-te-rone)

■ **Brand Name(s):** Halotestin
Chemical Class: Testosterone derivative

DEA Class: Schedule III

■ **Clinical Pharmacology:**
Mechanism of Action: An androgen that suppresses gonadotropin-releasing hormone, LH, and FSH. **Therapeutic Effect:** Stimulates spermatogenesis, development of male secondary sex characteristics, and sexual maturation at puberty. Stimulates production of red blood cells (RBCs).
Pharmacokinetics: Rapidly absorbed from the gastrointestinal (GI) tract. Protein binding: 98%. Metabolized in liver. Excreted in urine. **Half-life:** 9.2 hr.

■ **Available Forms:**
• *Tablets:* 2 mg, 5 mg, 10 mg (Halotestin).

■ **Indications and Dosages:**
Males (hypogonadism): PO 5-20 mg/day.
Females (inoperable breast cancer): PO 10-40 mg/day in divided doses for 1-3 mo.

■ **Contraindications:** Serious cardiac, renal, or hepatic dysfunction, men with carcinomas of the breast or prostate, hypersensitivity to fluoxymesterone or any component of the formulation including tartrazine

■ **Side Effects**
Frequent
Females: Virilism (e.g., acne, decreased breast size, enlarged clitoris, male pattern baldness), deepening voice
Males: UTI, breast soreness, gynecomastia, priapism, virilism (e.g., acne, early pubic hair growth)
Occasional
Edema, nausea, vomiting, mild acne, diarrhea, stomach pain
Males: Impotence, testicular atrophy

■ **Serious Reactions**
• Peliosis hepatitis (liver, spleen replaced with blood-filled cysts), hepatic neoplasms, and hepatocellular carcinoma have been associated with prolonged high dosage.

Patient/Family Education
- Weigh oneself each day and report to physician weight gains of 5 lb or more per week
- Notify the physician of acne, nausea, pedal edema, or vomiting
- The female patient should report deepening of voice or hoarsenes
- The male patient should report difficulty urinating, frequent erections, and gynecomastia

Monitoring Parameters
- Frequent urine and serum calcium determinations (breast cancer)
- Periodic LFTs, Hct, Hgb
- Electrolytes, cholesterol
- Signs of virilization, such as deepening of voice
- Sleep patterns

Geriatric side effects at a glance:
❏ CNS   ❏ Bowel Dysfunction   ❏ Bladder Dysfunction   ❏ Falls

U.S. Regulatory Considerations
❏ FDA Black Box   ❏ OBRA regulated in U.S. Long Term Care

fluphenazine hydrochloride

(floo-fen'-a-zeen hye-droe-klor'-ide)

Brand Name(s): Permitil, Prolixin
Chemical Class: Piperazine phenothiazine derivative

Clinical Pharmacology:
Mechanism of Action: A phenothiazine that antagonizes dopamine neurotransmission at synapses by blocking postsynaptic dopaminergic receptors in the brain.
Therapeutic Effect: Decreases psychotic behavior. Also produces weak anticholinergic, sedative, and antiemetic effects and strong extrapyramidal effects.
Pharmacokinetics: Erratic absorption. Protein binding: greater than 90%. Metabolized in liver. Excreted in urine. **Half-life:** 33 hr.

Available Forms:
- Elixir (Prolixin): 2.5 mg/5 ml.
- Oral Concentrate (Permitil): 5 mg/ml.
- Tablets (Prolixin): 1 mg, 2.5 mg, 5 mg, 10 mg.
- Injection: 2.5 mg/ml (Prolixin), 25 mg/ml (Prolixin Decanoate).

Indications and Dosages:
Psychosis: PO 0.5-10 mg/day in divided doses q6-8h.   IM 2.5-10 mg/day in divided doses q6-8h or 12.5 mg (decanoate) q2wk.

- **Unlabeled Uses:** Treatment of neurogenic pain (adjunct to tricyclic antidepressants)

- **Contraindications:** Angle-closure glaucoma, myelosuppression, severe cardiac or hepatic disease, severe hypertension or hypotension, subcortical brain damage

- **Side Effects**
  Frequent
  Hypotension, dizziness, and syncope (occur frequently after first injection, occasionally after subsequent injections, and rarely with oral doses)
  Occasional
  Somnolence (during early therapy), dry mouth, blurred vision, lethargy, constipation or diarrhea, nasal congestion, peripheral edema, urine retention
  Rare
  Ocular changes, altered skin pigmentation (with prolonged use of high doses)

- **Serious Reactions**
  - Extrapyramidal symptoms (EPS) appear to be related to high dosages and are divided into 3 categories: akathisia (inability to sit still, tapping of feet), parkinsonian symptoms (such as hypersalivation, masklike facial expression, shuffling gait, and tremors), and acute dystonias (such as torticollis, opisthotonos, and oculogyric crisis).
  - Tardive dyskinesia, manifested as tongue protrusion, puffing of the cheeks, and chewing or puckering of the mouth occurs rarely but may be irreversible.
  - Abrupt withdrawal after long-term therapy may precipitate dizziness, gastritis, nausea and vomiting, and tremors.
  - Blood dyscrasias, particularly agranulocytosis and mild leukopenia, may occur.
  - Fluphenzine use may lower the seizure threshold.

Special Considerations

  - Concentrate must be diluted prior to administration; use only the following diluents: water, saline, 7-Up, homogenized milk, carbonated orange beverage, and pineapple, apricot, prune, orange, V-8, tomato, and grapefruit juices; do not mix with beverages containing caffeine, tannics (tea), or pectinates (apple juice), as physical incompatibility may result

- **Patient/Family Education**
  - May cause drowsiness; use caution while driving or performing other tasks requiring alertness; drowsiness generally subsides during continued therapy
  - Avoid contact with skin when using concentrates
  - Avoid prolonged exposure to sunlight
  - May discolor urine pink or reddish-brown
  - Use caution in hot weather, heatstroke may result
  - Arise slowly from a reclining position
  - Full therapeutic effect may take up to 6 wk to appear
  - Do not abruptly discontinue fluphenazine

- **Monitoring Parameters**
  - Monitor closely for the appearance of tardive dyskinesia
  - Blood pressure for hypotension
  - CBC for blood dyscrasias
  - Closely supervise suicidal patients during early therapy
  - Therapeutic response, such as improvement in self-care, increased ability to concentrate and interest in surroundings, and relaxed facial expression

- **Geriatric side effects at a glance:**
  ☑ CNS   ☑ Bowel Dysfunction   ☐ Bladder Dysfunction   ☑ Falls
  Other: Orthostatic hypotension, cardiac conduction disturbances, anticholinergic side effects

- **Use with caution in older patients with:** Parkinson's disease (an atypical antipsychotic is recommended), seizure disorders, cardiovascular disease with conduction disturbance, hepatic encephalopathy, narrow-angle glaucoma

- **U.S. Regulatory Considerations**
  ☐ FDA Black Box   ☑ OBRA regulated in U.S. Long Term Care

- **Other Uses in Geriatric Patient:** Behavior disturbances in the setting of dementia

- **Side Effects:**
  Of particular importance in the geriatric patient: Tardive dyskinesia, akathisia (may appear to exacerbate behavioral disturbances), anticholinergic effects, may increase risk of sudden death

- **Geriatric Considerations - Summary:** Sink and colleagues' systematic review showed statistically significant improvements on neuropsychiatric and behavioral scales for some drugs, but improvements were small and unlikely to be clinically important. Because of documented risks, and uncertain benefits, these agents should be used with caution in demented elderly persons, with frequent monitoring for side effects and a low threshold for discontinuing use.

- **References:**
  1. Leipzig RM, Cumming RG, Tinetti ME. Drugs and falls in older people: a systematic review and meta-analysis: I. Psychotropic drugs. J Am Geriatr Soc 1999;47:30-39.
  2. Sink KM, Holden KF, Yaffe K. Pharmacological treatment of neuropsychiatric symptoms of dementia: a review of the evidence. JAMA 2005;293:596-608.
  3. Ray WA, Meredith S, Thapa PB, et al. Antipsychotics and the risk of sudden cardiac death. Arch Gen Psychiatry 2001;58:1161-1167.

flurandrenolide

(flure-an-dren'-oh-lide)

- **Brand Name(s):** Cordran, Cordran SP, Cordran Tape
  Chemical Class: Corticosteroid, synthetic

- **Clinical Pharmacology:**
  Mechanism of Action: A fluorinated corticosteroid that decreases inflammation by suppression of the migration of polymorphonuclear leukocytes and reversal of increased capillary permeability. *Therapeutic Effect:* Decreases tissue response to inflammatory process.

Pharmacokinetics: Repeated applications may lead to percutaneous absorption. Absorption is about 36% from scrotal area, 7% from the forehead, 4% from scalp, and 1% from forearm. Metabolized in liver. Excreted in urine. **Half-life:** Unknown.

■ **Available Forms:**
  - *Cream*: 0.025%, 0.05% (Cordran SP).
  - *Lotion*: 0.05% (Cordran).
  - *Ointment*: 0.025%, 0.05% (Cordran).
  - *Tape, Topical*: 4 mcg/cm^2 (Cordran Tape).

■ **Indications and Dosages:**
  Anti-inflammatory, immunosuppressant, corticosteroid replacement therapy: Topical
  Apply 2-3 times/day.

■ **Contraindications:** Hypersensitivity to flurandrenolide or any component of the formulation; viral, fungal, or tubercular skin lesions

■ **Side Effects**
  Occasional
  Itching, dry skin, folliculitis
  Rare
  Intracranial hemorrhage, acne, striae, miliaria, allergic contact dermatitis, telangiectasis or raised dark red spots on skin

■ **Serious Reactions**
  - When taken in excessive quantities, systemic hypercorticism and adrenal suppression may occur.

■ **Patient/Family Education**
  - Apply sparingly only to affected area
  - Avoid contact with the eyes
  - Do not put bandages or dressings over treated area unless directed by clinician
  - Do not use on weeping, denuded, or infected areas
  - Discontinue drug, notify clinician if local irritation or fever develops

■ **Monitoring Parameters**
  - Assess the patient for clinical signs of improvement

■ **Geriatric side effects at a glance:**
  ❑ CNS ❑ Bowel Dysfunction ❑ Bladder Dysfunction ❑ Falls

■ **U.S. Regulatory Considerations**
  ❑ FDA Black Box ❑ OBRA regulated in U.S. Long Term Care

flurazepam hydrochloride

(flure-az'-e-pam hye-droe-klor'-ide)

- **Brand Name(s):** Dalmane
  Chemical Class: Benzodiazepine

  DEA Class: Schedule IV

- **Clinical Pharmacology:**
  Mechanism of Action: A benzodiazepine that enhances action of inhibitory neu-rotransmitter gamma-aminobutyric acid (GABA). **Therapeutic Effect:** Produces hyp-notic effect due to CNS depression.
  Pharmacokinetics:

Route	Onset	Peak	Duration
PO	15-20 min	3-6 hr	7-8 hr

  Well absorbed from the GI tract. Protein binding: 97%. Crosses the blood-brain barrier. Widely distributed. Metabolized in liver to active metabolite. Primarily excreted in urine. Not removed by hemodialysis. **Half-life:** 2.3 hr; metabolite: 40-114 hr.

- **Available Forms:**
  - *Capsules:* 15 mg, 30 mg.

- **Indications and Dosages:**
  Insomnia: PO 15-30 mg at bedtime.

- **Contraindications:** Acute alcohol intoxication, acute angle-closure glaucoma, hyper-sensitivity to other benzodiazepines

- **Side Effects**
  Frequent
  Drowsiness, dizziness, ataxia, sedation. Morning drowsiness may occur initially.
  Occasional
  GI disturbances, nervousness, blurred vision, dry mouth, headache, confusion, skin rash, irritability, slurred speech
  Rare
  Paradoxical CNS excitement or restlessness, particularly noted in elderly or debili-tated

- **Serious Reactions**
  - Abrupt or too-rapid withdrawal after long-term use may result in pronounced rest-lessness and irritability, insomnia, hand tremors, abdominal or muscle cramps, vomiting, diaphoresis, and seizures.
  - Overdose results in somnolence, confusion, diminished reflexes, and coma.

Special Considerations
  - Poor choice for elderly patients

Patient/Family Education
- Avoid alcohol and other CNS depressants
- Do not discontinue abruptly after prolonged therapy
- May experience disturbed sleep for the first or second night after discontinuing the drug
- May cause drowsiness or dizziness; use caution while driving or performing other tasks requiring alertness; hangover daytime drowsiness possible secondary to long duration of action

Monitoring Parameters
- Assess patients for paradoxical reaction, such as excitability, particularly during early therapy
- Evaluate the patient for therapeutic response to insomnia, a decrease in number of nocturnal awakenings and an increase in length of sleep

Geriatric side effects at a glance:
☑ CNS ☐ Bowel Dysfunction ☐ Bladder Dysfunction ☑ Falls
Other: None

Use with caution in older patients with: COPD; untreated sleep apnea

U.S. Regulatory Considerations
☐ FDA Black Box ☑ OBRA regulated in U.S. Long Term Care

Other Uses in Geriatric Patient: Hypnotic

Side Effects:
Of particular importance in the geriatric patient: Sedation

Geriatric Considerations - Summary: Benzodiazepines are effective anxiolytic agents, and hypnotics. These drugs should be reserved for short-term use. SSRIs are preferred for long-term management of anxiety disorders in older adults, and sedating antidepressants (e.g., trazodone) or eszopiclone are preferred for long-term management of sleep problems. Long-acting benzodiazepines, including flurazepam, chlordiazepoxide, clorazepate, diazepam, clonazepam, and quazepam, should generally be avoided in older adults as these agents have been associated with oversedation. On the other hand, short-acting benzodiazepines (e.g., triazolam) have been associated with a higher risk of withdrawal symptoms. When initiating therapy, benzodiazepines should be titrated carefully to avoid oversedation. In addition, many of the drugs in this class have been associated with severe withdrawal symptoms (e.g., anxiety and/or agitation, seizures) when discontinued abruptly.

References:
1. Leipzig RM, Cumming RG, Tinetti ME. Drugs and falls in older people: a systematic review and meta-analysis: I. Psychotropic drugs. J Am Geriatr Soc 1999;47:30-39.
2. Shorr RI, Robin DW. Rational use of benzodiazepines in the elderly. Drugs Aging 1994;4:9-20.
3. Shader RI, Greenblatt DJ. Use of benzodiazepines in anxiety disorders. N Engl J Med 1993;328:1398-1405.

flurbiprofen

(flure-bi'-proe-fen)

- **Brand Name(s):** Ansaid, Ocufen (ophthalmic)
  Chemical Class: Propionic acid derivative

- **Clinical Pharmacology:**
  Mechanism of Action: A phenylalkanoic acid that produces analgesic and anti-inflammatory effect by inhibiting prostaglandin synthesis. Also relaxes the iris sphincter.
  Therapeutic Effect: Reduces the inflammatory response and intensity of pain. Prevents or decreases miosis during cataract surgery.
  Pharmacokinetics: Well absorbed from the GI tract; ophthalmic solution penetrates cornea after administration, and may be systemically absorbed. Protein binding: 99%. Widely distributed. Metabolized in the liver. Primarily excreted in urine. **Half-life:** 3-4 hr.

- **Available Forms:**
  - *Tablets* (*Ansaid*): 50 mg, 100 mg.
  - *Ophthalmic Solution* (*Ocufen*): 0.03%.

- **Indications and Dosages:**
  Rheumatoid arthritis, osteoarthritis: PO 200–300 mg/day in 2–4 divided doses. Maximum: 100 mg/dose or 300 mg/day.
  Usual ophthalmic dosage: Ophthalmic Apply 1 drop q30min starting 2 hr before surgery for total of 4 doses.

- **Unlabeled Uses:** Oral: Ankylosing spondylitis, dental pain, postoperative gynecologic pain

- **Contraindications:** Active peptic ulcer, chronic inflammation of GI tract, GI bleeding or ulceration, history of hypersensitivity to aspirin or NSAIDs

- **Side Effects**
  Occasional
  PO (9%-3%): Headache, abdominal pain, diarrhea, indigestion, nausea, fluid retention
  Ophthalmic: Burning or stinging on instillation, keratitis, elevated intraocular pressure
  Rare (less than 3%)
  PO: Blurred vision, flushed skin, dizziness, somnolence, nervousness, insomnia, unusual fatigue, constipation, decreased appetite, vomiting, confusion

- **Serious Reactions**
  - Overdose may result in acute renal failure.
  - Rare reactions with long-term use include peptic ulcer disease, GI bleeding, gastritis, severe hepatic reaction (jaundice), nephrotoxicity (hematuria, dysuria, proteinuria), a severe hypersensitivity reaction (angioedema, bronchospasm), and cardiac arrhythmias.

Patient/Family Education
- Avoid aspirin and alcoholic beverages
- Take with food, milk, or antacids to decrease GI upset
- Notify clinician if edema, black stools, or persistent headache occurs
- Swallow flurbiprofen tablets whole and do not chew or crush them
- The eyes may sting momentarily during drug instillation of ophth flurbiprofen

Monitoring Parameters
- Initial hematocrit and fecal occult blood test within 3 mo of starting regular chronic therapy; repeat every 6-12 mo (more frequently in high-risk patients (>65 years, peptic ulcer disease, concurrent steroids or anticoagulants); electrolytes, creatinine, and BUN within 3 mo of starting regular chronic therapy; repeat every 6-12 mo
- Pattern of daily bowel activity and stool consistency
- Periodic eye exams on patients using ophthalmic flurbiprofen
- Therapeutic response, such as improved grip strength, increased joint mobility, and decreased pain, stiffness, and swelling

Geriatric side effects at a glance:
☑ CNS (oral only)   ☐ Bowel Dysfunction   ☐ Bladder Dysfunction   ☐ Falls
☑ Other: Gastropathy

Use with caution in older patients with:
Renal impairment, Hepatic impairment, CHF, HTN, PUD, History of GI bleeding, GERD, Bleeding and platelet disorders, History of aspirin sensitivity reaction. Also use with caution in patients taking Anticoagulants, Aspirin, and Antihypertensive agents.

U.S. Regulatory Considerations
☑ FDA Black Box
- Cardiovascular risk
- Gastrointestinal risk
☐ OBRA regulated in U.S. Long Term Care

Other Uses in Geriatric Patient: Acute Gout

Side Effects:
Of particular importance in the geriatric patient: Confusion, cognitive impairment, delirium, dizziness, dyspepsia, fluid retention, renal impairment

Geriatric Considerations - Summary:
Use of NSAIDs in older adults increases the risk of GI complications including gastric ulceration, bleeding, and perforation. These complications are not necessarily preceded by less severe GI symptoms. Concomitant use of a proton pump inhibitor or misoprostol reduces the risk for gastric ulceration and bleeding, but may not prevent long-term GI toxicity.

References:
1. COX-2 alternatives and GI protection. Med Lett Drugs Ther 2004;46:91.
2. Drugs that may cause cognitive disorders in the elderly. Med Lett Drugs Ther 2000;42:111-112.

flutamide

(floo'-ta-mide)

■ **Brand Name(s):** Eulexin
Chemical Class: Acetanilid derivative

■ **Clinical Pharmacology:**
Mechanism of Action: An antiandrogen hormone that inhibits androgen uptake and prevents androgen from binding to androgen receptors in target tissue. Used in conjunction with leuprolide to inhibit the stimulant effects of flutamide on serum testosterone levels. **Therapeutic Effect:** Suppresses testicular androgen production and decreases growth of prostate carcinoma.
Pharmacokinetics: Completely absorbed from the GI tract. Protein binding: 94%-96%. Metabolized in the liver to active metabolite. Primarily excreted in urine. Not removed by hemodialysis. **Half-life:** 6 hr (increased in elderly).

■ **Available Forms:**
• *Capsules:* 125 mg.

■ **Indications and Dosages:**
Prostatic carcinoma (in combination with leuprolide): PO 250 mg q8h.

■ **Unlabeled Uses:** Female hirsutism

■ **Contraindications:** Hepatic impairment - ALT > 2 times upper limit of normal

■ **Side Effects**
Frequent
Hot flashes (50%); decreased libido, diarrhea (24%); generalized pain (23%); asthenia (17%); constipation (12%); nausea, nocturia (11%)
Occasional (8%-6%)
Dizziness, paresthesia, insomnia, impotence, peripheral edema, gynecomastia
Rare (5%-4%)
Rash, diaphoresis, hypertension, hematuria, vomiting, urinary incontinence, headache, flu-like syndromes, photosensitivity

■ **Serious Reactions**
• Hepatoxicity, including hepatic encephalopathy, and hemolytic anemia may be noted.

Special Considerations
• Begin 8 wk before radiation therapy in Stage B_2-C carcinoma, continue during radiation
• In metastatic carcinoma continue until progression noted

■ **Patient/Family Education**
• Feminization may occur during therapy
• Do not discontinue therapy without discussion with clinician

- Urine may become amber or yellow-green during flutamide therapy
- Avoid overexposure to the sun or ultraviolet light and wear protective clothing outdoors until tolerance of ultraviolet light is determined

■ **Monitoring Parameters**
- Monthly LFTs for the first 4 mo of therapy, then periodically thereafter

■ **Geriatric side effects at a glance:**
☐ CNS ☑ Bowel Dysfunction ☐ Bladder Dysfunction ☐ Falls

■ **U.S. Regulatory Considerations**
☑ FDA Black Box
Hepatic injury: hospitalization and rarely death have been reported. Half of cases occurred within 3 mo of therapy initiation.
☐ OBRA regulated in U.S. Long Term Care

fluticasone propionate

(flu-tic'-a-zone pro'pe-o-nate)

■ **Brand Name(s):** Cutivate, Flonase, Flovent, Flovent Diskus, Flovent HFA, Flovent Rotadisk

Combinations
Rx: with salmeterol (Advair Diskus)
Chemical Class: Corticosteroid, synthetic

■ **Clinical Pharmacology:**
Mechanism of Action: A corticosteroid that controls the rate of protein synthesis, depresses migration of polymorphonuclear leukocytes, reverses capillary permeability, and stabilizes lysosomal membranes. **Therapeutic Effect:** Prevents or controls inflammation.
Pharmacokinetics: Inhalation/intranasal: Protein binding: 91%. Undergoes extensive first-pass metabolism in liver. Excreted in urine. **Half-life:** 3-7.8 hr. Topical: Amount absorbed depends on affected area and skin condition (absorption increased with fever, hydration, inflamed or denuded skin).

■ **Available Forms:**
- *Aerosol for Oral Inhalation (Flovent, Flovent HFA):* 44 mcg/inhalation, 110 mcg/inhalation, 220 mcg/ inhalation.
- *Powder for Oral Inhalation (Flovent Diskus):* 50 mcg, 100 mcg, 250 mcg.
- *Intranasal Spray (Flonase):* 50 mcg/inhalation.
- *Topical Cream (Cutivate):* 0.05%.
- *Topical Ointment (Cutivate):* 0.005%.

■ **Indications and Dosages:**
Allergic rhinitis: Intranasal Initially, 200 mcg (2 sprays in each nostril once daily or 1 spray in each nostril q12h). Maintenance: 1 spray in each nostril once daily. Maximum: 200 mcg/day.

Relief of inflammation and pruritus associated with steroid-responsive disorders, such as contact dermatitis and eczema: Topical Apply sparingly to affected area once or twice a day.

Maintenance treatment for asthma for those previously treated with bronchodilators: Inhalation Powder (Flovent Diskus) Initially, 100 mcg q12h. Maximum: 500 mcg/day. Inhalation (Oral [Flovent]) 88 mcg twice a day. Maximum: 440 mcg twice a day.

Maintenance treatment for asthma for those previously treated with inhaled steroids: Inhalation Powder (Flovent Diskus) Initially, 100-250 mcg q12h. Maximum: 500 mcg q12h. Inhalation (Oral [Flovent]) 88-220 mcg twice a day. Maximum: 440 mcg twice a day.

Maintenance treatment for asthma for those previously treated with oral steroids: Inhalation Powder (Flovent Diskus) 500-1000 mcg twice a day. Inhalation (Oral [Flovent]) 880 mcg twice a day.

■ **Contraindications:** Primary treatment of status asthmaticus or other acute asthma episodes (inhalation); untreated localized infection of nasal mucosa

■ **Side Effects**
Frequent
Inhalation: Throat irritation, hoarseness, dry mouth, cough, temporary wheezing, oropharyngeal candidiasis (particularly if mouth is not rinsed with water after each administration)
Intranasal: Mild nasopharyngeal irritation; nasal burning, stinging, or dryness; rebound congestion; rhinorrhea; loss of taste
Occasional
Inhalation: Oral candidiasis
Intranasal: Nasal and pharyngeal candidiasis, headache
Topical: Skin burning, pruritus

■ **Serious Reactions**
• Deaths due to adrenal insufficiency have occurred in asthma patients during and after transfer from use of long-term systemic corticosteroids to less systemically available inhaled corticosteroids.

Special Considerations
• Improvement following inhalation, 24 hr to 1-2 wk
• Systemic corticosteroid effects from inhaled and nasal steroids inadequate to prevent adrenal insufficiency in most patients withdrawn abruptly from corticosteroids
• Observe for evidence of inadequate adrenal response following periods of stress

■ **Patient/Family Education**
• Rinsing the mouth following INH and using a spacer device reduces common EENT adverse effects
• Review proper MDI administration technique regularly
• Do not discontinue the drug abruptly or change the dosage schedule; the dosage must be tapered gradually under medical supervision
• Drink plenty of fluids to decrease the thickness of lung secretions
• If the patient is using a bronchodilator inhaler concomitantly with a steroid inhaler, use the bronchodilator several minutes before using the corticosteroid to help the steroid penetrate into the bronchial tree
• Clear nasal passages before use
• Notify the physician if nasal irritation occurs or if symptoms, such as sneezing, fail to improve

- Symptoms should improve in several days
- The patient using topical fluticasone should rub a thin film gently on the affected area
- Keep the preparation away from the eyes

■ Monitoring Parameters
- Pulse rate and quality and respiratory depth, rate, rhythm, and type
- ABG levels
- Breath sounds for rales, rhonchi, and wheezing
- Oral mucous membranes for evidence of candidiasis

■ Geriatric side effects at a glance:
❑ CNS ❑ Bowel Dysfunction ❑ Bladder Dysfunction ❑ Falls

■ U.S. Regulatory Considerations
❑ FDA Black Box ❑ OBRA regulated in U.S. Long Term Care

fluvastatin sodium

(floo'-va-sta-tin soe'-dee-um)

■ Brand Name(s): Lescol, Lescol XL
Chemical Class: Substituted hexahydronaphthalene

■ Clinical Pharmacology:
Mechanism of Action: An antihyperlipidemic that inhibits HMG-CoA reductase, the enzyme that catalyzes the early step in cholesterol synthesis. **Therapeutic Effect:** Decreases LDL cholesterol, VLDL, and plasma triglyceride levels. Slightly increases HDL cholesterol concentration.
Pharmacokinetics: Well absorbed from the GI tract and is unaffected by food. Does not cross the blood-brain barrier. Protein binding: greater than 98%. Primarily eliminated in feces. **Half-life:** 1.2 hr.

■ Available Forms:
- *Capsules (Lescol):* 20 mg, 40 mg.
- *Tablets (Extended-Release [Lescol XL]):* 80 mg.

■ Indications and Dosages:
Hyperlipoproteinemia: PO Initially, 20 mg/day (capsule) in the evening. May increase up to 40 mg/day. Maintenance: 20-40 mg/day in a single dose or divided doses. *Patients requiring more than a 25% decrease in* LDL *cholesterol.* 40 mg (capsule) 1-2 times a day or 80 mg tablet once a day.

■ Contraindications: Active hepatic disease, unexplained increased serum transaminase levels

■ Side Effects
Frequent (8%-5%)
Headache, dyspepsia, back pain, myalgia, arthralgia, diarrhea, abdominal cramping, rhinitis

Occasional (4%-2%)
Nausea, vomiting, insomnia, constipation, flatulence, rash, pruritus, fatigue, cough, dizziness

■ **Serious Reactions**
- Myositis (inflammation of voluntary muscle) with or without increased CK, and muscle weakness, occur rarely. These conditions may progress to frank rhabdomyolysis and renal impairment.

Special Considerations
- Statin selection based on lipid-lowering prowess, cost, and availability

■ **Patient/Family Education**
- Report symptoms of myalgia, muscle tenderness, or weakness
- Take daily doses in the evening for increased effect
- May take without regard to food
- Follow the prescribed diet
- Periodic laboratory tests are an essential part of therapy

■ **Monitoring Parameters**
- Cholesterol (max therapeutic response 4-6 wk)
- LFTs (AST, ALT) at baseline and at 12 wk of therapy; if no change, no further monitoring necessary (discontinue if elevations persist at >3 times upper limit of normal)
- CPK in patients complaining of diffuse myalgia, muscle tenderness, or weakness

■ **Geriatric side effects at a glance:**
  ❑ CNS   ❑ Bowel Dysfunction   ❑ Bladder Dysfunction   ❑ Falls

■ **U.S. Regulatory Considerations**
  ❑ FDA Black Box   ❑ OBRA regulated in U.S. Long Term Care

fluvoxamine maleate

(floo-vox'-a-meen mal'-ee-ate)

■ **Brand Name(s):** Luvox
  Chemical Class: Aralkylketone derivative

■ **Clinical Pharmacology:**
  Mechanism of Action: An antidepressant and antiobsessive agent that selectively inhibits neuronal reuptake of serotonin. **Therapeutic Effect:** Relieves depression and symptoms of obsessive-compulsive disorder.
  Pharmacokinetics: Well absorbed following PO administration. Protein binding: 77%. Metabolized in liver. Excreted in urine. **Half-life:** 15.6 hr.

- ■ **Available Forms:**
  - *Tablets*: 25 mg, 50 mg, 100 mg.

- ■ **Indications and Dosages:**
  Obsessive-compulsive disorder (OCD): PO 50 mg at bedtime; may increase by 50 mg every 4-7 days. Dosages greater than 100 mg/day given in 2 divided doses. Maximum: 300 mg/day.

- ■ **Unlabeled Uses:** Treatment of depression, panic disorder

- ■ **Contraindications:** Use within 14 days of MAOIs, co-administration of thioridazine, terfenadine, astemizole, cisapride, or pimozide with fluvoxamine

- ■ **Side Effects**
  Frequent
  Nausea (40%), headache, somnolence, insomnia (22%-21%)
  Occasional (14%-8%)
  Dizziness, diarrhea, dry mouth, asthenia, weakness, dyspepsia, constipation, abnormal ejaculation
  Rare (6%-3%)
  Anorexia, anxiety, tremor, vomiting, flatulence, urinary frequency, sexual dysfunction, altered taste

- ■ **Serious Reactions**
  - Overdose may produce seizures, nausea, vomiting, and extreme agitation and restlessness.

- ■ **Patient/Family Education**
  - May cause dizziness or drowsiness; use caution driving or performing tasks requiring alertness
  - Maximum therapeutic response may require 4 wk or more to appear
  - Do not discontinue the drug abruptly
  - Take sips of tepid water and chew sugarless gum to relieve dry mouth

- ■ **Monitoring Parameters**
  - Assess appearance, behavior, level of interest, mood, and sleep pattern
  - Assess pattern of daily bowel activity and stool consistency

- ■ **Geriatric side effects at a glance:**
  ❑ CNS   ☑ Bowel Dysfunction   ❑ Bladder Dysfunction   ☑ Falls
  Other: Hyponatremia, weight gain (long term)

- ■ **Use with caution in older patients with:** None

- ■ **U.S. Regulatory Considerations**
  ☑ FDA Black Box
  - Because there is an increased risk of suicide in children and adolescents, older adults should also be closely monitored for suicide ideation.
  ☑ OBRA regulated in U.S. Long Term Care

- ■ **Other Uses in Geriatric Patient:** Anxiety symptoms and related disorders

■ **Side Effects:**
Of particular importance in the geriatric patient: Hyponatremia, withdrawal symptoms when abruptly discontinued (e.g., during hospitalization) rather than tapered

■ **Geriatric Considerations - Summary:** These agents are now considered by many the first-line therapy for treatment of depression in older adults. They are also effective in the management of symptoms of anxiety. Although these agents appear to have a more favorable side-effect profile than tricyclic antidepressants for most older adults, it is important to note that some of these agents have the potential for significant drug interactions, have been associated with falls, and require careful attention to electrolyte status. In addition, many of the drugs in this class have been associated with severe withdrawal symptoms (e.g., nausea and/or vomiting, dizziness, headaches, lethargy or light-headedness, anxiety and/or agitation) when discontinued abruptly.

■ **References:**
1. Cadieux RJ. Antidepressant drug interactions in the elderly. Understanding the P-450 system is half the battle in reducing risks. Postgrad Med 1999;106:231-240, 245.
2. Roose SP, Laghrissi-Thode F, Kennedy JS, et al. Comparison of paroxetine and nortriptyline in depressed patients with ischemic heart disease. JAMA 1998;279:287-291.
3. Thapa PB, Gideon P, Cost TW, et al. Antidepressants and the risk of falls among nursing home residents. N Engl J Med 1998;339:875-882.
4. Bouman WP, Pinner G, Johnson H. Incidence of selective serotonin reuptake inhibitor (SSRI) induced hyponatraemia due to the syndrome of inappropriate antidiuretic hormone (SIADH) secretion in the elderly. Int J Geriatr Psychiatry 1998;13:12-15.

folic acid/sodium folate (NUTR-vitamin B₉)

(foe'-lik as'-id soe'-dee-um fo'-late)

■ **Brand Name(s):** (folic acid) Folvite
Chemical Class: NUTR-vitamin B complex

■ **Clinical Pharmacology:**
Mechanism of Action: A coenzyme that stimulates production of platelets, RBCs, and WBCs. **Therapeutic Effect:** Essential for nucleoprotein synthesis and maintenance of normal erythropoiesis.
Pharmacokinetics: PO form almost completely absorbed from the GI tract (upper duodenum). Protein binding: High. Metabolized in the liver and plasma to active form. Excreted in urine. Removed by hemodialysis.

■ **Available Forms:**
• *Tablets:* 0.4 mg, 0.8 mg, 1 mg.
• *Injection:* 5 mg/ml.

■ **Indications and Dosages:**
Dietary supplement (RDA): PO 400 mcg/day. Maximum: 0.1 mg/day.

Folic acid deficiency: PO, IV, IM, Subcutaneous Initially, 1 mg/day. Maintenance: 0.5 mg/day.

■ **Unlabeled Uses:** To decrease the risk of colon cancer

■ **Contraindications:** Anemias (aplastic, normocytic, pernicious, refractory)

■ **Side Effects**
None known.

■ **Serious Reactions**
  • Allergic hypersensitivity occurs rarely with parenteral form. Oral folic acid is non-toxic.

Special Considerations
  • Recent evidence supports the premise that lowering elevated plasma homocysteine levels may reduce the risk of coronary heart disease

■ **Patient/Family Education**
  • Take only under medical supervision
  • Eat foods rich in folic acid including fruits, vegetables, and organ meats

■ **Monitoring Parameters**
  • CBC; serum folate concentrations <0.005 mcg/ml indicate folic acid deficiency and concentrations <0.002 mcg/ml usually result in megaloblastic anemia
  • Therapeutic improvement, including improved sense of well-being and relief from iron deficiency symptoms, such as fatigue, headache, pallor, dyspnea, and sore tongue

■ **Geriatric side effects at a glance:**
  ❑ CNS ❑ Bowel Dysfunction ❑ Bladder Dysfunction ❑ Falls

■ **U.S. Regulatory Considerations**
  ❑ FDA Black Box ❑ OBRA regulated in U.S. Long Term Care

fomepizole

(foe-mep'-i-zoll)

■ **Brand Name(s):** Antizol
   Chemical Class: Pyrazole derivative

■ **Clinical Pharmacology:**
   Mechanism of Action: An alcohol dehydrogenase inhibitor that inhibits the enzyme that catalyzes the metabolism of ethanol, ethylene glycol, and methanol to their toxic metabolites. ***Therapeutic Effect:*** Inhibits conversion of ethylene glycol and methanol into toxic metabolites.

531

Pharmacokinetics: Protein binding: low. Rapidly distributes to total body water after IV infusion. Extensively metabolized by the liver. Minimal excretion in the urine. Removed by hemodialysis. **Half-life:** 5 hr.

■ **Available Forms:**
  • *Solution for Injection:* 1 g/ml (Antizol).

■ **Indications and Dosages:**
  Ethylene glycol or methanol intoxication: IV infusion 15 mg/kg as loading dose, followed by 10 mg/kg q12h for 4 doses, then 15 mg/kg q12h until ethylene glycol or methanol concentrations are below 20 mg/dl. All doses should be administered as a slow IV infusion over 30 min.
  Dosage in renal impairment: *During hemodialysis.* 15 mg/kg as a loading dose, followed by 10 mg/kg q4h for 4 doses, then 15 mg/kg q4h until ethylene glycol or methanol concentrations are below 20 mg/dL. *After hemodialysis.* If the time between the last dose and end of hemodialysis is less than 1 hour, do not give dose. If the time between is 1-3 hours, give 50% of next scheduled dose. If time is greater than 3 hours give next scheduled dose.

■ **Unlabeled Uses:** Butoxyethanol intoxication, diethylene glycol intoxication, ethanol sensitivity

■ **Contraindications:** Hypersensitivity to fomepizole or other pyrazoles

■ **Side Effects**
  Frequent
  Hypertriglyceridemia, headache, nausea, dizziness
  Occasional
  Abnormal sense of smell, nystagmus, visual disturbances, ringing in ears, agitation, seizures, anorexia, heartburn, anxiety, vertigo, light-headedness, altered sense of awareness
  Rare
  Anuria, disseminated intravascular coagulopathy

■ **Serious Reactions**
  • Mild allergic reactions including rash and eosinophilia occur rarely.
  • Overdose may cause nausea, dizziness, and vertigo.

■ **Patient/Family Education**
  • Common side effects are headache and nausea

■ **Monitoring Parameters**
  • Frequently monitor both ethylene glycol levels and acid-base balance, as determined by serum electrolyte (anion gap) or arterial blood gas analysis
  • In patients with high ethylene glycol levels ($\geq$50 mg/dl), significant metabolic acidosis or renal failure, consider hemodialysis to remove ethylene glycol and its toxic metabolites
  • Treatment with fomepizole may be discontinued when ethylene glycol levels have been reduced to <20 mg/dl

■ **Geriatric side effects at a glance:**
  ❏ CNS   ❏ Bowel Dysfunction   ❏ Bladder Dysfunction   ❏ Falls

fomivirsen sodium

(foh-mih-ver'-sen soe'-dee-um)

■ **Brand Name(s):** Vitravene
   Chemical Class: Antisense oligonucleotide

■ **Clinical Pharmacology:**
   Mechanism of Action: An antiviral that binds to messenger RNA, inhibiting the synthesis of viral proteins. **Therapeutic Effect:** Blocks replication of cytomegalovirus (CMV).
   Pharmacokinetics: Minimal systemic absorption following intravitreal injection.

■ **Available Forms:**
   • *Intravitreal Injection*: 6.6 mg/ml.

■ **Indications and Dosages:**
   CMV *retinitis*: Intravitreal injection   330 mcg (0.05 ml) every other week for 2 doses, then 330 mcg every 4 weeks.

■ **Contraindications:** None known.

■ **Side Effects**
   Frequent (10%-5%)
   Fever, headache, nausea, diarrhea, vomiting, abdominal pain, anemia, uveitis, abnormal vision
   Occasional (5%-2%)
   Chest pain, confusion, dizziness, depression, neuropathy, anorexia, weight loss, pancreatitis, dyspnea, cough

■ **Serious Reactions**
   • Thrombocytopenia may occur.

■ **Patient/Family Education**
   • Does not treat systemic aspects of CMV infection

■ **Monitoring Parameters**
   • Ophthalmologic examination
   • Monitor the patient for signs and symptoms of extraocular CMV infection, including pneumonitis and colitis. Also, assess for signs and symptoms of CMV infection in the untreated eye if only one eye is undergoing treatment

fondaparinux sodium

(fon-da-pa'-rin-ux soe'-dee-um)

■ **Brand Name(s):** Arixtra
   Chemical Class: Pentasaccharide

■ **Clinical Pharmacology:**
   Mechanism of Action: A factor Xa inhibitor and pentasaccharide that selectively binds to antithrombin, and increases its affinity for factor Xa, thereby inhibiting factor Xa and stopping the blood coagulation cascade. **Therapeutic Effect:** Indirectly prevents formation of thrombin and subsequently the fibrin clot.
   Pharmacokinetics: Well absorbed after subcutaneous administration. Undergoes minimal, if any, metabolism. Highly bound to antithrombin III. Distributed mainly in blood and to a minor extent in extravascular fluid. Excreted unchanged in urine. Removed by hemodialysis. **Half-life:** 17–21 hr (prolonged in patients with impaired renal function).:

Patient consideration	Reduction in total clearance
Creatinine clearance 50-80 ml/min	25%
Creatinine clearance 30-49 ml/min	40%
Creatinine clearance less than 30 ml/min	55%
Age - older than 75 years	25%
Weight - less than 50 kg	30%

■ **Available Forms:**
   • *Injection*: 2.5 mg/0.5 ml prefilled syringe.

■ **Indications and Dosages:**
   Prevention of venous thromboembolism: Subcutaneous 2.5 mg once a day for 5-9 days after surgery. Initial dose should be given 6-8 hr after surgery. Dosage should be adjusted in those older than 75 years of age and those with renal impairment.
   Treatment of venous thromboembolism, pulmonary embolism: Subcutaneous *Weight greater than 100 kg.* 10 mg once daily. *Weight 50-100 kg.* 7.5 mg once daily. *Weight less than 50 kg.* 5 mg once daily.

■ **Contraindications:** Active major bleeding, bacterial endocarditis, body weight less than 50 kg, severe renal impairment (with creatinine clearance less than 30 ml/min), thrombocytopenia associated with antiplatelet antibody formation in the presence of fondaparinux

■ **Side Effects**
   Occasional (14%)
   Fever

Rare (4%-1%)
Injection site hematoma, nausea, peripheral edema

■ **Serious Reactions**
- Accidental overdose may lead to bleeding complications ranging from local ecchymoses to major hemorrhage.
- Thrombocytopenia occurs rarely.

Special Considerations
- Slightly better at preventing DVT than enoxaparin; caused more bleeding than enoxaparin after knee replacement surgery; therapeutic niche not well defined

■ **Patient/Family Education**
- The usual length of therapy is 5-9 days
- Do not take other medications, including OTC drugs (especially aspirin and NSAIDs), without physician approval
- Report severe or sudden headache, swelling in the feet or hands, unusual back pain, or unusual bleeding, bruising, or weakness
- Report bleeding from surgical site, chest pain, or dyspnea
- Use an electric razor and soft toothbrush to prevent bleeding during therapy
- Give injection instructions

■ **Monitoring Parameters**
- Periodic CBC, serum Cr, stool occult blood; there is no need for daily monitoring in patients with normal presurgical coagulation parameters
- Blood pressure, pulse - hypotension and tachycardia may indicate bleeding
- Assess for signs of bleeding, including bleeding at injection or surgical sites or from gums, blood in stool, ecchymosis, hematuria, and petechiae

■ **Geriatric side effects at a glance:**
❑ CNS   ❑ Bowel Dysfunction   ❑ Bladder Dysfunction   ❑ Falls

■ **U.S. Regulatory Considerations**
☑ FDA Black Box
Increased risk of spinal/epidural hematomas with neuraxial anesthesia or spinal puncture. Risk is further increased by use of indwelling spinal catheters, repeated/traumatic epidural/spinal puncture, or use of drugs affecting hemostasis (NSAIDs, anticoagulants, platelet inhibitors).
❑ OBRA regulated in U.S. Long Term Care

formoterol fumarate

(for-moh'-te-role fyoo'-muh-rate)

■ **Brand Name(s):** Foradil Aerolizer
   Chemical Class: Sympathomimetic amine; β_2-adrenergic agonist

■ **Clinical Pharmacology:**
   Mechanism of Action: A long-acting bronchodilator that stimulates beta$_2$-adrenergic receptors in the lungs, resulting in relaxation of bronchial smooth muscle. Also inhibits release of mediators from various cells in the lungs, including mast cells, with little effect on heart rate. **Therapeutic Effect:** Relieves bronchospasm, reduces airway resistance. Improves bronchodilation, nighttime asthma control, and peak flow rates.
   Pharmacokinetics:

Route	Onset	Peak	Duration
Inhalation	1-3 min	0.5-1 hr	12 hr

Absorbed from bronchi after inhalation. Metabolized in the liver. Primarily excreted in urine. Unknown if removed by hemodialysis. **Half-life:** 10 hr.

■ **Available Forms:**
   • *Inhalation Powder in Capsules:* 12 mcg.

■ **Indications and Dosages:**
   Asthma, chronic obstructive pulmonary disease (COPD): Inhalation 12-mcg capsule q12h.
   Exercise-induced bronchospasm: Inhalation 12-mcg capsule at least 15 min before exercise. Do not repeat for another 12 hr.

■ **Contraindications:** None known.

■ **Side Effects**
   Occasional
   Tremor, muscle cramps, tachycardia, insomnia, headache, irritability, irritation of mouth or throat

■ **Serious Reactions**
   • Excessive sympathomimetic stimulation may produce palpitations, extrasystole, and chest pain.

Special Considerations
   • Not indicated for patients whose asthma can be managed by occasional use of inhaled, short-acting β_2-agonists
   • Can be used concomitantly with short-acting β_2-agonists, inhaled or systemic corticosteroids, and theophylline
   • Does not eliminate the need for treatment with an inhaled anti-inflammatory agent
   • Do not initiate therapy in patients with significantly worsening or acutely deteriorating asthma
   • For use only with the Aerolizer Inhaler

■ **Patient/Family Education**
- Should never be used more frequently than twice daily (morning and evening) at the recommended dose; do not use to treat acute symptoms
- Discontinue the regular use of short-acting β_2-agonists and use them only for symptomatic relief of acute asthma symptoms
- Seek medical advice immediately if a previously effective asthma medication regimen fails to provide the usual response
- For inhalation only, do not take orally
- Store in blister packaging, only remove immediately before use; handle capsules with dry hands
- Use the new Aerolizer Inhaler provided with each new prescription
- Drink plenty of fluids to decrease the thickness of lung secretions
- Avoid excessive use of caffeinated products, such as chocolate, cola, coffee, and tea

■ **Monitoring Parameters**
- Pulmonary function tests
- Serum potassium
- Pulse rate and quality and respiratory rate, depth, rhythm, and type
- ECG

■ **Geriatric side effects at a glance:**
❑ CNS ❑ Bowel Dysfunction ❑ Bladder Dysfunction ❑ Falls

■ **U.S. Regulatory Considerations**
❑ FDA Black Box ❑ OBRA regulated in U.S. Long Term Care

fosamprenavir calcium

(fos'-am-pren-a-veer kal'-see-um)

■ **Brand Name(s):** Lexiva
Chemical Class: HIV protease inhibitor

■ **Clinical Pharmacology:**
Mechanism of Action: An antiretroviral that is rapidly converted to amprenavir, which inhibits HIV-1 protease by binding to the enzyme's active site, thus preventing the processing of viral precursors and resulting in the formation of immature, noninfectious viral particles. **Therapeutic Effect:** Impairs HIV replication and proliferation.
Pharmacokinetics: Rapidly absorbed after PO administration. Protein binding: 90%. Metabolized in the liver. Excreted in urine and feces. **Half-life:** 7.7 hr.

■ **Available Forms:**
- *Tablets*: 700 mg (equivalent to 600 mg amprenavir).

■ **Indications and Dosages:**
HIV infection in patients who have not had previous protease inhibitor therapy: PO 1400 mg twice daily without ritonavir; or 1400 mg once daily plus ritonavir 200 mg once daily; or 700 mg twice daily plus ritonavir 100 mg twice daily.

HIV infection in patients who have had previous protease inhibitor therapy: PO 700 mg twice daily plus ritonavir 100 mg twice daily.

Concurrent therapy with efavirenz: PO In patients receiving fosamprenavir plus once-daily ritonavir in combination with efavirenz, an additional 100 mg/day ritonavir (300 mg total/day) should be given.

■ **Contraindications:** Concurrent use of amprenavir, dihydroergotamine, ergonovine, ergotamine, flecainide, methylergonovine, midazolam, pimozide, propafenone, ritonavir, triazolam

■ **Side Effects**
   Frequent (39%-35%)
   Nausea, rash, diarrhea
   Occasional (19%-8%)
   Headache, vomiting, fatigue, depression
   Rare (7%-2%)
   Pruritus, abdominal pain, perioral paresthesia

■ **Serious Reactions**
   • Severe and possibly life-threatening dermatologic reactions, including Stevens-Johnson syndrome, occur rarely.
   • New onset or exacerbation of diabetes mellitus has been reported.

Special Considerations
   • Fosamprenavir is a prodrug for amprenavir, and allows fewer capsules to be administered per day, due to improved absorption
   • Always check updated treatment guidelines before initiating or changing antiretroviral therapy. (http://AIDSinfo.nih.gov)

■ **Patient/Family Education**
   • Space doses evenly and continue taking fosamprenavir for the full course of treatment
   • Consume small, frequent meals to help offset nausea and vomiting; consider taking OTC antidiarrheals if diarrhea occurs
   • Fosamprenavir is not a cure for HIV infection, nor does it reduce the risk of transmitting HIV to others

■ **Monitoring Parameters**
   • HIV RNA level, CD4 count, CBC, metabolic panel, liver function tests, triglyceride and cholesterol levels
   • Pattern of daily bowel activity and stool consistency
   • Skin for rash

■ **Geriatric side effects at a glance:**
   ❑ CNS ☑ Bowel Dysfunction ❑ Bladder Dysfunction ❑ Falls

■ **U.S. Regulatory Considerations**
   ❑ FDA Black Box ❑ OBRA regulated in U.S. Long Term Care

foscarnet sodium

(foss-car'-net soe'-dee-um)

■ **Brand Name(s):** Foscavir
  Chemical Class: Pyrophosphate analog

■ **Clinical Pharmacology:**
  Mechanism of Action: An antiviral that selectively inhibits binding sites on virus-specific DNA polymerase and reverse transcriptase. **Therapeutic Effect:** Inhibits replication of herpesvirus.
  Pharmacokinetics: Sequestered into bone and cartilage. Protein binding: 14%-17%. Primarily excreted unchanged in urine. Removed by hemodialysis. **Half-life:** 3.3-6.8 hr (increased in impaired renal function).

■ **Available Forms:**
  • *Injection*: 24 mg/ml.

■ **Indications and Dosages:**
  Cytomegalovirus (CMV) retinitis: IV Initially, 60 mg/kg q8h or 100 mg/kg q12h for 2-3 wk. Maintenance: 90-120 mg/kg/day as a single IV infusion.
  Herpes infection: IV 40 mg/kg q8-12h for 2-3 wk or until healed.
  Dosage in renal impairment: Dosages are individualized based on creatinine clearance. Refer to the dosing guide provided by the manufacturer.

■ **Contraindications:** None known.

■ **Side Effects**
  Frequent
  Fever (65%); nausea (47%); vomiting, diarrhea (30%)
  Occasional (5% or greater)
  Anorexia, pain and inflammation at injection site, fever, rigors, malaise, headache, paresthesia, dizziness, rash, diaphoresis, abdominal pain
  Rare (5%-1%)
  Back or chest pain, edema, flushing, pruritus, constipation, dry mouth

■ **Serious Reactions**
  • Nephrotoxicity occurs to some extent in most patients.
  • Seizures and serum mineral or electrolyte imbalances may be life-threatening.

Special Considerations
  • Hydration to establish diuresis both prior to and during administration is recommended to minimize renal toxicity; the standard 24 mg/ml sol may be used undiluted via a central venous catheter, dilute to 12 mg/ml with D5W or NS when a peripheral vein catheter is used

■ **Patient/Family Education**
  • Foscarnet is not a cure for CMV retinitis

539

- Notify clinician of perioral tingling, numbness in the extremities, tremors, or paresthesias (could signify electrolyte imbalances)

■ **Monitoring Parameters**
- Serum creatinine, calcium, phosphorus, potassium, magnesium at baseline and 2-3 times/wk during induction and at least every 1-2 wk during maintenance
- Hemoglobin
- Regular ophthalmologic examinations
- Signs and symptoms of serum electrolyte imbalances, especially hypocalcemia (numbness or tingling in the extremities or around the mouth) and hypokalemia (irritability, muscle cramps, numbness or tingling of the extremities, and weakness)

■ **Geriatric side effects at a glance:**
  ❑ CNS   ☑ Bowel Dysfunction   ❑ Bladder Dysfunction   ❑ Falls

■ **U.S. Regulatory Considerations**
  ☑ FDA Black Box
  Nephrotoxicity, seizures related to electrolyte levels.
  ❑ OBRA regulated in U.S. Long Term Care

fosfomycin tromethamine

(fos-foe-mye'-sin troe-meth'-a-meen)

■ **Brand Name(s):** Monurol
  Chemical Class: Phosphoric acid derivative

■ **Clinical Pharmacology:**
  Mechanism of Action: An antibacterial that prevents bacterial cell wall formation by inhibiting the synthesis of peptidoglycan. *Therapeutic Effect:* Bactericidal.
  Pharmacokinetics: Rapidly absorbed following PO administration. Not bound to plasma proteins. Not metabolized. Partially excreted in urine; minimal elimination in feces. *Half-life:* 5.7 + 2.8 hr.

■ **Available Forms:**
- *Powder for Oral Solution:* 3 g.

■ **Indications and Dosages:**
  UTIs: PO (Uncomplicated) *Females.* 3g mixed in 4 oz water as a single dose. PO (Complicated) *Males.* 3 g/day q2-3days for 3 doses.

■ **Unlabeled Uses:** Serious UTI in men

■ **Contraindications:** None known.

■ **Side Effects**
  Occasional (9%-3%)
  Diarrhea, nausea, headache, back pain

Rare (less than 2%)
Pharyngitis, abdominal pain, rash

■ **Serious Reactions**
• None known.

Special Considerations

• Inferior 5- to 11-day post-therapy microbiologic eradication rates compared to ciprofloxacin and co-trimoxazole for acute cystitis; eradication rates comparable to nitrofurantoin
• Reserve for women unable to tolerate or unlikely to comply with 3-day courses of co-trimoxazole or trimethoprim

■ **Patient/Family Education**
• Always mix with water before ingesting
• Symptoms should improve 2-3 days after the initial dose of fosfomycin

■ **Geriatric side effects at a glance:**
❑ CNS   ❑ Bowel Dysfunction   ❑ Bladder Dysfunction   ❑ Falls

■ **U.S. Regulatory Considerations**
❑ FDA Black Box   ❑ OBRA regulated in U.S. Long Term Care

fosinopril

(foe-sin'-oh-pril)

■ **Brand Name(s):** Monopril
Chemical Class: Angiotensin-converting enzyme (ACE) inhibitor, nonsulfhydryl

■ **Clinical Pharmacology:**
Mechanism of Action: An ACE inhibitor that suppresses the renin-angiotensin-aldosterone system and prevents conversion of angiotensin I to angiotensin II, a potent vasoconstrictor; may also inhibit angiotensin II at local vascular and renal sites. Decreases plasma angiotensin II, increases plasma renin activity, and decreases aldosterone secretion. **Therapeutic Effect:** Reduces peripheral arterial resistance, pulmonary capillary wedge pressure; improves cardiac output, and exercise tolerance.
Pharmacokinetics:

Route	Onset	Peak	Duration
PO	1 hr	2-6 hr	24 hr

Slowly absorbed from the GI tract. Protein binding: 97%-98%. Metabolized in the liver and GI mucosa to active metabolite. Primarily excreted in urine. Minimal removal by hemodialysis. **Half-life:** 11.5 hr.

■ **Available Forms:**
• *Tablets:* 10 mg, 20 mg, 40 mg.

■ **Indications and Dosages:**
    Hypertension: PO Initially, 10 mg/day. Maintenance: 20–40 mg/day as a single or 2 divided doses. Maximum: 80 mg/day.
    Heart failure: PO Initially, 10 mg/day. Maintenance: 20–40 mg/day. Maximum: 40 mg/day.

■ **Unlabeled Uses:** Treatment of diabetic and nondiabetic nephropathy, post-MI left ventricular dysfunction, renal crisis in scleroderma

■ **Contraindications:** History of angioedema from previous treatment with ACE inhibitors

■ **Side Effects**
    Frequent (12%-9%)
    Dizziness, cough
    Occasional (4%-2%)
    Hypotension, nausea, vomiting, upper respiratory tract infection

■ **Serious Reactions**
- Excessive hypotension ("first-dose syncope") may occur in patients with CHF and in those who are severely salt and volume depleted.
- Angioedema (swelling of face and lips) and hyperkalemia occur rarely.
- Agranulocytosis and neutropenia may be noted in those with collagen vascular disease, including scleroderma and systemic lupus erythematosus, and impaired renal function.
- Nephrotic syndrome may be noted in those with history of renal disease.
- Hypoglycemia may occur in patients with diabetes using glucose-lowering drugs.

■ **Patient/Family Education**
- Caution with salt substitutes containing potassium chloride
- Rise slowly to sitting/standing position to minimize orthostatic hypotension
- Dizziness, fainting, light-headedness may occur during 1st few days of therapy
- May cause altered taste perception or cough; persistent dry cough usually does not subside unless medication is stopped; notify clinician if these symptoms persist
- Report any signs or symptoms of infection, such as fever or sore throat
- Full therapeutic effect of fosinopril may take several weeks to appear
- Noncompliance with drug therapy or skipping fosinopril doses may cause severe, rebound hypertension

■ **Monitoring Parameters**
- BUN, creatinine, potassium within 2 wk after initiation of therapy (increased levels may indicate acute renal failure)
- Blood pressure
- Intake and output
- In patients with CHF, assess for crackles and wheezes
- Urinalysis for proteinuria

■ **Geriatric side effects at a glance:**
    ❑ CNS ❑ Bowel Dysfunction ❑ Bladder Dysfunction ❑ Falls

■ **U.S. Regulatory Considerations**
    ☑ FDA Black Box

Although not relevant for geriatric patients, teratogenicity is associated with the use of ACE inhibitors.
❑ OBRA regulated in U.S. Long Term Care

frovatriptan succinate

(froe-va-trip'-tan suk'-si-nate)

■ **Brand Name(s):** Frova
Chemical Class: Serotonin derivative

■ **Clinical Pharmacology:**
Mechanism of Action: A serotonin receptor agonist that binds selectively to vascular receptors, producing a vasoconstrictive effect on cranial blood vessels. **Therapeutic Effect:** Relieves migraine headache.
Pharmacokinetics: Well absorbed after PO administration. Metabolized by the liver to inactive metabolite. Eliminated in urine. **Half-life:** 26 hr (increased in hepatic impairment).

■ **Available Forms:**
• *Tablets*: 2.5 mg.

■ **Indications and Dosages:**
Acute migraine attack: PO Initially 2.5 mg. If headache improves but then returns, dose may be repeated after 2 hr. Maximum: 7.5 mg/day.

■ **Contraindications:** Basilar or hemiplegic migraine, cerebrovascular or peripheral vascular disease, coronary artery disease, ischemic heart disease (including angina pectoris, history of MI, silent ischemia, and Prinzmetal's angina), severe hepatic impairment (Child-Pugh grade C), uncontrolled hypertension, use within 24 hours of ergotamine-containing preparations or another serotonin receptor agonist, use within 14 days of MAOIs

■ **Side Effects**
Occasional (8%-4%)
Dizziness, paresthesia, fatigue, flushing
Rare (3%-2%)
Hot or cold sensation, dry mouth, dyspepsia

■ **Serious Reactions**
• Cardiac reactions (including ischemia, coronary artery vasospasm, and MI), and noncardiac vasospasm-related reactions (such as cerebral hemorrhage and cerebrovascular accident [CVA]), occur rarely, particularly in patients with hypertension, diabetes, or a strong family history of coronary artery disease; obese patients; smokers; males older than 40 years; and postmenopausal women.

- Triptans and dihydroergotamine are drugs of choice for moderate to severe migraine attacks; nasal sumatriptan is usually considered the triptan of choice due to its rapid onset; there are a number of oral triptans, including frovatriptan, with more favorable biopharmaceutic profiles and high costs; comparisons not available
- There is no evidence that a second dose of frovatriptan is effective in patients who do not respond to a first dose of the drug for the same headache

■ **Patient/Family Education**
- Useful medication for treatment of acute migraine attacks, not prevention; take a single dose of frovatriptan as soon as migraine symptoms appear
- Do not crush or chew film-coated tablets
- If the headache improves but then recurs, take a second dose at least 2 hr after the first dose
- Avoid tasks that require mental alertness or motor skills until response to the drug has been established
- Notify the physician immediately if palpitations, pain or weakness in the extremities, pain or tightness in the chest or throat, or sudden or severe abdominal pain occurs
- Lie down in a dark, quiet room for additional benefit after taking frovatriptan

■ **Monitoring Parameters**
- Headache response 1-4 hr after a dose (reduction from moderate or severe pain to minimal or no pain), functional disability, need for a second dose, headache recurrence, pulse, blood pressure

■ **Geriatric side effects at a glance:**
  ❑ CNS ❑ Bowel Dysfunction ❑ Bladder Dysfunction ❑ Falls

■ **U.S. Regulatory Considerations**
  ❑ FDA Black Box ❑ OBRA regulated in U.S. Long Term Care

fulvestrant

(fool-ves'-trant)

■ **Brand Name(s):** Faslodex
  Chemical Class: Estrogen derivative

■ **Clinical Pharmacology:**
  Mechanism of Action: An estrogen antagonist that competes with endogenous estrogen at estrogen receptor binding sites. **Therapeutic Effect:** Inhibits tumor growth.
  Pharmacokinetics: Extensively and rapidly distributed after IM administration. Protein binding: 99%. Metabolized in the liver. Eliminated by hepatobiliary route; excreted in feces. **Half-life:** 40 days in postmenopausal women. Peak serum levels occur in 7-9 days.

■ **Available Forms:**
- *Prefilled Syringe*: 50 mg/ml in 2.5-ml and 5-ml syringes.

■ **Indications and Dosages:**
Breast cancer: IM 250 mg given once monthly.

■ **Unlabeled Uses:** Uterine bleeding

■ **Contraindications:** None known.

■ **Side Effects**
Frequent (26%-13%)
Nausea, hot flashes, pharyngitis, asthenia, vomiting, vasodilatation, headache
Occasional (12%-5%)
Injection site pain, constipation, diarrhea, abdominal pain, anorexia, dizziness, insomnia, paresthesia, bone or back pain, depression, anxiety, peripheral edema, rash, diaphoresis, fever
Rare (2%-1%)
Vertigo, weight gain

■ **Serious Reactions**
- UTIs, vaginitis, anemia, thromboembolic phenomena, and leukopenia occur rarely.

Special Considerations
- Store in refrigerator

■ **Patient/Family Education**
- Notify the physician if weakness, hot flashes, or nausea become unmanageable

■ **Monitoring Parameters**
- Blood chemistry and plasma lipid levels
- Evaluate the level of bone pain and ensure adequate pain relief if pain increases
- Assess for edema, especially in dependent areas
- Monitor for asthenia and dizziness and provide assistance with ambulation if these symptoms occur
- Assess for headache
- Offer an antiemetic, if ordered, to prevent or treat nausea and vomiting

■ **Geriatric side effects at a glance:**
❏ CNS   ❏ Bowel Dysfunction   ❏ Bladder Dysfunction   ❏ Falls

■ **U.S. Regulatory Considerations**
❏ FDA Black Box   ❏ OBRA regulated in U.S. Long Term Care

furosemide

(fur-oh'-se-mide)

■ **Brand Name(s):** Lasix
   Chemical Class: Anthranilic acid derivative

■ **Clinical Pharmacology:**
   Mechanism of Action: A loop diuretic that enhances excretion of sodium, chloride, and potassium by direct action at the ascending limb of the loop of Henle. **Therapeutic Effect:** Produces diuresis and lowers BP.
   Pharmacokinetics:

Route	Onset	Peak	Duration
PO	30-60 min	1-2 hr	6-8 hr
IV	5 min	20-60 min	2 hr
IM	30 min	N/A	N/A

   Well absorbed from the GI tract. Protein binding: 91%-97%. Partially metabolized in the liver. Primarily excreted in urine (nonrenal clearance increases in severe renal impairment). Not removed by hemodialysis. **Half-life:** 30-90 min (increased in renal or hepatic impairment).

■ **Available Forms:**
   • *Oral Solution*: 10 mg/ml, 40 mg/5 ml.
   • *Tablets*: 20 mg, 40 mg, 80 mg.
   • *Injection*: 10 mg/ml.

■ **Indications and Dosages:**
   Edema, hypertension: PO Initially, 20-80 mg/dose; may increase by 20-40 mg/dose q6-8h. May titrate up to 600 mg/day in severe edematous states. IV, IM 20-40 mg/dose; may increase by 20 mg/dose q1-2h. IV Infusion Bolus of 0.1 mg/kg, followed by infusion of 0.1 mg/kg/hr; may double q2h. Maximum: 0.4 mg/kg/hr.

■ **Unlabeled Uses:** Hypercalcemia

■ **Contraindications:** Anuria, hepatic coma, severe electrolyte depletion

■ **Side Effects**
   Expected
   Increased urinary frequency and urine volume
   Frequent
   Nausea, dyspepsia, abdominal cramps, diarrhea or constipation, electrolyte disturbances
   Occasional
   Dizziness, light-headedness, headache, blurred vision, paresthesia, photosensitivity, rash, fatigue, bladder spasm, restlessness, diaphoresis
   Rare
   Flank pain

546

■ Serious Reactions
- Vigorous diuresis may lead to profound water loss and electrolyte depletion, resulting in hypokalemia, hyponatremia, and dehydration.
- Sudden volume depletion may result in increased risk of thrombosis, circulatory collapse, and sudden death.
- Acute hypotensive episodes may occur, sometimes several days after beginning therapy.
- Ototoxicity - manifested as deafness, vertigo, or tinnitus - may occur, especially in patients with severe renal impairment.
- Furosemide use can exacerbate diabetes mellitus, systemic lupus erythematosus, gout, and pancreatitis.
- Blood dyscrasias have been reported.
- Use with caution in persons with sulfa allergy.

Special Considerations
- Although allergic cross-reactivity with sulfonamide antibiotics and sulfonamide nonantibiotics has not been demonstrated, use with caution in patients with a history of severe sulfa allergies.

■ Patient/Family Education
- May cause GI upset, take with food or milk
- Take early in the day
- Avoid prolonged exposure to sunlight
- Expect an increase in the frequency and volume of urination
- Notify the physician if hearing abnormalities (ringing, roaring, or sense of fullness in the ears) or signs of an electrolyte imbalance (irregular heartbeat, muscle cramps or weakness, tremor) occur
- Eat foods high in potassium, including apricots, bananas, orange juice, potatoes, raisins, legumes, meat, and whole grains (such as cereals)

■ Monitoring Parameters
- Urine volume, creatinine clearance, BUN, electrolytes, reduction in edema, increased diuresis, decrease in body weight, reduction in blood pressure, glucose, uric acid, serum calcium (tetany), tinnitus, vertigo, hearing loss (especially in those at risk for ototoxicity—IV doses >120 mg; concomitant ototoxic drugs; renal disease)

■ Geriatric side effects at a glance:
❑ CNS   ❑ Bowel Dysfunction   ❑ Bladder Dysfunction   ❑ Falls

■ U.S. Regulatory Considerations
❑ FDA Black Box   ❑ OBRA regulated in U.S. Long Term Care

gabapentin

(ga'-ba-pen-tin)

■ **Brand Name(s):** Neurontin
  Chemical Class: Cyclohexanacetic acid derivative

■ **Clinical Pharmacology:**
  Mechanism of Action: An anticonvulsant and antineuralgic agent whose exact mechanism is unknown. May increase the synthesis or accumulation of gamma-aminobutyric acid by binding to as-yet-undefined receptor sites in brain tissue. **Therapeutic Effect:** Reduces seizure activity and neuropathic pain.
  Pharmacokinetics: Well absorbed from the GI tract (not affected by food). Protein binding: less than 5%. Widely distributed. Crosses the blood-brain barrier. Primarily excreted unchanged in urine. Removed by hemodialysis. **Half-life:** 5-7 hr (increased in impaired renal function and the elderly).

■ **Available Forms:**
  - *Capsules (Neurontin):* 100 mg, 300 mg, 400 mg.
  - *Oral Solution (Neurontin):* 250 mg/5 ml.
  - *Tablets (Neurontin):* 100 mg, 300 mg, 400 mg, 600 mg, 800 mg.

■ **Indications and Dosages:**
  Adjunctive therapy for seizure control: PO Initially, 300 mg 3 times a day. May titrate dosage. Range: 900-1800 mg/day in 3 divided doses. Maximum: 3,600 mg/day.
  Adjunctive therapy for neuropathic pain: PO Initially, 100 mg 3 times a day; may increase by 300 mg/day at weekly intervals. Maximum: 3,600 mg/day in 3 divided doses.
  Postherpetic neuralgia: PO 300 mg on day 1, 300 mg twice a day on day 2, and 300 mg 3 times a day on day 3. Titrate up to 1,800 mg/day.
  Dosage in renal impairment: Dosage and frequency are modified based on creatinine clearance:

Creatinine Clearance	Dosage
60 ml/min or higher	400 mg q8h
30-59 ml/min	300 mg q12h
16-29 ml/min	300 mg daily
less than 16 ml/min	300 mg every other day
Hemodialysis	200-300 mg after each 4-hr hemodialysis session

■ **Unlabeled Uses:** Treatment of bipolar disorder, chronic pain, diabetic peripheral neuropathy, essential tremor, hot flashes, hyperhidrosis, migraines, psychiatric disorders (social phobia)

■ **Contraindications:** None known.

■ **Side Effects**
  Frequent (19%-10%)
  Fatigue, somnolence, dizziness, ataxia
  Occasional (8%-3%)
  Nystagmus, tremor, diplopia, rhinitis, weight gain

548

Rare (less than 2%)

Nervousness, dysarthria, memory loss, dyspepsia, pharyngitis, myalgia

■ **Serious Reactions**
- Abrupt withdrawal may increase seizure frequency.
- Overdosage may result in diplopia, slurred speech, drowsiness, lethargy, and diarrhea.

■ **Patient/Family Education**
- Do not stop abruptly; taper over 1 wk
- Take gabapentin only as prescribed
- Avoid tasks requiring mental alertness or motor skills until response to the drug is established
- Avoid alcohol while taking gabapentin
- Always carry an identification card or wear an identification bracelet that displays seizure disorder and anticonvulsant therapy

■ **Monitoring Parameters**
- Drug level monitoring not necessary
- Weight, renal function, and behavior (in children)
- Seizure duration and frequency

■ **Geriatric side effects at a glance:**
❑ CNS   ❑ Bowel Dysfunction   ❑ Bladder Dysfunction   ❑ Falls
Other: Weight gain

■ **Use with caution in older patients with:** Renal impairment, Urinary incontinence

■ **U.S. Regulatory Considerations**
❑ FDA Black Box   ❑ OBRA regulated in U.S. Long Term Care

■ **Other Uses in Geriatric Patient:** Neuropathic Pain, Post-Herpetic Neuralgia, Essential Tremor

■ **Side Effects:**
Of particular importance in the geriatric patient: Delirium, confusion, sedation, fatigue, dizziness, ataxia, asthenia, headache, weight gain

■ **Geriatric Considerations - Summary:** Dosage adjustments required in older adults with creatinine clearance < 60 ml/min. Gabapentin has been well-studied in older adults and is considered a first-line agent as a result of tolerability, small effects on cognition, and few drug interactions. Absorption is reduced by approximately 50% at doses > 3600 mg/day. Capsules are large and may be difficult to swallow, especially in patients with dysphagia or dry mouth.

■ **References:**
1. Brodie M, Kwan P. Epilepsy in elderly people. BMJ 2005;331:1317-1322.
2. Rowan AJ, Ramsay RE, Collins JF, et. al. New onset geriatric epilepsy: a randomized study of gabapentin, lamotrigine, and carbamazepine. Neurology 2005;64:1868-1873.
3. Arroyo S, Kramer G. Treating epilepsy in the elderly: safety considerations. Drug Safety 2001;24:991-1015.

4. Drugs that may cause cognitive disorders in the elderly. Med Lett 2000;42:111-112.
5. Willmore LJ. Choice and use of newer anticonvulsant drugs in older patients. Drugs Aging 2000;17:441-452.
6. Faught E. Epidemiolgy and drug treatment of epilepsy in elderly people. Drugs Aging 1999;15:255-269.

galantamine hydrobromide

(ga-lan'-ta-meen hye-droe-broe'-mide)

■ **Brand Name(s):** Razadyne, Razadyne ER
Chemical Class: Benzazepine derivative; cholinesterase inhibitor

■ **Clinical Pharmacology:**
Mechanism of Action: A cholinesterase inhibitor that inhibits the enzyme acetylcholinesterase, thus increasing the concentration of acetylcholine at cholinergic synapses and enhancing cholinergic function in the CNS. **Therapeutic Effect:** Slows the progression of Alzheimer's disease.
Pharmacokinetics: Rapidly absorbed from the GI tract. Protein binding: 18%. Distributed to blood cells; binds to plasma proteins, mainly albumin. Metabolized in the liver. Excreted in urine. **Half-life:** 7 hr.

■ **Available Forms:**
- *Capsules (Extended-Release [Razadyne ER]):* 8 mg, 16 mg, 24 mg.
- *Oral Solution (Razadyne):* 4 mg/ml.
- *Tablets (Razadyne):* 4 mg, 8 mg, 12 mg.

■ **Indications and Dosages:**
Alzheimer's disease: PO Initially, 4 mg twice a day (8 mg/day). After a minimum of 4 wk (if well tolerated), may increase to 8 mg twice a day (16 mg/day). After another 4 wk, may increase to 12 mg twice daily (24 mg/day). Range: 16-24 mg/day in 2 divided doses. PO (Extended Release) 8-24 mg/day as a single daily dose.
Dosage in renal or hepatic impairment: For moderate impairment, maximum dosage is 16 mg/day. Drug is not recommended for patients with severe impairment.

■ **Contraindications:** Severe hepatic or renal impairment

■ **Side Effects**
Frequent (17%-5%)
Nausea, vomiting, diarrhea, anorexia, weight loss
Occasional (9%-4%)
Abdominal pain, insomnia, depression, headache, dizziness, fatigue, rhinitis
Rare (less than 3%)
Tremors, constipation, confusion, cough, anxiety, urinary incontinence

■ **Serious Reactions**
- Overdose may cause cholinergic crisis, characterized by increased salivation, lacrimation, severe nausea and vomiting, bradycardia, respiratory depression, hypotension, and increased muscle weakness. Treatment usually consists of supportive measures and an anticholinergic such as atropine.

- Extracted from the bulbs of the daffodil, *Narcissus pseudonarcissus*

■ Patient/Family Education
- Patient and caregiver should be advised of high incidence of gastrointestinal effects and directions for resource and resolution
- Take galantamine with morning and evening meals to reduce the risk of nausea
- Avoid tasks that require mental alertness or motor skills until response to the drug has been established
- Notify the physician if excessive sweating, tearing, salivation, depression, dizziness, excessive fatigue, muscle weakness, insomnia, or persistent GI disturbances occur
- Galantamine is not a cure for Alzheimer's disease but may slow the progression of its symptoms

■ Monitoring Parameters
- Cognitive function (e.g., ADAS, Mini-Mental Status Exam [MMSE]), activities of daily living, global functioning, blood chemistry, complete blood counts, heart rate, blood pressure
- Periodically assess the 12-lead ECG and rhythm strips of patients with underlying arrhythmias
- Assess the patient for signs of GI distress, including nausea, vomiting, diarrhea, anorexia, and weight loss

■ Geriatric side effects at a glance:
☑ CNS   ☑ Bowel Dysfunction   ❏ Bladder Dysfunction   ❏ Falls
Other: Anorexia, weight loss, bradycardia

■ Use with caution in older patients with: None

■ U.S. Regulatory Considerations
❏ FDA Black Box   ❏ OBRA regulated in U.S. Long Term Care

■ Other Uses in Geriatric Patient: None

■ Side Effects:
Of particular importance in the geriatric patient: None

■ Geriatric Considerations - Summary: Galantamine, like other cholinesterase inhibitors, is modestly effective for treatment of cognitive decline associated with Alzheimer's disease. Compared to placebo, persons using galantamine have less decline in performance on cognitive tests, but most patients derive minimal clinical benefit, and there is no evidence the drug delays disability or institutionalization. Galantamine is expensive, and not cost-effective for this indication. Persons using drugs to treat Alzheimer's disease should be monitored closely, and prescribers should have a low threshold for discontinuing these agents if no clinical benefit is observed.

■ References:
1. Cummings JL. Alzheimer's disease. N Engl J Med 2004;351:56-67.
2. Kaduszkiewicz H, Zimmermann T, Beck-Bornholdt HP, et al. Cholinesterase inhibitors for patients with Alzheimer's disease: systematic review of randomised clinical trials. BMJ 2005;331:321-327.

ganciclovir sodium

(gan-sye'-kloe-veer soe'-dee-um)

■ **Brand Name(s):** Cytovene, Vitrasert
  Chemical Class: Acyclic purine nucleoside analog

■ **Clinical Pharmacology:**
  Mechanism of Action: This synthetic nucleoside competes with viral DNA polymerase and is incorporated into growing viral DNA chains. **Therapeutic Effect:** Interferes with synthesis and replication of viral DNA.
  Pharmacokinetics: Widely distributed. Protein binding: 1%-2%. Undergoes minimal metabolism. Excreted unchanged primarily in urine. Removed by hemodialysis. **Half-life:** 2.5-3.6 hr (increased in impaired renal function).

■ **Available Forms:**
  • *Capsules (Cytovene):* 250 mg, 500 mg.
  • *Powder for Injection (Cytovene):* 500 mg.
  • *Implant (Vitrasert):* 4.5 mg.

■ **Indications and Dosages:**
  Cytomegalovirus (CMV) retinitis: IV 10 mg/kg/day in divided doses q12h for 14-21 days, then 5 mg/kg/day as a single daily dose or 6 mg/kg 5 days a week.
  Prevention of CMV disease in transplant patients: IV 10 mg/kg/day in divided doses q12h for 7-14 days, then 5 mg/kg/day as a single daily dose.
  Other CMV infections: IV Initially, 10 mg/kg/day in divided doses q12h for 14-21 days, then 5 mg/kg/day as a single daily dose. Maintenance: 1000 mg 3 times a day or 500 mg q3h (6 times a day). Intravitreal implant 1 implant q6-9mo plus oral ganciclovir.
  Dosage in renal impairment: Dosage and frequency are modified based on creatinine clearance.

CrCl	Induction Dosage	Maintenance Dosage	Oral
50-69 ml/ min	2.5 mg/kg q12h	2.5 mg/kg q24h	1500 mg/day
25-49 ml/ min	2.5 mg/kg q24h	1.25 mg/ kg q24h	1000 mg/day
10-24 ml/ min	1.25 mg/kg q24h	0.625 mg/ kg q24h	500 mg/day
less than 10 ml/ min	1.25 mg/kg 3 times/wk	0.625 mg/kg 3 times/wk	500 mg 3 times/wk

■ **Unlabeled Uses:** Treatment of other CMV infections, such as gastroenteritis, hepatitis, and pneumonitis

■ **Contraindications:** Absolute neutrophil count less than 500/mm^3, platelet count less than 25,000/mm^3, hypersensitivity to acyclovir or ganciclovir, immunocompetent patients, patients with congenital CMV disease

■ **Side Effects**
  Frequent
  Diarrhea (41%), fever (40%), nausea (25%), abdominal pain (17%), vomiting (13%)
  Occasional (11%-6%)
  Diaphoresis, infection, paresthesia, flatulence, pruritus

552

Rare (4%-2%)
Headache, stomatitis, dyspepsia, phlebitis

■ **Serious Reactions**
- Hematologic toxicity occurs commonly: leukopenia in 41%-29% of patients and anemia in 25%-19%.
- Intra-ocular insertion occasionally results in visual acuity loss, vitreous hemorrhage, and retinal detachment.
- GI hemorrhage occurs rarely.

■ **Patient/Family Education**
- Compliance with laboratory monitoring is essential
- Promptly report any new symptom to the physician
- Male patients should be aware that ganciclovir may temporarily or permanently inhibit sperm production
- Male patients should use barrier contraception during ganciclovir therapy and for 90 days afterward because of the drug's mutagenic potential
- Ganciclovir suppresses but does not cure CMV retinitis

■ **Monitoring Parameters**
- CBC with differential and platelets q2 days during induction and weekly thereafter
- Serum creatinine q2wk
- Intake and output
- Signs and symptoms of infiltration, phlebitis, pruritus, and rash
- Vision

■ **Geriatric side effects at a glance:**
❑ CNS   ☑ Bowel Dysfunction   ❑ Bladder Dysfunction   ❑ Falls

■ **U.S. Regulatory Considerations**
☑ FDA Black Box
Risk for granulocytopenia, anemia, and thrombocytopenia. Oral capsules associated with risk of rapid rate of CMV retinitis progression and should be used as maintenance therapy in patients who benefit from avoiding daily IV infusions.
❑ OBRA regulated in U.S. Long Term Care

gatifloxacin

(ga-ti-flocks'-a-sin)

■ **Brand Name(s):** Tequin, Tequin Teqpaq, Zymar
Chemical Class: Fluoroquinolone derivative

■ **Clinical Pharmacology:**

Mechanism of Action: A fluoroquinolone that inhibits two enzymes, topoisomerase II and IV, in susceptible microorganisms. **Therapeutic Effect:** Interferes with bacterial DNA replication. Prevents or delays resistance emergence. Bactericidal.

Pharmacokinetics: Well absorbed from the GI tract after PO administration. Protein binding: 20%. Widely distributed. Metabolized in liver. Primarily excreted in urine. **Half-life:** 7-14 hr.

■ **Available Forms:**

- *Tablets (Tequin, Tequin Teqpaq):* 200 mg, 400 mg.
- *Injection (Tequin):* 200-mg, 400-mg vials.
- *Ophthalmic Solution (Zymar):* 0.3%.

■ **Indications and Dosages:**

Chronic bronchitis, complicated urinary tract infections, pyelonephritis, skin infections: PO, IV 400 mg/day for 7-10 days (5 days for chronic bronchitis).
Sinusitis: PO, IV 400 mg/day for 10 days.
Pneumonia: PO, IV 400 mg/day for 7-14 days.
Cystitis: PO, IV 400 mg as a single dose or 200 mg/day for 3 days.
Urethral gonorrhea in men and women, endocervical and rectal gonorrhea in women: PO, IV 400 mg as a single dose.
Topical treatment of bacterial conjunctivitis due to susceptible strains of bacteria: Ophthalmic 1 drop q2h while awake for 2 days, then 1 drop up to 4 times/day for days 3-7.
Dosage in renal impairment:

Creatinine Clearance	Dosage
40 ml/min	400 mg/day
less than 40 ml/min	Initially, 400 mg/day, then 200 mg/day
Hemodialysis	Initially, 400 mg/day, then 200 mg/day
Peritoneal dialysis	Initially, 400 mg/day, then 200 mg/day

■ **Contraindications:** Hypersensitivity to quinolones

■ **Side Effects**

Occasional (8%-3%)
Nausea, vaginitis, diarrhea, headache, dizziness
Ophthalmic: conjunctival irritation, increased tearing, corneal inflammation
Rare (3%-0.1%)
Abdominal pain, constipation, dyspepsia, stomatitis, edema, insomnia, abnormal dreams, diaphoresis, altered taste, rash
Ophthalmic: corneal swelling, dry eye, eye pain, eyelid swelling, headache, red eye, reduced visual acuity, altered taste

■ **Serious Reactions**

- Pseudomembranous colitis, as evidenced by severe abdominal pain and cramps, severe watery diarrhea, and fever, may occur.
- Superinfection, manifested as genital or anal pruritus, ulceration or changes in oral mucosa, and moderate to severe diarrhea, may occur.
- Symptomatic hyperglycemia and hypoglycemia may occur.
- Tendon effects, including ruptures of shoulder, hand, Achilles tendon or other tendons, may occur. Risk increases with concomitant corticosteroid use, especially in the elderly.

Patient/Family Education
- May be taken with or without meals
- Should be taken at least 4 hr before or 8 hr after multivitamins (containing iron or zinc), antacids (containing magnesium, calcium, or aluminum), sucralfate, or didanosine chewable/buffered tablets
- Discontinue treatment, rest and refrain from exercise, and inform prescriber if pain, inflammation, or rupture of a tendon occurs
- Test reaction to this drug before operating an automobile or machinery or engaging in activities requiring mental alertness or coordination
- Drink plenty of fluids
- Avoid exposure to direct sunlight as this may cause a photosensitivity reaction
- Take for the full course of therapy

Monitoring Parameters
- WBC count
- Signs of infection
- Evaluate for abdominal pain, altered sense of taste, dyspepsia (heartburn, indigestion), headache, and vomiting
- Daily bowel activity and stool consistency. Although mild GI effects may be tolerable, severe symptoms may indicate the onset of antibiotic-associated colitis.
- Signs and symptoms of superinfection include abdominal pain or cramping, anal or genital pruritus or discharge, moderate to severe diarrhea, severe mouth or tongue soreness, and new or increased fever.

Geriatric side effects at a glance:
☑ CNS   ☑ Bowel Dysfunction   ☐ Bladder Dysfunction   ☐ Falls

U.S. Regulatory Considerations
☐ FDA Black Box   ☐ OBRA regulated in U.S. Long Term Care

gemfibrozil

(jem-fi'-broe-zil)

■ **Brand Name(s):** Lopid
Chemical Class: Fibric acid derivative

■ **Clinical Pharmacology:**
Mechanism of Action: A fibric acid derivative that inhibits lipolysis of fat in adipose tissue; decreases liver uptake of free fatty acids and reduces hepatic triglyceride production. Inhibits synthesis of VLDL carrier apolipoprotein B. **Therapeutic Effect:** Lowers serum cholesterol and triglycerides (decreases VLDL, LDL; increases HDL).
Pharmacokinetics: Well absorbed from the GI tract. Protein binding: 99%. Metabolized in liver. Primarily excreted in urine. Not removed by hemodialysis. **Half-life:** 1.5 hr.

- **Available Forms:**
  - *Tablets*: 600 mg.

- **Indications and Dosages:**
  Hyperlipidemia: PO 1200 mg/day in 2 divided doses 30 min before breakfast and dinner.

- **Contraindications:** Liver dysfunction (including primary biliary cirrhosis), preexisting gallbladder disease, severe renal dysfunction

- **Side Effects**
  Frequent (20%)
  Dyspepsia
  Occasional (10%-2%)
  Abdominal pain, diarrhea, nausea, vomiting, fatigue
  Rare (less than 2%)
  Constipation, acute appendicitis, vertigo, headache, rash, pruritus, altered taste

- **Serious Reactions**
  - Cholelithiasis, cholecystitis, acute appendicitis, pancreatitis, and malignancy occur rarely.

- **Patient/Family Education**
  - May cause dizziness or blurred vision; use caution while driving or performing other tasks requiring alertness
  - Notify clinician if GI side effects become pronounced
  - Follow the prescribed diet
  - Take gemfibrozil before meals
  - Periodic laboratory tests are an essential part of therapy

- **Monitoring Parameters**
  - Serum CK level in patients complaining of muscle pain, tenderness, or weakness
  - Periodic CBC during first 12 mo of therapy
  - Periodic LFTs; discontinue therapy if abnormalities persist
  - Blood glucose
  - Pattern of daily bowel activity and stool consistency
  - Serum LDL, VLDL, triglyceride, and cholesterol levels for a therapeutic response
  - Evaluate the patient for dizziness and headache
  - Assess the patient for pain, especially in the right upper quadrant of the abdomen, because epigastric pain may indicate cholecystitis or cholelithiasis

- **Geriatric side effects at a glance:**
  ❏ CNS ❏ Bowel Dysfunction ❏ Bladder Dysfunction ❏ Falls

- **U.S. Regulatory Considerations**
  ❏ FDA Black Box ❏ OBRA regulated in U.S. Long Term Care

gemifloxacin mesylate

(gem-ah-flox'-a-sin mes'-sil-ate)

■ **Brand Name(s):** Factive
  Chemical Class: Fluoroquinolone derivative

■ **Clinical Pharmacology:**
  Mechanism of Action: A fluoroquinolone that inhibits the enzyme DNA gyrase in susceptible microorganisms, interfering with bacterial cell replication and repair. **Therapeutic Effect:** Bactericidal.
  Pharmacokinetics: Rapidly and well absorbed from the GI tract. Protein binding: 70%. Widely distributed. Penetrates well into lung tissue and fluid. Undergoes limited metabolism in the liver. Primarily excreted in feces; lesser amount eliminated in urine. Partially removed by hemodialysis. **Half-life:** 4-12 hr.

■ **Available Forms:**
  • *Tablets:* 320 mg.

■ **Indications and Dosages:**
  Acute bacterial exacerbation of chronic bronchitis: PO 320 mg once a day for 5 days.
  Community-acquired pneumonia: PO 320 mg once a day for 7 days.
  Dosage in renal impairment: Dosage and frequency are modified based on creatinine clearance.

Creatinine Clearance	Dosage
greater than 40 ml/min	320 mg once a day
40 ml/min or less	160 mg once a day

■ **Contraindications:** Concurrent use of amiodarone, quinidine, procainamide, or sotalol; history of prolonged QTc interval; hypersensitivity to fluoroquinolones; uncorrected electrolyte disorders (such as hypokalemia and hypomagnesemia)

■ **Side Effects**
  Occasional (4%-2%)
  Diarrhea, rash, nausea
  Rare (1% or less)
  Headache, abdominal pain, dizziness

■ **Serious Reactions**
  • Antibiotic-associated colitis may result from altered bacterial balance.
  • Hypersensitivity reactions, including photosensitivity (as evidenced by rash, pruritus, blisters, edema, and burning skin), have occurred.
  • Tendon effects, including ruptures of shoulder, hand, Achilles tendon or other tendons, may occur. Risk increases with concomitant corticosteroid use, especially in the elderly.

Special Considerations
  • Use with caution in pneumonia due to *Klebsiella pneumoniae.* In clinical trials, 2 treatment failures occurred out of 13 cases

■ Patient/Family Education
- May be taken with or without meals
- Do not chew pills
- Take for the full course of therapy
- Drink several glasses of water between meals
- Should not be taken within 3 hr of multivitamins (containing iron or zinc), antacids (containing magnesium, calcium, or aluminum), sucralfate, or didanosine chewable/buffered tablets
- Discontinue treatment, rest and refrain from exercise, and inform prescriber if pain, inflammation, or rupture of a tendon occurs
- Test reaction to this drug before operating an automobile or machinery or engaging in activities requiring mental alertness or coordination
- Your skin may be more sensitive to sunlight while taking this medication. Wear sunscreen when outdoors. Avoid sunlamps and tanning beds.

■ Monitoring Parameters
- Liver function test results and WBC count
- Signs and symptoms of infection
- Skin for rash
- Calculate the QT and QTc intervals to check for prolongation
- Daily bowel activity and stool consistency. Although mild GI effects may be tolerable, severe symptoms may indicate the onset of antibiotic-associated colitis.
- Signs and symptoms of superinfection include abdominal pain or cramping, anal or genital pruritus or discharge, moderate to severe diarrhea, severe mouth or tongue soreness, and new or increased fever.

■ Geriatric side effects at a glance:
☑ CNS   ☑ Bowel Dysfunction   ❑ Bladder Dysfunction   ❑ Falls

■ U.S. Regulatory Considerations
❑ FDA Black Box   ❑ OBRA regulated in U.S. Long Term Care

gentamicin sulfate

(jen-ta-mye'-sin sul'-fate)

■ Brand Name(s): Garamycin, Garamycin Ophthalmic, Garamycin Topical, Genoptic, Gentacidin, Gentak, Ocu-Mycin

Combinations
Rx: with prednisolone (Pred-G)
Chemical Class: Aminoglycoside

■ Clinical Pharmacology:
Mechanism of Action: An aminoglycoside antibacterial that irreversibly binds to the protein of bacterial ribosomes. *Therapeutic Effect:* Interferes with protein synthesis of susceptible microorganisms. Bactericidal.

Pharmacokinetics: Rapid, complete absorption after IM administration. Protein binding: less than 30%. Widely distributed (doesn't cross the blood-brain barrier, low concentrations in CSF). Excreted unchanged in urine. Removed by hemodialysis. **Half-life:** 2-4 hr (increased in impaired renal function; decreased in cystic fibrosis and burn or febrile patients).

■ **Available Forms:**
- *Injection*: 10 mg/ml, 40 mg/ml (Garamycin), 40 mg/50 ml-0.9%, 60 mg/50 ml-0.9%, 60 mg/100 ml-0.9%, 70 mg/50 ml-0.9%, 80 mg/50 ml-0.9%, 80 mg/100 ml-0.9%, 90 mg/100 ml-0.9%, 100 mg/50 ml-0.9%, 100 mg/100 ml-0.9%.
- *Ophthalmic Solution (Garamycin Ophthalmic, Genoptic, Gentacidin, Gentak, Ocu-Mycin)*: 0.3%.
- *Ophthalmic Ointment (Gentak)*: 0.3%.
- *Cream (Garamycin Topical)*: 0.1%.
- *Ointment*: 0.1%.

■ **Indications and Dosages:**
Acute pelvic, bone, intra-abdominal, joint, respiratory tract, burn wound, postoperative, and skin or skin-structure infections; complicated UTIs; septicemia; meningitis: IV, IM Usual dosage, 3-6 mg/kg/day in divided doses q8h or 4-6.6 mg/kg once a day.
Hemodialysis: IV, IM 0.5-0.7 mg/kg/dose after dialysis. Intrathecal 4-8 mg/day.
Superficial eye infections: Ophthalmic Ointment Usual dosage, apply thin strip to conjunctiva 2-3 times a day. Ophthalmic Solution Usual dosage, 1-2 drops q2-4h up to 2 drops/hr.
Superficial skin infections: Topical Usual dosage, apply 3-4 times/day.
Dosage in renal impairment: Creatinine clearance greater than 41-60 ml/min. Dosage interval q12h. *Creatinine clearance 20-40 ml/min.* Dosage interval q24h. *Creatinine clearance less than 20 ml/min.* Monitor levels to determine dosage interval.

■ **Unlabeled Uses:** *Topical:* Prophylaxis of minor bacterial skin infections, treatment of dermal ulcer

■ **Contraindications:** Hypersensitivity to other aminoglycosides (cross-sensitivity), or their components. Sulfite sensitivity may result in anaphylaxis, especially in asthmatic patients.

■ **Side Effects**
Occasional
IM: Pain, induration
IV: Phlebitis, thrombophlebitis, hypersensitivity reactions (fever, pruritus, rash, urticaria)
Ophthalmic: Burning, tearing, itching, blurred vision
Topical: Redness, itching
Rare
Alopecia, hypertension, weakness

■ **Serious Reactions**
- Nephrotoxicity (as evidenced by increased BUN and serum creatinine levels and decreased creatinine clearance) may be reversible if the drug is stopped at the first sign of symptoms.
- Irreversible ototoxicity (manifested as tinnitus, dizziness, ringing or roaring in the ears, and diminished hearing), and neurotoxicity (as evidenced by headache, dizziness, lethargy, tremor, and visual disturbances) occur occasionally. The risk of these effects increases with higher dosages or prolonged therapy and when the solution is applied directly to the mucosa.

- Superinfections, particularly with fungal infections, may result from bacterial imbalance no matter which administration route is used.
- Ophthalmic application may cause paresthesia of conjunctiva or mydriasis.

Special Considerations
- Individualize treatment based on local susceptibility patterns.

■ Patient/Family Education
- Report headache, dizziness, loss of hearing, ringing, roaring in ears, or feeling of fullness in head
- Tilt head back, place medication in conjunctival sac, and close eyes
- Apply light finger pressure on lacrimal sac for 1 min following instillation (gtt)
- May cause temporary blurring of vision following administration (ophth)
- Notify clinician if stinging, burning, or itching becomes pronounced or if redness, irritation, swelling, decreasing vision, or pain persists or worsens (ophth)
- Do not touch tip of container to any surface (ophth)
- For external use only (ophth)
- Cleanse affected area of skin prior to application (top)
- Notify clinician if condition worsens or if rash or irritation develops (top)
- IM injection may cause discomfort

■ Monitoring Parameters
- Urinalysis for proteinuria, cells, casts
- Urine output
- Serum peak, drawn at 30-60 min after IV INF or 60 min after IM inj, trough level drawn just before next dose; adjust dosage per levels (usual therapeutic plasma levels, peak 4-8 mcg/ml, trough ≤2 mcg/ml)
- Serum creatinine for CrCl calculation
- Serum calcium, magnesium, sodium
- Audiometric testing, assess hearing before, during, after treatment
- Evaluate the IV infusion site for signs and symptoms of phlebitis, such as heat, pain, and red streaking over the vein
- Skin for rash
- If giving ophthalmic gentamicin, monitor the patient's eye for burning, itching, redness, and tearing
- If giving topical gentamicin, monitor the patient for itching and redness
- Be alert for signs and symptoms of superinfection, particularly changes in the oral mucosa, diarrhea, and genital or anal pruritus
- In patients with neuromuscular disorders, assess the respiratory response carefully

■ Geriatric side effects at a glance:
❏ CNS ❏ Bowel Dysfunction ❏ Bladder Dysfunction ❏ Falls

■ U.S. Regulatory Considerations
☑ FDA Black Box
Neurotoxicity (both auditory and vestibular ototoxicity) and nephrotoxicity. Risk is increased in patients with impaired renal function and in those who receive high doses or prolonged therapy.
❏ OBRA regulated in U.S. Long Term Care

glatiramer acetate

(gla-teer'-a-mer as'-eh-tate)

- **Brand Name(s):** Copaxone
  Chemical Class: Polypeptide, synthetic

- **Clinical Pharmacology:**
  Mechanism of Action: An immunosuppressive whose exact mechanism is unknown. May act by modifying immune processes thought to be responsible for the pathogenesis of multiple sclerosis (MS). **Therapeutic Effect:** Slows progression of MS.
  Pharmacokinetics: Substantial fraction of glatiramer is hydrolyzed locally. Some fraction of injected material enters lymphatic circulation, reaching regional lymph nodes; some may enter systemic circulation intact.

- **Available Forms:**
  - Injection: 20 mg/ml in prefilled syringes.

- **Indications and Dosages:**
  MS: Subcutaneous 20 mg once a day.

- **Contraindications:** Hypersensitivity to mannitol

- **Side Effects**
  Expected (73%-40%)
  Pain, erythema, inflammation, or pruritus at injection site; asthenia
  Frequent (27%-18%)
  Arthralgia, vasodilation, anxiety, hypertonia, nausea, transient chest pain, dyspnea, flu-like symptoms, rash, pruritus
  Occasional (17%-10%)
  Palpitations, back pain, diaphoresis, rhinitis, diarrhea, urinary urgency
  Rare (8%-6%)
  Anorexia, fever, neck pain, peripheral edema, ear pain, facial edema, vertigo, vomiting

- **Serious Reactions**
  - Infection is a common effect.
  - Lymphadenopathy occurs occasionally.

Special Considerations

  - May be useful for relapsing-remitting multiple sclerosis in patients who are not benefiting from, or are intolerant of, interferon β-1 a/b; less effective in patients with advanced disease or chronic-progressive multiple sclerosis; not a cure for multiple sclerosis and benefits achieved are relatively modest
  - Sites for injection include arms, abdomen, hips, and thighs

- **Patient/Family Education**
  - Teach the patient and caregiver how to administer subcutaneous injections and properly dispose of needles

- Notify the physician if rash, weakness, difficulty breathing or swallowing, or itching or swelling of the legs occurs

■ **Monitoring Parameters**
  - Assess for injection site reactions
  - Monitor the patient for fever, chills, and other evidence of infection

■ **Geriatric side effects at a glance:**
  ❑ CNS ❑ Bowel Dysfunction ❑ Bladder Dysfunction ❑ Falls

■ **U.S. Regulatory Considerations**
  ❑ FDA Black Box ❑ OBRA regulated in U.S. Long Term Care

glimepiride

(glye'-meh-pye-ride)

■ **Brand Name(s):** Amaryl
  Chemical Class: Sulfonylurea (2nd generation)

■ **Clinical Pharmacology:**
  Mechanism of Action: A second-generation sulfonylurea that promotes release of insulin from beta cells of the pancreas and increases insulin sensitivity at peripheral sites. **Therapeutic Effect:** Lowers blood glucose concentration.
  Pharmacokinetics:

Route	Onset	Peak	Duration
PO	N/A	2-3 hr	24 hr

Completely absorbed from the GI tract. Protein binding: greater than 99%. Metabolized in the liver. Excreted in urine and eliminated in feces. **Half-life:** 5-9.2 hr.

■ **Available Forms:**
  - *Tablets*: 1 mg, 2 mg, 4 mg.

■ **Indications and Dosages:**
  Diabetes mellitus: PO Initially, 1-2 mg once a day, with breakfast or first main meal. Maintenance: 1-4 mg once a day. After dose of 2 mg is reached, dosage should be increased in increments of up to 2 mg q1-2wk, based on blood glucose response. Maximum: 8 mg/day.
  Dosage in renal impairment: PO 1 mg once/day.

■ **Contraindications:** Diabetic complications, such as ketosis, acidosis, and diabetic coma; monotherapy for type 1 diabetes mellitus; severe hepatic or renal impairment; stress situations, including severe infection, trauma, and surgery

■ **Side Effects**
  Frequent
  Altered taste sensation, dizziness, somnolence, weight gain, constipation, diarrhea, heartburn, nausea, vomiting, stomach fullness, headache

Occasional

Increased sensitivity of skin to sunlight, peeling of skin, itching, rash

■ **Serious Reactions**
- Overdose or insufficient food intake may produce hypoglycemia, especially with increased glucose demands.
- GI hemorrhage, cholestatic hepatic jaundice, leukopenia, thrombocytopenia, pancytopenia, agranulocytosis, and aplastic or hemolytic anemia occur rarely.

Special Considerations
- No demonstrated advantage over existing second-generation sulfonylureas
- Although allergic cross-reactivity with sulfonamide antibiotics and sulfonamide nonantibiotics has not been demonstrated, use with caution in patients with a history of severe sulfa allergies.

■ **Patient/Family Education**
- Multiple drug interactions, including alcohol and salicylates
- Symptoms of hypoglycemia: tingling lips/tongue, nausea, confusion, fatigue, sweating, hunger, visual changes (spots)
- A prescribed diet is a principal part of treatment; do not skip or delay meals
- Carry candy, sugar packets, or other sugar supplements for immediate response to hypoglycemia and urge the patient to wear medical alert identification stating he or she has diabetes
- Consult the physician when glucose demands are altered, such as with fever, heavy physical activity, infection, stress, or trauma
- Wear sunscreen and protective eyewear to prevent the effects of light sensitivity

■ **Monitoring Parameters**
- Self-monitored blood glucoses, glycosolated hemoglobin q3-6 mo
- Assess for signs and symptoms of hypoglycemia (anxiety, cool wet skin, diplopia, dizziness, headache, hunger, numbness in mouth, tachycardia, tremors), or hyperglycemia (deep rapid breathing, dim vision, fatigue, nausea, polydipsia, polyphagia, polyuria, vomiting)
- Be alert to conditions that alter blood glucose requirements, such as fever, increased activity, stress, or a surgical procedure

■ **Geriatric side effects at a glance:**
❑ CNS   ❑ Bowel Dysfunction   ❑ Bladder Dysfunction   ❑ Falls
Other: Hypoglycemia

■ **Use with caution in older patients with:** Hepatic impairment, Renal impairment, Hypoalbuminemia

■ **U.S. Regulatory Considerations**
❑ FDA Black Box   ❑ OBRA regulated in U.S. Long Term Care

■ **Other Uses in Geriatric Patient:** None

■ **Side Effects:**
Of particular importance in the geriatric patient: Hypoglycemia, dizziness, headaches, weight gain

- **Geriatric Considerations - Summary:** Lower risk of hypoglycemia when compared to glyburide.

- **References:**
  1. Haas L. Management of diabetes mellitus medications in the nursing home. Drugs Aging 2005;22:209-218.
  2. Chelliah A, Burge MR. Hypoglycemia in elderly patients with diabetes mellitus. Causes and strategies for prevention. Drugs Aging 2004;21:511-530.
  3. Rosenstock J. Management of type 2 diabetes mellitus in the elderly: special considerations. Drugs Aging 2001;18:31-44.
  4. Dills DG, Schneider J, et. al. Clinical evaluation of glimepiride versus glyburide in NIDDM in a double-blind comparative study. Horm Metab Res 1996;28:426-429.

glipizide

(glip'-i-zide)

- **Brand Name(s):** Glucotrol, Glucotrol XL

  Combinations
  Rx: with metformin (Metaglip)
  Chemical Class: Sulfonylurea (2nd generation)

- **Clinical Pharmacology:**
  Mechanism of Action: A second-generation sulfonylurea that promotes the release of insulin from beta cells of the pancreas and increases insulin sensitivity at peripheral sites. **Therapeutic Effect:** Lowers blood glucose concentration.
  Pharmacokinetics:

Route	Onset	Peak	Duration
PO	15-30 min	2-3 hr	12-24 hr
Extended-release	2-3 hr	6-12 hr	24 hr

  Well absorbed from the GI tract. Protein binding: 99%. Metabolized in the liver. Excreted in urine. **Half-life:** 2-4 hr.

- **Available Forms:**
  - *Tablets (Glucotrol):* 5 mg, 10 mg.
  - *Tablets (Extended-Release [Glucotrol XL]):* 2.5 mg, 5 mg, 10 mg.

- **Indications and Dosages:**
  Diabetes mellitus: PO Initially, 2.5-5 mg/day. May increase by 2.5-5 mg/day q1–2wk.

- **Contraindications:** Diabetic ketoacidosis with or without coma, type 1 diabetes mellitus

- **Side Effects**
  Frequent
  Altered taste sensation, dizziness, somnolence, weight gain, constipation, diarrhea, heartburn, nausea, vomiting, stomach fullness, headache

Occasional

Increased sensitivity of skin to sunlight, peeling of skin, itching, rash

■ **Serious Reactions**
- Overdose or insufficient food intake may produce hypoglycemia, especially with increased glucose demands.
- GI hemorrhage, cholestatic hepatic jaundice, leukopenia, thrombocytopenia, pancytopenia, agranulocytosis, and aplastic or hemolytic anemia occurs rarely.

Special Considerations
- Although allergic cross-reactivity with sulfonamide antibiotics and sulfonamide nonantibiotics has not been demonstrated, use with caution in patients with a history of severe sulfa allergies.

■ **Patient/Family Education**
- Administer 30 min ac
- Notify clinician of fever, sore throat, rash, unusual bruising, or bleeding
- Multiple drug interactions, including alcohol and salicylates
- Symptoms of hypoglycemia: tingling lips/tongue, nausea, confusion, fatigue, sweating, hunger, visual changes (spots)
- Carry candy, sugar packets, or other sugar supplements for immediate response to hypoglycemia
- Notify clinician of fever, sore throat, rash, unusual bruising, or bleeding
- Diet is a principal part of treatment; do not skip or delay meals
- Wear sunscreen and protective eyewear to prevent the effects of light sensitivity

■ **Monitoring Parameters**
- Self-monitored blood glucose; glycosylated hemoglobin q3-6 mo
- Assess the patient for signs and symptoms of hypoglycemia (anxiety, cool wet skin, diplopia, dizziness, headache, hunger, numbness in mouth, tachycardia, tremors), or hyperglycemia (deep rapid breathing, dim vision, fatigue, nausea, polydipsia, polyphagia, polyuria, vomiting)
- Be alert to conditions that alter blood glucose requirements, such as fever, increased activity, stress, or a surgical procedure

■ **Geriatric side effects at a glance:**
   ❑ CNS   ❑ Bowel Dysfunction   ❑ Bladder Dysfunction   ❑ Falls
   Other: Hypoglycemia

■ **Use with caution in older patients with:** Hepatic impairment

■ **U.S. Regulatory Considerations**
   ❑ FDA Black Box   ❑ OBRA regulated in U.S. Long Term Care

■ **Other Uses in Geriatric Patient:** None

■ **Side Effects:**
   Of particular importance in the geriatric patient: Hypoglycemia, weight gain

■ **Geriatric Considerations - Summary:** Glipizide is primarily metabolized in the liver to inactive metabolites, therefore may be safer in older adults. Elimination half-life in older adults is not increased as compared to younger adults. Hypoglycemia risk may be increased with use of the long-acting formulation of glipizide.

■ **References:**
1. Haas L. Management of diabetes mellitus medications in the nursing home. Drugs Aging 2005;22:209-218.
2. Chelliah A, Burge MR. Hypoglycemia in elderly patients with diabetes mellitus. Causes and strategies for prevention. Drugs Aging 2004;21:511-530.
3. Rosenstock J. Management of type 2 diabetes mellitus in the elderly: special considerations. Drugs Aging 2001;18:31-44.
4. Shorr RI, Ray WA, Daugherty JR, et. al. Incidence and risk factors for serious hypoglycemia in older persons using insulin or sulfonylureas. Arch Intern Med 1997;157:1681-1686.
5. Shorr RI, Ray WA, Daugherty JR, et. al. Individual sulfonylureas and serious hypoglycemia in older people. J Am Geriatr Soc 1996;44:751-755.
6. Jaber LA, Ducharme MP, Edwards DJ, et. al. The influence of multiple dosing and age on the pharmacokinetics and pharmacodynamics of glipizide in patients with diabetes. Pharmacotherapy 1996;16:760-768.

glucagon hydrochloride

(gloo'-ka-gon hye-dro-klor'-ide)

■ **Brand Name(s):** GlucaGen, GlucaGen Diagnostic Kit, Glucagon, Glucagon Diagnostic Kit, Glucagon Emergency Kit
Chemical Class: Polypeptide hormone

■ **Clinical Pharmacology:**
Mechanism of Action: A glucose elevating agent that promotes hepatic glycogenolysis, gluconeogenesis. Stimulates production of cyclic adenosine monophosphate (cAMP), which results in increased plasma glucose concentration, smooth muscle relaxation, and an inotropic myocardial effect. **Therapeutic Effect:** Increases plasma glucose level.
Pharmacokinetics: Onset of action occurs within 4-10 min following IM administration. Recovery occurs within 12-32 minutes. **Half-life:** 8-18 min.

■ **Available Forms:**
• *Powder for Injection (GlucaGen, GlucaGen Diagnostic Kit, Glucagon, Glucagon Diagnostic Kit, Glucagon Emergency Kit):* 1 mg.

■ **Indications and Dosages:**
Hypoglycemia: IV, IM, Subcutaneous 0.5-1 mg. May give 1 or 2 additional doses if response is delayed.
Diagnostic aid: IV, IM 0.25-2 mg 10 min prior to procedure.

■ **Unlabeled Uses:** Treatment of esophageal obstruction due to foreign bodies, toxicity associated with beta-blockers or calcium channel blockers

■ **Contraindications:** Hypersensitivity to glucagon or beef or pork proteins, known pheochromocytoma

■ **Side Effects**
Occasional
Nausea, vomiting

Rare

Allergic reaction, such as urticaria, respiratory distress, and hypotension

- **Serious Reactions**
  - Overdose may produce persistent nausea and vomiting and hypokalemia, marked by severe weakness, decreased appetite, irregular heartbeat, and muscle cramps.

- **Patient/Family Education**
  - Notify clinician when hypoglycemic reactions occur so that antidiabetic therapy can be adjusted
  - Treat early signs of hypoglycemia with a simple sugar first, such as hard candy, honey, orange juice, sugar cubes, or table sugar dissolved in water or juice, followed by a protein source, such as cheese and crackers, half a sandwich, or a glass of milk

- **Monitoring Parameters**
  - Blood sugar, level of consciousness
  - Have IV dextrose readily available in case the patient does not awaken within 20 min
  - Assess the patient for evidence of an allergic reaction, including hypotension, respiratory difficulty, and urticaria

- **Geriatric side effects at a glance:**
  - ❑ CNS ❑ Bowel Dysfunction ❑ Bladder Dysfunction ❑ Falls

- **U.S. Regulatory Considerations**
  - ❑ FDA Black Box ❑ OBRA regulated in U.S. Long Term Care

glyburide

(glye'-byoor-ide)

- **Brand Name(s):** DiaBeta, Glycron, Glynase, Glynase Pres-Tab, Micronase

  Combinations
  Rx: with metformin (Glucovance)
  Chemical Class: Sulfonylurea (2nd generation)

- **Clinical Pharmacology:**
  Mechanism of Action: A second-generation sulfonylurea that promotes release of insulin from beta cells of the pancreas and increases insulin sensitivity at peripheral sites. **Therapeutic Effect:** Lowers blood glucose concentration.
  Pharmacokinetics:

Route	Onset	Peak	Duration
PO	0.25-1 hr	1-2 hr	12-24 hr

  Well absorbed from the GI tract. Protein binding: 99%. Metabolized in the liver to weakly active metabolite. Primarily excreted in urine. Not removed by hemodialysis.
  Half-life: 1.4-1.8 hr.

■ **Available Forms:**
  • *Tablets (DiaBeta, Micronase)*: 1.25 mg, 2.5 mg, 5 mg.
  • *Tablets (Micronized [Glycron, Glynase])*: 1.5 mg, 3 mg, 4.5 mg, 6 mg.

■ **Indications and Dosages:**
  Diabetes mellitus: PO Initially, 1.25-2.5 mg/day. May increase by 1.25-2.5 mg/day at 1- to 3-wk intervals PO (micronized tablets) Initially 0.75-3 mg/day. May increase by 1.5 mg/day at weekly intervals. Maintenance: 0.75-12 mg/day as a single dose or in divided doses.
  Dosage in renal impairment: Glyburide is not recommended in patients with creatinine clearance less than 50 ml/min.

■ **Contraindications:** Diabetic ketoacidosis with or without coma, monotherapy for type 1 diabetes mellitus

■ **Side Effects**
  Frequent
  Altered taste sensation, dizziness, somnolence, weight gain, constipation, diarrhea, heartburn, nausea, vomiting, stomach fullness, headache
  Occasional
  Increased sensitivity of skin to sunlight, peeling of skin, itching, rash

■ **Serious Reactions**
  • Overdose or insufficient food intake may produce hypoglycemia, especially in patients with increased glucose demands.
  • Cholestatic jaundice, leukopenia, thrombocytopenia, pancytopenia, agranulocytosis, and aplastic or hemolytic anemia occur rarely.

Special Considerations
  • Micronized formulations do not provide bioequivalent serum concentrations to nonmicronized formulations; retitrate patients when transferring from any hypoglycemic to micronized glyburide
  • Although allergic cross-reactivity with sulfonamide antibiotics and sulfonamide nonantibiotics has not been demonstrated, use with caution in patients with a history of severe sulfa allergies.

■ **Patient/Family Education**
  • Multiple drug interactions including alcohol and salicylates
  • Notify clinician of fever, sore throat, rash, unusual bruising, or bleeding
  • Do not skip or delay meals
  • Be aware of signs and symptoms of hypoglycemia and hyperglycemia
  • Carry candy, sugar packets, or other sugar supplements for immediate response to hypoglycemia and wear medical alert identification stating that one has diabetes
  • Consult the physician when glucose demands are altered, such as with fever, heavy physical activity, infection, stress, or trauma
  • Wear sunscreen and protective eyewear to prevent the effects of light sensitivity

■ **Monitoring Parameters**
  • Self-monitored blood glucose; glycosylated Hgb q3-6 mo

- Assess the patient for signs and symptoms of hypoglycemia (anxiety, cool wet skin, diplopia, dizziness, headache, hunger, perioral numbness, tachycardia, tremors), or hyperglycemia (deep rapid breathing, dim vision, fatigue, nausea, polydipsia, polyphagia, polyuria, vomiting)
- Be alert to conditions that alter blood glucose requirements, such as fever, increased activity, stress, or a surgical procedure

■ **Geriatric side effects at a glance:**
❑ CNS ❑ Bowel Dysfunction ❑ Bladder Dysfunction ❑ Falls

■ **U.S. Regulatory Considerations**
❑ FDA Black Box ❑ OBRA regulated in U.S. Long Term Care

■ **Other Uses in Geriatric Patient:** None

■ **Side Effects:**
Of particular importance in the geriatric patient: Hypoglycemia, weight gain

■ **Geriatric Considerations - Summary:** Glyburide is metabolized in the liver to active metabolites that are renally eliminated, which may increase the risk of and prolong hypoglycemia in older adults. Hypoglycemics with inactive metabolites are preferred in older adults.

■ **References:**
1. Haas L. Management of diabetes mellitus medications in the nursing home. Drugs Aging 2005;22:209-218.
2. Chelliah A, Burge MR. Hypoglycemia in elderly patients with diabetes mellitus. Causes and strategies for prevention. Drugs Aging 2004;21:511-530.
3. Rosenstock J. Management of type 2 diabetes mellitus in the elderly: special considerations. Drugs Aging 2001;18:31-44.
4. Shorr RI, Ray WA, Daugherty JR, et al. Incidence and risk factors for serious hypoglycemia in older persons using insulin or sulfonylureas. Arch Intern Med 1997;157:1681-1686.
5. Shorr RI, Ray WA, Daugherty JR, et. al. Individual sulfonylureas and serious hypoglycemia in older people. J Am Geriatr Soc 1996;44:751-755.

glycerin

(gli'-ser-in)

■ **Brand Name(s):** Osmoglyn
OTC: Bausch & Lomb Computer Eye Drops, Fleet Liquid Glycerin Suppositories for Adults, Fleet Maximum-Strength Glycerin Suppositories, Fleet Glycerin Suppositories for Adults, Glyrol, Sani-Supp
Chemical Class: Trihydric alcohol

■ **Clinical Pharmacology:**
Mechanism of Action: An osmotic dehydrating agent that increases osmotic pressure and draws fluid into colon and stimulates evacuation of inspissated feces. Lowers

both intraocular and intracranial pressure by osmotic dehydrating effects. Increases blood flow to ischemic areas, decreases serum free fatty acids, and increases synthesis of glycerides in the brain. **Therapeutic Effect:** Aids in fecal evacuation. **Pharmacokinetics:** Well absorbed after PO administration but poorly absorbed after rectal administration. Widely distributed to extracellular space. Rapidly metabolized in liver. Primarily excreted in urine. **Half-life:** 30-45 min.

■ **Available Forms:**
- *Ophthalmic Solution:* 1% (Bausch & Lomb Computer Eye Drops).
- *Oral Solution:* 50% (Osmoglyn).
- *Rectal Solution:* 5.6g (Fleet Liquid Glycerin Suppositories).
- *Suppositories:* 2g (Fleet Glycerin Suppositories), 3g (Fleet Maximum-Strength Glycerin Suppositories), 82.5% (Sani-Supp).

■ **Indications and Dosages:**
Constipation: Rectal 3 g/day.
Ophthalmologic procedures: Ophthalmic 1 or 2 drops prior to examination q3-4h.
Reduction of intracranial pressure: PO 1.5 g/kg/day q4h or 1 g/kg/dose q6h.
Reduction of intraocular pressure: PO 1-1.8 g/kg 1-1.5 hr preoperatively.

■ **Unlabeled Uses:** Viral meningoencephalitis

■ **Contraindications:** Hypersensitivity to any component in the preparation, well-established anuria, severe dehydration, frank or impending acute pulmonary edema, severe cardiac decompensation

■ **Side Effects**
Frequent
Oral: Nausea, headache,vomiting
Rectal: Some degree of abdominal discomfort, nausea, mild cramps, headache,vomiting
Occasional
Oral: Diarrhea, dizziness, dry mouth or increased thirst
Ophthalmic: Pain and irritation may occur upon instillation
Rectal: Faintness, weakness, abdominal pain, bloating

■ **Serious Reactions**
- Laxative abuse includes symptoms of abdominal pain, weakness, fatigue, thirst, vomiting, edema, bone pain, fluid and electrolyte imbalance, hypoalbuminemia, and syndromes that mimic colitis.

■ **Patient/Family Education**
- Do not use laxative in the presence of abdominal pain, nausea, or vomiting
- Do not use longer than 1 wk
- Prolonged or frequent use may result in dependency or electrolyte imbalance
- Notify clinician if unrelieved constipation, rectal bleeding, muscle cramps, weakness, or dizziness occurs
- Institute measures to promote defecation such as increasing fluid intake, exercising, and eating a high-fiber diet

Monitoring Parameters
- Blood glucose, intraocular pressure
- Daily bowel activity and stool consistency
- Hydration status
- Serum electrolytes
- Abdominal disturbances

Geriatric side effects at a glance:
☐ CNS   ☑ Bowel Dysfunction   ☐ Bladder Dysfunction   ☐ Falls

U.S. Regulatory Considerations
☐ FDA Black Box   ☐ OBRA regulated in U.S. Long Term Care

glycopyrrolate

(glye-koe-pye'-roe-late)

Brand Name(s): Robinul, Robinul Forte
Chemical Class: Quaternary ammonium derivative

Clinical Pharmacology:
Mechanism of Action: A quaternary anticholinergic that inhibits action of acetylcholine at postganglionic parasympathetic sites in smooth muscle, secretory glands, and CNS. **Therapeutic Effect:** Reduces salivation and excessive secretions of respiratory tract; reduces gastric secretions and acidity.
Pharmacokinetics: Poorly and irregularly absorbed from GI tract after oral administration. Metabolized in the liver. Primarily excreted in urine. **Half-life:** 1.7 hr.

Available Forms:
- Injection (Robinul): 0.2 mg/ml.
- Tablets: 1 mg (Robinul), 2 mg (Robinul Forte).

Indications and Dosages:
Preoperative inhibition of salivation and excessive respiratory tract secretions: IM 4 mcg/kg 30-60 min before procedure.
To block effects of anticholinesterase agents: IV 0.2 mg for each 1 mg neostigmine or 5 mg pyridostigmine.
Peptic ulcer disease, adjunct: IV, IM 0.1 mg IV or IM 3-4 times/day. PO 1-2 mg 2-3 times/day. Maximum: 8 mg/day.

Contraindications: Acute hemorrhage, myasthenia gravis, narrow-angle glaucoma, obstructive uropathy, paralytic ileus, tachycardia, ulcerative colitis

Side Effects
Frequent
Dry mouth, decreased sweating, constipation

Occasional

Blurred vision, gastric bloating, urinary hesitancy, somnolence (with high dosage), headache, intolerance to light, loss of taste, nervousness, flushing, insomnia, impotence, mental confusion or excitement, temporary light-headedness (with parenteral form), local irritation (with parenteral form)

Rare

Dizziness, faintness

■ Serious Reactions

- Overdose may produce temporary paralysis of ciliary muscle; pupillary dilation; tachycardia; palpitations; hot, dry, or flushed skin; absence of bowel sounds; hyperthermia; increased respiratory rate; ECG abnormalities; nausea; vomiting; rash over face or upper trunk; CNS stimulation; and psychosis (marked by agitation, restlessness, rambling speech, visual hallucinations, paranoid behavior, and delusions, followed by depression).

■ Patient/Family Education

- Glycopyrrolate may cause dry mouth
- Do not become overheated while exercising in hot weather because this may cause heatstroke
- Avoid hot baths and saunas
- Avoid tasks that require mental alertness or motor skills until response to the drug has been established

■ Monitoring Parameters

- Blood pressure, body temperature, and heart rate
- Bowel sounds for peristalsis, and mucous membranes and skin turgor for hydration status
- Palpate the patient's bladder for signs of urine retention, and monitor urine output

■ Geriatric side effects at a glance:

☑ CNS ☑ Bowel Dysfunction ☑ Bladder Dysfunction ❑ Falls
Other: Confusion

■ Use with caution in older patients with: Possibly less likely to antagonize cholinergic drug therapy in the treatment of Alzheimer's disease.

■ U.S. Regulatory Considerations

❑ FDA Black Box ❑ OBRA regulated in U.S. Long Term Care

■ Other Uses in Geriatric Patient: Vertigo

■ Side Effects:
Of particular importance in the geriatric patient: None

■ Geriatric Considerations - Summary: Glycopyrrolate does not cross the blood-brain barrier so is less likely to cause the central effects seen with anticholinergics such as atropine. Other anticholinergic side effects such as blurred vision, dry mouth, urinary retention, and constipation do occur and can limit the usefulness of this drug in the older adult.

■ **References:**
1. Tune LE. Anticholinergic effects of medication in elderly patients. J Clin Psychiatry 2001;62(suppl 21):11-14.

goserelin acetate

(goe'-se-rel-in as'-eh-tate)

■ **Brand Name(s):** Zoladex
Chemical Class: Gonadotropin-releasing hormone analog

■ **Clinical Pharmacology:**
Mechanism of Action: A gonadotropin-releasing hormone analog and antineoplastic agent that stimulates the release of luteinizing hormone (LH) and follicle-stimulating hormone (FSH) from the anterior pituitary gland. In males, increases testosterone concentrations initially, then suppresses secretion of LH and FSH, resulting in decreased testosterone levels. **Therapeutic Effect:** In females, causes a reduction in ovarian size and function, reduction in uterine and mammary gland size, and regression of sex-hormone-responsive tumors. In males, produces pharmacologic castration and decreases the growth of abnormal prostate tissue.
Pharmacokinetics: Protein binding: 27%. Metabolized in liver. Excreted in urine. **Half-life:** 4.2 hr (male); 2.3 hr (female).

■ **Available Forms:**
• *Implant (Zoladex):* 3.6 mg, 10.8 mg.

■ **Indications and Dosages:**
Prostatic carcinoma: Implant 3.6 mg every 28 days or 10.8 mg q12wk subcutaneously into upper abdominal wall.
Breast carcinoma: Implant 3.6 mg every 28 days subcutaneously into upper abdominal wall.
Endometrial thinning: Implant 3.6 mg subcutaneously into upper abdominal wall as a single dose or in 2 doses 4 wk apart.

■ **Contraindications:** None known.

■ **Side Effects**
Frequent
Headache (60%), hot flashes (55%), depression (54%), diaphoresis (45%), sexual dysfunction (21%), decreased erection (18%), lower urinary tract symptoms (13%)
Occasional (10%-5%)
Pain, lethargy, dizziness, insomnia, anorexia, nausea, rash, upper respiratory tract infection, hirsutism, abdominal pain
Rare
Pruritus

■ **Serious Reactions**
• Arrhythmias, CHF, and hypertension occur rarely.

- Ureteral obstruction and spinal cord compression have been observed. An immediate orchiectomy may be necessary if these conditions occur.

■ **Patient/Family Education**
- An initial flare in bone pain may occur (prostate cancer therapy)

■ **Monitoring Parameters**
- Prostate-specific antigen, acid phosphatase, alk phosphatase
- Testosterone level (<25 ng/dl)
- Bone density if therapy prolonged

■ **Geriatric side effects at a glance:**
    ☑ CNS   ❑ Bowel Dysfunction   ☑ Bladder Dysfunction   ❑ Falls

■ **U.S. Regulatory Considerations**
    ❑ FDA Black Box   ❑ OBRA regulated in U.S. Long Term Care

granisetron hydrochloride

(gra-ni'-se-tron hye-droe-klor'-ide)

■ **Brand Name(s):** Kytril
   Chemical Class: Carbazole derivative

■ **Clinical Pharmacology:**
   Mechanism of Action: A $5\text{-}HT_3$ receptor antagonist that acts centrally in the chemoreceptor trigger zone or peripherally at the vagal nerve terminals. **Therapeutic Effect:** Prevents nausea and vomiting.
   Pharmacokinetics:

Route	Onset	Peak	Duration
IV	1-3 min	N/A	24 hr

Rapidly and widely distributed to tissues. Protein binding: 65%. Metabolized in the liver to active metabolite. Eliminated in urine and feces. **Half-life:** 10-12 hr (increased in the elderly).

■ **Available Forms:**
- *Oral Solution:* 2 mg/10 ml.
- *Tablets:* 1 mg.
- *Injection:* 0.1 mg/ml, 1 mg/ml.

■ **Indications and Dosages:**
   Prevention of chemotherapy-induced nausea and vomiting: PO 2 mg 1 hr before chemotherapy or 1 mg 1 hr before and 12 hr after chemotherapy. IV 10 mcg/kg/dose (or 1 mg/dose) within 30 min of chemotherapy.

Prevention of radiation-induced nausea and vomiting: PO 2 mg once a day, given 1 hr before radiation therapy.
Postoperative nausea or vomiting: PO 20-40 mcg/kg as a single postoperative dose. IV 1 mg as a single postoperative dose.

- **Unlabeled Uses:** PO: Prophylaxis of nausea or vomiting associated with radiation therapy

- **Contraindications:** None known.

- **Side Effects**
  Frequent (21%-14%)
  Headache, constipation, asthenia
  Occasional (8%-6%)
  Diarrhea, abdominal pain
  Rare (less than 2%)
  Altered taste, hypersensitivity reaction

- **Serious Reactions**
  - Hypertension, hypotension, arrhythmias such as sinus bradycardia, atrial fibrillation, varying degrees of AV block, ventricular ectopy including nonsustained tachycardia, and ECG abnormalities have been observed.
  - Rare cases of hypersensitivity reactions, sometimes severe (e.g., anaphylaxis, shortness of breath, hypotension, urticaria) have been reported.

- **Patient/Family Education**
  - Granisetron is effective shortly after administration in preventing nausea and vomiting
  - The drug may affect the sense of taste temporarily
  - Use other methods of reducing nausea and vomiting, such as lying quietly and avoiding strong odors

- **Monitoring Parameters**
  - Monitor for therapeutic effect
  - Assess for headache
  - Assess pattern of daily bowel activity and stool consistency

- **Geriatric side effects at a glance:**
  ❑ CNS ❑ Bowel Dysfunction ❑ Bladder Dysfunction ❑ Falls

- **U.S. Regulatory Considerations**
  ❑ FDA Black Box ❑ OBRA regulated in U.S. Long Term Care

griseofulvin

(gri-see-oh-ful'-vin)

- **Brand Name(s):** Fulvicin P/G, Fulvicin U/F, Grifulvin V, Grisactin 500, Griseofulicin, Gris-PEG
  Chemical Class: Penicillium griseofulvum derivative

- **Clinical Pharmacology:**
  Mechanism of Action: An antifungal that inhibits fungal cell mitosis by disrupting mitotic spindle structure. **Therapeutic Effect:** Fungistatic.
  Pharmacokinetics: Ultramicrosize is almost completely absorbed. Absorption is significantly enhanced after a fatty meal. Extensively metabolized in liver. Minimal excretion in urine. **Half-life:** 24 hr.

- **Available Forms:**
  - *Oral Suspension (Grifulvin V):* 125 mg/5 ml.
  - *Tablets (Microsize [Fulvicin-U/F, Grisactin 500, Grifulvin V]):* 250 mg, 500 mg.
  - *Tablets (Ultramicrosize):* 125 mg (Fulvicin P/G, Gris-PEG), 165 mg (Fulvicin P/G), 250 mg (Fulvicin P/G, Gris-PEG), 330 mg (Fulvicin P/G, Griseofulicin).

- **Indications and Dosages:**
  Tinea capitis, tinea corporis, tinea cruris, tinea pedis, tinea unguium: PO (Microsize Tablets, Oral Suspension) Usual dosage, 500-1,000 mg as a single dose or in divided doses. PO (Ultramicrosize Tablets) Usual dosage, 330-750 mg/day as a single dose or in divided doses.

- **Contraindications:** Hepatocellular failure, porphyria

- **Side Effects**
  Occasional
  Hypersensitivity reaction (including pruritus, rash, and urticaria), headache, nausea, diarrhea, excessive thirst, flatulence, oral thrush, dizziness, insomnia
  Rare
  Paresthesia of hands or feet, proteinuria, photosensitivity reaction

- **Serious Reactions**
  - Granulocytopenia occurs rarely.

Special Considerations
  - Prior to therapy, the type of fungus responsible for the infection should be identified

- **Patient/Family Education**
  - Response to therapy may not be apparent for some time; complete entire course of therapy
  - Avoid prolonged exposure to sunlight or sunlamps
  - Notify clinician if sore throat or skin rash occurs
  - Store oral suspensions at room temp in light-resistant container

- Avoid alcohol because flushing or tachycardia may occur
- Maintain good hygiene to help prevent superinfection
- Separate personal items that come in direct contact with affected areas
- Keep affected areas dry and wear light clothing for ventilation
- Take griseofulvin with foods high in fat, such as milk or ice cream, to reduce GI upset and assist in drug absorption

■ Monitoring Parameters
- Periodic assessments of renal, hepatic, and hematopoietic function during prolonged therapy
- Skin for a rash
- Therapeutic response to the drug
- Daily pattern of bowel activity and stool consistency
- Granulocyte count; if the patient develops granulocytopenia, notify the physician and expect to discontinue the drug
- In patients experiencing headache, establish and document the headache's location, onset, and type

■ Geriatric side effects at a glance:
❑ CNS ❑ Bowel Dysfunction ❑ Bladder Dysfunction ❑ Falls

■ U.S. Regulatory Considerations
❑ FDA Black Box ❑ OBRA regulated in U.S. Long Term Care

guaifenesin

(gwye-fen'-e-sin)

■ Brand Name(s): Allfen, Amibid LA, Drituss G, Duratuss G, Fenesin, Ganidin NR, GG 200 NR, Guaibid-LA, Guaifenex G, Guaifenex LA, Gua-SR, Guiadrine G-1200, Guiatuss, Humavent LA, Humibid LA, Iofen, Iophen NR, Liquidbid, Liquidbid 1200, Liquidbid LA, Mucinex, Mucobid-L.A., Muco-Fen, Muco-Fen 800, Muco-Fen 1200, Organ-1 NR, Organidin NR, Pneumomist, Q-Bid LA, Respa-GF, Touro EX, Tussin
OTC: Anti-Tuss, Breonesin, Genatuss, Glytuss, Guiatuss, Hytuss, Hytuss 2X, Mytussin, Naldecon Senior EX, Robitussin

Combinations
Rx: with codeine (Guiatussin AC); with dextromethorphan (Guaibid-DM); with hydrocodone (Hycotuss); with phenylpropanolamine (Entex LA)
Chemical Class: Glyceryl derivative

■ Clinical Pharmacology:
Mechanism of Action: An expectorant that stimulates respiratory tract secretions by decreasing adhesiveness and viscosity of phlegm. *Therapeutic Effect:* Promotes removal of viscous mucus.
Pharmacokinetics: Well absorbed from the GI tract. Metabolized in the liver. Excreted in urine. *Half-life:* 1 hr.

■ Available Forms:
- *Tablets (GG 200 NR, Iofen, Organ-1 NR, Organidin NR)*: 200 mg.
- *Tablets (Extended-Release)*: 575 mg (Touro EX), 600 mg (Amibid LA, Fenesin, Guaibid-LA, Guaifenex LA, Gua-SR, Humavent LA, Humibid LA, Liquidbid, Liquidbid LA, Mucinex, Mucobid-L.A., Pneumomist, Q-Bid LA, Respa-GF), 800 mg (Muco-Fen 800), 1000 mg (Allfen, Muco-Fen), 1200 mg (Duratuss G, Guaifenex G, Guiadrine G-1200, Liquidbid 1200, Muco-Fen 1200).
- *Syrup (Ganidin NR, Guiatuss, Iophen NR, Robitussin, Tussin)*: 100 mg/5 ml.

■ Indications and Dosages:
Expectorant: PO 200-400 mg q4h. PO (Extended-Release) 600-1200 mg q12h. Maximum: 2.4 g/day.

■ Contraindications: None known.

■ Side Effects
Rare
Dizziness, headache, rash, diarrhea, nausea, vomiting, abdominal pain

■ Serious Reactions
- Overdose may produce nausea and vomiting.

■ Patient/Family Education
- Drink a full glass of water with each dose to help further loosen mucus
- Notify clinician if cough persists after medication has been used for 7 days or cough is associated with headache, high fever, skin rash, or sore throat
- Do not take guaifenesin for chronic cough
- Avoid performing tasks that require mental alertness or motor skills until response to the drug has been established

■ Monitoring Parameters
- Increase environmental humidity and fluid intake to lower the viscosity of the patient's lung secretions
- Assess the patient for clinical improvement, and record the onset of cough relief

■ Geriatric side effects at a glance:
❑ CNS ❑ Bowel Dysfunction ❑ Bladder Dysfunction ❑ Falls

■ U.S. Regulatory Considerations
❑ FDA Black Box ❑ OBRA regulated in U.S. Long Term Care

guanabenz acetate

(gwan'-a-benz as'-eh-tayte)

■ **Brand Name(s):** Wytensin
Chemical Class: Dichlorobenzene derivative

■ **Clinical Pharmacology:**
Mechanism of Action: An alpha-adrenergic agonist that stimulates $alpha_2$-adrenergic receptors. Inhibits sympathetic cardioaccelerator and vasoconstrictor center to heart, kidneys, peripheral vasculature. **Therapeutic Effect:** Decreases systolic, diastolic blood pressure (BP). Chronic use decreases peripheral vascular resistance.
Pharmacokinetics: Well absorbed from gastrointestinal (GI) tract. Widely distributed. Protein binding: 90%. Metabolized in liver. Excreted in urine and feces. Not removed by hemodialysis. **Half-life:** 6 hr.

■ **Available Forms:**
• *Tablets*: 4 mg, 8 mg (Wytensin).

■ **Indications and Dosages:**
Hypertension: PO Initially, 4 mg 2 times/day. Increase by 4-8 mg at 1-2 wk intervals. Elderly. Initially, 4 mg/day. May increase q1-2 wk. Maintenance: 8-16 mg/day. Maximum: 32 mg/day.

■ **Contraindications:** History of hypersensitivity to guanabenz or any component of the formulation

■ **Side Effects**
Frequent
Drowsiness, dry mouth, dizziness
Occasional
Weakness, headache, nausea, decreased sexual ability
Rare
Ataxia, sleep disturbances, rash, itching, diarrhea, constipation, altered taste, muscle aches

■ **Serious Reactions**
• Abrupt withdrawal may result in rebound hypertension manifested as nervousness, agitation, anxiety, insomnia, hand tingling, tremor, flushing, and sweating.
• Overdosage produces hypotension, somnolence, lethargy, irritability, bradycardia, and miosis (pupillary constriction).

■ **Patient/Family Education**
• Avoid hazardous activities, since drug may cause drowsiness
• Do not discontinue drug abruptly, or withdrawal symptoms may occur (anxiety, increased BP, headache, insomnia, increased pulse, tremors, nausea, sweating)
• Do not use OTC (cough, cold, or allergy) products unless directed by clinician

- Rise slowly to sitting or standing position to minimize orthostatic hypotension, especially elderly
- May cause dizziness, fainting, light-headedness during first few days of therapy
- May cause dry mouth; use hard candy, saliva product, or frequent rinsing of mouth
- Avoid alcohol

■ **Monitoring Parameters**
- Blood pressure (posturally), mental depression

■ **Geriatric side effects at a glance:**
❏ CNS ❏ Bowel Dysfunction ❏ Bladder Dysfunction ❏ Falls

■ **U.S. Regulatory Considerations**
❏ FDA Black Box ❏ OBRA regulated in U.S. Long Term Care

guanfacine hydrochloride

(gwahn'-fa-seen hye-droe-klor'-ide)

■ **Brand Name(s):** Tenex
Chemical Class: Phenylacyl guanidine

■ **Clinical Pharmacology:**
Mechanism of Action: An alpha-adrenergic agonist that stimulates alpha$_2$-adrenergic receptors and inhibits sympathetic cardioaccelerator and vasoconstrictor center to heart, kidneys, peripheral vasculature. **Therapeutic Effect:** Decreases systolic, diastolic blood pressure (BP). Chronic use decreases peripheral vascular resistance.
Pharmacokinetics: Well absorbed from gastrointestinal (GI) tract. Widely distributed. Protein binding: 71%. Metabolized in liver. Excreted in urine and feces. Not removed by hemodialysis. **Half-life:** 17 hr.

■ **Available Forms:**
- *Tablets*: 1 mg, 2 mg (Tenex).

■ **Indications and Dosages:**
Hypertension: PO Initially, 1 mg/day. Increase by 1 mg/day at intervals of 3-4 wk up to 3 mg/day in single or divided doses.

■ **Unlabeled Uses:** Attention-deficit hyperactivity disorder (ADHD), tic disorders

■ **Contraindications:** History of hypersensitivity to guanfacine or any component of the formulation

■ **Side Effects**
Frequent
Dry mouth, somnolence

Occasional

Fatigue, headache, asthenia (loss of strength, energy), dizziness

- ### Serious Reactions
  - Overdosage may produce difficult breathing, dizziness, faintness, severe drowsiness, bradycardia.

- ### Patient/Family Education
  - Avoid hazardous activities, since drug may cause drowsiness
  - Do not discontinue oral drug abruptly, or withdrawal symptoms may occur after 3-4 days (anxiety, increased BP, headache, insomnia, increased pulse, tremors, nausea, sweating)
  - Do not use OTC (cough, cold, or allergy) products unless directed by clinician
  - Rise slowly to sitting or standing position to minimize orthostatic hypotension, especially elderly
  - Dizziness, fainting, light-headedness may occur during first few days of therapy
  - May cause dry mouth; use hard candy, saliva product, or frequent rinsing of mouth
  - Avoid alcohol

- ### Monitoring Parameters
  - Blood pressure (posturally), blood glucose in patients with diabetes mellitus; confusion, mental depression

- ### Geriatric side effects at a glance:
  ❑ CNS   ❑ Bowel Dysfunction   ❑ Bladder Dysfunction   ❑ Falls

- ### U.S. Regulatory Considerations
  ❑ FDA Black Box   ❑ OBRA regulated in U.S. Long Term Care

halcinonide

(hal-sin'-o-nide)

- ### Brand Name(s): Halog, Halog-E
  Chemical Class: Corticosteroid, synthetic

- ### Clinical Pharmacology:
  Mechanism of Action: A topical corticosteroid that has anti-inflammatory, antipruritic, and vasoconstrictive properties. The exact mechanism of the anti-inflammatory process is unclear. *Therapeutic Effect:* Reduces or prevents tissue response to the inflammatory process.
  Pharmacokinetics: Well absorbed systemically. Large variation in absorption among sites. Protein binding: varies. Metabolized in liver. Primarily excreted in urine.

■ **Available Forms:**
  • *Cream*: 0.1% (Halog).
  • *Cream (emollient base)*: 0.1% (Halog-E).
  • *Ointment*: 0.1% (Halog).
  • *Solution*: 0.1% (Halog).

■ **Indications and Dosages:**
  Dermatoses: Topical Apply sparingly 1-3 times/day.

■ **Contraindications:** History of hypersensitivity to halcinonide or other corticosteroids

■ **Side Effects**
  Occasional
  Itching, redness, irritation, burning at site of application, dryness, folliculitis, acnei-form eruptions, hypopigmentation
  Rare
  Allergic contact dermatitis, maceration of the skin, secondary infection, skin atrophy

■ **Serious Reactions**
  • The serious reactions of long-term therapy and the addition of occlusive dressings are reversible hypothalamic-pituitary-adrenal (HPA) axis suppression, manifestations of Cushing's syndrome, hyperglycemia, and glucosuria.

■ **Patient/Family Education**
  • Apply sparingly only to affected area
  • Avoid contact with the eyes
  • Do not put bandages or dressings over treated area unless directed by clinician
  • Do not use on weeping, denuded, or infected areas
  • Discontinue drug, notify clinician if local irritation or fever develops
  • Avoid exposure to sunlight

■ **Monitoring Parameters**
  • Skin for rash

■ **Geriatric side effects at a glance:**
  ❑ CNS ❑ Bowel Dysfunction ❑ Bladder Dysfunction ❑ Falls

■ **U.S. Regulatory Considerations**
  ❑ FDA Black Box ❑ OBRA regulated in U.S. Long Term Care

halobetasol

(hal-oh-bay'-ta-sol)

■ **Brand Name(s):** Ultravate
Chemical Class: Corticosteroid, synthetic

■ **Clinical Pharmacology:**
Mechanism of Action: A corticosteroid that inhibits accumulation of inflammatory cells at inflammation sites, phagocytosis, lysosomal enzyme release and synthesis or release of mediators of inflammation. **Therapeutic Effect:** Decreases or prevents tissue response to inflammatory process.
Pharmacokinetics: Variation in absorption among individuals and sites: scrotum 36%, forehead 7%, scalp 4%, forearm 1%.

■ **Available Forms:**
- *Cream:* 0.05% (Ultravate).
- *Ointment:* 0.05% (Ultravate).

■ **Indications and Dosages:**
Dermatoses, corticosteroid-unresponsive: Topical Apply 1-2 times/day. Maximum: 50 g for 2 wk.

■ **Contraindications:** Hypersensitivity to halobetasol or other corticosteroids.

■ **Side Effects**
Frequent
Burning, stinging, pruritus
Rare
Cushing's syndrome, hyperglycemia, glucosuria, hypothalamic-pituitary-adrenal axis suppression

■ **Serious Reactions**
- Overdosage can occur from topically applied halobetasol absorbed in sufficient amounts to produce systemic effects producing reversible adrenal suppression, manifestations of Cushing's syndrome, hyperglycemia, and glucosuria in some patients.

■ **Patient/Family Education**
- Apply sparingly only to affected area
- Avoid contact with the eyes
- Do not put bandages or dressings over treated area
- Do not use on weeping, denuded, or infected areas
- Discontinue drug, notify clinician if local irritation or fever develops
- Treatment should be limited to 2 wk, and amounts greater than 50 g/wk should not be used

■ **Monitoring Parameters**
- Therapeutic response
- Sign of contact dermatitis or worsening of condition

■ **Geriatric side effects at a glance:**
☐ CNS ☐ Bowel Dysfunction ☐ Bladder Dysfunction ☐ Falls

■ **U.S. Regulatory Considerations**
☐ FDA Black Box ☐ OBRA regulated in U.S. Long Term Care

haloperidol

(ha-loe-per'-idole)

■ **Brand Name(s):** Haldol, Haldol Decanoate
Chemical Class: Butyrophenone derivative

■ **Clinical Pharmacology:**
Mechanism of Action: An antipsychotic, antiemetic, and antidyskinetic agent that competitively blocks postsynaptic dopamine receptors, interrupts nerve impulse movement, and increases turnover of dopamine in the brain. Has strong extrapyramidal and antiemetic effects; weak anticholinergic and sedative effects. **Therapeutic Effect:** Produces tranquilizing effect.
Pharmacokinetics: Readily absorbed from the GI tract. Protein binding: 92%. Extensively metabolized in the liver. Primarily excreted in urine. Not removed by hemodialysis. **Half-life:** 12-37 hr PO; 10-19 hr IV; 17-25 hr IM.

■ **Available Forms:**
- *Oral Concentrate*: 1 mg/ml, 2 mg/ml.
- *Tablets (Haldol)*: 0.5 mg, 1 mg, 2 mg, 5 mg, 10 mg, 20 mg.
- *Injection (Lactate [Haldol])*: 5 mg/ml.
- *Injection (Decanoate [Haldol Decanoate])*: 50 mg/ml, 100 mg/ml.

■ **Indications and Dosages:**
Acute psychosis, delirium: IV 0.5-50 mg at a rate of 5 mg/min. May repeat as needed.
Psychotic disorder: PO Initially, 0.5-5 mg 2-3 times a day. Maximum: 100 mg/day.
Tourette's disorder: PO 6-15 mg/day. May increase by 2-mg increments as needed. Maintenance: 9 mg/day.

■ **Unlabeled Uses:** Treatment of Huntington's chorea, nausea or vomiting associated with cancer chemotherapy

■ **Contraindications:** Angle-closure glaucoma, CNS depression, myelosuppression, Parkinson's disease, severe cardiac or hepatic disease

■ **Side Effects**
Frequent
Blurred vision, constipation, orthostatic hypotension, dry mouth, swelling or soreness of female breasts, peripheral edema

Occasional

Allergic reaction, difficulty urinating, decreased thirst, dizziness, decreased sexual function, drowsiness, nausea, vomiting, photosensitivity, lethargy

■ Serious Reactions

- Extrapyramidal symptoms appear to be dose-related and typically occur in the first few days of therapy. Marked drowsiness and lethargy, excessive salivation, and fixed stare occur frequently. Less common reactions include severe akathisia (motor restlessness) and acute dystonias (such as torticollis, opisthotonos, and oculogyric crisis).
- Tardive dyskinesia (tongue protrusion, puffing of the cheeks, chewing or puckering of the mouth) may occur during long-term therapy or after discontinuing the drug and may be irreversible. Elderly female patients have a greater risk of developing this reaction.

■ Patient/Family Education

- Do not mix liquid formulation with coffee or tea
- Use calibrated dropper
- Take with food or milk
- Arise slowly from reclining position
- Do not discontinue abruptly
- Use a sunscreen during sun exposure to prevent burns
- Take special precautions to stay cool in hot weather
- The drug's full therapeutic effect may take up to 6 wk to appear
- Drowsiness generally subsides with continued therapy
- Avoid tasks that require mental alertness or motor skills until response to the drug has been established
- Notify the physician if muscle stiffness occurs
- Take sips of tepid water or chew sugarless gum to help relieve dry mouth

■ Monitoring Parameters

- Observe closely for signs of tardive dyskinesia
- Closely supervise suicidal patients during early therapy. As depression lessens, the patient's energy level improves, which increases the suicide potential
- Assess the patient for evidence of a therapeutic response, including improvement in self-care, increased interest in surroundings and ability to concentrate, and relaxed facial expression
- The therapeutic serum level for haloperidol is 0.2 to 1 mcg/ml, and the toxic serum level is greater than 1 mcg/ml

■ Geriatric side effects at a glance:

☑ CNS ☑ Bowel Dysfunction ☐ Bladder Dysfunction ☑ Falls

Other: Orthostatic hypotension, cardiac conduction disturbances, torsades de pointes, anticholinergic side effects.

■ Use with caution in older patients with:
Parkinson's disease (an atypical antipsychotic is recommended), seizure disorders, cardiovascular disease with conduction disturbance, hepatic encephalopathy, narrow-angle glaucoma, congenital prolonged Q-T syndrome or drugs which prolong Q-T interval, drugs which inhibit or utilize 26D substrate of cytochrome P450.

■ **U.S. Regulatory Considerations**
  ❏ FDA Black Box   ☑ OBRA regulated in U.S. Long Term Care

■ **Other Uses in Geriatric Patient:** Behavior disturbances in the setting of dementia

■ **Side Effects:**
  Of particular importance in the geriatric patient: Tardive dyskinesia, akathisia (may appear to exacerbate behavioral disturbances), anticholinergic effects, may increase risk of sudden death

■ **Geriatric Considerations - Summary:** Sink and colleagues' systematic review showed statistically significant improvements on neuropsychiatric and behavioral scales for some drugs, but improvements were small and unlikely to be clinically important. Because of documented risks, and uncertain benefits, these agents should be used with caution in demented elderly persons, with frequent monitoring for side effects and a low threshold for discontinuing use.

■ **References:**
  1. Leipzig RM, Cumming RG, Tinetti ME. Drugs and falls in older people: a systematic review and meta-analysis: I. Psychotropic drugs. J Am Geriatr Soc 1999;47:30-39.
  2. Sink KM, Holden KF, Yaffe K. Pharmacological treatment of neuropsychiatric symptoms of dementia: a review of the evidence. JAMA 2005;293:596-608.
  3. Ray WA, Meredith S, Thapa PB, Meador KG, Hall K, Murray KT. Antipsychotics and the risk of sudden cardiac death. Arch Gen Psychiatry 2001;58:1161-1167.

heparin sodium

(hep'-a-rin soe'-dee-um)

■ **Brand Name(s):** Hep-Lock, Hep-Pak CVC
  Chemical Class: Glycosaminoglycan, sulfated

■ **Clinical Pharmacology:**
  Mechanism of Action: A blood modifier that interferes with blood coagulation by blocking conversion of prothrombin to thrombin and fibrinogen to fibrin. **Therapeutic Effect:** Prevents further extension of existing thrombi or new clot formation. Has no effect on existing clots.
  Pharmacokinetics: Well absorbed following subcutaneous administration. Protein binding: Very high. Metabolized in the liver. Removed from the circulation via uptake by the reticuloendothelial system. Primarily excreted in urine. Not removed by hemodialysis. **Half-life:** 1-6 hr.

■ **Available Forms:**
  • Injection (Hep-Lock): 10 units/ml, 100 units/ml, 1000 units/ml, 2500 units/ml, 5000 units/ml, 7500 units/ml, 10,000 units/ml, 20,000 units/ml, 25,000 units/500 ml infusion.
  • Injectable Kit (Hep-Pak CVC): 20 units/ml, 100 units/ml.

■ **Indications and Dosages:**
Line flushing: IV 100 units q6-8h.
Treatment of venous thrombosis, pulmonary embolism, peripheral arterial embolism, atrial fibrillation with embolism: Intermittent IV Initially, 10,000 units, then 50-70 units/kg (5000–10,000 units) q4-6h. IV Infusion Loading dose: 80 units/kg, then 18 units/kg/hr, with adjustments based on aPTT. Range: 10-30 units/kg/hr.
Prevention of venous thrombosis, pulmonary embolism, peripheral arterial embolism, atrial fibrillation with embolism: Subcutaneous 5000 units q8-12h.

■ **Contraindications:** Intracranial hemorrhage, severe hypotension, severe thrombocytopenia, subacute bacterial endocarditis, uncontrolled bleeding

■ **Side Effects**
Occasional
Itching, burning (particularly on soles of feet) caused by vasospastic reaction
Rare
Pain, cyanosis of extremity 6-10 days after initial therapy lasting 4-6 hours; hypersensitivity reaction, including chills, fever, pruritus, urticaria, asthma, rhinitis, lacrimation, and headache

■ **Serious Reactions**
- Bleeding complications ranging from local ecchymoses to major hemorrhage occur more frequently in high-dose therapy, intermittent IV infusion, and in women 60 years of age and older.
- Antidote: Protamine sulfate 1-1.5 mg, IV, for every 100 units heparin subcutaneous within 30 min of overdose, 0.5-0.75 mg for every 100 units heparin subcutaneous if within 30-60 min of overdose, 0.25-0.375 mg for every 100 units heparin subcutaneous if 2 hr have elapsed since overdose, 25-50 mg if heparin was given by IV infusion.

■ **Patient/Family Education**
- Report any signs of bleeding: gums, under skin, urine, stools
- Use an electric razor and soft toothbrush, to prevent bleeding during heparin therapy
- Do not take other medications, including OTC drugs, especially aspirin and NSAIDs, without physician approval
- Inform the dentist and other physicians of heparin therapy

■ **Monitoring Parameters**
- aPTT (usual goal is to prolong aPTT to a value that corresponds to a plasma heparin level of 0.2-0.4 U/ml by protamine titration or to an antifactor Xa level of about 0.3-0.6 U/ml; this range must be determined for each individual laboratory), usually measure 6-8 hr after initiation of IV and 6-8 hr after INF rate changes; increase or decrease INF by 2-4 U/kg/hr dependent on aPTT
- For intermittent inj, measure aPTT 3.5-4 hr after IV inj; at midinterval after SC inj
- Platelet counts, signs of bleeding, Hgb,Hct, AST (SGOT) and ALT (SGPT) levels, and stool and urine cultures for occult blood
- Assess the patient's gums for erythema and gingival bleeding, skin for ecchymosis or petechiae, and urine for hematuria
- Evaluate the patient for abdominal or back pain, a decrease in blood pressure, an increase in pulse rate, and severe headache, which may be evidence of hemorrhage
- Check the patient's peripheral pulses for loss of peripheral circulation

- When converting to warfarin therapy, monitor the patient's PT/INR results, as ordered. PT/INR will be 10%-20% higher while heparin is being given concurrently

■ Geriatric side effects at a glance:
❑ CNS ❑ Bowel Dysfunction ❑ Bladder Dysfunction ❑ Falls

■ U.S. Regulatory Considerations
☑ FDA Black Box

Increased risk of spinal/epidural hematomas with neuraxial anesthesia or spinal puncture. Risk is further increased by use of indwelling spinal catheters, repeated/traumatic epidural/spinal puncture, or use of drugs affecting hemostasis (NSAIDs, anticoagulants, platelet inhibitors).

❑ OBRA regulated in U.S. Long Term Care

hydralazine hydrochloride

(hye-dral'-a-zeen hye-droe-klor'-ide)

■ Brand Name(s): Apresoline

Combinations
Rx: with hydrochlorothiazide (Apresazide); with hydrochlorothiazide, reserpine (Ser-Ap-Es)
Chemical Class: Phthalazine derivative

■ Clinical Pharmacology:
Mechanism of Action: An antihypertensive with direct vasodilating effects on arterioles. **Therapeutic Effect:** Decreases BP and systemic resistance.
Pharmacokinetics:

Route	Onset	Peak	Duration
PO	20-30 min	N/A	2-4 hr
IV	5-20 min	N/A	2-6 hr

Well absorbed from the GI tract. Widely distributed. Protein binding: 85%-90%. Metabolized in the liver to active metabolite. Primarily excreted in urine. Not removed by hemodialysis. **Half-life:** 3-7 hr (increased with impaired renal function).

■ Available Forms:
- *Tablets:* 10 mg, 25 mg, 50 mg, 100 mg.
- *Injection:* 20 mg/ml.

■ Indications and Dosages:
Moderate to severe hypertension: PO Initially, 10 mg 2-3 times a day. May increase by 10-25 mg q2-3days. IV, IM Initially, 10-20 mg/dose q4-6h. May increase to 40 mg/dose.

Dosage in renal impairment: Dosage interval is based on creatinine clearance.

Creatinine Clearance	Dosage Interval
10-50 ml/min	q8h
less than 10 ml/min	q8-24h

■ **Unlabeled Uses:** Treatment of CHF, hypertension secondary to eclampsia and pre-eclampsia, primary pulmonary hypertension.

■ **Contraindications:** Coronary artery disease, lupus erythematosus, rheumatic heart disease

■ **Side Effects**
Frequent
Headache, palpitations, tachycardia (generally disappears in 7–10 days)
Occasional
GI disturbance (nausea, vomiting, diarrhea), paresthesia, fluid retention, peripheral edema, dizziness, flushed face, nasal congestion

■ **Serious Reactions**
• High dosage may produce lupus erythematosus–like reaction, including fever, facial rash, muscle and joint aches, and splenomegaly.
• Severe orthostatic hypotension, skin flushing, severe headache, myocardial ischemia, and cardiac arrhythmias may develop.
• Profound shock may occur with severe overdosage.

Special Considerations
• Lupus-like syndrome more common in "slow acetylators" and following higher doses for prolonged periods

■ **Patient/Family Education**
• Take with meals
• Notify clinician of any unexplained prolonged general tiredness or fever, muscle or joint aching, or chest pain
• Stools may turn black
• Rise slowly from a lying to a sitting position and permit legs to dangle from the bed momentarily before standing to reduce the hypotensive effect of hydralazine

■ **Monitoring Parameters**
• CBC and ANA titer before and during prolonged therapy
• Pattern of daily bowel activity and stool consistency
• Monitor the patient for headache, palpitations, and tachycardia
• Assess for peripheral edema of the hands and feet

■ **Geriatric side effects at a glance:**
❏ CNS   ❏ Bowel Dysfunction   ❏ Bladder Dysfunction   ❏ Falls

■ **U.S. Regulatory Considerations**
❏ FDA Black Box   ❏ OBRA regulated in U.S. Long Term Care

hydrochlorothiazide

(hye-droe-klor-oh-thye'-a-zide)

■ **Brand Name(s):** Aquazide H, Esidrix, HydroDIURIL, Microzide, Oretic

Combinations

Rx: with ACE inhibitors: quinapril (Accuretic); captopril (Acediur, Capozide); lisino-pril (Prinzide, Zestoretic); benazepril (Lotensin HCT); moexipril (Uniretic); enalapril (Vaseretic); with spironolactone (Aldactazide, Spirozide); with methyl-dopa (Aldoril); with hydralazine (Apresazide); with reserpine (Aqwesine, Hydropres, Hydroserpine, Hydrotensin, Mallopres, Marpres, Unipres); with angio-tensin II receptor blockers: irbesartan (Avalide), valsartan (Diovan HCT), losartan (Hyzaar); with hydralazine and reserpine (Cam-ap-es, H.H.R., Hyserp, Lo-Ten, Ser-A-Gen, Seralazide, Ser-Ap-Es, Serpex, Uni-Serp); with triamterene (Dyazide, Maxzide); with potassium (Esidrix-K); with guanethidine (Esimil); with β-blockers: propranolol (Inderide); metoprolol (Lopressor HCT); labetalol (Normazide, Tran-date-HCT); timolol (Timolide); bisoprolol (Ziac); with amiloride (Moduretic)

Chemical Class: Sulfonamide derivative

■ **Clinical Pharmacology:**

Mechanism of Action: A sulfonamide derivative that acts as a thiazide diuretic and an-tihypertensive. As a diuretic, blocks reabsorption of water, sodium, and potassium at the cortical diluting segment of the distal tubule. As an antihypertensive, reduces plasma, extracellular fluid volume, and peripheral vascular resistance by direct effect on blood vessels. **Therapeutic Effect:** Promotes diuresis; reduces BP.

Pharmacokinetics:

Route	Onset	Peak	Duration
PO (diuretic)	2 hr	4-6 hr	6-12 hr

Variably absorbed from the GI tract. Primarily excreted unchanged in urine. Not re-moved by hemodialysis. **Half-life:** 5.6-14.8 hr.

■ **Available Forms:**
- *Capsules (Microzide)*: 12.5 mg.
- *Oral Solution*: 50 mg/5 ml.
- *Tablets (Aquazide, Oretic)*: 25 mg, 50 mg, 100 mg.

■ **Indications and Dosages:**

Edema: PO 25-100 mg/day as a single dose or in divided doses.

Hypertension: PO Initially, 12.5-25 mg once daily. May increase up to 50-100 mg/day as a single dose or in divided doses.

■ **Unlabeled Uses:** Treatment of diabetes insipidus, prevention of calcium-containing re-nal calculi

■ **Contraindications:** Anuria, history of hypersensitivity to sulfonamides or thiazide di-uretics, renal decompensation

■ **Side Effects**

Expected

Increase in urinary frequency and urine volume

Frequent
Potassium depletion
Occasional
Orthostatic hypotension, headache, GI disturbances, photosensitivity

■ **Serious Reactions**
- Vigorous diuresis may lead to profound water and electrolyte depletion, resulting in hypokalemia, hyponatremia, and dehydration.
- Acute hypotensive episodes may occur.
- Hyperglycemia may occur during prolonged therapy.
- Pancreatitis, blood dyscrasias, pulmonary edema, allergic pneumonitis, and dermatologic reactions occur rarely.
- Overdose can lead to lethargy and coma without changes in electrolytes or hydration.
- Use with caution in patients with sulfa allergy.

Special Considerations
- May protect against osteoporotic hip fractures
- Loop diuretics or metolazone more effective if CrCl less than 40-50 ml/min
- Combinations with triamterene, lisinopril have potassium-sparing effect
- Doses above 25 mg provide no further blood pressure reduction, but are more likely to induce metabolic disturbance (hypokalemia, hyperuricemia, etc.)
- Although allergic cross-reactivity with sulfonamide antibiotics and sulfonamide nonantibiotics has not been demonstrated, use with caution in patients with a history of severe sulfa allergies.

■ **Patient/Family Education**
- Will increase urination temporarily (for about 3 wk); take early in the day
- May cause sensitivity to sunlight; avoid prolonged exposure to the sun and other ultraviolet light
- May cause gout attacks; notify clinician if sudden joint pain occurs
- Change positions slowly and let legs dangle momentarily before standing to reduce the drug's hypotensive effect
- Eat foods high in potassium, including apricots, bananas, raisins, orange juice, potatoes, legumes, meat, and whole grains (such as cereals)

■ **Monitoring Parameters**
- Weight, urine output, serum electrolytes, BUN, creatinine, CBC, uric acid, glucose, lipids
- Blood pressure
- Be especially alert for signs of potassium depletion, such as cardiac arrhythmias, in patients taking digoxin
- Assess the patient for constipation, which may occur with exercise diuresis

■ **Geriatric side effects at a glance:**
  ❑ CNS   ❑ Bowel Dysfunction   ❑ Bladder Dysfunction   ❑ Falls

■ **U.S. Regulatory Considerations**
  ❑ FDA Black Box   ❑ OBRA regulated in U.S. Long Term Care

hydrocodone bitartrate

(high-drough-koe'-doan bi-tahr'trāt)

■ **Clinical Pharmacology:**
   Mechanism of Action: An opiate and antitussive that binds with opioid receptors in the CNS. **Therapeutic Effect:** Alters the perception of and emotional response to pain; suppresses cough reflex.
   Pharmacokinetics:

Route	Onset	Peak	Duration
PO (analgesic)	10-20 min	30-60 min	4-6 hr
PO (antitussive)	N/A	N/A	4-6 hr

   Well absorbed from the GI tract. Metabolized in the liver. Primarily excreted in urine. **Half-life:** 3.8 hr (increased in elderly).

■ **Indications and Dosages:**
   Analgesia: PO 2.5-10 mg q4-6h.
   Cough: PO 5-10 mg q4-6h as needed. Maximum: 15 mg/dose. PO (Extended-Release) 10 mg q12h.

■ **Contraindications:** None known.

■ **Side Effects**
   Frequent
   Sedation, hypotension, diaphoresis, facial flushing, dizziness, somnolence, constipation
   Occasional
   Urine retention, blurred vision, dry mouth, headache, nausea, vomiting, difficult or painful urination, euphoria, dysphoria

■ **Serious Reactions**
   • Overdose results in respiratory depression, skeletal muscle flaccidity, cold or clammy skin, cyanosis, and extreme somnolence progressing to seizures, stupor, and coma.
   • The patient who uses hydrocodone repeatedly may develop a tolerance to the drug's analgesic effect as well as physical dependence.
   • The drug may have a prolonged duration of action and cumulative effect in patients with hepatic or renal impairment.

■ **Geriatric side effects at a glance:**
   ☑ CNS ☑ Bowel Dysfunction ☑ Bladder Dysfunction ☑ Falls

■ **U.S. Regulatory Considerations**
   ☐ FDA Black Box ☑ OBRA regulated in U.S. Long Term Care

hydrocortisone

(hye-droe-kor'-ti-sone)

■ **Brand Name(s):** Acticort 100, Aeroseb-HC, A-Hydrocort, Ala-Cort, Ala-Scalp HP, Anucort-HC, Anumed-HC, Anusol-HC, Anutone-HC, Caldecort, Cetacort, Colocort, Cor-
tane, Cortaid, Cort-Dome High Potency, Cortef, Cortenema, Cortifoam, Cortizone-5,
Cortizone-10, Cotacort, Emcort, Gly-Cort, Hemorrhoidal HC, Hemril-30, Hemril-HC
Uniserts, Hydrocortone, Hydrocortone Phosphate, Hytone, Instacort 10, Lacticare-
HC, Locoid, Locoid Lipocream, Nupercainal Hydrocortisone Cream, Nutracort, Ora-
base HCA, Pandel, Penecort, Preparation H Hydrocortisone, Proctocort, Procto-
cream-HC, Procto-Kit 1%, Procto-Kit 2.5%, Proctosert HC, Proctosol-HC, Proctozone-
HC, Rectasol-HC, Rederm, Scalp-Aid, Solu-Cortef, Texacort, WestCort
OTC: Cortaid, Cortizone, Dermolate, Gynecort Female Creme, Lanacort-5, Tegrin-HC

Combinations
Rx: with chloramphenicol (Chloromycetin/HC suspension—ophthalmic); with neomycin and polymyxin B (Cortisporin Otic, Drotic, Otocort—otic); with neomycin,
polymyxin B, and bacitracin (Cortisporin Ointment, Neotricin HC—ophthalmic);
with oxytetracycline (Terra-Cortril—ophthalmic); with urea (Carmol HC)
Chemical Class: Glucocorticoid

■ **Clinical Pharmacology:**
Mechanism of Action: An adrenocortical steroid that inhibits accumulation of inflammatory cells at inflammation sites, phagocytosis, lysosomal enzyme release and synthesis, and release of mediators of inflammation. **Therapeutic Effect:** Prevents or suppresses cell-mediated immune reactions. Decreases or prevents tissue response to
inflammatory process.
Pharmacokinetics:

Route	Onset	Peak	Duration
IV	N/A	4-6 hr	8-12 hr

Well absorbed after IM administration. Widely distributed. Metabolized in the liver.
Half-life: Plasma, 1.5-2 hr; biologic, 8-12 hr.

■ **Available Forms:**
- *Tablets (Cortef)* : 5 mg, 10 mg, 20 mg.
- *Oral Suspension, cypionate (Cortef)*: 10 mg/5 ml
- *Cream (Rectal)*: 1% (Nupercainal Hydrocortisone Cream, Cortizone-10, Preparation
  H Hydrocortisone, Proctocort, Procto-Kit 1%), 2.5% (Anusol-HC, Hemorrhoidal HC,
  Procto-Kit 2.5%, Proctosol-HC, Proctozone-HC).
- *Cream, butyrate (Topical [Locoid, Locoid Lipocream])*: 0.1%.
- *Cream, probutate (Topical [Pandel])*: 0.1%.
- *Cream, valerate (Topical [WestCort])*: 0.2%.
- *Cream (Topical)*: 0.5% (Cortizone-5), 1% (Ala-Cort, Caldecort, Cortizone-10, Hycort,
  Hytone, Penecort), 2.5% (Hytone, Proctocream-HC).
- *Foam (Rectal [Cortifoam])*: 10%.
- *Gel (Topical [Instacort 10])*: 1%.

- *Lotion*: 0.5% (Cetacort), 1% (Ala-Cort, Cetacort, Cortone, Lacticare-HC, Nutracort), 2.5% (Hytone, Lacticare-HC, Nutracort).
- *Ointment, butyrate (Topical [Locoid])*: 0.1%.
- *Ointment, valerate (Topical [WestCort])*: 0.2%.
- *Ointment (Topical)*: 0.5% (Cortizone-5), 1% (Anusol-HC, Cortaid, Cortizone-10, Hydrocortisone 1%, Hytone), 2.5% (Hytone).
- *Paste (Topical [Orabase HCA])*: 0.5%.
- *Solution (Topical)*: 1% (Acticort 100, Gly-Cort, Penecort, Rederm, Scalp-Aid, Texacort), 2.5% (Texacort).
- *Solution, butyrate (Topical [Locoid])*: 0.1%.
- *Spray (Topical [Aeroseb-HC])*: 0.5%.
- *Suppositories*: 25 mg (Anucort-HC, Anumed-HC, Anusol-HC, Anutone-HC, Cort-Dome High Potency, Hemorrhoidal HC, Hemril-HC, Proctosol-HC, Rectasol-HC), 30 mg (Emcort, Hemril-30, Proctocort, Proctosert HC).
- *Suppositories (Rectal [Colocort, Cortenema])*: 100 mg/60 ml.
- *Injection (A-Hydrocort, Solu-Cortef)*: 100 mg, 250 mg, 500 mg, 1 g.
- *Injectable Solution, sodium phosphate (Hydrocortone Phosphate)*: 50 mg/ml.
- *Injectable Suspension, acetate*: 25 mg/ml, 50 mg/ml.

■ Indications and Dosages:
Acute adrenal insufficiency: IV 100 mg IV bolus; then 300 mg/day in divided doses q8h.
Anti-inflammation, immunosuppression: IV, IM 15-240 mg q12h. PO 15-240 mg q12h.
Status asthmaticus: IV 100-500 mg q6h.
Shock: IV 500 mg-2g q2-6h.
Adjunctive treatment of ulcerative colitis: Rectal 100 mg at bedtime for 21 nights or until clinical and proctologic remission occurs (may require 2-3 mo of therapy). Rectal (Cortifoam) 1 applicator 1-2 times a day for 2-3 wk, then every second day until therapy ends. Topical Apply sparingly 2-4 times a day.

■ Contraindications: Fungal, tuberculosis, or viral skin lesions; serious infections

■ Side Effects
Frequent
Insomnia, heartburn, nervousness, abdominal distention, diaphoresis, acne, mood swings, increased appetite, facial flushing, delayed wound healing, increased susceptibility to infection, diarrhea or constipation
Occasional
Headache, edema, change in skin color, frequent urination
Topical: Itching, redness, irritation
Rare
Tachycardia, allergic reaction (such as rash and hives), psychological changes, hallucinations, depression
Topical: Allergic contact dermatitis, purpura

■ Serious Reactions
- Long-term therapy may cause hypocalcemia, hypokalemia, muscle wasting (especially in arms and legs), osteoporosis, spontaneous fractures, amenorrhea, cataracts, glaucoma, peptic ulcer disease, and CHF.
- Abruptly withdrawing the drug after long-term therapy may cause anorexia, nausea, fever, headache, sudden severe joint pain, rebound inflammation, fatigue, weakness, lethargy, dizziness, and orthostatic hypotension.

■ Patient/Family Education
- May cause GI upset; take with meals or snacks
- Take single daily doses in AM
- Increased dose of rapidly acting corticosteroids may be necessary in patients subjected to unusual stress
- Signs of adrenal insufficiency include fatigue, anorexia, nausea, vomiting, diarrhea, weight loss, weakness, dizziness, and low blood sugar
- Avoid abrupt withdrawal of therapy following high-dose or long-term therapy
- May mask infections
- Do not give live virus vaccines to patients on prolonged therapy
- Patients on chronic steroid therapy should wear medical alert bracelet
- Avoid alcohol and limit caffeine intake during hydrocortisone therapy
- Notify the dentist and other physicians that he or she is taking hydrocortisone or has taken it within the past 12 mo
- Avoid contact with eyes
- Apply topical hydrocortisone valerate after a bath or shower for best absorption. Do not cover the affected area with plastic pants, tight diapers, or other types of coverings unless the physician instructs otherwise
- Steroids often cause mood swings, ranging from euphoria to depression

■ Monitoring Parameters
- Serum K and glucose
- Edema, blood pressure, CHF, mental status, weight
- Electrolytes
- Pattern of daily bowel activity and stool consistency
- Monitor the patient for signs and symptoms of hypocalcemia (such as cramps and muscle twitching), or hypokalemia (such as ECG changes, irritability, nausea and vomiting, numbness or tingling of lower extremities, and weakness)

■ Geriatric side effects at a glance:
❑ CNS ❑ Bowel Dysfunction ❑ Bladder Dysfunction ❑ Falls

■ U.S. Regulatory Considerations
❑ FDA Black Box ❑ OBRA regulated in U.S. Long Term Care

hydroflumethiazide

(hye-droe-floo-meth-eye'-a-zide)

■ Brand Name(s): Diucardin, Saluron

Combinations
Rx: reserpine (Salutensin, Salutensin-Demi)
Chemical Class: Sulfonamide derivative

Clinical Pharmacology:

Mechanism of Action: A diuretic that blocks reabsorption of water and the electrolytes sodium and potassium at cortical diluting segment of distal tubule. As an antihypertensive, it reduces plasma and extracellular fluid volume and decreases peripheral vascular resistance (PVR) by direct effect on blood vessels. **Therapeutic Effect:** Promotes diuresis, reduces blood pressure (BP).

Pharmacokinetics: Rapidly but incompletely absorbed from the gastrointestinal (GI) tract. Metabolized to metabolite that is extensively bound to red blood cells and has a longer half-life than parent compound. Primarily excreted in urine. Not removed by hemodialysis. **Half-life:** 2-17 hr.

Available Forms:

- *Tablets*: 50 mg (Diucardin, Saluron).

Indications and Dosages:

Edema: PO Initially, 50 mg 2 times/day. Maintenance: 25-200 mg/day.
Hypertension: PO 1 mg/kg/day.

Unlabeled Uses: Treatment of diabetes insipidus

Contraindications: Anuria, history of hypersensitivity to sulfonamides or thiazide diuretics, renal decompensation, pregnancy

Side Effects

Expected
Increase in urine frequency and volume
Frequent
Potassium depletion
Occasional
Postural hypotension, headache, gastrointestinal (GI) disturbances, photosensitivity reaction

Serious Reactions

- Vigorous diuresis may lead to profound water loss and electrolyte depletion, resulting in hypokalemia, hyponatremia, and dehydration.
- Acute hypotensive episodes may occur.
- Hyperglycemia may be noted during prolonged therapy.
- GI upset, pancreatitis, dizziness, paresthesias, headache, blood dyscrasias, pulmonary edema, allergic pneumonitis, and dermatologic reactions occur rarely.
- Overdosage can lead to lethargy and coma without changes in electrolytes or hydration.

Special Considerations

- May protect against osteoporotic hip fractures
- Loop diuretics or metolazone more effective if CrCl less than 40-50 ml/min
- Although allergic cross-reactivity with sulfonamide antibiotics and sulfonamide nonantibiotics has not been demonstrated, use with caution in patients with a history of severe sulfa allergies.

Patient/Family Education

- Will increase urination temporarily (approximately 3 wk); take early in the day to prevent sleep disturbance

- May cause sensitivity to sunlight; avoid prolonged exposure to the sun and other ultraviolet light
- May cause gout attacks; notify clinician if sudden joint pain occurs
- Change positions slowly and let legs dangle momentarily before standing to reduce the drug's hypotensive effect
- Eat foods high in potassium, including apricots, bananas, raisins, orange juice, potatoes, legumes, meat, and whole grains (such as cereals)

■ Monitoring Parameters
- Weight, urine output, serum electrolytes, BUN, creatinine, CBC, uric acid, glucose, lipids
- Blood pressure
- Be especially alert for signs of potassium depletion, such as cardiac arrhythmias, in patients taking digoxin
- Assess the patient for constipation, which may occur with exercise diuresis

■ Geriatric side effects at a glance:
❑ CNS   ❑ Bowel Dysfunction   ❑ Bladder Dysfunction   ❑ Falls

■ U.S. Regulatory Considerations
❑ FDA Black Box   ❑ OBRA regulated in U.S. Long Term Care

hydromorphone hydrochloride

(hye-droe-mor'-fone hye-droe-klor'-ide)

■ Brand Name(s): Dilaudid, Dilaudid-5, Dilaudid HP, Hydromorph, Hydrostat IR
Chemical Class: Opiate derivative; phenanthrene derivative

DEA Class: Schedule II

■ Clinical Pharmacology:
Mechanism of Action: An opioid agonist that binds to opioid receptors in the CNS, reducing the intensity of pain stimuli from sensory nerve endings. **Therapeutic Effect:** Alters the perception of and emotional response to pain; suppresses cough reflex.
Pharmacokinetics:

Route	Onset	Peak	Duration
PO	30 min	90-120 min	4 hr
IV	10-15 min	15-30 min	2-3 hr
IM	15 min	30-60 min	4-5 hr
Subcutaneous	15 min	30-90 min	4 hr
Rectal	15-30 min	N/A	N/A

Well absorbed from the GI tract after IM administration. Widely distributed. Metabolized in the liver. Excreted in urine. **Half-life:** 1-3 hr.

■ **Available Forms:**
- *Liquid:* 1 mg/ml (Dilaudid-5), 5 mg/5 ml (Dilaudid).
- *Tablets:* 2 mg (Dilaudid, Hydrostat IR), 3 mg (Dilaudid, Hydrostat IR), 4 mg (Dilaudid), 8 mg (Dilaudid).
- *Injection:* 1 mg/ml (Dilaudid), 2 mg/ml (Dilaudid), 4 mg/ml (Dilaudid), 10 mg/ml (Dilaudid HP).
- *Suppository (Dilaudid):* 3 mg.

■ **Indications and Dosages:**
Analgesia: PO 2-4 mg q3-4h. Range: 2-8 mg/dose. IV 0.2-0.6 mg q2-3h. Rectal 3 mg q4-8h.
Patient-controlled analgesia (PCA): IV 0.05-0.5 mg at 5-15 min lockout. Maximum (4-hr): 4-6 mg. Epidural Bolus dose of 1-1.5 mg at rate of 0.04-0.4 mg/hr. Demand dose of 0.15 mg at 30-min lockout.
Cough: PO 1 mg q3-4h.

■ **Contraindications:** Respiratory depression in the absence of resuscitative equipment, status asthmaticus

■ **Side Effects**
Frequent
Somnolence, dizziness, hypotension (including orthostatic hypotension), decreased appetite, constipation
Occasional
Confusion, diaphoresis, facial flushing, urine retention, dry mouth, nausea, vomiting, headache, pain at injection site
Rare
Allergic reaction, depression

■ **Serious Reactions**
- Overdose results in respiratory depression, skeletal muscle flaccidity, cold or clammy skin, cyanosis, and extreme somnolence progressing to seizures, stupor, and coma.
- The patient who uses hydromorphone repeatedly may develop a tolerance to the drug's analgesic effect as well as physical dependence.
- This drug may have a prolonged duration of action and cumulative effect in patients with hepatic or renal impairment.

Special Considerations
- Do not administer agonist/antagonist analgesics (i.e., pentazocine, nalbuphine, butorphanol, dezocine, buprenorphine) to patient who has received a prolonged course of hydromorphone (a pure agonist). In opioid-dependent patients, mixed agonist/antagonist analgesics may precipitate withdrawal symptoms.

■ **Patient/Family Education**
- Physical dependency may result when used for extended periods
- Avoid hazardous activities if drowsiness or dizziness occurs
- Avoid alcohol, other CNS depressants unless directed by clinician
- Minimize nausea by administering with food and remain lying down following dose
- Be alert to the onset of pain because the drug is less effective if a full pain response recurs before the next dose
- Change positions slowly to avoid orthostatic hypotension

Monitoring Parameters
- Vital signs
- Pattern of daily bowel activity and stool consistency, especially with long-term use
- Keep in mind that the drug's effect is reduced if the full pain response recurs before the next dose
- For patients being treated for a cough, auscultate the lungs for adventitious breath sounds and increase fluid intake and environmental humidity to decrease the viscosity of lung secretions
- Initiate deep-breathing and coughing exercises, particularly in patients with impaired respiratory function
- Clinical improvement and record the onset of pain or cough relief

Geriatric side effects at a glance:
☑ CNS   ☑ Bowel Dysfunction   ☑ Bladder Dysfunction   ☑ Falls

U.S. Regulatory Considerations
❑ FDA Black Box   ☑ OBRA regulated in U.S. Long Term Care

hydroquinone

(hye-droe-kwin'-one)

Brand Name(s):
Alphaquin HP, Alustra, Claripel, Eldopaque, Eldopaque Forte, Eldoquin, EpiQuin Micro, Esoterica Regular, Glyquin, Lustra, Lustra-AF, Melanex, Melpaque HP, Melquin-3, Melquin HP, Neostrata AHA, Neostrata HQ, Nuquin-HP, Palmer's Skin Success Fade Cream, Solaquin, Solaquin Forte

Combinations
Rx: with fluocinolone/tretinoin (Tri-Luma)
Chemical Class: Monobenzone derivative

Clinical Pharmacology:
Mechanism of Action: A depigmenting agent that suppresses melanocyte metabolic processes of the skin. Inhibits the enzymatic oxidation of tyrosine to DOPA (3, 4-dihydroxyphenylalanine). Sun exposure reverses this effect and causes repigmentation.
Therapeutic Effect: Lightens hyperpigmented areas.
Pharmacokinetics: Onset and duration of depigmentation vary among individuals. About 35% is absorbed.

Available Forms:
- *Cream*: 2% (Eldopaque, Esoterica Regular, Palmer's Skin Success Fade Cream), 4% (Alphaquin HP, Alustra, EpiQuin Micro, Lustra, Melquin HP, Nuquin HP).
- *Cream, with sunscreen*: 2% (Solaquin), 4% (Claripel, Glyquin, Solaquin, Solaquin Forte, Lustra-AF, Melpaque HP).
- *Gel*: 2% (NeoStrata AHA).
- *Gel, with sunscreen*: 4% (Nuquin HP, Solaquin Forte).

■ **Indications and Dosages:**
Hyperpigmentation, melanin: Topical Apply twice daily.

■ **Unlabeled Uses:** None known.

■ **Contraindications:** Hypersensitivity to hydroquinone, sulfites, or any other component of its formulation

■ **Side Effects**
Occasional
Burning, itching, stinging, erythema such as localized contact dermatitis
Rare
Conjunctival changes, fingernail staining

■ **Serious Reactions**
• Gradual blue-black darkening of skin has been reported.
• Occasional cutaneous hypersensitivity (localized contact dermatitis) may occur.

■ **Patient/Family Education**
• Apply small amount to an unbroken patch of skin and check in 24 hr; if vesicle formation, itching, or excessive inflammation occurs, further treatment not advised
• Positive response may require 3 wk-6 mo
• Protect the treated area from UV light by using a sunscreen, sun block, or protective clothing
• Avoid application to lips or near eyes

■ **Monitoring Parameters**
• Skin for any irritation or rash

■ **Geriatric side effects at a glance:**
❑ CNS   ❑ Bowel Dysfunction   ❑ Bladder Dysfunction   ❑ Falls

■ **U.S. Regulatory Considerations**
❑ FDA Black Box   ❑ OBRA regulated in U.S. Long Term Care

hydroxychloroquine sulfate

(hye-drox-ee-klor'-oh-kwin sul'-fate)

■ **Brand Name(s):** Plaquenil
Chemical Class: 4-Aminoquinoline derivative

■ **Clinical Pharmacology:**
Mechanism of Action: An antimalarial and antirheumatic that concentrates in parasite acid vesicles, increasing the pH of the vesicles and interfering with parasite pro-

tein synthesis. Antirheumatic action may involve suppressing formation of antigens responsible for hypersensitivity reactions. **Therapeutic Effect:** Inhibits parasite growth.
Pharmacokinetics: Variable rate of absorption. Widely distributed in body tissues (eyes, kidneys, liver, lungs). Protein binding: 45%. Partially metabolized in liver. Partially excreted in urine. **Half-life:** 32 days (in plasma); 50 days (in blood).

■ **Available Forms:**
- *Tablets*: 200 mg (155 mg base).

■ **Indications and Dosages:**
Rheumatoid arthritis: PO Initially, 400-600 mg (310-465 mg base) daily for 5-10 days, gradually increased to optimum response level. Maintenance (usually within 4-12 wk): Dosage decreased by 50% and then continued at maintenance dose of 200-400 mg/day. Maximum effect may not be seen for several months.
Systemic lupus erythematosus: PO Initially, 400 mg once or twice a day for several weeks or months. Maintenance: 200-400 mg/day.

■ **Unlabeled Uses:** Sarcoid-associated hypercalcemia

■ **Contraindications:** Porphyria, psoriasis, retinal or visual field changes

■ **Side Effects**
Frequent
Mild, transient headache; anorexia; nausea; vomiting
Occasional
Visual disturbances, nervousness, fatigue, pruritus (especially of palms, soles, and scalp), irritability, personality changes, diarrhea
Rare
Stomatitis, dermatitis, impaired hearing

■ **Serious Reactions**
- Ocular toxicity, especially retinopathy, may occur and may progress even after drug is discontinued.
- Prolonged therapy may result in peripheral neuritis, neuromyopathy, hypotension, ECG changes, agranulocytosis, aplastic anemia, thrombocytopenia, seizures, and psychosis.
- Overdosage may result in headache, vomiting, visual disturbances, drowsiness, seizures, and hypokalemia followed by cardiovascular collapse and death.

■ **Patient/Family Education**
- Report any muscle weakness, visual disturbances, difficulty hearing, or ringing in ears to clinician
- Continue taking hydroxychloroquine for the full course of treatment
- Therapeutic response may not be evident for up to 6 mo

■ **Monitoring Parameters**
- Baseline and periodic ophthalmologic examinations (visual acuity, slit lamp, funduscopic, and visual field tests); periodic tests of knee and ankle reflexes to detect muscular weakness
- Periodic CBCs during prolonged therapy
- Liver function test

- Assess the patient's buccal mucosa and skin, and check for pruritus
- Evaluate the patient for GI distress

■ **Geriatric side effects at a glance:**
  ❑ CNS ❑ Bowel Dysfunction ❑ Bladder Dysfunction ❑ Falls

■ **U.S. Regulatory Considerations**
  ☑ FDA Black Box
  - Prescribed by experienced physicians
  ❑ OBRA regulated in U.S. Long Term Care

hydroxyprogesterone

(hi-drox'-se-pro-jes'-ter-one)

■ **Brand Name(s):** Gestrol LA
  Chemical Class: ENDO-progestin derivative

■ **Clinical Pharmacology:**
  Mechanism of Action: A hormone that influences proliferative endometrium and transforms into secretory endometrium. Secretion of pituitary gonadotropins is inhibited which prevents follicular maturation and ovulation. ***Therapeutic Effect***: Facilitates ureteral dilatation associated with hydronephrosis of pregnancy.

■ **Available Forms:**
  - Injection: 250 mg/ml (Gestrol LA).

■ **Indications and Dosages:**
  Endogenous estrogen production : IM 125 to 250 mg beginning on the tenth day of cycle and repeated every 7 days until suppression is no longer desired.
  Endometrial carcinoma: IM 1,000 mg 1 or more times weekly.
  Abnormal uterine bleeding: IM 5-10 mg for 6 days. When estrogen is given concomitantly, begin progesterone after 2 wk of estrogen therapy; discontinue when menstrual flow begins.
  Prevention of endometrial hyperplasia: IM 200 mg in evening for 12 days per 28-day cycle in combination with daily conjugated estrogen.

■ **Unlabeled Uses:** Alopecia, stress incontinence, menopausal symptoms, treatment of prostatic hyperplasia, seborrhea, ureteral stones

■ **Contraindications:** Breast cancer, cerebral apoplexy or history of these conditions, severe liver dysfunction, thromboembolic disorders, thrombophlebitis, undiagnosed vaginal bleeding, genital malignancy

■ **Side Effects**
  Frequent
  Breast tenderness
  Occasional
  Edema, weight gain or loss, rash, pruritus, photosensitivity, skin pigmentation
  Rare
  Pain or swelling at injection site, acne, mental depression, alopecia, hirsutism

- **Serious Reactions**
  - Thrombophlebitis, cerebrovascular disorders, retinal thrombosis, and pulmonary embolism rarely occur.

- **Patient/Family Education**
  - Take protective measures against exposure to UV light or sunlight
  - Notify the physician of abnormal vaginal bleeding or other symptoms
  - Do not smoke tobacco

- **Monitoring Parameters**
  - Weight
  - Blood pressure
  - Skin for rash and urticaria

- **Geriatric side effects at a glance:**
  - ❑ CNS   ❑ Bowel Dysfunction   ❑ Bladder Dysfunction   ❑ Falls

- **U.S. Regulatory Considerations**
  - ❑ FDA Black Box   ❑ OBRA regulated in U.S. Long Term Care

hydroxyzine

(hye-drox'-i-zeen)

- **Brand Name(s):** Atarax, Hyzine, Vistacot, Vistaject-50, Vistaril, Vistaril IM
  Chemical Class: Piperidine derivative

- **Clinical Pharmacology:**
  Mechanism of Action: A piperazine derivative that competes with histamine for receptor sites in the GI tract, blood vessels, and respiratory tract. May exert CNS depressant activity in subcortical areas. Diminishes vestibular stimulation and depresses labyrinthine function. **Therapeutic Effect:** Produces anxiolytic, anticholinergic, antihistaminic, and analgesic effects; relaxes skeletal muscle; controls nausea and vomiting.
  Pharmacokinetics:

Route	Onset	Peak	Duration
PO	15-30 min	N/A	4-6 hr

  Well absorbed from the GI tract and after parenteral administration. Metabolized in the liver. Primarily excreted in urine. Not removed by hemodialysis. **Half-life:** 20-25 hr or greater.

- **Available Forms:**
  - *Capsules (Vistaril):* 25 mg, 50 mg, 100 mg.
  - *Oral Suspension (Vistaril):* 25 mg/5 ml.
  - *Syrup (Atarax):* 10 mg/5 ml.

- *Tablets* (*Atarax*): 10 mg, 25 mg, 50 mg, 100 mg.
- Injection (*Hyzine*, *Vistacot*, *Vistaject-50*, *Vistaril* IM): 25 mg/ml, 50 mg/ml.

■ Indications and Dosages:
Anxiety: PO 25-100 mg 4 times a day. Maximum: 600 mg/day.
Nausea and vomiting: IM 25-100 mg/dose q4-6h.
Pruritus: PO 25 mg 3-4 times a day.
Preoperative sedation: PO 50-100 mg. IM 25-100 mg.

■ Contraindications: None known.

■ Side Effects
Frequent
Side effects are generally mild and transient.
Occasional
Somnolence, dry mouth, marked discomfort with IM injection
Rare
Dizziness, ataxia, asthenia, slurred speech, headache, agitation, increased anxiety
Paradoxical CNS reactions, such as excitement or restlessness in elderly or debilitated patients (generally noted during first 2 wk of therapy, particularly in presence of uncontrolled pain)

■ Serious Reactions
- A hypersensitivity reaction, including wheezing, dyspnea, and chest tightness, may occur.

■ Patient/Family Education
- The IM injection may cause marked discomfort
- Drowsiness usually diminishes with continued therapy
- Avoid tasks that require mental alertness and motor skills until response to the drug has been established
- Take sips of tepid water and chew sugarless gum to help relieve dry mouth

■ Monitoring Parameters
- CBC and blood chemistry tests periodically for patients on long-term therapy
- Breath sounds for signs of a hypersensitivity reaction, such as wheezing
- Electrolytes
- Assess the patient for paradoxical CNS reactions, particularly early in therapy

■ Geriatric side effects at a glance:
☑ CNS ☑ Bowel Dysfunction ☑ Bladder Dysfunction ☐ Falls
Other: Dry mouth, somnolence, restlessness, confusion, psychoses

■ Use with caution in older patients with: Narrow-angle glaucoma, overflow incontinence, orthostatic hypotension.

■ U.S. Regulatory Considerations
☐ FDA Black Box ☑ OBRA regulated in U.S. Long Term Care

■ Other Uses in Geriatric Patient: Allergic rhinitis

■ **Side Effects:**
Of particular importance in the geriatric patient: Anticholinergic effects

■ **Geriatric Considerations - Summary:** Hydroxyzine is a first-generation piperazine antihistamine with potent H_1-receptor antagonism. It has CNS depressant effects, causing drowsiness and has anticholinergric properties. Older adults taking this drug are at risk of dizziness and hypotension. Hydroxyzine can have a prolonged elimination half-life of up to 30 hr in older adults. The use of hydroxyzine to treat anxiety in older adults is limited by the drug's potential for causing adverse effects.

■ **References:**

1. Juniper EF, Stahl E, Doty RL, et al. Clinical outcomes and adverse effect monitoring in allergic rhinitis 2005;115(suppl 1):390-413.
2. Tune LE. Anticholinergic effects of medication in elderly patients. J Clin Psychiatry 2001;62(suppl 21):11-14.

hyoscyamine sulfate

(hye-oh-sye'-a-meen sul'-fate)

■ **Brand Name(s):** A-Spas S/L, Anaspaz, Cystospaz, Cystospaz-M, Donnamar, Hyosine, IV-Stat, Levbid, Levsin, Levsin S/L, Levsinex, Neosol, NuLev, Spacol, Spacol T/S, Spasdel, Symax SL, Symax SR

Combinations
Rx: with phenobarbital (Levsin PB)
Chemical Class: Belladonna alkaloid

■ **Clinical Pharmacology:**
Mechanism of Action: A GI antispasmodic and anticholinergic agent that inhibits the action of acetylcholine at postganglionic (muscarinic) receptor sites. *Therapeutic Effect:* Decreases secretions (bronchial, salivary, sweat gland) and gastric juices and reduces motility of GI and urinary tract.
Pharmacokinetics: Completely absorbed following PO administration. Partially hydrolyzed. Majority of hyoscyamine dose is excreted unchanged in urine. Removed by hemodialysis. *Half-life:* 3.5 hr (immediate-release); 7 hr (sustained-release).

■ **Available Forms:**
• *Tablets (Anaspaz, Cystospaz, Levsin, Spacol):* 0.125 mg.
• *Tablets (Oral-Disintegrating [NuLev]):* 0.125 mg.
• *Tablets (Sublingual [Levsin S/L, Symax SL]):* 0.125 mg.
• *Tablets (Extended-Release [Levbid, Spacol T/S, Symax SR]):* 0.375 mg.
• *Capsules (Extended-Release [Cystospaz-M, Levsinex]):* 0.375 mg.
• *Liquid (Hyosine, Spacol):* 0.125 mg/5 ml.
• *Oral Drops (Hyosine, Levsin):* 0.125 mg/ml.
• *Oral Solution (Hyosine, Levsin):* 0.125 mg/5 ml

605

■ **Indications and Dosages:**
GI tract disorders: PO 0.125–0.25 mg q4h as needed. Extended-release: 0.375-0.75 mg q12h. Maximum: 1.5 mg/day. IV, IM 0.25–0.5 mg q4h for 1–4 doses.
Hypermotility of lower urinary tract: PO, Sublingual 0.15–0.3 mg 4 times a day; or extended-release 0.375 mg q12h.

■ **Contraindications:** GI or GU obstruction, myasthenia gravis, narrow-angle glaucoma, paralytic ileus, severe ulcerative colitis

■ **Side Effects**
Frequent
Dry mouth (sometimes severe), decreased sweating, constipation
Occasional
Blurred vision; bloated feeling; urinary hesitancy; somnolence (with high dosage); headache; intolerance to light; loss of taste; nervousness; flushing; insomnia; impotence; mental confusion or excitement; temporary light-headedness (with parenteral form); local irritation (with parenteral form)
Rare
Dizziness, faintness

■ **Serious Reactions**
• Overdose may produce temporary paralysis of ciliary muscle; pupillary dilation; tachycardia; palpitations; hot, dry, or flushed skin; absence of bowel sounds; hyperthermia; increased respiratory rate; ECG abnormalities; nausea; vomiting; rash over face or upper trunk; CNS stimulation; and psychosis (marked by agitation, restlessness, rambling speech, visual hallucinations, paranoid behavior, and delusions, followed by depression).

■ **Patient/Family Education**
• Dry mouth may occur during hyoscyamine therapy; maintain good oral hygiene because the lack of saliva may increase the risk of cavities
• Notify the physician if constipation, difficulty urinating, eye pain, or rash occurs
• Avoid hot baths and saunas
• Avoid tasks that require mental alertness or motor skills until response to the drug has been established

■ **Monitoring Parameters**
• Pattern of daily bowel activity and stool consistency
• Blood pressure, body temperature

■ **Geriatric side effects at a glance:**
☑ CNS ☑ Bowel Dysfunction ☑ Bladder Dysfunction ☑ Falls
Other: Dry mouth, blurred vision, confusion, psychoses

■ **Use with caution in older patients with:** Narrow-angle glaucoma, overflow incontinence, preexisting psychotic symptoms

■ **U.S. Regulatory Considerations**
❑ FDA Black Box ❑ OBRA regulated in U.S. Long Term Care

■ **Other Uses in Geriatric Patient:** Used to decrease salivation

- **Side Effects:**
  Of particular importance in the geriatric patient: Anticholinergic effects

- **Geriatric Considerations - Summary:** Hyoscyamine and related anticholingerics have limited benefits in the treatment of GI tract disorders and present significant risk to older adults. These drugs possess potent anticholinergic effects and can cause cognitive impairment, delirium, dry mouth, blurred vision, and increased risk of falls. The use of this drug and related compounds should be limited and when used, patients should be closely monitored.

- **References:**
  1. Vangala V, Tueth M. Chronic anticholinergic toxicity: Identification and management in older patients. Geriatrics 2003;58:36-37.
  2. Tune LE. Anticholinergic effects of medication in elderly patients. J Clin Psychiatry 2001;62(suppl 21):11-14.

ibandronate sodium

(i-ban'-droh-nate soe'-dee-um)

- **Brand Name(s):** Boniva
  Chemical Class: Pyrophosphate analog

- **Clinical Pharmacology:**
  Mechanism of Action: A bisphosphonate that binds to bone hydroxyapatite (part of the mineral matrix of bone) and inhibits osteoclast activity. *Therapeutic Effect:* Reduces rate of bone turnover and bone resorption, resulting in a net gain in bone mass. *Pharmacokinetics:* Absorbed in the upper GI tract. Extent of absorption impaired by food or beverages (other than plain water). Rapidly binds to bone. Unabsorbed portion is eliminated in urine. Protein binding: 90%. *Half-life:* 10–60 hr.

- **Available Forms:**
  - *Tablets:* 2.5 mg, 150 mg.

- **Indications and Dosages:**
  Osteoporosis: PO 2.5 mg daily. Alternatively, 150 mg once monthly.

- **Contraindications:** Hypersensitivity to other bisphosphonates, including alendronate, etidronate, pamidronate, risedronate, and tiludronate; inability to stand or sit upright for at least 60 min; severe renal impairment with creatinine clearance less than 30 ml/min; uncorrected hypocalcemia

- **Side Effects**
  Frequent (13%–6%)
  Back pain; dyspepsia, including epigastric distress and heartburn; peripheral discomfort; diarrhea; headache; myalgia
  Occasional (4%–3%)
  Dizziness, arthralgia, asthenia

Rare (2% or less)
Vomiting, hypersensitivity reaction

■ **Serious Reactions**
- Upper respiratory tract infection occurs occasionally.
- Overdose causes hypocalcemia, hypophosphatemia, and significant GI disturbances

Special Considerations
- Clinicians should remain alert to signs or symptoms signaling possible esophageal irritation reaction (dysphagia, retrosternal pain, or heartburn)

■ **Patient/Family Education**
- To maximize absorption and clinical benefit, patients should be instructed to take drug at least 60 min before first food or drink of the day or other oral medications (particularly calcium, antacids, or vitamins)
- To reduce potential for esophageal irritation, patients should be instructed to swallow tablets intact (not chew or suck) with a full glass of plain water (not mineral water) while remaining in the standing or sitting upright position for 60 min
- Patients should receive supplemental calcium and vitamin D if dietary intake is inadequate
- Consider beginning weight-bearing exercises and modifying behavioral factors, such as reducing alcohol consumption and stopping cigarette smoking

■ **Monitoring Parameters**
- Bone mass density (T-score, hip, spine), N-telopeptide; serum calcium (adjusted for hypoalbuminemia), phosphorus, magnesium, renal function, liver function, serum electrolytes, signs and symptoms of toxicity (i.e., esophageal irritation)

■ **Geriatric side effects at a glance:**
❑ CNS ❑ Bowel Dysfunction ❑ Bladder Dysfunction ❑ Falls

■ **U.S. Regulatory Considerations**
❑ FDA Black Box ❑ OBRA regulated in U.S. Long Term Care

ibuprofen

(eye-byoo'-proe-fen)

■ **Brand Name(s):** Advil, Ibu, Ibu-4, Ibu-6, Ibu-8, Ibu-Tab, Motrin
OTC: Advil, Advil Migraine, Arthritis Foundation Pain Reliever, Ibuprin, Menadol, Motrin IB, Nuprin

Combinations
Rx: with hydrocodone (Vicoprofen); with oxycodone (Combunox)
OTC: With pseudoephedrine (Sine-Aid IB, Motrin IB Sinus)
Chemical Class: Propionic acid derivative

■ Clinical Pharmacology:

Mechanism of Action: An NSAID that inhibits prostaglandin synthesis. Also produces vasodilation by acting centrally on the heat-regulating center of the hypothalamus. **Therapeutic Effect:** Produces analgesic and anti-inflammatory effects and decreases fever.

Pharmacokinetics:

Route	Onset	Peak	Duration
PO (analgesic)	0.5 hr	N/A	4–6 hr
PO (antirheumatic)	2 days	1–2 wk	N/A

Rapidly absorbed from the GI tract. Protein binding: greater than 90%. Metabolized in the liver. Primarily excreted in urine. Not removed by hemodialysis. **Half-life:** 2–4 hr.

■ Available Forms:

- *Caplets* (Advil, Menadol, Motrin): 200 mg.
- *Capsules* (Advil, Advil Migraine): 200 mg.
- *Gelcaps* (Advil, Motrin IB): 200 mg.
- *Tablets*: 200 mg (Advil, Motrin IB), 400 mg (Ibu, Ibu-4, Ibu-6, Ibu-8, Ibu-Tab, Motrin), 600 mg (Ibu, Ibu-4, Ibu-6, Ibu-8, Ibu-Tab, Motrin), 800 mg (Ibu, Ibu-4, Ibu-6, Ibu-8, Ibu-Tab, Motrin).
- *Oral Suspension* (Advil): 100 mg/5 ml.

■ Indications and Dosages:

Acute or chronic rheumatoid arthritis, osteoarthritis, migraine pain, gouty arthritis: PO 400–800 mg 3–4 times a day. Maximum: 3.2 g/day.
Mild to moderate pain: PO 200–400 mg q4–6h as needed. Maximum: 1.6 g/day.
Fever, minor aches or pain: PO 200–400 mg q4–6h. Maximum: 1.6 g/day.

■ Unlabeled Uses: Treatment of psoriatic arthritis, vascular headaches

■ Contraindications: Active peptic ulcer, chronic inflammation of GI tract, GI bleeding disorders or ulceration, history of hypersensitivity to aspirin or NSAIDs

■ Side Effects

Occasional (9%–3%)
Nausea with or without vomiting, dyspepsia, dizziness, rash
Rare (less than 3%)
Diarrhea or constipation, flatulence, abdominal cramps or pain, pruritus

■ Serious Reactions

- Acute overdose may result in metabolic acidosis.
- Rare reactions with long-term use include peptic ulcer disease, GI bleeding, gastritis, a severe hepatic reaction (cholestasis, jaundice), nephrotoxicity (dysuria, hematuria, proteinuria, nephrotic syndrome), and a severe hypersensitivity reaction (particularly in patients with systemic lupus erythematosus or other collagen diseases).

Special Considerations

- Administer with food or antacids if GI symptoms occur

■ Patient/Family Education

- Do not chew or crush enteric-coated ibuprofen tablets
- Ibuprofen may cause dizziness

- Avoid alcohol and aspirin during ibuprofen therapy because these substances increase the risk of GI bleeding
- Avoid performing tasks that require mental alertness or motor skills until response to the drug has been established

■ **Monitoring Parameters**
- Initial hematocrit and fecal occult blood test within 3 mo of starting regular chronic therapy; repeat every 6-12 mo (more frequently in high-risk patients, >65 years, peptic ulcer disease, concurrent steroids or anticoagulants); electrolytes, creatinine, and BUN within 3 mo of starting regular chronic therapy; repeat every 6-12 mo
- Body temperature for fever
- CBC, platelet count, serum alkaline phosphatase, bilirubin, AST (SGOT), and ALT (SGPT) levels
- Pattern of daily bowel activity and stool consistency
- Therapeutic response, such as improved grip strength, increased joint mobility, and decreased pain, tenderness, stiffness, and swelling

■ **Geriatric side effects at a glance:**
☑ CNS ☐ Bowel Dysfunction ☐ Bladder Dysfunction ☐ Falls
☑ Other: Gastropathy

■ **Use with caution in older patients with:** Renal impairment, Hepatic impairment, CHF, HTN, PUD, History of GI bleeding, GERD, Bleeding and platelet disorders, History of aspirin sensitivity reaction. Also use with caution in patients taking Anticoagulants, Aspirin, and Antihypertensive agents.

■ **U.S. Regulatory Considerations**
☑ FDA Black Box
- Cardiovascular problems
- Gastrointestinal problems
☐ OBRA regulated in U.S. Long Term Care

■ **Other Uses in Geriatric Patient:** Acute gout

■ **Side Effects:**
Of particular importance in the geriatric patient: Confusion, cognitive impairment, delirium, dizziness, dyspepsia, fluid retention, renal impairment

■ **Geriatric Considerations - Summary:** A preferred agent in older adults due to its association with fewer GI adverse effects. Use of NSAIDs in older adults increases the risk of GI complications including gastric ulceration, bleeding, and perforation. These complications are not necessarily preceded by less severe GI symptoms. Concomitant use of a proton pump inhibitor or misoprostol reduces the risk for gastric ulceration and bleeding, but may not prevent long-term GI toxicity.

■ **References:**
1. COX-2 alternatives and GI protection. Med Lett Drugs Ther 2004;46:91.
2. Drugs that may cause cognitive disorders in the elderly. Med Lett Drugs Ther 2000;42:111-112.

ibutilide fumarate

(eye-byoo'-ti-lide fyoo'-muh-rate)

- **Brand Name(s):** Corvert
  Chemical Class: Methanesulfonamide derivative

- **Clinical Pharmacology:**
  Mechanism of Action: An antiarrhythmic that prolongs both atrial and ventricular action potential duration and increases the atrial and ventricular refractory period. Activates slow, inward current (mostly of sodium), produces mild slowing of sinus node rate and AV conduction, and causes dose-related prolongation of QT interval. **Therapeutic Effect:** Converts arrhythmias to sinus rhythm.
  Pharmacokinetics: After IV administration, highly distributed, rapidly cleared. Protein binding: 40%. Primarily excreted in urine as metabolite. **Half-life:** 2–12 hr (average: 6 hr).

- **Available Forms:**
  - *Injection:* 0.1 mg/ml solution.

- **Indications and Dosages:**
  Rapid conversion of atrial fibrillation or flutter of recent onset to normal sinus rhythm: IV Infusion *Weight 60 kg and more.* One vial (1 mg) given over 10 min. If arrhythmia does not stop within 10 min after end of initial infusion, a second 1 mg/10-min infusion may be given. *Weight less than 60 kg.* 0.01 mg/kg given over 10 min. If arrhythmia does not stop within 10 min after end of initial infusion, a second 0.01 mg/kg, 10-min infusion may be given.

- **Contraindications:** None known.

- **Side Effects**
  Ibutilide is generally well tolerated.
  Occasional
  Ventricular extrasystoles (5.1%), ventricular tachycardia (4.9%), headache (3.6%), hypotension, orthostatic hypotension (2%)
  Rare
  Bundle-branch block, AV block, bradycardia, hypertension

- **Serious Reactions**
  - Sustained polymorphic ventricular tachycardia, occasionally with QT prolongation (torsades de pointes) occurs rarely.
  - Overdose results in CNS toxicity, including CNS depression, rapid gasping breathing, and seizures.
  - Expect that prolongation of repolarization may be exaggerated.
  - Existing arrhythmias may worsen or new arrhythmias may develop.

- **Patient/Family Education**
  - Blood pressure and ECG will be continuously monitored during therapy
  - Immediately report palpitations or other adverse reactions

611

■ **Monitoring Parameters**
  - Continuous ECG monitoring for at least 4 hr following infusion or until QTc returns to baseline (longer monitoring if dysrhythmic activity noted). Defibrillator must be available
  - Blood pressure

■ **Geriatric side effects at a glance:**
  ❑ CNS ❑ Bowel Dysfunction ❑ Bladder Dysfunction ❑ Falls

■ **U.S. Regulatory Considerations**
  ☑ FDA Black Box
  - Potentially fatal arrhythmias have occurred. This drug's administration requires a setting with continuous ECG monitoring and personnel trained in identification and treatment of acute ventricular arrhythmias.
  - Patients with chronic atrial fibrillation have a strong tendency to revert after conversion to sinus rhythm. Treatment to maintain sinus rhythms carries risks. Patients should be carefully selected for ibutilide therapy.
  ❑ OBRA regulated in U.S. Long Term Care

iloprost

(eye'-loe-prost)

■ **Brand Name(s):** Ventavis

■ **Clinical Pharmacology:**
  Mechanism of Action: A prostaglandin that dilates systemic and pulmonary arterial vascular beds, alters pulmonary vascular resistance, and suppresses vascular smooth muscle proliferation. **Therapeutic Effect:** Improves symptoms and exercise tolerance in patients with pulmonary hypertension; delays deterioration of condition.
  Pharmacokinetics: Protein binding: 60%. Metabolized in liver. Primarily excreted in urine; minimal elimination in feces. **Half-life:** 20-30 min.

■ **Available Forms:**
  - *Solution for Oral Inhalation*: 10 mcg/ml (2-ml ampule).

■ **Indications and Dosages:**
  Pulmonary hypertension in patients with NYHA Class III or IV symptoms: Oral Inhalation Initially, 2.5 mcg/dose; if tolerated, increased to 5 mcg/dose. Administer 6-9 times a day at intervals of 2 hr or longer while patient is awake. Maintenance: 5 mcg/dose. Maximum daily dose: 45 mcg.

■ **Contraindications:** None known.

■ **Side Effects**
  Frequent (39%-27%)
  Increased cough, headache, flushing

Occasional (13%-11%)
Flu-like symptoms, nausea, lockjaw, jaw pain, hypotension
Rare (8%-2%)
Insomnia, syncope, palpitations, vomiting, back pain, muscle cramps

- **Serious Reactions**
  - Hemoptysis and pneumonia occur occasionally.
  - CHF, renal failure, dyspnea, and chest pain occur rarely.

- **Geriatric side effects at a glance:**
  ❏ CNS ❏ Bowel Dysfunction ❏ Bladder Dysfunction ❏ Falls

- **U.S. Regulatory Considerations**
  ❏ FDA Black Box ❏ OBRA regulated in U.S. Long Term Care

imatinib mesylate

(im'-a-tin-ib mes'-sil-ate)

- **Brand Name(s):** Gleevec
  Chemical Class: Phenylaminopyrimidine derivative

- **Clinical Pharmacology:**
  Mechanism of Action: Inhibits Bcr-Abl tyrosine kinase, an enzyme created by the Philadelphia chromosome abnormality found in patients with chronic myeloid leukemia (CML). **Therapeutic Effect:** Suppresses tumor growth during the three stages of CML: blast crisis, accelerated phase, and chronic phase.
  Pharmacokinetics: Well absorbed after PO administration. Binds to plasma proteins, particularly albumin. Metabolized in the liver. Eliminated mainly in the feces as metabolites. **Half-life:** 18 hr.

- **Available Forms:**
  - *Tablets*: 100 mg, 400 mg.
  - *Capsules*: 100 mg.

- **Indications and Dosages:**
  CML: PO 400 mg/day for patients in chronic-phase CML; 600 mg/day for patients in accelerated phase or blast crisis. May increase dosage from 400-600 mg/day for patients in chronic phase or from 600-800 mg (given as 300-400 mg twice a day) for patients in accelerated phase or blast crisis in the absence of a severe drug reaction or severe neutropenia or thrombocytopenia in the following circumstances: progression of the disease, failure to achieve a satisfactory hematologic response after 3 mo or more of treatment, or loss of a previously achieved hematologic response.
  GI stromal tumors: PO 400 or 600 mg once daily

- **Contraindications:** None known.

■ **Side Effects**
Frequent (68%-24%)
Nausea, diarrhea, vomiting, headache, fluid retention (periorbital, lower extremities), rash, musculoskeletal pain, muscle cramps, arthralgia
Occasional (23%-10%)
Abdominal pain, cough, myalgia, fatigue, fever, anorexia, dyspepsia, constipation, night sweats, pruritus
Rare (less than 10%)
Nasopharyngitis, petechiae, asthenia, epistaxis

■ **Serious Reactions**
- Severe fluid retention (manifested as pleural effusion, pericardial effusion, pulmonary edema, and ascites) and hepatotoxicity occur rarely.
- Neutropenia and thrombocytopenia are expected responses to the drug.
- Respiratory toxicity, manifested as dyspnea and pneumonia, may occur.

Special Considerations
- Median time to hematologic response 1 mo
- Manage fluid retention with interruption of therapy, diuretics, dose reduction
- If bilirubin increases >3 × upper limits normal (ULN) or transaminases >5 × ULN, withhold until bilirubin <1.5 × ULN and transaminases <2.5 × ULN; reduce dose and continue treatment
- If in chronic phase and ANC <1 × 10^9/L and/or platelets <50 × 10^9/L, stop therapy until ANC = 1.5 × 10^9/L and platelets = 75 × 10^9/L, resume at reduced dose; if patient in accelerated phase or blast crisis, check if cytopenia related to leukemia

■ **Patient/Family Education**
- Take with food and large glass of water to minimize GI side effects
- Avoid acetaminophen (hepatotoxicity)
- Numerous drugs may interact with imatinib, discuss with prescriber
- Avoid receiving vaccinations and coming in contact with crowds, people with known infections, and anyone who has recently received a live-virus vaccine

■ **Monitoring Parameters**
- Follow weights and monitor for fluid retention
- LFTs before treatment and every month, CBC, serum chemistry, bone marrow assessment (including cytogenic analysis)
- Pattern of daily bowel activity and stool consistency

■ **Geriatric side effects at a glance:**
❑ CNS ☑ Bowel Dysfunction ❑ Bladder Dysfunction ❑ Falls

■ **U.S. Regulatory Considerations**
❑ FDA Black Box ❑ OBRA regulated in U.S. Long Term Care

imipenem cilastatin sodium

(i-mi-pen'-em sye-la-stat'-in soe'-dee-um)

- **Brand Name(s):** Primaxin IM, Primaxin IV
  Chemical Class: Carbapenem; renal dipeptidase inhibitor (cilistatin); thienamycin derivative

- **Clinical Pharmacology:**
  Mechanism of Action: A fixed-combination carbapenem. Imipenem penetrates the bacterial cell membrane and binds to penicillin-binding proteins, inhibiting cell wall synthesis. Cilastatin competitively inhibits the enzyme dehydropeptidase, preventing renal metabolism of imipenem. **Therapeutic Effect:** Produces bacterial cell death.
  Pharmacokinetics: Readily absorbed after IM administration. Protein binding: 13%-21%. Widely distributed. Metabolized in the kidneys. Primarily excreted in urine. Removed by hemodialysis. **Half-life:** 1 hr (increased in impaired renal function).

- **Available Forms:**
  - IV Injection (Primaxin IV): 250 mg, 500 mg.
  - IM Injection (Primaxin IM): 500 mg, 750 mg.

- **Indications and Dosages:**
  Serious respiratory tract, skin and skin-structure, gynecologic, bone, joint, intra-abdominal, nosocomial, and polymicrobic infections; UTIs; endocarditis; septicemia: IV 2-4 g/day in divided doses q6h.
  Mild to moderate respiratory tract, skin and skin-structure, gynecologic, bone, joint, intra-abdominal, and polymicrobic infections; UTIs; endocarditis; septicemia: IV 1-2 g/day in divided doses q6–8h. IM 500-750 mg q12h.
  Dosage in renal impairment: Dosage and frequency are modified based on creatinine clearance and the severity of the infection.

Creatinine Clearance	Dosage (IV)
31-70 ml/min	500 mg q8h
21-30 ml/min	500 mg q12h
5-20 ml/min	250 mg q12h

- **Contraindications:** IM: Severe shock or heart block, hypersensitivity to local anesthetics of the amide type.
  IV: Meningitis.

- **Side Effects**
  Occasional (3%-2%)
  Diarrhea, nausea, vomiting
  Rare (2%-1%)
  Rash

- **Serious Reactions**
  - Antibiotic-associated colitis and other superinfections may occur.
  - Anaphylactic reactions have been reported.

• Individualize treatment based on local susceptibility patterns.

■ **Patient/Family Education**
• Notify the physician if severe diarrhea occurs

■ **Monitoring Parameters**
• Liver and renal function
• Daily bowel activity and stool consistency. Although mild GI effects may be tolerable, severe symptoms may indicate the onset of antibiotic-associated colitis.
• Signs and symptoms of superinfection include abdominal pain or cramping, anal or genital pruritus or discharge, moderate to severe diarrhea, severe mouth or tongue soreness, and new or increased fever.

■ **Geriatric side effects at a glance:**
❑ CNS   ☑ Bowel Dysfunction   ❑ Bladder Dysfunction   ❑ Falls

■ **U.S. Regulatory Considerations**
❑ FDA Black Box   ❑ OBRA regulated in U.S. Long Term Care

imipramine

(im-ip'-ra-meen)

■ **Brand Name(s):** Tofranil, Tofranil PM
Chemical Class: Dibenzazepine derivative; tertiary amine

■ **Clinical Pharmacology:**
Mechanism of Action: A tricyclic antidepressant, antineuralgic, and antineuritic agent that blocks the reuptake of neurotransmitters, such as norepinephrine and serotonin, at presynaptic membranes, increasing their concentration at postsynaptic receptor sites. **Therapeutic Effect:** Relieves depression and controls nocturnal enuresis.
Pharmacokinetics: Rapidly, well absorbed following PO administration. Protein binding: more than 90%. Metabolized in liver, with first-pass effect. Excreted in urine as metabolites. **Half-life:** 6-18 hr.

■ **Available Forms:**
• *Tablets (Tofranil)*: 10 mg, 25 mg, 50 mg.
• *Capsules (Tofranil*-PM): 75 mg, 100 mg, 125 mg, 150 mg.

■ **Indications and Dosages:**
Depression: PO Initially, 10-25 mg/day at bedtime. May increase by 10-25 mg every 3-7 days. Range: 50-150 mg/day.

■ **Unlabeled Uses:** Treatment of cataplexy associated with narcolepsy, neurogenic pain, panic disorder

- **Contraindications:** Acute recovery period after MI, use within 14 days of MAOIs

- **Side Effects**
  Frequent
  Somnolence, fatigue, dry mouth, blurred vision, constipation, delayed micturition, orthostatic hypotension, diaphoresis, impaired concentration, increased appetite, urine retention, photosensitivity.
  Occasional
  GI disturbances (nausea, metallic taste).
  Rare
  Paradoxical reactions (agitation, restlessness, nightmares, insomnia), extrapyramidal symptoms (particularly fine hand tremor).

- **Serious Reactions**
  - Overdose may produce seizures; cardiovascular effects, such as severe orthostatic hypotension, dizziness, tachycardia, palpitations, and arrhythmias; and altered temperature regulation, including hyperpyrexia or hypothermia.
  - Abrupt discontinuation after prolonged therapy may produce headache, malaise, nausea, vomiting, and vivid dreams.

- **Patient/Family Education**
  - Withdrawal symptoms (headache, nausea, vomiting, muscle pain, weakness) may occur if drug discontinued abruptly
  - At doses of 20 mg/kg ventricular arrhythmias occur
  - Improvement may occur 2-5 days after starting therapy but the full therapeutic effect will likely occur within 2-3 wk
  - Change positions slowly to help prevent dizziness
  - The patient will develop tolerance to the drug's anticholinergic, hypotensive, and sedative effects during early therapy
  - Avoid tasks that require mental alertness or motor skills until response to the drug has been established
  - Take sips of tepid water and chew sugarless gum to relieve dry mouth

- **Monitoring Parameters**
  - Closely monitor suicidal patients during early therapy. As depression lessens, the patient's energy level generally improves, increasing the likelihood of suicide attempts
  - Assess the patient's appearance, behavior, level of interest, mood, and sleep pattern before and during therapy
  - Pattern of daily bowel activity and stool consistency
  - Blood pressure, pulse rate
  - Evidence of urine retention
  - Though not used clinically, the therapeutic serum level for imipramine is 225 to 300 ng/ml; the toxic serum level is greater than 500 ng/ml

- **Geriatric side effects at a glance:**
  ☑ CNS ☑ Bowel Dysfunction ☑ Bladder Dysfunction ☑ Falls
  Other: Orthostatic hypotension, cardiac conduction disturbances, anticholinergic side effects

- **Use with caution in older patients with:** Cardiovascular disease, prostatic hypertrophy or other conditions which increase the risk of urinary retention

- **U.S. Regulatory Considerations**
  - ☑ FDA Black Box
  - Because there is an increased risk of suicide in children and adolescents, older adults should also be closely monitored for suicide ideation.
  - ☑ OBRA regulated in U.S. Long Term Care

- **Other Uses in Geriatric Patient:** Neuropathic pain, urge urinary incontinence

- **Side Effects:**
  Of particular importance in the geriatric patient: Anticholinergic effects, extrapyramidal symptoms, high doses (>100 mg) may increase risk of sudden death

- **Geriatric Considerations - Summary:** Although tricyclic antidepressants are effective in the treatment of major depression in older adults, the side-effect profile and low toxic-to-therapeutic ratio relegate them to second-line agents (after serotonin reuptake inhibitors) for most older patients. These agents are effective in the treatment of urge urinary incontinence and neuropathic pain, but must be monitored closely. Of the tricyclic antidepressants, imipramine and amitryptyline have the highest anticholinergic activity and may be best choice in this class for management of incontinence, but should otherwise be avoided.

- **References:**
  1. Leipzig RM, Cumming RG, Tinetti ME. Drugs and falls in older people: a systematic review and meta-analysis: I. Psychotropic drugs. J Am Geriatr Soc 1999;47:30-39.
  2. Cadieux RJ. Antidepressant drug interactions in the elderly. Understanding the P-450 system is half the battle in reducing risks. Postgrad Med 1999;106:231-240, 245.
  3. Ray WA, Meredith S, Thapa PB, et al. Cyclic antidepressants and the risk of sudden cardiac death. Clin Pharmacol Ther 2004;75:234-241.
  4. Roose SP, Laghrissi-Thode F, Kennedy JS, et al. Comparison of paroxetine and nortriptyline in depressed patients with ischemic heart disease. JAMA 1998;279:287-291.

imiquimod

(i-mi-kwi'-mod)

- **Brand Name(s):** Aldara
  Chemical Class: Imidazoquinoline amine

- **Clinical Pharmacology:**
  Mechanism of Action: An immune response modifier whose mechanism of action is unknown. **Therapeutic Effect:** Reduces genital and perianal warts.
  Pharmacokinetics: Minimal absorption after topical administration. Minimal excretion in urine and feces.

- **Available Forms:**
  - *Cream:* 5% (Aldara).

- ■ **Indications and Dosages:**
  Warts/condylomata acuminata: Topical Apply 3 times/wk before normal sleeping hours; leave on skin 6-10 hr. Remove following treatment period. Continue therapy for maximum of 16 wk.

- ■ **Contraindications:** History of hypersensitivity to imiquimod

- ■ **Side Effects**
  Frequent
  Local skin reactions: erythema, itching, burning, erosion, excoriation /flaking, fungal infections (women)
  Occasional
  Pain, induration, ulceration, scabbing, soreness, headache, flulike symptoms

- ■ **Serious Reactions**
  - None reported.

Special Considerations
  - New option for treatment of genital and perianal warts which can be applied by patient at home and appears to have low toxicity compared to podofilox
  - Response rates approximately 50% and relapses are common

- ■ **Patient/Family Education**
  - Apply thin layer to wart(s) and rub in until cream is no longer visible
  - Do not occlude application site
  - Should severe local reaction occur, remove cream by washing with soap and water; treatment may be resumed once skin reaction has subsided
  - Wash hands before and after application

- ■ **Monitoring Parameters**
  - Skin for local reaction

- ■ **Geriatric side effects at a glance:**
  ❑ CNS   ❑ Bowel Dysfunction   ❑ Bladder Dysfunction   ❑ Falls

- ■ **U.S. Regulatory Considerations**
  ❑ FDA Black Box   ❑ OBRA regulated in U.S. Long Term Care

inamrinone lactate

(in-am'-ri-nohn lack'-tate)

- ■ **Brand Name(s):** Inamrinone
  Chemical Class: Bipyridine derivative

- ■ **Clinical Pharmacology:**
  Mechanism of Action: A positive inotropic agent that inhibits myocardial cyclic adenosine monophosphate (cAMP) phosphodiesterase activity and directly stimulates

cardiac contractility. Peripheral vasodilation reduces both preload and afterload. **Therapeutic Effect:** Reduces preload and afterload; increases cardiac output. **Pharmacokinetics:** After IV administration, rapidly absorbed from the gastrointestinal (GI) tract. Protein binding: 10%-49%. Partially metabolized in liver. Excreted in urine as both inamrinone and its metabolites. **Half-life:** 3-6 hr (half-life increased with congestive heart failure).

■ Available Forms:
- *Injection:* 5mg/ml (Inamrinone).

■ Indications and Dosages:
Short-term management of intractable heart failure: IV Infusion (Continuous) Initially, 0.75 mg/kg loading dose over 2-3 minutes followed by a maintenance infusion of 5 and 10 mcg/kg/min. A bolus dose of 0.75 mg/kg may be given 30 minutes after the initiation of therapy. Use within 24 hours and do not dilute with solutions that contain dextrose. Maximum: 10 mg/kg/day.

■ Contraindications:
Severe aortic or pulmonic valvular disease; hypersensitivity to inamrinone or bisulfites.

■ Side Effects
Occasional
Arrhythmia, nausea, hypotension, thrombocytopenia
Rare
Fever, vomiting, abdominal pain, anorexia, chest pain, decreased tear production, hepatotoxicity, and burning at the site of injection, hypersensitivity to inamrinone

■ Serious Reactions
- Overdose may cause severe hypotension.

■ Patient/Family Education
- Report dizziness or trouble swallowing

■ Monitoring Parameters
- BP and pulse q5 min during infusion; if BP drops 30 mm Hg, stop infusion
- Cardiac output and pulmonary capillary wedge pressure
- Monitor platelet count and serum K, Na, Cl, Ca, BUN, creatinine, ALT, AST, and bilirubin daily

■ Geriatric side effects at a glance:
❑ CNS ❑ Bowel Dysfunction ❑ Bladder Dysfunction ❑ Falls

■ U.S. Regulatory Considerations
❑ FDA Black Box ❑ OBRA regulated in U.S. Long Term Care

indapamide

(in-dap'-a-mide)

■ **Brand Name(s):** Lozol
Chemical Class: Indoline derivative

■ **Clinical Pharmacology:**
Mechanism of Action: A thiazide-like diuretic that blocks reabsorption of water, sodium, and potassium at the cortical diluting segment of the distal tubule; also reduces plasma and extracellular fluid volume and peripheral vascular resistance by direct effect on blood vessels. **Therapeutic Effect:** Promotes diuresis and reduces BP.
Pharmacokinetics: Almost completely absorbed following PO administration. Protein binding: 71%-79%. Extensively metabolized in liver. Excreted in urine. **Half-life:** 14-15 hr.

■ **Available Forms:**
• *Tablets*: 1.25 mg, 2.5 mg.

■ **Indications and Dosages:**
Edema: PO Initially, 2.5 mg/day, may increase to 5 mg/day after 1 wk.
Hypertension: PO Initially, 1.25 mg, may increase to 2.5 mg/day after 4 wk or 5 mg/day after additional 4 wk.

■ **Contraindications:** Anuria, hypersensitivity to sulfonamides

■ **Side Effects**
Frequent (5% and greater)
Fatigue, numbness of extremities, tension, irritability, agitation, headache, dizziness, light-headedness, insomnia, muscle cramps
Occasional (less than 5%)
Tingling of extremities, urinary frequency, urticaria, rhinorrhea, flushing, weight loss, orthostatic hypotension, depression, blurred vision, nausea, vomiting, diarrhea or constipation, dry mouth, impotence, rash, pruritus

■ **Serious Reactions**
• Vigorous diuresis may lead to profound water and electrolyte depletion, resulting in hypokalemia, hyponatremia, and dehydration.
• Acute hypotensive episodes may occur.
• Hyperglycemia may occur during prolonged therapy.
• Pancreatitis, blood dyscrasias, pulmonary edema, allergic pneumonitis, and dermatologic reactions occur rarely.
• Overdose can lead to lethargy and coma without changes in electrolytes or hydration.

■ **Patient/Family Education**
• May cause sensitivity to sunlight; avoid prolonged exposure to the sun and other ultraviolet light

- May cause gout attacks; notify clinician if sudden joint pain occurs
- May worsen control or increase requirements of hypoglycemic agents
- Take indapamide early in the day to avoid urination at night
- Change positions slowly and let legs dangle momentarily before standing to reduce the drug's hypotensive effect
- Eat foods high in potassium, such as apricots, bananas, raisins, orange juice, potatoes, legumes, meat, and whole grains (such as cereals)
- Although allergic cross-reactivity with sulfonamide antibiotics and sulfonamide nonantibiotics has not been demonstrated, use with caution in patients with a history of severe sulfa allergies.

■ **Monitoring Parameters**
- Weight, urine output, serum electrolytes, BUN, creatinine, CBC, uric acid, glucose, lipids
- Blood pressure

■ **Geriatric side effects at a glance:**
❑ CNS ❑ Bowel Dysfunction ❑ Bladder Dysfunction ❑ Falls

■ **U.S. Regulatory Considerations**
❑ FDA Black Box ❑ OBRA regulated in U.S. Long Term Care

indinavir

(in-din'-a-veer)

■ **Brand Name(s):** Crixivan
Chemical Class: Protease inhibitor, HIV

■ **Clinical Pharmacology:**
Mechanism of Action: A protease inhibitor that suppresses HIV protease, an enzyme necessary for splitting viral polyprotein precursors into mature and infectious viral particles. **Therapeutic Effect:** Interrupts HIV replication, slowing the progression of HIV infection.
Pharmacokinetics: Rapidly absorbed after PO administration. Protein binding: 60%. Metabolized in the liver. Primarily excreted in urine. Unknown if removed by hemodialysis. **Half-life:** 1.8 hr (increased in impaired hepatic function).

■ **Available Forms:**
- *Capsules:* 100 mg, 200 mg, 333 mg, 400 mg.

■ **Indications and Dosages:**
HIV infection (in combination with other antiretrovirals): PO 800 mg (two 400-mg capsules) q8h. Dosage adjustments when given concomitantly **Delavirdine, itraconazole, ketoconazole:** Reduce dose to 600 mg q8h. **Efavirenz:** Increase dose to 1,000 mg q8h. **Lopinavir/ritonavir:** Reduce dose to 600 mg twice a day. **Nevirapine:** Increase dose to 1,000 mg q8h. **Rifabutin:** Reduce rifabutin by ½ and increase indinavir to 1,000 mg q8h. **Ritonavir:** 100-200 mg twice a day and indinavir 800 mg twice a day or ritonavir 400 mg twice a day and indinavir 400 mg twice a day.

HIV *infection in patients with hepatic insufficiency*: PO 600 mg q8h.

■ **Unlabeled Uses:** Prophylaxis following occupational exposure to HIV

■ **Contraindications:** Concurrent use with terfenadine, cisapride, astemizole, triazolam, midazolam, pimozide, ergot derivatives; nephrolithiasis

■ **Side Effects**

Frequent
Nausea (12%), abdominal pain (9%), headache (6%), diarrhea (5%)
Occasional
Vomiting, asthenia, fatigue (4%); insomnia; accumulation of fat in waist, abdomen, or back of neck
Rare
Abnormal taste sensation, heartburn, symptomatic urinary tract disease, transient renal dysfunction

■ **Serious Reactions**
  • Nephrolithiasis (flank pain with or without hematuria) occurs in 4% of patients.

Special Considerations
  • Antiretroviral activity of indinavir may be increased when used in combination with reverse transcriptase inhibitors
  • Always check updated treatment guidelines before initiating or changing antiretroviral therapy. (http://AIDSinfo.nih.gov)

■ **Patient/Family Education**
  • Drink plenty of water, at least 48 oz/day
  • Take with water or light, low-fat meals (dry toast, apple juice, corn flakes, skim milk). High fat meals and grapefruit juice reduce absorption
  • Capsules sensitive to moisture. Keep desiccant in bottle
  • If dose is missed, take next dose on schedule; do not double this dose
  • Separate dosing with didanosine by 1 hr
  • Take 1 hr before or 2 hr after meals; may take with skim milk or low-fat meal

■ **Monitoring Parameters**
  • Serum amylase, bilirubin, cholesterol, lipase, and triglyceride levels; blood glucose level; CBC; CD4+ cell count; and liver function test results
  • Monitor for signs and symptoms of nephrolithiasis (flank pain and hematuria), and notify the physician if symptoms occur; if nephrolithiasis occurs, expect therapy to be interrupted for 1-3 days
  • Pattern of daily bowel activity and stool consistency

■ **Geriatric side effects at a glance:**
  ❑ CNS ☑ Bowel Dysfunction ❑ Bladder Dysfunction ❑ Falls

■ **U.S. Regulatory Considerations**
  ❑ FDA Black Box ❑ OBRA regulated in U.S. Long Term Care

indomethacin

(in-doe-meth'-a-sin)

■ **Brand Name(s):** Indocin, Indocin IV, Indocin SR, Indo-Lemmon
Chemical Class: Indole acetic acid derivative

■ **Clinical Pharmacology:**
Mechanism of Action: An NSAID that produces analgesic and anti-inflammatory effects by inhibiting prostaglandin synthesis. Also increases the sensitivity of the premature ductus to the dilating effects of prostaglandins. **Therapeutic Effect:** Reduces the inflammatory response and intensity of pain. Closure of the patent ductus arteriosus.
Pharmacokinetics: Rectal absorption more rapid than oral administration. Protein binding: 99%. Metabolized in liver. Excreted in urine. **Half-life:** 4.5 hr.

■ **Available Forms:**
- *Capsules (Indocin)*: 25 mg, 50 mg.
- *Capsules (Sustained-Release [Indocin SR])*: 75 mg.
- *Oral Suspension (Indocin)*: 25 mg/5 ml.
- *Powder for Injection (Indocin IV)*: 1 mg.
- *Suppositories*: 50 mg.

■ **Indications and Dosages:**
Moderate to severe rheumatoid arthritis, osteoarthritis, ankylosing spondylitis: PO Initially, 25 mg 2–3 times a day; increased by 25–50 mg/wk up to 150–200 mg/day. Or 75 mg/day (extended-release) up to 75 mg twice a day.
Acute gouty arthritis: PO Initially, 100 mg, then 50 mg 3 times a day.
Acute shoulder pain: PO 75–150 mg/day in 3–4 divided doses.
Usual rectal dosage: 50 mg 4 times a day.

■ **Unlabeled Uses:** Treatment of fever due to malignancy, pericarditis, psoriatic arthritis, rheumatic complications associated with Paget's disease of bone, vascular headache

■ **Contraindications:** Active GI bleeding or ulcerations; hypersensitivity to aspirin, indomethacin, or other NSAIDs; renal impairment, thrombocytopenia

■ **Side Effects**
Frequent (11%–3%)
Headache, nausea, vomiting, dyspepsia, dizziness
Occasional (less than 3%)
Depression, tinnitus, diaphoresis, somnolence, constipation, diarrhea, bleeding disturbances in patent ductus arteriosus
Rare
Hypertension, confusion, urticaria, pruritus, rash, blurred vision

■ **Serious Reactions**
- Paralytic ileus and ulceration of the esophagus, stomach, duodenum, or small intestine may occur.

- Patients with impaired renal function may develop hyperkalemia and worsening of renal impairment.
- Indomethacin use may aggravate epilepsy, parkinsonism, and depression or other psychiatric disturbances.
- Nephrotoxicity, including dysuria, hematuria, proteinuria, and nephrotic syndrome, occurs rarely.

■ Patient/Family Education
- Take with food
- No significant advantage over other oral NSAIDs; cost and clinical situation should govern use
- Swallow capsules whole and do not chew, open, or crush them
- Avoid tasks that require mental alertness or motor skills until response to the drug has been established
- Avoid alcohol and aspirin during indomethacin therapy because these substances increase the risk of GI bleeding

■ Monitoring Parameters
- Renal and hepatic function with prolonged use: check after 3 months, then q6-12 months
- Initial CBC and fecal occult blood test within 3 months of starting regular chronic therapy; repeat q6-12 months (more frequently in high-risk patients)
- Blood pressure, ECG, heart rate, platelet count, serum sodium and blood glucose levels, and urine output

■ Geriatric side effects at a glance:
☑ CNS ☐ Bowel Dysfunction ☐ Bladder Dysfunction ☐ Falls
☑ Other: Gastropathy

■ Use with caution in older patients with: Renal impairment, Hepatic impairment, CHF, HTN, PUD, History of GI bleeding, GERD, Bleeding and platelet disorders, History of aspirin sensitivity reaction. Also use with caution in patients taking Anticoagulants, Aspirin, and Antihypertensive agents.

■ U.S. Regulatory Considerations
☑ FDA Black Box
- Cardiovascular risk
- Gastrointestinal risk
☑ OBRA regulated in U.S. Long Term Care

■ Other Uses in Geriatric Patient: Acute Gout

■ Side Effects:
Of *particular importance in the geriatric patient*: Confusion, cognitive impairment, delirium, amnesia, depression, paranoia, psychosis, anxiety, dizziness, dyspepsia, fluid retention, renal impairment

■ Geriatric Considerations - Summary: Use with caution due to the higher risk of GI and CNS adverse events. Not a preferred NSAID in older adults. Use of NSAIDs in older adults increases the risk of GI complications including gastric ulceration, bleeding, and perforation. These complications are not necessarily preceded by less severe GI

symptoms. Concomitant use of a proton pump inhibitor or misoprostol reduces the risk for gastric ulceration and bleeding, but may not prevent long-term GI toxicity. The incidence of CNS effects is greatest for indomethacin as compared to other NSAIDs.

■ **References:**
1. COX-2 alternatives and GI protection. Med Lett Drugs Ther 2004;46:91.
2. Drugs that may cause cognitive disorders in the elderly. Med Lett Drugs Ther 2000;42:111-112.
3. Drugs that may cause psychiatric symptoms. Med Lett Drugs Ther 2002;44:59-62.

infliximab

(in-flix'-i-mab)

■ **Brand Name(s):** Remicade
Chemical Class: Monoclonal antibody

■ **Clinical Pharmacology:**
Mechanism of Action: A monoclonal antibody that binds to tumor necrosis factor (TNF), inhibiting functional activity of TNF. Reduces infiltration of inflammatory cells.
Therapeutic Effect: Decreases inflamed areas of the intestine.
Pharmacokinetics:

Route	Onset	Peak	Duration
IV (Crohn's disease)	1–2 wk	N/A	8–48 wk
IV (Rheumatoid arthritis [RA])	3–7 days	N/A	6–12 wk

Absorbed into the GI tissue; primarily distributed in the vascular compartment. **Half-life:** 9.5 days.

■ **Available Forms:**
• *Powder for Injection:* 100 mg.

■ **Indications and Dosages:**
Crohn's disease, moderate to severe, ulcerative colitis, psoriatic arthritis: IV Infusion Initially, 5 mg/kg at weeks 0, 2, and 6. Maintenance: 5 mg/kg q8wk thereafter.
Ankylosing spondylitis: IV Infusion Initially, 5 mg/kg at weeks 0, 2, and 6. Maintenance: 5 mg/kg q6wk thereafter.
Fistulizing Crohn's disease: IV Infusion Initially, 5 mg/kg followed by additional 5-mg/kg doses at 2 and 6 wk after first infusion.
Rheumatoid arthritis (RA): IV Infusion 3 mg/kg; followed by additional doses at 2 and 6 wk after first infusion: Then q8wk.

■ **Unlabeled Uses:** CHF, psoriasis, reactive arthritis, sciatica

■ **Contraindications:** Sensitivity to murine proteins, sepsis, serious active infection

■ **Side Effects**
Frequent (22%–10%)
Headache, nausea, fatigue, fever

Occasional (9%–5%)
Fever or chills during infusion, pharyngitis, vomiting, pain, dizziness, bronchitis, rash, rhinitis, cough, pruritus, sinusitis, myalgia, back pain
Rare (4%–1%)
Hypotension or hypertension, paresthesia, anxiety, depression, insomnia, diarrhea, urinary tract infection

■ Serious Reactions
- Serious infections, including sepsis, occur rarely.
- Hypersensitivity reaction, lupus-like syndrome, and severe hepatic reactions may occur.

Special Considerations
- Evaluate for risk of TB (TB skin test) prior to initiating therapy

■ Patient/Family Education
- More susceptible to infections; avoid crowds, people with URI, flu, etc.
- Expect follow-up tests, such as ESR, C-reactive protein measurement, and urinalysis
- Report signs of infection, such as fever
- The patient with rheumatoid arthritis should report increase in pain, stiffness, or swelling of joints
- The patient with Crohn's disease should report changes in stool color, consistency, or elimination pattern

■ Monitoring Parameters
- Decreased levels of serum IL-6, C-reactive protein, ESR, rheumatoid factor, signs and symptoms of disease, urinalysis, blood chemistry, human anti-cA2 titers, blood pressure (during and after infusion), temperature, body weight, signs and symptoms of infection (including TB)

■ Geriatric side effects at a glance:
❑ CNS   ❑ Bowel Dysfunction   ❑ Bladder Dysfunction   ❑ Falls

■ U.S. Regulatory Considerations
☑ FDA Black Box
- Increased risk of tuberculosis, fungal infections
- Evaluate patients for latent tuberculosis
❑ OBRA regulated in U.S. Long Term Care

insulin detemir (rDNA origin)

(in'-su-lin)

- **Brand Name(s):** Levemir

- **Clinical Pharmacology:**
  Mechanism of Action: A recombinant, soluble, long-acting insulin analog that binds to human albumin and provides slow absorption and a prolonged action. **Therapeutic Effect:** Controls glucose levels in diabetic patients.
  Pharmacokinetics:

Drug Form	Peak	Duration
Insulin detemir	6 hr	24 hr

- **Available Forms:**
  - *Cartridge*: 100 U/ml (Levemir).
  - *Prefilled Pen*: 100 U/ml (Levemir).

- **Indications and Dosages:**
  Diabetes mellitus (type 1 and type 2): Subcutaneous Individualize dose, administer 1 to 2 times daily. The average dose is 0.7 unit/kg.

- **Contraindications:** Hypersensitivity or insulin resistance

- **Side Effects**
  Occasional
  Hypoglycemia, nocturnal hypoglycemia
  Rare
  Insulin resistance

- **Serious Reactions**
  - Severe hypoglycemia caused by hyperinsulinism may occur in cases of insulin over-dose, when food intake is decreased or delayed, during periods of excessive exercise, or in patients with brittle diabetes.
  - Diabetic ketoacidosis may result from stress, illness, omission of insulin dose, or long-term poor insulin control.

- **Geriatric side effects at a glance:**
  ❏ CNS ❏ Bowel Dysfunction ❏ Bladder Dysfunction ❏ Falls

- **U.S. Regulatory Considerations**
  ❏ FDA Black Box   ❏ OBRA regulated in U.S. Long Term Care

insulin group

(in'-su-lin)

- **Brand Name(s):** Rapid-Acting: Insulin Lispro (Humalog), Insulin Aspart (Novolog)

- **Brand Name(s):** Regular Short-Acting: Humulin R, Novolin R, Regular Iletin II

- **Brand Name(s):** Intermediate-Acting: NPH (Humulin N, Novolin N, NPH Iletin II)

- **Brand Name(s):** Lente: Humulin L, Lente Iletin II, Novolin L

- **Brand Name(s):** Long-Acting: Insulin Glargine (Lantus Ultralente), Insulin Detemir (Levemir)

- **Brand Name(s):** Intermediate- and short-acting mixtures: Humulin 50/50, Humulin 70/30, Humalog Mix 75/25, Humalog Mix 50/50, Novolin 70/30, Novolog Mix 70/30
  Chemical Class: Exogenous insulin

- ## Clinical Pharmacology:
  Mechanism of Action: An exogenous insulin that facilitates passage of glucose, potassium, and magnesium across the cellular membranes of skeletal and cardiac muscle and adipose tissue. Controls storage and metabolism of carbohydrates, protein, and fats. Promotes conversion of glucose to glycogen in the liver. **Therapeutic Effect:** Controls glucose levels in diabetic patients.
  Pharmacokinetics:

Drug Form	Onset (hr)	Peak (hr)	Duration (hr)
Lispro	0.25	0.5–1.5	4–5
Insulin aspart	1/6	1–3	3–5
Regular	0.5–1	2–4	5–7
NPH	1–2	6–14	24+
Lente	1–3	6–14	24+
Insulin glargine	N/A	N/A	24

- ## Available Forms:
  - All insulins are available as 100 units/ml concentrations.
  - *Rapid Acting:* Humulin R, Novolin R, Novolog, Humalog, Regular Iletin II.
  - *Intermediate Acting:* Humulin L, Novolin L, Lente Iletin II, Humulin N, Novolin N, NPH Illetin II.
  - *Long Acting:* Lantus Ultralente, Levemir.
  - *Intermediate- and Short-Acting Mixtures:* Humulin 50/50, Humulin 70/30, Humalog Mix 75/25, Humalog Mix 50/50, Novolin 70/30, Novolog Mix 70/30.

- ## Indications and Dosages:
  Treatment of insulin-dependent type 1 diabetes mellitus and non–insulin-dependent type 2 diabetes mellitus when diet or weight control has failed to maintain satisfactory blood glucose levels or in event of fever, infection, surgery, or trauma, or severe endocrine, hepatic, or renal dysfunction; emergency treatment of ketoacidosis (regular insulin); to

promote passage of glucose across cell membrane in hyperalimentation (regular insulin); to facilitate intracellular shift of potassium in hyperkalemia (regular insulin): Subcutaneous 0.5–1 unit/kg/day.

■ **Contraindications:** Hypersensitivity or insulin resistance may require change of type or species source of insulin

■ **Side Effects**
Occasional
Localized redness, swelling, and itching caused by improper injection technique or allergy to cleansing solution or insulin
Infrequent
Somogyi effect, including rebound hyperglycemia with chronically excessive insulin dosages: systemic allergic reaction, marked by rash, angioedema, and anaphylaxis; lipodystrophy or depression at injection site due to breakdown of adipose tissue; lipohypertrophy or accumulation of subcutaneous tissue at injection site due to inadequate site rotation
Rare
Insulin resistance

■ **Serious Reactions**
- Severe hypoglycemia caused by hyperinsulinism may occur with insulin overdose, decrease or delay of food intake, or excessive exercise and in those with brittle diabetes.
- Diabetic ketoacidosis may result from stress, illness, omission of insulin dose, or long-term poor insulin control.

■ **Patient/Family Education**
- Symptoms of hypoglycemia include fatigue, weakness, confusion, headache, convulsions, hunger, nausea, pallor, sweating, rapid breathing
- For hypoglycemia, give 1 mg glucagon, glucose 25g IV (via dextrose 50% sol, 50 ml), or oral glucose if tolerated
- When mixing insulins, draw up short-acting first
- Dosage adjustment may be necessary when changing insulin products
- Human insulin considered insulin of choice secondary to antigenicity of animal insulins
- The regimen of exercise, good hygiene (including foot care), prescribed diet, and weight control is an integral part of treatment
- Carry candy, sugar packets, or other sugar supplements for immediate response to hypoglycemia

■ **Monitoring Parameters**
- Assess the patient for signs and symptoms of hypoglycemia (anxiety, cool wet skin, diplopia, dizziness, headache, hunger, numbness in mouth, tachycardia, tremors) or hyperglycemia (deep rapid breathing [Kussmaul's respirations], dim vision, fatigue, nausea, polydipsia, polyphagia, polyuria, vomiting)

- Be alert to conditions that alter blood glucose requirements, such as fever, increased activity, stress, or a surgical procedure
- Monitor the sleeping patient for diaphoresis and restlessness

■ **Geriatric side effects at a glance:**
❑ CNS ❑ Bowel Dysfunction ❑ Bladder Dysfunction ❑ Falls
Other: Hypoglycemia

■ **Use with caution in older patients with:** Impaired renal function

■ **U.S. Regulatory Considerations**
❑ FDA Black Box ❑ OBRA regulated in U.S. Long Term Care

■ **Other Uses in Geriatric Patient:** None

■ **Side Effects:**
Of particular importance in the geriatric patient: Hypoglycemia, weight gain

■ **Geriatric Considerations - Summary:** Ensure that the older adult can demonstrate the appropriate use of insulin by assessing his or her ability to draw up the correct dose from a multidose bottle, read syringe markings, and administer the dose subcutaneously. Comorbidities such as poor vision, arthritis, tremor, or cognitive impairment may impair this process. Insulin pens may be advantageous for some patients. Administration of insulin in the arm results in slower absorption than seen with abdominal administration.

■ **References:**
1. Haas L. Management of diabetes mellitus medications in the nursing home. Drugs Aging 2005;22:209-218.
2. Rosenstock J. Management of type 2 diabetes mellitus in the elderly: special considerations. Drugs Aging 2001;18:31-44.
3. Saudek CD, Golden SH. Feasibility and outcomes of insulin therapy in elderly patients with diabetes mellitus. Drugs Aging 1999;14:375-385.
4. Shorr RI, Ray WA, Daugherty JR, et al. Incidence and risk factors for serious hypoglycemia in older persons using insulin or sulfonylureas. Arch Intern Med 1997;157:1681-1686.

interferon alfa-2a/2b

(in-ter-feer'-on)

■ **Brand Name(s):** Roferon-A (alfa-2a), Intron-A (alfa-2b)

Combinations
Rx: Interferon alfa-2b with ribavirin (Rebetron Combination Therapy)
Chemical Class: Recombinant interferon

■ **Clinical Pharmacology:**

Mechanism of Action: A biologic response modifier that inhibits viral replication in virus-infected cells. **Therapeutic Effect:** Suppresses cell proliferation; increases phagocytic action of macrophages; augments specific lymphocytic cell toxicity.

Pharmacokinetics: Interferon alfa-2a: Well absorbed after IM, subcutaneous administration. Undergoes proteolytic degradation during reabsorption in kidney. **Half-life:** IM: 2 hr; Subcutaneous: 3 hr. Interferon alfa-2b: Well absorbed after IM, subcutaneous administration. Undergoes proteolytic degradation during reabsorption in kidney. **Half-life:** 2-3 hr.

■ **Available Forms:**

Interferon alfa-2a:
- Injection: 3 million units, 6 million units, 9 million units, 36 million units (Roferon-A).

Interferon alfa-2b:
- Injection Powder for Reconstitution: 3 million units, 5 million units, 6 million units, 10 million units, 18 million units, 25 million units, 50 million units (Intron-A).
- Injection, Prefilled Syringes: 3 million units, 5 million units, 6 million units, 10 million units, 18 million units, 25 million units, 50 million units (Intron-A).

■ **Indications and Dosages:**

Hairy cell leukemia: Interferon alfa-2a: Subcutaneous, IM Initially, 3 million units/day for 16-24 wk. Maintenance: 3 million units 3 times/wk. Do not use 36-million-unit vial. Interferon alfa-2b: Subcutaneous, IM 2 million units/m² 3 times/wk. If severe adverse reactions occur, modify dose or temporarily discontinue.

Chronic myelocytic leukemia (CML): Interferon alfa-2a: Subcutaneous, IM 9 million units daily.

Condylomata acuminata: Interferon alfa-2b: Intralesional 1 million units/lesion 3 times/wk for 3 wk. Use only 10-million-unit vial, reconstitute with no more than 1 ml diluent. Use tuberculin (TB) syringe with 25- or 26-gauge needle. Give in evening with acetaminophen, which alleviates side effects.

Melanoma: Interferon alfa-2a: Subcutaneous, IM 12 million units/m² 3 times/wk for 3 mo. Interferon alfa-2b: IV Initially, 20 million units/m² 5 times/wk for 4 wk. Maintenance: 10 million units IM/SC for 48 wk.

AIDS-related Kaposi's sarcoma: Interferon alfa-2a: Subcutaneous, IM Initially, 36 million units/day for 10-12 wk, may give 3 million units on day 1; 9 million units on day 2; 18 million units on day 3; then begin 36 million units/day for remainder of 10-12 wk. Maintenance: 36 million units/day 3 times/wk. Interferon alfa-2b: Subcutaneous/IM 30 million units/m² 3 times/wk. Use only 50-million-unit vials. If severe adverse reactions occur, modify dose or temporarily discontinue.

Chronic hepatitis B: Interferon alfa-2b: Subcutaneous, IM 30-35 million units/wk, 5 million units/day, or 10 million units 3 times/wk.

Chronic hepatitis C: Interferon alfa-2a: Subcutaneous, IM Initially, 6 million units once a day for 3 wk, then 3 million units 3 times/wk for 6 mo. Interferon alfa-2b: Subcutaneous, IM 3 million units 3 times/wk for up to 6 mo, for up to 18-24 mo for chronic hepatitis C.

■ **Unlabeled Uses**

Interferon alfa-2a: Treatment of active, chronic hepatitis, bladder or renal carcinoma, malignant melanoma, multiple myeloma, mycosis fungoides, non-Hodgkin's lymphoma

632

Interferon alfa-2b:
Treatment of bladder, cervical, renal carcinoma, chronic myelocytic leukemia, laryngeal papillomatosis, multiple myeloma, mycosis fungoides

■ **Contraindications:** Hypersensitivity to any component of the formulations

■ **Side Effects**
Frequent
Interferon alfa-2a: Flu-like symptoms, including fever, fatigue, headache, aches, pains, anorexia, and chills, nausea, vomiting, coughing, dyspnea, hypotension, edema, chest pain, dizziness, diarrhea, weight loss, taste change, abdominal discomfort, confusion, paresthesia, depression, visual and sleep disturbances, diaphoresis, lethargy
Interferon alfa-2b: Flu-like symptoms, including fever, fatigue, headache, aches, pains, anorexia, and chills, rash with hairy cell leukemia (Kaposi's sarcoma only)
Kaposi's sarcoma: All previously mentioned side effects plus depression, dyspepsia, dry mouth or thirst, alopecia, rigors
Occasional
Interferon alfa-2a: Partial alopecia, rash, dry throat or skin, pruritus, flatulence, constipation, hypertension, palpitations, sinusitis
Interferon alfa-2b: Dizziness, pruritus, dry skin, dermatitis, alteration in taste
Rare
Interferon alfa-2a: Hot flashes, hypermotility, Raynaud's syndrome, bronchospasm, earache, ecchymosis
Interferon alfa-2b: Confusion, leg cramps, back pain, gingivitis, flushing, tremor, nervousness, eye pain

■ **Serious Reactions**
- Arrhythmias, stroke, transient ischemic attacks, congestive heart failure (CHF), pulmonary edema, and myocardial infarction (MI) occur rarely with interferon alfa-2a.
- Hypersensitivity reaction occurs rarely with interferon alfa-2b.
- Severe adverse reactions of flu-like symptoms appear dose related with interferon alfa-2b.

Special Considerations
- Rebetron Combination Therapy (kit containing interferon alfa-2b inj plus ribavirin capsules) more effective than interferon alfa-2b monotherapy for chronic hepatitis C infection

■ **Patient/Family Education**
- Drink plenty of fluids
- Flu-like symptoms decrease during treatment. Acetaminophen (do not exceed recommended dose) may alleviate fever and headache
- The drug's therapeutic effects may take 1-3 mo to appear
- Avoid tasks that require mental alertness or motor skills until response to the drug has been established

- Notify the physician if nausea or vomiting continues at home
- Avoid consuming alcohol during drug therapy

■ **Monitoring Parameters**
- Monitor all levels of clinical function and assess for the numerous side effects

■ **Geriatric side effects at a glance:**
☑ CNS   ☑ Bowel Dysfunction   ☐ Bladder Dysfunction   ☐ Falls

■ **U.S. Regulatory Considerations**
☑ FDA Black Box
Interferons may cause or aggravate neuropsychiatric (depression), autoimmune, ischemic, and infectious disorders.
☐ OBRA regulated in U.S. Long Term Care

interferon alfa-n3

(in-ter-feer'-on)

■ **Brand Name(s):** Alferon N
Chemical Class: Human leukocyte interferon

■ **Clinical Pharmacology:**
Mechanism of Action: A biologic response modifier that inhibits viral replication in virus-infected cells, suppresses cell proliferation, increases phagocytic action of macrophages, and augments specific cytotoxicity of lymphocytes for target cells. **Therapeutic Effect:** Inhibits viral growth in condylomata acuminata.
Pharmacokinetics: Metabolized and excreted in kidney. **Half-life:** 4-7 hr.

■ **Available Forms:**
- Injection: 5 million international units/ml.

■ **Indications and Dosages:**
Condyloma acuminatum: Intralesional 0.05 ml (250,000 international units) per wart twice a week up to 8 wk. Maximum dose/treatment session: 0.5 ml (2.5 million international units). Do not repeat for 3 mo after initial 8-wk course unless warts enlarge or new warts appear.

■ **Unlabeled Uses:** Treatment of active chronic hepatitis, bladder carcinoma, chronic myelocytic leukemia, laryngeal papillomatosis, malignant melanoma, multiple myeloma, mycosis fungoides, non-Hodgkin's lymphoma

- **Contraindications:** Previous history of anaphylactic reaction to egg protein, mouse immunoglobulin, or neomycin

- **Side Effects**
  Frequent
  Flu-like symptoms
  Occasional
  Dizziness, pruritus, dry skin, dermatitis, altered taste
  Rare
  Confusion, leg cramps, back pain, gingivitis, flushing, tremor, nervousness, eye pain

- **Serious Reactions**
  - Hypersensitivity reaction occurs rarely.
  - Severe flu-like symptoms may occur at higher doses.

- **Patient/Family Education**
  - Flu-like symptoms may be alleviated or minimized by taking doses at bedtime and tend to diminish with continued therapy

- **Monitoring Parameters**
  - Assess for side effects

- **Geriatric side effects at a glance:**
  ☑ CNS ☑ Bowel Dysfunction ☐ Bladder Dysfunction ☐ Falls

- **U.S. Regulatory Considerations**
  ☑ FDA Black Box
  Interferons may cause or aggravate neuropsychiatric (depression), autoimmune, ischemic, and infectious disorders.
  ☐ OBRA regulated in U.S. Long Term Care

interferon alfacon-1

(in-ter-feer'-on al'-fa-kon one)

- **Brand Name(s):** Infergen
  Chemical Class: Recombinant interferon

- **Clinical Pharmacology:**
  Mechanism of Action: A biologic response modifier that stimulates the immune system. **Therapeutic Effect:** Inhibits hepatitis C virus.
  Pharmacokinetics: **Half-life:** 0.5-7 hr.

- **Available Forms:**
  - *Injection*: 9 mcg/0.3 ml, 15 mcg/0.5 ml.

■ **Indications and Dosages:**
Chronic hepatitis C: Subcutaneous 9 mcg 3 times/wk for 24 wk. May increase to 15 mcg 3 times/wk in patients who tolerate but fail to respond to 9-mcg dose.

■ **Unlabeled Uses:** Carcinoid tumors, chronic hepatitis B

■ **Contraindications:** History of autoimmune hepatitis or severe psychiatric disorders, hypersensitivity to alpha interferons

■ **Side Effects**
Frequent (greater than 50%)
Headache, fatigue, fever, depression

Special Considerations

- Response rates (normal ALT, HCV RNA negative) of 9-mcg dose approximately 35%; about half those have sustained response 24 wk after treatment
- Withold dosage temporarily if severe adverse reaction occurs; consider decreasing dose to 7.5 mcg

■ **Patient/Family Education**
- Needs to be refrigerated (36-46° F), may allow to reach room temp before injection; call manufacturer for advice if left out
- Notify the physician of side effects, including headache or injection site pain, as soon as possible

■ **Monitoring Parameters**
- CBC, platelets, TSH, triglycerides, LFTs initially, repeat after 2-wk treatment and periodically thereafter
- Withold for ANC $<0.5 \times 10^9$/L or platelets $<50 \times 10^9$/L

■ **Geriatric side effects at a glance:**
☑ CNS ☑ Bowel Dysfunction ☐ Bladder Dysfunction ☐ Falls

■ **U.S. Regulatory Considerations**
☑ FDA Black Box
Interferons may cause or aggravate neuropsychiatric (depression), autoimmune, ischemic, and infectious disorders.
☐ OBRA regulated in U.S. Long Term Care

interferon beta-1 a/b

(in-ter-feer'-on)

■ **Brand Name(s):** Avonex, Rebif, Betaferon, Betaseron
Chemical Class: Recombinant interferon

■ **Clinical Pharmacology:**
  Mechanism of Action: A biologic response modifier that interacts with specific cell receptors found on surface of human cells. **Therapeutic Effect:** Possesses antiviral and immunoregulatory activities.
  Pharmacokinetics: *Interferon beta-1a:* After IM administration, peak serum levels attained in 3-15 hr. Biologic markers increase within 12 hr and remain elevated for 4 days. **Half-life:** 10 hr (IM). *Interferon beta-1b:* **Half-life:** 8 min-4.3 hr.

■ **Available Forms:**
  Interferon beta-1a:
  • *Powder for Injection:* 22 mcg (Rebif), 30 mcg (Avonex), 44 mcg (Rebif).
  Interferon beta-1b:
  • *Powder for Injection:* 0.3 mg (9.6 million units) (Betaseron).

■ **Indications and Dosages:**
  Relapsing-remitting multiple sclerosis: *Interferon beta-1a:* IM 30 mcg Avonex once weekly. Subcutaneous Initially 8.8 mcg Rebif 3 times/wk, may increase over 4-6 wk to 44 mcg Rebif 3 times/wk. *Interferon beta-1b:* Subcutaneous 0.25 mg (8 million units) every other day.

■ **Unlabeled Uses:** Treatment of acquired immune deficiency syndrome (AIDS), AIDS-related Kaposi's sarcoma, malignant melanoma, renal cell carcinoma

■ **Contraindications:** Hypersensitivity to albumin, interferon

■ **Side Effects**
  Frequent
  Interferon beta-1a: Headache (67%), flu-like symptoms (61%), myalgia (34%), upper respiratory infection (31%), pain (24%), asthenia, chills (21%), sinusitis (18%), infection (11%)
  Interferon beta-1b: Injection site reaction (85%), headache (84%), flu-like symptoms (76%), fever (59%), pain (52%), asthenia (49%), myalgia (44%), sinusitis (36%), diarrhea, dizziness (35%), mental status changes (29%), constipation (24%), diaphoresis (23%), vomiting (21%)
  Occasional
  Interferon beta-1a: Abdominal pain, arthralgia (9%), chest pain, dyspnea (6%), malaise, syncope (4%)
  Interferon beta-1b: Malaise (15%), somnolence (6%), alopecia (4%)
  Rare
  Interferon beta-1a: Injection site reaction, hypersensitivity reaction (3%)

■ **Serious Reactions**
  • Anemia occurs in 8% of patients taking interferon beta-1a.
  • Seizures occur rarely in patients taking interferon beta-1b.

■ **Patient/Family Education**
  • Use acetaminophen for relief of flu-like symptoms
  • Avoid prolonged sun exposure (photosensitivity)

- Benefit in chronic progressive multiple sclerosis has not been evaluated
- Patients treated × 2 yr had significantly longer time to progression of disability compared with placebo group
- Do not change drug dosage or administration schedule without consulting the physician
- Document the type and severity of injection site reaction; these reactions will not require discontinuation of therapy, but should be reported immediately

■ **Monitoring Parameters**
- CBC, platelets, liver function tests, and blood chemistries q3mo
- Discontinue if ANC <750/m³, ALT/AST >10 × upper normal limits; when labs return to these levels, restart at 50% of dose
- Assess for flu-like symptoms, headache, and myalgia
- Evaluate for depression and suicidal ideation

■ **Geriatric side effects at a glance:**
❑ CNS ❑ Bowel Dysfunction ❑ Bladder Dysfunction ❑ Falls

■ **U.S. Regulatory Considerations**
❑ FDA Black Box ❑ OBRA regulated in U.S. Long Term Care

interferon gamma-1 b

(in-ter-feer'-on)

■ **Brand Name(s):** Actimmune
Chemical Class: Recombinant interferon

■ **Clinical Pharmacology:**
Mechanism of Action: A biologic response modifier that induces activation of macrophages in blood monocytes to phagocytes, which is necessary in the body's cellular immune response to intracellular and extracellular pathogens. Enhances phagocytic function and antimicrobial activity of monocytes. **Therapeutic Effect:** Decreases signs and symptoms of serious infections in chronic granulomatous disease.
Pharmacokinetics: Slowly absorbed after subcutaneous administration. **Half-life:** 0.5-1 hr.

■ **Available Forms:**
- **Injection:** 100 mcg (2 million units).

■ **Indications and Dosages:**
Chronic granulomatous disease; severe, malignant osteopetrosis: Subcutaneous 50 mcg/m² (1.5 million units/m²) in patients with body surface area (BSA) greater than 0.5 m²; 1.5 mcg/kg/dose in patients with BSA 0.5 m² or less. Give 3 times a week.

638

- **Contraindications:** Hypersensitivity to *Escherichia coli*-derived products

- **Side Effects**
  Frequent
  Fever (52%); headache (33%); rash (17%); chills, fatigue, diarrhea (14%)
  Occasional (13%–10%)
  Vomiting, nausea
  Rare (6%–3%)
  Weight loss, myalgia, anorexia

- **Serious Reactions**
  - Interferon gamma-1b may exacerbate preexisting CNS disturbances, including decreased mental status, gait disturbance, and dizziness, as well as cardiac disorders.

Special Considerations
  - Optimal sites for injection are the right and left deltoid and anterior thigh

- **Patient/Family Education**
  - Use acetaminophen to relieve fever, headache
  - Store vials in the refrigerator
  - Teach the patient how to properly administer the drug and dispose of needles and syringes
  - Flu-like symptoms may be alleviated or minimized by taking doses at bedtime and tend to diminish with continued therapy
  - Avoid performing tasks that require mental alertness or motor skills until response to the drug has been established

- **Monitoring Parameters**
  - Monitor the patient for flu-like symptoms, including chills, fatigue, fever, and myalgia
  - Skin for rash

- **Geriatric side effects at a glance:**
  ❑ CNS   ❑ Bowel Dysfunction   ❑ Bladder Dysfunction   ❑ Falls

- **U.S. Regulatory Considerations**
  ❑ FDA Black Box   ❑ OBRA regulated in U.S. Long Term Care

iodoquinol

(eye-oh-do-kwin'-ole)

- **Brand Name(s):** Yodoxin
  Chemical Class: Hydroxyquinoline derivative

- **Clinical Pharmacology:**
  Mechanism of Action: An antibacterial, antifungal, and antitrichomonal agent that works in the intestinal lumen by an unknown mechanism. **Therapeutic Effect:** Amebicidal.
  Pharmacokinetics: Partially and irregularly absorbed from the gastrointestinal (GI) tract. Metabolized in liver. Primarily excreted in feces.

- **Available Forms:**
  - *Tablets:* 210 mg, 650 mg (Yodoxin).
  - *Powder:* 25 g, 100 g (Yodoxin).

- **Indications and Dosages:**
  Intestinal amebiasis: PO 630-650 mg 3 times a day for 20 days.

- **Contraindications:** Hepatic impairment, renal impairment, chronic diarrhea, hypersensitivity to iodine and 8-hydroxyquinolones

- **Side Effects**
  Occasional
  Fever, chills, headache, nausea, vomiting, diarrhea, cramps, urticaria, pruritus

- **Serious Reactions**
  - Optic neuritis, atrophy, and peripheral neuropathy have been reported with high dosages and long-term use.

- **Patient/Family Education**
  - Take full course of therapy
  - Nausea, diarrhea or GI upset may occur
  - Skin, hair, and clothing may be temporarily stained yellow-brown following iodoquinol use

- **Monitoring Parameters**
  - Therapeutic response to therapy

- **Geriatric side effects at a glance:**
  ☐ CNS   ☐ Bowel Dysfunction   ☐ Bladder Dysfunction   ☐ Falls

- **U.S. Regulatory Considerations**
  ☐ FDA Black Box   ☐ OBRA regulated in U.S. Long Term Care

ipecac syrup

(ip'-e-kak)

OTC: Ipecac
Chemical Class: *Cephaelis ipecacuanha* derivative

■ **Clinical Pharmacology:**
Mechanism of Action: An antidote that acts centrally by stimulating medullary chemoreceptor trigger zone and locally by irritating gastric mucosa. **Therapeutic Effect:** Produces emesis.
Pharmacokinetics: Onset of action occurs within 20-30 min. Eliminated very slowly in urine.

■ **Available Forms:**
- *Syrup:* 70 mg/ml.

■ **Indications and Dosages:**
Poisoning, acute: PO 15-30 ml followed by 200-300 ml of water.

■ **Contraindications:** Ingestion of petroleum distillate, ingestion of strong acids or bases, ingestion of strychnine, unconsciousness or absence of gag reflex, hypersensitivity to ipecac or any component of the formulation

■ **Side Effects**
Expected response
Nausea, vomiting, drowsiness and mild CNS depression after vomiting
Occasional
Diarrhea, lethargy, muscle aching, stomach cramps

■ **Serious Reactions**
- Cardiotoxicity may occur if ipecac syrup is not vomited (noted as hypotension, tachycardia, precordial chest pain, pulmonary congestion, dyspnea, ventricular tachycardia and fibrillation, cardiac arrest).
- Overdose may produce diarrhea, fast/irregular heartbeat, nausea continuing >30 min, stomach pain, respiratory difficulty, unusually tired, and aching/stiff muscles.

■ **Geriatric side effects at a glance:**
❑ CNS   ❑ Bowel Dysfunction   ❑ Bladder Dysfunction   ❑ Falls

■ **U.S. Regulatory Considerations**
❑ FDA Black Box   ❑ OBRA regulated in U.S. Long Term Care

ipratropium bromide

(eye-pra-troep'-ee-um broe'-mide)

■ **Brand Name(s):** Atrovent, Atrovent Nasal

Combinations
Rx: with albuterol (Combivent)
Chemical Class: Quaternary ammonium compound

■ **Clinical Pharmacology:**
Mechanism of Action: An anticholinergic that blocks the action of acetylcholine at parasympathetic sites in bronchial smooth muscle. **Therapeutic Effect:** Causes bronchodilation and inhibits nasal secretions.
Pharmacokinetics:

Route	Onset	Peak	Duration
Inhalation	1–3 min	1–2 hr	4–6 hr

Minimal systemic absorption after inhalation. Metabolized in the liver (systemic absorption). Primarily eliminated in feces. **Half-life:** 1.5–4 hr.

■ **Available Forms:**
- *Oral Inhalation:* 18 mcg/actuation.
- *Aerosol Solution for Inhalation:* 0.02%.
- *Nasal Spray:* 0.03%, 0.06%.

■ **Indications and Dosages:**
Bronchospasm: Inhalation 2 inhalations 4 times a day. Maximum: 12 inhalations/day. Nebulization 500 mcg 3-4 times a day.
Rhinorrhea (perennial allergic and nonallergic rhinitis): Intranasal (0.03%) 2 sprays per nostril 2-3 times a day.
Rhinorrhea (common cold): Intranasal (0.06%) 2 sprays per nostril 3-4 times a day for up to 4 days.
Rhinorrhea (seasonal allergy): Intranasal (0.06%) 2 sprays per nostril 4 times a day for up to 3 wk.

■ **Contraindications:** History of hypersensitivity to atropine, soya lecithin, or related food products such as soybean and peanut

■ **Side Effects**
Frequent
Inhalation (6%–3%): Cough, dry mouth, headache, nausea
Nasal: Dry nose and mouth, headache, nasal irritation
Occasional
Inhalation (2%): Dizziness, transient increased bronchospasm
Rare (less than 1%)
Inhalation: Hypotension, insomnia, metallic or unpleasant taste, palpitations, urine retention
Nasal: Diarrhea or constipation, dry throat, abdominal pain, stuffy nose

■ Serious Reactions
- Worsening of angle-closure glaucoma, acute eye pain, and hypotension occur rarely.

Special Considerations
- Bronchodilator of choice for COPD

■ Patient/Family Education
- Do not take more than 2 inhalations at a time because excessive use decreases the drug's effectiveness and may cause paradoxical bronchoconstriction
- Rinse mouth with water immediately after inhalation to prevent mouth and throat dryness
- Drink plenty of fluids to decrease the thickness of lung secretions
- Avoid excessive use of caffeinated products, such as chocolate, cocoa, cola, coffee, and tea

■ Monitoring Parameters
- Pulse rate and quality and respiratory rate, depth, rhythm, and type
- Breath sounds for crackles, rhonchi, and wheezing
- ABG levels
- Examine the patient's lips and fingernails for a blue or gray color in light-skinned patients and a gray color in dark-skinned patients, which are signs of hypoxemia
- Observe the patient for clavicular, intercostal, and sternal retractions and a hand tremor
- Evaluate the patient for evidence of clinical improvement, such as cessation of retractions, quieter and slower respirations, and a relaxed facial expression

■ Geriatric side effects at a glance:
❑ CNS   ❑ Bowel Dysfunction   ❑ Bladder Dysfunction   ❑ Falls

■ U.S. Regulatory Considerations
❑ FDA Black Box   ❑ OBRA regulated in U.S. Long Term Care

irbesartan

(ir-be-sar'-tan)

■ Brand Name(s): Avapro
Combinations
Rx: with hydrochlorothiazide (Avalide)
Chemical Class: Angiotensin II receptor antagonist

■ Clinical Pharmacology:
Mechanism of Action: An angiotensin II receptor, type AT_1, antagonist that blocks the vasoconstrictor and aldosterone-secreting effects of angiotensin II, inhibiting the

binding of angiotensin II to the AT$_1$ receptors. **Therapeutic Effect:** Causes vasodilation, decreases peripheral resistance, and decreases BP.
Pharmacokinetics: Rapidly and completely absorbed after PO administration. Protein binding: 90%. Undergoes hepatic metabolism to inactive metabolite. Recovered primarily in feces and, to a lesser extent, in urine. Not removed by hemodialysis. **Half-life:** 11–15 hr.

■ **Available Forms:**
  • *Tablets*: 75 mg, 150 mg, 300 mg.

■ **Indications and Dosages:**
  Hypertension alone or in combination with other antihypertensives: PO Initially, 75–150 mg/day. May increase to 300 mg/day.
  Nephropathy: PO Target dose of 300 mg/day.

■ **Unlabeled Uses:** Treatment of atrial fibrillation, CHF

■ **Contraindications:** Bilateral renal artery stenosis, biliary cirrhosis or obstruction, primary hyperaldosteronism, severe hepatic insufficiency

■ **Side Effects**
  Occasional (9%–3%)
  Upper respiratory tract infection, fatigue, diarrhea, cough
  Rare (2%–1%)
  Heartburn, dizziness, headache, nausea, rash

■ **Serious Reactions**
  • Overdosage may manifest as hypotension and tachycardia. Bradycardia occurs less often.
  • Hypoglycemia may occur in patients with diabetes using glucose-lowering drugs.

Special Considerations
  • Potentially as or more effective than angiotensin-converting enzyme inhibitors, without cough; no evidence for reduction in morbidity and mortality as first-line agents in hypertension, yet; whether they provide the same cardiac and renal protection also still tentative; Like ACE inhibitors, less effective in black patients

■ **Patient/Family Education**
  • Call your clinician immediately if note following side effects: wheezing; lip, throat or face swelling; hives or rash
  • Avoid tasks that require mental alertness or motor skills until response to the drug has been established
  • Report signs and symptoms of infection, including fever and sore throat
  • Avoid outdoor exercise during hot weather to avoid the risks of dehydration and hypotension

■ **Monitoring Parameters**
  • Baseline electrolytes, urinalysis, blood urea nitrogen and creatinine with recheck at 2-4 wk after initiation (sooner in volume-depleted patients); monitor sitting blood pressure; watch for symptomatic hypotension, particularly in volume depleted patients

■ **Geriatric side effects at a glance:**
  ❏ CNS   ❏ Bowel Dysfunction   ❏ Bladder Dysfunction   ❏ Falls

    ☑ FDA Black Box
    Although not relevant for geriatric patients, teratogenicity is associated with the use
    of angiotensin II receptor antagonists.
    ❏ OBRA regulated in U.S. Long Term Care

iron dextran

(iron dex'-tran)

■ **Brand Name(s):** InFeD, DexFerrum
    Chemical Class: Ferric hydroxide complexed with dextran

■ **Clinical Pharmacology:**
    Mechanism of Action: A trace element and essential component in the formation of
    Hgb. Necessary for effective erythropoiesis and transport and utilization of oxygen.
    Serves as cofactor of several essential enzymes. **Therapeutic Effect:** Replenishes Hgb
    and depleted iron stores.
    Pharmacokinetics: Readily absorbed after IM administration. Most absorption oc-
    curs within 72 hr; remainder within 3–4 wk. Bound to protein to form hemosiderin, fer-
    ritin, or transferrin. No physiologic system of elimination. Small amounts lost daily in
    shedding of skin, hair, and nails and in feces, urine, and perspiration. **Half-life:** 5–20 hr.

■ **Available Forms:**
    • *Injection* (DexFerrum, InFeD): 50 mg/ml.

■ **Indications and Dosages:**
    Iron deficiency anemia (no blood loss): Dosage is expressed in terms of milligrams of
    elemental iron, degree of anemia, patient weight, and presence of any bleeding. Ex-
    pect to use periodic hematologic determinations as guide to therapy. IV, IM Mg iron
    $= 0.66 \times$ weight (kg) $\times$ (100 – Hgb [g/dl]/14.8)
    Iron replacement secondary to blood loss: IV, IM Replacement iron (mg) = blood loss
    (ml) $\times$ Hct.
    Maximum daily dosages: 100 mg.

■ **Contraindications:** All anemias except iron deficiency anemia, including pernicious,
    aplastic, normocytic, and refractory

■ **Side Effects**
    Frequent
    Allergic reaction (such as rash and itching), backache, myalgia, chills, dizziness, head-
    ache, fever, nausea, vomiting, flushed skin, pain or redness at injection site, brown
    discoloration of skin, metallic taste

■ **Serious Reactions**
    • Anaphylaxis has occurred during the first few minutes after injection, causing death
      rarely.
    • Leukocytosis and lymphadenopathy occur rarely.

- Use only in patients unable to take oral iron and with lab-confirmed iron deficiency.
- Discontinue oral iron before giving
- Delayed reaction (fever, myalgias, arthralgias, nausea) may occur 1-2 days after administration
- When giving IM, give only in gluteal muscle

■ **Patient/Family Education**
- Pain and brown staining of the skin may occur at the injection site
- Do not take oral iron while receiving iron injections
- Stools may become black during iron therapy; this side effect is harmless unless accompanied by abdominal cramping or pain and red streaking or sticky consistency of stool
- Report abdominal cramping or pain, back pain, fever, headache, or red streaking or a sticky consistency of stool
- Chew gum, suck on hard candy, and maintain good oral hygiene to prevent or reduce the metallic taste

■ **Geriatric side effects at a glance:**
☑ CNS   ☑ Bowel Dysfunction   ☐ Bladder Dysfunction   ☐ Falls

■ **U.S. Regulatory Considerations**
☑ FDA Black Box
Anaphylactic reactions that are sometimes fatal
☐ OBRA regulated in U.S. Long Term Care

iron sucrose

(iron sue'-crose)

■ **Brand Name(s):** Venofer

■ **Clinical Pharmacology:**
Mechanism of Action: A trace element that is an essential component in the formation of Hgb. It's necessary for effective erythropoiesis and oxygen transport capacity of blood, and transport and utilization of oxygen, and serves as cofactor of several essential enzymes. **Therapeutic Effect:** Replenishes body iron stores in patients who have iron deficiency anemia.
Pharmacokinetics: Distributed mainly in blood and to some extent in extravascular fluid. Iron sucrose is dissociated into iron and sucrose by the reticuloendothelial system. The sucrose component is eliminated mainly by urinary excretion. **Half-life:** 6 hr.

■ **Available Forms:**
- **Injection:** 20 mg/ml or 100 mg elemental iron in 5-ml single-dose vial.

■ **Indications and Dosages:**
Iron deficiency anemia: IV Dosage is expressed in terms of milligrams of elemental iron. 5 ml iron sucrose, or 100 mg elemental iron, delivered during dialysis; administer 1–3 times a wk to total dose of 1,000 mg in 10 doses. Give no more than 3 times a wk.

- **Unlabeled Uses:** Treatment of dystrophic epidermolysis bullosa

- **Contraindications:** All anemias except iron deficiency anemia, including pernicious, aplastic, normocytic, and refractory anemia; evidence of iron overload

- **Side Effects**
  Frequent (36%–23%)
  Hypotension, leg cramps, diarrhea

- **Serious Reactions**
  - Too-rapid IV administration may produce severe hypotension, headache, vomiting, nausea, dizziness, paresthesia, abdominal and muscle pain, edema, and cardiovascular collapse.
  - Hypersensitivity reaction occurs rarely.

- **Geriatric side effects at a glance:**
  ❑ CNS ❑ Bowel Dysfunction ❑ Bladder Dysfunction ❑ Falls

- **U.S. Regulatory Considerations**
  ❑ FDA Black Box ☑ OBRA regulated in U.S. Long Term Care

isocarboxazid

(eye-soe-kar-box′-a-zid)

- **Brand Name(s):** Marplan
  Chemical Class: Hydrazine derivative

- **Clinical Pharmacology:**
  Mechanism of Action: An antidepressant that inhibits the MAO enzyme system at central nervous system (CNS) storage sites. The reduced MAO activity causes an increased concentration in epinephrine, norepinephrine, serotonin, and dopamine at neuron receptor sites. **Therapeutic Effect:** Produces antidepressant effect.

- **Available Forms:**
  - *Tablets*: 10 mg (Marplan).

- **Indications and Dosages:**
  Depression refractory to other antidepressants or electroconvulsive therapy: PO Initially, 10 mg 3 times/day. May increase to 60 mg/day.

- **Unlabeled Uses:** Treatment of panic disorder, vascular or tension headaches

- **Contraindications:** Cardiovascular disease (CVD), cerebrovascular disease, liver impairment, pheochromocytoma

- **Side Effects**
  Frequent (more than 10%)
  Postural hypotension, drowsiness, decreased sexual ability, weakness, trembling, visual disturbances

Occasional (10%-1%)
Tachycardia, peripheral edema, nervousness, chills, diarrhea, anorexia, constipation, xerostomia
Rare (less than 1%)
Hepatitis, leukopenia, parkinsonian syndrome

- **Serious Reactions**
  - Hypertensive crisis, marked by severe hypertension, occipital headache radiating frontally, neck stiffness or soreness, nausea, vomiting, sweating, fever or chilliness, clammy skin, dilated pupils, palpitations, tachycardia or bradycardia, and constricting chest pain.

Special Considerations
  - Phentolamine for severe hypertension

- **Patient/Family Education**
  - Avoid high-tyramine foods: cheese (aged), sour cream, beer, wine, pickled products, liver, raisins, bananas, figs, avocados, meat tenderizers, chocolate, yogurt; soy sauce, caffeine
  - Do not discontinue medication quickly after long-term use
  - Notify the physician if headache or neck soreness or stiffness occurs
  - Avoid using OTC preparations for colds, hayfever, and weight reduction

- **Monitoring Parameters**
  - Blood pressure, heart rate, weight
  - Diet
  - Mood
  - Monitor the patient for occipital headache radiating frontally and neck stiffness or soreness, which may be the first sign of impending hypertensive crisis

- **Geriatric side effects at a glance:**
  ☐ CNS ☐ Bowel Dysfunction ☐ Bladder Dysfunction ☐ Falls
  Other: Orthostatic hypotension

- **Use with caution in older patients with:** None

- **U.S. Regulatory Considerations**
  ☑ FDA Black Box
  - Because there is an increased risk of suicide in children and adolescents, older adults should also be closely monitored for suicide ideation.
  ☑ OBRA regulated in U.S. Long Term Care

- **Other Uses in Geriatric Patient:** Depression refractory to other measures, anxiety symptoms and related disorders

- **Side Effects:**
  Of particular importance in the geriatric patient: None

- **Geriatric Considerations - Summary:** Because of the severe toxicity of these agents and the long list of potentially serious drug-drug and drug-food interactions, they are NOT recommended for routine treatment of depression in older adults. If prescribed, they require close monitoring by specialists.

■ **References:**
1. Boyer EW, Shannon M. The serotonin syndrome. N Engl J Med 2005;352:1112-1120.
2. Volz HP, Gleiter CH. Monoamine oxidase inhibitors. A perspective on their use in the elderly. Drugs Aging 1998;13:341-355.

isoetharine hydrochloride / isoetharine mesylate

(eye-soe-eth'-a-reen hye-droe-klor'-ide/eye-soe-eth'-a-reen mes'-sil-ate)

■ **Brand Name(s):** Beta-2, Bronkosol, Dey-Lute

■ **Brand Name(s):** Bronkometer
Chemical Class: Sympathomimetic amine; β_2-adrenergic agonist

■ **Clinical Pharmacology:**
Mechanism of Action: A sympathomimetic (adrenergic agonist) that stimulates beta$_2$-adrenergic receptors in the lungs, resulting in relaxation of bronchial smooth muscle. **Therapeutic Effect:** Relieves bronchospasm, reduces airway resistance.
Pharmacokinetics: Rapidly, well absorbed from the gastrointestinal (GI) tract. Extensive metabolism in GI tract. Unknown extent metabolized in liver and lungs. Excreted in urine. **Half-life:** 4 hr.

■ **Available Forms:**
• *Metered Spray*: 0.61% (Bronkometer).
• *Solution for Inhalation*: 0.08% (Dey-Lute), 0.1% (Dey-Lute), 0.17% (Dey-Lute), 1% (Beta-2, Bronkosol).

■ **Indications and Dosages:**
Bronchospasm: Hand-bulb Nebulizer   4 inhalations (range: 3-7 inhalations) undiluted. May be repeated up to 5 times/day.   Metered Dose Inhalation   1-2 inhalations q4h. Wait 1 min before administering 2nd inhalation.   IPPB, Oxygen Aerosolization 0.5-1 ml of a 0.5% or 0.5 ml of a 1% solution diluted 1:3.

■ **Contraindications:** History of hypersensitivity to sympathomimetics

■ **Side Effects**
Occasional
Tremor, nausea, nervousness, palpitations, tachycardia, peripheral vasodilation, dryness of mouth, throat, dizziness, vomiting, headache, increased BP, insomnia.

■ **Serious Reactions**
• Excessive sympathomimetic stimulation may produce palpitations, extrasystoles, tachycardia, chest pain, slight increase in BP followed by a substantial decrease, chills, sweating, and blanching of skin.

- Too frequent or excessive use may lead to loss of bronchodilating effectiveness and severe and paradoxical bronchoconstriction.

Special Considerations
- Inhalation technique critical
- Re-educate routinely

■ Patient/Family Education
- Increase fluid intake to decrease the viscosity of pulmonary secretions
- Rinse mouth with water immediately after inhalation
- Avoid excessive use of caffeine derivatives, such as chocolate, cocoa, coffee, cola, and tea

■ Monitoring Parameters
- Lung sounds for rhonchi, wheezing, and rales
- Clinical improvement (quieter, slower respirations, relaxed facial expression, cessation of clavicular retractions)

■ Geriatric side effects at a glance:
❑ CNS   ❑ Bowel Dysfunction   ❑ Bladder Dysfunction   ❑ Falls

■ U.S. Regulatory Considerations
❑ FDA Black Box   ❑ OBRA regulated in U.S. Long Term Care

isoniazid

(eye-soe-nye'-a-zid)

■ Brand Name(s): INH: Nydrazid

Combinations
Rx: with rifampin (Rifamate); with rifampin, pyrazinamide (Rifater)
Chemical Class: Isonicotinic acid derivative

■ Clinical Pharmacology:
Mechanism of Action: An isonicotinic acid hydrazide (INH) derivative that inhibits mycolic acid synthesis and causes disruption of the bacterial cell wall and loss of acid-fast properties in susceptible mycobacteria. Active only during bacterial cell division. **Therapeutic Effect:** Bactericidal against actively growing intracelleluar and extracellular susceptible mycobacteria.
Pharmacokinetics: Readily absorbed from the GI tract. Protein binding: 10%-15%. Widely distributed (including to CSF). Metabolized in the liver. Primarily excreted in urine. Removed by hemodialysis. **Half-life:** 0.5-5 hr.

■ Available Forms:
- *Tablets:* 100 mg, 300 mg.
- *Syrup:* 50 mg/5 ml.
- *Injection (Nydrazid):* 100 mg/ml.

- **Indications and Dosages:**
  Tuberculosis (in combination with one or more antituberculars): PO, IM 5 mg/kg/day as a single dose. Maximum 300 mg/day.
  Prevention of tuberculosis: PO, IM 300 mg/day as a single dose.

- **Contraindications:** Acute hepatic disease, history of hypersensitivity reactions or hepatic injury with previous isoniazid therapy

- **Side Effects**
  Frequent
  Nausea, vomiting, diarrhea, abdominal pain
  Rare
  Pain at injection site, hypersensitivity reaction

- **Serious Reactions**
  - Rare reactions include neurotoxicity (as evidenced by ataxia and paresthesia), optic neuritis, and hepatotoxicity.

- **Patient/Family Education**
  - Take on empty stomach if possible; however, may be taken with food to decrease GI upset
  - Minimize daily alcohol consumption to lessen the risk of hepatitis
  - Notify clinician of weakness, fatigue, loss of appetite, nausea and vomiting, yellowing of skin or eyes, darkening of urine, numbness or tingling of hands and feet
  - Do not skip doses and continue taking isoniazid for the full course of therapy (6-24 mo)
  - Avoid foods containing tyramine, including aged cheeses, sauerkraut, smoked fish, and tuna, because these foods may cause headache, a hot or clammy feeling, lightheadedness, pounding heartbeat, and red or itching skin

- **Monitoring Parameters**
  - Periodic ophthalmologic examinations even when visual symptoms do not occur
  - Periodic liver function tests
  - Assess the patient for burning, numbness, and tingling of the extremities. Be aware that patients at risk for neuropathy, such as alcoholics, those with chronic hepatic disease, diabetics, the elderly, and malnourished individuals, may receive pyridoxine prophylactically
  - Be alert for signs and symptoms of a hypersensitivity reaction, including fever and skin eruptions

- **Geriatric side effects at a glance:**
  ☐ CNS ☑ Bowel Dysfunction ☐ Bladder Dysfunction ☐ Falls
  Other: Hepatoxicity

- **Use with caution in older patients with:** Hepatic dysfunction, Daily alcohol use

- **U.S. Regulatory Considerations**
  ☑ FDA Black Box
  Hepatitis; risk related to age and increased with daily alcohol intake.
  ☐ OBRA regulated in U.S. Long Term Care

■ **Other Uses in Geriatric Patient:** None

■ **Side Effects:**
Of *particular importance in the geriatric patient*: Weakness, lethargy, dysphoria, inability to concentrate, irritability, dysarthria, dizziness, peripheral neuropathy (dose-related), asymptomatic increase of LFTs, decreased appetite, lupus-like syndrome; diarrhea with liquid preparations that contain sorbitol

■ **Geriatric Considerations - Summary:** Age is not a contraindication to INH prophylaxis or treatment of tuberculosis. Follow adult guidelines for treatment. INH may be used in patient with stable hepatic disease. The risk of clinical hepatitis increases with age and has been reported in 2% of adults aged greater than 50. INH interferes with the metabolism of pyridoxine; therefore concomitant pyridoxine therapy at 25mg/day is recommended to prevent neurotoxicity. INH is metabolized via acetylation in the liver. Older adults who are slow acetylators of the drug may require lower doses to achieve effective serum concentrations and prevent adverse effects. Food, especially high-fat meals, delays and reduces absorption; therefore administer INH on an empty stomach.

■ **References:**
1. American Thoracic Society. American Thoracic Society/ Centers for Disease Control and Prevention/Infectious Diseases Society of America: treatment of tuberculosis. Am J Respir Crit Care Med 2003;167:603-662.
2. Van der Brande P. Revised guidelines for the diagnosis and control of tuberculosis. Impact on management in the elderly. Drugs Aging 2005;22:663-688.

isoproterenol hydrochloride

(eye-soe-proe-ter'-e-nole hye-droe-klor'-ide)

■ **Brand Name(s):** Isuprel

Combinations
Rx: with phenylephrine (Duo-Medihaler)
Chemical Class: Catecholamine, synthetic

■ **Clinical Pharmacology:**
Mechanism of Action: A sympathomimetic (adrenergic agonist) that stimulates $beta_1$-adrenergic receptors. *Therapeutic Effect:* Increases myocardial contractility, stroke volume, cardiac output.
Pharmacokinetics: Readily absorbed. Metabolized in liver. Primarily excreted in urine. *Half-life:* 2.5-5 min.

■ **Available Forms:**
• *Injection:* 0.02 mg/ml (Isuprel).

■ **Indications and Dosages:**
Arrhythmias: IV Bolus Initially, 0.02-0.06 mg (1-3 ml of diluted solution). Subsequent dose range: 0.01-0.2 mg (0.5-10 ml of diluted solution). IV Infusion Initially, 5 mcg/min (1.25 ml/min of diluted solution). Subsequent dose range: 2-20 mcg/min.

Complete heart block following closure of ventricular septal defects: IV 0.04-0.06 mg (2-3 ml of diluted solution).

Shock: IV Infusion Rate of 0.5-5 mcg/min (0.25-2.5 ml of 1:500,000 dilution); rate of infusion based on clinical response (heart rate, central venous pressure, systemic BP, urine flow measurements).

■ **Contraindications:** Tachycardia due to digitalis toxicity, preexisting arrhythmias, angina, precordial distress, hypersensitivity to isoproterenol or any component of the formulation

■ **Side Effects**
Frequent
Palpitations, tachycardia, restlessness, nervousness, tremor, insomnia, anxiety
Occasional
Increased sweating, headache, nausea, flushed skin, dizziness, coughing

■ **Serious Reactions**
- Excessive sympathomimetic stimulation may cause palpitations, extrasystoles, tachycardia, chest pain, slight increase in BP followed by a substantial decrease, chills, sweating, and blanching of skin.
- Ventricular arrhythmias may occur if heart rate is above 130 beats/min.
- Parotid gland swelling may occur with prolonged use.

■ **Patient/Family Education**
- Notify the physician of chest pain, palpitations, or pain or burning at the injection site

■ **Monitoring Parameters**
- Blood pressure, pulse, urine output, ECG

■ **Geriatric side effects at a glance:**
❑ CNS ❑ Bowel Dysfunction ❑ Bladder Dysfunction ❑ Falls

■ **U.S. Regulatory Considerations**
❑ FDA Black Box ❑ OBRA regulated in U.S. Long Term Care

isosorbide dinitrate/ isosorbide mononitrate

(eye-soe-sore'-bide dye-nye'-trate/eye-soe-sore'-bide mon-oh-nye'-trate)

■ **Brand Name(s):** (isosorbide dinitrate) Dilatrate, Dilatrate-SR, ISDN, Isochron, Isordil, Isordil Tembids, Isordil Titradose, Sorbitrate

■ **Brand Name(s):** (isosorbide mononitrate) Imdur, ISMO, Monoket
   Chemical Class: Nitrate, organic

■ **Clinical Pharmacology:**
   Mechanism of Action: A nitrate that stimulates intracellular cyclic guanosine monophosphate. **Therapeutic Effect:** Relaxes vascular smooth muscle of both arterial and
   venous vasculature. Decreases preload and afterload.
   Pharmacokinetics:

Route	Onset	Peak	Duration
Dinitrate			
Sublingual	2–5 min	N/A	1–2 hr
Oral (Chewable)	2-5 min	N/A	1–2 hr
Oral	15-40 min	N/A	4–6 hr
Oral (Sustained-Release)	30 min	N/A	12 hr
Mononitrate			
Oral (Extended-Release)	60 min	N/A	N/A

Dinitrate poorly absorbed and metabolized in the liver to its active metabolite isosorbide mononitrate. Mononitrate well absorbed after PO administration. Excreted
in urine and feces. **Half-life:** Dinitrate, 1–4 hr; mononitrate, 4 hr.

■ **Available Forms:**
   • *Capsules (Sustained-Release [Dilatrate, Isordil Tembids]):* 40 mg.
   • *Tablets:* 5 mg (ISDN, Isordil, Isordil Titradose), 10 mg (ISDN, ISMO, Isordil, Isordil Ti-
     tradose, Monoket), 20 mg (ISDN, ISMO, Isordil, Isordil Titradose, Monoket), 30 mg
     (ISDN, Isordil, Isordil Titradose), 40 mg (ISDN, Isordil, Isordil Titradose).
   • *Tablets (Chewable [Sorbitrate]):* 5 mg, 10 mg.
   • *Tablets (Extended-Release [Imdur]):* 30 mg, 60 mg, 120 mg.
   • *Tablets (Sublingual [Isordil]):* 2.5 mg, 5 mg, 10 mg.

■ **Indications and Dosages:**
   Angina: PO (isosorbide dinitrate) 5-40 mg 4 times a day. Sustained-Release: 40 mg
   q8-12h. PO (isosorbide mononitrate) 5-10 mg twice a day given 7 hr apart. Sustained-Release: Initially, 30-60 mg/day in morning as a single dose. May increase dose
   at 3-day intervals. Maximum: 240 mg/day.

■ **Unlabeled Uses:** CHF, dysphagia, pain relief, relief of esophageal spasm with gastroesophageal reflux

■ **Contraindications:** Closed-angle glaucoma, GI hypermotility or malabsorption (extended-release tablets), head trauma, hypersensitivity to nitrates, increased intracranial pressure, orthostatic hypotension, severe anemia (extended-release tablets)

■ **Side Effects**
   Frequent
   Burning and tingling at oral point of dissolution (sublingual), headache (possibly severe) occurs mostly in early therapy, diminishes rapidly in intensity, and usually disappears during continued treatment, transient flushing of face and neck, dizziness
   (especially if patient is standing immobile or is in a warm environment), weakness, orthostatic hypotension, nausea, vomiting, restlessness
   Occasional
   GI upset, blurred vision, dry mouth

654

Serious Reactions

- Blurred vision or dry mouth may occur (drug should be discontinued).
- Isosorbide administration may cause severe orthostatic hypotension manifested by fainting, pulselessness, cold or clammy skin, and diaphoresis.
- Tolerance may occur with repeated, prolonged therapy, but may not occur with the extended-release form. Minor tolerance may be seen with intermittent use of sublingual tablets.
- High dosage tends to produce severe headache.

Patient/Family Education

- Headache may be a marker for drug activity; do not try to avoid by altering treatment schedule; contact clinician if severe or persistent; aspirin or acetaminophen may be used for relief
- Dissolve SL tablets under tongue; do not crush, chew, or swallow
- Do not crush chewable tablets before administering
- Avoid alcohol
- Make changes in position slowly to prevent fainting

Monitoring Parameters

- Monitor and document the number of anginal episodes and orthostatic blood pressure
- Assess for dizziness or light-headedness and facial or neck flushing

Geriatric side effects at a glance:
❑ CNS ❑ Bowel Dysfunction ❑ Bladder Dysfunction ❑ Falls

U.S. Regulatory Considerations
❑ FDA Black Box ❑ OBRA regulated in U.S. Long Term Care

isradipine

(is-rad'-i-peen)

Brand Name(s): DynaCirc, DynaCirc CR
Chemical Class: Dihydropyridine

Clinical Pharmacology:
Mechanism of Action: An antihypertensive that inhibits calcium movement across cardiac and vascular smooth-muscle cell membranes. Potent peripheral vasodilator that does not depress SA or AV nodes. **Therapeutic Effect:** Produces relaxation of coronary vascular smooth muscle and coronary vasodilation. Increases myocardial oxygen delivery to those with vasospastic angina.

Pharmacokinetics:

Route	Onset	Peak	Duration
PO	2–3 hr	2–4 wk (with multiple doses) 8-16 hr (with single dose)	N/A
PO (Controlled-release)	2 hr	8-10 hr	N/A

Well absorbed from the GI tract. Protein binding: 95%. Metabolized in the liver (undergoes first-pass effect). Primarily excreted in urine. Not removed by hemodialysis. **Half-life:** 8 hr.

■ **Available Forms:**
- *Capsules (DynaCirc):* 2.5 mg, 5 mg.
- *Capsules (Controlled-Release [DynaCirc-CR]):* 5 mg, 10 mg.

■ **Indications and Dosages:**
Hypertension: PO Initially 2.5 mg twice a day. May increase by 2.5 mg at 2- to 4-wk intervals. Range: 5–20 mg/day

■ **Unlabeled Uses:** Treatment of chronic angina pectoris, Raynaud's phenomenon

■ **Contraindications:** Cardiogenic shock, CHF, heart block, hypotension, sinus bradycardia, ventricular tachycardia

■ **Side Effects**
Frequent (7%–4%)
Peripheral edema, palpitations (higher frequency in females)
Occasional (3%)
Facial flushing, cough
Rare (2%–1%)
Angina, tachycardia, rash, pruritus

■ **Serious Reactions**
- Overdose produces nausea, drowsiness, confusion, and slurred speech.
- CHF occurs rarely.

■ **Patient/Family Education**
- Do not abruptly discontinue isradipine
- Compliance with the treatment regimen is essential to control hypertension
- Rise slowly from a lying to a sitting position and wait momentarily before standing to avoid isradipine's hypotensive effect
- Notify the physician if an irregular heartbeat, nausea, pronounced dizziness, or shortness of breath occurs
- Avoid grapefruit and grapefruit juice because these foods may increase the absorption of isradipine

■ **Monitoring Parameters**
- Blood pressure for hypotension and pulse for bradycardia
- Assess for peripheral edema behind the medial malleolus in ambulatory patients or in the sacral area in bedridden patients
- Observe the patient for signs and symptoms of CHF and examine the patient's skin for flushing

itraconazole

(it-ra-con'-a-zol)

■ **Brand Name(s):** Sporanox
Chemical Class: Triazole derivative

■ **Clinical Pharmacology:**
Mechanism of Action: A fungistatic antifungal that inhibits the synthesis of ergosterol, a vital component of fungal cell formation. **Therapeutic Effect:** Damages the fungal cell membrane, altering its function.
Pharmacokinetics: Moderately absorbed from the GI tract. Absorption is increased if the drug is taken with food. Protein binding: 99%. Widely distributed, primarily in the fatty tissue, liver, and kidneys. Metabolized in the liver to active metabolite. Primarily excreted in urine. Not removed by hemodialysis. **Half-life:** 21 hr; metabolite, 12 hr.

■ **Available Forms:**
• *Capsules:* 100 mg.
• *Oral Solution:* 10 mg/ml.
• *Injection:* 10 mg/ml (25-ml ampule).

■ **Indications and Dosages:**
Blastomycosis, histoplasmosis: PO Initially, 200 mg once a day. Maximum: 400 mg/day in 2 divided doses. IV 200 mg twice a day for 4 doses, then 200 mg once a day.
Aspergillosis: PO 600 mg/day in 3 divided doses for 3-4 days, then 200-400 mg/day in 2 divided doses. IV 200 mg twice a day for 4 doses, then 200 mg once a day.
Esophageal candidiasis: PO Swish 100-200 mg (10-20 ml) in mouth for several seconds, then swallow. Maximum: 200 mg/day.
Oropharyngeal candidiasis: PO 200 mg (10 ml) oral solution, swish and swallow once a day for 7-14 days.
Febrile neutropenia: IV 200 mg twice a day for 4 doses, then 200 mg for up to 14 days. Then give PO 200 mg twice a day until neutropenia resolves.
Onychomycosis (fingernail): PO 200 mg twice a day for 7 days, off for 21 days, repeat 200 mg twice a day for 7 days.
Onychomycosis (toenail): PO 200 mg once daily for 12 wk.

■ **Unlabeled Uses:** Suppression of histoplasmosis; treatment of disseminated sporotrichosis, fungal pneumonia and septicemia, or ringworm of the hand

■ **Contraindications:** Hypersensitivity to fluconazole, ketoconazole, or miconazole

■ **Side Effects**
Frequent (11%-9%)
Nausea, rash

Occasional (5%-3%)
Vomiting, headache, diarrhea, hypertension, peripheral edema, fatigue, fever
Rare (2% or less)
Abdominal pain, dizziness, anorexia, pruritus

■ **Serious Reactions**
  • Hepatitis (as evidenced by anorexia, abdominal pain, unusual fatigue or weakness, jaundiced skin or sclera, and dark urine) occurs rarely.

■ **Patient/Family Education**
  • Take with food to ensure maximal absorption
  • Avoid antacids within 2 hr of itraconazole administration
  • Report decreased appetite, dark urine, nausea, vomiting, pale stools, unusual fatigue, or yellow skin to the physician
  • Avoid grapefruit and grapefruit juice because they may alter itraconazole absorption

■ **Monitoring Parameters**
  • Liver function tests in patients with preexisting abnormalities

■ **Geriatric side effects at a glance:**
  ❑ CNS   ❑ Bowel Dysfunction   ❑ Bladder Dysfunction   ❑ Falls

■ **U.S. Regulatory Considerations**
  ☑ FDA Black Box
  Itraconazole contraindicated in patients with evidence of ventricular dysfunction (CHF) or a history of CHF. Itraconazole is also a potent inhibitor of cytochrome P450 3A4 isoenzyme, which may increase plasma concentrations of drugs metabolized by this pathway. Serious cardiovascular events have occurred in patients taking cisapride, pimozide, levomethadyl, or quinidine concomitantly with itraconazole.
  ❑ OBRA regulated in U.S. Long Term Care

ivermectin

(eye-ver-mek'-tin)

■ **Brand Name(s):** Stromectol
  Chemical Class: Avermectin derivative

■ **Clinical Pharmacology:**
  Mechanism of Action: Selectively binds to chloride ion channels in invertebrate nerve/muscle cells, increasing permeability to chloride ions. In general the following organisms are susceptible to ivermectin: *Onchocerca volvulus, Pediculosis capitis, Strongyloides stercoralis, Sarcoptes scabiei,* and *Wuchereria bancrofti.* **Therapeutic Effects:** Causes paralysis/death of parasites.

Pharmacokinetics: Does not readily cross the blood-brain barrier. Metabolized in the liver. Excreted in the feces. **Half-life:** 4 hours. Well absorbed with plasma concentrations proportional to the dose.

■ Available Forms:
- **Tablets:** 3 mg, 6 mg

■ Indications and Dosages:
Strongyloidiasis: PO 200 mcg/kg as a single dose.
Onchoceriasis: PO 150 mcg/kg as a single dose at 3- to 12-mo intervals.
Scabies: PO 200 mcg/kg as a single dose and repeat 2 wk later
Norwegian Scabies (crusted scabies infection), superinfected scabies, or resistant scabies: PO 200 mcg/kg with repeated treatments or combined with a topical scabicide
Pediculosis: PO A regimen of 2 doses of 200 mcg/kg with each dose separated by 10 days
Bancroft's filariasis: PO 150 mcg/kg as a single dose. May repeat 1 or 2 more times (each dose a week apart) if larva continues to migrate 1 wk after the previous dose.

■ Unlabeled Uses:
Cutaneous larva migrans, filariasis, pediculosis, scabies, Wuchereria bancrofti

■ Contraindications:
Hypersensitivity to ivermectin or to any one of its components.

■ Side Effects
Occasional
Abdominal pain, anorexia, arthralgia, constipation, diarrhea, dizziness, drowsiness, edema, fatigue, fever, lymphadenopathy, maculopapular or unspecified rash, nausea, vomiting, orthostatic hypotension, pruritus, Stevens-Johnson syndrome, toxic epidermal necrolysis, tremor, urticaria, vertigo, visual impairment, weakness

■ Patient/Family Education
- Rapid killing of microfilariae may induce systemic or ocular inflammatory response (Mazzotti reaction, manifest by pruritus, rash, lymphadenopathy, and fever)
- Complete full course of therapy
- Keep hands away from mouth

■ Monitoring Parameters
- Stool for parasites; blood for microfilaria and eosinophils

■ Geriatric side effects at a glance:
❏ CNS ❏ Bowel Dysfunction ❏ Bladder Dysfunction ❏ Falls

■ U.S. Regulatory Considerations
❏ FDA Black Box ❏ OBRA regulated in U.S. Long Term Care

kanamycin sulfate

(kan-a-mye'-sin sul'-fate)

■ **Brand Name(s):** Kantrex
   Chemical Class: Aminoglycoside

■ **Clinical Pharmacology:**
   Mechanism of Action: An aminoglycoside antibacterial that irreversibly binds to protein on bacterial ribosomes. **Therapeutic Effect:** Interferes with protein synthesis of susceptible microorganisms.
   Pharmacokinetics: Negligible amounts are absorbed through intact intestinal mucosa. Protein binding: 0%-3%. Minimally metabolized in liver. Partially excreted in feces; small amounts eliminated in urine. Removed by hemodialysis. **Half-life:** approximately 2 hr.

■ **Available Forms:**
   • *Injection*: 1 g/3 ml.

■ **Indications and Dosages:**
   Short-term treatment of serious infections: IV 15 mg/kg/day. IM 15 mg/kg/day in 2 divided dosages administered at equally divided intervals (75 mg/kg q12h). If continuously high blood levels are desired, the daily dose of 15 mg/kg may be given in equally divided doses q6-8h.
   Dosage in renal impairment: GFR > 50 *ml/min*. 60%-90% of normal dose q8-12h. GFR 10-50 *ml/min*. 30%-70% of normal dose q12h. GFR, 10 *ml/min*. 20%-30% of normal dose q24-48h.

■ **Contraindications:** Hypersensitivity to other aminoglycosides (cross-sensitivity), or their components, long-term therapy

■ **Side Effects**
   Occasional
   Hypersensitivity reactions (fever, pruritus, rash, urticaria)
   Rare
   Headache

■ **Serious Reactions**
   • Serious reactions may include nephrotoxicity (as evidenced by increased thirst, decreased appetite, nausea, vomiting, increased BUN and serum creatinine levels, and decreased creatinine clearance), neurotoxicity (manifested as muscle twitching, visual disturbances, seizures, and tingling), and ototoxicity (as evidenced by tinnitus, dizziness, and loss of hearing).

Special Considerations
   • Individualize treatment based on local susceptibility patterns.

■ **Patient/Family Education**
   • Report headache, dizziness, loss of hearing, ringing, roaring in ears, or feeling of fullness in head

660

Monitoring Parameters
- Urinalysis
- Urine output
- Serum peak drawn at 30-60 min after IV INF or 60 min after IM inj, trough level drawn just before next dose; adjust dosage per levels, especially in renal function impairment (usual therapeutic plasma levels; peak 15-30 mg/L, trough ≤10 mg/L)
- Serum creatinine for CrCl calculation
- Serum calcium, magnesium, sodium
- Audiometric testing; assess hearing before, during, after treatment
- RBCs, WBCs

Geriatric side effects at a glance:
❑ CNS   ❑ Bowel Dysfunction   ❑ Bladder Dysfunction   ❑ Falls

U.S. Regulatory Considerations
☑ FDA Black Box
Neurotoxicity (both auditory and vestibular ototoxicity) and nephrotoxicity. Risk is greater in patients with impaired renal function and in those who receive high doses or prolonged therapy.
❑ OBRA regulated in U.S. Long Term Care

ketoconazole

(kee-toe-kon'-na-zole)

Brand Name(s): Nizoral, Nizoral Topical
OTC: Nizoral AD
Chemical Class: Imidazole derivative

Clinical Pharmacology:
Mechanism of Action: A fungistatic antifungal that inhibits the synthesis of ergosterol, a vital component of fungal cell formation. **Therapeutic Effect:** Damages the fungal cell membrane, altering its function.
Pharmacokinetics: Well absorbed from GI tract following PO administration. Protein binding: 91%-99%. Metabolized in liver. Primarily excreted in bile with minimal elimination in urine. Negligible systemic absorption following topical absorption. Ketoconazole is not detected in plasma after shampooing or topical administration. **Half-life:** 2-12 hr.

Available Forms:
- *Tablets (Nizoral)*: 200 mg.
- *Cream (Nizoral Topical)*: 2%.
- *Shampoo (Nizoral AD)*: 1%.

Indications and Dosages:
Histoplasmosis, blastomycosis, systemic candidiasis, chronic mucocutaneous candidiasis, coccidioidomycosis, paracoccidioidomycosis, chromomycosis, seborrheic dermatitis,

tinea corporis, tinea capitis, tinea manus, tinea cruris, tinea pedis, tinea unguium (ony-chomycosis), oral thrush, candiduria: PO 200-400 mg/day. Topical Apply to affected area 1-2 times a day for 2-4 wk. Shampoo Use twice weekly for 4 wk, allowing at least 3 days between shampooing. Use intermittently to maintain control.

■ **Unlabeled Uses:** *Systemic:* Treatment of fungal pneumonia, prostate cancer, septicemia

■ **Contraindications:** None known.

■ **Side Effects**
Occasional (10%-3%)
Nausea, vomiting
Rare (less than 2%)
Abdominal pain, diarrhea, headache, dizziness, photophobia, pruritus
Topical: itching, burning, irritation

■ **Serious Reactions**
- Hematologic toxicity (as evidenced by thrombocytopenia, hemolytic anemia, and leukopenia) occurs occasionally.
- Hepatotoxicity may occur within 1 wk to several mo after starting therapy.
- Anaphylaxis occurs rarely.

■ **Patient/Family Education**
- For shampoo, moisten hair and scalp, apply shampoo, and gently massage over entire scalp for 1 min; rinse with warm water; repeat, leaving shampoo on scalp for additional 3 min
- Do not take tab with antacids or H_2-receptor antagonists; separate doses by at least 2 hr
- Take tablets with food
- Prolonged therapy over weeks or months is usually necessary
- Do not miss a dose and continue therapy for as long as directed
- Avoid alcohol to minimize the risk of liver damage
- Avoid tasks that require mental alertness or motor skills until response to the drug is established
- Notify the physician if dark urine, pale stools, yellow skin or eyes, increased irritation (with topical use), or other new symptoms occurs
- The patient using topical ketoconazole should avoid drug contact with the eyes, keep the skin clean and dry, rub the drug well into affected areas, and wear light clothing for ventilation
- Separate personal items that come in direct contact with the affected area

■ **Monitoring Parameters**
- Liver function tests at baseline and periodically during treatment
- CBC for evidence of hematologic toxicity
- Pattern of daily bowel activity and stool consistency
- Skin for rash, pruritus, urticaria, burning, or irritation

■ **Geriatric side effects at a glance:**
❑ CNS ❑ Bowel Dysfunction ❑ Bladder Dysfunction ❑ Falls

■ **U.S. Regulatory Considerations**
☑ FDA Black Box

Hepatotoxicity. Severe cardiovascular events have occurred when co-administered with cisapride, astemizole or terfenadine—concurrent use is contraindicated.

❑ OBRA regulated in U.S. Long Term Care

ketoprofen

(kee-toe-proe'-fen)

■ **Brand Name(s):** Oruvail
OTC: Actron, Orudis KT
Chemical Class: Propionic acid derivative

■ **Clinical Pharmacology:**
Mechanism of Action: An NSAID that produces analgesic and anti-inflammatory effects by inhibiting prostaglandin synthesis. **Therapeutic Effect:** Reduces the inflammatory response and intensity of pain.
Pharmacokinetics: Immediate-release capsules are rapidly and well-absorbed following PO administration; extended-release capsules are also well-absorbed. Protein binding: 99%. Metabolized in liver. Excreted in urine; less than 10% excreted as unchanged (unconjugated) drug. **Half-life:** 2.4 hr.

■ **Available Forms:**
• *Capsules:* 25 mg, 50 mg, 75 mg.
• *Capsules (Extended-Release [Oruvail]):* 100 mg, 150 mg, 200 mg.
• *Tablets (Orudis KT):* 12.5 mg.

■ **Indications and Dosages:**
Acute or chronic rheumatoid arthritis and osteoarthritis: PO Initially, 25–50 mg 3–4 times a day. Maintenance: 150–300 mg/day in 3–4 divided doses. PO (Extended-Release) 100–200 mg once a day.
Mild to moderate pain: PO 25–50 mg q6–8h. Maximum: 300 mg/day.
Over-the-counter (OTC) dosage: PO 12.5 mg q4-6h. Maximum: 6 tabs/day.
Dosage in renal impairment: Mild. 150 mg/day maximum. Severe. 100 mg/day maximum.

■ **Unlabeled Uses:** Treatment of acute gouty arthritis, psoriatic arthritis, ankylosing spondylitis, vascular headache

■ **Contraindications:** Active peptic ulcer disease, chronic inflammation of the GI tract, GI bleeding or ulceration, history of hypersensitivity to aspirin or NSAIDs

■ **Side Effects**
Frequent (11%)
Dyspepsia
Occasional (more than 3%)
Nausea, diarrhea or constipation, flatulence, abdominal cramps, headache
Rare (less than 2%)
Anorexia, vomiting, visual disturbances, fluid retention

■ **Serious Reactions**
- Rare reactions with long-term use include peptic ulcer disease, GI bleeding, gastritis, and severe hepatic reactions (cholestasis, jaundice), nephrotoxicity (dysuria, hematuria, proteinuria, nephrotic syndrome), and severe hypersensitivity reaction (bronchospasm, angioedema).

Special Considerations
- No significant advantage over other NSAIDs; cost should govern use

■ **Patient/Family Education**
- Avoid aspirin and alcoholic beverages
- Take with food, milk, or antacids to decrease GI upset
- Swallow capsules whole and do not chew or crush them

■ **Monitoring Parameters**
- Initial hematocrit and fecal occult blood test within 3 mo of starting regular chronic therapy; repeat every 6-12 mo (more frequently in high-risk patients (>65 years, peptic ulcer disease, concurrent steroids or anticoagulants); electrolytes, creatinine, and BUN within 3 mo of starting regular chronic therapy; repeat every 6-12 mo
- Therapeutic response, such as improved grip strength, increased mobility, improved range of motion, and decreased pain, tenderness, stiffness, and swelling

■ **Geriatric side effects at a glance:**
☑ CNS ❑ Bowel Dysfunction ❑ Bladder Dysfunction ❑ Falls
☑ Other: Gastropathy

■ **Use with caution in older patients with:** Renal impairment, Hepatic impairment, CHF, HTN, PUD, History of GI bleeding, GERD, Bleeding and platelet disorders, History of aspirin sensitivity reaction. Also use with caution in patients taking Anticoagulants, Aspirin, and Antihypertensive agents.

■ **U.S. Regulatory Considerations**
☑ FDA Black Box
- Cardiovascular risk
- Gastrointestinal risk
❑ OBRA regulated in U.S. Long Term Care

■ **Other Uses in Geriatric Patient:** Acute Gout

■ **Side Effects:**
Of particular importance in the geriatric patient: Confusion, cognitive impairment, delirium, dizziness, dyspepsia, fluid retention, renal impairment

■ **Geriatric Considerations - Summary:** A preferred agent in older adults due to its association with fewer GI adverse effects. Use of NSAIDs in older adults increases the risk of GI complications including gastric ulceration, bleeding, and perforation. These complications are not necessarily preceded by less severe GI symptoms. Concomitant use of a proton pump inhibitor or misoprostol reduces the risk for gastric ulceration and bleeding, but may not prevent long-term GI toxicity.

■ **References:**
1. COX-2 alternatives and GI protection. Med Lett Drugs Ther 2004;46:91.

2. Drugs that may cause cognitive disorders in the elderly. Med Lett Drugs Ther 2000;42:111-112.

ketorolac tromethamine

(kee-toe-role'-ak troe-meth'-a-meen)

■ **Brand Name(s):** Acular, Acular LS, Acular PF, Toradol, Toradol IM, Toradol IV/IM
Chemical Class: Acetic acid derivative

■ **Clinical Pharmacology:**
Mechanism of Action: An NSAID that inhibits prostaglandin synthesis and reduces prostaglandin levels in the aqueous humor. **Therapeutic Effect:** Relieves pain stimulus and reduces intraocular inflammation.
Pharmacokinetics:

Route	Onset	Peak	Duration
PO	30–60 min	1.5–4 hr	4–6 hr
IV/IM	30 min	1–2 hr	4–6 hr

Readily absorbed from the GI tract, after IM administration. Protein binding: 99%. Largely metabolized in the liver. Primarily excreted in urine. Not removed by hemodialysis. **Half-life:** 3.8–6.3 hr (increased with impaired renal function and in the elderly).

■ **Available Forms:**
- *Tablets* (Toradol): 10 mg.
- *Injection* (Toradol, Toradol IM, Toradol IV/IM): 15 mg/ml, 30 mg/ml.
- *Ophthalmic Solution*: 0.4% (Acular LS), 0.5% (Acular, Acular PF).

■ **Indications and Dosages:**
Short-term relief of mild to moderate pain (multiple doses): PO 10 mg q4–6h. Maximum: 40 mg/24 hr. IV, IM 15 mg q6h. Maximum: 60 mg/24 hr.
Short-term relief of mild to moderate pain (single dose): IV 15 mg. IM 30 mg.
Allergic conjunctivitis: Ophthalmic 1 drop 4 times a day.
Cataract extraction: Ophthalmic 1 drop 4 times a day. Begin 24 hr after surgery and continue for 2 wk.
Refractive surgery: Ophthalmic 1 drop 4 times a day for 3 days.

■ **Unlabeled Uses:** Prevention or treatment of ocular inflammation (ophthalmic form)

■ **Contraindications:** Active peptic ulcer disease, chronic inflammation of GI tract, GI bleeding or ulceration, history of hypersensitivity to aspirin or NSAIDs

■ **Side Effects**
Frequent (17%–12%)
Headache, nausea, abdominal cramps or pain, dyspepsia
Occasional (9%–3%)
Diarrhea
Ophthalmic: Transient stinging and burning

Rare (3%–1%)
Constipation, vomiting, flatulence, stomatitis, dizziness
Ophthalmic: Ocular irritation, allergic reactions, superficial ocular infection, keratitis

■ **Serious Reactions**
- Rare reactions with long-term use include peptic ulcer disease, GI bleeding, gastritis, severe hepatic reactions (cholestasis, jaundice), nephrotoxicity (glomerular nephritis, interstitial nephritis, nephrotic syndrome), and an acute hypersensitivity reaction (including fever, chills, and joint pain).

■ **Patient/Family Education**
- Not for chronic use
- No significant advantage over other oral NSAIDs; cost and clinical situation should govern use; no reason to continue parenteral course of therapy with oral ketorolac (more expensive, more toxic)
- Combined use of ketorolac parenteral and oral should not exceed 5 days
- Take ketorolac with food or milk if GI upset occurs
- Do not administer ketorolac ophthalmic solution while wearing soft contact lenses; transient burning and stinging may occur after instillation
- Avoid tasks that require mental alertness or motor skills until response to the drug has been established

■ **Monitoring Parameters**
- CBC, liver and renal function test results, urine output, BUN level, and serum alkaline phosphatase, bilirubin, and creatinine levels
- Be alert for signs of bleeding, which may also occur with ophthalmic use if systemic absorption occurs
- Therapeutic response, such as improved grip strength, increased joint mobility, and decreased pain, tenderness, stiffness, and swelling

■ **Geriatric side effects at a glance:**
☑ CNS ☐ Bowel Dysfunction ☐ Bladder Dysfunction ☐ Falls
☑ Other: Gastropathy

■ **Use with caution in older patients with:** Renal impairment, Hepatic impairment, CHF, HTN, PUD, History of GI bleeding, GERD, Bleeding and platelet disorders, History of aspirin sensitivity reaction. Also use with caution in patients taking Anticoagulants, Aspirin, and Antihypertensive agents.

■ **U.S. Regulatory Considerations**
☑ FDA Black Box
- Cardiovascular risk
- Gastrointestinal risk
☐ OBRA regulated in U.S. Long Term Care

■ **Other Uses in Geriatric Patient:** Acute Gout

■ **Side Effects:**
Of particular importance in the geriatric patient: Confusion, cognitive impairment, delirium, renal failure, dizziness, dyspepsia, fluid retention

- **Geriatric Considerations - Summary:** Older adults are at an increased risk of ketorolac-induced gastrointestinal bleeding and perforation. Adverse effects are increased with increasing dose, treatment 5 days longer and advancing age. GI complications can occur with short-term use (< 5 days) as well. Not a preferred agent for use in older adults.

- **References:**
  1. Drugs that may cause cognitive disorders in the elderly. Med Lett Drugs Ther 2000;42:111-112.
  2. Reinhart DJ. Minimising the adverse effects of ketorolac. Drug Saf 200;22:487-497.

labetalol hydrochloride

(la-bet'-a-lole hye-droe-klor'-ide)

- **Brand Name(s):** Normodyne, Trandate

  Combinations
  Rx: with hydrochlorothiazide (Normozide, Trandate HCT)
  Chemical Class: α-Adrenergic blocker, peripheral; β-adrenergic blocker, nonselective

- **Clinical Pharmacology:**
  Mechanism of Action: An antihypertensive that blocks $alpha_1$-, $beta_1$-, and $beta_2$- (large doses) adrenergic receptor sites. Large doses increase airway resistance. **Therapeutic Effect:** Slows sinus heart rate; decreases peripheral vascular resistance, cardiac output, and BP.
  Pharmacokinetics:

Route	Onset	Peak	Duration
PO	0.5–2 hr	2–4 hr	8–12 hr
IV	2–5 min	5–15 min	2–4 hr

  Completely absorbed from the GI tract. Protein binding: 50%. Undergoes first-pass metabolism. Metabolized in the liver. Primarily excreted in urine. Not removed by hemodialysis. **Half-life:** PO, 6–8 hr; IV, 5.5 hr.

- **Available Forms:**
  - *Tablets* (*Normodyne, Trandate*): 100 mg, 200 mg, 300 mg.
  - *Injection* (*Trandate*): 5 mg/ml.

- **Indications and Dosages:**
  Hypertension: PO Initially, 100 mg 1–2 times a day. May increase as needed.
  Severe hypertension, hypertensive emergency: IV Initially, 20 mg. Additional doses of 20–80 mg may be given at 10-min intervals, up to total dose of 300 mg. IV Infusion Initially, 2 mg/min up to total dose of 300 mg. PO (after IV therapy) Initially, 200 mg; then, 200–400 mg in 6–12 hr. Increase dose at 1-day intervals to desired level.

- **Unlabeled Uses:** Control of hypotension during surgery, treatment of chronic angina pectoris

- **Contraindications:** Bronchial asthma, cardiogenic shock, overt cardiac failure, second- or third-degree heart block, severe bradycardia, uncontrolled CHF, other conditions associated with severe and prolonged hypotension

Side Effects

Frequent
Drowsiness, difficulty sleeping, unusual fatigue or weakness, diminished sexual ability, transient scalp tingling

Occasional
Dizziness, dyspnea, peripheral edema, depression, anxiety, constipation, diarrhea, nasal congestion, nausea, vomiting, abdominal discomfort

Rare
Altered taste, dry eyes, increased urination, paresthesia

Serious Reactions
- Labetalol administration may precipitate or aggravate CHF because of decreased myocardial stimulation.
- Abrupt withdrawal may precipitate ischemic heart disease, producing sweating, palpitations, headache, and tremor.
- May mask signs and symptoms of acute hypoglycemia (tachycardia, BP changes) in patients with diabetes.

Patient/Family Education
- Do not discontinue abruptly; may require taper; rapid withdrawal may produce rebound hypertension or angina
- Transient scalp tingling may occur, especially when treatment is initiated
- May mask the symptoms of hypoglycemia, except for sweating, in diabetic patients
- Maintain compliance
- Avoid tasks that require mental alertness or motor skills until response to the drug has been established
- Notify the physician if excessive fatigue, headache, prolonged dizziness, shortness of breath, or weight gain occurs
- Do not take nasal decongestants and OTC cold preparations, especially those containing stimulants, without physician approval

Monitoring Parameters
- Angina: Reduction in nitroglycerin usage; frequency, severity, onset, and duration of angina pain; heart rate
- Arrhythmias: Heart rate
- Congestive heart failure: Functional status, cough, dyspnea on exertion, paroxysmal nocturnal dyspnea, exercise tolerance, and ventricular function
- Hypertension: Blood pressure
- Postmyocardial infarction: Left ventricular function, lower resting heart rate
- Toxicity: Blood glucose, bronchospasm, hypotension, bradycardia, depression, confusion, hallucination, sexual dysfunction

Geriatric side effects at a glance:
☐ CNS ☐ Bowel Dysfunction ☐ Bladder Dysfunction ☐ Falls

U.S. Regulatory Considarations
☑ FDA Black Box
In patients using orally administered beta-blockers, abrupt withdrawal may precipitate angina or lead to myocardial infarction or ventricular arrhythmias.
☐ OBRA regulated in U.S. Long Term Care

lactulose

(lak'-tyoo-lose)

■ **Brand Name(s):** Cholac, Constilac, Constulose, Enulose, Generlac, Kristalose
Chemical Class: Disaccharide lactose analog

■ **Clinical Pharmacology:**
Mechanism of Action: A lactose derivative that retains ammonia in colon and decreases serum ammonia concentration, producing osmotic effect. **Therapeutic Effect:** Promotes increased peristalsis and bowel evacuation, which expels ammonia from the colon.
Pharmacokinetics:

Route	Onset	Peak	Duration
PO	24–48 hr	N/A	N/A
Rectal	30–60 min	N/A	N/A

Poorly absorbed from the GI tract. Acts in the colon. Primarily excreted in feces.

■ **Available Forms:**
- *Syrup*: 10 g/15 ml.
- *Packets*: 10 g, 20 g.

■ **Indications and Dosages:**
Constipation: PO 15–30 ml(10-20 g)/day, up to 60 ml(40 g)/day.
Portal-systemic encephalopathy: PO Initially, 30–45 ml every hr. Then, 30–45 ml (20-30 g) 3–4 times a day. Adjust dose q 1–2 days to produce 2–3 soft stools a day. Rectal (as retention enema) 300 ml with 700 ml water or saline solution; patient should retain 30–60 min. Repeat q4–6h. If evacuation occurs too promptly, repeat immediately.

■ **Contraindications:** Abdominal pain, appendicitis, nausea, patients on a galactose-free diet, vomiting

■ **Side Effects**
Occasional
Abdominal cramping, flatulence, increased thirst, abdominal discomfort
Rare
Nausea, vomiting

■ **Serious Reactions**
- Diarrhea indicates overdose.
- Long-term use may result in GI-laxative dependence, chronic constipation, and loss of normal bowel function.

■ **Patient/Family Education**
- May be mixed with fruit juice, water, or milk to increase palatability
- Do not take other laxatives while on lactulose therapy

- When receiving lactulose rectally, retain the liquid until cramping is felt; evacuation occurs in 24-48 hr of the initial drug dose
- Institute measures to promote defecation, such as increasing fluid intake, exercising, and eating a high-fiber diet

■ Monitoring Parameters
- Serum electrolytes, carbon dioxide periodically during chronic treatment
- Daily bowel activity and stool consistency, record time of evacuation
- Serum ammonia levels, looking for a reduction
- Mental status, and watch for signs of reduced ammonia level, such as lessening of asterixis

■ Geriatric side effects at a glance:
❑ CNS ☑ Bowel Dysfunction ❑ Bladder Dysfunction ❑ Falls

■ U.S. Regulatory Considerations
❑ FDA Black Box ❑ OBRA regulated in U.S. Long Term Care

lamivudine

(la-mi'-vyoo-deen)

■ Brand Name(s): Epivir, Epivir-HBV

Combinations
Rx: with abacavir (Epzicom); with zidovudine: (Combivir)
Chemical Class: Nucleoside analog

■ Clinical Pharmacology:
Mechanism of Action: An antiviral that inhibits HIV reverse transcriptase by viral DNA chain termination. Also inhibits RNA- and DNA-dependent DNA polymerase, an enzyme necessary for HIV replication. **Therapeutic Effect:** Interrupts HIV replication, slowing the progression of HIV infection.
Pharmacokinetics: Rapidly and completely absorbed from the GI tract. Protein binding: less than 36%. Widely distributed (crosses the blood-brain barrier). Primarily excreted unchanged in urine. Not removed by hemodialysis or peritoneal dialysis. **Half-life:** 11-15 hr (intracellular), 2-11 hr (serum, adults), 1.7-2 hr (serum, children). (Increased in impaired renal function).

■ Available Forms:
- *Oral Solution*: 5 mg/ml (Epivir-HBV), 10 mg/ml (Epivir).
- *Tablets*: 100 mg (Epivir-HBV), 150 mg (Epivir), 300 mg (Epivir).

■ Indications and Dosages:
HIV *infection* (*in combination with other antiretrovirals*): PO *Weight 50 kg (100 lb) or more*. 150 mg twice a day or 300 mg once a day. *Weight less than 50 kg*. 2 mg/kg twice a day.
Chronic hepatitis B: PO 100 mg/day.

Dosage in renal impairment: Dosage and frequency are modified based on creatinine clearance.

Creatinine Clearance (ml/min)	Dosage
50 ml/min or higher	150 mg twice a day
30-49 ml/min	150 mg once a day
15-29 ml/min	150 mg first dose, then 100 mg once a day
5-14 ml/min	150 mg first dose, then 50 mg once a day
less than 5 ml/min	50 mg first dose, then 25 mg once a day

- **Unlabeled Uses:** Prophylaxis in health care workers at risk of acquiring HIV after occupational exposure

- **Contraindications:** None known.

- **Side Effects**
  Frequent
  Headache (35%), nausea (33%), malaise and fatigue (27%), nasal disturbances (20%), diarrhea, cough (18%), musculoskeletal pain, neuropathy (12%), insomnia (11%), anorexia, dizziness, fever or chills (10%)
  Occasional
  Depression (9%); myalgia (8%); abdominal cramps (6%); dyspepsia, arthralgia (5%)

- **Serious Reactions**
  - Lactic acidosis and severe hepatomegaly with steatosis, including fatal cases, have been reported.
  - Pancreatitis occurs in 13% of pediatric patients.
  - Anemia, neutropenia, and thrombocytopenia occur rarely.

Special Considerations
  - Always check updated treatment guidelines before initiating or changing antiretroviral therapy. (http://AIDSinfo.nih.gov)

- **Patient/Family Education**
  - Space lamivudine doses evenly around the clock and continue taking the drug for the full course of treatment
  - Avoid performing tasks that require mental alertness or motor skills until response to the drug has been established
  - Lamivudine is not a cure for HIV, nor does it reduce the risk of transmitting HIV to others

- **Monitoring Parameters**
  - Serum amylase, BUN, and serum creatinine levels
  - Pattern of daily bowel activity and stool consistency
  - Evaluate for altered sleep patterns, cough, dizziness, headache, and nausea

- **Geriatric side effects at a glance:**
  ☑ CNS ☐ Bowel Dysfunction ☐ Bladder Dysfunction ☐ Falls

- **U.S. Regulatory Considerations**
  ☑ FDA Black Box
  Lactic acidosis and hepatomegaly with steatosis. Severe acute exacerbations of hepatitis B have occurred in patients co-infected with HBV and HIV.
  ☐ OBRA regulated in U.S. Long Term Care

lamotrigine

(la-moe-trih'-jeen)

- **Brand Name(s):** Lamictal, Lamictal CD
  Chemical Class: Phenyltriazine derivative

- **Clinical Pharmacology:**
  Mechanism of Action: An anticonvulsant whose exact mechanism is unknown. May block voltage-sensitive sodium channels, thus stabilizing neuronal membranes and regulating presynaptic transmitter release of excitatory amino acids. **Therapeutic Effect:** Reduces seizure activity.
  Pharmacokinetics: Rapidly absorbed from the GI tract. Protein binding: 55%. Metabolized primarily by glucuronic acid conjugation. Excreted in the urine. **Half-life:** 13-30 hr.

- **Available Forms:**
  - *Tablets:* 25 mg, 100 mg, 150 mg, 200 mg.
  - *Tablets (Chewable):* 2 mg, 5 mg, 25 mg.

- **Indications and Dosages:**
  Seizure control in patients receiving enzyme-inducing antiepileptic drug (EIAEDs), but not valproic acid: PO Recommended as add-on therapy: 50 mg once a day for 2 wk, followed by 100 mg/day in 2 divided doses for 2 wk. Maintenance: Dosage may be increased by 100 mg/day every week, up to 300-500 mg/day in 2 divided doses.
  Seizure control in patients receiving combination therapy of EIAEDs and valproic acid: PO 25 mg every other day for 2 wk, followed by 25 mg once a day for 2 wk. Maintenance: Dosage may be increased by 25-50 mg/day q1-2wk, up to 150 mg/day in 2 divided doses.
  Conversion to monotherapy for patients receiving EIAED: PO 500 mg/day in 2 divided doses. Titrate to desired dose while maintaining EIAED at fixed level, then withdraw EIAED by 20% each wk over a 4-wk period.
  Conversion to monotherapy for patients receiving valproic acid: PO Titrate lamotrigine to 200 mg/day, maintaining valproic acid dose. Maintain lamotrigine dose and decrease valproic acid to 500 mg/day, no greater than 500 mg/day/wk, then maintain 500 mg/day for 1 wk. Increase lamotrigine to 300 mg/day and decrease valproic acid to 250 mg/day. Maintain for 1 wk, then discontinue valproic acid and increase lamotrigine by 100 mg/day each wk until maintenance dose of 500 mg/day reached.
  Bipolar disorder in patients receiving EIAED: PO 50 mg/day for 2 wk, then 100 mg/day for 2 wk, then 200 mg/day for 1 wk, then 300 mg/day for 1 wk, then up to usual maintenance dose 400 mg/day in divided doses.
  Bipolar disorder in patients receiving valproic acid: PO 25 mg/day every other day for 2 wk, then 25 mg/day for 2 wk, then 50 mg/day for 1 wk, then 100 mg/day. Usual maintenance dose with valproic acid: 100 mg/day.
  Discontinuation therapy: A dosage reduction of approximately 50% per week over at least 2 wk is recommended.

- **Contraindications:** None known.

- **Side Effects**
  Frequent
  Dizziness (38%), diplopia (28%), headache (29%), ataxia (22%), nausea (19%), blurred vision (16%), somnolence, rhinitis (14%)

Occasional (10%-5%)

Rash, pharyngitis, vomiting, cough, flu-like symptoms, diarrhea, fever, insomnia, dyspepsia

Rare

Constipation, tremor, anxiety, pruritus, vaginitis, hypersensitivity reaction

■ **Serious Reactions**
- Abrupt withdrawal may increase seizure frequency.
- Serious rashes, including Stevens-Johnson syndrome, requiring hospitalization and discontinuation of treatment have been reported.

■ **Patient/Family Education**
- Notify clinician immediately if a skin rash develops
- Avoid prolonged exposure to direct sunlight
- Do not discontinue the drug abruptly after long-term therapy; strict maintenance of drug therapy is essential for seizure control
- Avoid alcohol and tasks that require mental alertness or motor skills until response to the drug is established

■ **Monitoring Parameters**
- Notify the physician promptly if rash occurs, and expect to discontinue the drug
- Assess for signs of clinical improvement, including a decrease in the frequency and intensity of seizures
- Assess the patient for headache and visual abnormalities

■ **Geriatric side effects at a glance:**
☑ CNS ☐ Bowel Dysfunction ☐ Bladder Dysfunction ☐ Falls
Other: Skin Rash

■ **Use with caution in older patients with:** Cardiac disease (drug may have an effect on PR interval), Unsteady gait, Urinary incontinence

■ **U.S. Regulatory Considerations**
☑ FDA Black Box
Serious rashes including Stevens-Johnson syndrome, Toxic epidermal necrolysis
☐ OBRA regulated in U.S. Long Term Care

■ **Other Uses in Geriatric Patient:** Bipolar disorder, aggressive behavior in dementia

■ **Side Effects:**
Of particular importance in the geriatric patient: Delirium, confusion, cognitive impairment, amnesia, somnolence, insomnia, dizziness, ataxia, headache, nausea, dose-related rash, asthenia

■ **Geriatric Considerations - Summary:** Used as a first-line anticonvulsant due to lower incidence of CNS effects and good overall tolerance. Well-studied in older adults. Slow dosage titration is required to prevent adverse effects, especially rash. Rash is related to rate of titration, initial starting dose, and concomitant use of valproic acid. Discontinue drug if a rash develops and do not rechallenge. Lamotrigine tends to be less sedating than other anticonvulsants and is associated with a low incidence of

CNS effects. CNS side effects usually occur during titration and early in therapy, then subside. Minor vision changes often precede ataxia as signs of toxicity.

References:
1. Brodie M, Kwan P. Epilepsy in elderly people. BMJ 2005;331:1317-1322.
2. Rowan AJ, Ramsay RE, Collins JF, et al. New onset geriatric epilepsy: a randomized study of gabapentin, lamotrigine, and carbamazepine. Neurology 2005;64:1868-1873.
3. Arroyo S, Kramer G. Treating epilepsy in the elderly: safety considerations. Drug Saf 2001;24:991-1015.
4. Drugs that may cause cognitive disorders in the elderly. Med Let 2000;42:111-112.
5. Willmore LJ. Choice and use of newer anticonvulsant drugs in older patients. Drugs Aging 2000;17:441-452.
6. Faught E. Epidemiolgy and drug treatment of epilepsy in elderly people. Drugs Aging 1999;15:255-269.
7. Brodie MJ, Overstall PW, Giorgi L, The UK Lamotrigine Elderly Study Group. Multicentre, double-blind, randomized comparison between lamotrigine and carbamazepine in elderly patients with newly diagnosed epilepsy. Epilepsy Res 1999;37:81-87.

lansoprazole

(lan-soe-pra'-zole)

■ **Brand Name(s):** Prevacid, Prevacid IV, Prevacid Solu-Tab

Combinations
Rx: with naproxen (NapraPAC)
Chemical Class: Benzimidazole derivative

■ **Clinical Pharmacology:**
Mechanism of Action: A proton pump inhibitor that selectively inhibits the parietal cell membrane enzyme system (hydrogen-potassium adenosine triphosphatase) or proton pump. **Therapeutic Effect:** Suppresses gastric acid secretion.
Pharmacokinetics:

Route	Onset	Peak	Duration
PO (15 mg)	2–3 hr	N/A	24 hr
PO (30 mg)	1–2 hr	N/A	longer than 24 hr

Rapid and complete absorption (food may decrease absorption) once drug has left stomach. Protein binding: 97%. Distributed primarily to gastric parietal cells and converted to two active metabolites. Extensively metabolized in the liver. Eliminated in bile and urine. Not removed by hemodialysis. **Half-life:** 1.5 hr (increased in the elderly and in those with hepatic impairment).

■ **Available Forms:**
- *Capsules (Delayed-Release [Prevacid]):* 15 mg, 30 mg.
- *Granules for Oral Suspension (Prevacid):* 15 mg/pack; 30 mg/pack.
- *Injection Powder for Reconstitution (Prevacid IV):* 30 mg.
- *Orally-Disintegrating Tablets (Prevacid Solu-Tab):* 15 mg, 30 mg.

■ **Indications and Dosages:**
    Duodenal ulcer: PO 15 mg/day, before eating, preferably in the morning, for up to 4 wk. Maintenance: 15 mg/day.
    Erosive esophagitis: PO 30 mg/day, before eating, for up to 8 wk. If healing does not occur within 8 wk (in 5%–10% of cases), may give for additional 8 wk. Maintenance: 15 mg/day. IV 30 mg once a day for up to 7 days. Switch to oral lansoprazole therapy as soon as patient can tolerate oral route.
    Gastric ulcer: PO 30 mg/day for up to 8 wk.
    NSAID gastric ulcer: PO (Healing): 30 mg/day for up to 8 wk. (Prevention): 15 mg/day for up to 12 wk.
    Healed duodenal ulcer, gastroesophageal reflux disease: PO 15 mg/day.
    Helicobacter pylori infection: PO (Triple drug therapy) 30 mg q12h for 10-14 days. PO (Dual drug therapy) 30 mg q8h for 14 days.
    Pathologic hypersecretory conditions (including Zollinger-Ellison syndrome): PO 60 mg/day. Individualize dosage according to patient needs and for as long as clinically indicated. Administer up to 120 mg/day in divided doses.

■ **Contraindications:** None known.

■ **Side Effects**
    Occasional (3%–2%)
    Diarrhea, abdominal pain, rash, pruritus, altered appetite
    Rare (1%)
    Nausea, headache

■ **Serious Reactions**
    • Bilirubinemia, eosinophilia, and hyperlipemia occur rarely.

Special Considerations
    • For patients with a nasogastric tube, capsules may be opened and the intact granules mixed with 40 ml of apple juice and injected through tube into stomach
    • For patients unable to swallow capsules, capsule can be opened and the intact granules sprinkled on 1 tablespoon of applesauce and swallowed immediately; do not crush or chew granules
    • For oral suspension, empty contents of packet into 30 ml of water only, don't use other liquids, do not crush or chew granules; if material remains add more water, stir, and drink immediately

■ **Monitoring Parameters**
    • Monitor the patient's ongoing laboratory results
    • Assess for abdominal pain, diarrhea, and nausea and watch for therapeutic response (relief of GI symptoms)

■ **Geriatric side effects at a glance:**
    ❑ CNS   ❑ Bowel Dysfunction   ❑ Bladder Dysfunction   ❑ Falls

■ **U.S. Regulatory Considerations**
    ❑ FDA Black Box   ❑ OBRA regulated in U.S. Long Term Care

latanoprost

(la-ta'-noe-prost)

■ **Brand Name(s):** Xalatan
   Chemical Class: Prostaglandin F_2-alpha analog

■ **Clinical Pharmacology:**
   Mechanism of Action: An ophthalmic agent that is a prostanoid selective FP receptor agonist. **Therapeutic Effect:** Reduces intraocular pressure (IOP) by reducing aqueous humor production.
   Pharmacokinetics: Absorbed through the cornea where the isopropyl ester prodrug is hydrolyzed to acid form to become biologically active. Highly lipophilic. The acid of latanoprost can be measured in the aqueous humor during the first 4 hours and in the plasma only during the first hour after local administration. In cornea, latanoprost is hydrolyzed to the biologically active acid. Metabolized in liver if it reaches systemic circulation. Metabolized to 1,2-dinor metabolite and 1,2,3,4-tetranor metabolite. Primarily eliminated by the kidneys. **Half-life:** 17 min.

■ **Available Forms:**
   • *Ophthalmic Solution*: 0.005% (Xalatan).

■ **Indications and Dosages:**
   Glaucoma, ocular hypertension: Ophthalmic 1 drop (1.5 mcg) in affected eye(s) once daily, in the evening.

■ **Contraindications:** Hypersensitivity to latanoprost or benzalkonium chloride, or any other component of the formulation

■ **Side Effects**
   Frequent
   Blurred vision
   Occasional
   Eyelash changes, eyelid skin darkening, iris pigmentation
   Rare
   Macular edema

■ **Serious Reactions**
   • Pigmentation is expected to increase as long as latanoprost is administered but after discontinuation, pigmentation of the iris is likely to be permanent, while pigmentation of the periorbital tissue and eyelash changes has been reported as reversible.
   • Inflammation (iritis/uveitis) and macular edema, including cystoid macular edema, have been reported.

■ **Patient/Family Education**
   • Keep in the refrigerator.

■ **Geriatric side effects at a glance:**
  ❏ CNS ❏ Bowel Dysfunction ❏ Bladder Dysfunction ❏ Falls

■ **U.S. Regulatory Considerations**
  ❏ FDA Black Box ❏ OBRA regulated in U.S. Long Term Care

leflunomide

(leh-floo'-no-mide)

■ **Brand Name(s):** Arava
  Chemical Class: Isoxazole derivative

■ **Clinical Pharmacology:**
  Mechanism of Action: A DMARD that inhibits dihydroorotate dehydrogenase, the enzyme involved in autoimmune process that leads to rheumatoid arthritis. **Therapeutic Effect:** Reduces signs and symptoms of rheumatoid arthritis and slows structural damage.
  Pharmacokinetics: Well absorbed after PO administration. Protein binding: greater than 99%. Metabolized to active metabolite in the GI wall and liver. Excreted through both renal and biliary systems. Not removed by hemodialysis. **Half-life:** 16 days.

■ **Available Forms:**
  • **Tablets:** 10 mg, 20 mg.

■ **Indications and Dosages:**
  Rheumatoid arthritis: PO Initially, 100 mg/day for 3 days, then 10–20 mg/day.

■ **Side Effects**
  Frequent (20%–10%)
  Diarrhea, respiratory tract infection, alopecia, rash, nausea

■ **Serious Reactions**
  • Transient thrombocytopenia and leukopenia occur rarely.
  • Rare cases of severe hepatic injury, including cases with fatal outcome, have been reported during treatment.

■ **Monitoring Parameters**
  • **Efficacy:** ESR, C-reactive protein, platelet count, hemoglobin, improvement of RA; toxicity: LFTs (baseline, then monthly until stable)

■ **Geriatric side effects at a glance:**
  ❏ CNS ❏ Bowel Dysfunction ❏ Bladder Dysfunction ❏ Falls

☑ FDA Black Box
Although not relevant for geriatric patients, this drug is contraindicated in pregnancy.
❑ OBRA regulated in U.S. Long Term Care

lepirudin

(leh-peer'-yoo-din)

■ **Brand Name(s):** Refludan
Chemical Class: Hirudin derivative; thrombin inhibitor

■ **Clinical Pharmacology:**
Mechanism of Action: An anticoagulant that inhibits thrombogenic action of thrombin (independent of antithrombin II and not inhibited by platelet factor 4). One molecule of lepirudin binds to one molecule of thrombin. **Therapeutic Effect:** Produces dose-dependent increases in aPTT.
Pharmacokinetics: Distributed primarily in extracellular fluid. Primarily eliminated by the kidneys. **Half-life:** 1.3 hr (increased in impaired renal function).

■ **Available Forms:**
• *Powder for Injection*: 50 mg.

■ **Indications and Dosages:**
Heparin-induced thrombocytopenia and associated thromboembolic disease to prevent further thromboembolic complications: IV, IV Infusion 0.2–0.4 mg/kg, IV slowly over 15–20 sec, followed by IV infusion of 0.1–0.15 mg/kg/hr for 2–10 days or longer.
Dosage in renal impairment: Initial dose is decreased to 0.2 mg/kg, with infusion rate adjusted based on creatinine clearance.

Creatinine Clearance	% of standard infusion rate	Infusion rate (mg/kg/hr)
45–60 (ml/min)	50	0.075
30–44 (ml/min)	30	0.045
15–29 (ml/min)	15	0.0225

■ **Contraindications:** None known.

■ **Side Effects**
Frequent (14%–5%)
Bleeding from gums, puncture sites, or wounds; hematuria; fever; GI and rectal bleeding
Occasional (3%–1%)
Epistaxis; allergic reaction, such as rash and pruritus; vaginal bleeding

■ **Serious Reactions**
• Overdose is characterized by excessively high aPTT.
• Intracranial bleeding occurs rarely.
• Abnormal hepatic function occurs in 6% of patients.

- Untreated, HIT can lead to thrombosis, venous thromboembolism, acute MI, peripheral artery occlusion, and stroke; mortality rate approaches 20% to 30%
- All sources of heparin must be discontinued as soon as HIT is detected
- In clinical trials the cumulative risk of death 35 days after starting treatment was 9% in the lepirudin-treated patients, compared with 18% in historical controls; cumulative risk of new thromboembolic complications was 6% with lepirudin and 22% in historical controls

■ Patient/Family Education

- Report bleeding, breathing difficulty, bruising, dizziness, edema, fever, itching, light-headedness, or rash
- Use an electric razor and soft toothbrush to prevent bleeding during lepirudin therapy
- Do not take other medications, including OTC drugs (especially aspirin and NSAIDs), without physician approval

■ Monitoring Parameters

- aPTT ratio (patient aPTT over median of laboratory normal range for aPTT); target range 1.5-2.5; do not start in patients with baseline aPTT ratio ≥2.5; determine aPTT ratio 4 hr following start of INF and at least daily thereafter
- CBC with platelet count (to detect bleeding complications and monitor recovery of platelets)
- Hct; renal function studies; BUN, serum creatinine, AST and ALT levels; stool and urine specimen for occult blood
- Assess for abdominal or back pain, a decrease in BP, an increase in pulse rate, and severe headache, which may be evidence of hemorrhage

■ Geriatric side effects at a glance:

❏ CNS ❏ Bowel Dysfunction ❏ Bladder Dysfunction ❏ Falls

■ U.S. Regulatory Considerations

❏ FDA Black Box ❏ OBRA regulated in U.S. Long Term Care

letrozole

(let'-roe-zole)

■ Brand Name(s): Femara
Chemical Class: Benzhydryltriazole derivative

■ Clinical Pharmacology:

Mechanism of Action: Decreases the level of circulating estrogen by inhibiting aromatase, an enzyme that catalyzes the final step in estrogen production. **Therapeutic Effect:** Inhibits the growth of breast cancers that are stimulated by estrogens.

Pharmacokinetics: Rapidly and completely absorbed. Metabolized in the liver. Primarily eliminated by the kidneys. Unknown if removed by hemodialysis. **Half-life:** Approximately 2 days.

■ **Available Forms:**
- *Tablets*: 2.5 mg.

■ **Indications and Dosages:**
Breast cancer: PO 2.5 mg/day. Continue until tumor progression is evident.

■ **Contraindications:** None known.

■ **Side Effects**
Frequent (21%-9%)
Musculoskeletal pain (back, arm, leg), nausea, headache
Occasional (8%-5%)
Constipation, arthralgia, fatigue, vomiting, hot flashes, diarrhea, abdominal pain, cough, rash, anorexia, hypertension, peripheral edema
Rare (4%-1%)
Asthenia, somnolence, dyspepsia, weight gain, pruritus

■ **Serious Reactions**
- Pleural effusion, pulmonary embolism, bone fracture, thromboembolic disorder, and MI have been reported.

■ **Patient/Family Education**
- May take without regard to meals
- Notify the physician if weakness, hot flashes, or nausea becomes unmanageable

■ **Monitoring Parameters**
- Consider CBC, TFTs, electrolytes, serum transaminases, creatinine until more toxicity information available
- Monitor for asthenia and dizziness
- Assess the patient for headache
- Administer an antiemetic to prevent or treat nausea and vomiting
- Evaluate for evidence of musculoskeletal pain, and provide analgesics

■ **Geriatric side effects at a glance:**
❏ CNS ❏ Bowel Dysfunction ❏ Bladder Dysfunction ❏ Falls

■ **U.S. Regulatory Considerations**
❏ FDA Black Box ❏ OBRA regulated in U.S. Long Term Care

leucovorin calcium (folinic acid, citrovorum factor)

(loo-koe-vor'-in kal'-see-um)

- **Brand Name(s):** Wellcovorin
  Chemical Class: Folic acid derivative

- **Clinical Pharmacology:**
  Mechanism of Action: An antidote to folic acid antagonists that may limit methotrexate action on normal cells by competing with methotrexate for the same transport processes into the cells. **Therapeutic Effect:** Reverses toxic effects of folic acid antagonists. Reverses folic acid deficiency.
  Pharmacokinetics: Readily absorbed from the GI tract. Widely distributed. Primarily concentrated in the liver. Metabolized in the liver and intestinal mucosa to active metabolite. Primarily excreted in urine. **Half-life:** 15 min; metabolite, 30–35 min.

- **Available Forms:**
  - *Tablets*: 5 mg, 10 mg, 15 mg, 25 mg.
  - *Powder for Injection*: 50 mg, 100 mg, 200 mg, 350 mg, 500 mg.

- **Indications and Dosages:**
  Conventional rescue dosage in high-dose methotrexate therapy: PO, IV, IM 10 mg/m^2 IM or IV one time, then PO q6h until serum methotrexate level is less than 10^{-8} M. If 24-hr serum creatinine level increases by 50% or greater over baseline or methotrexate level exceeds 5×10^{-6} M or 48-hr level exceeds 9×10^{-7} M, increase to 100 mg/m^2 IV q3h until methotrexate level is less than 10^{-8} M.
  Folic acid antagonist overdose: PO 2–15 mg/day for 3 days or 5 mg every 3 days.
  Megaloblastic anemia secondary to folate deficiency: IM 1 mg/day.
  Colon cancer: IV 200 mg/m^2 followed by 370 mg/m^2 fluorouracil daily for 5 days. Repeat course at 4-wk intervals for 2 courses then 4-5 wk intervals or 20 mg/m^2 followed by 425 mg/m^2 fluorouracil daily for 5 days. Repeat course at 4-wk intervals for 2 courses then 4-5 wk intervals.

- **Unlabeled Uses:** Treatment of Ewing's sarcoma, non-Hodgkin's lymphoma; treatment adjunct for head and neck carcinoma

- **Contraindications:** Pernicious anemia, other megaloblastic anemias secondary to vitamin B$_{12}$ deficiency

- **Side Effects**
  Frequent
  When combined with chemotherapeutic agents: Diarrhea, stomatitis, nausea, vomiting, lethargy or malaise or fatigue, alopecia, anorexia
  Occasional
  Urticaria, dermatitis

Special Considerations
- Administer as soon as possible following overdoses of dihydrofolate reductase inhibitors

■ **Patient/Family Education**
  - Encourage the patient with folic acid deficiency to eat foods high in folic acid, including dried beans, meat proteins, and green leafy vegetables
  - Notify the physician if an allergic reaction or vomiting occurs

■ **Monitoring Parameters**
  - CBC with differential and platelets, electrolytes, and liver function tests prior to each treatment with leucovorin/5-fluorouracil combination
  - Plasma methotrexate concentrations as a therapeutic guide to high-dose methotrexate therapy with leucovorin rescue; continue leucovorin until plasma methotrexate concentrations are $<5 \times 10^{-8}$M (see dosage)
  - Serum creatinine
  - Monitor the patient for vomiting, which may require a change from oral to parenteral therapy

■ **Geriatric side effects at a glance:**
  ❏ CNS   ☑ Bowel Dysfunction   ❏ Bladder Dysfunction   ❏ Falls

■ **U.S. Regulatory Considerations**
  ❏ FDA Black Box   ❏ OBRA regulated in U.S. Long Term Care

leuprolide acetate

(loo'-proe-lide as'-eh-tayte)

■ **Brand Name(s):** Eligard, Lupron, Lupron Depot, Lupron Depot-Gyn, Lupron Depot-Ped, Viadur
  Chemical Class: Gonadotropin-releasing hormone (GnRH) analog

■ **Clinical Pharmacology:**
  Mechanism of Action: A gonadotropin-releasing hormone analog and ONC-antineoplastic agent that stimulates the release of luteinizing hormone (LH) and follicle-stimulating hormone (FSH) from the anterior pituitary gland. **Therapeutic Effect:** Produces pharmacologic castration and decreases the growth of abnormal prostate tissue in males; causes endometrial tissue to become inactive and atrophic in females. **Pharmacokinetics:** Rapidly and well absorbed after SC administration. Absorbed slowly after IM administration. Protein binding: 43%-49%. **Half-life:** 3-4 hr.

■ **Available Forms:**
  - Implant (Viadur): 65 mg.
  - Injection Depot Formulation: 3.75 (Lupron Depot), 7.5 mg (Eligard, Lupron Depot, Lupron Depot-Ped), 11.25 (Lupron Depot, Lupron Depot-Ped, Lupron Depot-Gyn), 15 mg (Lupron Depot-Ped), 22.5 mg (Eligard, Lupron Depot), 30 mg (Lupron Depot).
  - Injection Solution (Lupron): 5 mg/ml.

■ **Indications and Dosages:**

Advanced prostatic carcinoma: IM (Lupron Depot) 7.5 mg every month or 22.5 mg q3mo or 30 mg q4mo. Subcutaneous (Eligard) 7.5 mg every month or 22.5 mg q3mo or 30 mg q4mo. Subcutaneous (Lupron) 1 mg/day. Subcutaneous (Viadur) 65 mg implanted q12mo.

Uterine leiomyomata: IM (with iron [Lupron Depot]) 3.75 mg/mo for up to 3 mo or 11.25 mg as a single injection.

■ **Contraindications:** Pernicious anemia, undiagnosed vaginal bleeding.

Eligard 7.5 mg is contraindicated in patients with hypersensitivity to GnRH, GnRH agonist analogs or any of the components; 30 mg Lupron Depot and the implant form are contraindicated in women

■ **Side Effects**

Frequent

Hot flashes (ranging from mild flushing to diaphoresis)

Occasional

Arrhythmias; palpitations; blurred vision; dizziness; edema; headache; burning, itching, or swelling at injection site; nausea; insomnia; weight gain

Females: Deepening voice, hirsutism, decreased libido, increased breast tenderness, vaginitis, altered mood

Males: Constipation, decreased testicle size, gynecomastia, impotence, decreased appetite, angina

Rare

Males: Thrombophlebitis

■ **Serious Reactions**

• Signs and symptoms of metastatic prostatic carcinoma (such as bone pain, dysuria or hematuria, and weakness or paresthesia of the lower extremities) occasionally worsen 1 to 2 wk after the initial dose but then subside with continued therapy.

• Pulmonary embolism and MI occur rarely.

■ **Patient/Family Education**

• May cause increase in bone pain and difficulty urinating during first few weeks of treatment for prostate cancer, may also cause hot flashes

• Gonadotropin and sex steroids rise above baseline initially; side effects greatest in first weeks

• In the patient with prostate cancer, signs and symptoms of the disease may worsen temporarily during the first few weeks of leuprolide therapy

• Avoid performing tasks that require mental alertness or motor skills until response to the drug has been established

■ **Monitoring Parameters**

• Monitor response to therapy for prostate cancer by measuring prostate-specific antigen (PSA) levels

• Monitor the patient for arrhythmias and palpitations

• Assess the patient for peripheral edema

• Evaluate the patient's sleep pattern

• Monitor the patient for visual difficulties

■ **Geriatric side effects at a glance:**

❑ CNS ❑ Bowel Dysfunction ☑ Bladder Dysfunction ❑ Falls

levetiracetam

(lev-a-tear-as'-e-tam)

■ **Brand Name(s):** Keppra
   Chemical Class: Pyrrolidone derivative

■ **Clinical Pharmacology:**
   Mechanism of Action: An anticonvulsant that inhibits burst firing without affecting normal neuronal excitability. **Therapeutic Effect:** Prevents seizure activity.
   Pharmacokinetics: Rapidly and almost completely absorbed through the GI tract. Protein binding: less than 10%. Insignificant amount metabolized in liver. Excreted in urine. Removed by hemodialysis. **Half-life:** 7 hr.

■ **Available Forms:**
   • *Oral Solution*: 100 mg/ml.
   • *Tablets*: 250 mg, 500 mg, 750 mg.

■ **Indications and Dosages:**
   Partial-onset seizures: PO Initially, 500 mg q12h. May increase by 1,000 mg/day q2wk. Maximum: 3,000 mg/day.
   Dosage in renal impairment: Dosage is modified based on creatinine clearance.

Creatinine Clearance	Dosage
Higher than 80 ml/min	500-1500 mg q12h
50-80 ml/min	500-1000 mg q12h
30-50 ml/min	250-750 mg q12h
less than 30 ml/min	250-500 mg q12h
End-stage renal disease using dialysis	500-1,000 mg q12h; after dialysis, a 250- to 500-mg supplemental dose is recommended.

■ **Contraindications:** None known.

■ **Side Effects**
   Frequent (15%-10%)
   Somnolence, asthenia, headache, infection
   Occasional (9%-3%)
   Dizziness, pharyngitis, pain, depression, nervousness, vertigo, rhinitis, anorexia
   Rare (less than 3%)
   Amnesia, anxiety, emotional lability, cough, sinusitis, anorexia, diplopia

■ **Serious Reactions**
   • Acute psychosis and seizures have been reported. Sudden discontinuance increases the risk of seizure activity.

- Reserve as an alternative treatment for patients with partial-onset seizures not responding to first-line agents

■ **Patient/Family Education**
- Caution about common adverse effects, i.e., dizziness and somnolence; these side effects usually diminish with continued therapy
- Avoid tasks that require mental alertness or motor skills until response to the drug is established
- Do not discontinue levetiracetam therapy abruptly because this may precipitate seizures; strict maintenance of drug therapy is essential for seizure control

■ **Monitoring Parameters**
- Therapeutic plasma concentrations not established; base dosing on therapeutic response (reduction in severity and frequency of seizures)
- Renal function tests

■ **Geriatric side effects at a glance:**
  ❑ CNS ❑ Bowel Dysfunction ❑ Bladder Dysfunction ❑ Falls
  Other: Tremor

■ **Use with caution in older patients with:** Renal impairment, Unsteady gait

■ **U.S. Regulatory Considerations**
  ❑ FDA Black Box ❑ OBRA regulated in U.S. Long Term Care

■ **Other Uses in Geriatric Patient:** None

■ **Side Effects:**
  Of particular importance in the geriatric patient: Delirium, confusion, cognitive impairment, somnolence, insomnia, dizziness, asthenia, headache, weakness, agitation, sedation, behavioral problems, anorexia, weight loss, tremor

■ **Geriatric Considerations-Summary:** Levetiracetam is associated with few drug interactions and low incidence of cognitive impairment. Tremor and headache are more prevalent in older adults as compared to adults < 65 years of age. Hemodialysis reduces plasma concentrations.

■ **References:**
1. Drugs that may cause cognitive disorders in the elderly. Med Let 2000;42:111-112.
2. Brodie M, Kwan P. Epilepsy in elderly people. BMJ 2005;331:1317-1322.
3. Arroyo S, Kramer G. Treating epilepsy in the elderly: safety considerations. Drug Saf 2001;24:991-1015.
4. Cramer JA, Leppik IE, DeRue K, et. al. Tolerability of levetiracetam in elderly patients with CNS disorders. Epilepsy Res 2003;56:135-145.

levobetaxolol hydrochloride

(lee-voh-be-taks'-oh-lol hye-droe-klor'-ide)

- **Brand Name(s):** Betaxon
  Chemical Class: β_1-Adrenergic blocker, cardioselective

- **Clinical Pharmacology:**
  Mechanism of Action: An antiglaucoma agent that blocks beta$_1$-adrenergic receptors. Reduces aqueous humor production. **Therapeutic Effect:** Reduces intraocular pressure (IOP).
  Pharmacokinetics:

Route	Onset	Peak	Duration
Eye drops	30 min	2 hr	12 hr

  May be systemically absorbed.

- **Available Forms:**
  - *Ophthalmic Solution*: 0.5% (Betaxon).

- **Indications and Dosages:**
  Glaucoma, ocular hypertension: Ophthalmic Instill 1 drop 2 times/day.

- **Contraindications:** Sinus bradycardia, second- or third-degree atrioventricular (AV) block, cardiogenic shock, overt heart failure, hypersensitivity to betaxolol, levobetaxolol, or any component of levobetaxolol formulations

- **Side Effects**
  Frequent
  Ocular discomfort
  Occasional
  Blurred vision
  Rare
  Anxiety, dizziness, vertigo, headache

- **Serious Reactions**
  - Diabetes, hypothyroidism, bradycardia, tachycardia, hypertension, hypotension, heart block, alopecia, dermatitis, psoriasis, arthritis, tendinitis, dyspnea and other respiratory symptoms (e.g., bronchitis, pneumonia, rhinitis, sinusititis, pharyngitis) occur rarely.
  - Ophthalmic overdosage may produce bradycardia, hypotension, bronchospasm, and acute cardiac failure.

- **Geriatric side effects at a glance:**
  ❑ CNS ❑ Bowel Dysfunction ❑ Bladder Dysfunction ❑ Falls
  Other: Yes; see side effects, below

- **Use with caution in older patients with:** Cardiovascular disease, 2nd or 3rd degree heart block, Sinus bradycardia, Respiratory disease (asthma, COPD), Diabetes, Myasthenia gravis

■ **U.S. Regulatory Considerations**
❑ FDA Black Box   ❑ OBRA regulated in U.S. Long Term Care

■ **Other Uses in Geriatric Patient:** None (ophthalmic)

■ **Side Effects:**
Of particular importance in the geriatric patient: Due to systemic absorption: bradycardia, hypotension, dizziness, fatigue, depression, anxiety, hallucinations, bronchospasm, impotence; due to topical administration: stinging, tearing, blurred vision, light sensitivity/photophobia, dryness, decreased visual acuity

■ **Geriatric Considerations - Summary:** Levobetaxolol decreases IOP on average 16%-23%. Systemic absorption of ophthalmic drugs may occur and cause adverse effects in older adults. Since levobetaxolol is a nonselective beta-blocker, older adults may be more sensitive to the cardiovascular, CNS, and respiratory effects of the drug. Tachyphylaxis may occur after long-term therapy.

■ **References:**
1. Marquis RE, Whitson JT. Management of glaucoma: focus on pharmacological therapy. Drugs Aging 2005;22:1-22.
2. Camras CB, Toris CB, Tamesis RR. Efficacy and adverse effects of medications used in the treatment of glaucoma. Drugs Aging 1999;15:377-388.

levobunolol hydrochloride

(lee-voe-byoo'-no-lol hye-droe-klor'-ide)

■ **Brand Name(s):** AK-Beta, Betagan
Chemical Class: β-Adrenergic blocker, nonselective

■ **Clinical Pharmacology:**
Mechanism of Action: A nonselective beta-blocker that blocks beta$_1$- and beta$_2$-adrenergic receptors. *Therapeutic Effect:* Reduces intraocular pressure. Decreases production of aqueous humor.
Pharmacokinetics: Well absorbed after administration. Metabolized in liver. Primarily excreted in urine. *Half-life:* 6.1 hr.

■ **Available Forms:**
• *Ophthalmic Solution:* 0.25%, 0.5% (AK-Beta, Betagan).

■ **Indications and Dosages:**
Glaucoma, ocular hypertension: Ophthalmic Instill 1-2 drops in affected eye(s) once daily.

■ **Unlabeled Uses:** Bronchial asthma, chronic obstructive pulmonary disease (COPD), cardiogenic shock, overt cardiac failure, second or third degree AV block, severe sinus bradycardia

■ **Contraindications:** Hypersensitivity to levobunolol or any component of the formulation

■ **Side Effects**
Frequent
Burning/stinging, eye irritation, visual disturbances
Occasional
Increased light sensitivity, watering of eye
Rare
Dry eye, conjunctivitis, eye pain, diarrhea, dyspepsia

■ **Serious Reactions**
- Abrupt withdrawal may result in sweating, headache, and fatigue.
- Ophthalmic overdosage may produce bradycardia, hypotension, bronchospasm, and acute cardiac failure.

■ **Geriatric side effects at a glance:**
❏ CNS ❏ Bowel Dysfunction ❏ Bladder Dysfunction ❏ Falls
Other: None

■ **Use with caution in older patients with:** Cardiovascular disease, 2nd or 3rd degree heart block, Sinus bradycardia, Respiratory disease (asthma, COPD), Diabetes, Myasthenia gravis

■ **U.S. Regulatory Considerations**
❏ FDA Black Box ❏ OBRA regulated in U.S. Long Term Care

■ **Side Effects:**
Of particular importance in the geriatric patient: Due to systemic absorption: bradycardia, hypotension, dizziness, fatigue, depression, anxiety, hallucinations, bronchospasm, impotence; due to topical administration: stinging, tearing, blurred vision, light sensitivity/photophobia, dryness, decreased visual acuity

■ **Geriatric Considerations - Summary:** Levobunolol decreased IOP approximately 29%. Systemic absorption of ophthalmic drugs may occur and cause adverse effects in older adults. Since levobunolol is a nonselective beta-blocker, older adults may be more sensitive to the cardiovascular, CNS, and respiratory effects of the drug. Tachyphylaxis may occur after long-term therapy.

■ **References:**
1. Marquis RE, Whitson JT. Management of glaucoma: focus on pharmacological therapy. Drugs Aging 2005;22:1-22.
2. Camras CB, Toris CB, Tamesis RR. Efficacy and adverse effects of medications used in the treatment of glaucoma. Drugs Aging 1999;15:377-388.

levocabastine

(lee-voe-kab'-as-teen)

■ **Brand Name(s):** Livostin
Chemical Class: Phenylisonipecotic acid derivative

■ **Clinical Pharmacology:**
Mechanism of Action: An antiallergic agent that selectively antagonizes H_1 receptor.
Therapeutic Effect: Blocks histamine-associated symptoms of seasonal allergic conjunctivitis.
Pharmacokinetics: Duration of action is about 2 hr. Minimal systemic absorption.

■ **Available Forms:**
• *Ophthalmic Suspension:* 0.05% (Livostin).

■ **Indications and Dosages:**
Allergic conjunctivitis: Ophthalmic 1 drop 4 times/day, for up to 2 wk.

■ **Contraindications:** Wearing of soft contact lenses (product contains benzalkonium chloride), hypersensitivity to levocabastine or any component of the formulation

■ **Side Effects**
Frequent
Transient stinging, burning, discomfort, headache
Occasional
Dry mouth, fatigue, eye dryness, lacrimation/discharge, eyelid edema
Rare
Rash, erythema, nausea, dyspnea

■ **Serious Reactions**
• None reported.

Special Considerations
• Shake well before using
• Do not wear soft contact lenses during therapy
• Mild burning or stinging may occur upon instillation

■ **Monitoring Parameters**
• Therapeutic response to medication

■ **Geriatric side effects at a glance:**
❑ CNS ❑ Bowel Dysfunction ❑ Bladder Dysfunction ❑ Falls

■ **U.S. Regulatory Considerations**
❑ FDA Black Box ❑ OBRA regulated in U.S. Long Term Care

levodopa

(lee-voe-doe'-pa)

■ **Brand Name(s):** Dopar, Larodopa
Combinations
Rx: with Carbidopa (Sinemet, Sinemet CR)
Chemical Class: Catecholamine precursor

■ **Clinical Pharmacology:**
Mechanism of Action: A dopamine prodrug that is converted to dopamine in basal ganglia. Increases dopamine concentrations in the brain, inhibiting hyperactive cholinergic activity. **Therapeutic Effect:** Decreases signs and symptoms of Parkinson's disease.
Pharmacokinetics: About 30% absorbed. May be reduced with high-protein meal. Protein binding: minimal. Crosses blood-brain barrier. Converted to dopamine. Eliminated primarily in urine and to a lesser amount in feces and expired air. Not removed by hemodialysis. **Half-life:** 0.75 -1.5 hr.

■ **Available Forms:**
- *Capsules:* 100 mg, 250 mg, 500 mg (Dopar).
- *Tablets:* 100 mg, 250 mg, 500 mg (Larodopa).

■ **Indications and Dosages:**
Parkinsonism: PO Initially, 0.5-1g 2-4 times/day. May increase in increments not exceeding 0.75g every 3-7 days, up to a maximum of 8 g/day.

■ **Contraindications:** Nonselective MAOI therapy, hypersensitivity to levodopa or any component of its formulation.

■ **Side Effects**
Frequent
Uncontrolled body movements of the face, tongue, arms, and upper body; nausea and vomiting; anorexia
Occasional
Depression, anxiety, confusion, nervousness, difficulty urinating, irregular heartbeats, hiccoughs, dizziness, light-headedness, decreased appetite, blurred vision, constipation, dry mouth, flushed skin, headache, insomnia, diarrhea, unusual tiredness, darkening of urine, discolored sweat
Rare
Hypertension; ulcer; hemolytic anemia, marked by tiredness or weakness.

■ **Serious Reactions**
- High incidence of involuntary dystonic and dyskinetic movements may be noted in patients on long-term therapy.
- Mental changes, such as paranoid ideation, psychotic episodes, and depression, may be noted.

- Numerous mild to severe central nervous system (CNS) psychiatric disturbances may include reduced attention span, anxiety, nightmares, daytime somnolence, euphoria, fatigue, paranoia, and hallucinations.

Special Considerations
- Combination with carbidopa is preferred preparation

■ Patient/Family Education
- Full benefit may require up to 6 mo
- Take with food to minimize GI upset
- Avoid sudden changes in posture
- May cause darkening of the urine or sweat
- Avoid tasks that require mental alertness or motor skills until response to the drug is established
- Avoid alcohol
- Take sips of tepid water or chew sugarless gum to relieve dry mouth
- Avoid meals that are high in protein because it may delay the effects of levodopa

■ Monitoring Parameters
- CBC, renal function, liver function, ECG, intraocular pressure
- Be alert to neurologic effects including agitation, headache, lethargy, and mental confusion
- Monitor the patient for dyskinesia, characterized by difficulty with movement
- Assess the patient for clinical reversal of symptoms, such as improvement of mask-like facial expression, muscular rigidity, shuffling gait, and resting tremors of hands and head

■ Geriatric side effects at a glance:
☑ CNS   ☑ Bowel Dysfunction   ❑ Bladder Dysfunction   ☑ Falls
Other: Dyskinesias

■ Use with caution in older patients with: Psychosis

■ U.S. Regulatory Considerations
❑ FDA Black Box   ❑ OBRA regulated in U.S. Long Term Care

■ Other Uses in Geriatric Patient: None

■ Side Effects:
Of particular importance in the geriatric patient: Nausea/vomiting, psychotic symptoms

■ Geriatric Considerations - Summary: Levodopa is a percursor to dopamine and is converted to dopamine in the CNS. Clinical effectiveness is increased by taking in combination with carbidopa, a dopa decarboxylase inhibitor. This combination is often the initial treatment for Parkinson's disease.

■ References:
1. Miyasaki JM, Martin WRW, Suchowersky O, et al. Practice parameter: initiation of treatment for Parkinson disease: an evidence based review. Neurology 2002;58:11-17.
2. Fahn S, Oakes D, Shoulson I, et al. Levodopa and the progression of Parkinson's disease. N Engl J Med 2005;351:2498-2508.

levofloxacin

(lee-voe-flox'-a-sin)

- **Brand Name(s):** Iquix, Levaquin, Levaquin Leva-Pak, Quixin
  Chemical Class: Fluoroquinolone derivative

- **Clinical Pharmacology:**
  Mechanism of Action: A fluoroquinolone that inhibits the DNA enzyme gyrase in susceptible microorganisms, interfering with bacterial cell replication and repair. **Therapeutic Effect:** Bactericidal.
  Pharmacokinetics: Well absorbed after both PO and IV administration. Protein binding: 8%-24%. Penetrates rapidly and extensively into leukocytes, epithelial cells, and macrophages. Lung concentrations are 2-5 times higher than those of plasma. Eliminated unchanged in the urine. Partially removed by hemodialysis. **Half-life:** 8 hr.

- **Available Forms:**
  - *Oral Solution:* 25 mg/ml.
  - *Tablets (Levaquin, Levaquin Leva-Pak):* 250 mg, 500 mg, 750 mg.
  - *Injection (Levaquin):* 500-mg/20-ml vials.
  - *Premixed Solution (Levaquin):* 25 mg/ml, 250 mg/50 ml, 500 mg/100 ml, 750 mg/150 ml.
  - *Ophthalmic Solution:* 0.5% (Iquix), 1.5% (Quixin).

- **Indications and Dosages:**
  Bacterial sinusitis: PO 500 mg once daily for 10 days or 750 mg once daily for 5 days.
  Bronchitis: PO, IV 500 mg q24h for 7 days.
  Community-acquired pneumonia: PO 750 mg/day for 5 days or 500 mg for 7-14 days.
  Pneumonia, nosocomial: PO, IV 750 mg q24h for 7-14 days.
  Acute maxillary sinusitis: PO, IV 500 mg q24h for 10-14 days.
  Skin and skin-structure infections: PO, IV (Uncomplicated) 500 mg q24h for 7-10 days. (Complicated) 750 mg q24h for 7-14 days.
  Prostatitis: IV, PO 500 mg q24h for 28 days.
  Uncomplicated UTI: IV, PO 250 mg q24h for 3 days.
  UTIs, acute pyelonephritis: PO, IV 250 mg q24h for 10 days.
  Bacterial conjunctivitis: Ophthalmic 1-2 drops q2h for 2 days (up to 8 times a day), then 1-2 drops q4h for 5 days.
  Corneal ulcer: Ophthalmic Days 1-3: Instill 1-2 drops q30min to 2 hours while awake and 4-6 hours after retiring. Days 4 through completion: 1-2 drops q1-4h while awake.
  Dosage in renal impairment: For bronchitis, pneumonia, sinusitis, and skin and skin-structure infections, dosage and frequency are modified based on creatinine clearance.

Creatinine Clearance	Dosage
50-80 ml/min	No change
20-49 ml/min	500 mg initially, then 250 mg q24h
10-19 ml/min	500 mg initially, then 250 mg q48h

Dialysis 500 mg initially, then 250 mg q48h.
For UTIs and pyelonephritis, dosage and frequency are modified based on creatinine clearance.

Creatinine Clearance	Dosage
20 ml/min	No change
10-19 ml/min	250 mg initially, then 250 mg q48h

■ **Unlabeled Uses:** Anthrax, gonorrhea, pelvic inflammatory disease (PID)

■ **Contraindications:** Hypersensitivity to other fluoroquinolones or nalidixic acid

■ **Side Effects**
Occasional (3%-1%)
Diarrhea, nausea, abdominal pain, dizziness, drowsiness, headache, light-headedness
Ophthalmic: Local burning or discomfort, margin crusting, crystals or scales, foreign body sensation, ocular itching, altered taste
Rare (less than 1%)
Flatulence; altered taste; pain; inflammation or swelling in calves, hands, or shoulder; chest pain; difficulty breathing; palpitations; edema; tendon pain
Ophthalmic: Corneal staining, keratitis, allergic reaction, eyelid swelling, tearing, reduced visual acuity

■ **Serious Reactions**
- Antibiotic-associated colitis and other superinfections may occur from altered bacterial balance.
- Hypersensitivity reactions, including photosensitivity (as evidenced by rash, pruritus, blisters, edema, and burning skin), have occurred in patients receiving fluoroquinolones.
- Tendon effects, including ruptures of shoulder, hand, Achilles tendon or other tendons, may occur. Risk increases with concomitant corticosteroid use, especially in the elderly.
- Symptomatic hyperglycemia and hypoglycemia have occurred.

Special Considerations
- L-isomer of the racemate, ofloxacin (a commercially available quinolone antibiotic)
- Individualize treatment based on local susceptibility patterns.

■ **Patient/Family Education**
- Avoid direct exposure to sunlight (even when using sunscreen)
- Drink fluids liberally
- Avoid tasks that require mental alertness or motor skills until response to the drug is established
- Notify the physician if chest pain, difficulty breathing, palpitations, persistent diarrhea, edema, or tendon pain occurs

■ **Monitoring Parameters**
- Blood glucose levels and liver and renal function tests
- Assess for any hypersensitivity reactions, including photosensitivity, pruritus, skin rash, and urticaria
- Be alert for signs and symptoms of superinfection, such as anal or genital pruritus, moderate to severe diarrhea, new or increased fever, and ulceration or changes in the oral mucosa
- Evaluate food tolerance and change in taste sensation

■ **Geriatric side effects at a glance:**
☑ CNS ☐ Bowel Dysfunction ☐ Bladder Dysfunction ☐ Falls

levorphanol

(lee-vor'-fa-nole)

■ **Brand Name(s):** Levo-Dromoran
Chemical Class: Opiate derivative; phenanthrene derivative

DEA *Class*: Schedule II

■ **Clinical Pharmacology:**
Mechanism of Action: An opioid agonist that binds at opiate receptor sites in central nervous system (CNS). **Therapeutic Effect:** Reduced intensity of pain stimuli incoming from sensory nerve endings, altering pain perception and emotional response to pain. **Pharmacokinetics:** Rapidly absorbed. Protein binding: 40%-50%. Extensively distributed. Metabolized in liver. Excreted in urine. **Half-life:** 11 hr.

■ **Available Forms:**
- *Tablets*: 2 mg (Levo-Dromoran).
- *Injection*: 2 mg/ml (Levo-Dromoran).

■ **Indications and Dosages:**
Pain: PO 2 mg. May be increased to 3 mg, if needed. IM, Subcutaneous 1-2 mg as a single dose. May repeat in 6-8 hr as needed. Maximum: 3-8 mg/day. IV Up to 1 mg injection in divided doses. May repeat in 3-6 hr as needed. Maximum: 4-8 mg/day.
Preoperative: IM, Subcutaneous 1-2 mg as a single dose 60-90 min before surgery.

■ **Contraindications:** Hypersensitivity to levorphanol or any component of the formulation

■ **Side Effects**
Effects are dependent on dosage amount, route of administration. Ambulatory patients and those not in severe pain may experience dizziness, nausea, vomiting, hypotension more frequently than those in supine position or having severe pain
Frequent
Dizziness, drowsiness, hypotension, nausea, vomiting, constipation
Occasional
Shortness of breath, confusion, decreased urination, stomach cramps, altered vision, dry mouth, headache, difficult or painful urination
Rare
Allergic reaction (rash, itching), histamine reaction (decreased BP, increased sweating, flushed face, wheezing)

■ **Serious Reactions**
- Overdosage results in respiratory depression, skeletal muscle flaccidity, cold clammy skin, cyanosis, extreme somnolence progressing to convulsions, stupor, coma.

- Tolerance to analgesic effect; physical dependence may occur with repeated use.
- Paralytic ileus may occur with prolonged use.

■ **Geriatric side effects at a glance:**
☑ CNS   ☑ Bowel Dysfunction   ☑ Bladder Dysfunction   ☑ Falls

■ **U.S. Regulatory Considerations**
❑ FDA Black Box   ☑ OBRA regulated in U.S. Long Term Care

levothyroxine sodium

(lee-voe-thye-rox'-een soe'-dee-um)

■ **Brand Name(s):**   Levo-T, Levothroid, Levoxyl, Synthroid, Unithroid)

Combinations
Rx: with liothyronine (Euthroid, Thyrolar)
Chemical Class: Synthetic levo isomer of thyroxine (T_4)

■ **Clinical Pharmacology:**
Mechanism of Action: A synthetic isomer of thyroxine involved in normal metabolism, growth, and development, especially of the CNS in infants. Possesses catabolic and anabolic effects. **Therapeutic Effect:** Increases basal metabolic rate, enhances gluconeogenesis and stimulates protein synthesis.
Pharmacokinetics: Variable, incomplete absorption from the GI tract. Protein binding: greater than 99%. Widely distributed. Deiodinated in peripheral tissues, minimal metabolism in the liver. Eliminated by biliary excretion. **Half-life:** 6–7 days.

■ **Available Forms:**
- *Tablets (Levo-T, Levothroid, Levoxyl, Synthroid, Unithroid)*: 0.025 mg, 0.05 mg, 0.075 mg, 0.088 mg, 0.1 mg, 0.112 mg, 0.125 mg, 0.137 mg, 0.15 mg, 0.175 mg, 0.2 mg, 0.3 mg.
- *Injection (Synthroid)*: 200 mcg, 500 mcg.

■ **Indications and Dosages:**
Hypothyroidism: PO 1.7 mcg/kg/day as single daily dose. Usual maintenance: 100-200 mcg/day.
Myxedema coma: IV Initially, 300-500 mcg. Maintenance: 75-100 mcg/day.
Pituitary TSH suppression: PO Doses greater than 2 mcg/kg/day usually required to suppress TSH below 0.1 milliunit/liter.

■ **Contraindications:** Hypersensitivity to tablet components, such as tartrazine; allergy to aspirin; lactose intolerance; MI and thyrotoxicosis uncomplicated by hypothyroidism; treatment of obesity

■ **Side Effects**
Rare
Dry skin, GI intolerance

■ Serious Reactions
- Excessive dosage produces signs and symptoms of hyperthyroidism, including weight loss, palpitations, increased appetite, tremors, nervousness, tachycardia, hypertension, headache, insomnia, and menstrual irregularities.
- Cardiac arrhythmias occur rarely.

Special Considerations
- Bioequivalence problems have been documented in the past for products marketed by different manufacturers; however, studies in patients have shown comparable clinical efficacy between brands based on the results of thyroid function tests; brand interchange should be limited to products with demonstrated therapeutic equivalence

■ Patient/Family Education
- Take as a single daily dose, preferably before breakfast
- Do not abruptly discontinue the drug
- Maintain follow-up office visits; thyroid function tests are essential
- Report chest pain, insomnia, nervousness, tremors, or weight loss
- Full therapeutic effect of the drug may take 1-3 wk to appear

■ Monitoring Parameters
- TSH
- Pulse for rate and rhythm; report a marked increase in pulse rate or one that exceeds 100 beats/minute
- Evaluate the patient's appetite and sleep pattern

■ Geriatric side effects at a glance:
❏ CNS   ❏ Bowel Dysfunction   ❏ Bladder Dysfunction   ❏ Falls

■ U.S. Regulatory Considerations
☑ FDA Black Box
Thyroid hormones should not be used in the treatment of obesity.
❏ OBRA regulated in U.S. Long Term Care

lidocaine

(lye'-doe-kane)

■ Brand Name(s): Lidoderm, Xylocaine
OTC: DermaFlex, Solarcaine, Zilactin-L

Combinations
Rx: with epinephrine (LidoSite, Xylocaine with Epinephrine); Prilocaine (EMLA)
Chemical Class: Amide derivative

■ Clinical Pharmacology:
Mechanism of Action: An amide anesthetic that inhibits conduction of nerve impulses. **Therapeutic Effect:** Causes temporary loss of feeling and sensation. Also an

antiarrhythmic that decreases depolarization, automaticity, excitability of the ventricle during diastole by direct action. **Therapeutic Effect:** Inhibits ventricular arrhythmias.

Pharmacokinetics:

Route	Onset	Peak	Duration
IV	30-90 sec	N/A	10-20 min
Local anesthetic	2.5 min	N/A	30-60 min

Completely absorbed after IM administration. Protein binding: 60% to 80%. Widely distributed. Metabolized in the liver. Primarily excreted in urine. Minimally removed by hemodialysis. **Half-life:** 1-2 hr.

■ Available Forms:
- IM Injection: 300 mg/3 ml.
- Direct IV Injection: 10 mg/ml, 20 mg/ml.
- IV Admixture Injection: 40 mg/ml, 100 mg/ml, 200 mg/ml.
- IV Infusion: 2 mg/ml, 4 mg/ml, 8 mg/ml.
- Injection (anesthesia): 0.5%, 1%, 1.5%, 2%, 4%.
- Liquid: 2.5%, 5%.
- Ointment: 2.5%, 5%.
- Cream: 0.5%.
- Gel: 0.5%, 2.5%.
- Topical Spray: 0.5%.
- Topical Solution: 2%, 4%.
- Topical Jelly: 2%.
- Dermal Patch: 5%.

■ Indications and Dosages:
Rapid control of acute ventricular arrhythmias after an MI, cardiac catheterization, cardiac surgery, or digitalis-induced ventricular arrhythmias: IM 300 mg (or 4.3 mg/kg). May repeat in 60–90 min. IV Initially, 50–100 mg (1 mg/kg) IV bolus at rate of 25–50 mg/min. May repeat in 5 min. Give no more than 200–300 mg in 1 hr. Maintenance: 20–50 mcg/kg/min (1–4 mg/min) as IV infusion.

Dental or surgical procedures, childbirth: Infiltration or Nerve Block Local anesthetic dosage varies with procedure, degree of anesthesia, vascularity, duration. Maximum dose: 4.5 mg/kg. Do not repeat within 2 hr.

Local skin disorders (minor burns, insect bites, prickly heat, skin manifestations of chickenpox, abrasions), and mucous membrane disorders (local anesthesia of oral, nasal, and laryngeal mucous membranes; local anesthesia of respiratory, urinary tract; relief of discomfort of pruritus ani, hemorrhoids, pruritus vulvae): Topical Apply to affected areas as needed.

Treatment of shingles-related skin pain: Topical (Dermal patch) Apply to intact skin over most painful area (up to 3 applications once for up to 12 hr in a 24-hr period).

■ Contraindications:
Adams-Stokes syndrome, hypersensitivity to amide-type local anesthetics, septicemia (spinal anesthesia), supraventricular arrhythmias, Wolff-Parkinson-White syndrome

■ Side Effects
CNS effects are generally dose-related and of short duration.

Occasional

IM: Pain at injection site

Topical: Burning, stinging, tenderness at application site

Rare

Generally with high dose: Drowsiness; dizziness; disorientation; light-headedness; tremors; apprehension; euphoria; sensation of heat, cold, or numbness; blurred or double vision; ringing or roaring in ears (tinnitus); nausea

■ **Serious Reactions**
- Although serious adverse reactions to lidocaine are uncommon, high dosage by any route may produce cardiovascular depression, bradycardia, hypotension, arrhythmias, heart block, cardiovascular collapse, and cardiac arrest.
- Potential for malignant hyperthermia.
- CNS toxicity may occur, especially with regional anesthesia use, progressing rapidly from mild side effects to tremors, somnolence, seizures, vomiting, and respiratory depression.
- Methemoglobinemia (evidenced by cyanosis) has occurred following topical application of lidocaine for teething discomfort and laryngeal anesthetic spray.

■ **Geriatric side effects at a glance:**
☑ CNS ☐ Bowel Dysfunction ☐ Bladder Dysfunction ☐ Falls

■ **U.S. Regulatory Considerations**
☐ FDA Black Box ☐ OBRA regulated in U.S. Long Term Care

lindane (gamma benzene hexachloride)

(lin'-dane)

■ **Brand Name(s):** Lindane
Chemical Class: Cyclic chlorinated hydrocarbon

■ **Clinical Pharmacology:**
Mechanism of Action: A scabicidal agent that is directly absorbed by parasites and ova through the exoskeleton. **Therapeutic Effect:** Stimulates the nervous system resulting in seizures and death of parasitic arthropods.
Pharmacokinetics: May be absorbed systemically. Metabolized in liver. Excreted in the urine and feces. **Half-life:** 17-22 hr.

■ **Available Forms:**
- **Lotion:** 1% (Lindane).
- **Shampoo:** 1% (Lidane).

■ **Indications and Dosages:**
Treatment of scabies: Topical Apply thin layer. Massage on skin from neck to the toes. Bathe and remove drug after 8-12 hr.

Head lice, crab lice: Topical Apply about 30 ml of shampoo to dry hair and massage into hair for 4 min. Add small amounts of water to hair until lather forms, then rinse hair thoroughly and comb with a fine tooth comb to remove nits. Maximum: 60 ml of shampoo.

- **Contraindications:** Hypersensitivity to lindane or any component of the formulation; uncontrolled seizure disorders; crusted (Norwegian) scabies; acutely inflamed skin or raw, weeping surfaces; other skin conditions which may increase systemic absorption

- **Side Effects**
  Rare (less than 1%)
  Burning, stinging, cardiac arrhythmia, ataxia, dizziness, headache, restlessness, seizures, pain, alopecia, contact dermatitis, skin and adipose tissue may act as repositories, eczematous eruptions, pruritus, urticaria, nausea, vomiting, aplastic anemia, hepatitis, paresthesias, hematuria, pulmonary edema

- **Serious Reactions**
  - Seizures rarely occur.

- **Patient/Family Education**
  - Do not exceed prescribed dosage
  - Do not apply to face
  - Avoid getting in eyes
  - Wear rubber gloves for application
  - Do not use oil-based hair products (e.g., conditioners) after using product
  - Treat sexual and household contacts concurrently

- **Monitoring Parameters**
  - Skin for local burning, itching, and irritation

- **Geriatric side effects at a glance:**
  ❑ CNS ❑ Bowel Dysfunction ❑ Bladder Dysfunction ❑ Falls

- **U.S. Regulatory Considerations**
  ☑ FDA Black Box
  - Neurotoxicity, seizures, and death have been reported
  - Reserved for second-line therapy.
  ❑ OBRA regulated in U.S. Long Term Care

linezolid

(li-ne'-zoh-lid)

■ **Brand Name(s):** Zyvox
Chemical Class: Oxazolidinone derivative

■ **Clinical Pharmacology:**
Mechanism of Action: An oxalodinone anti-infective that binds to a site on bacterial 23S ribosomal RNA, preventing the formation of a complex that is essential for bacterial translation. **Therapeutic Effect:** Bacteriostatic against enterococci and staphylococci; bactericidal against streptococci.
Pharmacokinetics: Rapidly and extensively absorbed after PO administration. Protein binding: 31%. Metabolized in the liver by oxidation. Excreted in urine. **Half-life:** 4-5.4 hr.

■ **Available Forms:**
- *Powder for Oral Suspension:* 100 mg/5 ml.
- *Tablets:* 400 mg, 600 mg.
- *Injection:* 2 mg/ml in 100-ml, 200-ml, 300-ml bags.

■ **Indications and Dosages:**
Vancomycin-resistant infections (VRE): PO, IV 600 mg q12h for 14-28 days.
Pneumonia, complicated skin and skin-structure infections: PO, IV 600 mg q12h for 10-14 days.
Uncomplicated skin and skin-structure infections: PO 400 mg q12h for 10-14 days.

■ **Contraindications:** None known.

■ **Side Effects**
Occasional (5%-2%)
Diarrhea, nausea, headache
Rare (less than 2%)
Altered taste, vaginal candidiasis, fungal infection, dizziness, tongue discoloration

■ **Serious Reactions**
- Thrombocytopenia and myelosuppression occur rarely.
- Antibiotic-associated colitis and other superinfections may result from altered bacterial balance.

Special Considerations
- Most appropriate use is when vancomycin-resistant *Enterococcus faecium* infection is documented or strongly suspected, or for oral therapy of methicillin-resistant *Staphylococcus aureus* infection

■ **Patient/Family Education**
- Avoid high tyramine foods (consume less than 100 mg per meal)
- Space drug doses evenly around the clock and continue linezolid therapy for the full course of treatment
- Take with food or milk if GI upset occurs

Monitoring Parameters

- CBC weekly if treatment longer than 2 wk, ALT, AST, renal function
- Pattern of daily bowel activity and stool consistency; mild GI effects may be tolerable, but severe symptoms may indicate the onset of antibiotic-associated colitis
- Be alert for signs and symptoms of superinfection, such as abdominal pain, moderate to severe diarrhea, severe anal or genital pruritus, and severe mouth soreness

Geriatric side effects at a glance:

☐ CNS   ☐ Bowel Dysfunction   ☐ Bladder Dysfunction   ☐ Falls

U.S. Regulatory Considerations

☐ FDA Black Box   ☐ OBRA regulated in U.S. Long Term Care

liothyronine (T₃)

(lye-oh-thye'-roe-neen)

Brand Name(s): Cytomel, Triostat

Combinations
Rx: with levothyroxine (Euthroid, Thyrolar)
Chemical Class: Synthetic triiodothyronine (T$_3$)

Clinical Pharmacology:

Mechanism of Action: A synthetic form of triiodothyronine (T$_3$), a thyroid hormone involved in normal metabolism, growth, and development. Possesses catabolic and anabolic effects. *Therapeutic Effect:* Increases basal metabolic rate, enhances gluconeogenesis, and stimulates protein synthesis.
Pharmacokinetics: Almost completely absorbed following PO administration. Absorption is reduced to 43% in congestive heart failure (CHF) patients. Not firmly bound to serum protein. Excreted in urine. *Half-life:* 25 hr.

Available Forms:

- *Tablets* (*Cytomel*): 5 mcg, 25 mcg, 50 mcg.
- *Injection* (*Triostat*): 10 mcg/ml.

Indications and Dosages:

Hypothyroidism: PO Initially, 25 mcg/day. May increase in increments of 12.5–25 mcg/day q1–2wk. Maximum: 100 mcg/day.
Myxedema: PO Initially, 5 mcg/day. Increase by 5–10 mcg q1–2wk (after 25 mcg/day has been reached, may increase in 12.5-mcg increments). Maintenance: 50–100 mcg/day.
Nontoxic goiter: PO Initially, 5 mcg/day. Increase by 5–10 mcg/day q1–2wk. When 25 mcg/day has been reached, may increase by 12.5–25 mcg/day q1–2wk. Maintenance: 75 mcg/day.
T$_3$ suppression test: PO 75–100 mcg/day for 7 days; then repeat ^{131}I thyroid uptake test.

Myxedema coma, precoma: IV Initially, 25–50 mcg (10–20 mcg in patients with cardiovascular disease). Total dose at least 65 mcg/day.

■ **Contraindications:** MI and thyrotoxicosis uncomplicated by hypothyroidism; obesity; uncorrected adrenal cortical insufficiency

■ **Side Effects**
Rare
Dry skin, GI intolerance, rash, hives

■ **Serious Reactions**
- Excessive dosage produces signs and symptoms of hyperthyroidism, including weight loss, palpitations, increased appetite, tremors, nervousness, tachycardia, hypertension, headache, insomnia, and menstrual irregularities.
- Cardiac arrhythmias occur rarely.

■ **Patient/Family Education**
- Other thyroid products have longer half-lives. Take this into consideration when switching from them to liothyronine.
- Take as single daily dose, preferably before breakfast
- Do not discontinue this drug
- Do not change brands of the drug
- Promptly report chest pain, insomnia, nervousness, tremors, or weight loss

■ **Monitoring Parameters**
- TSH
- Pulse for rate and rhythm
- Appetite and sleep pattern

■ **Geriatric side effects at a glance:**
❑ CNS ❑ Bowel Dysfunction ❑ Bladder Dysfunction ❑ Falls

■ **U.S. Regulatory Considerations**
☑ FDA Black Box
Thyroid hormones should not be used in the treatment of obesity.
❑ OBRA regulated in U.S. Long Term Care

lisinopril

(ly-sin'-oh-pril)

■ **Brand Name(s):** Prinivil, Zestril

Combinations
Rx: with hydrochlorothiazide (Prinzide, Zestoretic)
Chemical Class: Angiotensin-converting enzyme (ACE) inhibitor, nonsulfhydryl

Clinical Pharmacology:

Mechanism of Action: This angiotensin-converting enzyme (ACE) inhibitor suppresses the renin-angiotensin-aldosterone system and prevents conversion of angiotensin I to angiotensin II, a potent vasoconstrictor; may also inhibit angiotensin II at local vascular and renal sites. Decreases plasma angiotensin II, increases plasma renin activity, and decreases aldosterone secretion. **Therapeutic Effect:** Reduces peripheral arterial resistance, BP, afterload, pulmonary capillary wedge pressure (preload), and pulmonary vascular resistance. In those with heart failure, also decreases heart size, increases cardiac output, and exercise tolerance time.

Pharmacokinetics:

Route	Onset	Peak	Duration
PO	1 hr	6 hr	24 hr

Incompletely absorbed from the GI tract. Protein binding: 25%. Primarily excreted unchanged in urine. Removed by hemodialysis. **Half-life:** 12 hr (half-life is prolonged in those with impaired renal function).

Available Forms:

- *Tablets* (*Prinivil*, *Zestril*): 2.5 mg, 5 mg, 10 mg, 20 mg, 30 mg, 40 mg.

Indications and Dosages:

Hypertension (used alone): PO Initially, 2.5–5 mg/day. May increase by 2.5–5 mg/day at 1- to 2-wk intervals. Maximum: 40 mg/day.

Hypertension (used in combination with other CV-antihypertensive-ACEs): PO Initially, 2.5–5 mg/day titrated to patient's needs.

Adjunctive therapy for management of heart failure: PO Initially, 2.5–5 mg/day. May increase by no more than 10 mg/day at intervals of at least 2 wk. Maintenance: 5–40 mg/day.

Improve survival in patients after a myocardial infarction (MI): PO Initially, 5 mg, then 5 mg after 24 hr, 10 mg after 48 hr, then 10 mg/day for 6 wk. For patients with low systolic BP, give 2.5 mg/day for 3 days, then 2.5–5 mg/day.

Dosage in renal impairment: Titrate to patient's needs after giving the following initial dose:

Creatinine Clearance	% Normal Dose
10–50 ml/min	50–75
less than 10 ml/min	25–50

Unlabeled Uses: Treatment of hypertension or renal crises with scleroderma

Contraindications: History of angioedema from previous treatment with ACE inhibitors

Side Effects

Frequent (12%–5%)
Headache, dizziness, postural hypotension

Occasional (4%–2%)
Chest discomfort, fatigue, rash, abdominal pain, nausea, diarrhea, upper respiratory infection

Rare (1% or less)
Palpitations, tachycardia, peripheral edema, insomnia, paresthesia, confusion, constipation, dry mouth, muscle cramps

Serious Reactions

- Excessive hypotension ("first-dose syncope") may occur in patients with CHF and severe salt and volume depletion.

- Angioedema (swelling of face and lips) and hyperkalemia occurs rarely.
- Agranulocytosis and neutropenia may be noted in patients with collagen vascular disease, including scleroderma and systemic lupus erythematosus, and impaired renal function.
- Nephrotic syndrome may be noted in patients with history of renal disease.
- Hypoglycemia may occur in patients with diabetes using glucose-lowering drugs.

■ Patient/Family Education
- Caution with salt substitutes containing potassium chloride
- Rise slowly to sitting/standing position to minimize orthostatic hypotension
- Dizziness, fainting, light-headedness may occur during first few days of therapy
- May cause altered taste perception or cough; persistent dry cough usually does not subside unless medication is stopped; notify clinician if these symptoms persist
- Do not skip doses or discontinue the drug
- Avoid taking OTC cold preparations or nasal decongestants

■ Monitoring Parameters
- BUN, creatinine, potassium within 2 wk after initiation of therapy (increased levels may indicate acute renal failure)
- Intake and output
- Daily weights
- Assess for edema
- Pattern of daily bowel activity and stool consistency

■ Geriatric side effects at a glance:
❑ CNS   ❑ Bowel Dysfunction   ❑ Bladder Dysfunction   ❑ Falls

■ U.S. Regulatory Considerations
☑ FDA Black Box
Although not relevant for geriatric patients, teratogenicity is associated with the use of ACE inhibitors.
❑ OBRA regulated in U.S. Long Term Care

lithium carbonate/lithium citrate

(lith'-ee-um car'-bo-nate/lith'-ee-um sit'-rate)

■ Brand Name(s): (lithium carbonate) Eskalith, Lithobid

■ Brand Name(s): (lithium citrate) Cibalith-S
Chemical Class: Monovalent cation

■ **Clinical Pharmacology:**
Mechanism of Action: A mood stabilizer that affects the storage, release, and reuptake of neurotransmitters. Antimanic effect may result from increased norepinephrine reuptake and serotonin receptor sensitivity. **Therapeutic Effect:** Produces antimanic and antidepressant effects.
Pharmacokinetics: Rapidly and completely absorbed from the GI tract. Primarily excreted unchanged in urine. Removed by hemodialysis. **Half-life:** 18–24 hr (increased in elderly).

■ **Available Forms:**
- *Capsules:* 150 mg, 300 mg, 600 mg.
- *Syrup:* 300 mg/ml.
- *Tablets:* 300 mg.
- *Tablets (Controlled-Release):* 450 mg.
- *Tablets (Slow-Release):* 300 mg.

■ **Indications and Dosages:** Alert During acute phase, a therapeutic serum lithium concentration of 1–1.4 mEq/L is required. For long-term control, the desired level is 0.5–1.3 mEq/L. Monitor serum drug concentration and clinical response to determine proper dosage.
Prevention or treatment of acute mania, manic phase of bipolar disorder (manic-depressive illness): PO 900–1,200 mg/day. Maintenance: 300 mg twice a day. May increase by 300 mg/day q1wk.

■ **Unlabeled Uses:** Prevention of vascular headache; treatment of depression, neutropenia

■ **Contraindications:** Debilitated patients, severe cardiovascular disease, severe dehydration, severe renal disease, severe sodium depletion

■ **Side Effects**
Alert Side effects are dose related and seldom occur at lithium serum levels less than 1.5 mEq/L.
Occasional
Fine hand tremor, polydipsia, polyuria, mild nausea
Rare
Weight gain, bradycardia or tachycardia, acne, rash, muscle twitching, cold and cyanotic extremities, pseudotumor cerebri (eye pain, headache, tinnitus, vision disturbances)

■ **Serious Reactions**
- A lithium serum concentration of 1.5–2.0 mEq/L may produce vomiting, diarrhea, drowsiness, confusion, incoordination, coarse hand tremor, muscle twitching, and T-wave depression on ECG.
- A lithium serum concentration of 2.0–2.5 mEq/L may result in ataxia, giddiness, tinnitus, blurred vision, clonic movements, and severe hypotension.
- Acute toxicity may be characterized by seizures, oliguria, circulatory failure, coma, and death.

■ **Patient/Family Education**
- Take with meals to avoid stomach upset

- Discontinue medication and contact clinician for diarrhea, vomiting, unsteady walking, coarse hand tremor, severe drowsiness, muscle weakness
- Lithium may cause excessive thirst and increased urination
- Drink 8-12 glasses of water or other liquid every day
- Do not restrict sodium in diet
- Regular monitoring of lithium blood levels is necessary to determine proper dosage
- Limit consumption of alcohol and caffeine
- Avoid tasks that require mental alertness or motor skills until response to the drug has been established

■ **Monitoring Parameters**
- Serum lithium concentrations drawn immediately prior to next dose (8-12 hr after previous dose), monitor biweekly until stable then q2-3mo; therapeutic range 1.0-1.5 mEq/L (acute), 0.6-1.2 mEq/L (maintenance)
- Serum creatinine, CBC, urinalysis, serum electrolytes, fasting glucose, ECG, TSH
- Assess for increased urine output and persistent thirst
- Therapeutic response to the drug, as characterized by increased ability to concentrate, improvement in self-care, interest in surroundings, and a relaxed facial expression

■ **Geriatric side effects at a glance:**
❑ CNS   ❑ Bowel Dysfunction   ❑ Bladder Dysfunction   ❑ Falls
Other: Cognitive impairment, Potential for increased fall risk

■ **Use with caution in older patients with:** Renal impairment, Hypothyroidism, Dehydration, Hyponatremia, Patients taking diuretics, NSAIDs or ACE Inhibitors

■ **U.S. Regulatory Considerations**
☑ FDA Black Box
- Toxicity related to serum concentrations and close monitoring required
- Prompt and accurate serum levels necessary
❑ OBRA regulated in U.S. Long Term Care

■ **Other Uses in Geriatric Patient:** Schizoaffective disorder, Aggressive behavior in organic brain syndromes

■ **Side Effects:**
Of particular importance in the geriatric patient: Case reports of organic brain syndrome, cognitive impairment, ataxia, cerebellar dysfunction, AV block, edema, tremor, renal impairment, nephrogenic diabetes insipidus, urinary frequency, hypothyroidism, leukocytosis, weight gain

■ **Geriatric Considerations - Summary:** Volume of distribution (Vd), clearance, and half-life are significantly altered in older adults. Lithium toxicity may occur within the usual adult therapeutic range. Older adults are likely to exhibit toxic effects at lower serum concentrations. Significantly lower doses are often efficacious for affective disorders than are used in younger adults. Monitor serum concentrations closely. Increased risk of lithium toxicity when a diuretic, NSAID, or ACE Inhibitor is started in a patient already taking lithium.

■ **References:**
1. Sajatovic M, Madhusoodanan S, Coconcea N. Managing bipolar disorder in the elderly. Defining the role of newer agents. Drugs Aging 2005;22:39-54.

2. Juurlink DN, Mamdani MM, Kopp A, et al. Drug-induced lithium toxicity in the elderly: a population-based study. J Am Geriatr Soc 2004;52:794-798.
3. Sproule BA, Hardy BG, Shulman KI. Differential pharmacokinetics of lithium in elderly patients. Drugs Aging 2000;16:165-177.
4. Drugs that may cause cognitive disorders in the elderly. Med Let 2000;42:111-112.

Iodoxamide tromethamine

(loe-dox'-a-mide tro-meth'-a-meen)

■ **Brand Name(s):** Alomide
Chemical Class: Dioxamic acid derivative; mast cell stabilizer

■ **Clinical Pharmacology:**
Mechanism of Action: A mast cell stabilizer that prevents increase in cutaneous vascular permeability, antigen-stimulated histamine release, and may prevent calcium influx into mast cells. **Therapeutic Effect:** Inhibits sensitivity reaction.
Pharmacokinetics: Nondetectable absorption. **Half-life:** 8.5 hr.

■ **Available Forms:**
  • *Ophthalmic Solution*: 0.1% (Alomide).

■ **Indications and Dosages:**
Treatment of vernal keratoconjunctivitis, conjunctivitis, and keratitis: Ophthalmic 1-2 drops 4 times/day, for up to 3 mo.

■ **Contraindications:** Wearing soft contact lenses (product contains benzalkonium chloride), hypersensitivity to Iodoxamide tromethamine or any component of the formulation

■ **Side Effects**
Frequent
Transient stinging, burning, instillation discomfort
Occasional
Ocular itching, blurred vision, dry eye, tearing/discharge/foreign body sensation, headache
Rare
Scales on lid/lash, ocular swelling, sticky sensation, dizziness, somnolence, nausea, sneezing, dry nose, rash

■ **Serious Reactions**
  • None reported.

■ **Patient/Family Education**
  • Do not wear soft contact lenses during therapy
  • Mild burning and stinging may occur upon instillation

■ **Monitoring Parameters**
  • Therapeutic response to medication

■ **Geriatric side effects at a glance:**
  ❑ CNS ❑ Bowel Dysfunction ❑ Bladder Dysfunction ❑ Falls

■ **U.S. Regulatory Considerations**
  ❑ FDA Black Box ❑ OBRA regulated in U.S. Long Term Care

lomefloxacin hydrochloride

(loe-me-flox'-a-sin hy-droe-klor'-ide)

■ **Brand Name(s):** Maxaquin
  Chemical Class: Fluoroquinolone derivative

■ **Clinical Pharmacology:**
  Mechanism of Action: A quinolone that inhibits the enzyme DNA gyrase in susceptible microorganisms, interfering with bacterial cell replication and repair. **Therapeutic Effect:** Bactericidal.
  Pharmacokinetics: Well absorbed from the GI tract. Protein binding: 10%. Widely distributed. Metabolized in the liver. Primarily excreted in urine. Not removed by hemodialysis. **Half-life:** 4-6 hr (increased with impaired renal function and in the elderly).

■ **Available Forms:**
  • *Tablets*: 400 mg.

■ **Indications and Dosages:**
  Complicated UTIs: PO 400 mg/day for 10-14 days.
  Uncomplicated UTIs: PO *Females*. 400 mg/day for 3 days.
  Lower respiratory tract infections: PO 400 mg/day for 10 days.
  Surgical prophylaxis: PO 400 mg 2-6 hr before surgery.
  Dosage in renal impairment: Dosage and frequency are modified based on creatinine clearance.

Creatinine Clearance	Dosage
41 ml/min and higher	No change
10-40 ml/min	400 mg initially, then 200 mg/day for 10–14 days

■ **Contraindications:** Hypersensitivity to quinolones

■ **Side Effects**
  Occasional (3%-2%)
  Nausea, headache, photosensitivity, dizziness
  Rare (1%)
  Diarrhea

708

- **Serious Reactions**
  - Antibiotic-associated colitis and other superinfections may result from altered bacterial balance.
  - Hypersensitivity reactions, including photosensitivity (as evidenced by rash, pruritus, blisters, edema, and burning skin), have occurred in patients receiving fluoroquinolones.
  - Tendon effects, including ruptures of shoulder, hand, Achilles tendon or other tendons, may occur. Risk increases with concomitant corticosteroid use, especially in the elderly.

Special Considerations
  - Individualize treatment based on local susceptibility patterns.

- **Patient/Family Education**
  - Avoid direct and indirect exposure to sunlight (even when using sunscreen), discontinue at first signs of phototoxicity, avoid re-exposure to sunlight until completely recovered from reaction
  - Take dose in the evening to reduce risk of phototoxicity
  - Take without regard to meals
  - Drink fluids liberally
  - Do not take antacids containing magnesium or aluminum or products containing iron or zinc within 4 hr before or 2 hr after dosing
  - Do not skip drug doses and continue taking lomefloxacin for the full course of therapy
  - Your tendons may be more easily injured while taking this medication. Monitor for pain or swelling in your knee, ankle, shoulder, elbow, or wrist.
  - This medication may make you dizzy or drowsy. Avoid driving or other activities requiring you to be alert.

- **Monitoring Parameters**
  - WBC count
  - Mental status
  - Monitor for dizziness, headache, and signs and symptoms of infection
  - Be alert for signs and symptoms of superinfection, such as anal or genital pruritus, fever, oral candidiasis, and vaginitis

- **Geriatric side effects at a glance:**
  ☑ CNS ❑ Bowel Dysfunction ❑ Bladder Dysfunction ❑ Falls

- **U.S. Regulatory Considerations**
  ❑ FDA Black Box ❑ OBRA regulated in U.S. Long Term Care

Ioperamide hydrochloride

(loe-per'-a-mide hye-droe-klor'-ide)

- **Brand Name(s):** Imodium
  OTC: Imodium A-D, Maalox Anti-Diarrheal

  Combinations
  OTC: with simethicone (Imodium Advanced)
  Chemical Class: Piperidine derivative

- **Clinical Pharmacology:**
  Mechanism of Action: An antidiarrheal that directly affects the intestinal wall muscles.
  Therapeutic Effect: Slows intestinal motility and prolongs transit time of intestinal contents by reducing fecal volume, diminishing loss of fluid and electrolytes, and increasing viscosity and bulk of stool.
  Pharmacokinetics: Poorly absorbed from the GI tract. Protein binding: 97%. Metabolized in the liver. Eliminated in feces and excreted in urine. Not removed by hemodialysis. **Half-life:** 9.1–14.4 hr.

- **Available Forms:**
  - *Capsules:* 2 mg.
  - *Liquid:* 1 mg/5 ml.
  - *Tablets:* 2 mg.

- **Indications and Dosages:**
  Acute diarrhea : PO (capsules) Initially, 4 mg; then 2 mg after each unformed stool. Maximum: 16 mg/day.
  Chronic diarrhea: PO Initially, 4 mg; then 2 mg after each unformed stool until diarrhea is controlled.
  Traveler's diarrhea: PO Initially, 4 mg; then 2 mg after each loose bowel movement (LBM). Maximum: 8 mg/day for 2 days.

- **Contraindications:** Acute ulcerative colitis (may produce toxic megacolon), diarrhea associated with pseudomembranous enterocolitis due to broad-spectrum antibiotics or to organisms that invade intestinal mucosa (such as *Escherichia coli*, shigella, and salmonella), patients who must avoid constipation

- **Side Effects**
  Rare
  Dry mouth, somnolence, abdominal discomfort, allergic reaction (such as rash and itching)

- **Serious Reactions**
  - Toxicity results in constipation, GI irritation, including nausea and vomiting, and CNS depression. Activated charcoal is used to treat loperamide toxicity.

- **Patient/Family Education**
  - Do not self-medicate diarrhea for >48 hr without consulting provider

- Notify the physician if abdominal distention and pain, diarrhea that does not stop within 3 days, or fever occurs
- Loperamide may cause dry mouth
- Avoid alcohol during loperamide therapy
- Avoid tasks that require mental alertness or motor skills until response to the drug has been established

■ **Monitoring Parameters**
  - Bowel sounds for peristalsis
  - Pattern of daily bowel activity and stool consistency

■ **Geriatric side effects at a glance:**
  ☑ CNS ☑ Bowel Dysfunction ☑ Bladder Dysfunction ☐ Falls

■ **U.S. Regulatory Considerations**
  ☐ FDA Black Box ☐ OBRA regulated in U.S. Long Term Care

lopinavir; ritonavir

(low-pin'-a-veer; ri-toe'-na-veer)

■ **Brand Name(s):** Kaletra
  Chemical Class: Protease inhibitor, HIV

■ **Clinical Pharmacology:**
  Mechanism of Action: A protease inhibitor combination drug in which lopinavir inhibits the activity of the enzyme protease late in the HIV replication process and ritonavir increases plasma levels of lopinavir. **Therapeutic Effect:** Formation of immature, noninfectious viral particles.
  Pharmacokinetics: Readily absorbed after PO administration (absorption increased when taken with food). Protein binding: 98%-99%. Metabolized in the liver. Eliminated primarily in feces. Not removed by hemodialysis. **Half-life:** 5-6 hr.

■ **Available Forms:**
  - *Capsules:* 133.3 mg lopinavir/33.3 mg ritonavir.
  - *Oral Solution:* 80 mg/ml lopinavir/20 mg/ml ritonavir.

■ **Indications and Dosages:**
  HIV infection: PO 3 capsules (400 mg lopinavir/100 mg ritonavir) or 5 ml twice a day. Increase to 4 capsules (533 mg lopinavir/133 mg ritonavir) or 6.5 ml when taken with efavirenz or nevirapine. PO (Once Daily) 6 capsules (800 mg lopinavir/200 mg ritonavir) or 10 ml once daily. Increase to 8 capsules (1066 mg lopinavir/266 mg ritonavir) or 13 ml when taken with efavirenz or nevirapine.

■ **Contraindications:** Concomitant use of ergot derivatives (causes peripheral ischemia of extremities and vasospasm), flecainide, midazolam, pimozide, propafenone (increases the risk of serious cardiac arrhythmias), or triazolam (increases sedation or respiratory depression); hypersensitivity to lopinavir or ritonavir

- **Side Effects**
  Frequent (14%)
  Mild to moderate diarrhea
  Occasional (6%-2%)
  Nausea, asthenia, abdominal pain, headache, vomiting
  Rare (less than 2%)
  Insomnia, rash

- **Serious Reactions**
  - Anemia, leukopenia, lymphadenopathy, deep vein thrombosis, Cushing's syndrome, pancreatitis, and hemorrhagic colitis occur rarely.

Special Considerations
  - Always check updated treatment guidelines before initiating or changing antiretroviral therapy. (http://AIDSinfo.nih.gov)

- **Patient/Family Education**
  - Take with food to improve bioavailability
  - Be aware of many potential drug interactions
  - This drug is not a cure for HIV infection, nor does it reduce the risk of transmitting HIV to others

- **Monitoring Parameters**
  - Plasma glucose, lipid levels, hepatic function tests
  - CBC with differential, CD4+ cell count, HIV RNA level (viral load), serum electrolytes
  - Weight
  - Pattern of daily bowel activity and stool consistency
  - Assess for signs and symptoms of opportunistic infections, such as fever, oral mucosa changes, and a cough or other respiratory symptoms

- **Geriatric side effects at a glance:**
  ❏ CNS ☑ Bowel Dysfunction ❏ Bladder Dysfunction ❏ Falls

- **U.S. Regulatory Considerations**
  ❏ FDA Black Box ❏ OBRA regulated in U.S. Long Term Care

loracarbef

(lor-a-kar'-bef)

- **Brand Name(s):** Lorabid, Lorabid Pulvules
  Chemical Class: Carbacephem derivative

- **Clinical Pharmacology:**
  Mechanism of Action: A second-generation cephalosporin that binds to bacterial cell membranes and inhibits cell wall synthesis. **Therapeutic Effect:** Bactericidal.

Pharmacokinetics: Well absorbed from GI tract. Protein binding: 25%. Widely distributed. Primarily excreted unchanged in urine. Moderately removed by hemodialysis. **Half-life:** 1 hr (increased in impaired renal function).

■ **Available Forms:**
- *Capsules* (*Lorabid Pulvules*): 200 mg, 400 mg.
- *Powder for Oral Suspension* (*Lorabid*): 100 mg/5 ml, 200 mg/5 ml.

■ **Indications and Dosages:**
Bronchitis: PO 200-400 mg q12h for 7 days.
Pharyngitis: PO 200 mg q12h for 10 days.
Pneumonia: PO 400 mg q12h for 14 days.
Sinusitis: PO 400 mg q12h for 10 days.
Skin and soft tissue infections: PO 200 mg q12h for 7 days.
UTIs: PO 200-400 mg q12h for 7-14 days.

■ **Contraindications:** History of anaphylactic reaction to penicillins or hypersensitivity to cephalosporins

■ **Side Effects**
Frequent
Abdominal pain, anorexia, nausea, vomiting, diarrhea
Occasional
Rash, pruritus
Rare
Dizziness, headache, vaginitis

■ **Serious Reactions**
- Antibiotic-associated colitis and other superinfections may result from altered bacterial balance.
- Hypersensitivity reactions (ranging from rash, urticaria, and fever to anaphylaxis) occur in fewer than 5% of patients, most commonly in patients with a history of drug allergies, especially to penicillins.

Special Considerations
- Essentially same spectrum and utility as cefaclor
- Take 1 hr before eating or 2 hr after eating
- Individualize treatment based on local susceptibility patterns.

■ **Monitoring Parameters**
- Skin for a rash, especially in the diaper area in infants and toddlers
- Intake and output, renal function reports, and urinalysis results for signs of nephrotoxicity
- Assess for nausea or vomiting
- Daily bowel activity and stool consistency. Although mild GI effects may be tolerable, severe symptoms may indicate the onset of antibiotic-associated colitis.
- Signs and symptoms of superinfection include abdominal pain or cramping, anal or genital pruritus or discharge, moderate to severe diarrhea, severe mouth or tongue soreness, and new or increased fever.

■ **Geriatric side effects at a glance:**
❑ CNS ☑ Bowel Dysfunction ❑ Bladder Dysfunction ❑ Falls

    ❑ FDA Black Box   ❑ OBRA regulated in U.S. Long Term Care

loratadine

(lor-at'-a-deen)

OTC: Alavert, Claritin, Claritin RediTabs, Tavist ND

Combinations
OTC: with pseudoephedrine (Claritin-D)
Chemical Class: Piperidine derivative

■ **Clinical Pharmacology:**
Mechanism of Action: A long-acting nonsedating antihistamine that competes with histamine for H_1-receptor sites on effector cells. **Therapeutic Effect:** Prevents allergic responses mediated by histamine, such as rhinitis, urticaria, and pruritus.
Pharmacokinetics:

Route	Onset	Peak	Duration
PO	1–3 hr	8–12 hr	longer than 24 hr

Rapidly and almost completely absorbed from the GI tract. Protein binding: 97%; metabolite, 73%–77%. Distributed mainly to the liver, lungs, GI tract, and bile. Metabolized in the liver to active metabolite; undergoes extensive first-pass metabolism. Eliminated in urine and feces. Not removed by hemodialysis. **Half-life:** 8.4 hr; metabolite, 28 hr (increased in elderly and hepatic impairment).

■ **Available Forms:**
- *Syrup (Claritin):* 10 mg/10 ml.
- *Tablets (Alavert, Claritin, Tavist ND):* 10 mg.
- *Tablets (Rapidly-Disintegrating [Alavert, Claritin RediTabs]):* 10 mg.

■ **Indications and Dosages:**
Allergic rhinitis, urticaria: PO 10 mg once a day.
Dosage in renal and hepatic impairment: PO 10 mg every other day.

■ **Unlabeled Uses:** Adjunct treatment of bronchial asthma

■ **Contraindications:** Hypersensitivity to loratadine or its ingredients

■ **Side Effects**
    Frequent (12%–8%)
    Headache, fatigue, somnolence
    Occasional (3%)
    Dry mouth, nose, or throat
    Rare
    Photosensitivity

■ **Serious Reactions**
- Abnormal hepatic function, including jaundice, hepatitis, and hepatic necrosis; alopecia; anaphylaxis; breast enlargement; erythema multiforme; peripheral edema; and seizures have been reported.

Special Considerations
- Effective, but expensive nonsedating antihistamine; reserve for patients unable to tolerate sedating antihistamines like chlorpheniramine

■ **Patient/Family Education**
- May cause drowsiness
- Avoid tasks requiring mental alertness or motor skills until response to the drug has been established
- Drink plenty of water to help prevent dry mouth
- Avoid direct exposure to sunlight and wear sunscreen outdoors to prevent a photosensitivity reaction
- Avoid alcohol during loratadine therapy

■ **Monitoring Parameters**
- Increase fluid intake in patients with upper respiratory allergies to decrease the viscosity of secretions, offset thirst, and replace fluids lost from diaphoresis
- Monitor for relief of symptoms, including rhinorrhea, sneezing, and itching, red, watery eyes

■ **Geriatric side effects at a glance:**
❏ CNS   ❏ Bowel Dysfunction   ❏ Bladder Dysfunction   ❏ Falls
Other: Cognitive impairment, Sedation

■ **Use with caution in older patients with:** Hepatic impairment, Renal impairment, Cognitive impairment

■ **U.S. Regulatory Considerations**
❏ FDA Black Box   ❏ OBRA regulated in U.S. Long Term Care

■ **Other Uses in Geriatric Patient:** None

■ **Side Effects:**
Of particular importance in the geriatric patient: Impaired attention, decreased concentration, sedation, potential for anticholinergic effects, cognitive impairment

■ **Geriatric Considerations - Summary:** One of the least likely antihistamines to cause CNS effects. Increased risk of sedation at higher doses.

■ **References:**
1. Hansen J, Klimek L, Hormann K. Pharmacological management of allergic rhinitis in the elderly. Safety issues with oral antihistamines. Drugs Aging 2005;22:289-296.
2. Newer Antihistamines. Med Lett 2001;43.
3. Drugs that may cause cognitive disorders in the elderly. Med Lett 2000;42:111-112.
4. Mann RD, Pearce GL, Dunn N, Shakir S. Sedation with non-sedating antihistamines: four prescription-event monitoring studies in general practice. BMJ 2000;320:1184-1187.
5. Simons FER, Fraser TG, Maher J, et al. Central nervous system effects of H1-receptor antagonists in the elderly. Ann Allergy Asthma Immunol 1999;82:157-160.

lorazepam

(lor-a'-ze-pam)

■ **Brand Name(s):** Ativan, Lorazepam Intensol
Chemical Class: Benzodiazepine

DEA Class: Schedule IV

■ **Clinical Pharmacology:**
Mechanism of Action: A benzodiazepine that enhances the action of the inhibitory neurotransmitter gamma-aminobutyric acid in the CNS, affecting memory, as well as motor, sensory, and cognitive function. **Therapeutic Effect:** Produces anxiolytic, anti-convulsant, sedative, muscle relaxant, and antiemetic effects.
Pharmacokinetics:

Route	Onset	Peak	Duration
PO	60 min	N/A	8-12 hr
IV	15-30 min	N/A	8-12 hr
IM	30-60 min	N/A	8-12 hr

Well absorbed after PO and IM administration. Protein binding: 85%. Widely distributed. Metabolized in the liver. Primarily excreted in urine. Not removed by hemodialysis. **Half-life:** 10-20 hr.

■ **Available Forms:**
  • *Tablets* (Ativan): 0.5 mg, 1 mg, 2 mg.
  • *Injection* (Ativan): 2 mg/ml, 4 mg/ml.
  • *Oral Solution* (Lorazepam Intensol): 2 mg/ml.

■ **Indications and Dosages:**
Anxiety: PO Initially, 0.5-1 mg/day. May increase gradually. Range: 0.5-4 mg. IV 0.02-0.06 mg/kg q2-6h. IV Infusion 0.01-0.1 mg/kg/hr.
Insomnia due to anxiety: PO 0.5-1 mg at bedtime.
Preoperative sedation: IV 0.044 mg/kg 15-20 min before surgery. Maximum total dose: 2 mg. IM 0.05 mg/kg 2 hr before procedure. Maximum total dose: 4 mg.
Status epilepticus: IV 4 mg over 2-5 min. May repeat in 10-15 min. Maximum: 8 mg in 12-hr period.

■ **Unlabeled Uses:** Treatment of alcohol withdrawal, panic disorders, skeletal muscle spasms, chemotherapy-induced nausea or vomiting, tension headache, tremors; adjunctive treatment before endoscopic procedures (diminishes patient recall)

■ **Contraindications:** Angle-closure glaucoma, preexisting CNS depression, severe hypotension, severe uncontrolled pain

■ **Side Effects**
Frequent
Somnolence (initially in the morning), ataxia, confusion
Occasional
Blurred vision, slurred speech, hypotension, headache

716

Rare

Paradoxical CNS restlessness or excitement in elderly or debilitated

■ **Serious Reactions**
- Abrupt or too-rapid withdrawal may result in pronounced restlessness, irritability, insomnia, hand tremor, abdominal or muscle cramps, diaphoresis, vomiting, and seizures.
- Overdose results in somnolence, confusion, diminished reflexes, and coma.

Special Considerations
- A good choice for elderly or patients with liver dysfunction who need benzodiazepines due to phase II metabolism to inactive metabolites (less likely to accumulate)

■ **Patient/Family Education**
- Do not discontinue abruptly after long-term use; withdrawal syndrome (seizures, anxiety, insomnia, nausea, vomiting, flu-like illness, confusion, hallucinations, memory impairment) can occur
- Drowsiness usually disappears with continued therapy
- Avoid tasks that require mental alertness or motor skills until response to the drug has been established
- Avoid smoking, drinking alcoholic beverages, and taking other CNS depressants; smoking reduces the effectiveness of lorazepam, and alcohol and CNS depressants increase sedation

■ **Monitoring Parameters**
- Blood pressure, heart rate, respiratory rate, CBC with differential, and hepatic function. For those on long-term therapy, expect blood chemistry studies and hepatic and renal function tests to be performed periodically
- Therapeutic response, such as a calm facial expression, and decreased restlessness and insomnia
- Though not used clinically, the therapeutic serum level for lorazepam is 50-240 ng/ml; the toxic serum level is unknown

■ **Geriatric side effects at a glance:**
☑ CNS   ☐ Bowel Dysfunction   ☐ Bladder Dysfunction   ☑ Falls
Other: Withdrawal symptoms after long-term use

■ **Use with caution in older patients with:** COPD; untreated sleep apnea

■ **U.S. Regulatory Considerations**
☐ FDA Black Box   ☑ OBRA regulated in U.S. Long Term Care

■ **Other Uses in Geriatric Patient:** Dementia-related behavior disorders, anxiety disorders

■ **Side Effects:**
Of particular importance in the geriatric patient: Sedation, withdrawal symptoms when abruptly discontinued (e.g., during hospitalization) rather than tapered

■ **Geriatric Considerations - Summary:** Benzodiazepines are effective anxiolytic agents, and hypnotics. These drugs should be reserved for short-term use. SSRIs are preferred for long-term management of anxiety disorders in older adults, and sedating antidepressants (e.g., trazodone or eszopiclone) are preferred for long-term management of sleep problems. Long-acting benzodiazepines, including: flurazepam, chlordiazepoxide, clorazepate, diazepam, clonazepam, and quazepam should generally be avoided in older adults as these agents have been associated with oversedation. On the other hand, short-acting benzodiazepines (e.g., triazolam) have been associated with a higher risk of withdrawal symptoms. When initiating therapy, benzodiazepines should be titrated carefully to avoid oversedation. In addition, many of the drugs in this class have been associated with severe withdrawal symptoms (e.g., anxiety and/or agitation, seizures) when discontinued abruptly.

■ **References:**
1. Leipzig RM, Cumming RG, Tinetti ME. Drugs and falls in older people: a systematic review and meta-analysis: I. Psychotropic drugs. J Am Geriatr Soc 1999;47:30-39.
2. Shorr RI, Robin DW. Rational use of benzodiazepines in the elderly. Drugs Aging 1994;4:9-20.
3. Shader RI, Greenblatt DJ. Use of benzodiazepines in anxiety disorders. N Engl J Med 1993;328:1398-1405.

losartan potassium

(lo-sar'-tan poe-tass'-ee-um)

■ **Brand Name(s):** Cozaar

Combinations
Rx: with hydrochlorothiazide (Hyzaar)
Chemical Class: Angiotensin II receptor antagonist

■ **Clinical Pharmacology:**
Mechanism of Action: An angiotensin II receptor, type AT_1, antagonist that blocks vasoconstrictor and aldosterone-secreting effects of angiotensin II, inhibiting the binding of angiotensin II to the AT_1 receptors. *Therapeutic Effect:* Causes vasodilation, decreases peripheral resistance, and decreases BP.
Pharmacokinetics:

Route	Onset	Peak	Duration
PO	N/A	6 hr	24 hr

Well absorbed after PO administration. Protein binding: 98%. Undergoes first-pass metabolism in the liver to active metabolites. Excreted in urine and via the biliary system. Not removed by hemodialysis. *Half-life:* 2 hr, metabolite: 6–9 hr.

■ **Available Forms:**
• *Tablets:* 25 mg, 50 mg, 100 mg.

■ **Indications and Dosages:**
Hypertension: PO Initially, 50 mg once a day. Maximum: May be given once or twice a day, with total daily doses ranging from 25–100 mg.
Nephropathy: PO Initially, 50 mg/day. May increase to 100 mg/day based on BP response.

Stroke reduction: PO 50 mg/day. Maximum: 100 mg/day.
Hypertension in patients with impaired hepatic function: PO Initially, 25 mg/day.

■ **Unlabeled Uses:** CHF, erythrocytosis

■ **Contraindications:** None known.

■ **Side Effects**
   Frequent (8%)
   Upper respiratory tract infection
   Occasional (4%–2%)
   Dizziness, diarrhea, cough
   Rare (1% or less)
   Insomnia, dyspepsia, heartburn, back and leg pain, muscle cramps, myalgia, nasal congestion, sinusitis

■ **Serious Reactions**
   • Overdosage may manifest as hypotension and tachycardia. Bradycardia occurs less often.
   • Hypoglycemia may occur in patients with diabetes using glucose-lowering drugs.

Special Considerations
   • Potentially as or more effective than angiotensin-converting enzyme inhibitors, without cough; no evidence for reduction in morbidity and mortality as first-line agents in hypertension, yet; whether they provide the same cardiac and renal protection also still tentative; like ACE inhibitors, less effective in black patients

■ **Patient/Family Education**
   • Call your clinician immediately if note following side effects: wheezing; lip, throat or face swelling; hives or rash
   • Avoid tasks that require mental alertness or motor skills until response to the drug has been established
   • Avoid cold preparations or nasal decongestants while on losartan therapy
   • Do not abruptly discontinue the drug

■ **Monitoring Parameters**
   • Baseline electrolytes, urinalysis, blood urea nitrogen and creatinine with recheck at 2-4 wk after initiation (sooner in volume-depleted patients); monitor sitting blood pressure; pulse rate; watch for symptomatic hypotension, particularly in volume-depleted patients
   • Pattern of daily bowel activity and stool consistency

■ **Geriatric side effects at a glance:**
   ❑ CNS   ❑ Bowel Dysfunction   ❑ Bladder Dysfunction   ❑ Falls

■ **U.S. Regulatory Considerations**
   ☑ FDA Black Box
   Although not relevant for geriatric patients, teratogenicity is associated with the use of angiotensin II receptor antagonists.
   ❑ OBRA regulated in U.S. Long Term Care

lovastatin

(loe'-va-sta-tin)

■ **Brand Name(s):** Altocor, Mevacor

Combinations
Rx: With niacin extended-release (Advicor)
Chemical Class: Substituted hexahydronaphthalene

■ **Clinical Pharmacology:**
Mechanism of Action: An antihyperlipidemic that inhibits HMG-CoA reductase, the enzyme that catalyzes the early step in cholesterol synthesis. **Therapeutic Effect:** Decreases LDL cholesterol, VLDL cholesterol, plasma triglycerides; increases HDL cholesterol.
Pharmacokinetics:

Route	Onset	Peak	Duration
PO	3 days	4–6 wk	N/A

Incompletely absorbed from the GI tract (increased on empty stomach). Protein binding: 95%. Hydrolyzed in the liver to active metabolite. Primarily eliminated in feces. Not removed by hemodialysis. **Half-life:** 1.1–1.7 hr.

■ **Available Forms:**
  • *Tablets (Mevacor)*: 10 mg, 20 mg, 40 mg.
  • *Tablets (Extended-Release [Altocor])*: 20 mg, 40 mg, 60 mg.

■ **Indications and Dosages:**
Atherosclerosis, coronary artery disease: PO Initially, 20 mg/day. Maintenance: 10–80 mg once daily or in 2 divided doses. Maximum: 80 mg/day.
Hypercholesterolemia: PO Initially, 20 mg/day. Maintenance: 10-80 mg once daily or in 2 divided doses. Maximum: 80 mg/day. PO (Extended-Release) Initially, 20-60 mg once daily at bedtime. Maintenance: 10-60 mg once daily at bedtime.

■ **Contraindications:** Active liver disease, unexplained elevated liver function tests

■ **Side Effects**
Frequent (9%–5%)
Generally well tolerated. Side effects usually mild and transient. Headache, flatulence, diarrhea, abdominal pain or cramps, rash and pruritus
Occasional (4%–3%)
Nausea, vomiting, constipation, dyspepsia
Rare (2%–1%)
Dizziness, heartburn, myalgia, blurred vision, eye irritation

■ **Serious Reactions**
  • There is a potential for cataract development.
  • Lovastatin occasionally produces myopathy manifested as muscle pain, tenderness, or weakness with elevated creatine kinase. Myopathy may take the form of rhabdomyolysis fatalities.

- Statin selection based on lipid-lowering prowess, cost, and availability

■ **Patient/Family Education**
- Report symptoms of myalgia, muscle tenderness, or weakness
- Take daily doses in the evening for increased effect
- Take with meals
- A prescribed diet and periodic laboratory tests are essential parts of therapy
- Avoid consuming grapefruit juice

■ **Monitoring Parameters**
- Cholesterol (maximum therapeutic response 4-6 wk)
- LFTs (AST, ALT) at baseline and at 12 wk of therapy; if no change, no further monitoring necessary (discontinue drug if elevations persist >3 × upper limit of normal)
- CPK in patients complaining of diffuse myalgia, muscle tenderness, or weakness
- Daily pattern of bowel activity
- Assess the patient for pruritus and rash

■ **Geriatric side effects at a glance:**
❑ CNS ❑ Bowel Dysfunction ❑ Bladder Dysfunction ❑ Falls

■ **U.S. Regulatory Considerations**
❑ FDA Black Box ❑ OBRA regulated in U.S. Long Term Care

loxapine succinate

(lox'-a-peen suk'-si-nate)

■ **Brand Name(s):** Loxitane
Chemical Class: Dibenzoxazepine derivative; tertiary amine

■ **Clinical Pharmacology:**
Mechanism of Action: A dibenzodiazepine derivative that interferes with the binding of dopamine at postysnaptic receptor sites in brain. Strong anticholinergic effects.
Therapeutic Effect: Suppresses locomotor activity, produces tranquilization.
Pharmacokinetics: Onset of action occurs within 1 hr. Metabolized to active metabolites 8-hydroxyloxapine, 7-hydroxyloxapine, and 8-hydroxyamoxapine. Excreted in urine. **Half-life:** 4 hr.

■ **Available Forms:**
- *Capsules:* 5 mg, 10 mg, 25 mg, 50 mg (Loxitane).

■ **Indications and Dosages:**
Psychotic disorders: PO 10 mg 2 times/day. Increase dosage rapidly during first week to 50 mg, if needed. Usual therapeutic, maintenance range: 60-100 mg daily in 2-4 divided doses. Maximum: 250 mg/day.

■ **Contraindications:** Severe central nervous system (CNS) depression, comatose states, hypersensivitiy to loxapine or any component of the formulation

■ **Side Effects**
Frequent
Blurred vision, confusion, drowsiness, dry mouth, dizziness, light-headedness
Occasional
Allergic reaction (rash, itching), decreased urination, constipation, decreased sexual ability, enlarged breasts, headache, photosensitivity, nausea, vomiting, insomnia, weight gain

■ **Serious Reactions**
• Extrapyramidal symptoms frequently noted are akathisia (motor restlessness, anxiety). Less frequently noted are akinesia (rigidity, tremor, salivation, mask-like facial expression, reduced voluntary movements). Infrequently noted dystonias: torticollis (neck muscle spasm), opisthotonos (rigidity of back muscles), and oculogyric crisis (rolling back of eyes). Tardive dyskinesia (protrusion of tongue, puffing of cheeks, chewing/puckering of mouth) occurs rarely but may be irreversible. Risk is greater in female elderly patients.

■ **Patient/Family Education**
• Avoid alcohol; caution with activities requiring mental alertness
• Mix oral concentrate in orange or grapefruit juice
• Full therapeutic effect may take up to 6 wk
• Report any visual disturbances
• Chew sugarless gum or take sips of tepid water to relieve dry mouth
• Do not abruptly discontinue loxapine
• Avoid tasks that require mental alertness or motor skills until response to the drug is established

■ **Monitoring Parameters**
• Therapeutic response including increased ability to concentrate, improvement in self-care, interest in surroundings, and relaxed facial expression

■ **Geriatric side effects at a glance:**
☑ CNS   ☑ Bowel Dysfunction   ☑ Bladder Dysfunction   ☑ Falls
Other: Orthostatic hypotension, cardiac conduction disturbances, anticholinergic side effects

■ **Use with caution in older patients with:** Parkinson's disease (an atypical antipsychotic is recommended), seizure disorders, cardiovascular disease with conduction disturbance, hepatic encephalopathy, narrow-angle glaucoma

■ **U.S. Regulatory Considerations**
☐ FDA Black Box   ☑ OBRA regulated in U.S. Long Term Care

■ **Other Uses in Geriatric Patient:** Behavior disturbances in the setting of dementia

■ **Side Effects:**
Of particular importance in the geriatric patient: Tardive dyskinesia, akathisia (may appear to exacerbate behavioral disturbances), anticholinergic effects, may increase risk of sudden death

- **Geriatric Considerations - Summary:** Sink and colleagues' systematic review showed statistically significant improvements on neuropsychiatric and behavioral scales for some drugs, but improvements were small and unlikely to be clinically important. Because of documented risks, and uncertain benefits, these agents should be used with caution in demented elderly persons, with frequent monitoring for side effects and a low threshold for discontinuing use.

- **References:**
  1. Leipzig RM, Cumming RG, Tinetti ME. Drugs and falls in older people: a systematic review and meta-analysis: I. Psychotropic drugs. J Am Geriatr Soc 1999;47:30-39.
  2. Sink KM, Holden KF, Yaffe K. Pharmacological treatment of neuropsychiatric symptoms of dementia: a review of the evidence. JAMA 2005;293:596-608.
  3. Ray WA, Meredith S, Thapa PB, et al. Antipsychotics and the risk of sudden cardiac death. Arch Gen Psychiatry 2001;58:1161-1167.

mafenide

(ma'-fe-nide)

- **Brand Name(s):** Sulfamylon
  Chemical Class: Sulfonamide derivative

- **Clinical Pharmacology:**
  Mechanism of Action: A topical anti-infective that decreases number of bacteria in avascular tissue of second- and third-degree burns. **Therapeutic Effect:** Bacteriostatic. Promotes spontaneous healing of deep partial-thickness burns.
  Pharmacokinetics: Absorbed through devascularized areas into systemic circulation following topical administration. Excreted in the form of its metabolite rho-carboxy-benzenesulfonamide

- **Available Forms:**
  - *Cream*: 85 mg base/g (Sulfamylon).

- **Indications and Dosages:**
  Burns: Topical Apply 1-2 times/day.

- **Contraindications:** Hypersensitivity to mafenide or sulfite or any other component of the formulation

- **Side Effects**
  Difficult to distinguish side effects and effects of severe burn
  Frequent
  Pain, burning upon application
  Occasional
  Allergic reaction (usually 10-14 days after initiation): itching, rash, facial edema, swelling; unexplained syndrome of marked hyperventilation with respiratory alkalosis

Rare
Delay in eschar separation, excoriation of new skin

■ **Serious Reactions**
- Hemolytic anemia, porphyria, bone marrow depression, superinfections (especially with fungi), metabolic acidosis occurs rarely.

■ **Patient/Family Education**
- Topical application may cause temporary pain or bruising
- Do not interrupt therapy
- Bathe burn area daily

■ **Monitoring Parameters**
- Assess burn area and surrounding skin

■ **Geriatric side effects at a glance:**
❑ CNS   ❑ Bowel Dysfunction   ❑ Bladder Dysfunction   ❑ Falls

■ **U.S. Regulatory Considerations**
❑ FDA Black Box   ❑ OBRA regulated in U.S. Long Term Care

magaldrate

(mag'-il-drate)

OTC: Iosopan Plus, Lowsium Plus, Riopan

Combinations
OTC: with simethicone (Riopan Plus)
Chemical Class: Aluminum and magnesium hydroxide and sulfate mixture

■ **Clinical Pharmacology:**
Mechanism of Action: An antacid that causes less hydrogen ion available for diffusion through the gastrointestinal (GI) mucosa. **Therapeutic Effect:** Reduces and neutralizes gastric acid.

■ **Available Forms:**
- *Suspension (Riopan Plus):* Magaldrate 540 mg and simethicone 20 mg/5ml, magaldrate 540 mg and simethicone 40 mg/5ml, magaldrate 1,080 mg and simethicone 40 mg/5ml.
- *Tablets (Chewable) (Riopan Plus):* Magaldrate 540 mg and simethicone 20 mg, magaldrate 1,080 mg and simethicone 20 mg.

■ **Indications and Dosages:**
Hyperacidity, gas: PO 540-1,080 mg between meals and at bedtime.

■ **Contraindications:** Hypersensitivity to magaldrate, colostomy or ileostomy, appendicitis, ulcerative colitis, diverticulitis

■ **Side Effects**

Rare

Constipation, diarrhea, fluid retention, dizziness or light-headedness, continuing discomfort, irregular heartbeat, loss of appetite, mood or mental changes, muscle weakness, unusual tiredness or weakness, weight loss, chalky taste

■ **Serious Reactions**
- None known.

■ **Patient/Family Education**
- Take other medications at least 2 hr before or after dosing with magaldrate
- Drink several glasses of water a day to help reduce possible constipation
- Notify the physician if diarrhea occurs

■ **Monitoring Parameters**
- Pattern of daily bowel activity and stool consistency

■ **Geriatric side effects at a glance:**
❑ CNS   ❑ Bowel Dysfunction   ❑ Bladder Dysfunction   ❑ Falls

■ **U.S. Regulatory Considerations**
❑ FDA Black Box   ❑ OBRA regulated in U.S. Long Term Care

magnesium salicylate

(mag-nee'-zhum sa-li'-si-late)

■ **Brand Name(s):** Mobidin
OTC: Backache Pain Relief Extra Strength, Doan's Original, Extra Strength Doan's, Keygesic-10, Momentum
Chemical Class: Salicylate derivative

■ **Clinical Pharmacology:**
Mechanism of Action: A nonsteroidal anti-inflammatory that inhibits cyclooxygenase and suppresses prostaglandin synthesis. **Therapeutic Effect:** Produces analgesic and anti-inflammatory effect.
Pharmacokinetics: Rapidly absorbed from the gastrointestinal (GI) tract. Widely distributed. Protein binding: 80%-90%. Metabolized in liver. Primarily excreted in urine. Removed by hemodialysis. **Half-life:** 2-3 hr.

■ **Available Forms:**
- **Tablets:** 467 mg (Backache Pain Relief Extra Strength, Momentum), 325 mg (Doan's Original), 500 mg (Extra Strength Doan's), 650 mg (Keygesic-10), 600 mg (Mobidin).

■ **Indications and Dosages:**
Arthritis, inflammation, musculoskeletal disorders (backache): PO 650 mg every 4 hours or 1,090 mg 3 times/day. May increase to 3.6-4.8 g/day in 3-4 divided doses.

■ **Contraindications:** Severe renal impairment, hypersensitivity to magnesium salicylate or any component of the formulation

■ **Side Effects**
Occasional
Gastric mucosal irritation, bleeding

■ **Serious Reactions**
• Overdosage may cause tinnitus.

Special Considerations
• Consider for patients with GI intolerance to aspirin or patients in whom interference with normal platelet function by aspirin or other NSAIDs is undesirable

■ **Patient/Family Education**
• Report ringing in ears or persistent GI pain

■ **Monitoring Parameters**
• AST, ALT, bilirubin, creatinine, CBC, if patient is on long-term therapy

■ **Geriatric side effects at a glance:**
❑ CNS ❑ Bowel Dysfunction ❑ Bladder Dysfunction ❑ Falls
☑ Other: Gastropathy

■ **Use with caution in older patients with:** Renal impairment, Hepatic impairment, CHF, HTN, PUD, History of GI bleeding, GERD, Gout, Bleeding and platelet disorders, History of aspirin sensitivity reaction. Also use with caution in patients taking Anticoagulants, Aspirin, and Antihypertensive agents.

■ **U.S. Regulatory Considerations**
❑ FDA Black Box ❑ OBRA regulated in U.S. Long Term Care

■ **Other Uses in Geriatric Patient:** None

■ **Side Effects:**
Of particular importance in the geriatric patient: Confusion, cognitive impairment, delirium, dizziness, dyspepsia, fluid retention, renal impairment

■ **Geriatric Considerations - Summary:** As a nonacetylated salicylate, magnesium salicylate does not adversely affect platelet function and is associated with fewer adverse GI and renal effects. A preferred analgesic and anti-inflammatory agent for use in older adults. Use of NSAIDs in older adults increases the risk of GI complications including gastric ulceration, bleeding, and perforation. These complications are not necessarily preceded by less severe GI symptoms. Concomitant use of a proton pump inhibitor or misoprostol reduces the risk for gastric ulceration and bleeding, but may not prevent long-term GI toxicity.

■ **References:**
1. COX-2 alternatives and GI protection. Med Lett Drugs Ther 2004;46:91.
2. Drugs that may cause cognitive disorders in the elderly. Med Lett Drugs Ther 2000;42:111-112.

mannitol

(man'-i-tall)

■ **Brand Name(s):** Osmitrol, Resectisol
Chemical Class: Hexahydric alcohol

■ **Clinical Pharmacology:**
Mechanism of Action: An osmotic diuretic, antiglaucoma, and antihemolytic agent that elevates osmotic pressure of the glomerular filtrate, inhibiting tubular reabsorption of water and electrolytes, resulting in increased flow of water into interstitial fluid and plasma. **Therapeutic Effect:** Produces diuresis; reduces IOP; reduces ICP and cerebral edema.
Pharmacokinetics:

Route	Onset	Peak	Duration
IV (diuresis)	15-30 min	N/A	2-8 hr
IV (Reduced ICP)	15-30 min	N/A	3-8 hr
IV (Reduced IOP)	N/A	30-60 min	4-8 hr

Remains in extracellular fluid. Primarily excreted in urine. Removed by hemodialysis.
Half-life: 100 min.

■ **Available Forms:**
• *Injection (Osmitrol)*: 5%, 10%, 15%, 20%, 25%.
• *Irrigation Solution (Resectisol)*: 5%.

■ **Indications and Dosages:**
Intracranial pressure: IV 0.25-1 g/kg q6-8h. Maximum: 6 g/24 hr.
Intraocular pressure (IOP): IV 1.5-2 g/kg as a 15%-20% solution. Maximum: 6 g/24 hr.
Renal impairment, oliguria: IV Use test dose. 300-400 mg/kg or up to 100 g given as a single dose.
Toxicity, poisoning: IV Continuous infusion as a 5%-20% solution.

■ **Contraindications:** Dehydration, intracranial bleeding, severe pulmonary edema and congestion; severe renal disease (anuria), increasing oliguria and azotemia

■ **Side Effects**
Frequent
Dry mouth, thirst
Occasional
Blurred vision, increased urinary frequency and urine volume, headache, arm pain, backache, nausea, vomiting, urticaria, dizziness, hypotension or hypertension, tachycardia, fever, angina-like chest pain

■ Serious Reactions
- Fluid and electrolyte imbalance may occur from rapid administration of large doses or inadequate urine output resulting in overexpansion of extracellular fluid.
- Circulatory overload may produce pulmonary edema and CHF.
- Excessive diuresis may produce hypokalemia and hyponatremia.
- Fluid loss in excess of electrolyte excretion may produce hypernatremia and hyperkalemia.

■ Patient/Family Education
- Expect an increase in the frequency and volume of urination
- Mannitol may cause dry mouth
- Weigh him- or herself daily

■ Monitoring Parameters
- Serum electrolytes, urine output
- BUN and liver function tests
- Weight

■ Geriatric side effects at a glance:
❑ CNS   ❑ Bowel Dysfunction   ❑ Bladder Dysfunction   ❑ Falls

■ U.S. Regulatory Considerations
❑ FDA Black Box   ❑ OBRA regulated in U.S. Long Term Care

maprotiline hydrochloride

(mah-pro'-tih-leen hye-dro-klor'-ide)

■ Brand Name(s): Ludiomil
Chemical Class: Dibenzo-bicyclo-octadiene derivative

■ Clinical Pharmacology:
Mechanism of Action: A tetracyclic compound that blocks reuptake norepinephrine by CNS presynaptic neuronal membranes, increasing availability at postsynaptic neuronal receptor sites, and enhances synaptic activity. **Therapeutic Effect:** Produces antidepressant effect, with prominent sedative effects and low anticholinergic activity. **Pharmacokinetics:** Slowly and completely absorbed after PO administration. Protein binding: 88%. Metabolized in liver by hydroxylation and oxidative modification. Excreted in urine. Unknown if removed by hemodialysis. **Half-life:** 27-58 hr.

■ Available Forms:
- **Tablets:** 25 mg, 50 mg, 75 mg (Ludiomil).

■ **Indications and Dosages:**
Usual elderly dosage: PO Initially, 25 mg at bedtime. May increase by 25 mg q3-7 days. Maintenance: 50-75 mg/day.

■ **Contraindications:** Acute recovery period following myocardial infarction (MI), within 14 days of MAOI ingestion, known or suspected seizure disorder, hypersensitivity to maprotiline or any component of the formulation

■ **Side Effects**
Frequent
Drowsiness, fatigue, dry mouth, blurred vision, constipation, delayed micturition, postural hypotension, excessive sweating, disturbed concentration, increased appetite, urinary retention
Occasional
GI disturbances (nausea, GI distress, metallic taste sensation), photosensitivity
Rare
Paradoxical reaction (agitation, restlessness, nightmares, insomnia), extrapyramidal symptoms (particularly fine hand tremor)

■ **Serious Reactions**
• Higher incidence of seizures than with tricyclic antidepressants, especially in those with no previous history of seizures.
• High dosage may produce cardiovascular effects, such as severe postural hypotension, dizziness, tachycardia, palpitations, and arrhythmias.
• May also result in altered temperature regulation (hyperpyrexia or hypothermia).
• Abrupt withdrawal from prolonged therapy may produce headache, malaise, nausea, vomiting, and vivid dreams.

Special Considerations
• Not first-line agent due to risk of seizures

■ **Patient/Family Education**
• Use caution in driving or other activities requiring alertness
• Do not discontinue abruptly after long-term use
• Wear protective clothing and use sunscreen to protect skin from ultraviolet light or sunlight
• Report visual disturbances
• Take sips of tepid water or chew sugarless gum to relieve dry mouth

■ **Monitoring Parameters**
• CBC
• Weight
• *Mental status*: Mood, sensorium, affect, suicidal tendencies
• Determination of maprotiline plasma concentrations is not routinely recommended, but may be useful in identifying toxicity, drug interactions, or noncompliance (adjustments in dosage should be made according to clinical response, not plasma concentrations); Though not used clinically, therapeutic plasma levels are 200-300 ng/ml (including active metabolite)
• Blood pressure, pulse

■ **Geriatric side effects at a glance:**
❑ CNS ❑ Bowel Dysfunction ❑ Bladder Dysfunction ❑ Falls
Other: Seizures, rash, cardiotoxic at high doses, withdrawal symptoms

■ **Use with caution in older patients with:** None

■ **U.S. Regulatory Considerations**
  ☑ FDA Black Box
  • Because there is an increased risk of suicide in children and adolescents, older adults should also be closely monitored for suicide ideation.
  ☐ OBRA regulated in U.S. Long Term Care

■ **Other Uses in Geriatric Patient:** None

■ **Side Effects:**
  Of particular importance in the geriatric patient: None

■ **Geriatric Considerations - Summary:** Given the side-effect profile, and potential drug interactions, maprotiline is not recommended for treatement of depression in older adults.

mazindol

(may'-zin-doll)

■ **Brand Name(s):** Sanorex
  Chemical Class: Imidazoline derivative

  DEA Class: Schedule IV

■ **Clinical Pharmacology:**
  Mechanism of Action: An isoindole that stimulates the central nervous system and primarily exerting its effect on the limbic system. ***Therapeutic Effect*:** Stimulates the hypothalamus to reduce appetite.
  Pharmacokinetics: Slow but complete absorption. Protein binding: greater than 99%. Metabolized in liver to metabolites. Primarily excreted in urine as well as feces. Unknown if removed by hemodialysis. ***Half-life*:** 30-50 hr.

■ **Available Forms:**
  • *Tablets*: 1 mg, 2 mg.

■ **Indications and Dosages:**
  Obesity: PO 1 mg/day. Maximum: 3 mg/day.

■ **Unlabeled Uses:** Narcolepsy

■ **Contraindications:** Agitated states, glaucoma, history of drug abuse, symptomatic cardiovascular disease (arrhythmias), co-administration with or within 14 days of MAOI therapy, hypersensitivity to mazindol

■ **Side Effects**
  Occasional
  Insomnia, headache, tachycardia, palpitations, tremors, nervousness, restlessness, dry mouth, constipation

730

Rare

Blurred vision, impotence, insulin sensitivity, rash, sweating, weakness

■ **Serious Reactions**
  • Overdosage includes symptoms of irritability, agitation, hyperactivity, tachycardia, arrhythmia, tachypnea.

■ **Patient/Family Education**
  • May cause insomnia; avoid taking late in the day
  • Use caution while driving or performing other tasks requiring alertness; may cause dizziness or blurred vision
  • Take with food if stomach upset occurs
  • Do not discontinue abruptly
  • Mazindol is not for long-term use

■ **Monitoring Parameters**
  • Blood glucose
  • Weight

■ **Geriatric side effects at a glance:**
  ❑ CNS   ❑ Bowel Dysfunction   ❑ Bladder Dysfunction   ❑ Falls

■ **U.S. Regulatory Considerations**
  ❑ FDA Black Box   ❑ OBRA regulated in U.S. Long Term Care

mebendazole

(me-ben'-da-zole)

■ **Brand Name(s):** Vermox
  Chemical Class: Benzimidazole derivative

■ **Clinical Pharmacology:**
  Mechanism of Action: A synthetic benzimidazole derivative that degrades parasite cytoplasmic microtubules and irreversibly blocks glucose uptake in helminths and larvae. Vermicidal. **Therapeutic Effect:** Depletes glycogen, decreases ATP, causes helminth death.
  Pharmacokinetics: Poorly absorbed from GI tract (absorption increases with food). Metabolized in liver. Primarily eliminated in feces. **Half-life:** 2.5-9 hr (half life increased with impaired renal function.

■ **Available Forms:**
  • *Tablets, Chewable*: 100 mg.

■ **Indications and Dosages:**

Trichuriasis, ascariasis, hookworm: PO 1 tablet in morning and at bedtime for 3 days.
Enterobiasis: PO 1 tablet one time.

■ **Unlabeled Uses:** *Ancylostoma duodenale* or *Necator americanus* infection

■ **Contraindications:** Hypersensitivity to mebendazole or any component of the formulation

■ **Side Effects**

Occasional

Nausea, vomiting, headache, dizziness, transient abdominal pain, diarrhea with massive infection and expulsion of helminths

Rare

Fever

■ **Serious Reactions**

- High dosage may produce reversible myelosuppression (granulocytopenia, leukopenia, neutropenia).

■ **Patient/Family Education**

- Chew or crush tablets and administer with food
- Parasite death and removal from digestive tract may take up to 3 days after treatment
- Consult clinician if not cured in 3 wk
- For pinworms, all household contacts of patient should be treated
- Strict hygiene essential to prevent reinfection; disinfect toilet facilities, change and launder undergarments, bed linens, towels, and nightclothes

■ **Monitoring Parameters**

- Collect stool or perianal specimens, as required
- CBC with high dosage

■ **Geriatric side effects at a glance:**

❑ CNS ❑ Bowel Dysfunction ❑ Bladder Dysfunction ❑ Falls

■ **U.S. Regulatory Considerations**

❑ FDA Black Box ❑ OBRA regulated in U.S. Long Term Care

mecamylamine hydrochloride

(mek-a-mill'-a-meen hye-droe-klor-ide)

- **Brand Name(s):** Inversine
  Chemical Class: CNS-smoking deterrent

- **Clinical Pharmacology:**
  Mechanism of Action: A smoking deterrent that inhibits acetylcholine at the autonomic ganglia. Blocks central nicotinic cholinergic receptors, which inhibits effects of nicotine. **Therapeutic Effect:** Reduces blood pressure; decreases desire to smoke.
  Pharmacokinetics: Completely absorbed following PO administration. Widely distributed. Excreted in urine. **Half-life:** 24 hr.

- **Available Forms:**
  - *Tablets:* 2.5 mg.

- **Indications and Dosages:**
  Hypertension: PO Initially, 2.5 mg q12h for 2 days, then increase by 2.5-mg increments at more than 2-day intervals until desired blood pressure is achieved. The average daily dose is 25 mg in 3 divided doses.
  Smoking cessation: PO Initially, 2.5 mg q12h for 2 days, then increase by 2.5-mg increments during the first week of therapy. Range: 10-20 mg in divided doses.

- **Unlabeled Uses:** Tourette's syndrome, hyperreflexia

- **Contraindications:** Coronary insufficiency, pyloric stenosis, glaucoma, uremia, recent myocardial infarction, unreliable patients

- **Side Effects**
  Occasional
  Nausea, diarrhea, orthostatic hypotension, tachycardia, drowsiness, urinary retention, blurred vision, dilated pupils, confusion, mental depression, decreased sexual ability, loss of appetite
  Rare
  Pulmonary edema, pulmonary fibrosis, paresthesias

- **Serious Reactions**
  - Overdosage includes symptoms such as hypotension, nausea, vomiting, urinary retention, and constipation.

- **Patient/Family Education**
  - Take after meals
  - Arise slowly from reclining position
  - Orthostatic changes are exacerbated by alcohol, exercise, hot weather

- Notify the physician if loose bowel movements occur

■ Monitoring Parameters
- Maintenance doses should be limited to dose that causes slight faintness or dizziness in the standing position
- Blood pressure
- Intake and output, urinary frequency

■ Geriatric side effects at a glance:
❑ CNS ❑ Bowel Dysfunction ❑ Bladder Dysfunction ❑ Falls

■ U.S. Regulatory Considerations
❑ FDA Black Box ❑ OBRA regulated in U.S. Long Term Care

meclizine hydrochloride

(mek'-li-zeen hye-droe-klor'-ide)

■ Brand Name(s): Antivert, Meclicot, Meni-D
OTC: Bonine
Chemical Class: Piperazine derivative

■ Clinical Pharmacology:
Mechanism of Action: An anticholinergic that reduces labyrinthine excitability and diminishes vestibular stimulation of the labyrinth, affecting the chemoreceptor trigger zone. **Therapeutic Effect:** Reduces nausea, vomiting, and vertigo.
Pharmacokinetics:

Route	Onset	Peak	Duration
PO	30–60 min	N/A	12–24 hr

Well absorbed from the GI tract. Widely distributed. Metabolized in the liver. Primarily excreted in urine. **Half-life:** 6 hr.

■ Available Forms:
- *Tablets (Antivert, Meclicot, Meni-D):* 12.5 mg, 25 mg, 50 mg.
- *Tablets (Chewable [Bonine]):* 25 mg.

■ Indications and Dosages:
Motion sickness: PO 12.5-25 mg 1 hr before travel. May repeat q12-24h. May require a dose of 50 mg.
Vertigo: PO 25-100 mg/day in divided doses, as needed.

■ Contraindications: None known.

■ Side Effects
Frequent
Drowsiness

Occasional
Blurred vision; dry mouth, nose, or throat

- **Serious Reactions**
  - A hypersensitivity reaction, marked by eczema, pruritus, rash, cardiac disturbances, and photosensitivity, may occur.
  - Overdose may produce CNS depression (manifested as sedation, apnea, cardiovascular collapse, or death) or severe paradoxical reactions (such as hallucinations, tremor, and seizures).

- **Patient/Family Education**
  - Meclizine commonly causes drowsiness and dry mouth
  - Avoid tasks that require mental alertness or motor skills until response to the drug has been established
  - Avoid alcohol during meclizine therapy
  - Take sips of tepid water and chew sugarless gum to help relieve dry mouth

- **Monitoring Parameters**
  - Blood pressure, especially in elderly patients, who are at increased risk for hypotension
  - Electrolytes
  - Hydration status

- **Geriatric side effects at a glance:**
  ☑ CNS ☑ Bowel Dysfunction ☑ Bladder Dysfunction ❑ Falls
  Other: Dry mouth, somnolence, restlessness, confusion, psychoses

- **Use with caution in older patients with:** Narrow-angle glaucoma, overflow incontinence, orthostatic hypotension.

- **U.S. Regulatory Considerations**
  ❑ FDA Black Box ❑ OBRA regulated in U.S. Long Term Care

- **Other Uses in Geriatric Patient:** Antiemetic, anthistamine

- **Side Effects:**
  Of particular importance in the geriatric patient: Anticholinergic effects

- **Geriatric Considerations - Summary:** Meclizine is a first-generation piperazine anthistiamine with potent H_1-receptor antagonism. It has CNS depressant effects, causing drowsiness and has anticholinergric properties. Older adults taking this drug are at risk of dizziness and hypotension. Its use in the older adult is limited by the potential for adverse effects.

- **References:**
  1. Tune LE. Anticholinergic effects of medication in elderly patients. J Clin Psychiatry 2001;62(suppl 21):11-14.
  2. Molloy DW: Memory loss, confusion, and disorientation in an elderly woman taking meclizine. J Am Geriatr Soc 1987; 35:454-456.

meclofenamate sodium

(me-kloe-fen'-a-mate soe'-dee-um)

Chemical Class: Anthranilic acid derivative

■ **Clinical Pharmacology:**
   Mechanism of Action: A nonsteroidal anti-inflammatory drug that inhibits prostaglandin synthesis by decreasing activity of the enzyme, cyclooxygenase, which results in decreased formation of prostaglandin precursors. **Therapeutic Effect:** Reduces inflammatory response and intensity of pain stimulus reaching sensory nerve endings. **Pharmacokinetics:** PO route, onset 15 min, peak 0.5-1.5 hr, duration 2-4 hr. Completely absorbed from the gastrointestinal (GI) tract. Widely distributed. Protein binding: greater than 99%. Metabolized in liver. Primarily excreted in urine and feces as metabolites. Not removed by hemodialysis. **Half-life:** 2-3.3 hr.

■ **Available Forms:**
   • *Capsules*: 50 mg, 100 mg.

■ **Indications and Dosages:**
   Mild to moderate pain: PO 50 mg q4-6h as needed.
   Rheumatoid arthritis, osteoarthritis: PO 200-400 mg 3-4 times/day.

■ **Contraindications:** Active peptic ulcer disease, chronic inflammation of GI tract, GI bleeding disorders, GI ulceration, history of hypersensitivity to aspirin or NSAIDs

■ **Side Effects**
   Frequent (33%-10%)
   Diarrhea, nausea, abdominal cramping/pain, dyspepsia (heartburn, indigestion, epigastric pain)
   Occasional (9%-1%)
   Flatulence, rash, dizziness
   Rare (less than 1%)
   Constipation, anorexia, stomatitis, headache, ringing in the ears, rash

■ **Serious Reactions**
   • Overdosage may result in headache, seizure, vomiting, and cerebral edema.
   • Peptic ulcer disease, GI bleeding, gastritis, severe hepatic reactions (such as jaundice), nephrotoxicity (marked by hematuria, dysuria, proteinuria), and severe hypersensitivity reaction, including bronchospasm and facial edema occur rarely.

Special Considerations
   • No significant advantage over other NSAIDs; cost should govern use

■ **Patient/Family Education**
   • Swallow capsules whole and do not open, chew, or crush capsules
   • Avoid alcohol and aspirin during meclofenamate therapy
   • Notify the physician if edema, GI distress, headache, rash, signs of bleeding, or visual disturbances occurs

Monitoring Parameters

- Initial hematocrit and fecal occult blood test within 3 mo of starting regular chronic therapy; repeat every 6-12 mo (more frequently in high-risk patients (>65 years, peptic ulcer disease, concurrent steroids or anticoagulants); electrolytes, creatinine, and BUN within 3 mo of starting regular chronic therapy; repeat every 6-12 mo

Geriatric side effects at a glance:

☑ CNS   ❑ Bowel Dysfunction   ❑ Bladder Dysfunction   ❑ Falls
☑ Other: Gastropathy

Use with caution in older patients with: Renal impairment, Hepatic impairment, CHF, HTN, PUD, History of GI bleeding, GERD, Bleeding and platelet disorders, History of aspirin sensitivity reaction. Also use with caution in patients taking Anticoagulants, Aspirin, and Antihypertensive agents.

U.S. Regulatory Considerations

❑ FDA Black Box   ❑ OBRA regulated in U.S. Long Term Care

Other Uses in Geriatric Patient: Acute gout

Side Effects:

Of particular importance in the geriatric patient: Confusion, cognitive impairment, delirium, diarrhea, dizziness, dyspepsia, fluid retention, renal impairment

Geriatric Considerations - Summary: Use of NSAIDs in older adults increases the risk of GI complications, including gastric ulceration, bleeding, and perforation. These complications are not necessarily preceded by less severe GI symptoms. Concomitant use of a proton pump inhibitor or misoprostol reduces the risk for gastric ulceration and bleeding, but may not prevent long-term GI toxicity.

References:

1. COX-2 alternatives and GI protection. Med Lett Drugs Ther 2004;46:91.
2. Drugs that may cause cognitive disorders in the elderly. Med Lett Drugs Ther 2000;42:111-112.

medroxyprogesterone acetate

(me-drox'-ee-proe-jes'-te-rone as'-eh-tayte)

■ **Brand Name(s):** Depo-Provera, Depo-Provera Contraceptive, Depo-SubQ-Provera 104, Provera

Combinations
Rx: with estradiol (Lunelle)
Chemical Class: 17α-Hydroxyprogesterone derivative

Clinical Pharmacology:

Mechanism of Action: A hormone that transforms endometrium from proliferative to secretory in an estrogen-primed endometrium. Inhibits secretion of pituitary gonadotropins. **Therapeutic Effect:** Prevents follicular maturation and ovulation. Stimulates growth of mammary alveolar tissue and relaxes uterine smooth muscle. Corrects hormonal imbalance.

Pharmacokinetics: Slowly absorbed after IM administration. Protein binding: 90%. Metabolized in the liver. Primarily excreted in urine. **Half-life:** 30 days.

Available Forms:

- *Tablets* (*Provera*): 2.5 mg, 5 mg, 10 mg.
- *Injection*: 104 mg/0.65 ml prefilled syringe (Depo-SubQ-Provera 104), 150 mg/ml (Depo-Provera Contraceptive), 400 mg/ml (Depo-Provera).

Indications and Dosages:

Hormone replacement therapy: PO 5–10 mg for 12–14 consecutive days a month, beginning on day 1 or 16 of cycle given as part of regimen with conjugated estrogens.
Endometrial hyperplasia: PO 2.5–10 mg/day for 14 days.
Abnormal uterine bleeding: PO 5–10 mg/day for 5–10 days, beginning on calculated day 16 or day 21 of menstrual cycle.
Endometrial, renal carcinoma: IM Initially, 400–1,000 mg; repeat at 1-wk intervals. If improvement occurs and disease is stabilized, begin maintenance with as little as 400 mg/mo.

Unlabeled Uses: Hormone replacement therapy in estrogen-treated menopausal women

Contraindications: Carcinoma of breast; estrogen-dependent neoplasm; history of or active thrombotic disorders, such as cerebral apoplexy, thrombophlebitis, or thromboembolic disorders; hypersensitivity to progestins; severe hepatic dysfunction; undiagnosed abnormal genital bleeding

Side Effects

Occasional
Edema, weight change, breast tenderness, nervousness, insomnia, fatigue, dizziness
Rare
Alopecia, depression, dermatologic changes, headache, fever, nausea

Serious Reactions

- Thrombophlebitis, pulmonary or cerebral embolism, and retinal thrombosis occur rarely.
- Women who use medroxyprogesterone injection may lose significant bone mineral density.

Patient/Family Education

- Take protective measures against exposure to ultraviolet light
- Diabetic patients must monitor blood glucose carefully during therapy
- Take with food if GI upset occurs
- Immediately report chest pain, migraine headache, numbness of an arm or leg, sudden decrease in vision, sudden shortness of breath, and pain, redness, swelling, or warmth in the calf

- **Monitoring Parameters**
  - Blood pressure
  - Skin for rash
  - Weight

- **Geriatric side effects at a glance:**
  ☐ CNS   ☐ Bowel Dysfunction   ☐ Bladder Dysfunction   ☐ Falls

- **U.S. Regulatory Considerations**
  ☑ FDA Black Box
  Bone loss
  ☐ OBRA regulated in U.S. Long Term Care

mefenamic acid

(me-fe-nam'-ik as'-id)

- **Brand Name(s):** Ponstel
  Chemical Class: Anthranilic acid derivative

- **Clinical Pharmacology:**
  Mechanism of Action: A nonsteroidal anti-inflammatory that produces analgesic and anti-inflammatory effect by inhibiting prostaglandin synthesis. **Therapeutic Effect:** Reduces inflammatory response and intensity of pain stimulus reaching sensory nerve endings.
  Pharmacokinetics: Rapidly absorbed from the gastrointestinal (GI) tract. Protein binding: high. Metabolized in liver. Partially excreted in urine and partially in the feces. Not removed by hemodialysis. **Half-life:** 3.5 hr.

- **Available Forms:**
  - **Capsules:** 250 mg.

- **Indications and Dosages:**
  Mild to moderate pain, lower back pain: PO Initially, 500 mg to start, then 250 mg q4h as needed. Maximum: 1 week of therapy.

- **Unlabeled Uses:** Cataract prevention, menorrhagia, osteoarthritis, rheumatoid arthritis

- **Contraindications:** History of hypersensitivity to aspirin or NSAIDs

- **Side Effects**
  Occasional (10%-1%)
  Dyspepsia, including heartburn, indigestion, flatulence, abdominal cramping, constipation, nausea, diarrhea, epigastric pain, vomiting, headache, nervousness, dizziness, bleeding, elevated liver function tests, tinnitus

Rare (less than 1%)
Fluid retention, arrhythmias, tachycardia, confusion, drowsiness, rash, dry eyes, blurred vision, hot flashes

■ **Serious Reactions**
- Peptic ulcer, GI bleeding, gastritis, and severe hepatic reaction, such as cholestasis and jaundice, occur rarely.
- Nephrotoxicity (including dysuria, hematuria, proteinuria, and nephrotic syndrome) and severe hypersensitivity reaction, marked by bronchospasm and angioedema occur rarely.

Special Considerations
- No significant advantage over other NSAIDs; cost should govern use
- Use beyond 1 wk is not recommended

■ **Patient/Family Education**
- Avoid alcohol and aspirin during mefenamic acid therapy
- Swallow capsules whole
- Take the drug with food if GI upset occurs

■ **Monitoring Parameters**
- Initial hematocrit and fecal occult blood test within 3 mo of starting regular chronic therapy; repeat 6-12 mo (more frequently in high-risk patients (>65 years, peptic ulcer disease, concurrent steroids or anticoagulants); electrolytes, creatinine, and BUN within 3 mo of starting regular chronic therapy; repeat every 6-12 mo

■ **Geriatric side effects at a glance:**
  ☑ CNS   ❑ Bowel Dysfunction   ❑ Bladder Dysfunction   ❑ Falls
  ☑ Other: Gastropathy

■ **Use with caution in older patients with:** Renal impairment, Hepatic impairment, CHF, HTN, PUD, History of GI bleeding, GERD, Bleeding and platelet disorders, History of aspirin sensitivity reaction. Also use with caution in patients taking Anticoagulants, Aspirin, and Antihypertensive agents.

■ **U.S. Regulatory Considerations**
  ☑ FDA Black Box
  - Cardiovascular risk
  - Gastrointestinal risk
  ❑ OBRA regulated in U.S. Long Term Care

■ **Other Uses in Geriatric Patient:** Acute gout

■ **Side Effects:**
  Of particular importance in the geriatric patient: Confusion, cognitive impairment, delirium, dizziness, dyspepsia, fluid retention, renal impairment

■ **Geriatric Considerations - Summary:** Use of NSAIDs in older adults increases the risk of GI complications, including gastric ulceration, bleeding, and perforation. These complications are not necessarily preceded by less severe GI symptoms. Concomitant use of a proton pump inhibitor or misoprostol reduces the risk for gastric ulceration and bleeding, but may not prevent long-term GI toxicity.

- **References:**
  1. COX-2 alternatives and GI protection. Med Lett Drugs Ther 2004;46:91.
  2. Drugs that may cause cognitive disorders in the elderly. Med Lett Drugs Ther 2000;42:111-112.

mefloquine hydrochloride

(me'-floe-kwin hye-droe-klor'-ide)

- **Brand Name(s):** Lariam
  Chemical Class: Quinolinemethanol derivative

- **Clinical Pharmacology:**
  Mechanism of Action: A quinolone-methanol compound structurally similar to quinine that destroys the asexual blood forms of malarial pathogens, *Plasmodium falciparum, P. vivax, P. malariae, P. ovale.* **Therapeutic Effect:** Inhibits parasite growth.
  Pharmacokinetics: Well absorbed from the gastrointestinal (GI) tract. Protein binding: 98%. Widely distributed, including cerebrospinal fluid (CSF). Metabolized in liver. Primarily excreted in urine. **Half-life:** 21-22 days.

- **Available Forms:**
  - *Tablets:* 250 mg.

- **Indications and Dosages:**
  Suppression of malaria: PO 250 mg base weekly starting 1 wk before travel, continuing weekly during travel and for 4 wk after leaving endemic area.
  Treatment of malaria: PO 1,250 mg as a single dose.

- **Contraindications:** Cardiac abnormalities, severe psychiatric disorders, epilepsy, history of hypersensitivity to mefloquine

- **Side Effects**
  Occasional
  Mild transient headache, difficulty concentrating, insomnia, light-headedness, vertigo, diarrhea, nausea, vomiting, visual disturbances, tinnitus
  Rare
  Aggressive behavior, anxiety, bradycardia, depression, hallucinations, hypotension, panic attacks, paranoia, psychosis, syncope, tremor

- **Serious Reactions**
  - Prolonged therapy may result in peripheral neuritis, neuromyopathy, hypotension, electrocardiographic changes, agranulocytosis, aplastic anemia, thrombocytopenia, seizures, and psychosis.
  - Overdosage may result in headache, vomiting, visual disturbance, drowsiness, and seizures.

- **Patient/Family Education**
  - Do not take on an empty stomach
  - Take medication with at least 8 oz water

- Caution, initially, when driving, operating machinery, where concentration necessary
- Promptly report any visual disturbances

■ **Monitoring Parameters**
- Liver function tests and ophthalmic examinations during prolonged therapy

■ **Geriatric side effects at a glance:**
☑ CNS ☐ Bowel Dysfunction ☐ Bladder Dysfunction ☐ Falls

■ **U.S. Regulatory Considerations**
☐ FDA Black Box ☐ OBRA regulated in U.S. Long Term Care

megestrol acetate

(me-jess'-trole as'-eh-tayte)

■ **Brand Name(s):** Megace, Megace ES
Chemical Class: Progestin derivative

■ **Clinical Pharmacology:**
Mechanism of Action: A hormone and antineoplastic agent that suppresses the release of luteinizing hormone from the anterior pituitary gland by inhibiting pituitary function. **Therapeutic Effect:** Shrinks tumors. Also increases appetite by an unknown mechanism.
Pharmacokinetics: Well absorbed from the GI tract. Metabolized in the liver; excreted in urine. **Half-life:** 13-105 hr (mean 34 hr).

■ **Available Forms:**
- *Tablets (Megace)*: 20 mg, 40 mg.
- *Suspension*: 40 mg/ml (Megace), 625 mg/5 ml (equivalent to 800 mg/20 ml) (Megace ES).

■ **Indications and Dosages:**
Palliative treatment of advanced breast cancer: PO 160 mg/day in 4 equally divided doses.
Palliative treatment of advanced endometrial carcinoma: PO 40-320 mg/day in divided doses. Maximum: 800 mg/day in 1-4 divided doses.
Anorexia, cachexia, weight loss: PO 800 mg (20 ml)/day. PO (Megace ES) 625 mg/day.

■ **Unlabeled Uses:** Appetite stimulant, treatment of hormone-dependent or advanced prostate carcinoma, treatment of uterine bleeding

■ **Contraindications:** None known.

■ **Side Effects**
Frequent
Weight gain secondary to increased appetite

Occasional
Nausea, backache, headache, breast tenderness, carpal tunnel syndrome
Rare
Feeling of coldness

■ **Serious Reactions**
- Thrombophlebitis and pulmonary embolism occur rarely.

Special Considerations
- Average weight gain in AIDS patients 11 lb in 12 wk. Begin therapy only after treatable causes of weight loss are sought and addressed
- Contraception is imperative during megestrol therapy
- Notify the physician if calf pain, difficulty breathing, or vaginal bleeding occurs
- Megestrol may cause backache, breast tenderness, headache, nausea, and vomiting

■ **Monitoring Parameters**
- Signs and symptoms of a therapeutic response to the drug

■ **Geriatric side effects at a glance:**
❑ CNS ❑ Bowel Dysfunction ❑ Bladder Dysfunction ❑ Falls

■ **U.S. Regulatory Considerations**
❑ FDA Black Box ❑ OBRA regulated in U.S. Long Term Care

meloxicam

(mel-ox'-i-kam)

■ **Brand Name(s):** Mobic
Chemical Class: Oxicam derivative

■ **Clinical Pharmacology:**
Mechanism of Action: An NSAID that produces analgesic and anti-inflammatory effects by inhibiting prostaglandin synthesis. **Therapeutic Effect:** Reduces the inflammatory response and intensity of pain.
Pharmacokinetics:

Route	Onset	Peak	Duration
PO (analgesic)	30 min	4–5 hr	N/A

Well absorbed after PO administration. Protein binding: 99%. Metabolized in the liver. Eliminated in urine and feces. Not removed by hemodialysis. **Half-life:** 15–20 hr.

■ **Available Forms:**
- *Tablets:* 7.5 mg, 15 mg.
- *Oral Suspension:* 7.5 mg/5 ml.

- **Indications and Dosages:**
  Osteoarthritis, rheumatoid arthritis: PO Initially, 7.5 mg/day. Maximum: 15 mg/day.

- **Unlabeled Uses:** Ankylosing spondylitis

- **Contraindications:** Aspirin-induced nasal polyps associated with bronchospasm

- **Side Effects**
  Frequent (9%–7%)
  Dyspepsia, headache, diarrhea, nausea
  Occasional (4%–3%)
  Dizziness, insomnia, rash, pruritus, flatulence, constipation, vomiting
  Rare (less than 2%)
  Somnolence, urticaria, photosensitivity, tinnitus

- **Serious Reactions**
  - Rare reactions with long-term use include peptic ulcer disease, GI bleeding, gastritis, severe hepatic reaction (jaundice), nephrotoxicity (hematuria, dysuria, proteinuria), and a severe hypersensitivity reaction (bronchospasm, angioedema).

Special Considerations
  - Partial, not pure, COX-2 selective inhibitor; most studies have compared it with nonselective agents, making final assessment of place in therapy difficult

- **Patient/Family Education**
  - Take with food or milk; report gastrointestinal adverse effects
  - Avoid tasks that require mental alertness or motor skills until response to the drug has been established

- **Monitoring Parameters**
  - Acute phase reactants for efficacy in rheumatoid arthritis; pain, stiffness, number of swollen joints, range of motion, functional capacity, structural damage; fecal occult blood, hematocrit, renal and hepatic function

- **Geriatric side effects at a glance:**
  ☑ CNS   ☐ Bowel Dysfunction   ☐ Bladder Dysfunction   ☐ Falls
  ☑ Other: Gastropathy

- **Use with caution in older patients with:** Renal impairment, Hepatic impairment, CHF, HTN, PUD, History of GI bleeding, GERD, Bleeding and platelet disorders, History of aspirin sensitivity reaction. Also use with caution in patients taking Anticoagulants, Aspirin, and Antihypertensive agents.

- **U.S. Regulatory Considerations**
  ☑ FDA Black Box
  - Cardiovascular risk
  - Gastrointestinal risk
  ☐ OBRA regulated in U.S. Long Term Care

- **Other Uses in Geriatric Patient:** Acute gout

- **Side Effects:**
  Of particular importance in the geriatric patient: Confusion, cognitive impairment, delirium, dyspepsia, nausea, diarrhea, increased LFTs, dizziness, dyspepsia, fluid retention, renal impairment

- **Geriatric Considerations - Summary:** Use of NSAIDs in older adults increases the risk of GI complications, including gastric ulceration, bleeding, and perforation. These complications are not necessarily preceded by less severe GI symptoms. Concomitant use of a proton pump inhibitor or misoprostol reduces the risk for gastric ulceration and bleeding, but may not prevent long-term GI toxicity. No clinical data exist to support reduced GI toxicity with the use of meloxicam.

- **References:**
  1. COX-2 alternatives and GI protection. Med Lett Drugs Ther 2004;46:91.
  2. Drugs that may cause cognitive disorders in the elderly. Med Lett Drugs Ther 2000;42:111-112.
  3. Meloxicam (Mobic) for osteoarthritis. Med Lett Drugs Ther 2000;42:47.

memantine hydrochloride

(mem'-an-teen hye-droe-klor'-ide)

- **Brand Name(s):** Namenda
  Chemical Class: Adamantane derivative; tricyclic amine

- **Clinical Pharmacology:**
  Mechanism of Action: A neurotransmitter inhibitor that decreases the effects of glutamate, the principal excitatory neurotransmitter in the brain. Persistent CNS excitation by glutamate is thought to cause the symptoms of Alzheimer's disease. **Therapeutic Effect:** May reduce clinical deterioration in moderate to severe Alzheimer's disease.
  Pharmacokinetics: Rapidly and completely absorbed after PO administration. Protein binding: 45%. Undergoes little metabolism; most of the dose is excreted unchanged in urine. **Half-life:** 60-80 hr.

- **Available Forms:**
  - *Tablets:* 5 mg, 10 mg.
  - *Oral Solution:* 2 mg/ml.

- **Indications and Dosages:**
  Alzheimer's disease: PO Initially, 5 mg once a day. May increase dosage at intervals of at least 1 wk in 5-mg increments to 10 mg/day (5 mg twice a day), then 15 mg/day (5 mg and 10 mg as separate doses), and finally 20 mg/day (10 mg twice a day). Target dose: 20 mg/day.
  Dosage in renal failure: PO *Creatinine clearance < 30 ml/min.* Reduce to 5 mg 2 times/day.

- **Contraindications:** Severe renal impairment

■ **Side Effects**
   Occasional (7%-4%)
   Dizziness, headache, confusion, constipation, hypertension, cough
   Rare (3%-2%)
   Back pain, nausea, fatigue, anxiety, peripheral edema, arthralgia, insomnia

■ **Serious Reactions**
   • None known.

Special Considerations

   • Combination memantine-donepezil more likely to show a smaller decline or an improvement

■ **Patient/Family Education**
   • Twice daily for doses above 5 mg and minimum interval; 1-wk dose escalation
   • Do not abruptly discontinue memantine or adjust the drug dosage
   • If therapy is interrupted for several days, restart the drug at the lowest dose and increase the dosage at intervals of at least 1 week to the most recent dose, as prescribed
   • Maintain adequate fluid intake

■ **Monitoring Parameters**
   • *Efficacy*: Improvement or maintenance of mental status and functional quality of life scales
   • *Toxicity*: Pharmacotoxic psychosis (hallucinations, nervousness, changes in behavior, tremor, akathisia, restlessness, increased motor activity, insomnia, depression
   • Renal function, urine pH because alkaline urine may lead to an accumulation of the drug and a possible increase in side effects

■ **Geriatric side effects at a glance:**
   ☑ CNS ☑ Bowel Dysfunction ☐ Bladder Dysfunction ☐ Falls
   Other: Anorexia, weight loss, bradycardia

■ **Use with caution in older patients with:** None

■ **U.S. Regulatory Considerations**
   ☐ FDA Black Box ☐ OBRA regulated in U.S. Long Term Care

■ **Other Uses in Geriatric Patient:** None

■ **Side Effects:**
   Of particular importance in the geriatric patient: None

■ **Geriatric Considerations - Summary:** Memantine is modestly effective for treatment of cognitive decline associated with moderate-to-severe Alzheimer's disease. Furthermore, for persons with moderate-to-severe Alzheimer's disease using cholinesterase inhibitors, there is some evidence that memantine confers some additional benefit. Memantine is expensive, and its cost-effectiveness has not been demonstrated. Persons using drugs to treat Alzheimer's should be monitored closely, and prescribers should have a low threshold for discontinuing these agents if no clinical benefit is observed.

References:

1. Reisberg B, Doody R, Stoffler A, et al. Memantine in moderate-to-severe Alzheimer's disease. N Engl J Med 2003;348:1333-1341.
2. Tariot PN, Farlow MR, Grossberg GT, et al. Memantine treatment in patients with moderate to severe Alzheimer disease already receiving donepezil: a randomized controlled trial. JAMA 2004;291:317-324.
3. Areosa SA, Sherriff F, McShane R. Memantine for dementia. Cochrane Database Syst Rev 2005;CD003154
4. Cummings JL. Alzheimer's disease. N Engl J Med 2004;351:56-67.

meperidine hydrochloride

(me-per'-i-deen hye-droe-klor'-ide)

■ **Brand Name(s):** Demerol

Combinations
Rx: with promethazine (Mepergan)
Chemical Class: Opiate derivative; phenylpiperidine derivative

DEA Class: Schedule II

■ **Clinical Pharmacology:**
Mechanism of Action: An opioid agonist that binds to opioid receptors in the CNS.
Therapeutic Effect: Alters the perception of and emotional response to pain.
Pharmacokinetics:

Route	Onset	Peak	Duration
PO	15 min	60 min	2–4 hr
IV	less than 5 min	5–7 min	2–3 hr
IM	10–15 min	30–50 min	2–4 hr
Subcutaneous	10–15 min	30–50 min	2–4 hr

Variably absorbed from the GI tract; well absorbed after IM administration. Protein binding: 60%–80%. Widely distributed. Metabolized in the liver to active metabolite. Primarily excreted in urine. Not removed by hemodialysis. **Half-life:** 2.4–4 hr; metabolite 8–16 hr (increased in hepatic impairment and disease).

■ **Available Forms:**
- *Syrup:* 50 mg/5 ml.
- *Tablets:* 50 mg, 100 mg.
- *Injection:* 10 mg/ml, 25 mg/ml, 50 mg/ml, 75 mg/ml, 100 mg/ml.

■ **Indications and Dosages:**
Analgesia: PO, IM, Subcutaneous 50–150 mg q3–4h.
Patient-controlled analgesia (PCA): IV Loading dose: 50–100 mg. Intermittent bolus: 5–30 mg. Lockout interval: 10–20 min. Continuous infusion: 5–40 mg/hr. Maximum (4-hr): 200–300 mg.

Dosage in renal impairment: Dosage is based on creatinine clearance.

Creatinine Clearance	Dosage
10–50 ml/min	75% of usual dose
less than 10 ml/min	50% of usual dose

■ **Contraindications:** Diarrhea due to poisoning, use within 14 days of MAOIs

■ **Side Effects**
Frequent
Sedation, hypotension (including orthostatic hypotension), diaphoresis, facial flushing, dizziness, nausea, vomiting, constipation
Occasional
Confusion, arrhythmias, tremors, urine retention, abdominal pain, dry mouth, headache, irritation at injection site, euphoria, dysphoria
Rare
Allergic reaction (rash, pruritus), insomnia

■ **Serious Reactions**
- Overdose results in respiratory depression, skeletal muscle flaccidity, cold or clammy skin, cyanosis, and extreme somnolence progressing to seizures, stupor, and coma. The antidote is 0.4 mg naloxone.
- The patient who uses meperidine repeatedly may develop a tolerance to the drug's analgesic effect and physical dependence.

■ **Patient/Family Education**
- Physical dependency may result when used for extended periods
- Do not administer agonist/antagonist analgesics (i.e., pentazocine, nalbuphine, butorphanol, dezocine, buprenorphine) to patient who has received a prolonged course of meperidine (a pure agonist). In opioid-dependent patients, mixed agonist/antagonist analgesics may precipitate withdrawal symptoms.
- Change position slowly; orthostatic hypotension may occur
- Avoid hazardous activities if drowsiness or dizziness occurs
- Avoid alcohol, other CNS depressants unless directed by clinician
- Minimize nausea by administering with food and remain lying down following dose
- The injection may cause discomfort
- Increase fluid intake and consumption of high-fiber foods to prevent constipation

■ **Monitoring Parameters**
- Monitor the patient's vital signs for 15 to 30 minutes after an IM or subcutaneous dose and for 5 to 10 minutes after an IV dose. Be alert for decreased blood pressure, as well as a change in quality and rate of pulse
- Level of pain and sedation
- Pattern of daily bowel activity and stool consistency
- Though not used clinically, therapeutic serum drug level is 100 to 550 ng/ml; toxic serum drug level is greater than 1,000 ng/ml

■ **Geriatric side effects at a glance:**
☑ CNS ☑ Bowel Dysfunction ☑ Bladder Dysfunction ☑ Falls

■ **U.S. Regulatory Considerations**
❏ FDA Black Box ☑ OBRA regulated in U.S. Long Term Care

mephobarbital

(me'-foe-bar'-bi-tal)

■ **Brand Name(s):** Mebaral
   Chemical Class: Barbituric acid derivative

   DEA Class: Schedule IV

■ **Clinical Pharmacology:**
   Mechanism of Action: A barbiturate that increases seizure threshold in the motor cortex. **Therapeutic Effect:** Depresses monosynaptic and polysynaptic transmission in the central nervous system (CNS).
   Pharmacokinetics: PO route onset 20-60 min, peak N/A, duration 6-8 hr. Well absorbed after PO administration. Widely distributed. Metabolized in liver to active metabolite, a form of phenobarbital. Minimally excreted in urine. Removed by hemodialysis. **Half-life:** 34 hr.

■ **Available Forms:**
   • *Tablets:* 32 mg, 50 mg, 100 mg.

■ **Indications and Dosages:**
   Epilepsy: PO   400-600 mg/day in divided doses or at bedtime.
   Sedation: PO   32-100 mg/day in 3-4 divided doses.

■ **Contraindications:** Porphyria, history of hypersensitivity to mephobarbital or other barbituates

■ **Side Effects**
   Frequent
   Dizziness, light-headedness, somnolence
   Occasional
   Confusion, headache, insomnia, depression, nervousness, nightmares, unusual excitement
   Rare
   Rash, paradoxical CNS excitement or restlessness, generally noted during first 2 weeks of therapy, particularly noted in presence of uncontrolled pain

■ **Serious Reactions**
   • Abrupt withdrawal after prolonged therapy may produce effects including markedly increased dreaming, nightmares or insomnia, tremor, sweating, vomiting, hallucinations, delirium, seizures, and status epilepticus.
   • Skin eruptions appear as hypersensitivity reaction.
   • Blood dyscrasias, liver disease, and hypocalcemia occur rarely.
   • Overdosage produces cold or clammy skin, hypothermia, severe CNS depression, cyanosis, rapid pulse, and Cheyne-Stokes respirations.
   • Toxicity may result in severe renal impairment.

■ **Patient/Family Education**
  • Avoid driving or other activities requiring alertness
  • Avoid alcohol ingestion or CNS depressants
  • Do not discontinue medication abruptly after long-term use
  • Notify clinician of fever, sore throat, mouth sores, easy bruising or bleeding, broken blood vessels under skin
  • Mephobarbital may be habit-forming

■ **Monitoring Parameters**
  • Periodic CBC, liver and renal function tests, serum folate, vitamin D during prolonged therapy
  • Blood pressure, heart rate, respiratory rate
  • CNS status

■ **Geriatric side effects at a glance:**
  ☑ CNS   ❑ Bowel Dysfunction   ❑ Bladder Dysfunction   ☑ Falls
  Other: Withdrawal symptoms after long-term use

■ **Use with caution in older patients with:** Not recommeded for use in older adults.

■ **U.S. Regulatory Considerations**
  ❑ FDA Black Box   ☑ OBRA regulated in U.S. Long Term Care

■ **Other Uses in Geriatric Patient:** Anxiety disorders, sleep disorders, seizure disorders

■ **Side Effects:**
  Of particular importance in the geriatric patient: Sedation, withdrawal symptoms when abruptly discontinued (e.g., during hospitalization) rather than tapered

■ **Geriatric Considerations - Summary:** Because barbiturates have a low therapeutic window, a wide range of drug interactions and rapid development of tolerance, great potential for abuse and dependence, these agents are not recommended for use in older adults.

■ **Reference:**
  1. Hypnotic drugs. Med Lett Drugs Ther 2000;42:71-72.

meprobamate

(me-proe'-ba-mate)

- **Brand Name(s):** Miltown
  Chemical Class: Carbamate derivative

  DEA Class: Schedule IV

- **Clinical Pharmacology:**
  Mechanism of Action: A carbamate derivative that affects the thalamus and limbic system. Appears to inhibit multineuronal spinal reflexes. **Therapeutic Effect:** Relieves pain or muscle spasms.
  Pharmacokinetics: Slowly absorbed from the gastrointestinal (GI) tract. Protein binding: 0%-30%. Metabolized in liver. Excreted in urine and feces. Moderately dialyzable.
  Half-life: 10 hr.

- **Available Forms:**
  - **Tablets:** 200 mg, 400 mg, 600 mg.

- **Indications and Dosages:**
  Anxiety disorders: PO Use lowest effective dose. 200 mg 2-3 times/day
  Dosage in renal impairment:

Creatinine Clearance	Dosage Interval
10-50 ml/min	every 9-12 hr
less than 10 ml/min	every 12-18 hr

- **Unlabeled Uses:** Muscle contraction, headache, external sphincter spasticity, muscle rigidity, opisthotonos-associated with tetanus

- **Contraindications:** Acute intermittent porphyria, hypersensitivity to meprobamate or related compounds

- **Side Effects**
  Frequent
  Drowsiness, dizziness
  Occasional
  Tachycardia, palpitations, headache, light-headedness, dermatitis, diarrhea, nausea, vomiting, dyspnea, rash, weakness, blurred vision, wheezing.

- **Serious Reactions**
  - Agranulocytosis, aplastic anemia, leukopenia, anaphylaxis, cardiac arrhythmias, hypotensive crisis, syncope, Stevens-Johnson syndrome, and bullous dermatitis have been reported.
  - Overdose may cause CNS depression, ataxia, coma, shock, hypotension, and death.

- **Patient/Family Education**
  - Avoid alcohol
  - Do not discontinue abruptly following long-term use

- This drug may cause dizziness or drowsiness

■ **Monitoring Parameters**
- Periodic CBC with differential and platelets during prolonged therapy
- Renal function tests, BUN, serum creatinine, liver function tests

■ **Geriatric side effects at a glance:**
☑ CNS ☐ Bowel Dysfunction ☐ Bladder Dysfunction ☑ Falls
Other: Withdrawal symptoms after long-term use

■ **Use with caution in older patients with:** Not recommeded for use in older adults

■ **U.S. Regulatory Considerations**
☐ FDA Black Box ☑ OBRA regulated in U.S. Long Term Care

■ **Other Uses in Geriatric Patient:** Anxiety disorders, sleep disorders

■ **Side Effects:**
Of particular importance in the geriatric patient: Sedation, withdrawal symptoms when abruptly discontinued (e.g., during hospitalization) rather than tapered

■ **Geriatric Considerations - Summary:** Because meprobamate has a low therapeutic window, rapid development of tolerance, and great potential for abuse and dependence, these agents are not recommended for use in older adults.

meropenem

(mer-oh-pen'-em)

■ **Brand Name(s):** Merrem
Chemical Class: Carbapenem

■ **Clinical Pharmacology:**
Mechanism of Action: A carbapenem that binds to penicillin-binding proteins and inhibits bacterial cell wall synthesis. **Therapeutic Effect:** Produces bacterial cell death. **Pharmacokinetics:** After IV administration, widely distributed into tissues and body fluids, including CSF. Protein binding: 2%. Primarily excreted unchanged in urine. Removed by hemodialysis. **Half-life:** 1 hr.

■ **Available Forms:**
- *Powder for Injection:* 500 mg, 1 g.

■ **Indications and Dosages:**
Intra-abdominal infections: IV 1g q8h.
Meningitis: IV 2g q8h.

Dosage in renal impairment: Dosage and frequency are modified based on creatinine clearance.

Creatinine Clearance	Dosage	Interval
26-49 ml/min	Recommended dose (1,000 mg)	q12h
10-25 ml/min	1/2 of recommended dose	q12h
less than 10 ml/min	1/2 of recommended dose	q24h

■ **Unlabeled Uses:** Lower respiratory tract infections, febrile neutropenia, gynecologic and obstetric infections, sepsis

■ **Contraindications:** History of seizures or CNS abnormality, hypersensitivity to penicillins.

■ **Side Effects**

Frequent (5%-3%)
Diarrhea, nausea, vomiting, headache, inflammation at injection site
Occasional (2%)
Oral candidiasis, rash, pruritus
Rare (less than 2%)
Constipation, glossitis

■ **Serious Reactions**
- Antibiotic-associated colitis and other superinfections may occur.
- Anaphylactic reactions have been reported.
- Seizures may occur in those with CNS disorders (including brain lesions and a history of seizures), bacterial meningitis, or impaired renal function.

Special Considerations
- Less likely to induce seizures than imipenem-cilastatin
- Individualize treatment based on local susceptibility patterns.

■ **Patient/Family Education**
- Immediately notify the physician if severe diarrhea occurs and avoid taking antidiarrheals until directed to do so
- Notify the physician of troublesome or serious adverse reactions, including infusion site pain, redness, or swelling; nausea or vomiting; or a rash or itching

■ **Monitoring Parameters**
- Renal, hepatic, and hematopoietic function during prolonged therapy
- Hydration status, and check for nausea and vomiting
- Check the IV injection site for inflammation
- Check skin for a rash
- Electrolyte levels (especially potassium), intake and output, and renal function test results
- Observe the patient's mental status, and be alert for seizures or tremors
- Blood pressure and body temperature at least twice a day
- Daily bowel activity and stool consistency. Although mild GI effects may be tolerable, severe symptoms may indicate the onset of antibiotic-associated colitis.
- Signs and symptoms of superinfection include abdominal pain or cramping, anal or genital pruritus or discharge, moderate to severe diarrhea, severe mouth or tongue soreness, and new or increased fever.

- **Geriatric side effects at a glance:**
  ☐ CNS ☑ Bowel Dysfunction ☐ Bladder Dysfunction ☐ Falls

- **U.S. Regulatory Considerations**
  ☐ FDA Black Box ☐ OBRA regulated in U.S. Long Term Care

mesalamine/5-aminosalicylic acid/5-ASA

(mez-al'-a-meen/5-a-me'-no-sal-i-sil'-ik as'-id)

- **Brand Name(s):** Asacol, Canasa, Pentasa, Rowasa
  Chemical Class: 5-Amino derivative of salicylic acid

- **Clinical Pharmacology:**
  Mechanism of Action: A salicylic acid derivative that locally inhibits arachidonic acid metabolite production, which is increased in patients with chronic inflammatory bowel disease. **Therapeutic Effect:** Blocks prostaglandin production and diminishes inflammation in the colon.
  Pharmacokinetics: Poorly absorbed from the colon. Moderately absorbed from the GI tract. Metabolized in the liver to active metabolite. Unabsorbed portion eliminated in feces; absorbed portion excreted in urine. Unknown if removed by hemodialysis. **Half-life:** 0.5–1.5 hr; metabolite, 5–10 hr.

- **Available Forms:**
  - *Tablets (Delayed-Release [Asacol]):* 400 mg.
  - *Capsules (Controlled-Release [Pentasa]):* 250 mg.
  - *Rectal Suspension (Rowasa):* 4 g/60 ml.
  - *Suppositories (Canasa):* 500 mg, 1 g.

- **Indications and Dosages:**
  Treatment of ulcerative colitis: PO (capsule) 1 g 4 times a day. PO (tablet) 800 mg 3 times a day.
  Maintenance of remission in ulcerative colitis: PO (capsule) 1 g 4 times a day. PO (tablet) 1.6 g/day in divided doses.
  Distal ulcerative colitis, proctosigmoiditis, proctitis: Rectal (retention enema) 60 ml (4 g) at bedtime; retained overnight for approximately 8 hr for 3–6 wk. Rectal (500-mg suppository) Twice a day. May increase to 3 times a day. Rectal (1,000-mg suppository) Once daily at bedtime. Continue therapy for 3–6 wk.

- **Contraindications:** None known.

- **Side Effects**
  Mesalamine is generally well tolerated, with only mild and transient effects.
  Frequent (greater than 6%)
  PO: Abdominal cramps or pain, diarrhea, dizziness, headache, nausea, vomiting, rhinitis, unusual fatigue

Rectal: Abdominal or stomach cramps, flatulence, headache, nausea
Occasional (6%–2%)
PO: Hair loss, decreased appetite, back or joint pain, flatulence, acne
Rectal: Hair loss
Rare (less than 2%)
Rectal: Anal irritation

■ **Serious Reactions**
- Sulfite sensitivity may occur in susceptible patients, manifested by cramping, headache, diarrhea, fever, rash, hives, itching, and wheezing. Discontinue drug immediately.
- Hepatitis, pancreatitis, and pericarditis occur rarely with oral forms.

■ **Patient/Family Education**
- Swallow tabs whole, do not break the outer coating
- Intact or partially intact tabs may be found in stool; notify clinician if this occurs repeatedly
- Avoid excess handling of suppositories
- Lie on left side during enema administration (to facilitate migration into the sigmoid colon)
- Avoid tasks that require mental alertness or motor skills until response to the drug has been established
- Mesalamine may discolor urine yellow-brown

■ **Monitoring Parameters**
- Pattern of daily bowel activity and stool consistency and record time of evacuation
- Skin for rash and urticaria

■ **Geriatric side effects at a glance:**
  ❏ CNS ❏ Bowel Dysfunction ❏ Bladder Dysfunction ❏ Falls

■ **U.S. Regulatory Considerations**
  ❏ FDA Black Box ❏ OBRA regulated in U.S. Long Term Care

mesna

(mes'-na)

■ **Brand Name(s):** Mesnex
  Chemical Class: Thiol derivative

■ **Clinical Pharmacology:**
  Mechanism of Action: An antineoplastic adjunct and cytoprotective agent that binds with and detoxifies urotoxic metabolites of ifosfamide and cyclophosphamide. **Therapeutic Effect:** Inhibits ifosfamide- and cyclophosphamide-induced hemorrhagic cystitis.

Pharmacokinetics: Rapidly metabolized after IV administration to mesna disulfide, which is reduced to mesna in kidney. Excreted in urine. **Half-life:** 24 min.

■ **Available Forms:**
  - *Tablets*: 400 mg.
  - *Injection*: 100 mg/ml.

■ **Indications and Dosages:**
  Prevention of hemorrhagic cystitis in patients receiving ifosfamide: IV 20% of ifosfamide dose at time of ifosfamide administration and 4 hr and 8 hr after each dose of ifosfamide. Total dose: 60% of ifosfamide dosage. Range: 60%-160% of the daily ifosfamide dose.
  Hemorrhagic cystitis (chronic low-dose cyclophosphamide): PO 20 mg/kg q3-4h.
  Hemorrhagic cystitis (high-dose cyclophosphamide): IV 40% of cyclophosphamide dose at 0, 3, 6, 9 hr and IV fluids.

■ **Contraindications:** None known.

■ **Side Effects**
  Frequent (more than 17%)
  Bad taste, soft stools
  Large doses: Diarrhea, myalgia, headache, fatigue, nausea, hypotension, allergic reaction

■ **Serious Reactions**
  - Hematuria occurs rarely.

■ **Patient/Family Education**
  - Notify the physician or nurse if headache, myalgia, or nausea occurs

■ **Monitoring Parameters**
  - Urinalysis each day prior to ifosfamide administration
  - Reduction or discontinuation of ifosfamide may be initiated in patients developing hematuria (>50 RBC/hpf)
  - Pattern of daily bowel activity and stool consistency; record the time of evacuation
  - Blood pressure for hypotension

■ **Geriatric side effects at a glance:**
  ❏ CNS ☑ Bowel Dysfunction ❏ Bladder Dysfunction ❏ Falls

■ **U.S. Regulatory Considerations**
  ❏ FDA Black Box ❏ OBRA regulated in U.S. Long Term Care

mesoridazine besylate

(mez-oh-rid'-a-zeen bess'-il-late)

- **Brand Name(s):** Serentil
  Chemical Class: Piperidine phenothiazine derivative

- **Clinical Pharmacology:**
  Mechanism of Action: A phenothiazine that blocks dopamine at postsynaptic receptor sites in the brain. **Therapeutic Effect:** Diminishes schizophrenic behavior. Also has anticholinergic and sedative effects.
  Pharmacokinetics: Absorption may be erratic. Protein binding: 75%-91%. Undergoes first-pass metabolism. Small portions are metabolized in liver. Excreted in urine and feces. **Half-life:** Unknown.

- **Available Forms:**
  - *Oral Solution:* 25 mg/ml.
  - *Tablets:* 10 mg, 25 mg, 50 mg, 100 mg.
  - *Injection:* 25 mg/ml.

- **Indications and Dosages:**
  Schizophrenia: PO 25-50 mg 3 times a day. Maximum: 400 mg/day. IM Initially, 25 mg. May repeat in 30-60 min. Range: 25-200 mg.
  Severe behavioral problems (combativeness or explosive, hyperexcitable behavior) associated with neurologic diseases: PO Initially, 10 mg once or twice a day. May increase at 4- to 7-day intervals. Maximum: 250 mg. IM Initially, 25 mg. May repeat in 30-60 min. Range: 25-200 mg.

- **Contraindications:** Coma, concurrent administration of drugs that cause QTc-interval prolongation, myelosuppression, severe cardiovascular disease, severe CNS depression, subcortical brain damage

- **Side Effects**
  Frequent
  Orthostatic hypotension, dizziness, syncope (occur frequently after first injection, occasionally after subsequent injections, and rarely with oral form)
  Occasional
  Somnolence (during early therapy), dry mouth, blurred vision, lethargy, constipation or diarrhea, nasal congestion, peripheral edema, urine retention
  Rare
  Ocular changes, altered skin pigmentation (in those taking high doses for prolonged periods), darkening of urine

- **Serious Reactions**
  - Abrupt withdrawal after long-term therapy may precipitate nausea, vomiting, gastritis, dizziness, and tremors.
  - Blood dyscrasias, particularly agranulocytosis and mild leukopenia may occur.
  - Mesoridazine use may lower the seizure threshold.

■ **Patient/Family Education**
- Do not discontinue abruptly
- Concentrate may be diluted just prior to administration with distilled water, acidified tap water, orange or grape juice
- Full therapeutic effect may take up to 6 wk to appear
- Drowsiness generally subsides with continued therapy
- The drug may darken the urine

■ **Monitoring Parameters**
- Observe closely for signs of tardive dyskinesia
- Periodic CBC with platelets during prolonged therapy
- Pattern of daily bowel activity and stool consistency
- Closely supervise suicidal patients during early therapy. As depression lessens, the patient's energy level improves, which increases the suicide potential

■ **Geriatric side effects at a glance:**
  ☑ CNS ☑ Bowel Dysfunction ☑ Bladder Dysfunction ☑ Falls
  Other: Orthostatic hypotension, cardiac conduction disturbances, torsades de pointes, anticholinergic side effects

■ **Use with caution in older patients with:** Parkinson's disease (an atypical antipsychotic is recommended), seizure disorders, cardiovascular disease with conduction disturbance, hepatic encephalopathy, narrow-angle glaucoma

■ **U.S. Regulatory Considerations**
  ☑ FDA Black Box
  QTc prolongation dose-related; risk of torsades de pointes and sudden death
  ☑ OBRA regulated in U.S. Long Term Care

■ **Other Uses in Geriatric Patient:** Behavior disturbances in the setting of dementia

■ **Side Effects:**
  Of *particular importance in the geriatric patient*: Tardive dyskinesia, akathisia (may appear to exacerbate behavioral disturbances), anticholinergic effects, may increase risk of sudden death

■ **Geriatric Considerations - Summary:** Sink and colleagues' systematic review showed statistically significant improvements on neuropsychiatric and behavioral scales for some drugs, but improvements were small and unlikely to be clinically important. Because of documented risks, and uncertain benefits, these agents should be used with caution in demented elderly persons, with frequent monitoring for side effects and a low threshold for discontinuing use.

■ **References:**
1. Leipzig RM, Cumming RG, Tinetti ME. Drugs and falls in older people: a systematic review and meta-analysis: I. Psychotropic drugs. J Am Geriatr Soc 1999;47:30-39.
2. Sink KM, Holden KF, Yaffe K. Pharmacological treatment of neuropsychiatric symptoms of dementia: a review of the evidence. JAMA 2005;293:596-608.
3. Ray WA, Meredith S, Thapa PB, et al. Antipsychotics and the risk of sudden cardiac death. Arch Gen Psychiatry 2001;58:1161-1167.

metaproterenol sulfate

(met-a-proe-ter'-e-nole sul'-fate)

- **Brand Name(s):** Alupent
  Chemical Class: Sympathomimetic amine; β_2-adrenergic agonist

- **Clinical Pharmacology:**
  Mechanism of Action: A sympathomimetic that stimulates beta$_2$-adrenergic receptors, resulting in relaxation of bronchial smooth muscle. **Therapeutic Effect:** Relieves bronchospasm and reduces airway resistance.
  Pharmacokinetics: Systemic absorption is rapid following aerosol administration; however, serum concentrations at recommended doses are very low. Metabolized in liver. Excreted in urine primarily as glucoside metabolite. **Half-life:** Unknown.

- **Available Forms:**
  - *Syrup*: 10 mg/5 ml.
  - *Tablets*: 10 mg, 20 mg.
  - *Aerosol Oral Inhalation*: 0.65 mg/inhalation.
  - *Solution for Oral Inhalation*: 0.4%, 0.6%, 5%.

- **Indications and Dosages:**
  Treatment of bronchospasm: PO 10 mg 3–4 times a day. May increase to 20 mg/dose. Inhalation 2–3 inhalations q3–4h. Maximum: 12 inhalations/24 hr. Nebulization 10–15 mg (0.2–0.3 ml) of 5% q4–6h.

- **Contraindications:** Angle-closure glaucoma, preexisting arrhythmias associated with tachycardia

- **Side Effects**
  Frequent (over 10%)
  Rigors, tremors, anxiety, nausea, dry mouth
  Occasional (9%–1%)
  Dizziness, vertigo, asthenia, headache, GI distress, vomiting, cough, dry throat
  Rare (less than 1%)
  Somnolence, diarrhea, altered taste

- **Serious Reactions**
  - Excessive sympathomimetic stimulation may cause palpitations, extrasystoles, tachycardia, chest pain, a slight increase in BP followed by a substantial decrease, chills, diaphoresis, and blanching of skin.
  - Too-frequent or excessive use may lead to decreased drug effectiveness and severe, paradoxical bronchoconstriction.

- **Patient/Family Education**
  - Proper inhalation technique is vital for MDIs
  - Excessive use may lead to adverse effects

- Notify clinician if no response to usual doses
- Drink plenty of fluids to decrease the thickness of lung secretions
- Notify the physician if chest pain, difficulty breathing, dizziness, flushing, headache, palpitations, tachycardia, or tremors occur
- Avoid use of caffeine derivatives such as chocolate, cocoa, cola, coffee, and tea

■ Monitoring Parameters
- Pulse rate and quality and respiratory rate, depth, rhythm, and type
- ABG levels and pulmonary function test results
- Evidence of cyanosis, a blue or a dusky color in light-skinned patients and a gray color in dark-skinned patients
- Evaluate the patient for signs of clinical improvement, such as cessation of retractions, quieter and slower respirations, and a relaxed facial expression

■ Geriatric side effects at a glance:
❏ CNS   ❏ Bowel Dysfunction   ❏ Bladder Dysfunction   ❏ Falls

■ U.S. Regulatory Considerations
❏ FDA Black Box   ❏ OBRA regulated in U.S. Long Term Care

metaraminol bitartrate

(met-ar-am'-e-nol bye-tar'-trate)

■ Brand Name(s): Aramine
Chemical Class: Catecholamine, synthetic

■ Clinical Pharmacology:
Mechanism of Action: An alpha-adrenergic receptor agonist that causes vasoconstriction, reflex bradycardia, inhibits GI smooth muscle and vascular smooth muscle supplying skeletal muscle and increases heart rate and force of heart muscle contraction.
Therapeutic Effect: Increases both systolic and diastolic pressure.
Pharmacokinetics:

Route	Onset	Peak	Duration
IM (pressor effect)	10 min	N/A	20-60 min
IV	1-2 min	N/A	
SC	5-20 min	N/A	

Metabolized in the liver. Excreted in the urine and the bile.

■ Available Forms:
- *Injection*: 10 mg/ml (Aramine).

■ Indications and Dosages:
Prevention of hypotension: IM, SC 2-10 mg as a single dose.
Adjunctive treatment of hypotension: IV 15-100 mg IV infusion, administered at a rate to maintain the desired blood pressure.

Severe shock: IV 0.5-5 mg direct IV injection followed by 15-100 mg IV infusion in 250-500 ml fluid for control of blood pressure.

- **Contraindications:** Cyclopropane or halothane anesthesia, use of MAOIs, hypersensitivity to metaraminol

- **Side Effects**
  Occasional
  Tachycardia, hypertension, cardiac arrhythmias, flushing, palpitations, hypotension, angina, tremors, nervousness, headache, dizziness, weakness, sloughing of skin, nausea, abscess formation, diaphoresis

- **Serious Reactions**
  - Overdosage produces hypertension, cerebral hemorrhage, cardiac arrest, and seizures.

- **Patient/Family Education**
  - Notify the physician immediately if increased heart rate or palpitations occurs

- **Monitoring Parameters**
  - Maximum effect is not immediately apparent; allow at least 10 min to elapse before increasing the dose
  - BP and pulse

- **Geriatric side effects at a glance:**
  ❑ CNS   ❑ Bowel Dysfunction   ❑ Bladder Dysfunction   ❑ Falls

- **U.S. Regulatory Considerations**
  ❑ FDA Black Box   ❑ OBRA regulated in U.S. Long Term Care

metaxalone

(me-tax'-a-lone)

- **Brand Name(s):** Skelaxin
  Chemical Class: Oxazolidinedione derivative

- **Clinical Pharmacology:**
  Mechanism of Action: A central depressant whose exact mechanism is unknown. Many effects due to its central depressant actions. **Therapeutic Effect:** Relieves pain or muscle spasms.
  Pharmacokinetics: PO route onset 1 hour, peak 3 hours, duration 4-6 hours. Well absorbed from the gastrointestinal (GI) tract. Metabolized in liver. Primarily excreted in urine. **Half-life:** 9 hr.

■ **Available Forms:**
- *Tablets*: 400 mg, 800 mg.

■ **Indications and Dosages:**
Muscle Relaxant: PO 800 mg 3-4 times/day.

■ **Contraindications:** Impaired renal or hepatic function, history of drug-induced hemolytic anemias or other anemias, history of hypersensitivity to metaxalone

■ **Side Effects**
Occasional
Drowsiness, headache, light-headedness, dermatitis, nausea, vomiting, stomach cramps, dyspnea

■ **Serious Reactions**
- Overdose may cause CNS depression, coma, shock, and respiratory depression.

■ **Patient/Family Education**
- Drowsiness usually diminishes with continued therapy
- Avoid tasks that require mental alertness or motor skills until response to the drug is established
- Avoid alcohol or other depressants while taking metaxalone
- Avoid sudden changes in posture to help avoid hypotensive effects

■ **Monitoring Parameters**
- Therapeutic response, decreased intensity of skeletal muscle pain, stiffness, and tenderness and improved mobility

■ **Geriatric side effects at a glance:**
❏ CNS ☑ Bowel Dysfunction ☑ Bladder Dysfunction ☑ Falls
Other: None

■ **Use with caution in older patients with:** None

■ **U.S. Regulatory Considerations**
❏ FDA Black Box ☑ OBRA regulated in U.S. Long Term Care

■ **Other Uses in Geriatric Patient:** None

■ **Side Effects:**
Of particular importance in the geriatric patient: Drowsiness, dizziness

■ **Geriatric Considerations - Summary:** Metaxalone is a skeletal muscle relaxant with a primary effect of general CNS depression. Older adults taking this drug are at risk of somnolence and injuries from falls.

metformin hydrochloride

(met-for'-min hye-droe-klor'-ide)

- **Brand Name(s):** Fortamet, Glucophage, Glucophage XL, Glumetza, Riomet
  Combinations
  Rx: with rosiglitazone (Avandamet); with glyburide (Glucovance)
  Chemical Class: Biguanide

- **Clinical Pharmacology:**
  Mechanism of Action: An antihyperglycemic that decreases hepatic production of glucose. Decreases absorption of glucose and improves insulin sensitivity. **Therapeutic Effect:** Improves glycemic control, stabilizes or decreases body weight, and improves lipid profile.
  Pharmacokinetics: Slowly, incompletely absorbed after oral administration. Food delays or decreases the extent of absorption. Protein binding: Negligible. Primarily distributed to intestinal mucosa and salivary glands. Primarily excreted unchanged in urine. Removed by hemodialysis. **Half-life:** 3–6 hr.

- **Available Forms:**
  - *Oral Solution (Riomet):* 100 mg/ml.
  - *Tablets (Glucophage):* 500 mg, 850 mg, 1000 mg.
  - *Tablets (Extended-Release):* 500 mg (Fortamet, Glucophage XL, Glumetza), 750 mg (Glucophage XL), 1,000 mg (Fortamet, Glumetza).

- **Indications and Dosages:**
  Diabetes mellitus : PO (Immediate-Release Tablets, Solution) Initially, 500 mg twice a day or 850 mg once daily. Maintenance: 1-2.55 g/day in 2-3 divided doses. Maximum: 2,500 mg/day. PO (Extended-Release Tablets [Glucophage XL]) Initially, 500 mg once daily. Maintenance: 1-2g daily. Maximum: 2,000 mg/day. PO (Extended-Release Tablets [Fortamet, Glumetza]) 500 mg - 1g once daily. Maintenance: 1-2.5g once daily. Maximum: 2,500 mg/day.

- **Unlabeled Uses:** Treatment of HIV lipodystrophy syndrome, metabolic complications of AIDS, polycystic ovary syndrome, prediabetes, weight reduction

- **Contraindications:** Acute CHF, MI, cardiovascular collapse, renal disease or dysfunction, respiratory failure, septicemia

- **Side Effects**
  Occasional (greater than 3%)
  GI disturbances (including diarrhea, nausea, vomiting, abdominal bloating, flatulence, and anorexia) that are transient and resolve spontaneously during therapy.
  Rare (3%–1%)
  Unpleasant or metallic taste that resolves spontaneously during therapy

763

■ Serious Reactions

- Lactic acidosis occurs rarely but is a fatal complication in 50% of cases. Lactic acidosis is characterized by an increase in blood lactate levels (greater than 5 mmol/L), a decrease in blood pH, and electrolyte disturbances. Signs and symptoms of lactic acidosis include unexplained hyperventilation, myalgia, malaise, and somnolence, which may advance to cardiovascular collapse (shock), acute CHF, acute MI, and prerenal azotemia.

Special Considerations

- May also lower triglycerides
- May decrease insulin requirement in insulin-requiring diabetics

■ Patient/Family Education

- Administer with food
- Avoid excessive alcohol
- Notify clinician of diarrhea, severe muscle pain or cramping, shallow and fast breathing, unusual tiredness and weakness, unusual sleepiness (signs of lactic acidosis)

■ Monitoring Parameters

- Glycosylated hemoglobin q3-6 mo (<7.0%); self-monitored preprandial blood sugars <150 mg/dL; absence of hyperglycemia (e.g., polyuria, polyphagia, polydipsia, blurred vision)
- Renal and hepatic function tests before and annually during therapy
- Serum vitamin B_{12} annually during chronic therapy
- Assess the patient concurrently taking oral sulfonylureas for signs and symptoms of hypoglycemia, including anxiety, cool wet skin, diplopia, dizziness, headache, hunger, numbness in mouth, tachycardia, and tremors
- Be alert to conditions that alter blood glucose requirements, such as fever, increased activity, stress, or a surgical procedure

■ Geriatric side effects at a glance:

☐ CNS   ☑ Bowel Dysfunction   ☐ Bladder Dysfunction   ☐ Falls
Other: None

■ Use with caution in older patients with: Hepatic impairment, Impaired renal function, CHF, Compromised cardiorespiratory function, Untreated vitamin B_{12} deficiency, Increased liver function tests (ALT, AST)

■ U.S. Regulatory Considerations

☑ FDA Black Box
Lactic acidosis
☐ OBRA regulated in U.S. Long Term Care

■ Other Uses in Geriatric Patient: None

■ Side Effects:

Of particular importance in the geriatric patient: Slight decrease in vitamin B_{12} levels, weight loss, weakness, diarrhea

■ Geriatric Considerations - Summary: Avoid in patients > 80 years old, or if used, verify good renal function by 24-hour urine assessment of creatinine clearance. Hold before radiologic studies using contrast dye. Use with caution in long-term-care patients. Diarrhea can be avoided or minimized by administering the dose after meals.

■ **References:**
1. Haas L. Management of diabetes mellitus medications in the nursing home. Drugs Aging 2005;22:209-218.
2. Rosenstock J. Management of type 2 diabetes mellitus in the elderly: special considerations. Drugs Aging 2001;18:31-44.

methacholine chloride

(meth-a-ko'-leen klor'-ide)

■ **Brand Name(s):** Provocholine
  Chemical Class: Choline ester

■ **Clinical Pharmacology:**
  Mechanism of Action: A cholinergic, parasympathomimetic, synthetic analog of acetylcholine that stimulates muscarinic, postganglionic parasympathetic receptors. **Therapeutic Effect:** Results in smooth muscle contraction of the airways and increased tracheobronchial secretions.
  Pharmacokinetics: PO route onset rapid, peak 1-4 minutes, duration 15-75 minutes or 5 minutes if methacholine challenge is followed with a beta-agonist agent. Undergoes rapid hydrolysis in the plasma by acetylcholinesterase.

■ **Available Forms:**
  • *Powder for Oral Inhalation:* 100 mg/5 ml.

■ **Indications and Dosages:**
  Asthma diagnosis: Inhalation *Challenge test:* Before inhalation challenge, perform baseline pulmonary function tests; the patient must have an FEV_1 of at least 70% of the predicted value. The following is a suggested schedule for administration of methacholine challenge. Calculate cumulative units by multiplying number of breaths by concentration given. Total cumulative units are the sum of cumulative units for each concentration given.
  Vial E:
  • Serial concentration: 0.025 mg/ml
  • No. of breaths: 5
  • Cumulative units per concentration: 0.125
  • Total cumulative units: 0.125
  Vial D:
  • Serial concentration: 0.25 mg/ml
  • No. of breaths: 5
  • Cumulative units per concentration: 1.25
  • Total cumulative units: 1.375
  Vial C:
  • Serial concentration: 2.5 mg/ml
  • No. of breaths: 5
  • Cumulative units per concentration: 12.5
  • Total cumulative units: 13.88

765

Vial B:
- Serial concentration: 10 mg/ml
- No. of breaths: 5
- Cumulative units per concentration: 50
- Total cumulative units: 63.88

Vial A:
- Serial concentration: 25 mg/ml
- No. of breaths: 5
- Cumulative units per concentration: 125
- Total cumulative units: 188.88. Determine FEV_1 within 5 minutes of challenge; a positive challenge is a 20% reduction in FEV_1.

■ **Unlabeled Uses:** Adie's syndrome diagnosis, familial dysautonomia diagnosis, peripheral ischemia, parotitis

■ **Contraindications:** Asthma, wheezing, or very low baseline pulmonary function tests; concomitant use of beta-blockers; hypersensitivity to the drug, because of the potential for severe bronchoconstriction

■ **Side Effects**
Occasional
Headache, light-headedness, itching, throat irritation, wheezing

■ **Serious Reactions**
- Severe bronchoconstriction and reduction in respiratory function can result. Patients with severe hyperreactivity of the airways can experience bronchoconstriction at a dosage as low as 0.025 mg/ml (0.125 cumulative units). If severe bronchoconstriction occurs, reverse immediately by administration of a rapid-acting inhaled bronchodilator (beta-agonist).

■ **Patient/Family Education**
- Notify the physician immediately of difficulty breathing

■ **Monitoring Parameters**
- FEV_1 3-5 min after administration of each serial concentration; procedure is complete when there is a $\geq$20% reduction in FEV_1 compared to baseline (positive response) or when 5 inhalations have been administered at each concentration and FEV_1 has been reduced by $\leq$14% (negative response)

■ **Geriatric side effects at a glance:**
❏ CNS ❏ Bowel Dysfunction ❏ Bladder Dysfunction ❏ Falls

■ **U.S. Regulatory Considerations**
❏ FDA Black Box ❏ OBRA regulated in U.S. Long Term Care

methadone hydrochloride

(meth'-a-done hye-droe-klor'-ide)

- **Brand Name(s):** Dolophine, Methadone Intensol, Methadose
  Chemical Class: Diphenylheptane derivative; opiate derivative

  DEA Class: Schedule II

- **Clinical Pharmacology:**
  Mechanism of Action: An opioid agonist that binds with opioid receptors in the CNS.
  Therapeutic Effect: Alters the perception of and emotional response to pain; reduces withdrawal symptoms from other opioid drugs.
  Pharmacokinetics:

Route	Onset	Peak	Duration
Oral	0.5–1 hr	1.5–2 hr	6–8 hr
IM	10–20 min	1–2 hr	4–5 hr
IV	N/A	15–30 min	3-4 hr

  Well absorbed after IM injection. Protein binding: 80%–85%. Metabolized in the liver. Primarily excreted in urine. Not removed by hemodialysis. **Half-life:** 15–25 hr.

- **Available Forms:**
  - *Oral Concentrate (Methadone Intensol, Methadose):* 10 mg/ml.
  - *Oral Solution:* 5 mg/5 ml, 10 mg/ 5 ml.
  - *Tablets (Dolophine, Methadose):* 5 mg, 10 mg.
  - *Tablets (Dispersible [Methadose]):* 40 mg.
  - *Injection (Dolophine):* 10 mg/ml.

- **Indications and Dosages:**
  Analgesia: PO Initially, 5-10 mg q3-4h. IV, IM, Subcutaneous Initially, 2.5-10 mg q3-4h.
  Narcotic addiction: IM, PO 15-40 mg once daily or as needed. Reduce dose at 1- to 2-day intervals based on patient response. Maintenance: Individualized.

- **Contraindications:** Diarrhea due to poisoning, hypersensitivity to narcotics

- **Side Effects**
  Frequent
  Sedation, decreased BP (including orthostatic hypotension), diaphoresis, facial flushing, constipation, dizziness, nausea, vomiting
  Occasional
  Confusion, urine retention, palpitations, abdominal cramps, visual changes, dry mouth, headache, decreased appetite, anxiety, insomnia
  Rare
  Allergic reaction (rash, pruritus)

- **Serious Reactions**
  - Overdose results in respiratory depression, skeletal muscle flaccidity, cold or clammy skin, cyanosis, and extreme somnolence progressing to seizures, stupor, and coma. The antidote is 0.4 mg naloxone.

- The patient who uses methadone long-term may develop a tolerance to the drug's analgesic effect and physical dependence.

Special Considerations
- When used for the treatment of narcotic addiction in detoxification or maintenance programs, can only be dispensed by approved hospital pharmacies, approved community pharmacies, and maintenance programs approved by the Food and Drug Administration and the designated state authority
- Do not administer agonist/antagonist analgesics (i.e., pentazocine, nalbuphine, butorphanol, dezocine, buprenorphine) to patient who has received a prolonged course of methadone (a pure agonist). In opioid-dependent patients, mixed agonist/antagonist analgesics may precipitate withdrawal symptoms

■ Patient/Family Education
- Change position slowly; orthostatic hypotension may occur
- Minimize nausea by administering with food and remain lying down following dose
- Avoid tasks that require mental alertness or motor skills until response to the drug has been established

■ Monitoring Parameters
- Vital signs
- Assess for adequate voiding
- Clinical improvement and onset of relief of pain

■ Geriatric side effects at a glance:
☑ CNS   ☑ Bowel Dysfunction   ☑ Bladder Dysfunction   ☑ Falls

■ U.S. Regulatory Considerations
☑ FDA Black Box
- Use in withdrawal limited to approved programs
- Use in treating opioid addiction limited to approved programs
- Tablets are not for IV use
☑ OBRA regulated in U.S. Long Term Care

methamphetamine hydrochloride

(meth-am-fet'-a-meen hye-droe-klor'-ide)

■ Brand Name(s): Desoxyn, Gradumet
Chemical Class: Amphetamine derivative

DEA Class: Schedule II

■ Clinical Pharmacology:
Mechanism of Action: A sympathomimetic amine related to amphetamine and ephedrine that enhances CNS stimulant activity. Peripheral actions include elevation of

systolic and diastolic blood pressure and weak bronchodilator and respiratory stimulant action. **Therapeutic Effect:** Increases motor activity, mental alertness; decreases drowsiness, fatigue.
Pharmacokinetics: Rapidly absorbed from the gastrointestinal (GI) tract. Metabolized in liver. Primarily excreted in the urine. Unknown if removed by hemodialysis. *Half-life*: 4-5 hr.

■ Available Forms:
- *Tablets*: 5 mg.
- *Tablets* (*Extended-Release*): 5 mg, 10 mg, 15 mg (Desoxyn, Gradumet).

■ Indications and Dosages:
Attention-deficit/hyperactivity disorder (ADHD): PO Initially, 2.5-5 mg 1-2 times/day. Increase by 5 mg/day at weekly intervals until therapeutic response achieved.
Appetite suppressant: PO 5 mg daily, given 30 min before meals. Extended-Release 10-15 mg in the morning.

■ Unlabeled Uses: Narcolepsy

■ Contraindications: Advanced arteriosclerosis, agitated states, glaucoma, history of drug abuse, history of hypersensitivity to sympathomimetic amines, hyperthyroidism, moderate to severe hypertension, symptomatic cardiovascular disease, within 14 days following discontinuation of an MAOI

■ Side Effects
Frequent
Irregular pulse, increased motor activity, talkativeness, nervousness, mild euphoria, insomnia
Occasional
Headache, chills, dry mouth, GI distress, worsening depression in patients who are clinically depressed, tachycardia, palpitations, chest pain

■ Serious Reactions
- Overdose may produce skin pallor, flushing, arrhythmias, and psychosis
- Abrupt withdrawal following prolonged administration of high dosage may produce lethargy which may last for weeks.

■ Patient/Family Education
- Take early in the day
- Do not discontinue abruptly
- Avoid hazardous activities until stabilized on medication
- Avoid OTC preparations unless approved by clinician

■ Geriatric side effects at a glance:
☑ CNS ☐ Bowel Dysfunction ☐ Bladder Dysfunction ☐ Falls

■ U.S. Regulatory Considerations
☑ FDA Black Box
- CNS stimulant use has a high abuse potential with the risk of dependence.
- Misuse may cause sudden death and serious cardiovascular adverse events.
☐ OBRA regulated in U.S. Long Term Care

methazolamide

(meth-a-zoe'-la-mide)

■ **Brand Name(s):** Glauctabs, Neptazane
  Chemical Class: Carbonic anhydrase inhibitor; sulfonamide derivative

■ **Clinical Pharmacology:**
  Mechanism of Action: A noncompetitive inhibitor of carbonic anhydrase that inhibits the enzyme at the luminal border of cells of the proximal tubule. Increases urine volume and changes to an alkaline pH with subsequent decreases in the excretion of titratable acid and ammonia. **Therapeutic Effect:** Produces a diuretic and antiglaucoma effect.
  Pharmacokinetics: PO Onset 2-4 hr, peak 6-8 hr, duration 10-18 hr. Well absorbed slowly from the GI tract. Protein binding: 55%. Distributed into the tissues (including CSF). Metabolized slowly from the GI tract. Partially excreted in urine. Not removed by hemodialysis. **Half-life:** 14 hr.

■ **Available Forms:**
  • *Tablets*: 25 mg, 50 mg.

■ **Indications and Dosages:**
  Glaucoma: PO 50-100 mg/day 2-3 times/day.

■ **Unlabeled Uses:** Motion sickness, essential tremor

■ **Contraindications:** Kidney or liver dysfunction, severe pulmonary obstruction, hypersensitivity to methazolamide or any component of the formulation

■ **Side Effects**
  Occasional
  Paresthesias, hearing dysfunction or tinnitus, fatigue, malaise, loss of appetite, taste alteration, nausea, vomiting, diarrhea, polyuria, drowsiness, confusion, hypokalemia
  Rare
  Metabolic acidosis, electrolyte imbalance, transient myopia, urticaria, melena, hematuria, glycosuria, hepatic insufficiency, flaccid paralysis, photosensitivity, convulsions, and rarely, crystalluria, renal calculi

■ **Serious Reactions**
  • Malaise and complaints of tiredness and myalgia are signs of excessive dosing and acidosis in the elderly.
  • Stevens-Johnson syndrome, toxic epidermal necrolysis, fulminant hepatic necrosis, agranulocytosis, aplastic anemia, and other blood dyscrasias have been reported and have caused fatalities.
  • Use with caution in patients with a history of sulfa allergy.

■ **Patient/Family Education**
  • Take with food if GI upset occurs
  • Methazolamide may cause drowsiness and impair judgment or coordination

- Methazolamide may cause altered taste

■ **Monitoring Parameters**
- Intraocular pressure, reduction in AMS symptoms, serum electrolytes, creatinine, CO_2

■ **Geriatric side effects at a glance:**
  ☐ CNS ☐ Bowel Dysfunction ☐ Bladder Dysfunction ☐ Falls

■ **U.S. Regulatory Considerations**
  ☐ FDA Black Box ☐ OBRA regulated in U.S. Long Term Care

methenamine

(meth-en'-a-meen)

■ **Brand Name(s):** Hiprex, Mandelamine, Urex
  Chemical Class: Formaldehyde precursors

■ **Clinical Pharmacology:**
  Mechanism of Action: A hippuric acid salt that hydrolyzes to formaldehyde and ammonia in acidic urine. **Therapeutic Effect:** Formaldehyde has antibacterial action. Bactericidal.
  Pharmacokinetics: Readily absorbed from the gastrointestinal (GI) tract. Partially metabolized by hydrolysis (unless protected by enteric coating) and partially by the liver. Primarily excreted in urine. **Half-life:** 3-6 hr.

■ **Available Forms:**
- *Oral Suspension, as mandelate*: 0.5 g/5 ml.
- *Tablets, as hippurate*: 1g (Urex, Hiprex).
- *Tablets, enteric coated, as mandelate*: 500 mg, 1g (Mandelamine).

■ **Indications and Dosages:**
  Urinary tract infection (UTI): PO 1g 2 times/day (as hippurate). 1g 4 times/day (as mandelate)

■ **Unlabeled Uses:** Hyperhidrosis

■ **Contraindications:** Moderate to severe renal impairment, hepatic impairment (hippurate salt), tartrazine sensitivity (Hiprex contains tartrazine), hypersensitivity to methenamine or any of its components

■ **Side Effects**
  Occasional
  Rash, nausea, dyspepsia, difficulty urinating
  Rare
  Bladder irritation, increased liver enzymes

771

Serious Reactions
- Crystalluria can occur when methenamine is given in large doses.

Patient/Family Education
- Keep urine acidic (pH <5.5) by eating food that acidifies urine (meats, eggs, fish, gelatin products, prunes, plums, cranberries); may need to add ascorbic acid
- Fluids must be increased to 3 L/day to avoid crystallization in kidneys
- Take at evenly spaced intervals around clock for best results
- Take with food to reduce GI upset

Monitoring Parameters
- Periodic liver function tests (hippurate); urine pH
- Renal function
- Skin for rash

Geriatric side effects at a glance:
❑ CNS ❑ Bowel Dysfunction ❑ Bladder Dysfunction ❑ Falls

U.S. Regulatory Considerations
❑ FDA Black Box ❑ OBRA regulated in U.S. Long Term Care

methimazole

(meth-im'-a-zole)

Brand Name(s): Tapazole
Chemical Class: Thioimidazole derivative

Clinical Pharmacology:
Mechanism of Action: A thioimidazole derivative that inhibits synthesis of thyroid hormone by interfering with the incorporation of iodine into tyrosyl residues. **Therapeutic Effect:** Effectively treats hyperthyroidism by decreasing thyroid hormone levels. **Pharmacokinetics:** Rapid absorption following PO administration. Protein binding: Not significant. Widely distributed throughout the body. Metabolized in liver. Excreted in urine. **Half-life:** 5–6 hr.

Available Forms:
- **Tablets:** 5 mg, 10 mg, 20 mg.

Indications and Dosages:
Hyperthyroidism: PO Initially, 15–60 mg/day in 3 divided doses. Maintenance: 5–15 mg/day.

Contraindications: None known.

- **Side Effects**
  Frequent (5%–4%)
  Fever, rash, pruritus
  Occasional (3%–1%)
  Dizziness, loss of taste, nausea, vomiting, stomach pain, peripheral neuropathy or numbness in fingers, toes, face
  Rare (less than 1%)
  Swollen lymph nodes or salivary glands

- **Serious Reactions**
  - Agranulocytosis as long as 4 mo after therapy, pancytopenia, and hepatitis have occurred.

Special Considerations

  - Methimazole is the thioamide of choice based on improved patient adherence and outcomes

- **Patient/Family Education**
  - Notify clinician of fever, sore throat, unusual bleeding or bruising, rash, yellowing of skin, vomiting
  - Do not exceed the prescribed dosage
  - Space doses evenly around the clock
  - Restrict consumption of iodine products and seafood

- **Monitoring Parameters**
  - CBC periodically during therapy (especially during initial 3 mo), TSH
  - Prothrombin time
  - Serum hepatic enzymes
  - Pulse
  - Weight
  - Skin for rash

- **Geriatric side effects at a glance:**
  ❑ CNS ❑ Bowel Dysfunction ❑ Bladder Dysfunction ❑ Falls

- **U.S. Regulatory Considerations**
  ❑ FDA Black Box ❑ OBRA regulated in U.S. Long Term Care

methocarbamol

(meth-oh-kar'-ba-mole)

- **Brand Name(s):** Carbacot, Robaxin

  Combinations
  Rx: with aspirin (Robaxisal)
  Chemical Class: Carbamate derivative

■ **Clinical Pharmacology:**
Mechanism of Action: A carbamate derivative of guaifenesin that causes skeletal muscle relaxation by general CNS depression. **Therapeutic Effect:** Relieves muscle spasticity.
Pharmacokinetics: Rapidly and almost completely absorbed from the gastrointestinal (GI) tract. Protein binding: 46%-50%. Metabolized in liver by dealkylation and hydroxylation. Primarily excreted in urine as metabolites. **Half-life:** 1-2 hr.

■ **Available Forms:**
- *Injection:* 100 mg/ml (Robaxin).
- *Tablets:* 325 mg, 500 mg (Carbacot, Robaxin), 750 mg (Carbacot).

■ **Indications and Dosages:**
Musculoskeletal spasm: IM, IV 1g q8h for no more than 3 consecutive days. May repeat course of therapy after a drug-free interval of 48 hr. PO Initially, 500 mg 4 times a day. May gradually increase dosage
Tetanus spasm: IV 1-3g q6h until oral dosing is possible. Injection should be used no more than 3 consecutive days.

■ **Contraindications:** Hypersensitivity to methocarbamol or any component of the formulation, renal impairment (injection formulation)

■ **Side Effects**
Frequent
Transient drowsiness, weakness, dizziness, light-headedness, nausea, vomiting.
Occasional
Headache, constipation, anorexia, hypotension, confusion, blurred vision, vertigo, facial flushing, rash
Rare
Paradoxical CNS excitement and restlessness, slurred speech, tremor, dry mouth, diarrhea, nocturia, impotence, bradycardia, hypotension, syncope

■ **Serious Reactions**
- Anaphylactoid reactions, leukopenia, and seizures (intravenous form) have been reported.
- Methocarbamol overdosage results in cardiac arrhythmias, nausea, vomiting, drowsiness, and coma.

■ **Patient/Family Education**
- Drowsiness usually diminishes with continued therapy
- Avoid tasks that require mental alertness or motor skills until response to the drug is established
- Do not abruptly discontinue methocarbamol after long-term therapy

■ **Monitoring Parameters**
- Therapeutic response, such as decreased intensity of skeletal muscle pain

■ **Geriatric side effects at a glance:**
☑ CNS ☑ Bowel Dysfunction ☑ Bladder Dysfunction ☑ Falls
Other: Decreased mental alertness

■ **Use with caution in older patients with:** Potential for falls

774

■ **U.S. Regulatory Considerations**
  ❑ FDA Black Box   ☑ OBRA regulated in U.S. Long Term Care

■ **Other Uses in Geriatric Patient:** None

■ **Side Effects:**
  Of particular importance in the geriatric patient: None

■ **Geriatric Considerations - Summary:** Methocarbamol is a skeletal muscle relaxant that at higher doses can cause CNS depression. It appears to have modest clinical benefits and is most often used for acute muscle discomfort as compared to chronic muscle pain. Transient CNS depressant effects place the older adult at risk for falls and related accidents when taking this drug.

methotrexate sodium

(meth-oh-trex'-ate soe'-dee-um)

■ **Brand Name(s):** Rheumatrex, Trexall
  Chemical Class: Dihydrofolate reductase inhibitor

■ **Clinical Pharmacology:**
  Mechanism of Action: An antimetabolite that competes with enzymes necessary to reduce folic acid to tetrahydrofolic acid, a component essential to DNA, RNA, and protein synthesis. This action inhibits DNA, RNA, and protein synthesis. **Therapeutic Effect:** Causes death of cancer cells.
  Pharmacokinetics: Variably absorbed from the GI tract. Completely absorbed after IM administration. Protein binding: 50%-60%. Widely distributed. Metabolized intracellularly in the liver. Primarily excreted in urine. Removed by hemodialysis but not by peritoneal dialysis. **Half-life:** 8-12 hr (large doses, 8-15 hr).

■ **Available Forms:**
  • *Tablets:* 2.5 mg (Rheumatrex), 5 mg (Trexall), 7.5 mg (Trexall), 10 mg (Trexall), 15 mg (Trexall).
  • *Injection Solution:* 25 mg/ml.
  • *Injection Powder for Reconstitution:* 20 mg, 50 mg, 1 g.

■ **Indications and Dosages:**
  Rheumatoid arthritis: PO 7.5 mg once weekly or 2.5 mg q12h for 3 doses once weekly. Maximum: 20 mg/wk.
  Psoriasis: PO 10-25 mg once weekly or 2.5-5 mg q12h for 3 doses once weekly. IM 10-25 mg once weekly.
  Dosage in renal impairment: *Creatinine clearance 61-80 ml/min.* Reduce dose by 25%. *Creatinine clearance 51-60 ml/min.* Reduce dose by 33%. *Creatinine clearance 10-50 ml/min.* Reduce dose by 50%-70%.

■ **Unlabeled Uses:** Treatment of acute myelocytic leukemia; bladder, cervical, ovarian, prostatic, renal, and testicular carcinomas; psoriatic arthritis; systemic dermatomyositis

■ **Contraindications:** Hepatic disease or renal impairment, preexisting myelosuppression, psoriasis or rheumatoid arthritis with alcoholism

■ **Side Effects**
Frequent (10%-3%)
Nausea, vomiting, stomatitis; burning and erythema at psoriatic site (in patients with psoriasis)
Occasional (3%-1%)
Diarrhea, rash, dermatitis, pruritus, alopecia, dizziness, anorexia, malaise, headache, drowsiness, blurred vision

■ **Serious Reactions**
- GI toxicity may produce gingivitis, glossitis, pharyngitis, stomatitis, enteritis, and hematemesis.
- Hepatotoxicity is more likely to occur with frequent small doses than with large intermittent doses.
- Pulmonary toxicity may be characterized by interstitial pneumonitis.
- Hematologic toxicity, which may develop rapidly from marked myelosuppression, may be manifested as leukopenia, thrombocytopenia, anemia, and hemorrhage.
- Dermatologic toxicity may produce a rash, pruritus, urticaria, pigmentation, photosensitivity, petechiae, ecchymosis, and pustules.
- Severe nephrotoxicity may produce azotemia, hematuria, and renal failure.

■ **Patient/Family Education**
- Notify clinician of black, tarry stools, chills, fever, sore throat, bleeding, bruising, cough, shortness of breath, dark or bloody urine
- Hair may be lost during treatment; alopecia is reversible but the new hair may have a different color or texture
- Drink 10-12 glasses of fluid/day
- Avoid alcohol, salicylates, and overexposure to sun or ultraviolet light during methotrexate therapy
- Avoid receiving vaccinations and contact with crowds and those with known infections
- Both male and female patients should use contraceptive methods during therapy and for a certain period afterward
- Maintain fastidious oral hygiene

■ **Monitoring Parameters**
- Tumor response: Objective remissions are usually associated with a 50% decrease in the size of solid tumor as measured by physical measurement or test parameter (e.g., chest X-ray). After intrathecal administration, clearing of malignant cells in the cerebrospinal fluid indicates a positive response
- Rheumatoid arthritis: Tender, swollen joints, visual analogue scale for pain; acute phase reactants (ESR, C-reactive protein), duration of early morning stiffness, preservation of function
- CBC and platelets at 7, 10, and 14 days postdrug administration/injection; due to the possibility of early-onset pancytopenia, a lower initial dose for rheumatoid arthritis treatment along with intensified monitoring during early therapy is recommended—CBCs at 1, 2, and 4 wk of treatment; if stable, dose may be increased and subsequent CBCs should be performed at monthly intervals
- BUN, serum uric acid, urine ClCr, electrolytes before and during therapy

- Liver function tests before and during therapy

■ **Geriatric side effects at a glance:**
  ❑ CNS ❑ Bowel Dysfunction ❑ Bladder Dysfunction ❑ Falls

■ **U.S. Regulatory Considerations**
  ☑ FDA Black Box
  - Bone marrow suppression
  - Hepatotoxicity
  - Should be administered by experienced provider
  ❑ OBRA regulated in U.S. Long Term Care

methoxsalen

(meth-ox'-a-len)

■ **Brand Name(s):** 8-MOP, Oxsoralen, Oxsoralen-Ultra, Uvadex
  Chemical Class: Psoralen derivative

■ **Clinical Pharmacology:**
  Mechanism of Action: A member of the family of psoralens that induces an augmented sunburn reaction followed by hyperpigmentation in the presence of long-wave ultraviolet radiation. Bonds covalently to pyrimidine bases in DNA, inhibits the synthesis of DNA, and suppresses cell division. The augmented sunburn reaction involves excitation of the methoxsalen molecule by radiation in the long-wave ultraviolet light (UVA), resulting in transference of energy to the methoxsalen molecule producing an excited state, or "triplet electronic state." The excited molecule then reacts with cutaneous DNA. **Therapeutic Effect:** Results in symptomatic control of severe, recalcitrant disabling psoriasis, repigmentation of idiopathic vitiligo, palliative treatment of skin manifestations of cutaneous T-cell lymphoma (CTCL), and repigmentation of idiopathic vitiligo.
  Pharmacokinetics: Absorption varies. Food increases peak serum levels. Reversibly bound to albumin. Metabolized in the liver. Excreted in the urine. **Half-life:** 2 hr.

■ **Available Forms:**
  - *Capsule*: 10 mg (8-MOP).
  - *Gelcap*: 10 mg (Oxsoralen-Ultra).
  - *Lotion*: 1% (Oxsoralen).
  - *Solution*: 20 mcg/ml (Uvadex).

■ **Indications and Dosages:**
  Psoriasis: PO 10-70 mg 1.5-2 hr before exposure to UVA light, repeated 2-3 times/week. Give at least 48 hr apart. Dosage is based upon patient's body weight and skin type: **Less than 30 kg:** 10 mg. **30-50 kg:** 20 mg. **51-65 kg:** 30 mg. **66-80 kg:** 40 mg. **81-90 kg:** 50 mg. **91-115 kg:** 60 mg. **More than 115 kg:** 70 mg.
  Vitiligo: PO 20 mg 2-4 hr before exposure to UVA light. Give at least 48 hr apart. Topical Apply 1-2 hr before exposure to UVA light, no more than once weekly.

CTCL: Extracorporeal Inject 200 mcg into the photoactivation bag during collection cycle using the UVAR photopheresis system, 2 consecutive days every 4 wk for a minimum of 7 treatment cycles.

■ **Unlabeled Uses:** Dermographism, eczema, hypereosinophilic syndrome, hypopigmented sarcoidosis, ichthyosis linearis circumflexa, lymphomatoid papulosis, mycosis fungoides, palmoplantar pustulosis, pruritus, scleromyxedema, systemic sclerosis

■ **Contraindications:** Cataract, invasive squamous cell cancer, aphakia, melanoma, diseases associated with photosensitivity, hypersensitivity to methoxsalen (psoralens) or any component of the formulation

■ **Side Effects**
Occasional
Nausea, pruritus, edema, hypotension, nervousness, vertigo, depression, dizziness, headache, malaise, painful blistering, burning, rash, urticaria, loss of muscle coordination, leg cramps

■ **Serious Reactions**
• Hypersensitivity reaction, such as nausea and severe burns, may occur.

Special Considerations
• Hard and soft caps are not equivalent

■ **Patient/Family Education**
• Do not sunbathe during 24 hr prior to methoxsalen ingestion and UVA exposure
• Wear UVA-absorbing sunglasses for 24 hr following treatment to prevent cataract
• Avoid sun exposure for at least 8 hr after methoxsalen ingestion
• Avoid concurrent photosensitizing drugs
• Avoid furocoumarin-containing foods (e.g., limes, figs, parsley, parsnips, mustard, carrots, celery)
• Repigmentation of vitiligo may require 6-9 mo

■ **Monitoring Parameters**
• Weight
• UVA exposure

■ **Geriatric side effects at a glance:**
❏ CNS ❏ Bowel Dysfunction ❏ Bladder Dysfunction ❏ Falls

■ **U.S. Regulatory Considerations**
☑ FDA Black Box
• Use should be reserved to experienced physicians
• Ocular damage, skin cancer (including melanoma)
❏ OBRA regulated in U.S. Long Term Care

methscopolamine bromide

(meth-scoe-pol-a-meen broe'-mide)

■ **Brand Name(s):** Pamine
  Chemical Class: Quaternary ammonium derivative

■ **Clinical Pharmacology:**
  Mechanism of Action: A peripheral anticholinergic agent that has limited ability to cross the blood-brain barrier and provides a peripheral blockade of muscarinic receptors. **Therapeutic Effect:** Reduces the volume and the total acid content of gastric secretions, inhibits salivation, and reduces gastrointestinal motility.
  Pharmacokinetics: Poorly and unreliably absorbed from the gastrointestinal (GI) tract. Limited ability to cross the blood-brain barrier. Primarily excreted in the urine and the bile. The effects of methscopolamine appear to occur within 1 hr and last for 4-6 hr. Primarily excreted in urine. **Half-life:** Unknown.

■ **Available Forms:**
  • *Tab-Oral*: 2.5 mg, 5 mg.

■ **Indications and Dosages:**
  Peptic ulcer: Initially, 2.5 mg 30 min before meals and 2.5-5 mg at bedtime. May increase dose to 5 mg every 12 hr.

■ **Unlabeled Uses:** Gastrointestinal spasm

■ **Contraindications:** Reflux esophagitis; glaucoma, obstructed uropathy, obstructed disease of the GI tract (pyloroduodenal stenosis), paralytic ileus, intestinal atony of elderly or debilitated individuals, unstable cardiovascular status in acute hemorrhage, severe ulcerative colitis, toxic megacolon, complicated ulcerative colitis, myasthenia gravis, hypersensitivity to methscopolamine, any component of the formulation, or related drugs.

■ **Side Effects**
  Occasional
  Dry mouth, throat, and nose, urinary hesitancy and/or retention, constipation, tachycardia, palpitations, headache, insomnia, dry skin, urticaria, weakness.

■ **Serious Reactions**
  • Overdosage may vary from CNS depression, including sedation, apnea, hypotension, cardiovascular collapse, or death to severe paradoxical reaction (such as hallucinations, tremor, and seizures).

Special Considerations
  • Has not been shown to be effective in contributing to the healing of peptic ulcer, decreasing the rate of recurrence, or preventing complications

- ■ **Patient/Family Education**
  - Avoid performing tasks that require mental alertness or motor skills until response to the drug is established
  - Notify the physician if blood in stool occurs

- ■ **Monitoring Parameters**
  - Upper gastrointestinal contrast radiology or endoscopy to ensure healing
  - Stool tests for occult blood and blood hemoglobin or hematocrit values to rule out bleeding from ulcer

- ■ **Geriatric side effects at a glance:**
  ☑ CNS   ☑ Bowel Dysfunction   ☑ Bladder Dysfunction   ☐ Falls
  Other: Dry mouth, blurred vision, constipation

- ■ **Use with caution in older patients with:** Narrow-angle glaucoma, overflow incontinence,

- ■ **U.S. Regulatory Considerations**
  ☐ FDA Black Box   ☐ OBRA regulated in U.S. Long Term Care

- ■ **Other Uses in Geriatric Patient:** To decrease salivation, irritable bowel syndrome

- ■ **Side Effects:**
  Of particular importance in the geriatric patient: Possibly less likely to antagonize cholinergic drug therapy in the treatment of Alzheimer's disease.

- ■ **Geriatric Considerations - Summary:** Methoscopolamine is a peripheral anticholinergic drug that does not cross the blood-brain barrier so should cause less risk of psychosis and other central effects. Other anticholinergic side effects such as urinary retention and decreased bowel motility do occur and can limit the usefulness of this drug.

- ■ **References:**
  1. Vangala V, Tueth M. Chronic anticholinergic toxicity: Identification and management in older patients. Geriatrics 2003;58:36-37.
  2. Tune LE. Anticholinergic effects of medication in elderly patients. J Clin Psychiatry 2001;62(suppl 21):11-14.

methsuximide

(meth-sux'-i-mide)

- ■ **Brand Name(s):** Celontin
  Chemical Class: Succinimide derivative

- ■ **Clinical Pharmacology:**
  Mechanism of Action: An anticonvulsant agent that increases the seizure threshold, suppresses paroxysmal spike-and-wave pattern in absence seizures and depresses nerve transmission in the motor cortex. **Therapeutic Effect:** Controls absence (petit mal) seizures.

Pharmacokinetics: Rapidly metabolized in liver to active metabolite, N-desmethyl-methsuximide. Primarily excreted in urine. Unknown if removed by hemodialysis. **Half-life:** 1.4 hr.

■ **Available Forms:**
  • *Capsules:* 150 mg, 300 mg.

■ **Indications and Dosages:**
  Absence seizures: PO Initially, 300 mg/day for the first week. Increase dosage by 300 mg/day at weekly intervals until response is attained. Maintenance: 1,200 mg/day at 2-4 times/day.

■ **Unlabeled Uses:** Partial complex (psychomotor) seizures

■ **Contraindications:** Hypersensitivity to succinimides or any component of the formulation

■ **Side Effects**
  Frequent
  Drowsiness, dizziness, nausea, vomiting
  Occasional
  Visual abnormalities, such as spots before eyes, difficulty focusing, blurred vision, dry mouth or pharynx, tongue irritation, nervousness, insomnia, headache, constipation or diarrhea, rash, weight loss, proteinuria, edema

■ **Serious Reactions**
  • Toxic reactions appear as blood dyscrasias, including aplastic anemia, agranulocytosis, thrombocytopenia, leukopenia, leukocytosis, eosinophilia, cardiovascular disturbances, such as congestive heart failure (CHF), hypotension or hypertension, thrombophlebitis, arrhythmias, and dermatologic effects, such as rash, urticaria, pruritus, photosensitivity.
  • Abrupt withdrawal may precipitate status epilepticus.

■ **Patient/Family Education**
  • Take with food or milk
  • Do not discontinue abruptly
  • Drowsiness usually subsides with continued therapy
  • Avoid tasks that require mental alertness and motor skills until response to the drug is established
  • Notify the physician of visual disturbances, rash, or unusual bleeding

■ **Monitoring Parameters**
  • CBC with differential; liver enzymes
  • Serum N-desmethylmethsuximide concentrations at trough for efficacy (range 10-40 mcg/ml) and 3 hr postdose for toxicity (>40 mcg/ml)
  • Clinical improvement

■ **Geriatric side effects at a glance:**
  ❏ CNS ❏ Bowel Dysfunction ❏ Bladder Dysfunction ❏ Falls

■ **U.S. Regulatory Considerations**
  ❏ FDA Black Box ❏ OBRA regulated in U.S. Long Term Care

methyclothiazide

(meth-i-kloe-thye'-ah-zide)

■ **Brand Name(s):** Aquatensen, Enduron

Combinations
Rx: with reserpine (Diutensen-R)
Chemical Class: Sulfonamide derivative

■ **Clinical Pharmacology:**
Mechanism of Action: A sulfonamide derivative that acts as a thiazide diuretic and antihypertensive. As a diuretic, it blocks the reabsorption of water, sodium, and potassium at cortical diluting segment of distal tubule. As an antihypertensive, it reduces plasma and extracellular fluid volume and decreases peripheral vascular resistance (PVR) by direct effect on blood vessels. **Therapeutic Effect:** Promotes diuresis, reduces blood pressure (BP).
Pharmacokinetics: Variably absorbed from the gastrointestinal (GI) tract. Primarily excreted unchanged in urine. Not removed by hemodialysis. **Half-life:** 24 hr.

■ **Available Forms:**
  • *Tablets*: 2.5 mg, 5 mg (Aquatensen, Enduron).

■ **Indications and Dosages:**
Edema: PO 2.5-10 mg/day.
Hypertension: PO 2.5-5 mg/day.

■ **Unlabeled Uses:** Treatment of diabetes insipidus, prevention of calcium-containing renal stones

■ **Contraindications:** Anuria, history of hypersensitivity to sulfonamides or thiazide diuretics, renal decompensation

■ **Side Effects**
Expected
Increase in urinary frequency and volume
Frequent
Potassium depletion
Occasional
Postural hypotension, headache, GI disturbances, photosensitivity reaction, anorexia

■ **Serious Reactions**
  • Vigorous diuresis may lead to profound water loss and electrolyte depletion leading to hypokalemia, hyponatremia, and dehydration.
  • Acute hypotensive episodes may occur.
  • Hyperglycemia may be noted during prolonged therapy.
  • GI upset, pancreatitis, dizziness, paresthesias, headache, blood dyscrasias, pulmonary edema, allergic pneumonitis, and dermatologic reactions occur rarely.

- Overdosage can lead to lethargy and coma without changes in electrolytes or hydration.
- Use with caution in patients with sulfa allergy.

Special Considerations

- Doses above 2.5 mg provide no further blood pressure reduction, but are more likely to induce metabolic disturbance (hypokalemia, hyperuricemia, etc.)
- May protect against osteoporotic hip fractures
- Loop diuretics or metolazone more effective if CrCl <40-50 ml/min
- Although allergic cross-reactivity with sulfonamide antibiotics and sulfonamide nonantibiotics has not been demonstrated, use with caution in patients with a history of severe sulfa allergies.

■ Patient/Family Education

- Will increase urination temporarily (approx. 3 weeks); take early in the day to prevent sleep disturbance
- May cause sensitivity to sunlight; avoid prolonged exposure to the sun and other ultraviolet light
- May cause gout attacks; notify clinician if sudden joint pain occurs
- Rise slowly from lying to sitting position and permit legs to dangle momentarily before standing to reduce the drug's hypotensive effect

■ Monitoring Parameters

- Weight, urine output, serum electrolytes, BUN, creatinine, CBC, uric acid, glucose, lipids

■ Geriatric side effects at a glance:

❑ CNS   ❑ Bowel Dysfunction   ❑ Bladder Dysfunction   ❑ Falls

■ U.S. Regulatory Considerations

❑ FDA Black Box   ❑ OBRA regulated in U.S. Long Term Care

methylcellulose

(meth-ill-sell'-you-lose)

OTC: Citrucel, Cologel
Chemical Class: Hydrophilic semisynthetic cellulose derivative

■ Clinical Pharmacology:

Mechanism of Action: A bulk-forming laxative that dissolves and expands in water.
Therapeutic Effect: Provides increased bulk and moisture content in stool, increasing peristalsis and bowel motility.
Pharmacokinetics:

Route	Onset	Peak	Duration
PO	12–24 hr	N/A	N/A

Acts in small and large intestines. Full effect may not be evident for 2–3 days.

■ **Available Forms:**
  • *Powder (Citrucel, Cologel).*

■ **Indications and Dosages:**
  Constipation: PO 1 tbsp (15 ml) in 8 oz water 1–3 times a day.

■ **Contraindications:** Abdominal pain, dysphagia, nausea, partial bowel obstruction, symptoms of appendicitis, vomiting

■ **Side Effects**
  Rare
  Some degree of abdominal discomfort, nausea, mild cramps, griping, faintness

■ **Serious Reactions**
  • Esophageal or bowel obstruction may occur if administered with less than 250 ml or 1 full glass of liquid.

■ **Patient/Family Education**
  • Notify clinician of unrelieved constipation, rectal bleeding
  • Ensure adequate fluids, proper dietary fiber intake, and regular exercise
  • Take each dose with a full glass of water; taking methylcellulose with an inadequate amount of fluid may cause choking or swelling in the throat

■ **Monitoring Parameters**
  • Pattern of daily bowel activity and stool consistency, time of evacuation
  • Electrolytes

■ **Geriatric side effects at a glance:**
  ☐ CNS ☑ Bowel Dysfunction ☐ Bladder Dysfunction ☐ Falls

■ **U.S. Regulatory Considerations**
  ☐ FDA Black Box ☐ OBRA regulated in U.S. Long Term Care

methyldopa

(meth-ill-doe'-pa)

■ **Brand Name(s):** Aldomet, Methyldopate

  Combinations
  Rx: with HCTZ (Aldoril); with chlorothiazide (Aldoclor)
  Chemical Class: Catecholamine, synthetic

■ **Clinical Pharmacology:**
  Mechanism of Action: An antihypertensive agent that stimulates central inhibitory alpha-adrenergic receptors, lowers arterial pressure, and reduces plasma renin activity.
  Therapeutic Effect: Reduces BP.

Pharmacokinetics: Absorption from GI tract is variable. Protein binding: Negligible. Metabolized in liver. Excreted in urine. Removed by hemodialysis. **Half-life:** 1.7 hr.

■ **Available Forms:**
- *Tablets* (Aldomet): 125 mg, 250 mg, 500 mg.
- *Oral Suspension* (Methyldopate): 250 mg/5 ml.
- *Injection:* 50 mg/ml.

■ **Indications and Dosages:**
Hypertension: IV 250–500 mg q6h. Maximum: 1g q6h. PO Initially, 250 mg 2–3 times a day. May increase at 2-day intervals up to 3 g/day. Range: 250-1,000 mg/day in 2 divided doses.

■ **Contraindications:** Hepatic disease, hepatic disorders previously associated with methyldopa therapy, MAOIs, pheochromocytoma

■ **Side Effects**
Frequent
Peripheral edema, somnolence, headache, dry mouth
Occasional
Mental changes (such as anxiety, depression), decreased sexual function or libido, diarrhea, swelling of breasts, nausea, vomiting, light-headedness, paresthesia, rhinitis

■ **Serious Reactions**
- Hepatotoxicity (abnormal liver function test results, jaundice, hepatitis), hemolytic anemia, unexplained fever, and flu-like symptoms may occur. If these conditions appear, discontinue the medication and contact the physician.

Special Considerations
- Perform both direct and indirect Coombs test if blood transfusion needed. If indirect Coombs test positive, interference may occur with crossmatch. Positive direct Coombs test will not interfere

■ **Patient/Family Education**
- Urine exposed to air after voiding may darken
- Do not discontinue abruptly
- Initial sedation usually improves
- Avoid tasks requiring mental alertness and motor skills until response to the drug has been established

■ **Monitoring Parameters**
- CBC, liver function tests periodically during therapy
- Direct Coombs test before therapy and after 6-12 mo. If positive, rule out hemolytic anemia
- Blood pressure, pulse
- Weight

■ **Geriatric side effects at a glance:**
☑ CNS   ☐ Bowel Dysfunction   ☐ Bladder Dysfunction   ☐ Falls

■ **U.S. Regulatory Considerations**
☑ FDA Black Box

Do not use fixed combinations of methyldopa and thiazide diuretics for initial management of hypertension.
❑ OBRA regulated in U.S. Long Term Care

methylene blue

(meth'-i-leen bloo)

■ **Brand Name(s):** Urolene Blue
  Chemical Class: Thiazine dye

■ **Clinical Pharmacology:**
  Mechanism of Action: A weak germicide which hastens the conversion of methemoglobin to hemoglobin in low concentrations. At high concentrations, it has the opposite effect by converting ferrous ion of reduced hemoglobin to ferric iron to form methemoglobin. In cyanide toxicity, it combines with cyanide to form cyanmethemoglobin preventing interference of cyanide with the cytochrome system. **Therapeutic Effect:** Antidote for drug-induced methemoglobinemia.
  Pharmacokinetics: Erratic absorption. Protein binding: unknown. Metabolized in tissues to leucomethylene blue. Excreted unchanged in urine and feces. Unknown if removed by hemodialysis. **Half-life:** Unknown.

■ **Available Forms:**
  • *Injection*: 10 mg/ml.
  • *Tablets*: 65 mg (Urolene Blue).

■ **Indications and Dosages:**
  Methemoglobinemia, drug-induced: IV 1-2 mg/kg (0.1-0.2 ml/kg of 1% solution) injected very slowly over several minutes.
  Genitourniary antiseptic: PO 65-130 mg 3 times/day. Maximum: 390 mg/day.
  Dosage in renal impairment: Specific guidelines are unavailable although dosage adjustment should be considered.

■ **Contraindications:** Hypersensitivity to methylene blue or any component of its formulation, glucose-6-phosphate dehydrogenase (G6PD) deficiency, intraspinal injection, severe renal insufficiency, treatment of methemoglobinemia in cyanide poisoning

■ **Side Effects**
  Occasional
  Dizziness, headache, mental confusion, abdominal pain, diarrhea, nausea, vomiting, hypertension, hypotension, sweating
  Rare
  Arrhythmias, hemolytic anemia, methemoglobinemia

■ **Serious Reactions**
  • Hemolytic anemia and methemoglobinemia occur rarely.

Patient/Family Education
- Photosensitivity may occur
- Methylene blue may discolor urine and feces blue-green
- Take after meals with a full glass of water
- Remove any stains from methylene blue using hypochlorite solution

Monitoring Parameters
- Hct
- Blood pressure
- CBC

Geriatric side effects at a glance:
❑ CNS ❑ Bowel Dysfunction ❑ Bladder Dysfunction ❑ Falls

U.S. Regulatory Considerations
❑ FDA Black Box ❑ OBRA regulated in U.S. Long Term Care

methylphenidate hydrochloride

(meth-ill-fen'-i-date hye-dro-klor'-ide)

■ **Brand Name(s):** Concerta, Metadate CD, Metadate ER, Methylin, Methylin ER, Ritalin, Ritalin LA, Ritalin SR
Chemical Class: Piperidine derivative of amphetamine

DEA Class: Schedule II

■ Clinical Pharmacology:
Mechanism of Action: A CNS stimulant that blocks the reuptake of norepinephrine and dopamine into presynaptic neurons. **Therapeutic Effect:** Decreases motor restlessness and fatigue; increases motor activity, attention span, and mental alertness; produces mild euphoria.
Pharmacokinetics:

Onset	Peak	Duration
Immediate-release	2 hr	3-5 hr
Sustained-release	4-7 hr	3-8 hr
Extended-release	N/A	8-12 hr

Slowly and incompletely absorbed from the GI tract. Protein binding: 15%. Metabolized in the liver. Eliminated in urine and in feces by biliary system. Unknown if removed by hemodialysis. **Half-life:** 2-4 hr.

■ Available Forms:
- *Capsules (Extended-Release [Metadate CD]):* 10 mg, 20 mg, 30 mg.
- *Capsules (Extended-Release [Ritalin LA]):* 10 mg, 20 mg, 30 mg, 40 mg.

- *Tablets (Ritalin)*: 5 mg, 10 mg, 20 mg.
- *Tablets (Extended-Release [Metadate ER, Methylin ER])*: 10 mg, 20 mg.
- *Tablets (Extended-Release [Concerta])*: 18 mg, 27 mg, 36 mg, 54 mg, 72 mg.
- *Tablets (Sustained-Release [Ritalin SR])*: 20 mg.
- *Tablets (Chewable [Methylin])*: 2.5 mg, 5 mg, 10 mg.
- *Oral Solution (Methylin)*: 5 mg/5 ml, 10 mg/5 ml.

■ Indications and Dosages:
Narcolepsy: PO 10 mg 2-3 times a day. Range: 10-60 mg/day.

■ Unlabeled Uses: Treatment of disease-related fatigue, secondary mental depression

■ Contraindications: Use within 14 days of MAOIs

■ Side Effects
Frequent
Anxiety, insomnia, anorexia
Occasional
Dizziness, drowsiness, headache, nausea, abdominal pain, fever, rash, arthralgia, vomiting
Rare
Blurred vision, Tourette's syndrome (marked by uncontrolled vocal outbursts, repetitive body movements, and tics), palpitations

■ Serious Reactions
- Overdose may produce tachycardia, palpitations, arrhythmias, chest pain, psychotic episode, seizures, and coma.
- Hypersensitivity reactions and blood dyscrasias occur rarely.

Special Considerations
- Overdosage may cause vomiting, agitation, tremor, muscle twitching, seizures, confusion, tachycardia, hypertension, arrhythmias

■ Patient/Family Education
- Take last daily dose prior to 6 PM to avoid insomnia
- Do not discontinue abruptly
- Avoid OTC preparations unless approved by clinician
- Do not crush or chew sustained-release formulation
- Avoid performing tasks that require mental alertness or motor skills until response to the drug is established
- Dry mouth may be relieved by sugarless gum and sips of tepid water
- Report nervousness, palpitations, fever, vomiting, or skin rash

■ Monitoring Parameters
- Periodic CBC with differential and platelet count

■ Geriatric side effects at a glance:
☑ CNS ☐ Bowel Dysfunction ☐ Bladder Dysfunction ☐ Falls

■ U.S. Regulatory Considerations
☑ FDA Black Box
- CNS stimulant use has a high abuse potential with the risk of dependence.
- Misuse may cause sudden death and serious cardiovascular adverse events.
☑ OBRA regulated in U.S. Long Term Care

methylprednisolone/ methylprednisolone acetate/methylprednisolone sodium succinate

(meth-ill-pred-niss'-oh-lone)

- **Brand Name(s):** Adlone-40, Adlone-80, A-Methapred, Depmedalone, Dep Medalone 80, Depoject-80, Depo-Medrol, Depopred, Med-Jec-40, Medralone 80, Medrol, Medrol Dosepak, Methacort 40, Methacort 80, Methylcotol, Methylcotolone, Methylpred DP, Solu-Medrol
  Chemical Class: Glucocorticoid, synthetic

- **Clinical Pharmacology:**
  Mechanism of Action: An adrenocortical steroid that suppresses migration of poly-morphonuclear leukocytes and reverses increased capillary permeability. **Therapeutic Effect:** Decreases inflammation.
  Pharmacokinetics:

Route	Onset	Peak	Duration
PO	N/A	1–2 hr	30–36 hr
IM	N/A	4–8 days	1–4 wk

  Well absorbed from the GI tract after IM administration. Widely distributed. Metabolized in the liver. Excreted in urine. Removed by hemodialysis. **Half-life:** 3.5 hr.

- **Available Forms:**
  - *Tablets (Medrol, Medrol Dosepak, Methylpred DP):* 2 mg, 4 mg, 8 mg, 16 mg, 32 mg.
  - *Injection Powder for Reconstitution (A-Methapred, Solu-Medrol):* 40 mg, 125 mg, 500 mg, 1 g.
  - *Injection Suspension:* 20 mg/ml (Depo-Medrol), 40 mg/ml (Adlone-40, Depo-Medrol, Depopred, Depmedalone, Med-Jec-40, Methylcotol), 80 mg/ml (Adlone-80, Depmedalone, Dep Medalone 80, Depoject-80, Depopred, Depo-Medrol, Medralone 80, Methacort 80, Methylcotolone).

- **Indications and Dosages:**
  Anti-inflammatory, immunosuppressive: IV 10-40 mg. May repeat as needed. PO 2-60 mg/day in 1-4 divided doses.
  Status asthmaticus: IV Initially, 2 mg/kg/dose, then 0.5-1 mg/kg/dose q6h for up to 5 days.
  Spinal cord injury: IV Bolus 30 mg/kg over 15 min. Maintenance dose: 5.4 mg/kg/hr over 23 hr, to be given within 45 min of bolus dose. IM (methylprednisolone acetate) 10–80 mg/day. Intra-articular, Intralesional 4–40 mg, up to 80 mg q1–5wk.

- **Contraindications:** Administration of live virus vaccines, systemic fungal infection

■ Side Effects
Frequent
Insomnia, heartburn, anxiety, abdominal distention, diaphoresis, acne, mood swings, increased appetite, facial flushing, GI distress, delayed wound healing, increased susceptibility to infection, diarrhea or constipation
Occasional
Headache, edema, tachycardia, change in skin color, frequent urination, depression
Rare
Psychosis, increased blood coagulability, hallucinations

■ Serious Reactions
- Long-term therapy may cause hypocalcemia, hypokalemia, muscle wasting (especially in arms and legs), osteoporosis, spontaneous fractures, amenorrhea, cataracts, glaucoma, peptic ulcer disease, and CHF.
- Abruptly withdrawing the drug after long-term therapy may cause anorexia, nausea, fever, headache, sudden severe myalgia, rebound inflammation, fatigue, weakness, lethargy, dizziness, and orthostatic hypotension.

■ Patient/Family Education
- Take single daily doses in AM
- May mask infections
- Increased dose of rapidly acting corticosteroids may be necessary in patients subjected to unusual stresses
- Signs of adrenal insufficiency include fatigue, anorexia, nausea, vomiting, diarrhea, weight loss, weakness, dizziness, and low blood sugar
- Avoid abrupt withdrawal of therapy following high dose or long-term therapy. Relative insufficiency may exist for up to 1 yr after discontinuation
- Patients on chronic steroid therapy should wear Medic Alert bracelet
- Do not give live virus vaccines to patients on prolonged therapy
- Take oral methylprednisolone with food or milk

■ Monitoring Parameters
- Serum K and glucose
- Intake and output
- Weight
- Pattern of daily bowel activity
- Vital signs
- Signs and symptoms of hypocalcemia (such as cramps and muscle twitching), or hypokalemia (such as ECG changes, irritability, nausea and vomiting, numbness or tingling of lower extremities, and weakness)

■ Geriatric side effects at a glance:
☑ CNS ☐ Bowel Dysfunction ☐ Bladder Dysfunction ☐ Falls

■ U.S. Regulatory Considerations
☐ FDA Black Box ☑ OBRA regulated in U.S. Long Term Care

methyltestosterone

(meth-il-tes-tos'-te-rone)

- **Brand Name(s):** Android, Android-10, Android-25, Oreton Methyl, Testred, Virilon
  Chemical Class: Androgen; testosterone derivative

  DEA Class: Schedule III

- **Clinical Pharmacology:**
  Mechanism of Action: A synthetic testosterone derivative with androgen activity that promotes growth and development of male sex organs and maintains secondary sex characteristics in androgen-deficient males. **Therapeutic Effect:** Treats hypogonadism in males.
  Pharmacokinetics: Well absorbed from the gastrointestinal (GI) tract. Protein binding: 98%. Metabolized in liver. Primarily excreted in urine. Unknown if removed by hemodialysis. **Half-life:** 10-100 min.

- **Available Forms:**
  - *Capsules:* 10 mg (Android, Testred, Virilon).
  - *Tablets:* 10 mg (Android-10, Oreton Methyl), 25 mg (Android-25).

- **Indications and Dosages:**
  Breast cancer: PO 50-200 mg/day.
  Hypogonadism: PO 10-50 mg/day.

- **Unlabeled Uses:** Hereditary angiodema

- **Contraindications:** Prostatic or breast cancer in males, hypersensitivity to methyltestosterone or any other component of its formulation

- **Side Effects**
  Frequent
  Gynecomastia, acne
  Females: Hirsutism, deepening of voice, clitoral enlargement that may not be reversible when drug is discontinued.
  Occasional
  Edema, nausea, insomnia, oligospermia, priapism, male pattern of baldness, bladder irritability, hypercalcemia in immobilized patients or those with breast cancer, hypercholesterolemia
  Rare
  Polycythemia

- **Serious Reactions**
  - Cholestatic jaundice, hepatocellular neoplasms, peliosis hepatis, edema with or without congestive heart failure, and suppression of clotting factors II, V, VII, and X have been reported.

- **Patient/Family Education**
  - Do not swallow buccal tablets, allow to dissolve between cheek and gum
  - Avoid eating, drinking, or smoking while buccal tablet in place

■ **Monitoring Parameters**
  - LFTs, lipids, Hct, Hgb
  - Report weight gains of 5 lb or more
  - Weight
  - Blood pressure

■ **Geriatric side effects at a glance:**
  ❑ CNS ❑ Bowel Dysfunction ❑ Bladder Dysfunction ❑ Falls

■ **U.S. Regulatory Considerations**
  ❑ FDA Black Box ❑ OBRA regulated in U.S. Long Term Care

metoclopramide hydrochloride

(met'-oh-kloe-pra'-mide hye-droe-klor'-ide)

■ **Brand Name(s):** Reglan
  Chemical Class: Para-aminobenzoic acid derivative

■ **Clinical Pharmacology:**
  Mechanism of Action: A dopamine receptor antagonist that stimulates motility of the upper GI tract and decreases reflux into the esophagus. Also raises the threshold of activity in the chemoreceptor trigger zone. **Therapeutic Effect:** Accelerates intestinal transit and gastric emptying; relieves nausea and vomiting.
  Pharmacokinetics:

Route	Onset	Peak	Duration
PO	30-60 min	N/A	N/A
IV	1-3 min	N/A	N/A
IM	10-15 min	N/A	N/A

Well absorbed from the GI tract. Metabolized in the liver. Protein binding: 30%. Primarily excreted in urine. Not removed by hemodialysis. **Half-life:** 4-6 hr.

■ **Available Forms:**
  - *Syrup:* 5 mg/5 ml.
  - *Tablets:* 5 mg, 10 mg.
  - *Injection:* 5 mg/ml.

■ **Indications and Dosages:**
  Prevention of chemotherapy-induced nausea and vomiting: IV 1-2 mg/kg 30 min before chemotherapy; repeat q2h for 2 doses, then q3h as needed for total of 5 doses/day.
  Postoperative nausea, vomiting: IV 10-20 mg q4-6h as needed.
  Diabetic gastroparesis: PO Initially, 5 mg 30 min before meals and at bedtime. May increase to 10 mg. IV 5 mg over 1-2 min. May increase to 10 mg.
  Symptomatic gastroesophageal reflux: PO Initially, 5 mg 4 times a day. May increase to 10 mg.

To facilitate small bowel intubation (single dose): IV 10 mg as a single dose.
Dosage in renal impairment: Dosage is modified based on creatinine clearance.

Creatinine Clearance	% of normal dose
40-50 ml/min	75%
10-40 ml/min	50%
less than 10 ml/min	25%-50%

- **Unlabeled Uses:** Prevention of aspiration pneumonia; treatment of drug-related post-operative nausea and vomiting, persistent hiccups, slow gastric emptying, vascular headaches

- **Contraindications:** Concurrent use of medications likely to produce extrapyramidal reactions, GI hemorrhage, GI obstruction or perforation, history of seizure disorders, pheochromocytoma

- **Side Effects**
  Frequent (10%)
  Somnolence, restlessness, fatigue, lethargy
  Occasional (3%)
  Dizziness, anxiety, headache, insomnia, breast tenderness, constipation, rash, dry mouth, galactorrhea, gynecomastia
  Rare (less than 3%)
  Hypotension or hypertension, tachycardia

- **Serious Reactions**
  - Extrapyramidal reactions have been described in older adults.

Special Considerations
  - Dystonic reactions can be managed with 50 mg diphenhydramine or 1-2 mg benztropine IM

- **Patient/Family Education**
  - Use caution while driving or during other activities requiring alertness; may cause drowsiness
  - Notify the physician if involuntary eye, facial, or limb movement occurs
  - Avoid alcohol during metoclopramide therapy

- **Monitoring Parameters**
  - Blood pressure, heart rate, BUN, and serum creatinine levels to assess renal function

- **Geriatric side effects at a glance:**
  ☑ CNS ☑ Bowel Dysfunction ❑ Bladder Dysfunction ❑ Falls
  Other: Extrapyramidal symptoms (EPS), parkinsonism

- **Use with caution in older patients with:** Parkinson's disease or parkinsonism, Psychosis, Renal impairment, Cognitive impairment

- **U.S. Regulatory Considerations**
  ❑ FDA Black Box ❑ OBRA regulated in U.S. Long Term Care

- **Other Uses in Geriatric Patient:** Diabetic gastroparesis, Chemotherapy-induced nausea and vomiting, Postoperative nausea and vomiting

- **Side Effects:**
  Of particular importance in the geriatric patient: Confusion, drowsiness, extrapyramidal symptoms (parkinsonism, tremor), tardive dyskinesia (TD), restlessness, weakness, diarrhea

- **Geriatric Considerations - Summary:** Older adults are at high risk for EPS and TD. Adjust dose based on creatinine clearance. Long-term use (>3 mo) is not recommended. Adverse effects can occur at any time during therapy.

- **References:**
  1. Gawrich S, Shaker R. Medical management of nocturnal symptoms of gastro-oesophageal reflux disease in the elderly. Drugs Aging 2003;20:509-516.
  2. Thomson ABR. Gastro-oesophageal reflux in the elderly. Role of drug therapy in management. Drugs Aging 2001;18:409-414.
  3. Drugs that may cause cognitive disorders in the elderly. Med Let 2000;42:111-112.

metolazone

(me-tole'-a-zone)

- **Brand Name(s):** Mykrox (rapid acting), Zaroxolyn (slow acting)
  Chemical Class: Quinazoline derivative

- **Clinical Pharmacology:**
  Mechanism of Action: A thiazide-like diuretic and antihypertensive. As a diuretic, blocks reabsorption of sodium, potassium, and chloride at the distal convoluted tubule, increasing renal excretion of sodium and water. As an antihypertensive, reduces plasma and extracellular fluid volume and peripheral vascular resistance. **Therapeutic Effect:** Promotes diuresis and reduces BP.
  Pharmacokinetics:

Route	Onset	Peak	Duration
PO (diuretic)	1 hr	2 hr	12–24 hr

  Incompletely absorbed from the GI tract. Protein binding: 95%. Primarily excreted unchanged in urine. Not removed by hemodialysis. **Half-life:** 14 hr.

- **Available Forms:**
  - *Tablets (Prompt-Release [Mykrox]):* 0.5 mg.
  - *Tablets (Extended-Release [Zaroxolyn]):* 2.5 mg, 5 mg, 10 mg.

- **Indications and Dosages:**
  Edema: PO (Zaroxolyn) 5-10 mg/day. May increase to 20 mg/day in edema associated with renal disease or heart failure.
  Hypertension: PO (Zaroxolyn) 2.5-5 mg/day. PO (Mykrox) Initially, 0.5 mg/day. May increase up to 1 mg/day.

- **Contraindications:** Anuria, hepatic coma or precoma, history of hypersensitivity to sulfonamides or thiazide diuretics, renal decompensation

Side Effects
Expected
Increase in urinary frequency and urine volume
Frequent (10%–9%)
Dizziness, light-headedness, headache
Occasional (6%–4%)
Muscle cramps and spasm, fatigue, lethargy
Rare (less than 2%)
Asthenia, palpitations, depression, nausea, vomiting, abdominal bloating, constipation, diarrhea, urticaria

Serious Reactions
- Vigorous diuresis may lead to profound water and electrolyte depletion, resulting in hypokalemia, hyponatremia, and dehydration.
- Acute hypotensive episodes may occur.
- Hyperglycemia may occur during prolonged therapy.
- Pancreatitis, paresthesia, blood dyscrasias, pulmonary edema, allergic pneumonitis, and dermatologic reactions occur rarely.
- Overdose can lead to lethargy and coma without changes in electrolytes or hydration.

Special Considerations
- More effective than other thiazide-type diuretics in patients with impaired renal function
- Metolazone formulations are not bioequivalent or therapeutically equivalent at the same doses. Mykrox is more rapidly and completely bioavailable; Do not interchange brands.
- Although allergic cross-reactivity with sulfonamide antibiotics and sulfonamide nonantibiotics has not been demonstrated, use with caution in patients with a history of severe sulfa allergies.

Patient/Family Education
- Will increase urination; take early in the day to prevent sleep disturbance
- May cause sensitivity to sunlight; avoid prolonged exposure to the sun and other ultraviolet light
- May cause gout attacks; notify clinician if sudden joint pain occurs
- Change position slowly and let legs dangle momentarily before standing to reduce the drug's hypotensive effect
- Eat foods high in potassium such as apricots, bananas, raisins, orange juice, potatoes, legumes, meat, and whole grains (such as cereals)

Monitoring Parameters
- Weight, urine output, serum electrolytes, BUN, creatinine, CBC, uric acid, glucose, lipids

Geriatric side effects at a glance:
❏ CNS ❏ Bowel Dysfunction ❏ Bladder Dysfunction ❏ Falls

U.S. Regulatory Considerations
❏ FDA Black Box ❏ OBRA regulated in U.S. Long Term Care

metoprolol tartrate

(me-toe-proe'-lole tar'-trāt)

■ **Brand Name(s):** Lopressor, Toprol XL

Combinations
Rx: with hydrochlorothiazide (Lopressor HCT)
Chemical Class: β_1-Adrenergic blocker, cardioselective

■ **Clinical Pharmacology:**
Mechanism of Action: An antianginal, antihypertensive, and MI adjunct that selectively blocks beta$_1$-adrenergic receptors; high dosages may block beta$_2$-adrenergic receptors. Decreases oxygen requirements. Large doses increase airway resistance.
Therapeutic Effect: Slows sinus node heart rate, decreases cardiac output, and reduces BP. Also decreases myocardial ischemia severity.
Pharmacokinetics:

Route	Onset	Peak	Duration
PO	10–15 min	N/A	6 hr
PO (extended release)	N/A	6–12 hr	24 hr
IV	Immediate	20 min	5–8 hr

Well absorbed from the GI tract. Protein binding: 12%. Widely distributed. Metabolized in the liver (undergoes significant first-pass metabolism). Primarily excreted in urine. Removed by hemodialysis. **Half-life:** 3–7 hr.

■ **Available Forms:**
- *Tablets (Lopressor):* 25 mg, 50 mg, 100 mg.
- *Tablets (Extended-Release [Toprol XL]):* 25 mg, 50 mg, 100 mg, 200 mg.
- *Injection (Lopressor):* 1 mg/ml.

■ **Indications and Dosages:**
Mild to moderate hypertension: PO Initially, 100 mg/day as single or divided dose. Increase at weekly (or longer) intervals. Maintenance: 100–450 mg/day. Elderly. Initially, 25 mg/day. Range: 25–300 mg/day. PO (Extended-Release) Initially, 25-50 mg/day as a single dose. May increase at 1-2 week intervals.
Chronic, stable angina pectoris: PO Initially, 100 mg/day as single or divided dose. Increase at weekly (or longer) intervals. Maintenance: 100–450 mg/day. PO (Extended-Release) Initially, 100 mg/day as single dose. May increase at least at weekly intervals until optimum clinical response achieved. Maximum: 200 mg/day.
Congestive heart failure: PO (Extended-Release) Initially, 25 mg/day. May double dose q2wk. Maximum: 200 mg/day.
Early treatment of MI: IV 5 mg q2min for 3 doses, followed by 50 mg orally q6h for 48 hr. Begin oral dose 15 min after last IV dose. Or, in patients who do not tolerate full IV dose, give 25–50 mg orally q6h, 15 min after last IV dose.
Late treatment and maintenance after an MI: PO 100 mg twice a day for at least 3 mo.

■ **Unlabeled Uses:** To increase survival rate in diabetic patients with coronary artery disease (CAD); treatment or prevention of anxiety; cardiac arrhythmias; hypertrophic cardiomyopathy; mitral valve prolapse syndrome; pheochromocytoma; tremors; thyrotoxicosis; vascular headache

- **Contraindications:** Cardiogenic shock, MI with a heart rate less than 45 beats/minute or systolic BP less than 100 mm Hg, overt heart failure, second- or third-degree heart block, sinus bradycardia

- **Side Effects**

  Metoprolol is generally well tolerated, with transient and mild side effects.

  Frequent

  Diminished sexual function, drowsiness, insomnia, unusual fatigue or weakness

  Occasional

  Anxiety, nervousness, diarrhea, constipation, nausea, vomiting, nasal congestion, abdominal discomfort, dizziness, difficulty breathing, cold hands or feet

  Rare

  Altered taste, dry eyes, nightmares, paresthesia, allergic reaction (rash, pruritus)

- **Serious Reactions**
  - Overdose may produce profound bradycardia, hypotension, and bronchospasm.
  - Abrupt withdrawal of metoprolol may result in diaphoresis, palpitations, headache, tremulousness, exacerbation of angina, MI, and ventricular arrhythmias.
  - Metoprolol administration may precipitate CHF and MI in patients with heart disease; thyroid storm in those with thyrotoxicosis; and peripheral ischemia in those with existing peripheral vascular disease.
  - Hypoglycemia may occur in patients with previously controlled diabetes mellitus.

- **Patient/Family Education**
  - Do not discontinue abruptly; may require taper; rapid withdrawal may produce rebound hypertension or angina
  - Avoid driving or other activities requiring alertness until response to therapy is determined
  - Take with or immediately following meals
  - Extended-release tablets are scored and can be divided; whole or half tablet should be swallowed whole and not chewed or crushed

- **Monitoring Parameters**
  - Angina: Reduction in nitroglycerin usage; frequency, severity, onset, and duration of angina pain; heart rate
  - Arrhythmias: heart rate
  - Congestive heart failure: Functional status, cough, dyspnea on exertion, paroxysmal nocturnal dyspnea, exercise tolerance, and ventricular function
  - Hypertension: Blood pressure
  - Migraine headache: Reduction in the frequency, severity, and duration of attacks
  - Postmyocardial infarction: Left ventricular function, lower resting heart rate
  - Toxicity: Blood glucose, bronchospasm, hypotension, bradycardia, depression, confusion, hallucination, sexual dysfunction

- **Geriatric side effects at a glance:**
  ❑ CNS ❑ Bowel Dysfunction ❑ Bladder Dysfunction ❑ Falls

- **U.S. Regulatory Considerations**
  ☑ FDA Black Box

  In patients using <u>orally administered</u> beta-blockers, abrupt withdrawal may precipitate angina or lead to myocardial infarction or ventricular arrhythmias.

  ❑ OBRA regulated in U.S. Long Term Care

metronidazole

(me-troe-ni'-da-zole)

■ **Brand Name(s):** Flagyl, Flagyl 375, Flagyl ER, Flagyl I.V. RTU, MetroCream, MetroGel, MetroGel-Vaginal, Metro I.V., MetroLotion, Metronidazole Benzoate, Noritate, Protostat, Rozex
Chemical Class: Nitroimidazole derivative

■ **Clinical Pharmacology:**
Mechanism of Action: A nitroimidazole derivative that disrupts bacterial and protozoal DNA, inhibiting nucleic acid synthesis. **Therapeutic Effect:** Produces bactericidal, ID-antibacterial, amebicidal, and trichomonacidal effects. Produces anti-inflammatory and immunosuppressive effects when applied topically.
Pharmacokinetics: Well absorbed from the GI tract; minimally absorbed after topical application. Protein binding: less than 20%. Widely distributed; crosses blood-brain barrier. Metabolized in the liver to active metabolite. Primarily excreted in urine; partially eliminated in feces. Removed by hemodialysis. **Half-life:** 8 hr (increased in alcoholic hepatic disease).

■ **Available Forms:**
- *Capsules (Flagyl 375):* 375 mg.
- *Tablets (Flagyl, Protostat):* 250 mg, 500 mg.
- *Tablets (Extended-Release [Flagyl ER]):* 750 mg.
- *Injection (Infusion [Flagyl I.V. RTU]):* 500 mg/100 ml.
- *Topical Cream:* 0.75% (MetroCream, Rozex), 1% (Noritate).
- *Topical Gel (MetroGel):* 0.75%, 1%.
- *Topical Lotion (MetroLotion):* 0.75%.
- *Vaginal Gel (MetroGel-Vaginal):* 0.75%.

■ **Indications and Dosages:**
Anaerobic infections: PO, IV Initially, 15 mg/kg once, then 7.5 mg/kg/dose q6h. Maximum: 4 g/day.
Amebic dysentery: PO 750 mg 3 times a day for 5-10 days.
Amebic liver abscess: PO 500-750 mg 3 times a day for 5-10 days.
Giardiasis: PO 250 mg 3 times a day for 5 days.
Pseudomembranous colitis: PO 500-750 mg 3 times a day or 250-500 mg 4 times a day.
Trichomoniasis: PO 250 mg 3 times a day or 375 mg twice a day or 500 mg twice a day or 2g as a single dose.
Bacterial vaginosis: PO 500 mg twice a day for 7 days or 750 mg (extended-release) once daily for 7 days or 2g as a single dose. (pregnant): 250 mg 3 times a day for 7 days. Intravaginal 0.75% apply twice a day for 5 days. Centers for Disease Control and Prevention (CDC) does not recommend the use of topical agents during pregnancy.
Rosacea: Topical Apply to affected area once daily. (0.75%): Apply to affected area twice a day.

■ **Unlabeled Uses:** Treatment of bacterial vaginosis, grade III-IV decubitus ulcers with anaerobic infection, *Helicobacter pylori*–associated gastritis and duodenal ulcer, inflammatory bowel disease; topical treatment of acne rosacea

- **Contraindications:** Hypersensitivity to other nitroimidazole derivatives (also parabens with topical application)

- **Side Effects**

  Frequent

  Systemic: Anorexia, nausea, dry mouth, metallic taste

  Vaginal: Symptomatic cervicitis and vaginitis, abdominal cramps, uterine pain

  Occasional

  Systemic: Diarrhea or constipation, vomiting, dizziness, erythematous rash, urticaria, reddish brown urine

  Topical: Transient erythema, mild dryness, burning, irritation, stinging, tearing when applied too close to eyes

  Vaginal: Vaginal, perineal, or vulvar itching; vulvar swelling

  Rare

  Mild, transient leukopenia; thrombophlebitis with IV therapy

- **Serious Reactions**
  - Oral therapy may result in furry tongue, glossitis, cystitis, dysuria, pancreatitis, and flattening of T waves on ECG readings.
  - Peripheral neuropathy, manifested as numbness and tingling in hands or feet, is usually reversible if treatment is stopped immediately after neurologic symptoms appear.
  - Seizures occur occasionally.

Special Considerations
  - Treat sexual partner(s) for trichomoniasis
  - Individualize treatment based on local susceptibility patterns.

- **Patient/Family Education**
  - Drug may cause GI upset; take with food
  - Avoid alcoholic beverages during therapy and for at least 24 hr following last dose (disulfiram-like reaction possible)
  - Drug may cause darkening of urine
  - May cause an unpleasant metallic taste
  - H_2 blocker must be prescribed with Helidac kit
  - Avoid tasks requiring mental alertness or motor skills until response to the drug is established
  - The patient taking metronidazole for trichomoniasis should refrain from sexual intercourse until the full treatment is completed
  - The patient using topical metronidazole should avoid drug contact with eyes

- **Monitoring Parameters**
  - CBC
  - Intake and output and assess for urinary problems
  - Skin for rash and urticaria
  - Daily bowel activity and stool consistency. Although mild GI effects may be tolerable, severe symptoms may indicate the onset of antibiotic-associated colitis.
  - Signs and symptoms of superinfection include abdominal pain or cramping, anal or genital pruritus or discharge, moderate to severe diarrhea, severe mouth or tongue soreness, and new or increased fever.

- **Geriatric side effects at a glance:**
  ☐ CNS   ☑ Bowel Dysfunction   ☐ Bladder Dysfunction   ☐ Falls

■ **U.S. Regulatory Considerations**
◻ FDA Black Box
Carcinogenic in rodents
◻ OBRA regulated in U.S. Long Term Care

metyrosine

(me-tye'-roe-seen)

■ **Brand Name(s):** Demser
Chemical Class: α-Methyl-L-tyrosine

■ **Clinical Pharmacology:**
Mechanism of Action: A tyrosine hydroxylase inhibitor that blocks conversion of tyrosine to dihydroxyphenylalanine, the rate limiting step in the biosynthetic pathway of catecholamines. **Therapeutic Effect:** Reduces levels of endogenous catecholamines.
Pharmacokinetics: Well absorbed from the gastrointestinal (GI) tract. Metabolized in the liver. Excreted primarily in the urine. **Half-life:** 7.2 hr.

■ **Available Forms:**
• *Capsule*: 250 mg.

■ **Indications and Dosages:**
Pheochromocytoma (preoperative): PO Initially, 250 mg 4 times/day. Increase by 250-500 mg/day up to 4 g/day. Maintenance: 2-4 g/day in 4 divided doses for 5-7 days.

■ **Unlabeled Uses:** Tourette's syndrome

■ **Contraindications:** Hypertension of unknown etiology, hypersensitivity to metyrosine or any component of the formulation

■ **Side Effects**
Frequent
Drowsiness, extrapyramidal symptoms, diarrhea
Occasional
Galactorrhea, edema of the breasts, nausea, vomiting, dry mouth, impotence, nasal congestion
Rare
Lower extremity edema, urinary problems, urticaria, anemia, depression, disorientation

■ **Serious Reactions**
• Serious or life-threatening allergic reaction characterized by hallucinations, hematuria, hyperstimulation after withdrawal, severe lower extremity edema, and parkinsonism.

■ **Patient/Family Education**
- Maintain a daily liberal fluid intake
- Avoid alcohol or CNS depressants
- Avoid tasks that require mental alertness or motor skills until response to the drug is established

■ **Monitoring Parameters**
- Blood pressure, ECG

■ **Geriatric side effects at a glance:**
❑ CNS   ❑ Bowel Dysfunction   ❑ Bladder Dysfunction   ❑ Falls

■ **U.S. Regulatory Considerations**
❑ FDA Black Box   ❑ OBRA regulated in U.S. Long Term Care

mexiletine hydrochloride

(mex'-i-le-teen hye-droe-klor'-ide)

■ **Brand Name(s):** Mexitil
Chemical Class: Lidocaine derivative

■ **Clinical Pharmacology:**
Mechanism of Action: An antiarrhythmic that shortens duration of action potential and decreases effective refractory period in the His-Purkinje system of the myocardium by blocking sodium transport across myocardial cell membranes. **Therapeutic Effect:** Suppresses ventricular arrhythmias.
Pharmacokinetics: Well absorbed from the GI tract. Protein binding: 50%-60%. Metabolized in liver. Approximately 10% is excreted unchanged in urine. **Half-life:** 10-12 hr.

■ **Available Forms:**
- **Capsules:** 150 mg, 200 mg, 250 mg.

■ **Indications and Dosages:**
Arrhythmia: PO Initially, 200 mg q8h. Adjust dosage by 50-100 mg at 2- to 3-day intervals. **Maximum:** 1,200 mg/day.

■ **Unlabeled Uses:** Treatment of diabetic neuropathy

■ **Contraindications:** Cardiogenic shock, preexisting second- or third-degree AV block, right bundle-branch block without presence of pacemaker

■ **Side Effects**
Frequent (greater than 10%)
GI distress, including nausea, vomiting, and heartburn; dizziness; light-headedness; tremor
Occasional (10%–1%)
Nervousness, change in sleep habits, headache, visual disturbances, paresthesia, diarrhea or constipation, palpitations, chest pain, rash, respiratory difficulty, edema

801

- **Serious Reactions**
  - Mexiletine has the ability to worsen existing arrhythmias or produce new ones.
  - CHF may occur and existing CHF may worsen.
  - Abnormal liver function tests have been reported, some in the first few weeks of therapy with mexiletine.

Special Considerations
  - Because of proarrhythmic effects, not recommended for non–life threatening arrhythmias
  - Antiarrhythmic drugs have not been shown to increase survival of patients with ventricular arrhythmias
  - Initiate therapy in facilities capable of providing continuous ECG monitoring and managing life-threatening dysrhythmias

- **Patient/Family Education**
  - Take with food or antacid
  - Notify the physician if dark urine, cough, generalized fatigue, nausea, pale stools, severe or persistent abdominal pain, shortness of breath, unexplained sore throat or fever, vomiting, or yellowing of the eyes or skin occurs
  - Do not use nasal decongestants and OTC cold preparations without physician approval

- **Monitoring Parameters**
  - Therapeutic mexiletine concentrations 0.5-2 mcg/ml
  - ECG and vital signs for cardiac side effects
  - Pulse for rate, quality, and irregularity
  - Pattern of bowel activity and stool consistency
  - Signs and symptoms of CHF

- **Geriatric side effects at a glance:**
  ❑ CNS   ❑ Bowel Dysfunction   ❑ Bladder Dysfunction   ❑ Falls

- **U.S. Regulatory Considerations**
  ☑ FDA Black Box   ❑ OBRA regulated in U.S. Long Term Care
  - An excessive mortality or non-fatal cardiac arrest rate was observed in patients with non–life-threatening ventricular arrhythmias who had a recent MI.
  - Ventricular proarrhythmic effects have been observed in patients with atrial fibrillation/flutter. This drug is not recommended in patients with chronic atrial fibrillation.

miconazole

(mye-con'-a-zole)

- **Brand Name(s):** Monistat-Derm
  OTC: Femizol-M, Lotrimin-AF, Micatin, Monistat-3, Monistate-7
  Chemical Class: Imidazole derivative

Clinical Pharmacology:

Mechanism of Action: An imidazole derivative that inhibits synthesis of ergosterol (vital component of fungal cell formation), damaging cell membrane. **Therapeutic Effect:** Fungistatic; may be fungicidal, depending on concentration.
Pharmacokinetics: Parenteral: Widely distributed in tissues. Metabolized in liver. Primarily excreted in urine. **Half-life:** 24 hr. Topical: No systemic absorption following application to intact skin. Intravaginally: Small amount absorbed systemically.

Available Forms:

- *Injection:* 10 mg/ml.
- *Vaginal Suppository:* 100 mg (Monistat-7), 200 mg (Monistat-3).
- *Topical Cream:* 2% (Micatin, Monistat-Derm).
- *Vaginal Cream:* 2% (Femizol-M).
- *Topical Powder:* 2% (Micatin).
- *Topical Spray:* 2% (Lotrimin-AF).

Indications and Dosages:

Coccidioidomycosis: IV 1.8-3.6 g/day for 3-20 wk or longer.
Cryptococcosis: IV 1.2-2.4 g/day for 3-12 wk or longer.
Petriellidiosis: IV 0.6-3.0 g/day for 5-20 wk or longer.
Candidiasis: IV 0.6-1.8 g/day for 1-20 wk or longer.
Paracoccidioidomycosis: IV 0.2-1.2 g/day for 2-16 wk or longer.
Vulvovaginal candidiasis: Intravaginally One 200-mg suppository at bedtime for 3 days; one 100-mg suppository or one applicatorful at bedtime for 7 days.
Topical fungal infections, cutaneous candidiasis: Topical Apply liberally 2 times/day, morning and evening.

Contraindications: None known.

Side Effects

Frequent
Phlebitis, fever, chills, rash, itching, nausea, vomiting
Occasional
Dizziness, drowsiness, headache, flushed face, abdominal pain, constipation, diarrhea, decreased appetite
Topical: Itching, burning, stinging, erythema, urticaria
Vaginal: Vulvovaginal burning, itching, irritation, headache, skin rash

Serious Reactions

- Anemia, thrombocytopenia, and liver toxicity occur rarely

Patient/Family Education

- Avoid getting into eyes
- Continue for the full length of treatment

Monitoring Parameters

- Assess for vaginal burning and itching
- Pattern of daily bowel activity and stool consistency

Geriatric side effects at a glance:

❑ CNS ❑ Bowel Dysfunction ❑ Bladder Dysfunction ❑ Falls

midazolam hydrochloride

(mid'-ay-zoe-lam hye-droe-klor'-ide)

■ **Brand Name(s):** Versed
Chemical Class: Benzodiazepine

DEA Class: Schedule IV

■ **Clinical Pharmacology:**
Mechanism of Action: A benzodiazepine that enhances the action of gamma-aminobutyric acid, one of the major inhibitory neurotransmitters in the brain. **Therapeutic Effect:** Produces anxiolytic, hypnotic, anticonvulsant, muscle relaxant, and amnestic effects.
Pharmacokinetics:

Route	Onset	Peak	Duration
PO	10-20 min	N/A	N/A
IV	1-5 min	5-7 min	20-30 min
IM	5-15 min	15-60 min	2-6 hr

Well absorbed after IM administration. Protein binding: 97%. Metabolized in the liver to active metabolite. Primarily excreted in urine. Not removed by hemodialysis. **Half-life:** 1-5 hr.

■ **Available Forms:**
• **Syrup:** 2 mg/ml.
• **Injection:** 1 mg/ml, 5 mg/ml.
• **Injection (Preservative-free):** 1 mg/ml, 5 mg/ml.

■ **Indications and Dosages:**
Preoperative sedation: IV 0.02-0.04 mg/kg. IM 0.07-0.08 mg/kg 30-60 min before surgery.
Conscious sedation for diagnostic, therapeutic, and endoscopic procedures: IV 1-2.5 mg over 2 min. Titrate as needed. Maximum total dose: 2.5-5 mg.
Conscious sedation during mechanical ventilation: IV Initially, 0.02-0.08 mg/kg. May repeat at 5-15 minute intervals or continuous infusion rate of 0.04-0.2 mg/kg/hr and titrated to desired effect.

■ **Unlabeled Uses:** Anxiety, status epilepticus

■ **Contraindications:** Acute alcohol intoxication, acute angle-closure glaucoma, allergies to cherries, coma, shock

■ **Side Effects**
Frequent (10%-4%)
Decreased respiratory rate, tenderness at IM or IV injection site, pain during injection, oxygen desaturation, hiccups

Occasional (3%-2%)
Hypotension, paradoxical CNS reaction
Rare (less than 2%)
Nausea, vomiting, headache, coughing

■ **Serious Reactions**
  • Inadequate or excessive dosage or improper administration may result in cerebral hypoxia, agitation, involuntary movements, hyperactivity, and combativeness.
  • A too-rapid IV rate, excessive doses, or a single large dose increases the risk of respiratory depression or arrest.
  • Respiratory depression or apnea may produce hypoxia and cardiac arrest.

■ **Patient/Family Education**
  • Midazolam produces an amnesic effect

■ **Monitoring Parameters**
  • Monitor the patient's respiratory rate and oxygen saturation continuously during parenteral administration to detect apnea and respiratory depression
  • Monitor the patient's level of sedation every 3 to 5 min, and assess vital signs during the recovery period

■ **Geriatric side effects at a glance:**
  ☑ CNS   ☐ Bowel Dysfunction   ☐ Bladder Dysfunction   ☑ Falls
  Other: Paradoxical response (e.g., agitation)

■ **Use with caution in older patients with:** Concurrent treatment with potent CYP 3A4 inhibitors (e.g., nefazodone) leads to increased plasma concentrations of midazolam; COPD; untreated sleep apnea

■ **U.S. Regulatory Considerations**
  ☑ FDA Black Box
  • Respiratory depression/arrest, most often with concurrent CNS depressants
  • Continuous monitoring for respiratory and cardiac function
  ☑ OBRA regulated in U.S. Long Term Care

■ **Other Uses in Geriatric Patient:** Conscious sedation, status epilepticus

■ **Side Effects:**
  Of particular importance in the geriatric patient: Sedation

■ **Geriatric Considerations - Summary:** Midazolam is effective for oral or intravenous administration for short-term sedation, older adults require lower doses.

■ **References:**
  1. Eilers H, Niemann C. Clinically important drug interactions with intravenous anaesthetics in older patients. Drugs Aging 2003;20:969-980.
  2. Weinbroum AA, Szold O, Ogorek D, Flaishon R. The midazolam-induced paradox phenomenon is reversible by flumazenil. Epidemiology, patient characteristics and review of the literature. Eur J Anaesthesiol 2001;18:789-797.
  3. Waterhouse EJ, DeLorenzo RJ. Status epilepticus in older patients: epidemiology and treatment options. Drugs Aging 2001;18:133-142.

midodrine hydrochloride

(mye'-doe-drene hye-droe-klor'-ide)

■ **Brand Name(s):** ProAmatine
   Chemical Class: Catecholamine, synthetic

■ **Clinical Pharmacology:**
   Mechanism of Action: A vasopressor that forms the active metabolite desglymidodrine, an alpha$_1$-agonist, activating alpha receptors of the arteriolar and venous vasculature. **Therapeutic Effect:** Increases vascular tone and BP.
   Pharmacokinetics: Rapid absorption from the GI tract following PO administration. Protein binding: Low. Undergoes enzymatic hydrolysis (deglycination) in the systemic circulation. Excreted in urine. **Half-life:** 0.5 hr.

■ **Available Forms:**
   • **Tablets:** 2.5 mg, 5 mg, 10 mg.

■ **Indications and Dosages:**
   Orthostatic hypotension: PO 10 mg 3 times a day. Give during the day when patient is upright, such as upon arising, midday, and late afternoon. Do not give later than 6 PM.
   Dosage in renal impairment: Give 2.5 mg 3 times a day; increase gradually, as tolerated.

■ **Unlabeled Uses:** Infection-related hypotension, intradialytic hypotension, psychotropic agent-induced hypotension, urinary incontinence

■ **Contraindications:** Acute renal function impairment, persistent hypertension, pheochromocytoma, severe cardiac disease, thyrotoxicosis, urine retention

■ **Side Effects**
   Frequent (20%–7%)
   Paresthesia, piloerection, pruritus, dysuria, supine hypertension
   Occasional (less than 7%–1%)
   Pain, rash, chills, headache, facial flushing, confusion, dry mouth, anxiety

■ **Serious Reactions**
   • Increased systolic arterial pressure has been reported.

Special Considerations
   • Advantages include rapid and nearly complete absorption, a long elimination t$_{1/2}$, lack of central nervous system (CNS) penetration, and minimal to no cardiac effects
   • Supine hypertension has been a therapy-limiting complication

■ **Patient/Family Education**
   • To minimize supine hypertension, avoid taking drug after the evening meal
   • Use OTC medications, such as cough, cold, and diet preparations, cautiously because they may affect blood pressure

Monitoring Parameters
- Blood pressure, liver and renal function

Geriatric side effects at a glance:
❑ CNS ❑ Bowel Dysfunction ☑ Bladder Dysfunction ❑ Falls

U.S. Regulatory Considerations
❑ FDA Black Box ❑ OBRA regulated in U.S. Long Term Care

milrinone lactate

(mill'-re-none)

- **Brand Name(s):** Primacor, Primacor I.V.
  Chemical Class: Bipyridine derivative

- **Clinical Pharmacology:**
  Mechanism of Action: A cardiac inotropic agent that inhibits phosphodiesterase, which increases cyclic adenosine monophosphate and potentiates the delivery of calcium to myocardial contractile systems. **Therapeutic Effect:** Relaxes vascular muscle, causing vasodilation. Increases cardiac output; decreases pulmonary capillary wedge pressure and vascular resistance.
  Pharmacokinetics:

Route	Onset	Peak	Duration
IV	5–15 min	N/A	N/A

  Protein binding: 70%. Primarily excreted unchanged in urine. **Half-life:** 2.4 hr.

- **Available Forms:**
  - Injection (Primacor, Primacor I.V.): 1 mg/ml, 10-ml single-dose vial, 20-ml single-dose vial, 50-ml single-dose vial, 5-ml sterile cartridge unit.
  - Injection (Premix [Primacor]): 200 mcg/ml.

- **Indications and Dosages:**
  Short-term management of CHF: IV Initially, 50 mcg/kg over 10 min. Continue with maintenance infusion rate of 0.375–0.75 mcg/kg/min based on hemodynamic and clinical response. Total daily dosage: 0.59–1.13 mg/kg.
  Dosage in renal impairment: For patients with severe renal impairment, reduce dosage to 0.2–0.43 mcg/kg/min.

- **Contraindications:** None known.

- **Side Effects**
  Occasional (3%–1%)
  Headache, hypotension
  Rare (less than 1%)
  Angina, chest pain

Serious Reactions
- Supraventricular and ventricular arrhythmias (12%), nonsustained ventricular tachycardia (2%), and sustained ventricular tachycardia (1%) may occur.

Patient/Family Education
- Immediately report palpitations or chest pain
- Milrinone is not a cure for CHF but will help relieve symptoms

Monitoring Parameters
- Fluid and electrolyte changes, renal function
- Improvement in cardiac output may increase diuresis, and K^+ loss
- Blood pressure, ECG, heart rate, serum potassium levels
- Signs and symptoms of CHF

Geriatric side effects at a glance:
❏ CNS ❏ Bowel Dysfunction ❏ Bladder Dysfunction ❏ Falls

U.S. Regulatory Considerations
❏ FDA Black Box ❏ OBRA regulated in U.S. Long Term Care

minocycline hydrochloride

(mi-noe-sye'-kleen hye-droe-klor'-ide)

■ **Brand Name(s):** Arestin, Dynacin, Minocin, Myrac, Vectrin
Chemical Class: Tetracycline derivative

■ **Clinical Pharmacology:**
Mechanism of Action: A tetracycline antibacterial that inhibits bacterial protein synthesis by binding to ribosomes. **Therapeutic Effect:** Bacteriostatic.
Pharmacokinetics: Protein binding: 76%. Partial elimination in feces; minimal excretion in urine. Not removed by hemodialysis. **Half-life:** 11-12 hr (oral capsule).

■ **Available Forms:**
- *Capsules (Dynacin, Minocin, Vectrin):* 50 mg, 75 mg, 100 mg.
- *Capsules (Pellet-filled [Minocin]):* 50 mg, 100 mg.
- *Tablets (Minocin, Myrac):* 50 mg, 75 mg, 100 mg.
- *Powder for Injection (Minocin, Myrac):* 100 mg.

■ **Indications and Dosages:**
Mild, moderate, or severe prostate, urinary tract, and CNS infections (excluding meningitis); uncomplicated gonorrhea; inflammatory acne; brucellosis; skin granulomas; cholera; trachoma; nocardiasis; yaws; and syphilis when penicillins are contraindicated: PO Initially, 100-200 mg, then 100 mg q12h or 50 mg q6h. IV Initially, 200 mg, then 100 mg q12h up to 400 mg/day.

- **Unlabeled Uses:** Treatment of atypical mycobacterial infections, rheumatoid arthritis, scleroderma

- **Contraindications:** Hypersensitivity to tetracyclines

- **Side Effects**
  Frequent
  Dizziness, light-headedness, diarrhea, nausea, vomiting, abdominal cramps, possibly severe photosensitivity, drowsiness, vertigo
  Occasional
  Altered pigmentation of skin or mucous membranes, rectal or genital pruritus, stomatitis

- **Serious Reactions**
  - Superinfection (especially fungal), anaphylaxis, and benign intracranial hypertension may occur.

Special Considerations
  - Individualize treatment based on local susceptibility patterns.

- **Patient/Family Education**
  - May take with food
  - Avoid sun exposure
  - Drink a full glass of water
  - Space doses evenly around the clock and continue taking minocycline for the full course of treatment
  - Avoid tasks that require mental alertness or motor skills until response to the drug is established
  - Notify the physician if diarrhea, rash, or other new symptoms occur

- **Monitoring Parameters**
  - Skin for rash
  - Blood pressure
  - Daily bowel activity and stool consistency. Although mild GI effects may be tolerable, severe symptoms may indicate the onset of antibiotic-associated colitis.
  - Signs and symptoms of superinfection include abdominal pain or cramping, anal or genital pruritus or discharge, moderate to severe diarrhea, severe mouth or tongue soreness, and new or increased fever.

- **Geriatric side effects at a glance:**
  ☑ CNS ☑ Bowel Dysfunction ❑ Bladder Dysfunction ❑ Falls

- **U.S. Regulatory Considerations**
  ❑ FDA Black Box ❑ OBRA regulated in U.S. Long Term Care

minoxidil

(min-nox'-i-dill)

■ **Brand Name(s):** Loniten
　　OTC: Rogaine
　　Chemical Class: Piperidinopyrimidine derivative

■ **Clinical Pharmacology:**
　　Mechanism of Action: An antihypertensive and hair growth stimulant that has direct action on vascular smooth muscle, producing vasodilation of arterioles. **Therapeutic Effect:** Decreases peripheral vascular resistance and BP; increases cutaneous blood flow; stimulates hair follicle epithelium and hair follicle growth.
　　Pharmacokinetics:

Route	Onset	Peak	Duration
PO	0.5 hr	2–8 hr	2–5 days

Well absorbed from the GI tract; minimal absorption after topical application. Protein binding: None. Widely distributed. Metabolized in the liver to active metabolite. Primarily excreted in urine. Removed by hemodialysis. **Half-life:** 4.2 hr.

■ **Available Forms:**
　　• *Tablets (Loniten):* 2.5 mg, 10 mg.
　　• *Topical Solution:* 2% (20 mg/ml) (Rogaine), 5% (50 mg/ml) (Rogaine ExtraStrength).

■ **Indications and Dosages:**
　　Severe symptomatic hypertension, hypertension associated with organ damage, hypertension that has failed to respond to maximal therapeutic dosages of a diuretic or two other antihypertensives: PO Initially, 2.5 mg/day. May increase gradually. Maintenance: 10–40 mg/day. Maximum: 100 mg/day.
　　Hair regrowth: Topical 1 ml to affected areas of scalp 2 times a day. Total daily dose not to exceed 2 ml.

■ **Contraindications:** Pheochromocytoma

■ **Side Effects**
　　Frequent
　　PO: Edema with concurrent weight gain, hypertrichosis (elongation, thickening, increased pigmentation of fine body hair; develops in 80% of patients within 3–6 wk after beginning therapy)

　　Occasional
　　PO: T-wave changes (usually revert to pretreatment state with continued therapy or drug withdrawal)
　　Topical: Pruritus, rash, dry or flaking skin, erythema

　　Rare
　　PO: Breast tenderness, headache, photosensitivity reaction
　　Topical: Allergic reaction, alopecia, burning sensation at scalp, soreness at hair root, headache, visual disturbances

■ **Serious Reactions**
- Tachycardia and angina pectoris may occur because of increased oxygen demands associated with increased heart rate and cardiac output.
- Fluid and electrolyte imbalance and CHF may occur, especially if a diuretic is not given concurrently with minoxidil.
- Too-rapid reduction in BP may result in syncope, cerebrovascular accident (CVA), MI, and ocular or vestibular ischemia.
- Pericardial effusion and tamponade may be seen in patients with impaired renal function who are not on dialysis.

Special Considerations
- Must be used in conjunction with diuretic (except dialysis patients) and beta-blocker or other sympathetic nervous system depressant (to prevent reflex tachycardia)

■ **Patient/Family Education**
- At least 4 mo of bid application necessary before evidence of hair growth with topical solution
- Continued treatment necessary to maintain or increase hair growth with topical solution
- Maximum blood pressure response occurs 3–7 days after initiation of minoxidil therapy
- Avoid exposure to sunlight and artificial light sources

■ **Geriatric side effects at a glance:**
   ❑ CNS ❑ Bowel Dysfunction ❑ Bladder Dysfunction ❑ Falls

■ **U.S. Regulatory Considerations**
   ☑ FDA Black Box
- Oral minoxidil is a potent agent which has significant side effects including pericardial effusion leading to tamponade and angina pectoris.
- Oral minoxidil administration should be closely monitored, usually given with a beta-blocker to prevent tachycardia and a diuretic to prevent fluid accumulation.
   ❑ OBRA regulated in U.S. Long Term Care

mirtazapine

(mir-taz'-a-peen)

■ **Brand Name(s):** Remeron, Remeron Soltab
   Chemical Class: Tetracyclic piperazino-azepine derivative

■ **Clinical Pharmacology:**
   Mechanism of Action: A tetracyclic compound that acts as an antagonist at presynaptic alpha$_2$-adrenergic receptors, increasing both norepinephrine and serotonin neurotransmission. Has low anticholinergic activity. **Therapeutic Effect:** Relieves depression and produces sedative effects.

Pharmacokinetics: Rapidly and completely absorbed after PO administration; absorption not affected by food. Protein binding: 85%. Metabolized in the liver. Primarily excreted in urine. Unknown if removed by hemodialysis. **Half-life:** 20-40 hr (longer in males [37 hr] than females [26 hr]).

■ **Available Forms:**
- *Tablets*: 7.5 mg, 15 mg, 30 mg, 45 mg.
- *Tablets* (*Disintegrating*): 15 mg, 30 mg, 45 mg.

■ **Indications and Dosages:**
Depression: PO Initially, 7.5 mg at bedtime. May increase by 7.5-15 mg/day q1-2wk. Maximum: 45 mg/day.

■ **Contraindications:** Use within 14 days of MAOIs

■ **Side Effects**
Frequent
Somnolence (54%), dry mouth (25%), increased appetite (17%), constipation (13%), weight gain (12%)
Occasional
Asthenia (8%), dizziness (7%), flu-like symptoms (5%), abnormal dreams (4%)
Rare
Abdominal discomfort, vasodilation, paresthesia, acne, dry skin, thirst, arthralgia

■ **Serious Reactions**
- Mirtazapine poses a higher risk of seizures than tricyclic antidepressants, especially in those with no previous history of seizures.
- Overdose may produce cardiovascular effects, such as severe orthostatic hypotension, dizziness, tachycardia, palpitations, and arrhythmias.
- Abrupt discontinuation after prolonged therapy may produce headache, malaise, nausea, vomiting, and vivid dreams.
- Agranulocytosis occurs rarely.

Special Considerations
- Chemical structure unrelated to TCAs, SSRIs, MAOIs
- Shown to be an effective antidepressant in several trials but place in therapy not yet determined
- Manufacturer recommends stopping MAOI 14 days before initiating therapy secondary to interactions between MAOIs and other antidepressants

■ **Patient/Family Education**
- Take mirtazapine as a single bedtime dose
- Avoid alcohol and other sedating medications during therapy
- Avoid tasks that require mental alertness or motor skills until response to the drug has been established

■ **Monitoring Parameters**
- Assess appearance, behavior, level of interest, mood, and sleep pattern to determine the drug's therapeutic effect
- Closely supervise suicidal patients during early therapy; as depression lessens, the patient's energy level improves, increasing the suicide potential
- Monitor for signs and symptoms of hypotension and arrhythmias

- **Geriatric side effects at a glance:**
  ☐ CNS   ☐ Bowel Dysfunction   ☐ Bladder Dysfunction   ☑ Falls
  Other: Seizures (rare), agranulocytosis (rare), weight gain (long term)

- **Use with caution in older patients with:** None

- **U.S. Regulatory Considerations**
  ☑ FDA Black Box
  - Because there is an increased risk of suicide in children and adolescents, older adults should also be closely monitored for suicide ideation.
  ☐ OBRA regulated in U.S. Long Term Care

- **Other Uses in Geriatric Patient:** Anxiety symptoms and related disorders

- **Side Effects:**
  Of particular importance in the geriatric patient: None

- **Geriatric Considerations - Summary:** A novel compound, mirtazapine is an effective antidepressant which is highly sedating, and may be useful in the treatment of depressed elderly with anxiety or sleep disturbance. Sexual side effects, common with SSRIs, occur rarely among users of mirtazapine. Like SSRIs, however, weight gain may occur. This drug has not been well studied with respect to fall risk.

- **References:**
  1. Anttila SA, Leinonen EV. A review of the pharmacological and clinical profile of mirtazapine. CNS Drug Rev 2001;7:249-264.
  2. Holm KJ, Markham A. Mirtazapine: a review of its use in major depression. Drugs 1999;57:607-631.

misoprostol

(mye-soe-prost'-ol)

- **Brand Name(s):** Cytotec

  Combinations
  Rx: with diclofenac (Arthrotec)
  Chemical Class: Prostaglandin E_1 analog

- **Clinical Pharmacology:**
  Mechanism of Action: A prostaglandin that inhibits basal, nocturnal gastric acid secretion via direct action on parietal cells. **Therapeutic Effect:** Increases production of protective gastric mucus.
  Pharmacokinetics: Rapidly absorbed from gastrointestinal (GI) tract. Rapidly converted to active metabolite. Primarily excreted in urine. **Half-life:** 20-40 min.

- **Available Forms:**
  - *Tablets:* 100 mcg, 200 mcg (Cytotec).

- **Indications and Dosages:**
  Prevention of NSAID-induced gastric ulcer: PO 100-200 mcg 4 times/day with food.

- **Unlabeled Uses:** Treatment of duodenal ulcer

- **Contraindications:** Hypersensitivity to misoprostol or any component of the formulation

- **Side Effects**
  Frequent
  Abdominal pain, diarrhea
  Occasional
  Nausea, flatulence, dyspepsia, headache
  Rare
  Vomiting, constipation

- **Serious Reactions**
  - Overdosage may produce sedation, tremor, convulsions, dyspnea, palpitations, hypotension, and bradycardia.

Special Considerations
  - Reserve use for those patients at high risk for NSAID-induced ulcer (e.g., history of previous ulcer)
  - Does not prevent NSAID-associated GI pain or discomfort

- **Patient/Family Education**
  - Avoid magnesium-containing antacids

- **Monitoring Parameters**
  - Therapeutic response to therapy

- **Geriatric side effects at a glance:**
  ☐ CNS ☐ Bowel Dysfunction ☐ Bladder Dysfunction ☐ Falls

- **U.S. Regulatory Considerations**
  ☑ FDA Black Box
  - Although not relevant to geriatric patients, this drug is an abortificient.
  ☐ OBRA regulated in U.S. Long Term Care

modafinil

(moe-daf'-ih-nil)

- **Brand Name(s):** Provigil
  Chemical Class: Benzhydrylsulfinylacetamide compound

Clinical Pharmacology:
Mechanism of Action: An alpha$_1$-agonist that may bind to dopamine reuptake carrier sites, increasing alpha activity and decreasing delta, theta, and beta brain wave activity. **Therapeutic Effect:** Reduces the number of sleep episodes and total daytime sleep. **Pharmacokinetics:** Well absorbed. Protein binding: 60%. Widely distributed. Metabolized in the liver. Excreted by the kidneys. Unknown if removed by hemodialysis. **Half-life:** 8-10 hr.

Available Forms:
- *Tablets:* 100 mg, 200 mg.

Indications and Dosages:
Narcolepsy, other sleep disorders: PO 200 mg/day.

Unlabeled Uses:
Treatment of attention-deficit/hyperactivity disorder, brain injury-related underarousal, depression, endozepine stupor, multiple sclerosis-related fatigue, parkinson-related fatigue, seasonal affective disorder

Contraindications:
None known.

Side Effects
Frequent
Anxiety, insomnia, nausea
Occasional
Anorexia, diarrhea, dizziness, dry mouth or skin, muscle stiffness, polydipsia, rhinitis, paresthesia, tremor, headache, vomiting

Serious Reactions
- Agitation, excitation, hypertension, and insomnia may occur.

Special Considerations
- Comparisons of modafinil with agents that have proven effective in narcolepsy, including methylphenidate, pemoline, and dextroamphetamine, are needed to clarify its relative safety and efficacy, and place in therapy

Patient/Family Education
- Do not increase the drug dose without physician approval
- Avoid tasks that require mental alertness or motor skills until response to the drug has been established
- Take sips of tepid water and chew sugarless gum to relieve dry mouth

Monitoring Parameters
- *Efficacy:* Daytime sleepiness, daytime sleep episodes, and overall daily performance
- *Toxicity:* Blood pressure

Geriatric side effects at a glance:
☐ CNS ☐ Bowel Dysfunction ☐ Bladder Dysfunction ☐ Falls

U.S. Regulatory Considerations
☑ FDA Black Box
- CNS stimulant use has a high abuse potential with the risk of dependence.
- Misuse may cause sudden death and serious cardiovascular adverse events.
☐ OBRA regulated in U.S. Long Term Care

moexipril hydrochloride

(moe-ex'-i-pril hye-droe-klor'-ide)

■ **Brand Name(s):** Univasc

Combinations
Rx: with hydrochlorothiazide (Uniretic)
Chemical Class: Angiotensin-converting enzyme (ACE) inhibitor, nonsulfhydryl

■ **Clinical Pharmacology:**
Mechanism of Action: An ACE inhibitor that suppresses the renin-angiotensin-aldosterone system and prevents conversion of angiotensin I to angiotensin II, a potent vasoconstrictor; may also inhibit angiotensin II at local vascular and renal sites. **Therapeutic Effect:** Reduces peripheral arterial resistance and lowers BP.
Pharmacokinetics:

Route	Onset	Peak	Duration
PO	1 hr	3–6 hr	24 hr

Incompletely absorbed from the GI tract. Food decreases drug absorption. Rapidly converted to active metabolite. Protein binding: 50%. Primarily recovered in feces, partially excreted in urine. Unknown if removed by dialysis. **Half-life:** 1 hr, metabolite 2–9 hr.

■ **Available Forms:**
- *Tablets:* 7.5 mg, 15 mg.

■ **Indications and Dosages:**
Hypertension: PO For patients not receiving diuretics, initial dose is 7.5 mg once a day 1 hr before meals. Adjust according to BP effect. Maintenance: 7.5–30 mg a day in 1–2 divided doses 1 hr before meals.
Hypertension in patients with impaired renal function: PO 3.75 mg once a day in patients with creatinine clearance of 40 ml/min. Maximum: May titrate up to 15 mg/day.

■ **Contraindications:** History of angioedema from previous treatment with ACE inhibitors

■ **Side Effects**
Occasional
Cough, headache (6%); dizziness (4%); fatigue (3%)
Rare
Flushing, rash, myalgia, nausea, vomiting

■ **Serious Reactions**
- Excessive hypotension ("first-dose syncope") may occur in patients with CHF and in those who are severely salt or volume depleted.
- Angioedema (swelling of face and lips) and hyperkalemia occur rarely.
- Agranulocytosis and neutropenia may be noted in those with collagen vascular disease, including scleroderma and systemic lupus erythematosus, and impaired renal function.

- Nephrotic syndrome may be noted in those with history of renal disease.
- Hypoglycemia may occur in patients with diabetes using glucose-lowering drugs.

■ Patient/Family Education
- Caution with salt substitutes containing potassium chloride
- Rise slowly to sitting/standing position to minimize orthostatic hypotension
- Dizziness, fainting, light-headedness may occur during first few days of therapy
- May cause altered taste perception or cough; persistent dry cough usually does not subside unless medication is stopped; notify clinician if these symptoms persist
- Do not abruptly discontinue the drug
- Notify the physician if chest pain, cough, difficulty breathing, fever, sore throat, or swelling of the eyes, face, feet, hands, lips, or tongue occurs

■ Monitoring Parameters
- BUN, creatinine, potassium within 2 wk after initiation of therapy (increased levels may indicate acute renal failure)
- Blood pressure, WBC count

■ Geriatric side effects at a glance:
❑ CNS   ❑ Bowel Dysfunction   ❑ Bladder Dysfunction   ❑ Falls

■ U.S. Regulatory Considerations
☑ FDA Black Box

Although not relevant for geriatric patients, teratogenicity is associated with the use of ACE inhibitors.

❑ OBRA regulated in U.S. Long Term Care

molindone hydrochloride

(moe-lin'-done hye-droe-klor'-ide)

■ Brand Name(s): Moban
Chemical Class: Dihydroindolone derivative

■ Clinical Pharmacology:
Mechanism of Action: An indole derivative of dihydroindole compounds that reduces spontaneous locomotion and aggressiveness. Therapeutic Effect: Suppresses behavioral response in psychosis.

Pharmacokinetics: Rapidly absorbed from the gastrointestinal (GI) tract. Metabolized in liver. Excreted in feces, and a small amount excreted via lungs as carbon dioxide. Not removed by dialysis. Half-life: unknown.

■ Available Forms:
- Oral Solution: 20 mg/ml.
- Tablets: 5 mg, 10 mg, 25 mg, 50 mg, 100 mg.

- **Indications and Dosages:**
    Schizophrenia: PO Initially, 50-75 mg/day, increased to 100 mg/day in 3-4 days (mild psychosis): Maintenance 5-15 mg 3-4 times/day (moderate psychosis): Maintenance 10-25 mg 3-4 times/day (severe psychosis): Maintenance 225 mg/day maximum in divided doses.

- **Contraindications:** Severe central nervous system (CNS) depression, hypersensitivity to molindone or any component of the formulation

- **Side Effects**
    Frequent
    Blurred vision, constipation, drowsiness, headache, extrapyramidal symptoms
    Occasional
    Mental depression
    Rare
    Skin rash, hot and dry skin, inability to sweat, muscle weakness, confusion, jaundice, convulsions

- **Serious Reactions**
    - Neuroleptic malignant syndrome or tardive dyskinesia has been reported.

Special Considerations

  - Neuroleptic structurally different from the phenothiazines, thioxanthenes, and butyrophenones
  - High potency with high incidence of EPS, but a low incidence of sedation, anticholinergic effects, and cardiovascular effects

- **Patient/Family Education**
    - Do not abruptly discontinue molindone after long-term therapy
    - Notify the physician if high fever, muscle stiffness, fast or irregular heartbeat, unexplained weakness or tiredness, muscle spasms, twitching, or uncontrolled tongue movements occur
    - Drowsiness usually subsides with continued therapy
    - Avoid alcohol and CNS depressants

- **Monitoring Parameters**
    - CBC
    - Liver and renal function tests

- **Geriatric side effects at a glance:**
    ☑ CNS   ☑ Bowel Dysfunction   ☐ Bladder Dysfunction   ☑ Falls
    Other: Orthostatic hypotension, cardiac conduction disturbances, anticholinergic side effects

- **Use with caution in older patients with:** Parkinson's disease (an atypical antipsychotic is recommended), seizure disorders, cardiovascular disease with conduction disturbance, hepatic encephalopathy, narrow-angle glaucoma

- **U.S. Regulatory Considerations**
    ☐ FDA Black Box   ☑ OBRA regulated in U.S. Long Term Care

- **Other Uses in Geriatric Patient:** Behavior disturbances in the setting of dementia

Side Effects:

Of particular importance in the geriatric patient: Tardive dyskinesia, akathisia (may appear to exacerbate behavioral disturbances), anticholinergic effects, may increase risk of sudden death

Geriatric Considerations - Summary:
Sink and colleagues' systematic review showed statistically significant improvements on neuropsychiatric and behavioral scales for some drugs, but improvements were small and unlikely to be clinically important. Because of documented risks, and uncertain benefits, these agents should be used with caution in demented elderly persons, with frequent monitoring for side effects and a low threshold for discontinuing use.

References:
1. Leipzig RM, Cumming RG, Tinetti ME. Drugs and falls in older people: a systematic review and meta-analysis: I. Psychotropic drugs. J Am Geriatr Soc 1999;47:30-39.
2. Sink KM, Holden KF, Yaffe K. Pharmacological treatment of neuropsychiatric symptoms of dementia: a review of the evidence. JAMA 2005;293:596-608.
3. Ray WA, Meredith S, Thapa PB, et al. Antipsychotics and the risk of sudden cardiac death. Arch Gen Psychiatry 2001;58:1161-1167.

mometasone furoate monohydrate

(mo-met'-a-zone fyoo-roe'-ate mon-oh-hi'-drayte)

Brand Name(s): Asmanex Twisthaler, Elocon, Nasonex
Chemical Class: Corticosteroid, synthetic

Clinical Pharmacology:
Mechanism of Action: An adrenocorticosteroid that inhibits the release of inflammatory cells into nasal tissue, preventing early activation of the allergic reaction. **Therapeutic Effect:** Decreases response to seasonal and perennial rhinitis.
Pharmacokinetics: Undetectable in plasma. Protein binding: 98%–99%. The swallowed portion undergoes extensive metabolism. Excreted primarily through bile and, to a lesser extent, urine. **Half-life:** 5.8 hr (nasal).

Available Forms:
- *Nasal Spray (Nasonex):* 50 mcg/spray.
- *Cream (Elocon):* 0.1%.
- *Lotion (Elocon):* 0.1%.
- *Ointment (Elocon):* 0.1%.
- *Oral Inhaler (Asmanex Twisthaler):* 220 mcg.

Indications and Dosages:
Allergic rhinitis: Nasal Spray 2 sprays in each nostril once a day.

819

Asthma: Inhalation Initially, inhale 220 mcg (1 puff) once a day. Maximum: 880 mcg once a day.
Skin disease: Topical Apply cream, lotion, or ointment to affected area once a day.
Nasal polyp: Nasal spray 2 sprays in each nostril twice a day.

■ **Contraindications:** Hypersensitivity to any corticosteroid, persistently positive sputum cultures for *Candida albicans*, status asthmaticus (inhalation), systemic fungal infections, untreated localized infection involving nasal mucosa.

■ **Side Effects**
Occasional
Inhalation: Headache, allergic rhinitis, upper respiratory infection, muscle pain, fatigue
Nasal: Nasal irritation, stinging
Topical: Burning
Rare
Inhalation: Abdominal pain, dyspepsia, nausea
Nasal: Nasal or pharyngeal candidiasis
Topical: Pruritus

■ **Serious Reactions**
- An acute hypersensitivity reaction, including urticaria, angioedema, and severe bronchospasm, occurs rarely.
- Transfer from systemic to local steroid therapy may unmask previously suppressed bronchial asthma condition.

■ **Patient/Family Education**
- Symptoms should start to improve within 2 days of the first dose but the drug's maximum benefit may take up to 2 wk to appear
- Notify the physician of nasal irritation or if symptoms, such as sneezing, fail to improve

■ **Monitoring Parameters**
- Pulse rate and quality, ABG levels, and respiratory rate, depth, rhythm, and type

■ **Geriatric side effects at a glance:**
❏ CNS   ❏ Bowel Dysfunction   ❏ Bladder Dysfunction   ❏ Falls

■ **U.S. Regulatory Considerations**
❏ FDA Black Box   ❏ OBRA regulated in U.S. Long Term Care

monobenzone

(mon-oh-benz'-one)

■ **Brand Name(s):** Benoquin
  Chemical Class: Hydroquinone derivative

■ **Clinical Pharmacology:**
  Mechanism of Action: The mechanism of action is not fully understood. Monobenzone may be converted to hydroquinone, which inhibits the enzymatic oxidation of tyrosine to DOPA; it may have a direct action on tyrosinase, or it may act as an antioxidant to prevent SH-group oxidation so that more SH groups are available to inhibit tyrosinase. **Therapeutic Effect:** Depigmentation in extensive vitiligo.
  Pharmacokinetics: Not fully understood. Initial response occurs in 1-4 mo.

■ **Available Forms:**
  • *Cream*: 20%.

■ **Indications and Dosages:**
  Vitiligo: Topical Apply 2-3 times/day to affected area.

■ **Contraindications:** History of hypersensitivity to monobenzone or any of its components.

■ **Side Effects**
  Occasional
  Irritation, burning sensation, dermatitis

■ **Serious Reactions**
  • None known.

■ **Patient/Family Education**
  • Drug is not a mild cosmetic bleach; treated areas should not be exposed to sunlight (protect with a topical sunscreen)
  • Notify the physician of irritation or burning
  • Monobenzone is for external use only

■ **Monitoring Parameters**
  • Skin for irritation

■ **Geriatric side effects at a glance:**
  ❑ CNS ❑ Bowel Dysfunction ❑ Bladder Dysfunction ❑ Falls

■ **U.S. Regulatory Considerations**
  ❑ FDA Black Box ❑ OBRA regulated in U.S. Long Term Care

montelukast sodium

(mon-te'-loo-kast soe'-dee-um)

■ **Brand Name(s):** Singulair
  Chemical Class: Cyclopropaneacetic acid derivative

■ **Clinical Pharmacology:**
  Mechanism of Action: An antiasthmatic that binds to cysteinyl leukotriene receptors, inhibiting the effects of leukotrienes on bronchial smooth muscle. **Therapeutic Effect:** Decreases bronchoconstriction, vascular permeability, mucosal edema, and mucus production.
  Pharmacokinetics:

Route	Onset	Peak	Duration
PO	N/A	N/A	24 hr
PO (chewable)	N/A	N/A	24 hr

  Rapidly absorbed from the GI tract. Protein binding: 99%. Extensively metabolized in the liver. Excreted almost exclusively in feces. **Half-life:** 2.7–5.5 hr (slightly longer in the elderly).

■ **Available Forms:**
  • *Oral Granules:* 4 mg.
  • *Tablets:* 10 mg.
  • *Tablets (Chewable):* 4 mg, 5 mg.

■ **Indications and Dosages:**
  Bronchial asthma, perennial allergic rhinitis, seasonal allergic rhinitis: PO One 10-mg tablet a day, taken in the evening.

■ **Contraindications:** None known.

■ **Side Effects**
  Frequent (18%)
  Headache
  Occasional (4%)
  Influenza
  Rare (3%–2%)
  Abdominal pain, cough, dyspepsia, dizziness, fatigue, dental pain

■ **Serious Reactions**
  • None known.

■ **Patient/Family Education**
  • Take regularly, even during symptom-free periods
  • Do not alter the dosage or abruptly discontinue other asthma medications
  • Montelukast is not intended to treat acute asthma attacks
  • Drink plenty of fluids to decrease the thickness of lung secretions

- Patients with aspirin sensitivity should avoid aspirin and NSAIDs while taking montelukast

■ **Monitoring Parameters**
- Pulmonary function tests
- Pulse rate and quality as well as respiratory depth, rate, rhythm, and type
- Auscultate the patient's breath sounds for crackles, rhonchi, and wheezing
- Observe the patient's fingernails and lips for a blue or dusky color in light-skinned patients and a gray color in dark-skinned patients, which may be signs of hypoxemia

■ **Geriatric side effects at a glance:**
  ❑ CNS ❑ Bowel Dysfunction ❑ Bladder Dysfunction ❑ Falls

■ **U.S. Regulatory Considerations**
  ❑ FDA Black Box ❑ OBRA regulated in U.S. Long Term Care

moricizine hydrochloride

(mor-i'-siz-een hye-droe-klor'-ide)

■ **Brand Name(s):** Ethmozine
  Chemical Class: Phenothiazine derivative

■ **Clinical Pharmacology:**
  Mechanism of Action: An antiarrhythmic that prevents sodium current across myocardial cell membranes. Has potent local anesthetic activity and membrane stabilizing effects. Slows AV and His-Purkinje conduction and decreases action potential duration and effective refractory period. **Therapeutic Effect:** Suppresses ventricular arrhythmias.
  Pharmacokinetics: Almost completely absorbed from the GI tract. Protein binding: 92%-95%. Extensively metabolized in liver. Excreted in urine. **Half-life:** 2 hr.

■ **Available Forms:**
- *Tablets:* 200 mg, 250 mg, 300 mg.

■ **Indications and Dosages:**
  Arrhythmias: PO 200–300 mg q8h. May increase by 150 mg/day at no less than 3-day intervals.

■ **Unlabeled Uses:** Atrial arrhythmias, complete and nonsustained ventricular arrhythmias, premature ventricular contractions (PVCs)

■ **Contraindications:** Cardiogenic shock, preexisting second- or third-degree AV block or right bundle-branch block without pacemaker

■ **Side Effects**
  Frequent (15%–6%)
  Dizziness, nausea, headache, fatigue, dyspnea

823

Occasional (5%–2%)
Nervousness, paresthesia, sleep disturbances, dyspepsia, vomiting, diarrhea

■ **Serious Reactions**
  • Moricizine may worsen existing arrhythmias or produce new ones.
  • Jaundice with hepatitis occurs rarely.
  • Overdosage produces vomiting, lethargy, syncope, hypotension, conduction disturbances, exacerbation of CHF, MI, and sinus arrest.

Special Considerations
  • Antidysrhythmic therapy has not been proven to be beneficial in terms of improving survival among patients with asymptomatic or mildly symptomatic ventricular dysrhythmias
  • Studied in the CAST (Cardiac Arrhythmia Suppression Trial, I and II) with findings of excessive cardiac mortality and no benefit on long-term survival compared to placebo
  • Initiate therapy in facilities capable of providing continuous ECG monitoring and managing life-threatening dysrhythmias

■ **Patient/Family Education**
  • Do not abruptly discontinue the drug
  • Notify the physician if chest pain or irregular heartbeats occur

■ **Monitoring Parameters**
  • ECG for cardiac changes, especially increase in PR and QRS intervals
  • Pulse rate for quality and irregularity
  • Electrolytes, intake and output
  • Liver and renal function

■ **Geriatric side effects at a glance:**
  ❑ CNS   ❑ Bowel Dysfunction   ❑ Bladder Dysfunction   ❑ Falls

■ **U.S. Regulatory Considerations**
  ☑ FDA Black Box
  Because of proarrhythmic effects demonstrated in CAST trials, this agent should be used only in patients with life-threatening arrhythmias.
  ❑ OBRA regulated in U.S. Long Term Care

morphine sulfate

(mor'-feen sul'-fate)

■ **Brand Name(s):** Astramorph PF, Avinza, DepoDur, Duramorph PF, Infumorph, Kadian, M-Eslon, MS Contin, MSIR, MS/S, Oramorph SR, Rapi-Ject, RMS, Roxanol, Roxanol-T
  Chemical Class: Natural opium alkaloid; phenanthrene derivative

Clinical Pharmacology:

Mechanism of Action: An opioid agonist that binds with opioid receptors in the CNS. **Therapeutic Effect:** Alters the perception of and emotional response to pain; produces generalized CNS depression.

Pharmacokinetics:

Route	Onset	Peak	Duration
Oral Solution	N/A	1 hr	3–5 hr
Tablets	N/A	1 hr	3–5 hr
Tablets (ER)	N/A	3–4 hr	8–12 hr
IV	Rapid	0.3 hr	3–5 hr
IM	5–30 min	0.5–1 hr	3–5 hr
Epidural	N/A	1 hr	12–20 hr
Subcutaneous	N/A	1.1–5 hr	3–5 hr
Rectal	N/A	0.5–1 hr	3–7 hr

Variably absorbed from the GI tract. Readily absorbed after IM or subcutaneous administration. Protein binding: 20%–35%. Widely distributed. Metabolized in the liver. Primarily excreted in urine. Removed by hemodialysis. **Half-life:** 2–3 hr (increased in patients with hepatic disease)

Available Forms:

- *Capsules (Extended-Release):* 20 mg (Kadian), 30 mg (Avinza, Kadian), 50 mg (Kadian), 60 mg (Avinza, Kadian), 90 mg (Avinza), 100 mg (Kadian), 120 mg (Avinza).
- *Capsules (MSIR):* 15 mg, 30 mg.
- *Solution for Injection:* 0.5 mg/ml, 1 mg/ml, 2 mg/ml, 4 mg/ml, 5 mg/ml, 8 mg/ml, 10 mg/ml, 15 mg/ml, 25 mg/ml, 50 mg/ml.
- *Solution for Injection:* 5% dextrose-20 mg morphine/100 ml, 5% dextrose-100 mg morphine/100 ml.
- *Solution for Injection (Preservative-Free):* 0.5 mg/ml (Astramorph PF, Duramorph PF), 1 mg/ml (Astramorph PF, Duramorph PF), 10 mg/ml (Infumorph), 15 mg/ml, 25 mg/ml (Infumorph), 50 mg/ml.
- *Epidural and Intrathecal via Infusion Device (Infumorph):* 10 mg/ml, 25 mg/ml.
- *Oral Solution:* 10 mg/ml (MSIR), 20 mg/ml (MSIR, Roxanol), 100 mg/ml (Roxanol).
- *Suppositories (RMS):* 5 mg, 10 mg, 20 mg, 30 mg.
- *Tablets (MSIR):* 15 mg, 30 mg.
- *Tablets (Extended-Release):* 15 mg (MS Contin, Oramorph SR), 30 mg (MS Contin, Oramorph SR), 60 mg (MS Contin, Oramorph SR), 100 mg (MS Contin, Oramorph SR), 200 mg (MS Contin).
- *Liposomal Injection (DepoDur):* 10 mg/ml, 15 mg/1.5 ml, 20 mg/2 ml.

Indications and Dosages: Alert Dosage should be titrated to desired effect.

Analgesia: PO (Prompt-release) 10–30 mg q3-4h as needed. **Alert** For the Avinza dosage information below, be aware that this drug is to be administered once a day only **Alert** For the Kadian dosage information below, be aware that this drug is to be administered q12h or once a day only. **Alert** Be aware that pediatric dosages of extended-release preparations Kadian and Avinza have not been established. **Alert** For the MS Contin and Oramorph SR dosage information below, be aware that the daily dosage is divided and given q8h or q12h. PO (Extended-Release [Avinza]) Dosage requirement should be established using prompt-release formulations and is based on total daily dose. Avinza is given once a day only. PO (Extended-Release [Kadian]) Dosage requirement should be established using prompt-release formulations and is based on total daily dose. Dose is given once a day or divided and given q12h. PO (Extended-Release [MS Contin, Oramorph SR]) Dosage requirement should be established using prompt-release formulations and is based on total daily dose. Daily dose is divided and given q8h or q12h. IV 2.5-5 mg q3-4h as needed. Note: Repeated doses (e.g. 1-2 mg) may be given more frequently (e.g., every hour) if needed. IV Continuous Infusion 0.8-10 mg/h. Range: Up to 80 mg/h. IM 5-10 mg q3-4h as needed. Epidural Initially, 1-6 mg bolus, infusion rate: 0.1-1 mg/h. Maximum: 10 mg/24 h. Intrathecal One-tenth of the epidural dose: 0.2–1 mg/dose.

PCA: IV Loading dose: 5–10 mg. Intermittent bolus: 0.5–3 mg. Lockout interval: 5–12 min. Continuous infusion: 1–10 mg/h. 4-hr limit: 20–30 mg.

■ **Contraindications:** Acute or severe asthma, GI obstruction, paralytic ileus, severe hepatic or renal impairment, severe respiratory depression

■ **Side Effects**

Frequent

Sedation, decreased BP (including orthostatic hypotension), diaphoresis, facial flushing, constipation, dizziness, somnolence, nausea, vomiting

Occasional

Allergic reaction (rash, pruritus), dyspnea, confusion, palpitations, tremors, urine retention, abdominal cramps, vision changes, dry mouth, headache, decreased appetite, pain or burning at injection site

Rare

Paralytic ileus

■ **Serious Reactions**

- Overdose results in respiratory depression, skeletal muscle flaccidity, cold or clammy skin, cyanosis, and extreme somnolence progressing to seizures, stupor, and coma.
- The patient who uses morphine repeatedly may develop a tolerance to the drug's analgesic effect and physical dependence.
- The drug may have a prolonged duration of action and cumulative effect in those with hepatic and renal impairment.

Special Considerations

- *Treatment of overdose:* Naloxone (Narcan) 0.2-0.8 mg IV
- Remains the strong analgesic of choice for acute, severe pain, acute MI pain, and the agent of choice for chronic cancer pain
- 200-mg sustained-action tablet for use only in opioid-tolerant patients
- Do not administer agonist/antagonist analgesics (i.e., pentazocine, nalbuphine, butorphanol, dezocine, buprenorphine) to patient who has received a prolonged course of morphine (a pure agonist). In opioid-dependent patients, mixed agonist/anagonist analgesics may precipitate withdrawal symptoms

■ **Patient/Family Education**

- Change position slowly to avoid orthostasis
- Avoid alcohol and other CNS depressants
- Physical dependency may result
- Do not chew or crush sustained-action preparations
- Injection of morphine may cause discomfort
- Avoid tasks that require mental alertness or motor skills until response to the drug has been established

- Vital signs for 5 to 10 minutes after IV administration and 15 to 30 minutes after IM or subcutaneous injection
- Pattern of daily bowel activity and stool consistency
- Clinical improvement, and record the onset of pain relief

■ **Geriatric side effects at a glance:**
☑ CNS ☑ Bowel Dysfunction ☑ Bladder Dysfunction ☑ Falls

■ **U.S. Regulatory Considerations**
☑ FDA Black Box
Extended-release formulation (Avinza) is once daily only and must be swallowed whole and not taken with alcohol.
☑ OBRA regulated in U.S. Long Term Care

moxifloxacin hydrochloride

(mox-ee-flox'-a-sin hye-droe-klor'-ide)

■ **Brand Name(s):** Avelox, Avelox IV, Vigamox
Chemical Class: Fluoroquinolone derivative

■ **Clinical Pharmacology:**
Mechanism of Action: A fluoroquinolone that inhibits two enzymes, topoisomerase II and IV, in susceptible microorganisms. **Therapeutic Effect:** Interferes with bacterial DNA replication. Prevents or delays emergence of resistant organisms. Bactericidal. **Pharmacokinetics:** Well absorbed from the GI tract after PO administration. Protein binding: 50%. Widely distributed throughout body with tissue concentration often exceeding plasma concentration. Metabolized in liver. Primarily excreted in urine with a lesser amount in feces. **Half-life:** 10.7–13.3 hr.

■ **Available Forms:**
- *Tablets* (*Avelox*) : 400 mg.
- *Injection* (*Avelox* IV): 400 mg.
- *Ophthalmic Solution* (*Vigamox*): 0.5%.

■ **Indications and Dosages:**
Acute bacterial sinusitis: PO, IV 400 mg q24h for 10 days.
Acute bacterial exacerbation of chronic bronchitis: PO, IV 400 mg q24h for 5 days.
Community-acquired pneumonia: IV, PO 400 mg q24h for 7-14 days.
Skin and skin-structure infection: PO, IV 400 mg once a day for 7 days.
Topical treatment of bacterial conjunctivitis due to susceptible strains of bacteria: Ophthalmic 1 drop 3 times a day for 7 days.

■ **Contraindications:** Hypersensitivity to quinolones

■ **Side Effects**
Frequent (8%–6%)
Nausea, diarrhea

Occasional (3%–2%)
Dizziness, headache, abdominal pain, vomiting
Ophthalmic (6%–1%): conjunctival irritation, reduced visual acuity, dry eye, keratitis, eye pain, ocular itching, swelling of tissue around cornea, eye discharge, fever, cough, pharyngitis, rash, rhinitis
Rare (1%)
Change in sense of taste, dyspepsia (heartburn, indigestion), photosensitivity

■ **Serious Reactions**
- Pseudomembranous colitis as evidenced by fever, severe abdominal cramps or pain, and severe watery diarrhea may occur.
- Superinfection manifested as anal or genital pruritus, moderate to severe diarrhea, and stomatitis may occur.
- Tendon effects, including ruptures of shoulder, hand, Achilles tendon or other tendons, may occur. Risk increases with concomitant corticosteroid use, especially in the elderly.

■ **Patient/Family Education**
- May be taken with or without meals
- Should be taken at least 4 hr before or 8 hr after multivitamins (containing iron or zinc), antacids (containing magnesium, calcium, or aluminum), sucralfate, or didanosine chewable/buffered tablets
- Discontinue treatment, rest and refrain from exercise, and inform prescriber if pain, inflammation, or rupture of a tendon occurs
- Test reaction to this drug before operating an automobile or machinery or engaging in activities requiring mental alertness or coordination
- Drink plenty of fluids
- Avoid exposure to direct sunlight as this may cause a photosensitivity reaction
- Take for the full course of therapy

■ **Monitoring Parameters**
- WBC count
- Signs of infection
- Pattern of daily bowel activity and stool consistency
- Evaluate for abdominal pain, altered sense of taste, dyspepsia (heartburn, indigestion), headache, and vomiting

■ **Geriatric side effects at a glance:**
☑ CNS ☑ Bowel Dysfunction ☐ Bladder Dysfunction ☐ Falls

■ **U.S. Regulatory Considerations**
☐ FDA Black Box ☐ OBRA regulated in U.S. Long Term Care

mupirocin

(myoo-pye'-roe-sin)

■ **Brand Name(s):** Bactroban
   Chemical Class: Pseudomonic acid derivative

■ **Clinical Pharmacology:**
   Mechanism of Action: An antibacterial agent that inhibits bacterial protein, RNA synthesis. Less effective on DNA synthesis. Nasal: Eradicates nasal colonization of MRSA. **Therapeutic Effect:** Prevents bacterial growth and replication. Bacteriostatic.
   Pharmacokinetics: Metabolized in skin to inactive metabolite. Transported to skin surface; removed by normal skin desquamation.

■ **Available Forms:**
   • *Ointment*: 2% (Bactroban).
   • *Nasal Ointment*: 2% (Bactroban).

■ **Indications and Dosages:**
   Impetigo, infected traumatic skin lesions: Topical Apply 3 times/day (may cover w/gauze).
   Nasal colonization of resistant Staphylococcus aureus: Intranasal Apply 2 times/day for 5 days.

■ **Unlabeled Uses:** Treatment of infected eczema, folliculitis, minor bacterial skin infections.

■ **Contraindications:** Hypersensitivity to mupirocin or any component of the formulation

■ **Side Effects**
   Frequent
   Nasal: Headache, rhinitis, upper respiratory congestion, pharyngitis, altered taste
   Occasional
   Nasal: Burning, stinging, cough
   Topical: Pain, burning, stinging, itching
   Rare
   Nasal: Pruritus, diarrhea, dry mouth, epistaxis, nausea, rash
   Topical: Rash, nausea, dry skin, contact dermatitis

■ **Serious Reactions**
   • Superinfection may result in bacterial or fungal infections, especially with prolonged or repeated therapy.

Special Considerations
   • Comparable efficacy to systemic semisynthetic penicillins and erythromycin in impetigo and infected wounds

Patient/Family Education
- For external use only
- Notify the physician if skin reaction or irritation occurs
- If there is no improvement in 3-5 days, see the physician to be reevaluated

Monitoring Parameters
- Skin for irritation

Geriatric side effects at a glance:
❑ CNS ❑ Bowel Dysfunction ❑ Bladder Dysfunction ❑ Falls

U.S. Regulatory Considerations
❑ FDA Black Box ❑ OBRA regulated in U.S. Long Term Care

mycophenolate mofetil

(mye-koe-fen'-oh-late moe'-feh-till)

■ **Brand Name(s):** CellCept, Myfortic
Chemical Class: Mycophenolic acid derivative

■ **Clinical Pharmacology:**
Mechanism of Action: An immunologic agent that suppresses the immunologically mediated inflammatory response by inhibiting inosine monophosphate dehydrogenase, an enzyme that deprives lymphocytes of nucleotides necessary for DNA and RNA synthesis, thus inhibiting the proliferation of T and B lymphocytes. **Therapeutic Effect:** Prevents transplant rejection.
Pharmacokinetics: Rapidly and extensively absorbed after PO administration (food decreases drug plasma concentration but doesn't affect absorption). Protein binding: 97%. Completely hydrolyzed to active metabolite mycophenolic acid. Primarily excreted in urine. Not removed by hemodialysis. **Half-life:** 17.9 hr.

■ **Available Forms:**
- *Capsules (Cellcept)* : 250 mg.
- *Oral Suspension (Cellcept)*: 200 mg/ml.
- *Tablets (Cellcept)*: 500 mg.
- *Tablets (Delayed-Release [Myfortic])*: 180 mg, 360 mg.
- *Injection (Cellcept)*: 500 mg.

■ **Indications and Dosages:**
Prevention of renal transplant rejection: PO, IV (Cellcept) 1g twice a day. PO (Myfortic) 720 mg twice a day.
Prevention of heart transplant rejection: PO, IV (Cellcept) 1.5g twice a day.
Prevention of liver transplant rejection: PO (Cellcept) 1.5g twice a day. IV (Cellcept) 1g twice a day.

■ **Unlabeled Uses:** Treatment of liver transplantation rejection, mild heart transplant rejection, moderate to severe psoriasis

- **Contraindications:** Hypersensitivity to mycophenolic acid or polysorbate 80 (IV formulation)

- **Side Effects**

    Frequent (37%–20%)
    UTI, hypertension, peripheral edema, diarrhea, constipation, fever, headache, nausea
    Occasional (18%–10%)
    Dyspepsia; dyspnea; cough; hematuria; asthenia; vomiting; edema; tremors; abdominal, chest, or back pain; oral candidiasis; acne
    Rare (9%–6%)
    Insomnia, respiratory tract infection, rash, dizziness

- **Serious Reactions**
    - Significant anemia, leukopenia, thrombocytopenia, neutropenia, and leukocytosis may occur, particularly in those undergoing reanl transplant rejection.
    - Sepsis and infection occur occasionally.
    - GI tract hemorrhage occurs rarely.
    - Patients receiving mycophenolate have an increased risk of developing neoplasms.
    - Immunosuppression may result in an increased susceptibility to infection and the development of lymphoma.

Special Considerations
    - Drug can be given concurrently with cyclosporine, which may enable reduced cyclosporine doses and lower toxicity, or potential cyclosporine substitute in patients developing cyclosporine toxicity
    - Drug is less likely than azathioprine to induce severe bone marrow depression, and may replace azathioprine in conventional maintenance immunosuppression regimens
    - IV can be administered for up to 14 days; switch to PO as soon as possible

- **Patient/Family Education**
    - Notify the physician if abdominal pain, fever, sore throat, or unusual bleeding or bruising occurs
    - Regular laboratory tests during mycophenolate therapy are essential
    - Malignancies may occur; be prepared to answer questions and provide additional information

- **Monitoring Parameters**
    - CBC qwk × 1 mo, then q2wk × 2 mo, then monthly
    - Reduce the dosage or discontinue the drug if the patient experiences a rapid fall in WBC count

- **Geriatric side effects at a glance:**
    ❑ CNS ❑ Bowel Dysfunction ❑ Bladder Dysfunction ❑ Falls

- **U.S. Regulatory Considerations**
    ☑ FDA Black Box
    - Increased risk of infection
    - Increased risk of lymphoma
    - Should be administered by experienced personnel
    ❑ OBRA regulated in U.S. Long Term Care

nabumetone

(na-byoo'-me-tone)

■ **Brand Name(s):** Relafen
Chemical Class: Acetic acid derivative

■ **Clinical Pharmacology:**
Mechanism of Action: An NSAID that produces analgesic and anti-inflammatory effects by inhibiting prostaglandin synthesis. **Therapeutic Effect:** Reduces the inflammatory response and intensity of pain.
Pharmacokinetics: Readily absorbed from the GI tract. Protein binding: 99%. Widely distributed. Metabolized in the liver to active metabolite. Primarily excreted in urine. Not removed by hemodialysis. **Half-life:** 22–30 hr.

■ **Available Forms:**
• *Tablets*: 500 mg, 750 mg.

■ **Indications and Dosages:**
Acute or chronic rheumatoid arthritis and osteoarthritis: PO Initially, 1,000 mg as a single dose or in 2 divided doses. May increase up to 2,000 mg/day as a single or in 2 divided doses.

■ **Contraindications:** Active peptic ulcer disease, chronic inflammation of GI tract, GI bleeding or ulceration, history of hypersensitivity to aspirin or NSAIDs, history of significant renal impairment

■ **Side Effects**
Frequent (14%–12%)
Diarrhea, abdominal cramps or pain, dyspepsia
Occasional (9%–4%)
Nausea, constipation, flatulence, dizziness, headache
Rare (3%–1%)
Vomiting, stomatitis, confusion

■ **Serious Reactions**
• Overdose may result in acute hypotension and tachycardia.
• Rare reactions with long-term use include peptic ulcer disease, GI bleeding, gastritis, nephrotoxicity (dysuria, cystitis, hematuria, proteinuria, nephrotic syndrome), severe hepatic reactions (cholestasis, jaundice), and severe hypersensitivity reactions (bronchospasm, angioedema).

Special Considerations
• No significant advantage over other NSAIDs; cost should govern use

■ **Patient/Family Education**
• Take nabumetone with food if GI upset occurs
• Nabumetone may cause serious GI bleeding with or without pain; avoid aspirin during nabumetone therapy because it increases the risk of GI bleeding

- Nabumetone may cause confusion or dizziness; avoid performing tasks that require mental alertness or motor skills until response to the drug has been established

■ Monitoring Parameters
- Initial hematocrit and fecal occult blood test within 3 months of starting regular chronic therapy; repeat every 6-12 months (more frequently in high-risk patients (>65 years, peptic ulcer disease, concurrent steroids or anticoagulants); electrolytes, creatinine, and BUN within 3 months of starting regular chronic therapy; repeat every 6-12 months
- Pattern of daily bowel activity
- Therapeutic response, such as improved grip strength, increased joint mobility, and decreased pain, tenderness, stiffness, and swelling

■ Geriatric side effects at a glance:
☑ CNS ☐ Bowel Dysfunction ☐ Bladder Dysfunction ☐ Falls
☑ Other: Gastropathy

■ Use with caution in older patients with: Renal impairment, Hepatic impairment, CHF, HTN, PUD, History of GI bleeding, GERD, Bleeding and platelet disorders, History of aspirin sensitivity reaction. Also use with caution in patients taking Anticoagulants, Aspirin, and Antihypertensive agents.

■ U.S. Regulatory Considerations
☑ FDA Black Box
- Cardiovascular risk
- Gastrointestinal risk
☐ OBRA regulated in U.S. Long Term Care

■ Other Uses in Geriatric Patient: Acute gout

■ Side Effects:
Of particular importance in the geriatric patient: Confusion, cognitive impairment, delirium, dizziness, dyspepsia, fluid retention, renal impairment

■ Geriatric Considerations - Summary: A preferred agent in older adults due to its association with fewer GI adverse effects. Use of NSAIDs in older adults increases the risk of GI complications including gastric ulceration, bleeding, and perforation. These complications are not necessarily preceded by less severe GI symptoms. Concomitant use of a proton pump inhibitor or misoprostol reduces the risk for gastric ulceration and bleeding, but may not prevent long-term GI toxicity. No clinical data exist to support reduced GI toxicity with the use of nabumetone.

■ References:
1. COX-2 alternatives and GI protection. Med Lett Drugs Ther 2004;46:91.
2. Drugs that may cause cognitive disorders in the elderly. Med Lett Drugs Ther 2000;42:111-112.

nadolol

(nay-doe'-lole)

■ **Brand Name(s):** Corgard

    Combinations
    Rx: with Bendroflumethiazide (Corzide)
    Chemical Class: β-Adrenergic blocker, nonselective

■ **Clinical Pharmacology:**
    Mechanism of Action: A nonselective beta-blocker that blocks beta$_1$- and beta$_2$-adrenergic receptors. Large doses increase airway resistance. **Therapeutic Effect:** Slows sinus heart rate, decreases cardiac output and BP. Decreases myocardial ischemia severity by decreasing oxygen requirements.
    Pharmacokinetics: Variable absorption after PO administration. Protein binding: 28%-30%. Not metabolized. Excreted unchanged in feces. **Half-life:** 20-24 hr.

■ **Available Forms:**
    • *Tablets:* 20 mg, 40 mg, 80 mg, 120 mg, 160 mg.

■ **Indications and Dosages:**
    Mild to moderate hypertension, angina: PO Initially, 20 mg/day. May increase gradually. Range: 20–240 mg/day.
    Dosage in renal impairment: Dosage is modified based on creatinine clearance.

Creatinine Clearance	% Usual Dosage
10–50 ml/min	50
less than 10 ml/min	25

■ **Unlabeled Uses:** Treatment of arrhythmias, hypertrophic cardiomyopathy, MI, mitral valve prolapse syndrome, neuroleptic-induced akathisia, pheochromocytoma, tremors, thyrotoxicosis, vascular headaches

■ **Contraindications:** Bronchial asthma, cardiogenic shock, CHF secondary to tachyarrhythmias, chronic obstructive pulmonary disease (COPD), patients receiving MAOI therapy, second- or third-degree heart block, sinus bradycardia, uncontrolled cardiac failure

■ **Side Effects**
    Frequent
    Nadolol is generally well tolerated, with transient and mild side effects.
    Diminished sexual ability, drowsiness, unusual fatigue or weakness
    Occasional
    Bradycardia, difficulty breathing, depression, cold hands or feet, diarrhea, constipation, anxiety, nasal congestion, nausea, vomiting
    Rare
    Altered taste, dry eyes, itching

■ **Serious Reactions**
    • Overdose may produce profound bradycardia and hypotension.

- Abrupt withdrawal of nadolol may result in diaphoresis, palpitations, headache, tremors, exacerbation of angina, MI, and ventricular arrhythmias.
- Nadolol administration may precipitate CHF and MI in patients with cardiac disease; thyroid storm in those with thyrotoxicosis; and peripheral ischemia in those with existing peripheral vascular disease.
- Hypoglycemia may occur in patients with previously controlled diabetes.

Special Considerations
- No unique advantage over less expensive β-blockers

■ Patient/Family Education
- Do **not** discontinue abruptly; may require taper; rapid withdrawal may produce rebound hypertension or angina
- Notify the physician if confusion, depression, difficulty breathing, dizziness, fever, night cough, rash, slow pulse, sore throat, swelling of arms and legs, or unusual bleeding or bruising occurs
- Avoid tasks that require mental alertness or motor skills until response to the drug has been established

■ Monitoring Parameters
- Angina: reduction in nitroglycerin usage; frequency, severity, onset, and duration of angina pain; heart rate
- Arrhythmias: heart rate
- Congestive heart failure: functional status, cough, dyspnea on exertion, paroxysmal nocturnal dyspnea, exercise tolerance, and ventricular function
- Hypertension: blood pressure
- Migraine headache: reduction in the frequency, severity, and duration of attacks
- Post myocardial infarction: left ventricular function, lower resting heart rate
- Toxicity: blood glucose, bronchospasm, hypotension, bradycardia, depression, confusion, hallucination, sexual dysfunction

■ Geriatric side effects at a glance:
❑ CNS ❑ Bowel Dysfunction ❑ Bladder Dysfunction ❑ Falls

■ U.S. Regulatory Considerations
☑ FDA Black Box
In patients using orally administered beta blockers, abrupt withdrawal may precipitate angina or lead to myocardial infarction or ventricular arrhythmias.
❑ OBRA regulated in U.S. Long Term Care

nafcillin sodium

(naf-sill'-in soe'-dee-um)

- **Brand Name(s):** Nafcil, Nallpen, Unipen
  Chemical Class: Penicillin derivative, penicillinase-resistant

- **Clinical Pharmacology:**
  Mechanism of Action: A penicillin that acts as a bactericidal in susceptible microorganisms. **Therapeutic Effect:** Inhibits bacterial cell wall synthesis. Bactericidal.
  Pharmacokinetics: Poorly absorbed from gastrointestinal (GI) tract. Protein binding: 87%-90%. Metabolized in liver. Primarily excreted in urine. Not removed by hemodialysis. **Half-life:** 10.5-1 hr (half-life increased with imparied renal function).

- **Available Forms:**
  - *Tablets:* 500 mg (Unipen).
  - *Capsules:* 250 mg (Unipen).
  - *Powder for Injection:* 1 g, 2 g, 10g (Nafcil, Nallpen, Unipen).

- **Indications and Dosages:**
  Staphylococcal infections: IV 3-6 g/24 hr in divided doses. IM 500 mg q4-6h. PO 250 mg to 1g q4-6h.

- **Unlabeled Uses:** Surgical prophylaxis

- **Contraindications:** Hypersensitivity to any penicillin

- **Side Effects**
  Frequent
  Mild hypersensitivity reaction (fever, rash, pruritus), GI effects (nausea, vomiting, diarrhea) more frequent w/oral administration
  Occasional
  Hypokalemia with high IV doses, phlebitis, thrombophlebitis
  Rare
  Extravasation with IV administration

- **Serious Reactions**
  - Superinfections, potentially fatal antibacterial-associated colitis may result from altered bacterial balance.
  - Hematologic effects (especially involving platelets, WBCs), severe hypersensitivity reactions, and anaphylaxis occur rarely.

Special Considerations
  - Individualize treatment based on local susceptibility patterns.

- **Patient/Family Education**
  - Take for the full length of treatment
  - Notify the physician if diarrhea, rash, or other new symptoms occur

Monitoring Parameters
- Oral nafcillin absorption is erratic (consider alternate oral penicillinase-resistant penicillins)
- CBC, creatinine, and UA for eosinophils during therapy to monitor for adverse effects
- Daily bowel activity and stool consistency. Although mild GI effects may be tolerable, severe symptoms may indicate the onset of antibiotic-associated colitis.
- Signs and symptoms of superinfection include abdominal pain or cramping, anal or genital pruritus or discharge, moderate to severe diarrhea, severe mouth or tongue soreness, and new or increased fever.

Geriatric side effects at a glance:
❑ CNS ☑ Bowel Dysfunction ❑ Bladder Dysfunction ❑ Falls

U.S. Regulatory Considerations
❑ FDA Black Box ❑ OBRA regulated in U.S. Long Term Care

naftifine hydrochloride

(naf'-ti-feen hye-droe-klor'-ide)

Brand Name(s): Naftin
Chemical Class: Allylamine derivative

Clinical Pharmacology:
Mechanism of Action: An antifungal that selectively inhibits the enzyme squalene epoxidase in a dose-dependent manner, which results in the primary sterol, ergosterol, within the fungal membrane not being synthesized. **Therapeutic Effect:** Results in fungal cell death. Fungistatic and fungicidal.
Pharmacokinetics: Minimal systemic absorption. Metabolized in the liver. Excreted in the urine as well as the feces and bile. **Half-life:** 48-72 hr.

Available Forms:
- **Gel:** 1% (Naftin).
- **Cream:** 1% (Naftin).

Indications and Dosages:
Tinea pedis, T. cruris, T. corporis: Topical Apply cream 1 time a day for 4 weeks or until signs and symptoms significantly improve. Apply gel 2 times a day for 4 weeks or until signs and symptoms significantly improve.

Unlabeled Uses: Trichomycosis

Contraindications: Hypersensitivity to naftifine or any of its components

Side Effects
Frequent
Burning, stinging

Occasional
Erythema, itching, dryness, irritation

■ **Serious Reactions**
  • Excessive irritation may indicate hypersensitivity reaction.

Special Considerations
  • First of a new class of antifungals (allylamine derivatives) unrelated to imidazoles
  • Because of fungicidal activity at low concentrations, may provide quicker onset of healing, enhance patient compliance with qd therapy

■ **Patient/Family Education**
  • Wash hands after application
  • Do not use occlusive dressings unless directed to do so

■ **Monitoring Parameters**
  • Skin for signs of therapeutic response

■ **Geriatric side effects at a glance:**
  ❑ CNS ❑ Bowel Dysfunction ❑ Bladder Dysfunction ❑ Falls

■ **U.S. Regulatory Considerations**
  ❑ FDA Black Box ❑ OBRA regulated in U.S. Long Term Care

nalbuphine hydrochloride

(nal'-byoo-feen hye-droe-klor'-ide)

■ **Brand Name(s):** Nubain
  Chemical Class: Opiate derivative; phenanthrene derivative

■ **Clinical Pharmacology:**
  Mechanism of Action: A narcotic agonist-antagonist that binds with opioid receptors in the CNS. May displace opioid agonists and competitively inhibit their action; may precipitate withdrawal symptoms. **Therapeutic Effect:** Alters the perception of and emotional response to pain.
  Pharmacokinetics:

Route	Onset	Peak	Duration
IV	2- 3 min	30 min	3-6 hr
IM	less than 15 min	60 min	3-6 hr
Subcutaneous	less than 15 min	N/A	3-6 hr

  Well absorbed after IM or subcutaneous administration. Protein binding: 50%. Metabolized in the liver. Primarily eliminated in feces by biliary secretion. **Half-life:** 3.5-5 hr.

■ **Available Forms:**
  • *Injection*: 10 mg/ml, 20 mg/ml.

■ Indications and Dosages:
Analgesia: IV, IM, Subcutaneous 10 mg q3-6h as needed. Don't exceed maximum single dose of 20 mg or daily dose of 160 mg. For patients receiving long-term narcotic analgesics of similar duration of action, give 25% of usual dose.
Supplement to anesthesia: IV Induction: 0.3-3 mg/kg over 10-15 min. Maintenance: 0.25-0.5 mg/kg as needed.

■ Contraindications: Respiratory rate less than 12 breaths/minute

■ Side Effects
Frequent (35%)
Sedation
Occasional (9%-3%)
Diaphoresis, cold and clammy skin, nausea, vomiting, dizziness, vertigo, dry mouth, headache
Rare (less than 1%)
Restlessness, emotional lability, paresthesia, flushing, paradoxical reaction

■ Serious Reactions
- Abrupt withdrawal after prolonged use may produce symptoms of narcotic withdrawal, such as abdominal cramping, rhinorrhea, lacrimation, anxiety, fever, and piloerection (goose bumps).
- Overdose results in severe respiratory depression, skeletal muscle flaccidity, cyanosis, and extreme somnolence progressing to seizures, stupor, and coma.
- Repeated use may result in drug tolerance and physical dependence.

Special Considerations
- Proposed, but not significant, advantages include low abuse potential, low respiratory depressant effects, low incidence of psychomimetic toxicity, and a lower incidence of hemodynamic toxicity

■ Patient/Family Education
- The patient should alert you as soon as pain occurs and should not wait until the pain is unbearable because nalbuphine is more effective when given at the onset of pain
- Nalbuphine may be habit-forming
- Avoid alcohol and CNS depressants
- Avoid tasks that require mental alertness or motor skills until response to the drug has been established
- Nalbuphine may cause dry mouth

■ Monitoring Parameters
- Blood pressure, pulse rate, respiratory rate
- Pattern of daily bowel activity and stool consistency
- Clinical improvement, record the onset of relief of pain

■ Geriatric side effects at a glance:
❏ CNS ☑ Bowel Dysfunction ❏ Bladder Dysfunction ❏ Falls

■ U.S. Regulatory Considerations
❏ FDA Black Box ❏ OBRA regulated in U.S. Long Term Care

nalmefene hydrochloride

(nal'-me-feen hye-droe-klor'-ide)

■ **Brand Name(s):** Revex
   Chemical Class: Thebaine derivative

■ **Clinical Pharmacology:**
   Mechanism of Action: A narcotic antagonist that binds to opioid receptors. **Therapeutic Effect:** Prevents and reverses effects of opioids (respiratory depression, sedation, hypotension).
   Pharmacokinetics: Well absorbed. Protein binding: 45%. Metabolized primarily via glucuronidation. Excreted in urine and feces. **Half-life:** 8.5-10.8 hr.

■ **Available Forms:**
   • *Solution for Injection*: 100 mcg/ml ([blue label] Revex), 1,000 mcg/ml ([green label] Revex)

■ **Indications and Dosages:**
   Solution for Injection: 100 mcg/ml ([blue label] Revex), 1,000 mcg/ml ([green label] Revex): IV, IM, Subcutaneous Initially, 0.25 mcg/kg followed by additional 0.25 mcg doses at 2- to 5-min intervals until desired response. Cumulative doses >1 mcg/kg do not provide additional therapeutic effect.
   Known or suspected opioid overdose: IV, IM, Subcutaneous Initially, 0.5 mg/70 kg. May give 1 mg/70 kg in 2-5 min. If physical opioid dependence suspected, initial dose is 0.1 mg/70 kg.

■ **Contraindications:** Hypersensitivity to nalmefene

■ **Side Effects**
   Frequent
   Nausea, headache, hypertension
   Occasional
   Postop pain, fever, dizziness, headache, chills, hypotension, vasodilation

■ **Serious Reactions**
   • Signs and symptoms of opioid withdrawal include stuffy or runny nose, tearing, yawning, sweating, tremor, vomiting, piloerection, feeling of temperature change, joint, bone or muscle pain, abdominal cramps, and feeling of skin crawling.

Special Considerations
   • Longer duration of action than naloxone at fully reversing doses; agent of choice in instances where prolonged opioid effects are predicted, including overdose with longer-acting opioids (e.g., methadone, propoxyphene), patients given large doses of opioids, and those with liver disease or renal failure (eliminating the need for continuous infusions of naloxone and prolonged observation periods after outpatient procedures)

■ **Patient/Family Education**
   • Notify the physician of abdominal pain, dark-colored urine, white bowel movements, or yellow coloration of sclerae

- **Monitoring Parameters**
  - Observe patient until there is no reasonable risk of recurrent respiratory depression

- **Geriatric side effects at a glance:**
  - ❏ CNS   ❏ Bowel Dysfunction   ❏ Bladder Dysfunction   ❏ Falls

- **U.S. Regulatory Considerations**
  - ❏ FDA Black Box   ❏ OBRA regulated in U.S. Long Term Care

naloxone hydrochloride

(nal-oks'-one hye-droe-klor'-ide)

- **Brand Name(s):** Narcan

  Combinations
  Rx: with pentazocine (Talwin NX); with buprenorphine (Suboxone)
  Chemical Class: Thebaine derivative

- **Clinical Pharmacology:**
  Mechanism of Action: A narcotic antagonist that displaces opioids at opioid-occupied receptor sites in the CNS. *Therapeutic Effect:* Reverses opioid-induced sleep or sedation, increases respiratory rate, raises BP to normal range.
  Pharmacokinetics:

Route	Onset	Peak	Duration
IV	1-2 min	N/A	20-60 min
IM	2-5 min	N/A	20-60 min
Subcutaneous	2-5 min	N/A	20-60 min

  Well absorbed after IM or subcutaneous administration. Metabolized in the liver. Primarily excreted in urine. *Half-life:* 60-100 min.

- **Available Forms:**
  - *Injection:* 0.02 mg/ml, 0.4 mg/ml, 1 mg/ml.

- **Indications and Dosages:**
  Opioid toxicity: IV, IM, Subcutaneous 0.4-2 mg q2-3min as needed. May repeat q20-60min.

- **Unlabeled Uses:** Treatment of ethanol ingestion, *Pneumocystitis carinii* pneumonia (PCP)

- **Contraindications:** Respiratory depression due to nonopioid drugs

- **Side Effects**
  None known; little or no pharmacologic effect in absence of narcotics.

- **Serious Reactions**
  - Too-rapid reversal of narcotic-induced respiratory depression may result in nausea, vomiting, tremors, increased BP, and tachycardia.

- Excessive dosage in postoperative patients may produce significant excitement, tremors, and reversal of analgesia.
- Patients with cardiovascular disease may experience hypotension or hypertension, ventricular tachycardia and fibrillation, and pulmonary edema.

Special Considerations
- Duration of action of some narcotics may exceed that of naloxone; repeat doses prn

■ Patient/Family Education
- Notify the physician if pain or increased sedation occurs

■ Monitoring Parameters
- ECG, blood pressure, respiratory rate, mental status, pupil dilation
- Continue to monitor the patient even after a satisfactory response has been achieved. If the duration of action of the opioid exceeds that of naloxone, respiratory depression may recur

■ Geriatric side effects at a glance:
❑ CNS   ❑ Bowel Dysfunction   ❑ Bladder Dysfunction   ❑ Falls

■ U.S. Regulatory Considerations
❑ FDA Black Box   ❑ OBRA regulated in U.S. Long Term Care

naltrexone hydrochloride

(nal-trex'-one hye-droe-klor'-ide)

■ Brand Name(s): ReVia
Chemical Class: Thebaine derivative

■ Clinical Pharmacology:
Mechanism of Action: A narcotic antagonist that displaces opioids at opioid-occupied receptor sites in the CNS. **Therapeutic Effect:** Blocks physical effects of opioid analgesics; decreases craving for alcohol and relapse rate in alcoholism.
Pharmacokinetics: Well absorbed following oral administration. Metabolized in liver; undergoes first-pass metabolism. Excreted primarily in urine; partial elimination in feces. **Half-life:** 4 hr.

■ Available Forms:
- *Tablets:* 50 mg.

■ Indications and Dosages:
Naloxone challenge test to determine if patient is opioid dependent: IV Alert Expect to perform the naloxone challenge test if there is any question that the patient is opioid dependent. Don't administer naltrexone until the naloxone challenge test is negative.

Draw 2 ml (0.8 mg) of naloxone into syringe. Inject 0.5 ml (0.2 mg); while needle is still in vein, observe patient for 30 sec for withdrawal signs or symptoms. If no evidence of withdrawal, inject remaining 1.5 ml (0.6 mg); observe patient for additional 20 min for withdrawal signs or symptoms. Subcutaneous Inject 2 ml (0.8 mg) of naloxone; observe patient for 45 min for withdrawal signs or symptoms.

Treatment of opioid dependence in patients who have been opioid free for at least 7-10 days: PO Initially, 25 mg. Observe patient for 1 hr. If no withdrawal signs or symptoms appear, give another 25 mg. May be given as 100 mg every other day or 150 mg every 3 days.

Adjunctive treatment of alcohol dependence: PO 50 mg once a day.

■ **Unlabeled Uses:** Treatment of eating disorders, postconcussional syndrome unresponsive to other treatments

■ **Contraindications:** Acute hepatitis, acute opioid withdrawal, failed naloxone challenge test, hepatic failure, history of hypersensitivity to naltrexone, opioid dependence, positive urine screen for opioids

■ **Side Effects**

Frequent

Alcoholism (10%-7%): Nausea, headache, depression

Narcotic addiction (10%-5%): Insomnia, anxiety, nervousness, headache, low energy, abdominal cramps, nausea, vomiting, arthralgia, myalgia

Occasional

Alcoholism (4%-2%): Dizziness, nervousness, fatigue, insomnia, vomiting, anxiety, suicidal ideation

Narcotic addiction (5%-2%): Irritability, increased energy, dizziness, anorexia, diarrhea or constipation, rash, chills, increased thirst

■ **Serious Reactions**

- Signs and symptoms of opioid withdrawal include stuffy or runny nose, tearing, yawning, diaphoresis, tremor, vomiting, piloerection, feeling of temperature change, bone pain, arthralgia, myalgia, abdominal cramps, and feeling of skin crawling.
- Accidental naltrexone overdose produces withdrawal symptoms within 5 minutes of ingestion that may last for up to 48 hours. Symptoms include confusion, visual hallucinations, somnolence, and significant vomiting and diarrhea.
- Hepatocellular injury may occur with large doses.

■ **Patient/Family Education**

- Wear ID tag indicating naltrexone use
- Do not try to overcome reversal of opiate effects by self-administration of large doses of narcotic
- Do not exceed recommended dose
- Take naltrexone tablets with antacids, after meals, or with food to avoid GI upset
- Notify the physician if abdominal pain that lasts longer than 3 days, dark urine, white stools, or yellowing of the sclerae occurs

■ **Monitoring Parameters**

- Liver function tests
- Creatinine clearance

- **Geriatric side effects at a glance:**
  - ❏ CNS ❏ Bowel Dysfunction ❏ Bladder Dysfunction ❏ Falls

- **U.S. Regulatory Considerations**
  - ☑ FDA Black Box
    - Hepatocellular injury in excessive doses
    - Naltrexone is **contraindicated** in hepatitis or liver failure.
  - ❏ OBRA regulated in U.S. Long Term Care

nandrolone decanoate

(nan'-droe-lone)

- **Brand Name(s):** Deca-Durabolin, Durabolin
  Chemical Class: Anabolic steroid; testosterone derivative

  DEA Class: Schedule III

- **Clinical Pharmacology:**
  Mechanism of Action: An anabolic steroid that promotes tissue-building processes, increases production of erythropoietin, causes protein anabolism, and increases hemoglobin and red blood cell volume. **Therapeutic Effect:** Controls metastatic breast cancer and helps manage anemia of renal insufficiency.
  Pharmacokinetics: Well absorbed after IM administration (about 77%). Metabolized in liver. Primarily excreted in urine. **Half-life:** 6-8 days.

- **Available Forms:**
  - Injection, as decanoate (in sesame oil): 100 mg/ml, 200 mg/ml (Deca-Durabolin).

- **Indications and Dosages:**
  Breast cancer: IM 50-100 mg/week.
  Anemia of renal insufficiency: IM Male. 100-200 mg/week. Female. 50-100 mg/week.

- **Unlabeled Uses:** Hyperlipidemia, lung cancer, male contraception, malnutrition, postmenopausal osteoporosis, rheumatoid arthritis, Sjögren's syndrome, trauma/surgery

- **Contraindications:** Nephrosis, carcinoma of breast or prostate, hypersensitivity to nandrolone or any component of the formulation such as sesame oil

- **Side Effects**
  Frequent
  Male: Gynecomastia, acne, bladder irritability, priapism
  Females: Virilism
  Occasional
  Male: Insomnia, chills, decreased libido, hepatic dysfunction, nausea, diarrhea, prostatic hyperplasia (elderly), iron deficiency anemia, suppression of clotting factors

Female: Chills, insomnia, hypercalcemia, nausea, diarrhea, iron deficiency anemia, suppression of clotting factors, hepatic dysfunction
Rare
Hepatic necrosis, hepatocellular carcinoma

- ■ **Serious Reactions**
  - • Peliosis hepatis of liver, spleen replaced with blood-filled cysts; hepatic neoplasms, and hepatocellular carcinoma have been associated with prolonged high-dosage; anaphylactic reactions.

Special Considerations
- • Anabolic steroids have potential for abuse

- ■ **Patient/Family Education**
  - • Do not take any other medications, including OTC drugs, without first consulting the physician
  - • Weigh yourself each day
  - • Notify the physician if acne, nausea, pedal edema, or vomiting occurs
  - • Female patients should report deepening of voice and hoarseness
  - • Male patients should report difficulty urinating, frequent erections, and gynecomastia

- ■ **Monitoring Parameters**
  - • Women should be observed for signs of virilization
  - • Liver function tests, lipids, Hct
  - • Blood pressure
  - • Intake and output
  - • Sleep patterns

- ■ **Geriatric side effects at a glance:**
  - ❑ CNS ❑ Bowel Dysfunction ❑ Bladder Dysfunction ❑ Falls

- ■ **U.S. Regulatory Considerations**
  - ❑ FDA Black Box ❑ OBRA regulated in U.S. Long Term Care

naproxen/naproxen sodium

(na-prox'-en; na-prox'-en soe'-dee-um)

- ■ **Brand Name(s):** (naproxen) EC-Naprosyn, Naprelan, Naprelan 375, Naprelan 500

- ■ **Brand Name(s):** (naproxen sodium) Aflaxen, Aleve, Anaprox, Anaprox DS, Pamprin

  Combinations
  Rx: with lansoprazole (NapraPAC)
  Chemical Class: Propionic acid derivative

Clinical Pharmacology:

Mechanism of Action: An NSAID that produces analgesic and anti-inflammatory effects by inhibiting prostaglandin synthesis. **Therapeutic Effect:** Reduces the inflammatory response and intensity of pain.

Pharmacokinetics:

Route	Onset	Peak	Duration
PO (analgesic)	less than 1 hr	N/A	7 hr or less
PO (antirheumatic)	less than 14 days	2–4 wk	N/A

Completely absorbed from the GI tract. Protein binding: 99%. Metabolized in the liver. Primarily excreted in urine. Not removed by hemodialysis. **Half-life:** 13 hr.

Available Forms:

- *Gelcaps (Aleve):* 220 mg naproxen sodium (equivalent to 200 mg naproxen).
- *Oral Suspension (Naprosyn):* 125 mg/5 ml naproxen.
- *Tablets:* 220 mg naproxen (Aleve), 250 mg (Naprosyn), 275 mg naproxen sodium (equivalent to 250 mg naproxen) (Anaprox), 550 mg naproxen sodium (equivalent to 500 mg naproxen) (Aflaxen, Anaprox DS).
- *Tablets (Controlled-Release):* 375 mg naproxen (EC-Naprosyn), 421 mg naproxen (Naprelan), 500 mg naproxen (EC-Naprosyn), 550 mg naproxen sodium (equivalent to 500 mg naproxen) (Naprelan).

Indications and Dosages:

Rheumatoid arthritis, osteoarthritis, ankylosing spondylitis: PO 250–500 mg naproxen (275–550 mg naproxen sodium) twice a day or 250 mg naproxen (275 mg naproxen sodium) in morning and 500 mg naproxen (550 mg naproxen sodium) in evening. Naprelan: 750–1,000 mg once a day.

Acute gouty arthritis: PO Initially, 750 mg naproxen (825 mg naproxen sodium), then 250 mg naproxen (275 mg naproxen sodium) q8h until attack subsides. Naprelan: Initially, 1,000–1,500 mg, then 1,000 mg once a day until attack subsides.

Mild to moderate pain, bursitis, tendinitis: PO Initially, 500 mg naproxen (550 mg naproxen sodium), then 250 mg naproxen (275 mg naproxen sodium) q6–8h as needed. Maximum: 1.25 g/day naproxen (1.375 g/day naproxen sodium). Naprelan: 1,000 mg once a day.

OTC uses: PO 220 mg (200 mg naproxen sodium) q12h.

Unlabeled Uses: Treatment of vascular headaches

Contraindications: Hypersensitivity to aspirin, naproxen, or other NSAIDs

Side Effects

Frequent (9%–4%)
Nausea, constipation, abdominal cramps or pain, heartburn, dizziness, headache, somnolence
Occasional (3%–1%)
Stomatitis, diarrhea, indigestion
Rare (less than 1%)
Vomiting, confusion

Serious Reactions

- Rare reactions with long-term use include peptic ulcer disease, GI bleeding, gastritis, severe hepatic reactions (cholestasis, jaundice), nephrotoxicity (dysuria, hematuria, proteinuria, nephrotic syndrome), and a severe hypersensitivity reaction (fever, chills, bronchospasm).

- No significant advantage over other NSAIDs; cost should govern use

■ Patient/Family Education

- Avoid concurrent use of aspirin and alcoholic beverages
- Take with food, milk, or antacids to decrease GI upset
- Notify clinician if edema, black stools, or persistent headache occurs
- Avoid tasks that require mental alertness or motor skills until response to the drug has been established

■ Monitoring Parameters

- Initial hematocrit and fecal occult blood test within 3 mo of starting regular chronic therapy; repeat every 6-12 mo (more frequently in high-risk patients (>65 years, peptic ulcer disease, concurrent steroids or anticoagulants); electrolytes, creatinine, and BUN within 3 mo of starting regular chronic therapy; repeat every 6-12 mo
- CBC (particularly Hgb, Hct, and platelet count)
- Serum alkaline phosphatase, bilirubin, AST (SGOT), and ALT (SGPT) levels to assess hepatic and renal function
- Pattern of daily bowel activity and stool consistency
- Therapeutic response, such as improved grip strength, increased joint mobility, and decreased pain, tenderness, stiffness, and swelling

■ Geriatric side effects at a glance:

☑ CNS ☐ Bowel Dysfunction ☐ Bladder Dysfunction ☐ Falls
☑ Other: Gastropathy

■ Use with caution in older patients with:
Renal impairment, Hepatic impairment, CHF, HTN, PUD, History of GI bleeding, GERD, Bleeding and platelet disorders, History of aspirin sensitivity reaction. Also use with caution in patients taking Anticoagulants, Aspirin, and Antihypertensive agents.

■ U.S. Regulatory Considerations

☑ FDA Black Box
- Increased cardiovascular risk
- Increased gastrointestinal risk
☐ OBRA regulated in U.S. Long Term Care

■ Other Uses in Geriatric Patient: Acute gout

■ Side Effects:
Of particular importance in the geriatric patient: Confusion, cognitive impairment, delirium, dizziness, dyspepsia, fluid retention, renal impairment

■ Geriatric Considerations - Summary:
A preferred agent in older adults due to its association with fewer GI adverse effects. Use of NSAIDs in older adults increases the risk of GI complications including gastric ulceration, bleeding, and perforation. These complications are not necessarily preceded by less severe GI symptoms. Concomitant use of a proton pump inhibitor or misoprostol reduces the risk for gastric ulceration and bleeding, but may not prevent long-term GI toxicity.

■ **References:**
1. COX-2 alternatives and GI protection. Med Lett Drugs Ther 2004;46:91.
2. Drugs that may cause cognitive disorders in the elderly. Med Lett Drugs Ther 2000;42:111-112.

naratriptan hydrochloride

(nar-a-trip'-tan hye-droe-klor'-ide)

■ **Brand Name(s):** Amerge
Chemical Class: Serotonin derivative

■ **Clinical Pharmacology:**
Mechanism of Action: A serotonin receptor agonist that binds selectively to vascular receptors producing a vasoconstrictive effect on cranial blood vessels. **Therapeutic Effect:** Relieves migraine headache.
Pharmacokinetics: Well absorbed after PO administration. Protein binding: 28%-31%. Metabolized by the liver to inactive metabolite. Eliminated primarily in urine and, to a lesser extent, in feces. **Half-life:** 6 hr (increased in hepatic or renal impairment).

■ **Available Forms:**
• *Tablets:* 1 mg, 2.5 mg.

■ **Indications and Dosages:**
Acute migraine attack: PO 1 mg or 2.5 mg. If headache improves but then returns, dose may be repeated after 4 hr. Maximum: 5 mg/24 hr.
Dosage in mild to moderate hepatic or renal impairment: A lower starting dose is recommended. Don't exceed 2.5 mg/24 hr.

■ **Contraindications:** Basilar or hemiplegic migraine, cerebrovascular or peripheral vascular disease, coronary artery disease, ischemic heart disease (including angina pectoris, history of MI, silent ischemia, and Prinzmetal's angina), severe hepatic impairment (Child-Pugh grade C), severe renal impairment (serum creatinine less than 15 ml/min), uncontrolled hypertension, use within 24 hours of ergotamine-containing preparations or another serotonin receptor agonist, use within 14 days of MAOIs

■ **Side Effects**
Occasional (5%)
Nausea
Rare (2%)
Paresthesia; dizziness; fatigue; somnolence; jaw, neck, or throat pressure

■ **Serious Reactions**
• Corneal opacities and other ocular defects may occur.
• Cardiac reactions (including ischemia, coronary artery vasospasm, and MI) and noncardiac vasospasm-related reactions (such as hemorrhage and cerebrovascular accident |CVA|), occur rarely, particularly in patients with hypertension, diabetes, or a strong family history of coronary artery disease; obese patients; smokers; males older than 40 years; and postmenopausal women.

- Longer acting than sumatriptan and zolmitriptan so recurrent headaches requiring a second dose less likely; slower onset than sumatriptan and zolmitriptan; should probably be reserved for patients who get recurrent headaches
- Safety of treating, on average, more than 4 headaches in a 30-day period has not been established

■ Patient/Family Education
- Use only to treat migraine headache, not for prevention
- Swallow tablets whole with water; do not crush or chew them
- Take another dose of naratriptan, if needed, 4 hr after the first dose for a maximum of 5 mg/24 hr
- May cause dizziness, drowsiness, and fatigue
- Avoid tasks that require mental alertness or motor skills until response to the drug has been established
- Notify the physician if anxiety, chest pain, palpitations, or tightness in the throat occurs
- Lie down in dark, quiet room for additional benefit after taking naratriptan

■ Monitoring Parameters
- Assess for relief of migraines and associated symptoms, including nausea and vomiting, photophobia, and phonophobia (sound sensitivity)

■ Geriatric side effects at a glance:
❑ CNS   ❑ Bowel Dysfunction   ❑ Bladder Dysfunction   ❑ Falls

■ U.S. Regulatory Considerations
❑ FDA Black Box   ❑ OBRA regulated in U.S. Long Term Care

natamycin

(na-ta-mye'-sin)

■ Brand Name(s): Natacyn
Chemical Class: Tetraene polyene derivative

■ Clinical Pharmacology:
Mechanism of Action: A polyene antifungal agent that increases cell membrane permeability in susceptible fungi. **Therapeutic Effect:** Fungicidal.
Pharmacokinetics: Minimal systemic absorption. Adheres to cornea and retained in conjunctival fornices.

■ Available Forms:
- *Ophthalmic Suspension*: 5% (Natacyn).

■ Indications and Dosages:
Fungal keratitis, ophthalmic fungal infections: Ophthalmic Instill 1 drop in conjunctival sac every 1-2 hr. After 3-4 days, reduce to 1 drop 6-8 times daily. Usual course of therapy is 2-3 wk.

- **Unlabeled Uses:** Oral and vaginal candidiasis, onychomycosis, pulmonary aspergillosis

- **Contraindications:** Hypersensitivity to natamycin or any component of the formulation

- **Side Effects**
  Occasional (10%-3%)
  Blurred vision, eye irritation, eye pain, photophobia

- **Serious Reactions**
  - Vomiting and diarrhea have occurred with large doses in the treatment of systemic mycoses.

- **Patient/Family Education**
  - Shake well before using
  - Do not touch dropper to eye
  - Notify the physician if the condition worsens or does not improve after 3-4 days

- **Monitoring Parameters**
  - Failure of keratitis to improve following 7-10 days of administration suggests infection not susceptible to natamycin

- **Geriatric side effects at a glance:**
  ☐ CNS ☐ Bowel Dysfunction ☐ Bladder Dysfunction ☐ Falls

- **U.S. Regulatory Considerations**
  ☐ FDA Black Box ☐ OBRA regulated in U.S. Long Term Care

nateglinide

(na-teg'-lin-ide)

- **Brand Name(s):** Starlix
  Chemical Class: Amino acid derivative; meglitinide

- **Clinical Pharmacology:**
  Mechanism of Action: An antihyperglycemic that stimulates release of insulin from beta cells of the pancreas by depolarizing beta cells, leading to an opening of calcium channels. Resulting calcium influx induces insulin secretion. **Therapeutic Effect:** Lowers blood glucose concentration.
  Pharmacokinetics: Absolute bioavailability is approximately 73%. Protein binding: 98%. Extensive metabolism in liver. Primarily excreted in urine; minimal elimination in feces. **Half-life:** 1.5 hr.

- ■ **Available Forms:**
  - • *Tablets:* 60 mg, 120 mg.

- ■ **Indications and Dosages:**
  Diabetes mellitus: PO 120 mg 3 times a day before meals. Initially, 60 mg may be given.

- ■ **Contraindications:** Diabetic ketoacidosis, type 1 diabetes mellitus

- ■ **Side Effects**
  Frequent (10%)
  Upper respiratory tract infection
  Occasional (4%–3%)
  Back pain, flu symptoms, dizziness, arthropathy, diarrhea
  Rare (3% or less)
  Bronchitis, cough

- ■ **Serious Reactions**
  - • Hypoglycemia occurs in less than 2% of patients.

Special Considerations

- • *Pharmacodynamics* (60-120 mg tid ac for 24 wk): HbA_{1c} change—0.5%; fasting plasma glucose change—15 mg/dl; weight change—0.3-0.9 kg

- ■ **Patient/Family Education**
  - • Review signs and symptoms and management of hypoglycemia
  - • Drug administration timing (i.e., before meals)
  - • The prescribed diet is a principal part of treatment
  - • Carry candy, sugar packets, or other sugar supplements for immediate response to hypoglycemia and wear medical alert identification stating that he or she has diabetes
  - • Consult the physician when glucose demands are altered, such as with fever, heavy physical activity, infection, stress, or trauma

- ■ **Monitoring Parameters**
  - • Home/self blood glucose monitoring, HbA_{1c}, signs and symptoms of hyper/hypoglycemia, complete blood count, routine blood chemistry

- ■ **Geriatric side effects at a glance:**
  - ❑ CNS   ❑ Bowel Dysfunction   ❑ Bladder Dysfunction   ❑ Falls
  - ☑ Other: Hypoglycemia

- ■ **Use with caution in older patients with:** Hepatic impairment, Severe renal impairment

- ■ **U.S. Regulatory Considerations**
  - ❑ FDA Black Box   ❑ OBRA regulated in U.S. Long Term Care

- ■ **Other Uses in Geriatric Patient:** None

- ■ **Side Effects:**
  Of particular importance in the geriatric patient: Hypoglycemia, dizziness, weight gain

- **Geriatric Considerations - Summary:** Older adults may be at a greater risk of hypoglycemia. Metabolized in the liver to potentially active metabolites that are renally eliminated; therefore, may increase the risk for and prolong hypoglycemia in older adults. Because of its short half-life and pre-meal administration, nateglinide can be held if the patient does not eat a meal in order to prevent hypoglycemia. May be less effective than sulfonylureas.

- **References:**
  1. Haas L. Management of diabetes mellitus medications in the nursing home. Drugs Aging 2005;22:209-218.
  2. Chelliah A, Burge MR. Hypoglycemia in elderly patients with diabetes mellitus. Causes and strategies for prevention. Drugs Aging 2004;21:511-530.
  3. Nateglinide for type 2 diabetes. Med Let 2001;43:29-31.

nedocromil sodium

(ne-doe-kroe'-mil soe'-dee-um)

- **Brand Name(s):** *Oral:* Tilade

- **Brand Name(s):** *Ophth:* Alocril
  Chemical Class: Mast cell stabilizer; pyranoquinoline dicarboxylic acid derivative

- **Clinical Pharmacology:**
  Mechanism of Action: A mast cell stabilizer that prevents the activation and release of inflammatory mediators, such as histamine, leukotrienes, mast cells, eosinophils, and monocytes. **Therapeutic Effect:** Prevents both early and late asthmatic responses. **Pharmacokinetics:** The extent of absorption is 7% to 9% of a single inhaled dose of 3.5 to 4 mg and 17% of multiple inhaled doses, with absorption largely from the respiratory tract. Although most of the inhaled dose is subsequently swallowed, only 2% to 3% is absorbed from the GI tract. Less than 4% of the total dose is systemically absorbed following multiple doses of ophthalmic solution. Protein binding: 89%. Not metabolized. Excreted in urine. **Half-life:** 1.5-3.3 hr.

- **Available Forms:**
  - *Aerosol for Inhalation (Tilade):* 1.75 mg/activation.
  - *Ophthalmic Solution (Alocril):* 2%.

- **Indications and Dosages:**
  Mild to moderate asthma: Oral Inhalation 2 inhalations 4 times a day. May decrease to 3 times a day, then twice a day as asthma becomes controlled.
  Allergic conjunctivitis: Ophthalmic 1–2 drops in each eye twice a day.

- **Unlabeled Uses:** Prevention of bronchospasm in patients with reversible obstructive airway disease

- **Contraindications:** None known.

Side Effects

Frequent (10%–6%)

Inhalation: Cough, pharyngitis, bronchospasm, headache, altered taste

Ophthalmic: Burning sensation in eye

Occasional (5%–1%)

Inhalation: Rhinitis, upper respiratory tract infection, abdominal pain, fatigue

Rare (less than 1%)

Inhalation: Diarrhea, dizziness

Ophthalmic: Conjunctivitis, light intolerance

Serious Reactions

- None known.

Patient/Family Education

- Must be used regularly to achieve benefit, even during symptom-free periods
- Therapeutic effect may take up to 4 wk
- Not to be used to treat acute asthmatic symptoms
- Administer nedocromil at regular intervals, even when symptom-free, to achieve optimal results
- Rinse mouth with water immediately after inhalation to help relieve unpleasant taste
- Drink plenty of fluids to decrease the thickness of lung secretions

Monitoring Parameters

- Therapeutic response, such as less frequent or severe asthmatic attacks or reduced dependence on antihistamines

Geriatric side effects at a glance:

❏ CNS ❏ Bowel Dysfunction ❏ Bladder Dysfunction ❏ Falls

U.S. Regulatory Considerations

❏ FDA Black Box ❏ OBRA regulated in U.S. Long Term Care

nefazodone hydrochloride

(neh-faz'-oh-doan hye-droe-klor'-ide)

Brand Name(s): Serzone

Chemical Class: Phenylpiperazine derivative

Clinical Pharmacology:

Mechanism of Action: Exact mechanism is unknown. Appears to inhibit neuronal uptake of serotonin and norepinephrine and to antagonize alpha$_1$-adrenergic receptors.

Therapeutic Effect: Relieves depression.

Pharmacokinetics: Rapidly and completely absorbed from the GI tract; food delays absorption. Protein binding: 99%. Widely distributed in body tissues, including CNS. Extensively metabolized to active metabolites. Excreted in urine and eliminated in feces. Unknown if removed by hemodialysis. **Half-life:** 2-4 hr.

■ **Available Forms:**
  • *Tablets:* 50 mg, 100 mg, 150 mg, 200 mg, 250 mg.

■ **Indications and Dosages:**
  Depression, prevention of relapse of acute depressive episode: PO Initially, 100 mg/day in 2 divided doses. Subsequent dosage titration based on clinical response. Range: 200-400 mg/day.

■ **Contraindications:** Co-administration of terfenadine, astemizole, cisapride, pimozide, or carbamazepine; hypersensitivity to other phenylpiperazine antidepressants; those who were withdrawn from nefazodone due to evidence of hepatic injury; use within 14 days of MAOIs

■ **Side Effects**
  Frequent
  Headache (36%); dry mouth, somnolence (25%); nausea (22%); dizziness (17%); constipation (14%); insomnia, asthenia, light-headedness (10%).
  Occasional
  Dyspepsia, blurred vision (9%); diarrhea, infection (8%); confusion, abnormal vision (7%); pharyngitis (6%); increased appetite (5%); orthostatic hypotension, flushing, feeling of warmth (4%); peripheral edema, cough, flu-like symptoms (3%).

■ **Serious Reactions**
  • *Alert* Cases of life-threatening hepatic failures have been reported.
  • Serious reactions, such as hyperthermia, rigidity, myoclonus, extreme agitation, delirium, and coma, will occur if the patient takes an MAOI concurrently or fails to let enough time elapse when switching from an MAOI to nefazodone or vice versa.

Special Considerations
  • Priapism has been reported; educate and monitor appropriately

■ **Patient/Family Education**
  • Therapeutic effect may not be apparent for several weeks
  • Drug may cause drowsiness, use caution driving or performing other tasks where alertness is required
  • Notify the physician if headache, nausea, or visual disturbances occurs
  • Avoid tasks that require mental alertness or motor skills until response to the drug has been established
  • Avoid alcohol while taking nefazodone
  • Take sips of tepid water or chew sugarless gum to help relieve dry mouth

■ **Monitoring Parameters**
  • Blood pressure and pulse rate
  • Pattern of daily bowel activity and stool consistency
  • Assess appearance, behavior, level of interest, mood, and sleep pattern before and during therapy

- **Geriatric side effects at a glance:**
  - ☑ CNS   ☐ Bowel Dysfunction   ☐ Bladder Dysfunction   ☑ Falls
  - ☑ Other: Priapism

- **Use with caution in older patients with:** Using interacting medications, liver abnormalities

- **U.S. Regulatory Considerations**
  - ☑ FDA Black Box
  - Because there is an increased risk of suicide in children and adolescents, older adults should also be closely monitored for suicide ideation.
  - ☐ OBRA regulated in U.S. Long Term Care

- **Other Uses in Geriatric Patient:** Sleep disturbance

- **Side Effects:**
  Of particular importance in the geriatric patient: None

- **Geriatric Considerations - Summary:** Nefazodone is an effective antidepressant, with less cardiotoxicity than other antidepressants. Although nefazodone has not been well studied with respect to fall risk, older adults using nefazodone, like other psychotropic drugs, should still be carefully monitered for falls. This agent is a potent inhibitor of CYP3A, and thus doses of many drugs (e.g., alprazolam, triazolam, buspirone) should be reduced by 50%-75% if co-administered. Due to the risk of hepatotoxicity this drug is rarely used.

- **References:**
  1. Richelson E. Pharmacokinetic interactions of antidepressants. J Clin Psychiatry 1998;59 (Suppl 10):22-26.
  2. Goldberg RJ. Antidepressant use in the elderly. Current status of nefazodone, venlafaxine and moclobemide. Drugs Aging 1997;11:119-131.

nelfinavir mesylate

(nel-fin'-a-veer mes'-sil-ate)

- **Brand Name(s):** Viracept
  Chemical Class: Protease inhibitor, HIV

- **Clinical Pharmacology:**
  Mechanism of Action: Inhibits the activity of HIV-1 protease, the enzyme necessary for the formation of infectious HIV. *Therapeutic Effect:* Formation of immature noninfectious viral particles rather than HIV replication.
  Pharmacokinetics: Well absorbed after PO administration (absorption increased with food). Protein binding: 98%. Metabolized in the liver. Highly bound to plasma proteins. Eliminated primarily in feces. Unknown if removed by hemodialysis. *Half-life:* 3.5-5 hr.

Available Forms:
- *Powder for Oral Suspension*: 50 mg/g.
- *Tablets*: 250 mg, 625 mg.

Indications and Dosages:
HIV *infection*: PO 750 mg (three 250-mg tablets) 3 times a day or 1,250 mg twice a day in combination with nucleoside analogs (enhances antiviral activity).

Unlabeled Uses: HIV, postexposure prophylaxis

Contraindications: Concurrent administration with midazolam, rifampin, or triazolam

Side Effects
Frequent (20%)
Diarrhea
Occasional (7%-3%)
Nausea, rash
Rare (2%-1%)
Flatulence, asthenia

Serious Reactions
- Diabetes mellitus and hyperglycemia occur rarely.

Special Considerations
- Positive results of treatment are based on surrogate markers only
- Take with meal or snack
- Always check updated treatment guidelines before initiating or changing antiretroviral therapy. (http://AIDSinfo.nih.gov)

Patient/Family Education
- Contains phenylalanine, take with food
- Space drug doses evenly around the clock and take the drug every day as prescribed
- Do not alter the dose or discontinue the drug without first notifying the physician
- Nelfinavir is not a cure for HIV infection, nor does it reduce the risk of transmitting HIV to others; the patient may continue to experience illnesses associated with advanced HIV infection, including opportunistic infections

Monitoring Parameters
- CBC, electrolytes, renal function, liver enzymes, CPK
- Pattern of daily bowel activity and stool consistency
- Signs and symptoms of opportunistic infections, such as chills, cough, fever, and myalgia

Geriatric side effects at a glance:
❏ CNS ☑ Bowel Dysfunction ❏ Bladder Dysfunction ❏ Falls

U.S. Regulatory Considerations
❏ FDA Black Box ❏ OBRA regulated in U.S. Long Term Care

neomycin sulfate

(nee-oh-mye'-sin sul'-fayte)

- **Brand Name(s):** Myciguent, Neo-Fradin, Neo-Rx, Neo-Tab

  Combinations
  Rx: with polymyxin B (Neosporin G.U. irrigant)
  OTC: with polymyxin B, bacitracin (Neosporin, Mycitracin)
  Chemical Class: Aminoglycoside

- **Clinical Pharmacology:**
  Mechanism of Action: An aminoglycoside antibacterial that binds to bacterial micro-organisms. **Therapeutic Effect:** Interferes with bacterial protein synthesis.
  Pharmacokinetics: Poorly absorbed from the GI tract following PO administration. Protein binding: Low. Primarily eliminated unchanged in the feces; minimal excretion in urine. Removed by hemodialysis. **Half-life:** 3 hr.

- **Available Forms:**
  - *Tablets (Neo-Tab):* 500 mg.
  - *Ointment (Myciguent):* 0.5%.
  - *Cream (Myciguent):* 0.5%.
  - *Oral Solution (Neo-Fradin):* 125 mg/5 ml.
  - *Powder for Compounding (Neo-Rx):* 100%.

- **Indications and Dosages:**
  Preoperative bowel antisepsis: PO 1 g/hr for 4 doses; then 1g q4h for 5 doses or 1g at 1 p.m., 2 p.m., and 10 p.m. (with erythromycin) on day before surgery.
  Hepatic encephalopathy: PO 4-12 g/day in divided doses q4-6h.
  Diarrhea caused by Escherichia coli: PO 3 g/day in divided doses q6h.
  Minor skin infections: Topical Usual dosage, apply to affected area 1-3 times a day.

- **Contraindications:** Hypersensitivity to neomycin, other aminoglycosides (cross-sensitivity), or their components

- **Side Effects**
  Frequent
  Systemic: Nausea, vomiting, diarrhea, irritation of mouth or rectal area
  Topical: Itching, redness, swelling, rash
  Rare
  Systemic: Malabsorption syndrome, neuromuscular blockade (difficulty breathing, drowsiness, weakness)

- **Serious Reactions**
  - Nephrotoxicity (as evidenced by increased BUN and serum creatinine levels and decreased creatinine clearance) may be reversible if the drug is stopped at the first sign of nephrotoxic symptoms.
  - Irreversible ototoxicity (manifested as tinnitus, dizziness, and impaired hearing) and neurotoxicity (as evidenced by headache, dizziness, lethargy, tremor, and visual disturbances) occur occasionally.

- Severe respiratory depression and anaphylaxis occur rarely.
- Superinfections, particularly fungal infections, may occur.

Special Considerations
- Inform patient and family about possible toxic effects on the 8th cranial nerve; monitor for loss of hearing, ringing or roaring in ears, or a feeling of fullness in head

■ Patient/Family Education
- Drink plenty of fluids
- Continue taking neomycin for the full course of treatment and space doses evenly around the clock
- Notify the physician if dizziness, impaired hearing, or ringing in the ears occurs
- The patient using topical neomycin should clean the affected area gently before applying the drug and should notify the physician if itching or redness occurs

■ Monitoring Parameters
- Renal function, audiometric testing during extended therapy or with application to extensive burns or large surface area
- Evaluate the patient for signs and symptoms of a hypersensitivity reaction. With topical application, symptoms may include a rash, redness, or itching
- Watch the patient for signs and symptoms of superinfection, particularly diarrhea, genital or anal pruritus, and stomatitis

■ Geriatric side effects at a glance:
❑ CNS ☑ Bowel Dysfunction ❑ Bladder Dysfunction ❑ Falls

■ U.S. Regulatory Considerations
❑ FDA Black Box ❑ OBRA regulated in U.S. Long Term Care

neostigmine bromide

(nee-oh-stig'-meen bro'-mide)

■ Brand Name(s): Prostigmin, Prostigmin Bromide
Chemical Class: Cholinesterase inhibitor; quaternary ammonium derivative

■ Clinical Pharmacology:
Mechanism of Action: A cholinergic drug that prevents destruction of acetylcholine by inhibiting the enzyme acetylcholinesterase, thus enhancing impulse transmission across the myoneural junction. *Therapeutic Effect:* Improves intestinal and skeletal muscle tone; stimulates salivary and sweat gland secretions.
Pharmacokinetics: Poorly absorbed from the GI tract following oral administration. Partially eliminated in urine. *Half-life:* 52 min.

■ Available Forms:
- *Tablets (Prostigmin Bromide):* 15 mg.
- *Injection (Prostigmin):* 0.25 mg/ml, 0.5 mg/ml, 1 mg/ml.

■ Indications and Dosages:

Myasthenia gravis: PO Initially, 15–30 mg 3–4 times a day. Increase as necessary. Maintenance: 150 mg/day (range of 15–375 mg). IV, IM, Subcutaneous 0.5–2.5 mg as needed.

Diagnosis of myasthenia gravis: IM 0.022 mg/kg. If CNS-cholinergic-myasthenia reaction occurs, discontinue tests and administer 0.4–0.6 mg or more atropine sulfate IV.

Prevention of postoperative urinary retention: IM, Subcutaneous 0.25 mg q4–6h for 2–3 days.

Postoperative abdomonial distention and urine retention: IM, Subcutaneous 0.5–1 mg. Catheterize patient if voiding does not occur within 1 hr. After voiding, administer 0.5 mg q3h for 5 injections.

Reversal of neuromuscular blockade: IV 0.5–2.5 mg given slowly.

■ Contraindications: GI or GU obstruction, history of hypersensitivity reaction to bromides, peritonitis

■ Side Effects

Frequent

Muscarinic effects (diarrhea, diaphoresis, increased salivation, nausea, vomiting, abdominal cramps or pain)

Occasional

Muscarinic effects (urinary urgency or frequency, increased bronchial secretions, miosis, lacrimation)

■ Serious Reactions

- Overdose produces a cholinergic crisis manifested as abdominal discomfort or cramps, nausea, vomiting, diarrhea, flushing, facial warmth, excessive salivation, diaphoresis, lacrimation, pallor, bradycardia or tachycardia, hypotension, bronchospasm, urinary urgency, blurred vision, miosis, and fasciculation (involuntary muscular contractions visible under the skin).

■ Patient/Family Education

- Notify the physician if diarrhea, difficulty breathing, increased salivation, irregular heartbeat, muscle weakness, nausea and vomiting, severe abdominal pain, or increased sweating occurs
- Log energy level and muscle strength as a guide for drug dosing

■ Monitoring Parameters

- Vital signs
- Intake and output

Myasthenia gravis

- *Therapeutic response*: Increased muscle strength, improved gait, absence of labored breathing
- *Toxicity*: Narrow margin between first appearance of side effects and serious toxicity

■ Geriatric side effects at a glance:

❑ CNS   ☑ Bowel Dysfunction   ❑ Bladder Dysfunction   ❑ Falls

■ U.S. Regulatory Considerations

❑ FDA Black Box   ❑ OBRA regulated in U.S. Long Term Care

nesiritide

(ni-sir'-i-tide)

■ **Brand Name(s):** Natrecor
Chemical Class: Recombinant human peptide

■ **Clinical Pharmacology:**
Mechanism of Action: A brain natriuretic peptide that facilitates cardiovascular homeostasis and fluid status through counterregulation of the renin-angiotensin-aldosterone system, stimulating cyclic guanosine monophosphate, thereby leading to smooth-muscle cell relaxation. **Therapeutic Effect:** Promotes vasodilation, natriuresis, and diuresis, correcting CHF.
Pharmacokinetics:

Route	Onset	Peak	Duration
IV	15–30 min	1–2 hr	4 hr

Excreted primarily in the heart by the left ventricle. Metabolized by the natriuretic neutral endopeptidase enzymes on the vascular luminal surface. **Half-life:** 18–23 min.

■ **Available Forms:**
- *Injection Powder for Reconstitution:* 1.5 mg/5-ml vial.

■ **Indications and Dosages:**
Treatment of acutely decompensated CHF in patients with dyspnea at rest or with minimal activity: IV bolus 2 mcg/kg followed by a continuous IV infusion of 0.01 mcg/kg/min. At intervals of 3 hr or longer, may be increased by 0.005 mcg/kg/min (preceded by a bolus of 1 mcg/kg), up to a maximum of 0.03 mcg/kg/min.

■ **Contraindications:** Cardiogenic shock, systolic BP less than 90 mm Hg

■ **Side Effects**
Frequent (11%)
Hypotension
Occasional (8%–2%)
Headache, nausea, bradycardia
Rare (1% or less)
Confusion, paresthesia, somnolence, tremor

■ **Serious Reactions**
- Ventricular arrhythmias, including ventricular tachycardia, atrial fibrillation, AV node conduction abnormalities, and angina pectoris, occur rarely.

Special Considerations
- Limited experience in administration for longer than 48 hr
- If hypotension occurs, discontinue and subsequently restart at dose reduced by 30% (no bolus) once patient has stabilized

■ **Patient/Family Education**
- Nesiritide is not a cure for CHF but it will help relieve symptoms
- Immediately report chest pain or palpitations

Monitoring Parameters

- Plasma brain natriuretic peptide concentrations, plasma aldosterone, heart failure hemodynamic measurements, clinical symptoms of heart failure, routine blood chemistries, blood pressure for hypotension and pulse rate for abnormalities (hypotension is dose-limiting/dose-dependent)

Geriatric side effects at a glance:

❑ CNS   ❑ Bowel Dysfunction   ❑ Bladder Dysfunction   ❑ Falls

U.S. Regulatory Considerations

❑ FDA Black Box   ❑ OBRA regulated in U.S. Long Term Care

nevirapine

(ne-vye'-ra-peen)

Brand Name(s): Viramune
Chemical Class: Dipyridodiazepinone derivative; nonnucleoside reverse transcriptase inhibitor

Clinical Pharmacology:
Mechanism of Action: A nonnucleoside reverse transcriptase inhibitor that binds directly to HIV-1 reverse transcriptase, thus changing the shape of this enzyme and blocking RNA- and DNA-dependent polymerase activity. **Therapeutic Effect:** Interferes with HIV replication, slowing the progression of HIV infection.
Pharmacokinetics: Readily absorbed after PO administration. Protein binding: 60%. Widely distributed. Extensively metabolized in the liver. Excreted primarily in urine. **Half-life:** 45 hr (single dose), 25-30 hr (multiple doses).

Available Forms:
- *Tablets:* 200 mg.
- *Oral Suspension:* 50 mg/5 ml.

Indications and Dosages:
HIV infection: PO 200 mg once a day for 14 days (to reduce the risk of rash). Maintenance: 200 mg twice a day in combination with nucleoside analogs.

Contraindications: None known.

Side Effects
Frequent (8%-3%)
Rash, fever, headache, nausea, granulocytopenia
Occasional (3%-1%)
Stomatitis (burning, erythema, or ulceration of the oral mucosa; dysphagia)
Rare (less than 1%)
Paresthesia, myalgia, abdominal pain

Serious Reactions
- Hepatitis and rash may become severe and life-threatening.

Special Considerations
- 2-week lead in period with qd dosing decreases the potential for development of rash; stop therapy in any patient developing a severe rash or rash with constitutional symptoms
- Always check updated treatment guidelines before initiating or changing antiretroviral therapy (http://AIDSinfo.nih.gov)

Patient/Family Education
- Space drug doses evenly around the clock and continue nevirapine therapy for the full course of treatment
- If the patient fails to take nevirapine for longer than 7 days, instruct him or her to restart therapy by taking one 200-mg tablet each day for the first 14 days, and then one 200 mg tablet twice a day
- Stop therapy and notify the physician if a rash occurs
- Nevirapine is not a cure for HIV infection, nor does it reduce the risk of transmitting HIV to others

Monitoring Parameters
- CBC, ALT, AST, renal function
- Closely monitor for evidence of rash, which usually appears on the extremities, face, or trunk within the first 6 wk of drug therapy
- Evaluate for a rash accompanied by blistering, conjunctivitis, fever, general malaise, muscle or joint aches, oral lesions, and edema, which may indicate a severe, life-threatening skin or hypersensitivity reaction

Geriatric side effects at a glance:
☐ CNS   ☐ Bowel Dysfunction   ☐ Bladder Dysfunction   ☐ Falls

U.S. Regulatory Considerations
☑ FDA Black Box
Hepatotoxicity—women and patients with higher CD4 counts are at increased risk. Severe, life-threatening skin reactions including Stevens-Johnson syndrome, TEN, and hypersensitivity reactions.
☐ OBRA regulated in U.S. Long Term Care

niacin, nicotinic acid

(nye'-a-sin; nik'-oh-tin'ik as'-id)

- **Brand Name(s):** Niacor, Niaspan ER, Nicotinex, Slo-Niacin

    Combinations
    Rx: with lovastatin (Advicor)
    Chemical Class: vitamin B complex

- **Clinical Pharmacology:**

    Mechanism of Action: An antihyperlipidemic, water-soluble vitamin that is a component of two coenzymes needed for tissue respiration, lipid metabolism, and glycogenolysis. Inhibits synthesis of VLDLs. **Therapeutic Effect:** Reduces total, LDL, and VLDL cholesterol levels and triglyceride levels; increases HDL cholesterol concentration.

    Pharmacokinetics: Readily absorbed from the GI tract. Widely distributed. Metabolized in the liver. Primarily excreted in urine. **Half-life:** 45 min.

- **Available Forms:**
    - *Capsules (Timed-Release):* 125 mg, 250 mg, 400 mg, 500 mg.
    - *Tablets (Niacor):* 50 mg, 100 mg, 250 mg, 500 mg.
    - *Tablets (Timed-Release [Slo-Niacin]):* 250 mg, 500 mg, 750 mg.
    - *Tablets (Timed-Release [Niaspan]):* 500 mg, 750 mg, 1,000 mg.
    - *Elixir (Nicotinex):* 50 mg/5 ml.

- **Indications and Dosages:**

    Hyperlipidemia: PO (Immediate-Release) Initially, 50–100 mg twice a day for 7 days. Increase gradually by doubling dose qwk up to 1–1.5 g/day in 2–3 doses. Maximum: 3 g/day. PO (Niaspan) Initially, 500 mg/day at bedtime for 4 weeks; then increase to 1,000 mg/day at bedtime. Maximum dose: 2,000 mg/day at bedtime.
    Nutritional supplement: PO 10–20 mg/day. Maximum: 100 mg/day.
    Pellegra: PO 50-100 mg 3-4 times a day. Maximum: 500 mg/day.

- **Contraindications:** Active peptic ulcer disease, arterial hemorrhaging, hepatic dysfunction, hypersensitivity to niacin or tartrazine (frequently seen in patients sensitive to aspirin), severe hypotension

- **Side Effects**

    Frequent
    Flushing (especially of the face and neck) occurring within 20 min of drug administration and lasting for 30–60 min, GI upset, pruritus
    Occasional
    Dizziness, hypotension, headache, blurred vision, burning or tingling of skin, flatulence, nausea, vomiting, diarrhea
    Rare
    Hyperglycemia, glycosuria, rash, hyperpigmentation, dry skin

- **Serious Reactions**
    - Arrhythmias occur rarely.

- In 1-g doses: 10%-20% reduction of total plus LDL-cholesterol, 30%-70% reduction in triglycerides, and a 20%-35% increase in HDL-cholesterol
- Increased risk of hepatotoxicity with smoking cessation sustained-release products.
- Do not administer Niaspan in divided doses.
- OTC smoking cessation and prescription sustained-release products are not interchangeable.

■ Patient/Family Education
- Gradual dosage titration lessens flushing, adverse effects
- Avoid alcohol and hot beverages (increases flushing)
- Administer with meals and 2 glasses of water
- 125-350 mg of aspirin 20-30 min prior to dose may lessen flushing
- Do not miss any doses (flushing may return)
- If dizziness occurs, avoid sudden posture changes and activities that require steady and alert responses
- Flushing may decrease with continued therapy

■ Monitoring Parameters
- Liver function tests, blood glucose, uric acid regularly
- Fasting lipid profile q3-6mo
- Pattern of bowel activity
- Skin for rash or dryness

■ Geriatric side effects at a glance:
❑ CNS   ❑ Bowel Dysfunction   ❑ Bladder Dysfunction   ❑ Falls

■ U.S. Regulatory Considerations
❑ FDA Black Box   ❑ OBRA regulated in U.S. Long Term Care

nicardipine hydrochloride

(nye-kar'-de-peen hye-dro-klor'-ide)

■ Brand Name(s): Cardene, Cardene IV, Cardene SR
Chemical Class: Dihydropyridine

■ Clinical Pharmacology:
Mechanism of Action: An antianginal and antihypertensive agent that inhibits calcium ion movement across cell membranes, depressing contraction of cardiac and vascular smooth muscle. **Therapeutic Effect:** Increases heart rate and cardiac output. Decreases systemic vascular resistance and BP.

Pharmacokinetics:

Route	Onset	Peak	Duration
PO	N/A	1–2 hr	8 hr

Rapidly, completely absorbed from the GI tract. Protein binding: 95%. Undergoes first-pass metabolism in the liver. Primarily excreted in urine. Not removed by hemodialysis. **Half-life:** 2–4 hr.

■ Available Forms:
- *Capsules (Cardene):* 20 mg, 30 mg.
- *Capsules (Sustained-Release [Cardene* SR]): 30 mg, 45 mg, 60 mg.
- *Injection (Cardene* IV): 2.5 mg/ml.

■ Indications and Dosages:
Chronic stable (effort-associated) angina: PO Initially, 20 mg 3 times a day. Range: 20–40 mg 3 times a day.
Essential hypertension: PO Initially, 20 mg 3 times a day. Range: 20–40 mg 3 times a day. PO (Sustained-Release) Initially, 30 mg twice a day. Range: 30–60 mg twice a day.
Short-term treatment of hypertension when oral therapy isn't feasible or desirable (substitute for oral nicardipine): IV 0.5 mg/hr (for patient receiving 20 mg PO q8h); 1.2 mg/hr (for patient receiving 30 mg PO q8h); 2.2 mg/hr (for patient receiving 40 mg PO q8h).
Patients not already receiving nicardipine: IV *Gradual* BP *decrease.* Initially, 5 mg/hr. May increase by 2.5 mg/hr q15min. After BP goal is achieved, decrease rate to 3 mg/hr. *Rapid* BP *decrease.* Initially, 5 mg/hr. May increase by 2.5 mg/hr q5min. Maximum: 15 mg/hr until desired BP attained. After BP goal achieved, decrease rate to 3 mg/hr.
Changing from IV to oral antihypertensive therapy: Begin antihypertensives other than nicardipine when IV has been discontinued; for nicardipine, give first dose 1 hr before discontinuing IV.
Dosage in hepatic impairment: Initially give 20 mg twice a day; then titrate.
Dosage in renal impairment: Initially give 20 mg q8h (30 mg twice a day [sustained-release capsules]); then titrate.

■ Unlabeled Uses:
Treatment of associated neurologic deficits, Raynaud's phenomenon, subarachnoid hemorrhage, vasospastic angina

■ Contraindications:
Atrial fibrillation or flutter associated with accessory conduction pathways, cardiogenic shock, CHF, second- or third-degree heart block, severe hypotension, sinus bradycardia, ventricular tachycardia, within several hours of IV beta-blocker therapy

■ Side Effects
Frequent (10%–7%)
Headache, facial flushing, peripheral edema, light-headedness, dizziness
Occasional (6%–3%)
Asthenia (loss of strength, energy), palpitations, angina, tachycardia
Rare (less than 2%)
Nausea, abdominal cramps, dyspepsia, dry mouth, rash

■ Serious Reactions
- Overdose produces confusion, slurred speech, somnolence, marked hypotension, and bradycardia.

■ Patient/Family Education
- Take nicardipine's sustained-release form with food and do not crush or open the capsules
- Avoid alcohol and limit caffeine

- Notify the physician if anginal pain is not relieved by the medication or if constipation, dizziness, irregular heartbeat, nausea, shortness of breath, swelling, or symptoms of hypotension such as light-headedness occurs

■ **Monitoring Parameters**
- Blood pressure
- Liver function test
- ECG and pulse for tachycardia
- Skin for dermatitis, facial flushing, or rash

■ **Geriatric side effects at a glance:**
☐ CNS ☐ Bowel Dysfunction ☐ Bladder Dysfunction ☐ Falls

■ **U.S. Regulatory Considerations**
☐ FDA Black Box ☐ OBRA regulated in U.S. Long Term Care

nicotine

(nik'-oh-teen)

■ **Brand Name(s):** Nicotrol, Nicotrol Inhaler, Nicotrol NS
  OTC: Commit, NicoDerm CQ, NicoDerm CQ Clear, Nicorette
  Chemical Class: Pyridine alkaloid

■ **Clinical Pharmacology:**
  Mechanism of Action: A cholinergic-receptor agonist that binds to acetylcholine receptors, producing both stimulating and depressant effects on the peripheral and central nervous systems. **Therapeutic Effect:** Provides a source of nicotine during nicotine withdrawal and reduces withdrawal symptoms.
  Pharmacokinetics: Absorbed slowly after transdermal administration. Protein binding: 5%. Metabolized in the liver. Excreted primarily in urine. **Half-life:** 4 hr.

■ **Available Forms:**
- *Chewing Gum (Nicorette):* 2 mg, 4 mg.
- *Lozenge (Commit):* 2 mg, 4 mg.
- *Transdermal Patch (NicoDerm CQ, Nicotrol):* 5 mg/16 hr, 7 mg/24 hr, 10 mg/16 hr, 14 mg/24 hr, 21 mg/24 hr mg.
- *Nasal Spray (Nicotrol NS):* 0.5 mg/spray.
- *Inhalation (Nicotrol Inhaler):* 10-mg cartridge.

■ **Indications and Dosages:**
  Smoking cessation aid to relieve nicotine withdrawal symptoms: PO (Chewing gum) Usually, 10–12 pieces/day. Maximum: 30 pieces/day. PO (Lozenge) **Alert** For those who smoke the first cigarette within 30 min of waking, administer the 4 mg-lozenge; otherwise administer the 2-mg lozenge. One 4-mg or 2-mg lozenge q1-2h for the first 6 wk; one lozenge q2-4h for wk 7-9; and one lozenge q4-8h for wk 10-12. Maximum:

one lozenge at a time, 5 lozenges/6 hr, 20 lozenges/day. Transdermal *Those who smoke 10 cigarettes or more per day.* Follow the guidelines below. **Step 1:** 21 mg/day for 4–6 wk. **Step 2:** 14 mg/day for 2 wk. **Step 3:** 7 mg/day for 2 wk. *Those who smoke less than 10 cigarettes per day.* Follow the guidelines below. **Step 1:** 14 mg/day for 6 wk. **Step 2:** 7 mg/day for 2 wk. **Weight less than 100 lb, history of cardiovascular disease.** Initially, 14 mg/day for 4–6 wk, then 7 mg/day for 2–4 wk. Transdermal (Nicotrol) One patch a day for 6 wk. Nasal 1–2 doses/hr (1 dose = 2 sprays [1 in each nostril] = 1 mg). Maximum: 5 doses (5 mg)/hr; 40 doses (40 mg) /day. Inhaler (Nicotrol) Puff on nicotine cartridge mouth-piece for about 20 min as needed.

■ **Contraindications:** Immediate post MI period, life-threatening arrhythmias, severe or worsening angina

■ **Side Effects**
Frequent
All forms: Hiccups, nausea
Gum: Mouth or throat soreness, nausea, hiccups
Transdermal: Erythema, pruritus, or burning at application site
Occasional
All forms: Eructation, GI upset, dry mouth, insomnia, diaphoresis, irritability
Gum: Hiccups, hoarseness
Inhaler: Mouth or throat irritation, cough
Rare
All forms: Dizziness, myalgia, arthralgia

■ **Serious Reactions**
• Overdose produces palpitations, tachyarrhythmias, seizures, depression, confusion, diaphoresis, hypotension, rapid or weak pulse, and dyspnea. Lethal dose is 40–60 mg. Death results from respiratory paralysis.

Special Considerations
• Drugs that may require dosage reduction with smoking cessation: acetaminophen, caffeine, imipramine, oxazepam, pentazocine, propranolol, theophylline, insulin, prazocin, labetalol
• Drugs that may require an increase in dose with smoking cessation: isoproterenol, phenylephrine

■ **Patient/Family Education**
• Chew gum slowly until burning or tingling sensation is felt, then park gum between cheek and gum until tingling sensation goes away
• Chew <30 min/piece
• Avoid coffee and cola drinks while chewing gum or using inhaler
• Do not smoke while utilizing nicotine replacement therapy
• Apply new transdermal system daily
• Rotate sites; apply to nonhairy area on upper torso
• Notify the physician if itching or a persistent rash occurs during treatment with the transdermal patch

■ **Monitoring Parameters**
• Blood pressure, pulse rate
• If the transdermal system is used, monitor the application site for burning, erythema, and pruritus

nifedipine

(nye-fed'-i-peen)

■ **Brand Name(s):** Adalat CC, Nifedical XL, Procardia, Procardia XL
Chemical Class: Dihydropyridine

■ **Clinical Pharmacology:**
Mechanism of Action: An antianginal and antihypertensive agent that inhibits calcium ion movement across cell membranes, depressing contraction of cardiac and vascular smooth muscle. **Therapeutic Effect:** Increases heart rate and cardiac output. Decreases systemic vascular resistance and BP.
Pharmacokinetics:

Route	Onset	Peak	Duration
Sublingual	1–5 min	N/A	N/A
PO	20–30 min	N/A	4–8 hr
PO (extended release)	2 hr	N/A	24 hr

Rapidly, completely absorbed from the GI tract. Protein binding: 92%–98%. Undergoes first-pass metabolism in the liver. Primarily excreted in urine. Not removed by hemodialysis. **Half-life:** 2–5 hr.

■ **Available Forms:**
- *Capsules* (*Procardia*): 10 mg.
- *Tablets* (*Extended-Release*): 30 mg (Adalat CC, Nifedical XL, Procardia XL), 60 mg (Adalat CC, Nifedical XL, Procardia XL), 90 mg (Adalat CC, Procardia XL).

■ **Indications and Dosages:**
Prinzmetal's variant angina, chronic stable (effort-associated) angina: PO Initially, 10 mg 3 times a day. Increase at 7- to 14-day intervals. Maintenance: 10 mg 3 times a day up to 30 mg 4 times a day. PO (Extended-Release) Initially, 30–60 mg/day. Maintenance: Up to 120 mg/day.
Essential hypertension: PO (Extended-Release) Initially, 30–60 mg/day. Maintenance: Up to 120 mg/day.

■ **Unlabeled Uses:** Treatment of Raynaud's phenomenon

■ **Contraindications:** Advanced aortic stenosis, severe hypotension

■ **Side Effects**
Frequent (30%–11%)
Peripheral edema, headache, flushed skin, dizziness

Occasional (12%–6%)
Nausea, shakiness, muscle cramps and pain, somnolence, palpitations, nasal congestion, cough, dyspnea, wheezing
Rare (5%–3%)
Hypotension, rash, pruritus, urticaria, constipation, abdominal discomfort, flatulence, sexual difficulties

■ **Serious Reactions**
- Nifedipine may precipitate CHF and MI in patients with cardiac disease and peripheral ischemia.
- Overdose produces nausea, somnolence, confusion, and slurred speech.

Special Considerations
- Given the seriousness of the reported adverse events and the lack of any clinical documentation attesting to a benefit, the use of nifedipine capsules for hypertensive urgencies or emergencies should be abandoned (JAMA 1996; 276:1328-1331)

■ **Patient/Family Education**
- Administer Adalat CC on an empty stomach
- Do not crush or chew sustained-release dosage forms
- Empty Procardia XL tablets may appear in stool, this is no cause for concern
- Rise slowly from a lying to a sitting position and permit legs to dangle from bed momentarily before standing to reduce nifedipine's hypotensive effect
- Notify the physician if irregular heartbeat, prolonged dizziness, nausea, or shortness of breath occurs
- Avoid alcohol, grapefruit and grapefruit juice

■ **Monitoring Parameters**
- Skin for flushing
- Liver function tests

■ **Geriatric side effects at a glance:**
   ❑ CNS   ❑ Bowel Dysfunction   ❑ Bladder Dysfunction   ❑ Falls

■ **U.S. Regulatory Considerations**
   ❑ FDA Black Box   ❑ OBRA regulated in U.S. Long Term Care

nimodipine

(nye-moe'-di-peen)

■ **Brand Name(s):** Nimotop
   Chemical Class: Dihydropyridine

■ **Clinical Pharmacology:**
   Mechanism of Action: A cerebral vasospasm agent that inhibits movement of calcium ions across vascular smooth-muscle cell membranes. **Therapeutic Effect:** Produces fa-

vorable effect on severity of neurologic deficits due to cerebral vasospasm. Exerts greatest effect on cerebral arteries; may prevent cerebral spasm.
Pharmacokinetics: Rapidly absorbed from the GI tract. Protein binding: 95%. Metabolized in the liver. Excreted in urine; eliminated in feces. Not removed by hemodialysis. **Half-life:** terminal, 3 hr.

■ Available Forms:
- *Capsules*: 30 mg.

■ Indications and Dosages:
Improvement of neurologic deficits after subarachnoid hemorrhage from ruptured congenital aneurysms: PO 60 mg q4h for 21 days. Begin within 96 hr of subarachnoid hemorrhage.

■ Unlabeled Uses: Treatment of chronic and classic migraine, chronic cluster headaches

■ Contraindications: Atrial fibrillation or flutter, cardiogenic shock, CHF, heart block, sinus bradycardia, ventricular tachycardia, within several hours of IV beta-blocker therapy

■ Side Effects
Occasional (6% –2%)
Hypotension, peripheral edema, diarrhea, headache
Rare (less than 2%)
Allergic reaction (rash, hives), tachycardia, flushing of skin

■ Serious Reactions
- Overdose produces nausea, weakness, dizziness, somnolence, confusion, and slurred speech.

■ Patient/Family Education
- Do not crush or chew capsules
- Notify the physician if constipation, dizziness, irregular heartbeat, nausea, shortness of breath, or swelling occurs

■ Monitoring Parameters
- Blood pressure
- CNS response
- Heart rate for signs and symptoms of CHF and hypotension

■ Geriatric side effects at a glance:
❏ CNS   ❏ Bowel Dysfunction   ❏ Bladder Dysfunction   ❏ Falls

■ U.S. Regulatory Considerations
❏ FDA Black Box   ❏ OBRA regulated in U.S. Long Term Care

nisoldipine

(nye-sole'-di-peen)

■ **Brand Name(s):** Sular
   Chemical Class: Dihydropyridine

■ **Clinical Pharmacology:**
   Mechanism of Action: An antihypertensive that inhibits calcium ion movement across cell membrane, depressing contraction of cardiac and vascular smooth muscle. **Therapeutic Effect:** Increases heart rate and cardiac output. Decreases systemic vascular resistance and blood pressure (BP).
   Pharmacokinetics: Poor absorption from the gastrointestinal (GI) tract. Food increases bioavailability. Protein binding: more than 99%. Metabolism occurs in the gut wall. Primarily excreted in urine. Not removed by hemodialysis. **Half-life:** 7-12 hr.

■ **Available Forms:**
   • *Tablets (Extended-Release)*: 10 mg, 20 mg, 30 mg, 40 mg (Sular).

■ **Indications and Dosages:**
   Hypertension: PO Initially, 10 mg once daily. Increase by 10 mg per week to therapeutic response. Maintenance: 20-40 mg once daily. Maximum: 60 mg once daily.

■ **Unlabeled Uses:** Stable angina pectoris, CHF

■ **Contraindications:** Sick sinus syndrome/second- or third-degree AV block (except in presence of pacemaker), hypersensitivity to nisoldipine or any component of the formulation

■ **Side Effects**
   Frequent
   Giddiness, dizziness, light-headedness, peripheral edema, headache, flushing, weakness, nausea
   Occasional
   Transient hypotension, heartburn, muscle cramps, nasal congestion, cough, wheezing, sore throat, palpitations, nervousness, mood changes
   Rare
   Increase in frequency, intensity, duration of anginal attack during initial therapy

■ **Serious Reactions**
   • May precipitate congestive heart failure (CHF) and myocardial infarction (MI) in patients with cardiac disease and peripheral ischemia.
   • Overdose produces nausea, drowsiness, confusion, and slurred speech.

Special Considerations
   • No significant advantages over other dihydropyridine calcium channel blockers

■ **Patient/Family Education**
   • Do not take with high-fat meal or grapefruit juice

- Rise slowly from lying to sitting position and permit legs to dangle from bed momentarily before standing to reduce the drug's hypotensive effect

■ **Monitoring Parameters**
  - Blood pressure

■ **Geriatric side effects at a glance:**
  ❑ CNS   ❑ Bowel Dysfunction   ❑ Bladder Dysfunction   ❑ Falls

■ **U.S. Regulatory Considerations**
  ❑ FDA Black Box   ❑ OBRA regulated in U.S. Long Term Care

nitazoxanide

(nye-ta-zox'-ah-nide)

■ **Brand Name(s):** Alinia
  Chemical Class: Benzamide derivative

■ **Clinical Pharmacology:**
  Mechanism of Action: An antiparasitic that interferes with the body's reaction to pyruvate ferredoxin oxidoreductase, an enzyme essential for anaerobic energy metabolism. **Therapeutic Effect:** Produces antiprotozoal activity, reducing or terminating diarrheal episodes.
  Pharmacokinetics: Rapidly hydrolyzed to an active metabolite. Protein binding: 99%. Excreted in the urine, bile, and feces. **Half-life:** 2–4 hr.

■ **Available Forms:**
  - *Powder for Oral Suspension*: 100 mg/5 ml.
  - *Tablets*: 500 mg.

■ **Indications and Dosages:**
  Diarrhea caused by Giardia lamblia: PO 500 mg q12h for 3 days.

■ **Contraindications:** History of sensitivity to aspirin and salicylates

■ **Side Effects**
  Occasional (8%)
  Abdominal pain
  Rare (2%–1%)
  Diarrhea, vomiting, headache

■ **Serious Reactions**
  - None known.

Special Considerations
  - Efficacy in adults or immunocompromised patients not known
  - Efficacy for **G.** *lamblia* 90% (equal to metronidazole)

Patient/Family Education
- Take with food
- Oral suspension of nitazoxanide contains 1.48g of sucrose per 5 ml
- Nitazoxanide therapy should significantly improve diarrhea

Monitoring Parameters
- Blood glucose level in the patient with diabetes
- Electrolyte levels for abnormalities that may have been caused by diarrhea
- Weigh each day and encourage him or her to maintain adequate fluid intake
- Bowel sounds for peristalsis; pattern of daily bowel activity and stool consistency

Geriatric side effects at a glance:
❑ CNS ❑ Bowel Dysfunction ❑ Bladder Dysfunction ❑ Falls

U.S. Regulatory Considerations
❑ FDA Black Box ❑ OBRA regulated in U.S. Long Term Care

nitrofurantoin sodium

(nye-troe-fyoor-an'-toyn)

Brand Name(s): Furadantin, Macrobid, Macrodantin, Nitro Macro

Combinations
Rx: Nitrofurantoin macrocrystals with nitrofurantoin monohydrate (Macrobid)
Chemical Class: Nitrofuran derivative

Clinical Pharmacology:
Mechanism of Action: An antibacterial UTI agent that inhibits the synthesis of bacterial DNA, RNA, proteins, and cell walls by altering or inactivating ribosomal proteins.
Therapeutic Effect: Bacteriostatic (bactericidal at high concentrations).
Pharmacokinetics: Microcrystalline form rapidly and completely absorbed; macrocrystalline form more slowly absorbed. Food increases absorption. Protein binding: 40%. Primarily concentrated in urine and kidneys. Metabolized in most body tissues. Primarily excreted in urine. Removed by hemodialysis. **Half-life:** 20-60 min.

Available Forms:
- *Capsules (Macrocrystalline, monohydrate [Macrobid]):* 100 mg.
- *Capsules (Macrocrystalline [Macrodantin, Nitro Macro]):* 25 mg, 50 mg, 100 mg
- *Oral Suspension (Microcrystalline [Furadantin]):* 25 mg/5 ml.

Indications and Dosages:
UTIs: PO (Furadantin, Macrodantin) 50-100 mg q6h. Maximum: 400 mg/day. PO (Macrobid) 100 mg twice a day. Maximum: 400 mg/day.
Long-term prevention of UTIs: PO 50-100 mg at bedtime.

Unlabeled Uses: Prevention of bacterial UTIs

- **Contraindications:** Anuria, oliguria, substantial renal impairment (creatinine clearance less than 40 ml/min)

- **Side Effects**

  Frequent

  Anorexia, nausea, vomiting, dark urine

  Occasional

  Abdominal pain, diarrhea, rash, pruritus, urticaria, hypertension, headache, dizziness, drowsiness

  Rare

  Photosensitivity, transient alopecia, asthmatic exacerbation in those with history of asthma

- **Serious Reactions**
  - Superinfection, hepatotoxicity, peripheral neuropathy (may be irreversible), Stevens-Johnson syndrome, permanent pulmonary function impairment, and anaphylaxis occur rarely.

Special Considerations
  - Individualize treatment based on local susceptibility patterns.

- **Patient/Family Education**
  - Food or milk may decrease GI upset
  - May cause brown discoloration of urine
  - Continue taking nitrofurantoin for the full course of therapy
  - Avoid exposure to the sun and ultraviolet light and use sunscreen and wear protective clothing when outdoors
  - Notify the physician if chest pain, cough, difficult breathing, fever, or numbness and tingling of fingers or toes occurs
  - Hair loss may occur but is only temporary

- **Monitoring Parameters**
  - Periodic liver function tests during prolonged therapy
  - CBC with differential and platelets during prolonged therapy
  - Pulmonary review of systems
  - Intake and output and renal function test results
  - Pattern of daily bowel activity and stool consistency
  - Be alert for signs and symptoms of peripheral neuropathy, such as numbness or tingling, especially in the lower extremities

- **Geriatric side effects at a glance:**
  - ❑ CNS   ❑ Bowel Dysfunction   ❑ Bladder Dysfunction   ❑ Falls

- **U.S. Regulatory Considerations**
  - ❑ FDA Black Box   ❑ OBRA regulated in U.S. Long Term Care

nitrofurazone

(nye-troe-fyoor'-a-zone)

- **Brand Name(s):** Furacin
  Chemical Class: Nitrofuran derivative

- **Clinical Pharmacology:**
  Mechanism of Action: A synthetic nitrofuran that inhibits bacterial enzymes involved in carbohydrate metabolism. **Therapeutic Effect:** Inhibits a variety of enzymes. Bactericidal.
  Pharmacokinetics: Not known.

- **Available Forms:**
  - *Cream*: 0.2% (Furacin).
  - *Ointment*: 0.2% (Furacin).
  - *Solution*: 0.2% (Furacin).

- **Indications and Dosages:**
  Burns, catheter-related urinary tract infection, skin grafts: Topical Apply directly on lesion with spatula or place on a piece of gauze first. Use of a bandage is optional. Preparation should remain on lesion for at least 24 hours. Dressing may be changed several times daily or left on the lesion for a longer period.

- **Unlabeled Uses:** Fire and ant bites, scabies, urethritis, vaginal malodor, vasectomy, wounds

- **Contraindications:** Hypersensitivity to nitrofurazone or any of its components

- **Side Effects**
  Occasional
  Itching, rash, swelling

- **Serious Reactions**
  - Use of nitrofurazone may result in bacterial or fungal overgrowth of nonsusceptible pathogens, which may lead to secondary infection.

- **Patient/Family Education**
  - Avoid contact with eye
  - Notify the physician if irritation, inflammation, or rash occurs

- **Monitoring Parameters**
  - Skin for irritation

- **Geriatric side effects at a glance:**
  ❑ CNS ❑ Bowel Dysfunction ❑ Bladder Dysfunction ❑ Falls

nitroglycerin

(nye-troe-gli'-ser-in)

■ **Brand Name(s):** Minitran, Nitrek, Nitro-Bid, Nitro-Bid IV, Nitrocot, Nitro-Dur, Nitrogard, Nitroglyn E-R, Nitrol Appli-Kit, Nitrolingual, Nitrong, NitroQuick, Nitrostat, Nitro-Tab, Nitro TD Patch-A, Nitro-Time, Tridil
Chemical Class: Nitrate, organic

■ **Clinical Pharmacology:**
Mechanism of Action: A nitrate that decreases myocardial oxygen demand. Reduces left ventricular preload and afterload. **Therapeutic Effect:** Dilates coronary arteries and improves collateral blood flow to ischemic areas within myocardium. IV form produces peripheral vasodilation.
Pharmacokinetics:

Route	Onset	Peak	Duration
Sublingual	1–3 min	4–8 min	30–60 min
Translingual Spray	2 min	4-10 min	30-60 min
Buccal Tablet	2–5 min	4–10 min	2 hr
PO(Extended-Release)	20–45 min	45-120 min	4–8 hr
Topical	15–60 min	30-120 min	2–12 hr
Transdermal Patch	40–60 min	60-180 min	18–24 hr
IV	1–2 min	Immediate	3–5 min

Well absorbed after PO, sublingual, and topical administration. Undergoes extensive first-pass metabolism. Metabolized in the liver and by enzymes in the bloodstream. Primarily excreted in urine. Not removed by hemodialysis. **Half-life:** 1–4 min.

■ **Available Forms:**
- *Capsules (Extended-Release [NitroBid, Nitrocot, Nitroglyn E-R, Nitro-Time]):* 2.5 mg, 6.5 mg, 9 mg.
- *Tablets (Extended-Release, Oral Transmucosal):* 1 mg (Nitrogard), 2.6 mg (Nitrong), 3 mg (Nitrogard), 6.5 mg (Nitrong).
- *Tablets (Sublingual [NitroQuick, Nitrostat, Nitro-Tab]):* 0.3 mg, 0.4 mg, 0.6 mg.
- *Spray (Translingual [Nitrolingual]):* 0.4 mg/spray.
- *Infusion Solution:* 0.1 mg/ml, 0.2 mg/ml, 0.4 mg/ml.
- *Intravenous Solution (Nitro-Bid IV, Tridil):* 5 mg/ml.
- *Intravenous Solution:* 5% dextrose-10 mg nitroglycerin/100 ml, 5% dextrose-20 mg nitroglycerin/100 ml, 5% dextrose-40 mg nitroglycerin/100 ml.
- *Topical Ointment (Nitro-Bid, Nitrol, Nitrol Appli-Kit):* 2%.
- *Transdermal Patch (Minitran):* 0.1 mg/h (Minitran, Nitro-Dur), 0.2 mg/h (Minitran, Nitrek, Nitro-Dur), 0.3 mg/h (Minitran, Nitro-Dur), 0.4 mg/h (Minitran, Nitrek, Nitro-Dur), 0.6 mg/h (Nitrek, Nitro-Dur), 0.8 mg/h (Nitro-Dur).

- ■ **Indications and Dosages:**

  Acute relief of angina pectoris, acute prophylaxis: Lingual Spray 1 spray onto or under tongue q3–5min until relief is noted (no more than 3 sprays in 15-min period). Sublingual 0.4 mg q5min until relief is noted (no more than 3 doses in 15-min period). Use prophylactically 5–10 min before activities that may cause an acute attack.

  Long-term prophylaxis of angina: PO (Extended-Release) 2.5–9 mg 2–4 times a day. Maximum: 26 mg 4 times a day. Topical Initially, ½ inch q8h. Increase by ½ inch with each application. Range: 1–2 inches q8h up to 4–5 inches q4h. Transdermal Patch Initially, 0.2–0.4 mg/h. Maintenance: 0.4–0.8 mg/h. Consider patch on for 12–14 h, patch off for 10–12 h (prevents tolerance).

  CHF *associated with acute MI:* IV Initially, 5 mcg/min via infusion pump. Increase in 5-mcg/min increments at 3- to 5-min intervals until BP response is noted or until dosage reaches 20 mcg/min; then increase as needed by 10 mcg/min. Dosage may be further titrated according to clinical, therapeutic response up to 200 mcg/min.

- ■ **Contraindications:** Allergy to adhesives (transdermal), closed-angle glaucoma, constrictive pericarditis (IV), early MI (sublingual), GI hypermotility or malabsorption (extended-release), head trauma, hypotension (IV), inadequate cerebral circulation (IV), increased intracranial pressure (ICP), nitrates, orthostatic hypotension, pericardial tamponade (IV), severe anemia, uncorrected hypovolemia (IV)

- ■ **Side Effects**

  Frequent

  Headache (possibly severe; occurs mostly in early therapy, diminishes rapidly in intensity, and usually disappears during continued treatment), transient flushing of face and neck, dizziness (especially if patient is standing immobile or is in a warm environment), weakness, orthostatic hypotension

  Sublingual: Burning, tingling sensation at oral point of dissolution

  Ointment: Erythema, pruritus

  Occasional

  GI upset

  Transdermal: Contact dermatitis

- ■ **Serious Reactions**

  - Nitroglycerin should be discontinued if blurred vision or dry mouth occurs.
  - Severe orthostatic hypotension may occur, manifested by fainting, pulselessness, cold or clammy skin, and diaphoresis.
  - Tolerance may occur with repeated, prolonged therapy; minor tolerance may occur with intermittent use of sublingual tablets.
  - High doses of nitroglycerin tend to produce severe headache.

Special Considerations

- Ten- to 12-hr drug-free intervals prevent development of tolerance
- Remove the transdermal patch before cardioversion or defibrillation because the electrical current may cause arcing which can burn the patient and damage the paddles

- ■ **Patient/Family Education**

  - Avoid alcohol
  - Notify clinician if persistent headache occurs
  - Take oral nitrates on empty stomach with full glass of water
  - Keep tablets and capsules in original container, keep container closed tightly

- Dissolve SL tablets under tongue, lack of burning does not indicate loss of potency, use when seated, take at first sign of anginal attack, activate emergency response system if no relief after 3 tablets spaced 5 min apart
- Spray translingual spray onto or under tongue, do not inhale spray
- Place buccal tablets under upper lip or between cheek and gum, let dissolve slowly over 3-5 min, do not chew or swallow
- Spread thin layer of ointment on skin using applicator or dose-measuring papers, do not use fingers, do not rub or massage
- Apply transdermal systems to nonhairy area on upper torso, remove for 10-12 hr/day (usually hs)

■ **Monitoring Parameters**
- Blood pressure, heart rate at peak effect times
- ECG during IV administration
- Examine the patient for facial or neck flushing

■ **Geriatric side effects at a glance:**
❑ CNS ❑ Bowel Dysfunction ❑ Bladder Dysfunction ❑ Falls

■ **U.S. Regulatory Considerations**
❑ FDA Black Box ❑ OBRA regulated in U.S. Long Term Care

nitroprusside sodium

(nye-troe-pruss'-ide soe'-dee-um)

■ **Brand Name(s):** Nitropress
Chemical Class: Cyanonitrosylferrate derivative

■ **Clinical Pharmacology:**
Mechanism of Action: A potent vasodilator used to treat emergent hypertensive conditions; acts directly on arterial and venous smooth muscle. Decreases peripheral vascular resistance, preload and afterload; improves cardiac output. **Therapeutic Effect:** Dilates coronary arteries, decreases oxygen consumption, and relieves persistent chest pain.
Pharmacokinetics:

Route	Onset	Peak	Duration
IV	1–10 min	Dependent on infusion rate	Dissipates rapidly after stopping IV

Reacts with Hgb in erythrocytes, producing cyanmethemoglobin, and cyanide ions. Primarily excreted in urine. **Half-life:** less than 10 min.

■ **Available Forms:**
- *Injection*: 25 mg/ml.
- *Powder for Injection*: 50 mg.

- **Indications and Dosages:**

  Immediate reduction of BP in hypertensive crisis; to produce controlled hypotension in surgical procedures to reduce bleeding; treatment of acute **CHF:** IV Infusion Initially, 0.3-0.5 mcg/kg/min. May increase by 0.5 mcg/kg/min to desired hemodynamic effect or appearance of headache or nausea. Usual dose: 3 mcg/kg/min. Maximum: 10 mcg/kg/min.

- **Unlabeled Uses:** Control of paroxysmal hypertension before and during surgery for pheochromocytoma, peripheral vasospasm caused by ergot alkaloid overdose, treatment adjunct for MI, valvular regurgitation

- **Contraindications:** Compensatory hypertension (atrioventricular [AV] shunt or coarctation of aorta), congenital (Leber's) optic atrophy, inadequate cerebral circulation, moribund patients, tobacco amblyopia

- **Side Effects**

  Occasional

  Flushing of skin, increased intracranial pressure, rash, pain or redness at injection site

- **Serious Reactions**
  - A too-rapid IV infusion rate reduces BP too quickly.
  - Nausea, vomiting, diaphoresis, apprehension, headache, restlessness, muscle twitching, dizziness, palpitations, retrosternal pain, and abdominal pain may occur. Symptoms disappear rapidly if rate of administration is slowed or drug is temporarily discontinued.
  - Overdose produces metabolic acidosis and tolerance to therapeutic effect.

- **Patient/Family Education**
  - Immediately report dizziness, headache, nausea, palpitations, or other unusual signs or symptoms

- **Monitoring Parameters**
  - Blood pressure, arterial blood gases, oxygen saturation, cyanide and thiocyanate concentrations, anion gap, lactate levels
  - Intake and output
  - Monitor the rate of infusion frequently
  - Therapeutic response—expect to discontinue nitroprusside if the therapeutic response is not achieved within 10 minutes after IV infusion at 10 mcg/kg/min is initiated

- **Geriatric side effects at a glance:**
  ❑ CNS ❑ Bowel Dysfunction ❑ Bladder Dysfunction ❑ Falls

- **U.S. Regulatory Considerations**
  ☑ FDA Black Box
  - Requires dilution
  - Cyanide toxicity
  - Hypotension
  ❑ OBRA regulated in U.S. Long Term Care

nizatidine

(nye-za'-ti-deen)

■ **Brand Name(s):** Axid
   OTC: Axid AR
   Chemical Class: Ethenediamine derivative

■ **Clinical Pharmacology:**
   Mechanism of Action: An H_2 blocker and gastric acid secretion inhibitor that inhibits histamine action at histamine-2 receptors of parietal cells. **Therapeutic Effect:** Inhibits basal and nocturnal gastric acid secretion.
   Pharmacokinetics: Rapidly, well absorbed from the GI tract. Protein binding: 35%. Metabolized in the liver. Primarily excreted in urine. Not removed by hemodialysis. **Half-life:** 1–2 hr (increased with impaired renal function).

■ **Available Forms:**
   • *Capsules:* 75 mg (Axid AR), 150 mg (Axid), 300 mg (Axid).
   • *Oral Solution (Axid):* 15 mg/ml.

■ **Indications and Dosages:**
   Active duodenal ulcer: PO 300 mg at bedtime or 150 mg twice a day.
   Prevention of duodenal ulcer recurrence: PO 150 mg at bedtime.
   Gastroesophageal reflux disease: PO 150 mg twice a day.
   Active benign gastric ulcer: PO 150 mg twice a day or 300 mg at bedtime.
   Dyspepsia: PO 75 mg 30–60 min before meals; no more than 2 tablets a day.
   Dosage in renal impairment: Dosage adjustment is based on creatinine clearance.

Creatinine Clearance	Active Ulcer	Maintenance Therapy
20–50 ml/min	150 mg at bedtime	150 mg every other day
less than 20 ml/min	150 mg every other day	150 mg q3 days

■ **Unlabeled Uses:** Gastric hypersecretory conditions, multiple endocrine adenoma, Zollinger-Ellison syndrome, weight gain reduction in patients taking Zyprexa

■ **Contraindications:** Hypersensitivity to other H_2-antagonists

■ **Side Effects**
   Occasional (2%)
   Somnolence, fatigue
   Rare (1%)
   Diaphoresis, rash

■ **Serious Reactions**
   • Asymptomatic ventricular tachycardia, hyperuricemia not associated with gout, and nephrolithiasis occur rarely.

Special Considerations
   • No advantage over other agents of this class; base selection on cost

■ **Patient/Family Education**
  • Stagger doses of nizatidine and antacids
  • Avoid tasks that require mental alertness or motor skills until response to the drug has been established
  • Avoid alcohol, aspirin, and smoking during nizatidine therapy
  • Notify the physician if acid indigestion, gastric distress, or heartburn occurs after 2 weeks of continuous nizatidine therapy

■ **Monitoring Parameters**
  • Serum alkaline phosphatase, bilirubin, AST (SGOT), and ALT (SGPT) levels
  • Assess the patient for abdominal pain and GI bleeding. Observe for overt blood in emesis or stool and for tarry stools

■ **Geriatric side effects at a glance:**
  ☑ CNS ❑ Bowel Dysfunction ❑ Bladder Dysfunction ❑ Falls
  Other: Cognitive impairment

■ **Use with caution in older patients with:** Renal impairment, Cognitive impairment

■ **U.S. Regulatory Considerations**
  ❑ FDA Black Box ❑ OBRA regulated in U.S. Long Term Care

■ **Other Uses in Geriatric Patient:** None

■ **Side Effects:**
  Of particular importance in the geriatric patient: Delirium, confusion, dizziness, headache, constipation, diarrhea

■ **Geriatric Considerations - Summary:** Adjust dose based on creatinine clearance. Not effective in preventing NSAID-induced gastric ulceration and bleeding; proton pump inhibitors should be used for this indication instead.

■ **References:**
  1. Gawrich S, Shaker R. Medical management of nocturnal symptoms of gastro-oesophageal reflux disease in the elderly. Drugs Aging 2003;20:509-516.
  2. Thomson ABR. Gastro-oesophageal reflux in the elderly. Role of drug therapy in management. Drugs Aging 2001;18:409-414.
  3. Drugs that may cause cognitive disorders in the elderly. Med Lett 2000;42:111-112.

norepinephrine bitartrate

(nor-ep-i-nef'-rin bye-tar'-trate)

■ **Brand Name(s):** Levophed
  Chemical Class: Catecholamine, synthetic

■ **Clinical Pharmacology:**
  Mechanism of Action: A sympathomimetic that stimulates beta$_1$-adrenergic receptors and alpha-adrenergic receptors, increasing peripheral resistance. Enhances con-

tractile myocardial force, increases cardiac output. Constricts resistance and capacitance vessels. **Therapeutic Effect:** Increases systemic BP and coronary blood flow.
Pharmacokinetics:

Route	Onset	Peak	Duration
IV	Rapid	1–2 min	N/A

Localized in sympathetic tissue. Metabolized in the liver. Primarily excreted in urine.

■ **Available Forms:**
- *Injection*: 1-mg/ml ampules.

■ **Indications and Dosages:**
Acute hypotension unresponsive to fluid volume replacement: IV Initially, administer at 0.5–1 mcg/min. Adjust rate of flow to establish and maintain desired BP (40 mm Hg below preexisting systolic pressure). Average maintenance dose: 8–30 mcg/min.

■ **Contraindications:** Hypovolemic states (unless as an emergency measure), mesenteric or peripheral vascular thrombosis, profound hypoxia

■ **Side Effects**
Norepinephrine produces less pronounced and less frequent side effects than epinephrine.
Occasional (5%–3%)
Anxiety, bradycardia, palpitations
Rare (2%–1%)
Nausea, anginal pain, shortness of breath, fever

■ **Serious Reactions**
- Extravasation may produce tissue necrosis and sloughing.
- Overdose is manifested as severe hypertension with violent headache (which may be the first clinical sign of overdose), arrhythmias, photophobia, retrosternal or pharyngeal pain, pallor, excessive sweating, and vomiting.
- Prolonged therapy may result in plasma volume depletion. Hypotension may recur if plasma volume is not restored.

Special Considerations
- Antidote for extravasation ischemia: Infiltrate with 10-15 ml of saline containing 5-10 mg of phentolamine

■ **Patient/Family Education**
- Immediately report burning, pain, or coolness at the IV site

■ **Monitoring Parameters**
- Blood pressure, heart rate, ECG, urine output, peripheral perfusion
- Assess the patient for extravasation. If extravasation occurs, expect to infiltrate the affected area with 10 to 15 ml sterile saline containing 5 to 10 mg phentolamine. Know that phentolamine does not alter the pressor effects of norepinephrine

■ **Geriatric side effects at a glance:**
❑ CNS ❑ Bowel Dysfunction ❑ Bladder Dysfunction ❑ Falls

■ **U.S. Regulatory Considerations**
❑ FDA Black Box ❑ OBRA regulated in U.S. Long Term Care

norfloxacin

(nor-flox'-a-sin)

- **Brand Name(s):** Noroxin
  Chemical Class: Fluoroquinolone derivative

- **Clinical Pharmacology:**
  Mechanism of Action: A quinolone that inhibits DNA gyrase in susceptible microorganisms, interfering with bacterial cell replication and repair. **Therapeutic Effect:** Bactericidal.
  Pharmacokinetics: Well absorbed following oral administration. Protein binding: 10%-15%. Eliminated through metabolism, biliary excretion, and renal excretion. **Half-life:** 3-4 hr.

- **Available Forms:**
  - *Tablets:* 400 mg.

- **Indications and Dosages:**
  UTIs: PO 400 mg twice a day for 3-21 days.
  Prostatitis: PO 400 mg twice a day for 28 days.
  Uncomplicated gonococcal infections: PO 800 mg as a single dose.
  Dosage in renal impairment: Dosage and frequency are modified based on creatinine clearance.

Creatinine Clearance	Dosage
30 ml/min or higher	400 mg twice a day
less than 30 ml/min	400 mg once a day

- **Contraindications:** Hypersensitivity to other quinolones or their components

- **Side Effects**
  Frequent
  Nausea, headache, dizziness
  Rare
  Vomiting, diarrhea, dry mouth, bitter taste, nervousness, drowsiness, insomnia, photosensitivity, tinnitus, crystalluria, rash, fever, seizures

- **Serious Reactions**
  - Superinfection, anaphylaxis, Stevens-Johnson syndrome, and arthropathy occur rarely.
  - Hypersensitivity reactions, including photosensitivity (as evidenced by rash, pruritus, blisters, edema, and burning skin), have occurred in patients receiving fluoroquinolones.
  - Tendon effects, including ruptures of shoulder, hand, Achilles tendon or other tendons, may occur. Risk increases with concomitant corticosteroid use, especially in the elderly.

Special Considerations
  - Individualize treatment based on local susceptibility patterns.

883

Patient/Family Education
- Administer on an empty stomach (1 hr before or 2 hr after meals)
- Drink fluids liberally
- Do not take antacids containing magnesium or aluminum or products containing iron or zinc within 4 hr before or 2 hr after dosing
- Avoid excessive exposure to sunlight
- Take for the full course of therapy
- May cause dizziness or drowsiness
- Take sips of tepid water or chew sugarless gum to relieve dry mouth
- Your tendons may be more easily injured while taking this medication. Monitor for pain or swelling in your knee, ankle, shoulder, elbow, or wrist.

Monitoring Parameters
- Assess the patient for chest pain, dizziness, headache, joint pain, and nausea
- Evaluate the patient's food tolerance

Geriatric side effects at a glance:
☑ CNS ❑ Bowel Dysfunction ❑ Bladder Dysfunction ❑ Falls

U.S. Regulatory Considerations
❑ FDA Black Box ❑ OBRA regulated in U.S. Long Term Care

nortriptyline hydrochloride

(noor-trip'-ti-leen hye-droe-klor'-ide)

Brand Name(s): Aventyl, Pamelor
Chemical Class: Dibenzocycloheptene derivative; secondary amine

Clinical Pharmacology:
Mechanism of Action: A tricyclic antidepressant that blocks reuptake of the neurotransmitters norepinephrine and serotonin at neuronal presynaptic membranes, increasing their availability at postsynaptic receptor sites. **Therapeutic Effect:** Relieves depression.
Pharmacokinetics: Well absorbed from the GI tract. Protein binding: 86%-95%. Metabolized in the liver. Primarily excreted in urine. **Half-life:** 17.6 hr.

Available Forms:
- *Capsules (Aventyl):* 10 mg, 25 mg.
- *Capsules (Pamelor):* 10 mg, 25 mg, 50 mg, 75 mg.
- *Oral Solution (Aventyl, Pamelor):* 10 mg/5 ml .

Indications and Dosages:
Depression: PO Initially, 10-25 mg at bedtime. May increase by 25 mg every 3-7 days. Maximum: 150 mg/day.

■ **Unlabeled Uses:** Treatment of neurogenic pain, panic disorder; prevention of migraine headache

■ **Contraindications:** Acute recovery period after MI, use within 14 days of MAOIs

■ **Side Effects**

Frequent

Somnolence, fatigue, dry mouth, blurred vision, constipation, delayed micturition, orthostatic hypotension, diaphoresis, impaired concentration, increased appetite, urine retention

Occasional

GI disturbances (nausea, GI distress, metallic taste), photosensitivity

Rare

Paradoxical reactions (agitation, restlessness, nightmares, insomnia), extrapyramidal symptoms (particularly fine hand tremor)

■ **Serious Reactions**

- Overdose may produce seizures; cardiovascular effects, such as severe orthostatic hypotension, dizziness, tachycardia, palpitations, and arrhythmias; and altered temperature regulation, such as hyperpyrexia or hypothermia.
- Abrupt discontinuation after prolonged therapy may produce headache, malaise, nausea, vomiting, and vivid dreams.

■ **Patient/Family Education**

- Therapeutic effects may take 2-3 wk
- Avoid rising quickly from sitting to standing
- Avoid alcohol and other CNS depressants
- Do not discontinue abruptly after long-term use
- Wear sunscreen or large hat to prevent sunburn
- Avoid tasks that require mental alertness or motor skills until response to the drug has been established
- Notify the physician of visual disturbances
- Take sips of tepid water or chew sugarless gum to relieve dry mouth

■ **Monitoring Parameters**

- CBC, weight, ECG, mental status (mood, sensorium, affect, suicidal tendencies)
- Determination of nortriptyline plasma concentrations is not routinely recommended but may be useful in identifying toxicity, drug interactions, or noncompliance (adjustments in dosage should be made according to clinical response, not plasma concentrations); therapeutic range is 50-150 ng/ml
- Blood pressure, pulse rate
- Pattern of daily bowel activity and stool consistency

■ **Geriatric side effects at a glance:**

☑ CNS ☑ Bowel Dysfunction ☑ Bladder Dysfunction ☑ Falls
☐ Other: Orthostatic hypotension, cardiac conduction disturbances, anticholinergic side effects

■ **Use with caution in older patients with:** Cardiovascular disease, prostatic hyptertrophy or other conditions which increase the risk of urinary retention

■ U.S. Regulatory Considerations
  - FDA Black Box
    - Because there is an increased risk of suicide in children and adolescents, older adults should also be closely monitored for suicide ideation.
  - OBRA regulated in U.S. Long Term Care

■ Other Uses in Geriatric Patient: Neuropathic pain, urge urinary incontinence

■ Side Effects:
Of particular importance in the geriatric patient: Anticholinergic effects, extrapyramidal symptoms, high doses (>100 mg) may increase risk of sudden death

■ Geriatric Considerations - Summary: Although tricyclic antidepressants are effective in the treatment of major depression in older adults, the side-effect profile and low toxic-to-therapeutic ratio relegate them to second-line agents (after serotonin reuptake inhibitors) for most older patients. These agents are effective in the treatment of urge urinary incontinence and neuropathic pain, but must be monitored closely. Of the tricyclic antidepressants, imipramine and amitryptyline have the highest anticholinergic activity and may be useful for management of incontinence, but should otherwise be avoided.

■ References:
  1. Leipzig RM, Cumming RG, Tinetti ME. Drugs and falls in older people: a systematic review and meta-analysis: I. Psychotropic drugs. J Am Geriatr Soc 1999;47:30-39.
  2. Cadieux RJ. Antidepressant drug interactions in the elderly. Understanding the P-450 system is half the battle in reducing risks. Postgrad Med 1999;106:231-240, 245.
  3. Ray WA, Meredith S, Thapa PB, et al. Cyclic antidepressants and the risk of sudden cardiac death. Clin Pharmacol Ther 2004;75:234-241.
  4. Roose SP, Laghrissi-Thode F, Kennedy JS, et al. Comparison of paroxetine and nortriptyline in depressed patients with ischemic heart disease. JAMA 1998;279:287-291.

NUTR-vitamin A

(vye'-tah-min A)

■ Brand Name(s): Aquasol A, Palmitate A
Chemical Class: NUTR-vitamin, fat soluble

■ Clinical Pharmacology:
Mechanism of Action: A fat-soluble vitamin that may act as a cofactor in biochemical reactions. *Therapeutic Effect:* Is essential for normal function of retina, visual adaptation to darkness, bone growth, and testicular and ovarian function; preserves integrity of epithelial cells.
Pharmacokinetics: Rapidly absorbed from the GI tract if bile salts, pancreatic lipase, protein, and dietary fat are present. Transported in blood to the liver, where it's metabolized; stored in parenchymal hepatic cells, then transported in plasma as retinol, as needed. Excreted primarily in bile and, to a lesser extent, in urine.

■ Available Forms:
- *Capsules*: 10,000 units, 25,000 units.
- *Injection* (*Aquasol* A): 50,000 units/ml .
- *Tablets* (*Palmitate* A): 5,000 units, 15,000 units.

■ Indications and Dosages:
Severe vitamin A deficiency: PO 500,000 units/day for 3 days; then 50,000 units/day for 14 days, then 10,000–20,000 units/day for 2 mo. IM 100,000 units/day for 3 days; then 50,000 units/day for 14 days.
Malabsorption syndrome: PO 10,000-50,000 units/day.
Dietary supplement: PO *Males:* 3000 units/day. Maximum: 10,000 units/day. *Females:* 2,310 units/day. Maximum: 10,000 units/day.

■ Contraindications: Hypervitaminosis A, oral use in malabsorption syndrome

■ Side Effects
None known.

■ Serious Reactions
- Chronic overdose produces malaise, nausea, vomiting, drying or cracking of skin or lips, inflammation of tongue or gums, irritability, alopecia, and night sweats.

■ Patient/Family Education
- Administer with food for better PO absorption
- Foods high in vitamin A: yellow and dark green vegetables, yellow and orange fruits, A-fortified foods, liver, egg yolks

■ Geriatric side effects at a glance:
❑ CNS   ❑ Bowel Dysfunction   ❑ Bladder Dysfunction   ❑ Falls

■ U.S. Regulatory Considerations
❑ FDA Black Box   ❑ OBRA regulated in U.S. Long Term Care

NUTR-vitamin D

(vye'-ta-min D)

■ Brand Name(s): Calciferol, Drisdol
Chemical Class: NUTR-vitamin, fat soluble

■ Clinical Pharmacology:
Mechanism of Action: A fat-soluble vitamin that stimulates calcium and phosphate absorption from small intestine, promotes secretion of calcium from bone to blood, and promotes resorption of phosphate in renal tubules; also acts on bone cells to stimulate skeletal growth and on parathyroid gland to suppress hormone synthesis

and secretion. **Therapeutic Effect:** Essential for absorption and utilization of calcium and phosphate and normal bone calcification. Reduces parathyroid hormone level. Improves phosphorus and calcium homeostasis in chronic renal failure.
Pharmacokinetics: Readily absorbed from small intestine. Concentrated primarily in liver and fat deposits. Activated in the liver and kidneys. Eliminated by biliary system; excreted in urine. **Half-life:** 19–48 hr for ergocalciferol.

■ **Available Forms:**
- *Capsules (Drisdol):* 50,000 units (1.25 mg).
- *Injection (Calciferol):* 500,000 units/ml (12.5 mg).
- *Oral Liquid Drops (Calciferol, Drisdol):* 8,000 units/ml.

■ **Indications and Dosages:** Alert Oral dosing is preferred. Administer the drug IM only in patients with GI, hepatic, or biliary disease associated with malabsorption of vitamin D.
Dietary supplement: PO 10 mcg (400 units)/day.
Renal failure: PO 0.5 mg/day.
Hypoparathyroidism: PO 625 mcg–5 mg/day (with calcium supplements).
Nutritional rickets, osteomalacia: PO 25–125 mcg/day for 8–12 wk. *Those with malabsorption syndrome.* 250–7,500 mcg/day.
Vitamin D–dependent rickets: PO 250 mcg–1.5 mg/day.
Vitamin D–resistant rickets: PO 250–1,500 mcg/day (with phosphate supplements).
Osteoporosis prevention: PO 400-600 units/day. Maximum: 2,000 units/day.

■ **Contraindications:** Abnormal sensitivity to toxic effects of hypervitaminosis D, hypercalcemia, malabsorption syndrome

■ **Side Effects**
Frequency not defined
Nausea, constipation, stiffness, weakness, weight loss

■ **Serious Reactions**
- Early signs and symptoms of overdose are weakness, headache, somnolence, nausea, vomiting, dry mouth, constipation, muscle and bone pain, and metallic taste.
- Later signs and symptoms of overdose include polyuria, polydipsia, anorexia, weight loss, nocturia, photophobia, rhinorrhea, pruritus, disorientation, hallucinations, hyperthermia, hypertension, and cardiac arrhythmias.

Special Considerations
- IM therapy should be reserved for patients with GI, liver, or biliary disease associated with vitamin D malabsorption
- Ensure adequate calcium intake; maintain serum calcium levels between 9-10 mg/dl

■ **Patient/Family Education**
- Encourage the patient to consume foods rich in vitamin D, including milk, eggs, leafy vegetables, margarine, meats, and vegetable oils and shortening
- Do not take mineral oil during vitamin D therapy
- The patient receiving chronic renal dialysis should not take magnesium-containing antacids during vitamin D therapy
- Drink plenty of fluids

■ **Monitoring Parameters**
- Serum calcium and phosphorus levels (vitamin D levels also helpful, although less frequently)

- X-ray bones monthly until condition is corrected and stabilized (rickets)
- Periodically determine magnesium and alk phosphatase
- Serum calcium times phosphorous should not exceed 70 mg/dl to avoid ectopic calcification

■ **Geriatric side effects at a glance:**
  ❏ CNS ❏ Bowel Dysfunction ❏ Bladder Dysfunction ❏ Falls

■ **U.S. Regulatory Considerations**
  ❏ FDA Black Box ❏ OBRA regulated in U.S. Long Term Care

NUTR-vitamin E

(vye'-tah-min E)

■ **Brand Name(s):** Aqua Gem E, Aquasol E, E-Gems, Key-E, Key-E Kaps
  Chemical Class: NUTR-vitamin, fat soluble

■ **Clinical Pharmacology:**
  Mechanism of Action: An antioxidant that prevents oxidation of vitamins A and C, protects fatty acids from attack by free radicals, and protects RBCs from hemolysis by oxidizing agents. *Therapeutic Effect:* Prevents and treats vitamin E deficiency.
  Pharmacokinetics: Variably absorbed from the GI tract (requires bile salts, dietary fat, and normal pancreatic function). Primarily concentrated in adipose tissue. Metabolized in the liver. Primarily eliminated by biliary system.

■ **Available Forms:**
  - *Capsules* (E-Gems): 100 units, 600 units, 800 units, 1,000 units, 1,200 units.
  - *Capsules* (Aqua-Gem E, Key-E Kaps): 200 units, 400 units.
  - *Tablets* (Key-E): 100 units, 200 units, 400 units, 800 units.

■ **Indications and Dosages:**
  Dietary supplement (RDA): PO 15 mg/day. Maximum: 1,000 mg/day.
  Vitamin E deficiency: PO 60–75 units/day.

■ **Unlabeled Uses:** To decrease severity of tardive dyskinesia

■ **Contraindications:** None known.

■ **Side Effects**
  None known.

■ **Serious Reactions**
  - Chronic overdose may produce fatigue, weakness, nausea, headache, blurred vision, flatulence, and diarrhea.

- Recommended daily allowance: adult male 15 IU, adult female 12 IU

■ **Patient/Family Education**
- Swallow tablets and capsules whole; do not chew, open, or crush them
- Notify the physician if signs and symptoms of toxicity, including blurred vision, diarrhea, nausea, dizziness, flu-like symptoms, or headache
- Consume foods rich in vitamin E, including eggs, meats, milk, leafy vegetables, margarine, and vegetable oils and shortening

■ **Monitoring Parameters**
- Signs and symptoms of hypervitaminosis E, including headache, fatigue, nausea, weakness, and diarrhea

■ **Geriatric side effects at a glance:**
❑ CNS ❑ Bowel Dysfunction ❑ Bladder Dysfunction ❑ Falls

■ **U.S. Regulatory Considerations**
❑ FDA Black Box ❑ OBRA regulated in U.S. Long Term Care

NUTR-vitamin K

(vye'-ta-min K)

■ **Brand Name(s):** AquaMEPHYTON, Mephyton, Vitamin K1
  Chemical Class: Naphthoquinone derivative

■ **Clinical Pharmacology:**
  Mechanism of Action: A fat-soluble vitamin that promotes hepatic formation of coagulation factors II, VII, IX, and X. **Therapeutic Effect:** Essential for normal clotting of blood.
  Pharmacokinetics: Readily absorbed from the GI tract (duodenum) after IM or subcutaneous administration. Metabolized in the liver. Excreted in urine; eliminated by biliary system. **Onset of action:** with PO form, 6-10 hr; with parenteral form, hemorrhage controlled in 3–6 hr and PT returns to normal in 12–14 hr.

■ **Available Forms:**
- *Tablets* (*Mephyton*): 5 mg .
- *Injection* (AquaMEPHYTON, *Vitamin K1*): 1 mg/0.5 ml, 10 mg/ml.

■ **Indications and Dosages:**
  Oral anticoagulant overdose: PO, IV, Subcutaneous 2.5–10 mg/dose. May repeat in 12–48 hr if given orally and in 6–8 hr if given by IV or subcutaneous route.
  Vitamin K deficiency: PO 2.5–25 mg/24 hr. IV, IM, Subcutaneous 10 mg/dose.

■ **Contraindications:** None known.

■ Side Effects
Occasional
Pain, soreness, and swelling at IM injection site; pruritic erythema (with repeated injections); facial flushing; unusual taste

■ Serious Reactions
- A severe reaction (cramplike pain, chest pain, dyspnea, facial flushing, dizziness, rapid or weak pulse, rash, diaphoresis, hypotension progressing to shock, cardiac arrest) occurs rarely just after IV administration.

Special Considerations
- IV doses should be diluted and infused slowly over 20-30 min
- Avoid using IM administration for overanticoagulation to avoid hematoma

■ Patient/Family Education
- Avoid taking any other medications, including OTC preparations, without the physician's approval because they may interfere with platelet aggregation
- Use an electric razor and soft toothbrush to prevent bleeding
- Consuming foods high in vitamin K, including milk, egg yolks, leafy green vegetables, meat, tomatoes, and vegetable oil, is encouraged
- Notify the physician of abdominal or back pain, severe headache, black or red stool, coffee-ground vomitus, red or dark urine, or red-speckled mucus from a cough

■ Monitoring Parameters
- PT and international normalized ratio, Hct
- Stool and urine specimens for occult blood

■ Geriatric side effects at a glance:
❑ CNS   ❑ Bowel Dysfunction   ❑ Bladder Dysfunction   ❑ Falls

■ U.S. Regulatory Considerations
☑ FDA Black Box
Severe reactions, including death, have occurred with IV use. Avoid rapid infusion. Restrict IV use; use only when other routes of administration are unavailable and risk/benefit has been assessed.
❑ OBRA regulated in U.S. Long Term Care

nystatin

(nye-stat'-in)

■ Brand Name(s): Bio-Statin, Mycostatin, Mycostatin Pastilles, Mycostatin Topical, Nyaderm, Nystat-Rx, Nystex, Nystop

Combinations
Rx: *Topical:* with triamcinolone (Mycolog-II, Mycomer, Mycasone, Myco Biotic II, Tri-Statin II, Mytrex, Myco-Triacet II, Mycogen II)

Chemical Class: Amphoteric polyene macrolide

■ **Clinical Pharmacology:**
Mechanism of Action: A fungistatic antifungal that binds to sterols in the fungal cell membrane. **Therapeutic Effect:** Increases fungal cell-membrane permeability, allowing loss of potassium and other cellular components.
Pharmacokinetics: PO: Poorly absorbed from the GI tract. Eliminated unchanged in feces. Topical: Not absorbed systemically from intact skin.

■ **Available Forms:**
- *Oral Suspension (Mycostatin)*: 100,000 units/ml.
- *Tablets (Mycostatin)*: 500,000 units.
- *Capsules (Bio-Statin)*: 500,000 units, 1,000,000 units.
- *Oral Lozenge (Mycostatin Pastilles)*: 200,000 units.
- *Vaginal Tablets*: 100,000 units.
- *Cream (Mycostatin Topical)*: 100,000 units/g.
- *Ointment*: 100,000 units/g.
- *Topical Powder (Mycostatin Topical, Nystop)*: 100,000 units/g.
- *Powder (Compounding)*: 50,000,000 units (Nystat-Rx), 150,000,000 units (Bio-Statin, Nystat-Rx), 500,000,000 units (Nystat-Rx), 1,000,000,000 units, 2,000,000,000 units (Bio-Statin, Nystat-Rx).

■ **Indications and Dosages:**
Intestinal infections: PO 500,000-1,000,000 units q8h.
Oral candidiasis: PO 400,000-600,000 units 4 times/day.
Vaginal infections: Vaginal 1 tablet/day at bedtime for 14 days.
Cutaneous candidal infections: Topical Apply 2-4 times/day.

■ **Unlabeled Uses:** Prophylaxis and treatment of oropharyngeal candidiasis, tinea barbae, tinea capitis

■ **Contraindications:** None known.

■ **Side Effects**
Occasional
Topical: Skin irritation
Vaginal: Vaginal irritation

■ **Serious Reactions**
- High dosages of oral form may produce nausea, vomiting, diarrhea, and GI distress.

■ **Patient/Family Education**
- Do not miss a dose and complete the full course of treatment
- Swish the oral suspension in the mouth for as long as possible before swallowing
- Insert the vaginal form high into the vagina
- Do not let the topical form come in contact with the eyes
- Rub the topical form well into affected areas, keep affected areas clean and dry, and wear light clothing for ventilation

  • Assess the patient for increased irritation with topical application or increased vaginal discharge with vaginal application

■ **Geriatric side effects at a glance:**
  ❑ CNS   ❑ Bowel Dysfunction   ❑ Bladder Dysfunction   ❑ Falls

■ **U.S. Regulatory Considerations**
  ❑ FDA Black Box   ❑ OBRA regulated in U.S. Long Term Care

octreotide acetate

(ok-tree'-oh-tide as'-eh-tayte)

■ **Brand Name(s):** Sandostatin, Sandostatin LAR Depot
  Chemical Class: Somatostatin analog

■ **Clinical Pharmacology:**
  Mechanism of Action: An antidiarrheal and growth hormone suppressant that suppresses the secretion of serotonin and gastroenteropancreatic peptides and enhances fluid and electrolyte absorption from the GI tract. **Therapeutic Effect:** Prolongs intestinal transit time.
  Pharmacokinetics:

Route	Onset	Peak	Duration
Subcutaneous	N/A	N/A	Up to 12 hr

Rapidly and completely absorbed from injection site. Excreted in urine. Removed by hemodialysis. **Half-life:** 1.5 hr.

■ **Available Forms:**
  • Injection (*Sandostatin*): 0.05 mg/ml, 0.1 mg/ml, 0.2 mg/ml, 0.5 mg/ml, 1 mg/ml.
  • Suspension for Injection (*Sandostatin* LAR Depot): 10-mg, 20-mg, 30-mg vials.

■ **Indications and Dosages:**
  Diarrhea: IV (Sandostatin) Initially, 50–100 mcg q8h. May increase by 100 mcg/dose q48h. Maximum: 500 mcg q8h. Subcutaneous (Sandostatin) 50 mcg 1–2 times a day.
  Carcinoid tumors: IV, Subcutaneous (Sandostatin) 100–600 mcg/day in 2–4 divided doses. IM (Sandostatin LAR Depot) 20 mg q4wk.
  Vipomas: IV, Subcutaneous (Sandostatin) 200–300 mcg/day in 2–4 divided doses. IM (Sandostatin LAR Depot) 20 mg q4wk.
  Esophageal varices: IV (Sandostatin) Bolus of 25–50 mcg followed by IV infusion of 25–50 mcg/hr for 48 hr.
  Acromegaly: IV, Subcutaneous (Sandostatin) 50 mcg 3 times a day. Increase as needed. Maximum: 500 mcg 3 times a day. IM (Sandostatin LAR Depot) 20 mg q4wk for 3 mo. Maximum: 40 mg q4wk.

■ **Unlabeled Uses:** Control of bleeding esophageal varices, treatment of AIDS-associated secretory diarrhea, chemotherapy-induced diarrhea, insulinomas, small-bowel fistulas, control of bleeding esophageal varices

■ **Contraindications:** None known.

■ **Side Effects**
Frequent (10%–6%, 58%–30% in acromegaly patients)
Diarrhea, nausea, abdominal discomfort, headache, injection site pain
Occasional (5%–1%)
Vomiting, flatulence, constipation, alopecia, facial flushing, pruritus, dizziness, fatigue, arrhythmias, ecchymosis, blurred vision
Rare (less than 1%)
Depression, diminished libido, vertigo, palpitations, dyspnea

■ **Serious Reactions**
- Patients using octreotide may develop cholelithiasis or, with prolonged high dosages, hypothyroidism.
- GI bleeding, hepatitis, and seizures occur rarely.

Special Considerations
- Octreotide is incompatible in TPN solutions
- Patient tolerance to ocreotide should be determined with 2 wk SC/IV therapy before switching to depot therapy
- Only give depot intragluteally, avoid deltoid injections due to pain at injection site
- Withdraw octreotide yearly for 4 wk in acromegaly patients who have received irradiation to assess disease activity
- Notify the physician about any unusual signs or symptoms, such as palpitations or unusual bleeding
- Weigh himself or herself daily; and report a weight gain of more than 5 lb per week

■ **Monitoring Parameters**
- Thyroid function, serum glucose (especially in drug-treated diabetics), vitamin B_{12} levels
- Heart rate (especially in persons taking β-blockers and calcium channel blockers)
- Periodic zinc levels in patients receiving TPN
- Blood pressure
- Weight

■ **Geriatric side effects at a glance:**
☐ CNS   ☑ Bowel Dysfunction   ☐ Bladder Dysfunction   ☐ Falls

■ **U.S. Regulatory Considerations**
☐ FDA Black Box   ☐ OBRA regulated in U.S. Long Term Care

ofloxacin

(oh-floks'-a-sin)

- **Brand Name(s):** Floxin, Floxin Otic, Ocuflox
  Chemical Class: Fluoroquinolone derivative

- **Clinical Pharmacology:**
  Mechanism of Action: A fluoroquinolone antibacterial that inhibits DNA gyrase in susceptible microorganisms, interfering with bacterial cell replication and repair. **Therapeutic Effect:** Bactericidal.
  Pharmacokinetics: Rapidly and well absorbed from the GI tract. Protein binding: 20%-25%. Widely distributed (including to cerebrospinal fluid [CSF]). Metabolized in the liver. Primarily excreted in urine. Removed by hemodialysis. **Half-life:** 4.7-7 hr (increased in impaired renal function, cirrhosis, and the elderly).

- **Available Forms:**
  - *Tablets* (*Floxin*): 200 mg, 300 mg, 400 mg.
  - *Ophthalmic Solution* (*Ocuflox*): 0.3%.
  - *Otic Solution* (*Floxin Otic*): 0.3%.

- **Indications and Dosages:**
  UTIs: PO 200 mg q12h.
  Lower respiratory tract, skin, and skin-structure infections: PO 400 mg q12h for 10 days.
  Prostatitis, sexually transmitted diseases (cervicitis, urethritis): PO 300 mg q12h.
  Acute, uncomplicated gonorrhea: PO 400 mg 1 time.
  Bacterial conjunctivitis: Ophthalmic 1-2 drops q2-4h for 2 days, then 4 times a day for 5 days.
  Corneal ulcers: Ophthalmic 1-2 drops q30min while awake for 2 days, then q60min while awake for 5-7 days, then 4 times a day.
  Otitis externa: Otic 10 drops into the affected ear once a day for 7 days.
  Dosage in renal impairment: After a normal initial dose, dosage and frequency are based on creatinine clearance.

Creatinine Clearance	Adjusted Dose	Dosage Interval
greater than 50 ml/min	None	q12h
10-50 ml/min	None	q24h
less than 10 ml/min	½	q24h

- **Contraindications:** Hypersensitivity to any quinolones

- **Side Effects**
  Frequent (10%-7%)
  Nausea, headache, insomnia
  Occasional (5%-3%)
  Abdominal pain, diarrhea, vomiting, dry mouth, flatulence, dizziness, fatigue, drowsiness, rash, pruritus, fever
  Rare (less than 1%)
  Constipation, paresthesia

Serious Reactions
- Antibiotic-associated colitis and other superinfections may occur from altered bacterial balance.
- Hypersensitivity reactions, including photosensitivity (as evidenced by rash, pruritus, blisters, edema, and burning skin), have occurred in patients receiving fluoroquinolones.
- Arthropathy (swelling, pain, and clubbing of fingers and toes, degeneration of stress-bearing portion of a joint) may occur if the drug is given to children.
- There is a risk of peripheral neuropathy and torsades de pointes.
- Tendon effects, including ruptures of shoulder, hand, Achilles tendon or other tendons, may occur. Risk increases with concomitant corticosteriod use, especially in the elderly.
- Symptomatic hyperglycemia and hypoglycemia have occurred.

Patient/Family Education
- Administer on an empty stomach (1 hr before or 2 hr after meals)
- Drink fluids liberally
- Do not take antacids containing magnesium or aluminum or products containing iron or zinc within 4 hr before or 2 hr after dosing
- Avoid excessive exposure to sunlight
- Ofloxacin may cause dizziness, drowsiness, headache, and insomnia
- Avoid tasks requiring mental alertness or motor skills until response to ofloxacin is established
- Your tendons may be more easily injured while taking this medication. Monitor for pain or swelling in your knee, ankle, shoulder, elbow, or wrist.

Monitoring Parameters
- Signs and symptoms of infection
- Mental status and WBC count
- Skin for rash; withhold the drug and promptly notify the physician at the first sign of a rash or another allergic reaction
- Evaluate the patient for dizziness, headache, tremors, and visual difficulties
- Daily bowel activity and stool consistency. Although mild GI effects may be tolerable, severe symptoms may indicate the onset of antibiotic-associated colitis.
- Signs and symptoms of superinfection include abdominal pain or cramping, anal or genital pruritus or discharge, moderate to severe diarrhea, severe mouth or tongue soreness, and new or increased fever.

Geriatric side effects at a glance:
☑ CNS ☐ Bowel Dysfunction ☐ Bladder Dysfunction ☐ Falls

U.S. Regulatory Considerations
☐ FDA Black Box ☐ OBRA regulated in U.S. Long Term Care

olanzapine

(oh-lan'-zah-peen)

■ **Brand Name(s):** Zyprexa, Zyprexa Intramuscular, Zyprexa Zydis

Combinations
Rx: with fluoxetine (Symbyax)
Chemical Class: Thienbenzodiazepine derivative

■ **Clinical Pharmacology:**
Mechanism of Action: A thienobenzodiazepine derivative that antagonizes alpha$_1$-adrenergic, dopamine, histamine, muscarinic, and serotonin receptors. Produces anticholinergic, histaminic, and CNS depressant effects. **Therapeutic Effect:** Diminishes manifestations of psychotic symptoms.
Pharmacokinetics: Well absorbed after PO administration. Protein binding: 93%. Extensively distributed throughout the body. Undergoes extensive first-pass metabolism in the liver. Excreted primarily in urine and, to a lesser extent, in feces. Not removed by dialysis. **Half-life:** 21-54 hr.

■ **Available Forms:**
• *Tablets (Zyprexa)*: 2.5 mg, 5 mg, 7.5 mg, 10 mg, 15 mg, 20 mg.
• *Tablets (Orally-Disintegrating [Zyprexa Zydis])*: 5 mg, 10 mg, 15 mg, 20 mg.
• *Injection (Zyprexa Intramuscular)*: 10 mg.

■ **Indications and Dosages:**
Schizophrenia: PO Initially, 2.5 mg/day. May increase as indicated. Range: 2.5-10 mg/day.
Bipolar mania: PO Initially, 10-15 mg/day. May increase by 5 mg/day at intervals of at least 24 hr. Maximum: 20 mg/day.
Control agitation in schizophrenic or bipolar patients: IM 2.5-10 mg. May repeat 2 hr after first dose and 4 hr after 2nd dose. Maximum: 30 mg/day.

■ **Unlabeled Uses:** Treatment of anorexia, apathy, borderline personality disorder, Huntington's disease; maintenance of long-term treatment response in schizophrenic patients; nausea; vomiting

■ **Contraindications:** None known.

■ **Side Effects**
Frequent
Somnolence (26%), agitation (23%), insomnia (20%), headache (17%), nervousness (16%), hostility (15%), dizziness (11%), rhinitis (10%)
Occasional
Anxiety, constipation (9%); nonaggressive atypical behavior (8%); dry mouth (7%); weight gain (6%); orthostatic hypotension, fever, arthralgia, restlessness, cough, pharyngitis, visual changes (dim vision) (5%)
Rare
Tachycardia; back, chest, abdominal, or extremity pain; tremor

■ Serious Reactions

- Rare reactions include seizures and neuroleptic malignant syndrome, a potentially fatal syndrome characterized by hyperpyrexia, muscle rigidity, irregular pulse or BP, tachycardia, diaphoresis, and cardiac arrhythmias.
- Extrapyramidal symptoms and dysphagia may also occur.
- Overdose (300 mg) produces drowsiness and slurred speech.

■ Patient/Family Education

- Avoid exposure to extreme heat
- Take olanzapine as ordered; do not abruptly discontinue the drug or increase the dosage
- Drowsiness generally subsides with continued therapy
- Avoid tasks requiring mental alertness or motor skills until response to the drug has been established
- Take sips of tepid water and chew sugarless gum to help relieve dry mouth
- Maintain a healthy diet and exercise program to prevent weight gain

■ Monitoring Parameters

- Periodic assessment of liver transaminases in patients with significant hepatic disease
- Blood pressure
- Closely supervise suicidal patients during early therapy; as depression lessens, the patient's energy level improves, which increases the suicide potential
- Assess for evidence of a therapeutic response, such as improvement in self-care, increased interest in surroundings and ability to concentrate, and relaxed facial expression
- Assess the patient's sleep pattern
- Monitor the patient for extrapyramidal symptoms, and notify the physician if they occur

■ Geriatric side effects at a glance:

☑ CNS   ☑ Bowel Dysfunction   ☑ Bladder Dysfunction   ☑ Falls

☑ Other: Weight gain, glucose intolerance, diabetes, orthostatic hypotension, extrapyramidal symptoms

■ Use with caution in older patients with: Diabetes, glucose intolerance, cardiovascular disease

■ U.S. Regulatory Considerations

☑ FDA Black Box

There is an increased risk of death in older patients with dementia. Although the causes of death were varied, most of the deaths appeared to be either cardiovascular (e.g., heart failure, sudden death) or infectious (e.g., pneumonia) in nature. This drug is not approved for treatment of patients with dementia-related psychosis.

☑ OBRA regulated in U.S. Long Term Care

■ Other Uses in Geriatric Patient: Behavior disturbances in the setting of dementia

■ Side Effects:

Of particular importance in the geriatric patient: Weight gain, glucose intolerance, diabetes, increased risk of death (see FDA black box warning)

- **Geriatric Considerations - Summary:** Direct comparisons between older and newer antipsychotic drugs in demented elderly persons are scarce. Newer agents have the theoretical advantage of a lower incidence of tardive dyskinesia but may cause weight gain, impaired glycemic control, and increased risk for cardiovascular events. These agents should be used with caution in demented elderly persons, with frequent monitoring for side effects and a low threshold for discontinuing use. Indeed, the Food and Drug Administration has recently released an advisory about these medications outlining the risk for increased mortality.

- **References:**

1. Sink KM, Holden KF, Yaffe K. Pharmacological treatment of neuropsychiatric symptoms of dementia: a review of the evidence. JAMA 2005;293:596-608.
2. Alexopoulos GS, Streim J, Carpenter D, Docherty JP. Using antipsychotic agents in older patients. J Clin Psychiatry 2004;65 (Suppl 2):5-99.
3. Cohen D. Atypical antipsychotics and new onset diabetes mellitus. An overview of the literature. Pharmacopsychiatry 2004;37:1-11.
4. Deaths with antipsychotics in elderly patients with behavioral disturbances. Available at: www.fda.gov/cder/drug/advisory/antipsychotics.htm.
5. Katz IR. Optimizing atypical antipsychotic treatment strategies in the elderly. J Am Geriatr Soc 2004;52:S272-S277.

olsalazine sodium

(ole-sal'-a-zeen soe'-dee-um)

- **Brand Name(s):** Dipentum
  Chemical Class: Salicylate derivative

- **Clinical Pharmacology:**
  Mechanism of Action: A salicylic acid derivative that is converted to mesalamine in the colon by bacterial action. Blocks prostaglandin production in bowel mucosa. **Therapeutic Effect:** Reduces colonic inflammation in inflammatory bowel disease.
  Pharmacokinetics: Small amount absorbed. Protein binding: 99%. Metabolized by bacteria in the colon. Minimal elimination in urine and feces. **Half-life:** 0.9 hr.

- **Available Forms:**
  - *Capsules:* 250 mg.

- **Indications and Dosages:**
  Maintenance of controlled ulcerative colitis: PO 1 g/day in 2 divided doses, preferably q12h.

- **Unlabeled Uses:** Treatment of inflammatory bowel disease

- **Contraindications:** History of hypersensitivity to salicylates

- **Side Effects**
  Frequent (10%–5%)
  Headache, diarrhea, abdominal pain or cramps, nausea

Occasional (5%–1%)
Depression, fatigue, dyspepsia, upper respiratory tract infection, decreased appetite, rash, itching, arthralgia
Rare (1%)
Dizziness, vomiting, stomatitis

■ **Serious Reactions**
- Sulfite sensitivity may occur in susceptible patients, manifested by cramping, headache, diarrhea, fever, rash, hives, itching, and wheezing. Discontinue drug immediately.
- Excessive diarrhea associated with extreme fatigue is noted rarely.

■ **Patient/Family Education**
- Take with food. Notify clinician if diarrhea occurs
- Notify physician if persistent or increasing cramping, diarrhea, fever, pruritus, and rash occurs
- Maintain adequate fluid intake

■ **Monitoring Parameters**
- BUN, urinalysis, serum creatinine in patients with preexisting renal disease
- Pattern of daily bowel activity and stool consistency; record time of evacuation
- Skin for hives and rash

■ **Geriatric side effects at a glance:**
❑ CNS   ❑ Bowel Dysfunction   ❑ Bladder Dysfunction   ❑ Falls

■ **U.S. Regulatory Considerations**
❑ FDA Black Box   ❑ OBRA regulated in U.S. Long Term Care

omalizumab

(oh-mah-lye-zoo'-mab)

■ **Brand Name(s):** Xolair
Chemical Class: Monoclonal antibody

■ **Clinical Pharmacology:**
Mechanism of Action: A monoclonal antibody that selectively binds to human immunoglobulin E (IgE) preventing it from binding to the surface of mast cells and basophils. **Therapeutic Effect:** Prevents or reduces the number of asthmatic attacks.
Pharmacokinetics: Absorbed slowly after subcutaneous administration, with peak concentration in 7–8 days. Excreted in the liver, reticuloendothelial system, and endothelial cells. **Half-life:** 26 days.

- ■ **Available Forms:**
  - • *Powder for Injection*: 202.5 mg/1.2 ml or 150 mg/1.2 ml after reconstitution.

- ■ **Indications and Dosages:**

  Moderate to severe persistent asthma in patients who are reactive to a perennial allergen and whose asthma symptoms have been inadequately controlled with inhaled corticosteroids: Subcutaneous 150–375 mg every 2 or 4 wk; dose and dosing frequency are individualized based on weight and pretreatment IgE level (as shown below).

  4-week dosing table:

Pretreatment Serum IgE Levels (units/ml)	Weight 30–60 kg	Weight 61–70 kg	Weight 71–90 kg	Weight 91–150 kg
30 to 100	150 mg	150 mg	150 mg	300 mg
101-200	300 mg	300 mg	300 mg	See next table
201–300	300 mg	See next table	See next table	See next table

  2-week dosing table:

Pretreatment Serum IgE Levels (units/ml)	Weight 30–60 kg	Weight 61–70 kg	Weight 71–90 kg	Weight 91–150 kg
101-200	See preceding table	See preceding table	See preceding table	225 mg
201–300	See previous table	225 mg	225 mg	300 mg
301–400	225 mg	225 mg	300 mg	Do not dose
401–500	300 mg	300 mg	375 mg	Do not dose
501–600	300 mg	375 mg	Do not dose	Do not dose
601–700	375 mg	Do not dose	Do not dose	Do not dose

- ■ **Unlabeled Uses:** Treatment of seasonal allergic rhinitis

- ■ **Contraindications:** None known.

- ■ **Side Effects**

  Frequent (45%–11%)

  Injection site ecchymosis, redness, warmth, stinging, and urticaria; viral infections; sinusitis; headache; pharyngitis

  Occasional (8%–3%)

  Arthralgia, leg pain, fatigue, dizziness

  Rare (2%)

  Arm pain, earache, dermatitis, pruritus

- ■ **Serious Reactions**
  - • Anaphylaxis occurs within 2 hr of the first dose or subsequent doses in 0.1% of patients.
  - • Malignant neoplasms occur in 0.5% of patients.

Special Considerations

  - • In clinical studies, a reduction of asthma exacerbations was not observed in omalizumab-treated patients who had FEV_1 >80% at the time of randomization; reductions in exacerbations were not seen in patients who required oral steroids as maintenance therapy

- ■ **Patient/Family Education**
  - • Systemic or inhaled corticosteroids should not be abruptly discontinued upon initiation of omalizumab therapy

- Do not decrease the dose of, or stop taking, any other asthma medications unless otherwise instructed by clinician
- Immediate improvement in asthma symptoms may not be apparent after beginning omalizumab therapy
- Because the solution is slightly viscous, the injection may take 5-10 sec to administer
- Should be stored under refrigerated conditions 2-8°C (36-46°F)
- Drink plenty of fluids to decrease the thickness of lung secretions

■ Monitoring Parameters
- Patient should be observed after injection of omalizumab, and medications for the treatment of severe hypersensitivity reactions, including anaphylaxis, should be available
- Total IgE levels are elevated during treatment and remain elevated for up to 1 yr after the discontinuation of treatment; re-testing of IgE levels during omalizumab treatment cannot be used as a guide for dose determination; dose determination after treatment interruptions lasting <1 yr should be based on serum IgE levels obtained at the initial dose determination
- Doses should be adjusted for significant changes in body weight
- Pulse rate and quality as well as respiratory rate, depth, rhythm, and type
- Observe fingernails and lips for cyanosis characterized by a blue or dusky color in light-skinned patients or a gray color in dark-skinned patients

■ Geriatric side effects at a glance:
❑ CNS   ❑ Bowel Dysfunction   ❑ Bladder Dysfunction   ❑ Falls

■ U.S. Regulatory Considerations
❑ FDA Black Box   ❑ OBRA regulated in U.S. Long Term Care

omega-3-acid ethyl esters

(oh-meg'-a-three-as'-id eth'-ul es'-terz)

Combinations
Rx: Omacor

■ Clinical Pharmacology:
Mechanism of Action: A combination of ethyl esters of eicosapentaenoic acid (EPA) and docosahexaenoic acid (DHA) that inhibits acyl coenzyme A:1,2-diacylglycerol acyltransferase and increases peroxisomal oxidation in the liver. **Therapeutic Effect:** Reduces the synthesis of triglycerides in the liver.
Pharmacokinetics: EPA and DHA are absorbed well when given orally as ethyl esters.

■ Available Forms:
- *Capsules:* 1g of ethyl esters of omega-3 fatty acids (Omacor).

■ Indications and Dosages:
Hypertriglyceridemia : PO   4g (4 capsules) once daily or two 2-g doses (2 capsules) twice daily.

- **Contraindications:** Hypersensitivity to any component of the formulation

- **Side Effects**
  Occasional
  Back pain, excess air or gas in stomach, belching, flu syndrome, infection, rash, taste perversion

- **Serious Reactions**
  - Angina pectoris and shortness of breath have been reported.

- **Geriatric side effects at a glance:**
  ☐ CNS ☐ Bowel Dysfunction ☐ Bladder Dysfunction ☐ Falls

- **U.S. Regulatory Considerations**
  ☐ FDA Black Box ☐ OBRA regulated in U.S. Long Term Care

omeprazole

(oh-me'-pray-zol)

- **Brand Name(s):** Prilosec, Zegerid
  OTC: Prilosec OTC
  Chemical Class: Benzimidazole derivative

- **Clinical Pharmacology:**
  Mechanism of Action: A benzimidazole that is converted to active metabolites that irreversibly bind to and inhibit hydrogen-potassium adenosine triphosphatase, an enzyme on the surface of gastric parietal cells. Inhibits hydrogen ion transport into gastric lumen. **Therapeutic Effect:** Increases gastric pH, reduces gastric acid production.
  Pharmacokinetics:

Route	Onset	Peak	Duration
PO	1 hr	2 hr	72 hr

  Rapidly absorbed from the GI tract. Protein binding: 99%. Primarily distributed into gastric parietal cells. Metabolized extensively in the liver. Primarily excreted in urine. Unknown if removed by hemodialysis. **Half-life:** 0.5–1 hr (increased in patients with hepatic impairment).

- **Available Forms:**
  - *Capsules (Delayed-Release [Prilosec])*: 10 mg, 20 mg, 40 mg.
  - *Oral Suspension (Zegerid)*: 20 mg, 40 mg.

- **Indications and Dosages:**
  Erosive esophagitis, poorly responsive gastroesophageal reflux disease, active duodenal ulcer, prevention and treatment of NSAID-induced ulcers: PO 20 mg/day.
  To maintain healing of erosive esophagitis: PO 20 mg/day.
  Pathologic hypersecretory conditions: PO Initially, 60 mg/day up to 120 mg 3 times a day.

Helicobacter pylori duodenal ulcer: PO 20 mg once daily or 40 mg/day as a single or in 2 divided doses in combination therapy with antibiotics. Dose varies with regimen used.
Active benign gastric ulcer: PO 40 mg/day for 4–8 wk.
OTC use (frequent heartburn): PO 20 mg/day for 14 days. May repeat after 4 mo if needed.

■ **Unlabeled Uses:** H. *pylori*–associated duodenal ulcer (with amoxicillin and clarithromycin), prevention and treatment of NSAID-induced ulcers, treatment of active benign gastric ulcers

■ **Contraindications:** None known.

■ **Side Effects**
Frequent (7%)
Headache
Occasional (3%–2%)
Diarrhea, abdominal pain, nausea
Rare (2%)
Dizziness, asthenia or loss of strength, vomiting, constipation, upper respiratory tract infection, back pain, rash, cough

■ **Serious Reactions**
• Pancreatitis, hepatotoxicity, and interstitial nephritis have been reported.

Special Considerations
• Some patients on maintenance therapy may respond to 10 mg qd or 20 mg qod

■ **Patient/Family Education**
• Take before eating
• Swallow capsule whole; do not open, chew, or crush
• Notify the physician if headache occurs during omeprazole therapy

■ **Monitoring Parameters**
• Therapeutic response (relief of GI symptoms)

■ **Geriatric side effects at a glance:**
❑ CNS ❑ Bowel Dysfunction ❑ Bladder Dysfunction ❑ Falls

■ **U.S. Regulatory Considerations**
❑ FDA Black Box ❑ OBRA regulated in U.S. Long Term Care

904

ondansetron hydrochloride

(on-dan-seh'-tron hye-droe-klor'-ide)

■ **Brand Name(s):** Zofran, Zofran ODT
  Chemical Class: Carbazole derivative

■ **Clinical Pharmacology:**
  Mechanism of Action: An antiemetic that blocks serotonin, both peripherally on vagal nerve terminals and centrally in the chemoreceptor trigger zone. **Therapeutic Effect:** Prevents nausea and vomiting.
  Pharmacokinetics: Readily absorbed from the GI tract. Protein binding: 70%-76%. Metabolized in the liver. Primarily excreted in urine. Unknown if removed by hemodialysis. **Half-life:** 4 hr.

■ **Available Forms:**
  • *Oral Solution (Zofran)*: 4 mg/5 ml.
  • *Tablets (Zofran)*: 4 mg, 8 mg, 24 mg.
  • *Tablets (Orally Disintegrating [Zofran ODT])*: 4 mg, 8 mg.
  • *Injection (Zofran)*: 2 mg/ml.
  • *Injection (Zofran Premixed)*: 32 mg/50 ml.

■ **Indications and Dosages:**
  Chemotherapy-induced emesis: IV 0.15 mg/kg 3 times a day beginning 30 minutes before chemotherapy or 0.45 mg/kg once daily or 8-10 mg 1-2 times/day or 24-32 mg once daily. PO (Highly emetogenic) 24 mg 30 minutes before start of chemotherapy. (Moderately emetogenic): 8 mg q12h beginning 30 minutes before chemotherapy and continuing for 1-2 days after completion of chemotherapy.
  Prevention of postoperative nausea and vomiting: IV, IM 4 mg as a single dose PO 16 mg 1 hour before induction of anesthesia.
  Prevention of radiation-induced nausea and vomiting: PO (Total body irradiation): 8 mg 1-2 hours daily before each fraction of radiotherapy. (Single high-dose radiotherapy to abdomen): 8 mg 1-2 hours before irradiation, then 8 mg q8h after first dose for 1-2 days after completion of radiotherapy. (Daily fractionated radiotherapy to abdomen): 8 mg 1-2 hours before irradiation, then 8 mg 8 hours after first dose for each day of radiotherapy.

■ **Unlabeled Uses:** Treatment of postoperative nausea and vomiting

■ **Contraindications:** None known.

■ **Side Effects**
  Frequent (13%-5%)
  Anxiety, dizziness, somnolence, headache, fatigue, constipation, diarrhea, hypoxia, urine retention
  Occasional (4%-2%)
  Abdominal pain, xerostomia, fever, feeling of cold, redness and pain at injection site, paresthesia, asthenia
  Rare (1%)
  Hypersensitivity reaction (including rash and pruritus), blurred vision

Serious Reactions
- Overdose may produce a combination of CNS stimulant and depressant effects.

Patient/Family Education
- Nausea and vomiting should be relieved shortly after drug administration; notify the physician if vomiting persists
- Ondansetron may cause dizziness or drowsiness
- Avoid alcohol and barbiturates while taking ondansetron
- Use other methods of reducing nausea and vomiting, including lying quietly and avoiding strong odors
- Avoid performing tasks that require mental alertness or motor skills until response to ondansetron has been established

Monitoring Parameters
- Pattern of daily bowel activity and stool consistency

Geriatric side effects at a glance:
☐ CNS ☑ Bowel Dysfunction ☐ Bladder Dysfunction ☐ Falls

U.S. Regulatory Considerations
☐ FDA Black Box ☐ OBRA regulated in U.S. Long Term Care

opium tincture

(oh'-pee-um tink'-chur)

Brand Name(s): Opium Tincture

Combinations
Rx: with belladonna alkaloids (B & O Suppositories)
Chemical Class: Natural alkaloid

DEA Class: Schedule II

Clinical Pharmacology:
Mechanism of Action: An opioid agonist that contains many narcotic alkaloids including morphine. It inhibits gastric motility due to its morphine content. **Therapeutic Effect:** Decreases digestive secretions, increases gastrointestinal (GI) muscle tone, and reduces GI propulsion.
Pharmacokinetics: Duration of action is 4-5 hr. Variably absorbed from the GI tract. Protein binding: unknown. Metabolized in liver. Primarily excreted in urine. Unknown if removed by hemodialysis. **Half-life:** unknown.

Available Forms:
- Liquid: 10%.

- ■ **Indications and Dosages:**
  Analgesia: PO 0.6-1.5 ml q3-4h. Maximum: 6 ml/day.
  Antidiarrheal: PO 0.3-1 ml q2-6h. Maximum: 6 ml/day.

- ■ **Unlabeled Uses:** None known.

- ■ **Contraindications:** Hypersensitivity to morphine sulfate or any component of the formulation, increased intracranial pressure, severe respiratory depression, severe hepatic or renal insufficiency, pregnancy (prolonged use or high dosages near term)

- ■ **Side Effects**
  Frequent
  Constipation, drowsiness, nausea, vomiting
  Occasional
  Paradoxical excitement, confusion, pounding heartbeat, facial flushing, decreased urination, blurred vision, dizziness, dry mouth, headache, hypotension, decreased appetite, redness, burning, pain at injection site
  Rare
  Hallucinations, depression, stomach pain, insomnia

- ■ **Serious Reactions**
  - Overdosage results in cold or clammy skin, confusion, convulsions, decreased blood pressure (BP), restlessness, pinpoint pupils, bradycardia, respiratory depression, decreased level of consciousness (LOC), and severe weakness.
  - Tolerance to analgesic effect and physical dependence may occur with repeated use.

Special Considerations
  - Opium has been replaced by safer, more effective analgesics and sedative/hypnotics for diagnostic or operative medication; useful as an antidiarrheal
  - Do not administer agonist/antagonist analgesics (i.e., pentazocine, nalbuphine, butorphanol, dezocine, buprenorphine) to patient who has received a prolonged course of opium (a pure agonist). In opioid-dependent patients, mixed agonist/antagonist analgesics may precipitate withdrawal symptoms

- ■ **Patient/Family Education**
  - Drug may be addictive if used for prolonged periods
  - Do not exceed the prescribed dose
  - Change positions slowly
  - Avoid tasks that require mental alertness or motor skills until response to the drug is established
  - Avoid alcohol

- ■ **Monitoring Parameters**
  - Daily pattern of bowel activity and stool consistency
  - Clinical improvement

- ■ **Geriatric side effects at a glance:**
  ☑ CNS ☑ Bowel Dysfunction ☑ Bladder Dysfunction ☑ Falls

- ■ **U.S. Regulatory Considerations**
  ❑ FDA Black Box ☑ OBRA regulated in U.S. Long Term Care

orlistat

(or'-li-stat)

■ **Brand Name(s):** Xenical
Chemical Class: Lipase inhibitor

■ **Clinical Pharmacology:**
Mechanism of Action: A gastric and pancreatic lipase inhibitor that inhibits absorption of dietary fats by inactivating gastric and pancreatic enzymes. **Therapeutic Effect:** Resulting caloric deficit may positively affect weight control.
Pharmacokinetics: Minimal absorption after administration. Protein binding: 99%. Primarily eliminated unchanged in feces. Unknown if removed by hemodialysis. **Half-life:** 1–2 hr.

■ **Available Forms:**
• *Capsules*: 120 mg.

■ **Indications and Dosages:**
Weight reduction: PO 120 mg 3 times a day with each main meal containing fat (omit if meal is occasionally missed or contains no fat).

■ **Unlabeled Uses:** Type 2 diabetes

■ **Contraindications:** Cholestasis, chronic malabsorption syndrome

■ **Side Effects**
Frequent (30%–20%)
Headache, abdominal discomfort, flatulence, fecal urgency, fatty or oily stool
Occasional (14%–5%)
Back pain, nausea, fatigue, diarrhea, dizziness
Rare (less than 4%)
Anxiety, rash, myalgia, dry skin, vomiting

■ **Serious Reactions**
• Hypersensitivity reaction occurs rarely.

Special Considerations
• Standard weight loss maintained over 2 years is approximately 10% of initial weight

■ **Patient/Family Education**
• If a meal contains no fat, the dose of orlistat can be omitted
• Supplement with fat-soluble vitamin, vitamin D, and beta-carotene
• Psyllium laxative may decrease GI adverse effects
• Unpleasant side effects, such as flatulence and urgency, should diminish with time

■ **Monitoring Parameters**
• Lipids, weight, plasma levels of vitamins A, D, E
• Blood glucose

- **Geriatric side effects at a glance:**
  - ❑ CNS ☑ Bowel Dysfunction ❑ Bladder Dysfunction ❑ Falls

- **U.S. Regulatory Considerations**
  - ❑ FDA Black Box ❑ OBRA regulated in U.S. Long Term Care

oseltamivir phosphate

(os-el-tam'-i-vir foss'-fate)

- **Brand Name(s):** Tamiflu
  Chemical Class: Carboxylic acid ethyl ester

- **Clinical Pharmacology:**
  Mechanism of Action: A selective inhibitor of influenza virus neuraminidase, an enzyme essential for viral replication. Acts against both influenza A and B viruses. **Therapeutic Effect:** Suppresses the spread of infection within the respiratory system and reduces the duration of clinical symptoms.
  Pharmacokinetics: Readily absorbed. Protein binding: 3%. Extensively converted to active drug in the liver. Primarily excreted in urine. **Half-life:** 6-10 hr.

- **Available Forms:**
  - *Capsules*: 75 mg.
  - *Oral Suspension*: 12 mg/ml.

- **Indications and Dosages:**
  Influenza: PO 75 mg 2 times a day for 5 days.
  Prevention of influenza: PO 75 mg once daily for at least 7 days.
  Dosage in renal impairment: PO Dosage is decreased to 75 mg once a day for at least 7 days and possibly up to 6 wk.

- **Contraindications:** None known.

- **Side Effects**
  Frequent (10%-7%)
  Nausea, vomiting, diarrhea
  Rare (2%-1%)
  Abdominal pain, bronchitis, dizziness, headache, cough, insomnia, fatigue, vertigo

- **Serious Reactions**
  - Colitis, pneumonia, tympanic membrane disorder, and pyrexia occur rarely.

- **Patient/Family Education**
  - May administer without regard for food

- When started within 40 hr of onset of symptoms, there was a 1.3-day reduction in the median time to improvement in influenza-infected subjects receiving oseltamivir compared to subjects receiving placebo

■ **Monitoring Parameters**
- Renal function
- Blood glucose levels of diabetic patients

■ **Geriatric side effects at a glance:**
   ☑ CNS   ☑ Bowel Dysfunction   ☐ Bladder Dysfunction   ☐ Falls

■ **U.S. Regulatory Considerations**
   ☐ FDA Black Box   ☐ OBRA regulated in U.S. Long Term Care

oxacillin sodium

(ox-a-sill'-in soe'-dee-um)

■ **Brand Name(s):** Bactocill
   Chemical Class: Penicillin derivative, penicillinase-resistant

■ **Clinical Pharmacology:**
   Mechanism of Action: A penicillin that binds to bacterial membranes. **Therapeutic Effect:** Bactericidal.
   Pharmacokinetics: Rapid and incomplete absorption following PO administration. Protein binding: 94%. Rapidly excreted as unchanged drug in urine. **Half-life:** 30 min.

■ **Available Forms:**
- *Capsules:* 250 mg, 500 mg.
- *Powder for Reconstitution (Oral):* 250 mg/5 ml.
- *Powder for Injection:* 500-mg vials, 1-g vials, 2-g vials, 4-g vials, 10-g vials.
- *Intravenous Solution:* 1 g/50 ml.

■ **Indications and Dosages:**
   Upper respiratory tract, skin, and skin-structure infections: IV, IM 250-500 mg q4-6h.
   Lower respiratory tract and other serious infections: IV, IM 1g q4-6h. Maximum: 12 g/day.
   Mild to moderate infections: PO 500 mg q4-6h.
   Severe infections: PO 1g q4-6h.

■ **Contraindications:** Hypersensitivity to any penicillin

■ **Side Effects**
   Frequent
   Mild hypersensitivity reaction (fever, rash, pruritus), GI effects (nausea, vomiting, diarrhea)
   Occasional
   Phlebitis, thrombophlebitis, hepatotoxicity (with high IV dosage)

910

Serious Reactions
- Antibiotic-associated colitis and other superinfections may result from altered bacterial balance.
- A mild to severe hypersensitivity reaction may occur in those allergic to penicillins.

Special Considerations
- Sodium content of 1g = 2.8-3.1 mEq
- Individualize treatment based on local susceptibility patterns.

Patient/Family Education
- Administer on an empty stomach (1 hr before or 2 hr after meals)
- Report burning or pain at IV site
- Immediately report signs of an allergic reaction, such as shortness of breath, chest tightness, or hives
- Practice good oral hygiene

Monitoring Parameters
- Urinalysis, BUN, serum creatinine, CBC with differential, periodic liver function tests
- Withhold oxacillin as prescribed, and promptly notify the physician if the patient experiences a rash or diarrhea with abdominal pain, blood or mucus in stools, fever
- Assess the patient for signs and symptoms of superinfection, such as anal or genital pruritus, black hairy tongue, oral ulceration or pain, diarrhea, increased fever, sore throat, and vomiting

Geriatric side effects at a glance:
☐ CNS ☑ Bowel Dysfunction ☐ Bladder Dysfunction ☐ Falls

U.S. Regulatory Considerations
☐ FDA Black Box ☐ OBRA regulated in U.S. Long Term Care

oxaliplatin

(ox-al'-i-pla-tin)

Brand Name(s): Eloxatin
Chemical Class: Organoplatinum complex

Clinical Pharmacology:
Mechanism of Action: A platinum-containing complex that cross-links with DNA strands, preventing cell division. Cell cycle–phase nonspecific. **Therapeutic Effect:** Inhibits DNA replication.
Pharmacokinetics: Rapidly distributed. Protein binding: 90%. Undergoes rapid, extensive nonenzymatic biotransformation. Excreted in urine. **Half-life:** 70 hr.

Available Forms:
- Injection Solution: 50-mg, 100-mg vials 5 mg/ml.

■ **Indications and Dosages:**

Metastatic colon or rectal cancer in patients whose disease has recurred or progressed during or within 6 months of completing first-line therapy with bolus 5-fluorouracil (5-FU), leucovorin, and irinotecan: IV Day 1: Oxaliplatin 85 mg/m² in 250-500 ml D₅W and leucovorin 200 mg/m², both given simultaneously over more than 2 hr in separate bags using a Y-line, followed by 5-FU 400 mg/m² IV bolus given over 2-4 min, followed by 5-FU 600 mg/m² in 500 ml D₅W as a 22-hr continuous IV infusion. Day 2: Leucovorin 200 mg/m² IV infusion given over more than 2 hr, followed by 5-FU 400 mg/m² IV bolus given over 2-4 min, followed by 5-FU 600 mg/m² in 500 ml D₅W as a 22-hr continuous IV infusion.

Ovarian cancer: IV Cisplatin 100 mg/m² and oxaliplatin 130 mg/m² q3wk.

■ **Unlabeled Uses:** Treatment of germ cell cancer, ovarian cancer, pancreatic cancer, renal cell cancer, solid tumors

■ **Contraindications:** History of allergy to other platinum compounds

■ **Side Effects**

Frequent (76%-20%)
Peripheral or sensory neuropathy (usually occurs in hands, feet, perioral area, and throat but may present as jaw spasm, abnormal tongue sensation, eye pain, chest pressure, or difficulty walking, swallowing, or writing), nausea (64%), fatigue, diarrhea, vomiting, constipation, abdominal pain, fever, anorexia

Occasional (14%-10%)
Stomatitis, earache, insomnia, cough, difficulty breathing, backache, edema

Rare (7%-3%)
Dyspepsia, dizziness, rhinitis, flushing, alopecia

■ **Serious Reactions**
• Peripheral or sensory neuropathy can occur, sometimes precipitated or exacerbated by drinking or holding a glass of cold liquid during the IV infusion.
• Pulmonary fibrosis, characterized by a nonproductive cough, dyspnea, crackles, and radiologic pulmonary infiltrates, may require drug discontinuation.
• Hypersensitivity reaction (rash, urticaria, pruritus) occurs rarely.

Special Considerations
• Extravasation may lead to tissue necrosis

■ **Patient/Family Education**
• Neurotoxicity may be acute and aggravated by exposure to cold
• Promptly report easy bruising, fever, signs of local infection, sore throat, or unusual bleeding from any site
• Do not receive vaccinations during therapy and avoid contact with anyone who has recently received an oral polio vaccine

■ **Monitoring Parameters**
• CBC with platelets, hepatic and renal function
• Intake and output
• Evaluate for diarrhea and signs of GI bleeding, such as bright red or tarry stools
• Signs and symptoms of stomatitis, including erythema of the oral mucosa, sore throat, and ulceration of the lips or mouth

■ **Geriatric side effects at a glance:**
❑ CNS ☑ Bowel Dysfunction ❑ Bladder Dysfunction ❑ Falls

912

■ **U.S. Regulatory Considerations**
  ❑ FDA Black Box ❑ OBRA regulated in U.S. Long Term Care

oxandrolone

(ox-an'-droe-lone)

■ **Brand Name(s):** Oxandrin
  Chemical Class: Anabolic steroid; testosterone derivative

  DEA Class: Schedule III

■ **Clinical Pharmacology:**
  Mechanism of Action: A synthetic testosterone derivative that promotes growth and development of male sex organs, maintains secondary sex characteristics in androgen-deficient males. **Therapeutic Effect:** Androgenic and anabolic actions.
  Pharmacokinetics: Well absorbed from the gastrointestinal (GI) tract. Protein binding: 94%-97%. Metabolized in liver. Primarily excreted in urine. Unknown if removed by hemodialysis. **Half-life:** 5-13 hr.

■ **Available Forms:**
  • *Tablets*: 2.5 mg, 10 mg.

■ **Indications and Dosages:**
  Weight gain: 2.5-20 mg in divided doses 2-4 times/day usually for 2-4 weeks. Course of therapy is based on individual response. Repeat intermittently as needed.

■ **Unlabeled Uses:** AIDS wasting syndrome, alcoholic hepatitis, burns, Turner syndrome

■ **Contraindications:** Nephrosis, carcinoma of breast or prostate hypercalcemia, hypersensitivity to oxandrolone or any component of the formulation

■ **Side Effects**
  Frequent
  Gynecomastia, acne
  Females: Hirsutism, deepening of voice, clitoral enlargement that may not be reversible when drug is discontinued
  Occasional
  Edema, nausea, insomnia, oligospermia, priapism, male pattern of baldness, bladder irritability, hypercalcemia in immobilized patients or those with breast cancer, hypercholesterolemia
  Rare
  Polycythemia with high dosage

■ **Serious Reactions**
  • Peliosis hepatis of the liver, spleen replaced with blood-filled cysts, hepatic neoplasms, and hepatocellular carcinoma have been associated with prolonged high-dosage; anaphylactic reactions.

- Anabolic steroids have potential for abuse

Patient/Family Education
- Adequate dietary intake of calories and protein essential for successful treatment
- Reduce salt intake
- Notify the physician if acne, nausea, pedal edema, or vomiting occurs.
- The female patient should promptly report deepening of voice and hoarseness
- The male patient should report difficulty urinating, frequent erections, and gynecomastia

Monitoring Parameters
- LFTs, lipids
- Serum calcium in breast cancer patients
- Weight
- Intake and output
- Sleep patterns
- Blood pressure

Geriatric side effects at a glance:
❑ CNS   ❑ Bowel Dysfunction   ❑ Bladder Dysfunction   ❑ Falls

U.S. Regulatory Considerations
❑ FDA Black Box   ❑ OBRA regulated in U.S. Long Term Care

oxaprozin

(ox-a-proe'-zin)

Brand Name(s): Daypro
Chemical Class: Propionic acid derivative

Clinical Pharmacology:
Mechanism of Action: An NSAID that produces analgesic and anti-inflammatory effects by inhibiting prostaglandin synthesis. **Therapeutic Effect:** Reduces the inflammatory response and intensity of pain.
Pharmacokinetics: Well absorbed from the GI tract. Protein binding: 99%. Widely distributed. Metabolized in the liver. Primarily excreted in urine; partially eliminated in feces. Not removed by hemodialysis. **Half-life:** 42–50 hr.

Available Forms:
- *Tablets*: 600 mg.

Indications and Dosages:
Osteoarthritis: PO 1,200 mg once a day (600 mg in patients with low body weight or mild disease). Maximum: 1,800 mg/day.
Rheumatoid arthritis: PO 1,200 mg once a day. Range: 600–1,800 mg/day.

Dosage in renal impairment: For patients with renal impairment, the recommended initial dose is 600 mg/day; may be increased up to 1,200 mg/day.

■ **Contraindications:** Active peptic ulcer disease, chronic inflammation of GI tract, GI bleeding or ulceration, history of hypersensitivity to aspirin or NSAIDs

■ **Side Effects**
Occasional (9%–3%)
Nausea, diarrhea, constipation, dyspepsia, edema
Rare (less than 3%)
Vomiting, abdominal cramps or pain, flatulence, anorexia, confusion, tinnitus, insomnia, somnolence

■ **Serious Reactions**
- Hypertension, acute renal failure, respiratory depression, GI bleeding, and coma occur rarely.

Special Considerations
- No significant advantage over other NSAIDs; cost should govern use

■ **Patient/Family Education**
- Avoid aspirin and alcoholic beverages
- Take with food, milk, or antacids to decrease GI upset
- Avoid performing tasks that require mental alertness or motor skills until response to the drug has been established
- Notify the physician if persistent GI effects, especially black, tarry stools occur

■ **Monitoring Parameters**
- Initial hematocrit and fecal occult blood test within 3 mo of starting regular chronic therapy; repeat every 6-12 mo (more frequently in high-risk patients (>65 years, peptic ulcer disease, concurrent steroids or anticoagulants); electrolytes, creatinine, and BUN within 3 mo of starting regular chronic therapy; repeat every 6-12 mo
- Therapeutic response, such as improved grip strength, increased joint mobility, and decreased pain, tenderness, stiffness, and swelling

■ **Geriatric side effects at a glance:**
☑ CNS ☐ Bowel Dysfunction ☐ Bladder Dysfunction ☐ Falls
☑ Other: Gastropathy

■ **Use with caution in older patients with:** Renal impairment, Hepatic impairment, CHF, HTN, PUD, History of GI bleeding, GERD, Bleeding and platelet disorders, History of aspirin sensitivity reaction. Also use with caution in patients taking Anticoagulants, Aspirin, and Antihypertensive agents.

■ **U.S. Regulatory Considerations**
☐ FDA Black Box ☐ OBRA regulated in U.S. Long Term Care

■ **Other Uses in Geriatric Patient:** Acute gout

■ **Side Effects:**
Of particular importance in the geriatric patient: Confusion, cognitive impairment, delirium, dizziness, dyspepsia, fluid retention, renal impairment

■ **Geriatric Considerations - Summary:** A preferred agent in older adults due to its association with fewer GI adverse effects. Use of NSAIDs in older adults increases the risk of GI complications including gastric ulceration, bleeding and perforation. These complications are not necessarily preceded by less severe GI symptoms. Concomitant use of a proton pump inhibitor or misoprostol reduces the risk for gastric ulceration and bleeding, but may not prevent long-term GI toxicity.

■ **References:**

1. COX-2 alternatives and GI protection. Med Lett Drugs Ther 2004;46:91.
2. Drugs that may cause cognitive disorders in the elderly. Med Lett Drugs Ther 2000;42:111-112.

oxazepam

(ox-a'-ze-pam)

■ **Brand Name(s):** Serax
Chemical Class: Benzodiazepine

DEA Class: Schedule IV

■ **Clinical Pharmacology:**
Mechanism of Action: A benzodiazepine that potentiates the effects of gamma-aminobutyric acid and other inhibitory neurotransmitters by binding to specific receptors in the CNS. **Therapeutic Effect:** Produces sedative effect and skeletal muscle relaxation.
Pharmacokinetics: Well absorbed from the GI tract. Protein binding: 97%. Metabolized in the liver. Primarily excreted in urine. Not removed by hemodialysis. **Half-life:** 5-20 hr.

■ **Available Forms:**
- *Capsules*: 10 mg, 15 mg, 30 mg.
- *Tablets*: 15 mg.

■ **Indications and Dosages:**
Anxiety: PO 10 mg 2-3 times a day.
Alcohol withdrawal: PO 15-30 mg 3-4 times a day.

■ **Contraindications:** Angle-closure glaucoma; preexisting CNS depression; severe, uncontrolled pain

■ **Side Effects**
Frequent
Mild, transient somnolence at beginning of therapy
Occasional
Dizziness, headache
Rare
Paradoxical CNS reactions, such as excitement or restlessness (generally noted during the first 2 weeks of therapy)

- **Serious Reactions**
  - Abrupt or too-rapid withdrawal may result in pronounced restlessness, irritability, insomnia, hand tremor, abdominal or muscle cramps, diaphoresis, vomiting, and seizures.
  - Overdose results in somnolence, confusion, diminished reflexes, and coma.

Special Considerations

  - Useful for treatment of anxiety in patients with hepatic disease; consider for alcohol withdrawal
  - Tablet form contains tartrazine; risk of allergic-type reactions, especially in patients with aspirin hypersensitivity

- **Patient/Family Education**
  - Avoid alcohol and other CNS depressants
  - Do not discontinue abruptly after prolonged therapy
  - Oxazepam may cause drowsiness. Avoid tasks requiring mental alertness or motor skills until response to the drug has been established
  - May be habit forming

- **Monitoring Parameters**
  - Periodic CBC, UA, blood chemistry analyses during prolonged therapy
  - Hepatic and renal function periodically
  - Therapeutic response, such as a calm facial expression and decreased restlessness and diminished insomnia

- **Geriatric side effects at a glance:**
  ☑ CNS   ❑ Bowel Dysfunction   ❑ Bladder Dysfunction   ☑ Falls
  Other: Withdrawal symptoms after long-term use

- **Use with caution in older patients with:** COPD; untreated sleep apnea

- **U.S. Regulatory Considerations**
  ❑ FDA Black Box   ☑ OBRA regulated in U.S. Long Term Care

- **Other Uses in Geriatric Patient:** Anxiety symptoms and related disorders, dementia-related behavioral problems

- **Side Effects:**
  Of particular importance in the geriatric patient: Sedation, withdrawal symptoms when abruptly discontinued (e.g., during hospitalization) rather than tapered

- **Geriatric Considerations - Summary:** Benzodiazepines are effective anxiolytic agents, and hypnotics. These drugs should be reserved for short-term use. SSRIs are preferred for long-term management of anxiety disorders in older adults, and sedating antidepressants (e.g., trazodone) or eszopiclone are preferred for long-term management of sleep problems. Long-acting benzodiazepines, including: flurazepam, chlordiazepoxide, clorazepate, diazepam, clonazepam, and quazepam should generally be avoided in older adults as these agents have been associated with oversedation. On the other hand, short-acting benzodiazepines (e.g., triazolam) have been associated with a higher risk of withdrawal symptoms. When initiating therapy, benzodiazepines should be titrated carefully to avoid oversedation. In addition, many of the drugs in this class have been associated with severe withdrawal symptoms (e.g., anxiety and/or agitation, seizures) when discontinued abruptly.

■ **References:**
1. Leipzig RM, Cumming RG, Tinetti ME. Drugs and falls in older people: a systematic review and meta-analysis: I. Psychotropic drugs. J Am Geriatr Soc 1999;47:30-39.
2. Shorr RI, Robin DW. Rational use of benzodiazepines in the elderly. Drugs Aging 1994;4:9-20.
3. Shader RI, Greenblatt DJ. Use of benzodiazepines in anxiety disorders. N Engl J Med 1993;328:1398-1405.

oxcarbazepine

(ox-car-baz'-e-peen)

■ **Brand Name(s):** Trileptal
Chemical Class: Dibenzazepine derivative

■ **Clinical Pharmacology:**
Mechanism of Action: An anticonvulsant that blocks sodium channels, resulting in stabilization of hyperexcited neural membranes, inhibition of repetitive neuronal firing, and diminishing synaptic impulses. **Therapeutic Effect:** Prevents seizures.
Pharmacokinetics: Completely absorbed from GI tract and extensively metabolized in the liver to active metabolite. Protein binding: 40%. Primarily excreted in urine. **Half-life:** 2 hr; metabolite, 6-10 hr.

■ **Available Forms:**
• *Oral Suspension*: 300 mg/5 ml.
• *Tablets*: 150 mg, 300 mg, 600 mg.

■ **Indications and Dosages:**
Adjunctive treatment of seizures: PO Initially, 600 mg/day in 2 divided doses. May increase by up to 600 mg/day at weekly intervals. Maximum: 2,400 mg/day.
Conversion to monotherapy: PO 600 mg/day in 2 divided doses (while decreasing concomitant CNS-anticonvulsant-new over 3-6 wk). May increase by 600 mg/day at weekly intervals up to 2,400 mg/day.
Initiation of monotherapy: PO 600 mg/day in 2 divided doses. May increase by 300 mg/day every 3 days up to 1,200 mg/day.
Dosage in renal impairment: For patients with creatinine clearance less than 30 ml/min, give 50% of normal starting dose, then titrate slowly to desired dose.

■ **Unlabeled Uses:** Atypical panic disorder, bipolar disorders, neuralgia/neuropathy

■ **Contraindications:** None known.

■ **Side Effects**
Frequent (22%-13%)
Dizziness, nausea, headache
Occasional (7%-5%)
Vomiting, diarrhea, ataxia, nervousness, heartburn, indigestion, epigastric pain, constipation

918

Rare (4%)
Tremor, rash, back pain, epistaxis, sinusitis, diplopia

■ **Serious Reactions**
  • Clinically significant hyponatremia may occur.

Special Considerations
  • Considered an alternative to carbamazepine in intolerant patients

■ **Patient/Family Education**
  • Review and reinforce prevalence of CNS adverse effects early in treatment (reason for gradual titration regimens) with tolerance developing with continued adherence
  • Risk of recurrent seizures with missed doses
  • Periodic blood tests are necessary

■ **Monitoring Parameters**
  • Seizure frequency and electroencephalogram changes in patients with seizure disorder; a reduction or elimination of pain in patients with trigeminal neuralgia; therapeutic serum levels not adequately established; use estimates of therapeutic serum concentrations of the active metabolite (MHD) in the 50-110 µmol range; serum electrolytes (especially sodium), LFTs, blood counts, serum lipids

■ **Geriatric side effects at a glance:**
  ❑ CNS ❑ Bowel Dysfunction ❑ Bladder Dysfunction ❑ Falls
  Other: Hyponatremia

■ **Use with caution in older patients with:** Hepatic impairment, Renal impairment, Patients taking diuretics, NSAIDs, or with nephropathy (increased risk of hyponatremia), Unsteady gait, Urinary incontinence

■ **U.S. Regulatory Considerations**
  ❑ FDA Black Box ❑ OBRA regulated in U.S. Long Term Care

■ **Other Uses in Geriatric Patient:** None

■ **Side Effects:**
  Of particular importance in the geriatric patient: Delirium, confusion, cognitive impairment, sedation, dizziness, fatigue, nausea/vomiting, hyponatremia (usually dose dependent)

■ **Geriatric Considerations - Summary:** Well-tolerated in older adults. Adjust dose based on creatinine clearance. Autoinduction of metabolism does not occur as seen with carbamazepine, but drug interactions are still an issue. Many of the CNS effects occur early in treatment and are transitory. One-third of patients with hypersensitivity reactions to carbamazepine will experience cross-sensitivity to oxcarbazepine.

■ **References:**
  1. Brodie M, Kwan P. Epilepsy in elderly people. BMJ 2005;331:1317-1322.
  2. Kutluay E, McCague K, D'Souza JD, Beydoun A. Safety and tolerability of oxcarbazepine in elderly patients with epilepsy. Epilepsy & Behavior 2003;4:108-175.
  3. Arroyo S, Kramer G. Treating epilepsy in the elderly: safety considerations. Drug Saf 2001;24:991-1015.

4. Drugs that may cause cognitive disorders in the elderly. Med Let 2000;42:111-112.
5. Willmore LJ. Choice and use of newer anticonvulsant drugs in older patients. Drugs Aging 2000;17:441-452.

oxiconazole nitrate

(ox-i-kon'-a-zole nye'-trate)

- **Brand Name(s):** Oxistat
  Chemical Class: Imidazole derivative

- **Clinical Pharmacology:**
  Mechanism of Action: An antifungal agent that inhibits ergosterol synthesis. **Therapeutic Effect:** Destroys cytoplasmic membrane integrity of fungi. Fungicidal.
  Pharmacokinetics: Low systemic absorption. Absorbed and distributed in each layer of the dermis. Excreted in the urine.

- **Available Forms:**
  - *Cream*: 1% (Oxistat).
  - *Lotion*: 1% (Oxistat).

- **Indications and Dosages:**
  Tinea pedis: Topical Apply 1-2 times daily for 1 mo or until signs and symptoms significantly improve.
  Tinea cruris, tinea corporis: Topical Apply 1-2 times daily for 2 wk or until signs and symptoms significantly improve.

- **Contraindications:** Not for ophthalmic use; hypersensitivity to oxiconazole or any other azole fungals

- **Side Effects**
  Occasional
  Itching, local irritation, stinging, dryness

- **Serious Reactions**
  - Hypersensitivity reactions characterized by rash, swelling, pruritus, maceration, and a sensation of warmth may occur.

Special Considerations
  - **Niche**: Once daily imadazole; base choice on cost and convenience

- **Patient/Family Education**
  - For external use only, avoid contact with eyes or vagina
  - Separate personal items that come in contact with affected areas
  - Rub topical form well into the affected and surrounding area
  - Notify the physician if skin irritation occurs

oxtriphylline

(ox-trye'-fi-lin)

■ **Brand Name(s):** Choledyl SA
  Chemical Class: Xanthine derivative (64% theophylline)

■ **Clinical Pharmacology:**
  Mechanism of Action: A choline salt of theophylline which acts as a bronchodilator by directly relaxing smooth muscle of the bronchial airway and pulmonary blood vessels. **Therapeutic Effect:** Relieves bronchospasm, increases vital capacity. Produces cardiac skeletal muscle stimulation.
  Pharmacokinetics: Absorbed slowly due to extended-release formulation. Protein binding: 40%. Distributed rapidly into peripheral nonadipose tissues and body water, including cerebrospinal fluid (CSF). Metabolized in liver. Eliminated in urine. **Half-life:** Adults, 6-12 hr.

■ **Available Forms:**
  • *Tablet* (*Extended Release*): 400 mg, 600 mg.

■ **Indications and Dosages:**
  Asthma: PO 400-600 mg q12h

■ **Contraindications:** Active peptic ulcer disease, seizure disorder (unless receiving appropriate anticonvulsant medication), history of hypersensitivity to xanthines

■ **Side Effects**
  Frequent
  Headache, shakiness, restlessness, tachycardia, trembling
  Occasional
  Nausea, vomiting, epigastric pain, diarrhea, headache, mild diuresis, insomnia
  Rare
  Alopecia, hyperglycemia, SIADH, rash

■ **Serious Reactions**
  • Nausea, vomiting, seizures, and coma can result from overdosage.

Special Considerations

- Touted to produce less GI side effects; if dosed equipotently based on theophylline equivalents (oxtriphylline = 64% theophylline), no difference; compare costs as well as other characteristics

■ **Patient/Family Education**
- Avoid large amounts of caffeine-containing products (tea, coffee, chocolate, colas)
- Increase fluid intake
- Smoking and charcoal-broiled food may decrease drug level

■ **Monitoring Parameters**
- Serum theophylline concentrations (therapeutic level is 8-20 mcg/ml); toxicity may occur with small increase above 20 mcg/ml, especially in the elderly
- Rate, depth, rhythm, and type of breathing
- ABGs

■ **Geriatric side effects at a glance:**
  ☐ CNS ☑ Bowel Dysfunction ☐ Bladder Dysfunction ☐ Falls

■ **U.S. Regulatory Considerations**
  ☐ FDA Black Box ☐ OBRA regulated in U.S. Long Term Care

oxybutynin

(ox-i-byoo'-ti-nin)

■ **Brand Name(s):** Ditropan, Ditropan XL, Oxytrol, Urotrol
  Chemical Class: Tertiary amine

■ **Clinical Pharmacology:**
  Mechanism of Action: An anticholinergic that exerts antispasmodic (papaverine-like) and antimuscarinic (atropine-like) action on the detrusor smooth muscle of the bladder. **Therapeutic Effect:** Increases bladder capacity and delays desire to void.
  Pharmacokinetics:

Route	Onset	Peak	Duration
PO	0.5–1 hr	3–6 hr	6–10 hr

  Rapidly absorbed from the GI tract. Metabolized in the liver. Primarily excreted in urine. Unknown if removed by hemodialysis. **Half-life:** 1–2.3 hr.

■ **Available Forms:**
- *Syrup (Ditropan):* 5 mg/5 ml .
- *Tablets (Ditropan, Urotrol):* 5 mg.
- *Tablets (Extended-Release [Ditropan XL]):* 5 mg, 10 mg, 15 mg.
- *Transdermal (Oxytrol):* 3.9 mg.

922

- **Indications and Dosages:**
  Neurogenic bladder: PO 2.5–5 mg twice a day. May increase by 2.5 mg/day every 1–2 days. PO (Extended-Release) 5–10 mg/day up to 30 mg/day. Transdermal 3.9 mg applied twice a week. Apply every 3–4 days.

- **Contraindications:** GI or GU obstruction, glaucoma, myasthenia gravis, toxic megacolon, ulcerative colitis

- **Side Effects**
  Frequent
  Constipation, dry mouth, somnolence, decreased perspiration
  Occasional
  Decreased lacrimation or salivation, impotence, urinary hesitancy and retention, suppressed lactation, blurred vision, mydriasis, nausea or vomiting, insomnia, cognitive impairment, delirium

- **Serious Reactions**
  - Overdose produces CNS excitation (including nervousness, restlessness, hallucinations, and irritability), hypotension or hypertension, confusion, tachycardia, facial flushing, and respiratory depression.

Special Considerations
  - Reported anticholinergic side effects not clinically or significantly different from other agents (i.e., propantheline); compare costs

- **Patient/Family Education**
  - Avoid prolonged exposure to hot environments; heat prostration may result
  - Use caution in driving or other activities requiring alertness
  - Swallow extended-release tablets whole; do not chew or crush
  - Extended release tablet shell not absorbable
  - Apply patch to dry, intact skin on abdomen, hip, or buttock; select new side with each new patch to avoid re-application to the same site within 7 days
  - May cause drowsiness and dry mouth
  - Avoid alcohol

- **Monitoring Parameters**
  - Intake and output
  - Pattern of daily bowel activity and stool consistency
  - Symptomatic relief

- **Geriatric side effects at a glance:**
  ☑ CNS   ☑ Bowel Dysfunction   ☑ Bladder Dysfunction   ☑ Falls
  Other: Dry mouth, blurred vision, dizziness, somnolence

- **Use with caution in older patients with:** Tachyarrhythmias, overflow incontinence.

- **U.S. Regulatory Considerations**
  ☐ FDA Black Box   ☑ OBRA regulated in U.S. Long Term Care

- **Other Uses in Geriatric Patient:** None

■ **Side Effects:**
  Of particular importance in the geriatric patient: Delirium, possible antagonism of cholinergic drug therapy in the treatment of Alzheimer's disease.

■ **Geriatric Considerations - Summary:** Oxybutynin and related muscarinic drugs are moderately effective in the treatment of urge urinary incontinence. The effectiveness of these agents must be balanced against anticholinergic side effects including cognitive impairment, delirium, dry mouth, blurred vision, and increased risk of falls. Long-acting preparations may cause less adverse effects. Newer medications in this class include tolterodine, trospium, solifenacin, and darifenacin and offer the potential benefit of selective antagonism of muscarinic receptors with less potental to induce CNS side effects. The relative safety and efficacy of these agents, which are significantly more expensive, has not been well studied to determine if they are superior to longer-acting anticholinergics.

■ **References:**
  1. Hay-Smith J, Herbison P, Ellis G, Moore K. Anticholinergic drugs versus placebo for overactive bladder syndrome in adults. Cochrane Database System Rev 2003;3.
  2. Vangala V, Tueth M. Chronic anticholinergic toxicity: identification and management in older patients. Geriatrics 2003;58:36-37.
  3. Tune LE. Anticholinergic effects of medication in elderly patients. J Clin Psychiatry 2001;62(suppl 21):11-14.
  4. Solifenacin and Darifenacin for overactive bladder. Med Let 2005;47:23-24.
  5. Ouslander JG. Management of overactive bladder. N Engl J Med 2004;350:786-799.

oxycodone hydrochloride

(ox-i-koe'-done hye-droe-klor'-ide)

■ **Brand Name(s):** M-Oxy, OxyContin, Oxydose, OxyFast, OxyIR, Percolone, Roxicodone, Roxicodone Intensol

  Combinations
  Rx: with aspirin (Percodan, Endodan, Roxiprin); with acetaminophen (Percocet, Endocet, Tylox, Roxicet, Roxilox)
  Chemical Class: Opiate derivative; phenanthrene derivative

  DEA Class: Schedule II

■ **Clinical Pharmacology:**
  Mechanism of Action: An opioid analgesic that binds with opioid receptors in the CNS. **Therapeutic Effect:** Alters the perception of and emotional response to pain.
  Pharmacokinetics:

Route	Onset	Peak	Duration
PO, Immediate-release	N/A	N/A	4-5 hr
PO, Controlled-release	N/A	N/A	12 hr

  Moderately absorbed from the GI tract. Protein binding: 38%-45%. Widely distributed. Metabolized in the liver. Excreted in urine. Unknown if removed by hemodialysis. **Half-life:** 2-3 hr (3.2 hr controlled-release).

■ Available Forms:

- *Capsules (Immediate-Release [OxyIR])*: 5 mg.
- *Oral Concentrate (Oxydose, OxyFast, Roxicodone Intensol)*: 20 mg/ml.
- *Oral Solution (Roxicodone)*: 5 mg/5ml.
- *Tablets (M-Oxy, Percolone, Roxicodone)*: 5 mg, 15 mg, 30 mg.
- *Tablets (Extended-Release [OxyContin])*: 10 mg, 20 mg, 40 mg, 80 mg, 160 mg.

■ Indications and Dosages:

Analgesia: PO (Controlled-Release) Initially, 10 mg q12h. May increase every 1-2 days by 25%-50%. Usual: 40 mg/day (100 mg/day for cancer pain). PO (Immediate-Release) Initially, 5 mg q6h as needed. May increase up to 30 mg q4h. Usual: 10-30 mg q4h as needed.

■ Contraindications: Acute bronchial asthma or hypercarbia, paralytic ileus, respiratory depression

■ Side Effects

Frequent

Somnolence, dizziness, hypotension (including orthostatic hypotension), anorexia

Occasional

Confusion, diaphoresis, facial flushing, urine retention, constipation, dry mouth, nausea, vomiting, headache

Rare

Allergic reaction, depression, paradoxical excitement and restlessness

■ Serious Reactions

- Overdose results in respiratory depression, skeletal muscle flaccidity, cold or clammy skin, cyanosis, and extreme somnolence progressing to seizures, stupor, and coma.
- Hepatotoxicity may occur with overdose of the acetaminophen component of fixed-combination products.
- The patient who uses oxycodone repeatedly may develop a tolerance to the drug's analgesic effect and physical dependence.

■ Patient/Family Education

- Physical dependency may result when used for extended periods
- Change position slowly, orthostatic hypotension may occur
- Do not administer agonist/antagonist analgesics (i.e., pentazocine, nalbuphine, butorphanol, dezocine, buprenorphine) to patient who has received a prolonged course of oxycodone (a pure agonist). In opioid-dependent patients, mixed agonist/antagonist analgesics may precipitate withdrawal symptoms
- Do not break, chew, or crush controlled-release tablets (OxyContin)
- Take oxycodone before the pain returns
- Avoid performing tasks that require mental alertness or motor skills until response to the drug has been established
- Avoid alcohol

■ Monitoring Parameters

- Blood pressure, respiratory rate
- Mental status
- Pattern of daily bowel activity and stool consistency
- Clinical improvement and onset of pain relief

oxymetazoline

(ox-i-met-az'-oh-leen)

OTC: Afrin, Afrin 12-Hour, Ocuclear, Sinex 12 Hour Long-Acting
Chemical Class: Imidazoline derivative

- **Clinical Pharmacology:**
  Mechanism of Action: A direct-acting sympathomimetic amine that acts on alpha-adrenergic receptors in arterioles of the nasal mucosa to produce constriction. **Therapeutic Effect:** Causes vasoconstriction resulting in decreased blood flow and decreased nasal congestion.
  Pharmacokinetics: Onset of action is about 10 min and duration of action is 7 hr or more. Absorption occurs from the nasal mucosa and can produce systemic effects, primarily following overdose or excessive use. Excreted mostly in the urine as well as the feces. **Half-life:** 5-8 hr.

- **Available Forms:**
  - **Eye Drops:** 0.025% (Ocuclear).
  - **Nasal Drops:** 0.05% (Afrin).
  - **Nasal Spray:** 0.05% (Afrin, Afrin 12-Hour, Sinex 12 Hour Long-Acting).

- **Indications and Dosages:**
  Rhinitis: Intranasal 2-3 drops/sprays (0.05% nasal solution) in each nostril q12h.
  Conjunctivitis: Ophthalmic 1-2 drops (0.025% ophthalmic solution) q6h for 3-4 days.

- **Unlabeled Uses:** Otitis media surgical procedures

- **Contraindications:** Narrow-angle glaucoma or other serious eye diseases, hypersensitivity to oxymetazoline or other adrenergic agents

- **Side Effects**
  Occasional
  Intranasal: Transient burning, stinging, sneezing, dryness of mucosa. Prolonged use may result in rebound congestion
  Ophthalmic: Irritation, blurred vision, mydriasis

Systemic sympathomimetic effects may occur with either route: headache, hypertension, weakness, sweating, palpitations, tremors

■ **Serious Reactions**
- Large doses may produce tachycardia, hypertension, arrhythmias, palpitations, light-headedness, nausea, and vomiting.
- Overdosage may produce hallucinations, CNS depression, and seizures.

Special Considerations
- Manage rebound congestion by stopping oxymetazoline: one nostril at a time, substitute systemic decongestant and/or substitute inhaled steroid

■ **Patient/Family Education**
- Do not use for longer than 3-5 days or rebound congestion may occur
- Discontinue and consult physician immediately if ocular pain or visual changes occur or if condition worsens or continues for more than 72 hr

■ **Geriatric side effects at a glance:**
  ❏ CNS ❏ Bowel Dysfunction ❏ Bladder Dysfunction ❏ Falls

■ **U.S. Regulatory Considerations**
  ❏ FDA Black Box ❏ OBRA regulated in U.S. Long Term Care

oxymorphone hydrochloride

(ox-ee-mor'-fone hye-droe-klor'-ide)

■ **Brand Name(s):** Numorphan
  Chemical Class: Opiate derivative; phenanthrene derivative

  DEA Class: Schedule II

■ **Clinical Pharmacology:**
  Mechanism of Action: An opioid agonist, similar to morphine, that binds at opiate receptor sites in the central nervous system (CNS). **Therapeutic Effect:** Reduces intensity of pain stimuli incoming from sensory nerve endings, altering pain perception and emotional response to pain; suppresses cough reflex.
  Pharmacokinetics:

Route	Onset	Peak	Duration
Subcutaneous	5-10 min	30-90 min	4-6 hr
IM	5-10 min	30-60 min	3-6 hr
IV	5-10 min	15-30 min	3-6 hr
Rectal	15-30 min	N/A	3-6 hr

Well absorbed from the gastrointestinal (GI) tract, after IM administration. Widely distributed. Metabolized in liver via glucuronidation. Excreted in urine. **Half-life:** 1-2 hr.

■ **Available Forms:**
- *Injection*: 1 mg/ml, 1.5 mg/ml (Numorphan).
- *Suppository*: 5 mg (Numorphan).

■ **Indications and Dosages:**
  Analgesic, Anxiety, Preanesthesia: IV Initially 0.5 mg. SC, IM 1-1.5 mg q4-6h as needed Rectal 0.5-1 mg q4-6h.

■ **Unlabeled Uses:** Cancer pain, intractable pain in narcotic-tolerant patients

■ **Contraindications:** Paralytic ileus, acute asthma attack, pulmonary edema secondary to chemical respiratory irritant, severe respiratory depression, upper airway obstruction

■ **Side Effects**
  Frequent
  Drowsiness, dizziness, hypotension, decreased appetite, tolerance or dependence
  Occasional
  Confusion, diaphoresis, facial flushing, urinary retention, constipation, dry mouth, nausea, vomiting, headache, pain at injection site, abdominal cramps
  Rare
  Allergic reaction, depression

■ **Serious Reactions**
- Hypotension, paralytic ileus, respiratory depression, and toxic megacolon rarely occur.
- Overdosage results in respiratory depression, skeletal muscle flaccidity, cold or clammy skin, cyanosis, extreme somnolence progressing to seizures, stupor, and coma.
- Tolerance to analgesic effect and physical dependence may occur with repeated use.
- Prolonged duration of action and cumulative effect may occur in patients with impaired liver or renal function.

Special Considerations
- Do not administer agonist/antagonist analgesics (i.e., pentazocine, nalbuphine, butorphanol, dezocine, buprenorphine) to patient who has received a prolonged course of oxymorphone (a pure agonist). In opioid-dependent patients, mixed agonist/antagonist analgesics may precipitate withdrawal symptoms.

■ **Patient/Family Education**
- Physical dependency may result when used for extended periods
- Change position slowly, orthostatic hypotension may occur
- Avoid alcohol
- Avoid tasks that require mental alertness and motor skills until response to the drug is established

■ **Monitoring Parameters**
- Vital signs
- Pattern of daily bowel activity and stool consistency
- Clinical improvement, onset of relief of cough or pain

oxytetracycline hydrochloride

(ox'-ee-tet-tra-sye'-kleen hye-droe-klor'-ide)

■ **Brand Name(s):** Terramycin IM

  Combinations
  Rx: with polymyxin (Terek); with phenazopyridine, sulfamethizole (Urobiotic-250, Tija)
  Chemical Class: Tetracycline derivative

■ **Clinical Pharmacology:**
  Mechanism of Action: A tetracycline antibacterial that inhibits bacterial protein synthesis by binding to ribosomes. Cell wall synthesis is not affected. **Therapeutic Effect:** Prevents bacterial cell growth. Bacteriostatic.
  Pharmacokinetics: Poorly absorbed after IM administration. Protein binding: 27%-35%. Metabolized in liver. Excreted in urine. Eliminated in feces via biliary system. Not removed by hemodialysis. **Half-life:** 8.5-9.6 hr (half-life is increased with impaired renal function).

■ **Available Forms:**
  • *Injection, Solution:* 5% (Terramycin IM).

■ **Indications and Dosages:**
  Treatment of inflammatory acne, anthrax, gonorrhea, skin infections, urinary tract infection (UTI): IM   250 mg/day or 300 mg/day divided q8-12h
  Dosage in renal impairment:

Creatinine Clearance	Dosage Interval
less than 10 ml/min	q24h

■ **Unlabeled Uses:** Chlamydia infection, nonspecific urethritis, peptic ulcer

■ **Contraindications:** Hypersensitivity to tetracyclines or any component of the formulation

■ **Side Effects**
  Frequent
  Dizziness, light-headedness, diarrhea, nausea, vomiting, stomach cramps, increased sensitivity of skin to sunlight

Occasional
Pigmentation of skin, mucous membranes, itching in rectal or genital area, sore mouth or tongue, increased BUN, irritation at injection site

■ **Serious Reactions**
- Superinfection (especially fungal), anaphylaxis, and increased intracranial pressure may occur.

Special Considerations
- Offers no significant advantage over tetracycline; shares similar spectrum of activity (may be slightly less active than tetracycline and has longer dosage interval)
- Individualize treatment based on local susceptibility patterns.

■ **Patient/Family Education**
- Avoid milk products, take with a full glass of water
- Take for the full length of treatment and space doses around the clock
- Notify the physician if diarrhea, rash, or any other new symptoms occur
- Protect skin from sun exposure and avoid overexposure to sun or ultraviolet light to prevent photosensitivity reactions

■ **Monitoring Parameters**
- Blood pressure
- Skin for rash
- Daily bowel activity and stool consistency. Although mild GI effects may be tolerable, severe symptoms may indicate the onset of antibiotic-associated colitis.
- Signs and symptoms of superinfection include abdominal pain or cramping, anal or genital pruritus or discharge, moderate to severe diarrhea, severe mouth or tongue soreness, and new or increased fever.

■ **Geriatric side effects at a glance:**
☑ CNS   ☑ Bowel Dysfunction   ❑ Bladder Dysfunction   ❑ Falls

■ **U.S. Regulatory Considerations**
❑ FDA Black Box   ❑ OBRA regulated in U.S. Long Term Care

palifermin

(pal-ee-fer'-min)

■ **Brand Name(s):** Kepivance

■ **Clinical Pharmacology:**
Mechanism of Action: An antineoplastic adjunct that binds to the keratinocyte growth factor receptor, present on epithelial cells of the buccal mucosa and tongue, resulting in the proliferation, differentiation, and migration of epithelial cells. **Therapeutic Effect:** Reduces incidence and duration of severe oral mucositis.

Pharmacokinetics: Clearance is higher in cancer patients compared to healthy subjects. **Half-life:** 4.5 hr.

■ **Available Forms:**
- *Injection*: 6.25-mg vials.

■ **Indications and Dosages:**
Mucositis (*premyelotoxic therapy*): IV 60 mcg/kg/day for 3 consecutive days, with the 3rd dose 24-48 hr before chemotherapy.
Mucositis (*postmyelotoxic therapy*): IV The last 3 doses should be administered after myelotoxic therapy; the first of these doses should be administered after, but on the same day of, hematopoietic stem cell infusion and at least 4 days after the most recent administration of palifermin.

■ **Contraindications:** Patients allergic to *Escherichia coli*-derived proteins

■ **Side Effects**
Frequent
Rash (62%), fever (39%), pruritus (35%), erythema (32%), edema (28%)
Occasional
Mouth and tongue thickness or discoloration (17%), altered taste (16%), dysesthesia manifested as hyperesthesia, hypoesthesia, paresthesia (12%), arthralgia (10%)

■ **Serious Reactions**
- Transient hypertension occurs occasionally.

■ **Geriatric side effects at a glance:**
❑ CNS ❑ Bowel Dysfunction ❑ Bladder Dysfunction ❑ Falls

■ **U.S. Regulatory Considerations**
❑ FDA Black Box ❑ OBRA regulated in U.S. Long Term Care

palonosetron hydrochloride

(pal-oh-noe'-se-tron hye-droe-klor'-ide)

■ **Brand Name(s):** Aloxi
Chemical Class: Isoquinoline derivative

■ **Clinical Pharmacology:**
Mechanism of Action: A 5-HT$_3$ receptor antagonist that acts centrally in the chemoreceptor trigger zone and peripherally at the vagal nerve terminals. **Therapeutic Effect:** Prevents nausea and vomiting associated with chemotherapy.
Pharmacokinetics: *Protein binding*: 52%. Metabolized in liver. Eliminated in urine. **Half-life:** 40 hr.

■ **Available Forms:**
- *Injection*: 0.25 mg/5 ml.

- **Indications and Dosages:**
  Chemotherapy-induced nausea and vomiting: IV 0.25 mg as a single dose 30 min before starting chemotherapy.

- **Unlabeled Uses:** Prevention of postoperative bleeding

- **Contraindications:** None known.

- **Side Effects**
  Occasional (9%-5%)
  Headache, constipation
  Rare (less than 1%)
  Diarrhea, dizziness, fatigue, abdominal pain, insomnia

- **Serious Reactions**
  - Overdose may produce a combination of CNS stimulant and depressant effects.
  - Cardiac dysrhythmia has been reported.

Special Considerations
  - Clinical superiority over other 5-HT$_3$ receptor antagonists (e.g., ondansetron, dolasetron) has not been adequately demonstrated

- **Patient/Family Education**
  - Nausea and vomiting should be relieved shortly after drug administration; notify the physician if vomiting persists
  - Avoid alcohol and barbiturates during palonosetron therapy
  - Other methods of reducing nausea and vomiting include lying quietly and avoiding strong odors

- **Monitoring Parameters**
  - Pattern of daily bowel activity and stool consistency and record time of evacuation

- **Geriatric side effects at a glance:**
  ❑ CNS ❑ Bowel Dysfunction ❑ Bladder Dysfunction ❑ Falls

- **U.S. Regulatory Considerations**
  ❑ FDA Black Box ❑ OBRA regulated in U.S. Long Term Care

pamidronate disodium

(pa-mi-droe'-nate dye-soe'-dee-um)

- **Brand Name(s):** Aredia, Pamidronate Disodium Novaplus
  Chemical Class: Pyrophosphate analog

- **Clinical Pharmacology:**
  Mechanism of Action: A bisphosphate that binds to bone and inhibits osteoclast-mediated calcium resorption. **Therapeutic Effect:** Lowers serum calcium concentrations.

Pharmacokinetics:

Route	Onset	Peak	Duration
IV	24–48 hr	5–7 days	N/A

After IV administration, rapidly absorbed by bone. Slowly excreted unchanged in urine. Unknown if removed by hemodialysis. **Half-life:** bone, 300 days; unmetabolized, 2.5 hr.

■ **Available Forms:**
- *Powder for Injection (Aredia, Pamidronate Disodium Novaplus):* 30 mg, 90 mg.
- *Injection Solution:* 3 mg/ml, 6 mg/ml, 9 mg/ml.

■ **Indications and Dosages:**
Hypercalcemia: IV Infusion Moderate hypercalcemia (corrected serum calcium level 12–13.5 mg/dl): 60–90 mg. Severe hypercalcemia (corrected serum calcium level greater than 13.5 mg/dl): 90 mg.
Paget's disease: IV Infusion 30 mg/day for 3 days.
Osteolytic bone lesion: IV Infusion 90 mg over 2–4 hr once a month.

■ **Contraindications:** Hypersensitivity to other bisphosphonates, such as etidronate, tiludronate, risedronate, and alendronate

■ **Side Effects**
Frequent (greater than 10%)
Temperature elevation (at least 1°C) 24–48 hr after administration (27%); redness, swelling, induration, pain at catheter site in patients receiving 90 mg (18%); anorexia, nausea, fatigue
Occasional (10%–1%)
Constipation, rhinitis
Rare
Osteonecrosis of the jaw

■ **Serious Reactions**
- Hypophosphatemia, hypokalemia, hypomagnesemia, and hypocalcemia occur more frequently with higher dosages.
- Anemia, hypertension, tachycardia, atrial fibrillation, and somnolence occur more frequently with 90-mg doses.
- GI hemorrhage occurs rarely.

Special Considerations

- "Second-generation" bisphosphonate that offers potential advantages over etidronate (as does alendronate) in that it inhibits bone resorption at doses that do not impair bone mineralization, and is less likely than etidronate to produce osteomalacia
- Allow at least 7 days between initial treatment for patients requiring retreatment for hypercalcemia
- A dental examination with appropriate preventive dentistry should be considered prior to treatment with bisphosphonates in patients with concomitant risk factors (e.g., cancer, chemotherapy, corticosteroid use, poor oral hygiene). While on bisphosphonate treatment, patients with concomitant risk factors should avoid invasive dental procedures if possible. For patients who develop osteonecrosis of the jaw while on bisphosphonate therapy, dental surgery may exacerbate the condition. For patients requiring dental procedures, there are no data available to suggest whether discontinuation of bisphosphonate treatment reduces the risk of osteonecrosis of the jaw.

Patient/Family Education
- Avoid drugs containing calcium and vitamin D, such as antacids, because they might antagonize the effects of pamidronate
- Inform your dentist if you are taking this drug.
- If you develop jaw pain, loose teeth, or signs of oral infection, immediately inform your doctor.

Monitoring Parameters
- Hct, Hgb, and serum magnesium and creatinine levels
- Fluid intake and output carefully
- Examine lungs for crackles and dependent body parts for edema
- Blood pressure, pulse, temperature

Geriatric side effects at a glance:
❑ CNS ❑ Bowel Dysfunction ❑ Bladder Dysfunction ❑ Falls

U.S. Regulatory Considerations
❑ FDA Black Box ❑ OBRA regulated in U.S. Long Term Care

pancreatin/pancrelipase

(pan-kree-ah'-tin/pan-kre-li'-pase)

■ **Brand Name(s):** (pancreatin) Ku-Zyme, Pancreatin

■ **Brand Name(s):** (pancrelipase) Cotazym-S, Creon 5, Creon 10, Creon 20, Ilozyme, Kutrase, Ku-Zyme, Ku-Zyme HP, Lipram, Lipram-CR, Lipram-CR 5, Lipram-CR 20, Lipram-PN, Lipram-UL 12, Lipram-UL 18, Lipram-UL 20, Panase, Pancrease, Pancrease MT 4, Pancrease MT 10, Pancrease MT 16, Pancrease MT 20, Pancreatic EC, Pancreatil-UL 12, Pancrecarb MS-4, Pancrecarb MS-8, Pangestyme CN 10, Pangestyme CN 20, Pangestyme EC, Pangestyme MT 16, Pangestyme NL 18, Panokase, Plaretase, Protilase, Ultrase, Ultrase MT 12, Ultrase MT 18, Ultrase MT 20, Viokase, Viokase 8, Viokase 16, Zymase
Chemical Class: Pancreatic enzymes

■ **Clinical Pharmacology:**
Mechanism of Action: Digestive enzymes that replace endogenous pancreatic enzymes. **Therapeutic Effect:** Assist in digestion of protein, starch, and fats.
Pharmacokinetics: Not absorbed systemically. Released at the duodenojejunal junction.

■ **Available Forms:**
- *Capsules:* 15,000 units-12,000 units-15,000 units (Ku-Zyme), 30,000 units-24,000 units-30,000 units (Kutrase), 30,000 units-8,000 units-30,000 units (Panokase, Cotazym, Ku-Zyme HP).
- *Capsules (Extended-Release):* 33,200 units-10,000 units-37,500 units (Creon 10, Lipram-CR), 30,000 units-10,000 units-30,000 units (Pangestyme CN 10, Lipram, Pancrease MT 10), 39,000 units-12,000 units-39,000 units (Lipram-UL 12, Pancreatil-UL

934

12, Ultrase MT 12), 12,000 units-4,000 units-12,000 units (Pancrease MT 4), 48,000 units-16,000 units-48,000 units (Lipram-PN, Pancrease MT 16, Pangestyme MT 16), 16,600 units-5,000 units-18,750 units (Creon 5, Lipram-CR5), 59,000 units-18,000 units-59,000 units (Pangestyme NL 18, Lipram-UL 18, Ultrase MT 18), 20,000 units-5,000 units-20,000 units (Cotazym-S), 66,400 units-20,000 units-75,000 units (Creon 20, Lipram-CR 20), 20,000 units-4,500 units-25,000 units (Lipram, Pancrease, Pangestyme EC, Ultrase), 56,000 units-20,000 units-44,000 units (Lipram-PN, Pancrease MT 20), 65,000 units-20,000 units-65,000 units (Lipram-UL 20, Pangestyme NL 18, Pangestyme CN 20, Ultrase MT 20), 20,000 units-4,000 units-25,000 units (Panase, Pancreatic EC, Protilase), 25,000 units-4,000 units-25,000 units (Pancrecarb MS-4), 40,000 units-8,000 units-45,000 units (Pancrecarb MS-8).
- *Powder for Reconstitution, Oral (Viokase):* 70,000 units-16,800 units-70,000 units/0.7 g.
- *Tablets:* 30,000 units-11,000 units-30,000 units (Ilozyme), 60,000 units-16,000 units-60,000 units (Viokase 16), 30,000 units-8,000 units-30,000 units (Panokase, Plaretase, Viokase 8).

■ Indications and Dosages:
Pancreatic enzyme replacement or supplement when enzymes are absent or deficient, such as with chronic pancreatitis, cystic fibrosis, or ductal obstruction from cancer of the pancreas or common bile duct; to reduce malabsorption; treatment of steatorrhea associated with bowel resection or postgastrectomy syndrome: PO 1–3 capsules or tablets before or with meals or snacks. May increase to 8 tablets/dose.

■ Unlabeled Uses: Treatment of occluded feeding tubes

■ Contraindications: Acute pancreatitis, exacerbation of chronic pancreatitis, hypersensitivity to pork protein

■ Side Effects
Rare
Allergic reaction, mouth irritation, shortness of breath, wheezing

■ Serious Reactions
- Excessive dosage may produce nausea, cramping, and diarrhea.
- Hyperuricosuria and hyperuricemia have occurred with extremely high dosages.

Special Considerations
- Substitution at dispensing should be avoided
- Enteric-coated pancreatic enzymes are more effective than regular formulations; individual variations may require trials with several enzymatic preparations
- For patients who do not respond appropriately, adding antacid or H_2-antagonist may provide better results
- Preparations high in lipase concentration seem to be more effective for reducing steatorrhea

■ Patient/Family Education
- Advise patient to take before or with meals
- Protect enteric coating; advise patient not to crush or chew microspheres in caps or tabs
- Do not spill Viokase powder on the hands because it may irritate the skin
- Avoid inhaling powder because it may irritate mucous membranes and produce bronchospasm
- Do not change brands of the drug without first consulting the physician

■ **Monitoring Parameters**
  • Therapeutic response

■ **Geriatric side effects at a glance:**
  ❏ CNS ❏ Bowel Dysfunction ❏ Bladder Dysfunction ❏ Falls

■ **U.S. Regulatory Considerations**
  ❏ FDA Black Box ❏ OBRA regulated in U.S. Long Term Care

pantoprazole sodium

(pan-toe-pra'-zole soe'-dee-um)

■ **Brand Name(s):** Protonix, Protonix IV
  Chemical Class: Benzimidazole derivative

■ **Clinical Pharmacology:**
  Mechanism of Action: A benzimidazole that is converted to active metabolites that irreversibly bind to and inhibit hydrogen-potassium adenosine triphosphate, an enzyme on the surface of gastric parietal cells. Inhibits hydrogen ion transport into gastric lumen. **Therapeutic Effect:** Increases gastric pH and reduces gastric acid production.
  Pharmacokinetics:

Route	Onset	Peak	Duration
PO	N/A	N/A	24 hr

  Rapidly absorbed from the GI tract. Protein binding: 98%. Primarily distributed into gastric parietal cells. Metabolized extensively in the liver. Primarily excreted in urine. Not removed by hemodialysis. **Half-life:** 1 hr.

■ **Available Forms:**
  • *Tablets (Delayed-Release [Protonix]):* 20 mg, 40 mg.
  • *Powder for Injection (Protonix IV):* 40 mg.

■ **Indications and Dosages:**
  Erosive esophagitis: PO 40 mg/day for up to 8 wk. If not healed after 8 wk, may continue an additional 8 wk. IV 40 mg/day for 7–10 days.
  Hypersecretory conditions: PO Initially, 40 mg twice a day. May increase to 240 mg/day. IV 80 mg twice a day. May increase to 80 mg q8h.

■ **Unlabeled Uses:** Peptic ulcer disease, active ulcer bleeding (injection), adjunct in treatment of *Helicobacter pylori* infection.

■ **Contraindications:** None known.

■ **Side Effects**
  Rare (less than 2%)
  Diarrhea, headache, dizziness, pruritus, rash

- **Serious Reactions**
  - Hyperglycemia occurs rarely.

- **Patient/Family Education**
  - Caution patients not to split, crush, or chew delayed-release tablets; swallow whole
  - Notify the physician if headache occurs during pantoprazole therapy
  - Take tablets before eating

- **Monitoring Parameters**
  - Symptom relief, mucosal healing

- **Geriatric side effects at a glance:**
  - ❑ CNS   ❑ Bowel Dysfunction   ❑ Bladder Dysfunction   ❑ Falls

- **U.S. Regulatory Considerations**
  - ❑ FDA Black Box   ❑ OBRA regulated in U.S. Long Term Care

paregoric

(par-e-gor'-ik)

- **Brand Name(s):** Paregoric
  Chemical Class: Opiate (most preparations also contain camphor and ethanol)
  DEA Class: Schedule III

- **Clinical Pharmacology:**
  Mechanism of Action: An opioid agonist that contains many narcotic alkaloids including morphine. It inhibits gastric motility due to its morphine content. **Therapeutic Effect:** Decreases digestive secretions, increases gastrointestinal (GI) muscle tone, and reduces GI propulsion.
  Pharmacokinetics: Variably absorbed from the GI tract. Protein binding: low. Metabolized in liver. Primarily excreted in urine as morphine glucuronide conjugates and unchanged drug—morphine, codeine, papaverine, etc. Unknown if removed by hemodialysis. **Half-life:** 2-3 hr.

- **Available Forms:**
  - *Tincture:* 2 mg/5 ml (Paregoric).

- **Indications and Dosages:**
  Antidiarrheal: PO 5-10 ml 1-4 times/day.

- **Unlabeled Uses:** None known.

- **Contraindications:** Diarrhea caused by poisoning until the toxic material is removed, hypersensitivity to morphine sulfate or any component of the formulation

Side Effects
Frequent
Constipation, drowsiness, nausea, vomiting
Occasional
Paradoxical excitement, confusion, pounding heartbeat, facial flushing, decreased urination, blurred vision, dizziness, dry mouth, headache, hypotension, decreased appetite, redness, burning, pain at injection site
Rare
Hallucinations, depression, stomach pain, insomnia

■ Serious Reactions
- Overdosage results in cold or clammy skin, confusion, convulsions, decreased blood pressure (BP), restlessness, pinpoint pupils, bradycardia, respiratory depression, decreased level of consciousness (LOC), and severe weakness.
- Tolerance to analgesic effect and physical dependence may occur with repeated use.

Special Considerations
- Contains ethanol

■ Patient/Family Education
- Avoid performing tasks that require mental alertness or motor skills until response to the drug has been established
- Avoid alcohol
- Drug dependence or tolerance may occur with prolonged use of high dosages

■ Monitoring Parameters
- Pattern of bowel activity and stool consistency

■ Geriatric side effects at a glance:
☑ CNS   ☑ Bowel Dysfunction   ☑ Bladder Dysfunction   ☐ Falls

■ U.S. Regulatory Considerations
☐ FDA Black Box   ☐ OBRA regulated in U.S. Long Term Care

paricalcitol

(par-i-kal'-si-tole)

■ Brand Name(s): Zemplar
Chemical Class: NUTR-vitamin D analog

■ Clinical Pharmacology:
Mechanism of Action: A fat-soluble vitamin that is essential for absorption, utilization of calcium phosphate, and normal calcification of bone. **Therapeutic Effect:** Stimulates calcium and phosphate absorption from small intestine, promotes secretion of

calcium from bone to blood, promotes renal tubule phosphate resorption, acts on bone cells to stimulate skeletal growth and on parathyroid gland to suppress hormone synthesis and secretion.

Pharmacokinetics: Protein binding: more than 99%. Metabolized in liver. Primarily eliminated in feces; minimal excretion in urine. Not removed by hemodialysis. **Half-life:** 14-15 hr.

■ **Available Forms:**
  • *Injection*: 5 mcg/ml (Zemplar).

■ **Indications and Dosages:**
  Hypoparathyroidism: IV 0.04-0.1 mcg/kg (2.8-7 mcg) given as a bolus dose no more frequently than every other day at any time during dialysis; dose as high as 0.24 mcg/kg (16.8 mcg) has been administered safely. Usually start with 0.04 mcg/kg 3 times/week as a bolus, increased by 0.04 mcg/kg every 2 weeks. Adjust dose based on serum PTH levels. *Same or increasing serum* PTH *level*: Increase dose. *Serum* PTH *level decreased by* <30%: Increase dose. *Serum* PTH *level decreased by* >30% *and* <60%: Maintain dose. *Serum* PTH *level decreased by* >60%: Decrease dose. *Serum* PTH *level 1.5-3 times upper limit of normal*: Maintain dose.

■ **Contraindications:** Hypercalcemia, malabsorption syndrome, vitamin D toxicity, hypersensitivity to other vitamin D products or analogs

■ **Side Effects**
  Occasional
  Edema, nausea, vomiting, headache, dizziness
  Rare
  Palpitations

■ **Serious Reactions**
  • Early signs of overdosage are manifested as weakness, headache, somnolence, nausea, vomiting, dry mouth, constipation, muscle and bone pain, and metallic taste sensation.
  • Later signs of overdosage are evidenced by polyuria, polydipsia, anorexia, weight loss, nocturia, photophobia, rhinorrhea, pruritus, disorientation, hallucinations, hyperthermia, hypertension, and cardiac arrhythmias.
  • Hypercalcemia occurs rarely.

Special Considerations
  • Phosphate-binding compounds may be needed to control serum phosphorus levels

■ **Patient/Family Education**
  • Adhere to a dietary regimen of calcium supplementation and phosphorus restriction; avoid excessive use of aluminum-containing compounds
  • Consume foods rich in vitamin D including eggs, leafy vegetables, margarine, meats, milk, vegetable oils, and vegetable shortening
  • Drink plenty of fluids

■ **Monitoring Parameters**
  • Serum calcium and phosphorus twice weekly during initial phase of therapy, then at least monthly once dosage has been established; if an elevated calcium level or a Ca × P product > 75 is noted, immediately reduce or interrupt dosage until parameters are normalized, then reinitiate at lower dose; intact PTH assay every 3 mo (target range in CRF patients ≤ 1.5-3 × the nonuremic upper limit of normal)

- Serum alkaline phosphatase, BUN, serum creatinine

- **Geriatric side effects at a glance:**
  - ❏ CNS ❏ Bowel Dysfunction ❏ Bladder Dysfunction ❏ Falls

- **U.S. Regulatory Considerations**
  - ❏ FDA Black Box ❏ OBRA regulated in U.S. Long Term Care

paromomycin sulfate

(par-oh-moe-mye'-sin sul'-fate)

- **Brand Name(s):** Humatin
  Chemical Class: Aminoglycoside

- **Clinical Pharmacology:**
  Mechanism of Action: An antibacterial agent that acts directly on amebas and against normal and pathogenic organisms in the GI tract. Interferes with bacterial protein synthesis by binding to 30S ribosomal subunits. **Therapeutic Effect:** Produces amebicidal effects.
  Pharmacokinetics: Poorly absorbed from the GI tract and most of the dose is eliminated unchanged in feces.

- **Available Forms:**
  - *Capsules*: 250 mg.

- **Indications and Dosages:**
  Intestinal amebiasis: PO 25-35 mg/kg/day q8h for 5-10 days.
  Hepatic coma: PO 4 g/day q6-12h for 5-6 days.

- **Unlabeled Uses:** Cryptosporidiosis, giardiasis, leishmaniasis, microsporidiosis, mycobacterial infections, tapeworm infestation, trichomoniasis, typhoid carriers.

- **Contraindications:** Intestinal obstruction, renal failure, hypersensitivity to paromomycin or any of its components

- **Side Effects**
  Occasional
  Diarrhea, abdominal cramps, nausea, vomiting, heartburn
  Rare
  Rash, pruritus, vertigo

- **Serious Reactions**
  - Overdosage may result in nausea, vomiting, and diarrhea.

- **Patient/Family Education**
  - Report any audio disturbances
  - Do not skip doses

940

Monitoring Parameters
- Skin for rash
- Renal function

Geriatric side effects at a glance:
❑ CNS ❑ Bowel Dysfunction ❑ Bladder Dysfunction ❑ Falls

U.S. Regulatory Considerations
❑ FDA Black Box ❑ OBRA regulated in U.S. Long Term Care

paroxetine hydrochloride

(par-ox'-e-teen hye-droe-klor'-ide)

- **Brand Name(s):** Paxeva, Paxil, Paxil CR
  Chemical Class: Phenylpiperidine derivative

- **Clinical Pharmacology:**
  Mechanism of Action: An antidepressant, anxiolytic, and antiobsessional agent that selectively blocks uptake of the neurotransmitter serotonin at neuronal presynaptic membranes, thereby increasing its availability at postsynaptic receptor sites. **Therapeutic Effect:** Relieves depression, reduces obsessive-compulsive behavior, decreases anxiety.
  Pharmacokinetics: Well absorbed from the GI tract. Protein binding: 95%. Widely distributed. Metabolized in the liver. Excreted in urine. Not removed by hemodialysis. **Half-life:** 24 hr.

- **Available Forms:**
  - *Oral Suspension* (Paxil): 10 mg/5 ml.
  - *Tablets* (Paxil, Paxeva): 10 mg, 20 mg, 30 mg, 40 mg.
  - *Tablets* (Controlled-Release [Paxil CR]): 12.5 mg, 25 mg, 37.5 mg.

- **Indications and Dosages:**
  Depression and anxiety disorders: PO Initially, 10 mg/day. May increase by 10 mg/day at intervals of more than 1 wk. Maximum: 40 mg/day. (Controlled-Release): Initially, 12.5 mg/day. May increase by 12.5 mg/day at intervals of more than 1 wk. Maximum: 50 mg/day.

- **Unlabeled Uses:** Eating disorders, impulse disorders

- **Contraindications:** Use within 14 days of MAOIs

- **Side Effects**
  Frequent
  Nausea (26%); somnolence (23%); headache, dry mouth (18%); asthenia (15%); constipation (15%); dizziness, insomnia (13%); diarrhea (12%); diaphoresis (11%); tremor (8%)

941

Occasional

Decreased appetite, respiratory disturbance (such as increased cough) (6%); anxiety, nervousness (5%); flatulence, paresthesia, yawning (4%); decreased libido, sexual dysfunction, abdominal discomfort (3%)

Rare

Palpitations, vomiting, blurred vision, altered taste, confusion

■ **Serious Reactions**
- Abnormal bleeding, hyponatremia, seizures, hypomania, and suicidal thoughts have been reported.

Special Considerations
- Somewhat sedating compared to fluoxetine and sertraline

■ **Patient/Family Education**
- Avoid alcohol
- May take 1-4 wk to see improvement of symptoms
- Do not abruptly discontinue paroxetine
- Avoid tasks that require mental alertness or motor skills until response to the drug has been established
- Take sips of tepid water or chew sugarless gum to help relieve dry mouth

■ **Monitoring Parameters**
- CBC and hepatic and renal function tests periodically, as ordered, for patients on long-term therapy
- Closely supervise suicidal patients during early therapy; as depression lessens, energy level improves, increasing the suicide potential
- Assess appearance, behavior, level of interest, mood, and sleep pattern to determine the drug's therapeutic effect

■ **Geriatric side effects at a glance:**
  ☐ CNS ☑ Bowel Dysfunction ☐ Bladder Dysfunction ☑ Falls
  Other: Hyponatremia, weight gain (long term)

■ **Use with caution in older patients with:** None

■ **U.S. Regulatory Considerations**
  ☑ FDA Black Box
  - Because there is an increased risk of suicide in children and adolescents, older adults should also be closely monitored for suicide ideation.
  ☑ OBRA regulated in U.S. Long Term Care

■ **Other Uses in Geriatric Patient:** Anxiety symptoms and related disorders

■ **Side Effects:**
  Of *particular importance* in the *geriatric patient*: Hyponatremia, withdrawal symptoms when abruptly discontinued (e.g., during hospitalization) rather than tapered

■ **Geriatric Considerations - Summary:** These agents are now considered by many the first-line therapy for treatment of depression in older adults. They are also effective in the management of symptoms of anxiety. Although these agents appear to have a more favorable side-effect profile than tricyclic antidepressants for most older adults, it is important to note that some of these agents have the potential for significant drug interactions, have been associated with falls, and require careful attention to electrolyte status. In addition, many of the drugs in this class have been associated with severe withdrawal symptoms (e.g., nausea and/or vomiting, dizziness, headaches, lethargy or light-headedness, anxiety, and/or agitation) when discontinued abruptly.

■ **References:**
1. Cadieux RJ. Antidepressant drug interactions in the elderly. Understanding the P-450 system is half the battle in reducing risks. Postgrad Med 1999;106:231-240, 245.
2. Roose SP, Laghrissi-Thode F, Kennedy JS, et al. Comparison of paroxetine and nortriptyline in depressed patients with ischemic heart disease. JAMA 1998;279:287-291.
3. Thapa PB, Gideon P, Cost TW, et al. Antidepressants and the risk of falls among nursing home residents. N Engl J Med 1998;339:875-882.
4. Bouman WP, Pinner G, Johnson H. Incidence of selective serotonin reuptake inhibitor (SSRI) induced hyponatraemia due to the syndrome of inappropriate antidiuretic hormone (SIADH) secretion in the elderly. Int J Geriatr Psychiatry 1998;13:12-15.

pegaptanib sodium

(peg-apt'-i-nib soe'-dee-um)

■ **Brand Name(s):** Macugen

■ **Clinical Pharmacology:**
Mechanism of Action: A selective vascular endothelial growth factor (VEGF) antagonize that selectively binds and activates receptors located on the surface of vascular endothelial cells. **Therapeutic Effect:** Blocks angiogenesis and vascular permeability and inflammation which contribute to the progression of the neovascular (wet) form of age-related macular degeneration (AMD).
Pharmacokinetics: Human pharmacokinetics data are limited. Based on preclinical data, it is slowly absorbed into systemic circulation from the eye after intravitreous administration. Metabolized by endo- and exonucleases. Excreted in urine. **Half-life:** 10 days (plasma).

■ **Available Forms:**
• *Syringe for Injection:* 0.3 mg (Macugen).

■ **Indications and Dosages:**
Neovascular (wet) age-related macular degeneration: Injection, intravitreous 0.3 mg every 6 weeks.

■ **Contraindications:** Ocular or periocular infections, hypersensitivity to pegaptanib or any component of the formulation

■ **Side Effects**
Occasional
Corneal edema, eye discharge, eye irritation, eye pain, increased intraocular pressure, ocular discomfort, punctate keratitis, reduced visual acuity, visual disturbance, vitreous floater, vitreous opacities

Rare
Dizziness, dull nervousness, eye pain, fainting, tachycardia, bradycardia, itching, redness or other eye irritation, pale skin, pounding in ears, trouble breathing on exertion, weakness

■ **Serious Reactions**
- Endophthalmitis, retinal detachment, and iatrogenic traumatic cataract have been reported.

■ **Geriatric side effects at a glance:**
❏ CNS ❏ Bowel Dysfunction ❏ Bladder Dysfunction ❏ Falls

■ **U.S. Regulatory Considerations**
❏ FDA Black Box ❏ OBRA regulated in U.S. Long Term Care

pegfilgrastim

(peg-fil-gra'-stim)

■ **Brand Name(s):** Neulasta
Chemical Class: Amino acid glycoprotein

■ **Clinical Pharmacology:**
Mechanism of Action: A colony-stimulating factor that regulates production of neutrophils within bone marrow. Also a glycoprotein that primarily affects neutrophil progenitor proliferation, differentiation, and selected end-cell functional activation. **Therapeutic Effect:** Increases phagocytic ability and antibody-dependent destruction; decreases incidence of infection.
Pharmacokinetics: Readily absorbed after subcutaneous administration. **Half-life:** 15–80 hr.

■ **Available Forms:**
- *Solution for Injection:* 6 mg/0.6 ml syringe.

■ **Indications and Dosages:**
Myelosuppression: Subcutaneous Give as a single 6-mg injection once per chemotherapy cycle.

■ **Contraindications:** Hypersensitivity to *Escherichia coli*–derived proteins; do not administer within 14 days before and 24 hours after cytotoxic chemotherapy

■ **Side Effects**
Frequent (72%–15%)
Bone pain, nausea, fatigue, alopecia, diarrhea, vomiting, constipation, anorexia, abdominal pain, arthralgia, generalized weakness, peripheral edema, dizziness, stomatitis, mucositis, neutropenic fever

944

■ Serious Reactions
- Allergic reactions, such as anaphylaxis, rash, and urticaria, occur rarely.
- Cytopenia resulting from an antibody response to growth factors occurs rarely.
- Splenomegaly occurs rarely; assess for left upper abdominal or shoulder pain.
- Adult respiratory distress syndrome (ARDS) may occur in patients with sepsis.
- Severe sickle cell crisis has been reported.

Special Considerations
- Do not administer in the period between 14 days before and 24 hr after administration of cytotoxic chemotherapy
- Reduces duration of severe neutropenia from 6 days to 2 days, and incidence of febrile neutropenia from 30%-40% to 10%-20%

■ Patient/Family Education
- Compliance is important, including regular monitoring of blood counts
- Be aware of signs and symptoms of allergic reactions that may occur with pegfilgrastim

■ Monitoring Parameters
- CBC with platelets
- Monitor for allergic reactions
- Examine for peripheral edema, particularly behind the medial malleolus, which is usually the first area to show peripheral edema
- Assess mucous membranes for evidence of mucositis (such as red mucous membranes, white patches, and extreme mouth soreness), and stomatitis
- Evaluate muscle strength
- Pattern of daily bowel activity and stool consistency
- Evaluate patients with sepsis for signs and symptoms of ARDS, such as dyspnea

■ Geriatric side effects at a glance:
☑ CNS ☑ Bowel Dysfunction ☐ Bladder Dysfunction ☐ Falls

■ U.S. Regulatory Considerations
☐ FDA Black Box ☐ OBRA regulated in U.S. Long Term Care

peginterferon alfa-2a

(peg-in-ter-feer'-on alfa-2a)

■ Brand Name(s): Pegasys
Chemical Class: Recombinant interferon

■ Clinical Pharmacology:
Mechanism of Action: An immunomodulator that binds to specific membrane receptors on the cell surface, inhibiting viral replication in virus-infected cells, suppressing cell proliferation, and producing reversible decreases in leukocyte and platelet counts. **Therapeutic Effect:** Inhibits hepatitis C virus.

Pharmacokinetics: Readily absorbed after subcutaneous administration. Excreted by the kidneys. **Half-life:** 80 hr.

■ **Available Forms:**
- Injection Solution: 180 mcg/ml.
- Injection, Prefilled Syringe: 180 mcg/0.5 ml.

■ **Indications and Dosages:**
Hepatitis C: Subcutaneous 180 mcg (1 ml) injected in abdomen or thigh once weekly for 48 wk.
Dosage in renal impairment: For patients who require hemodialysis, dosage is 135 mg injected in abdomen or thigh once weekly for 48 wk.
Dosage in hepatic impairment: For patients with progressive ALT increases above baseline values, dosage is 90 mcg injected in abdomen or thigh once weekly for 48 wk.

■ **Contraindications:** Autoimmune hepatitis, decompensated hepatic disease

■ **Side Effects**
Frequent (54%)
Headache
Occasional (23%–13%)
Alopecia, nausea, insomnia, anorexia, dizziness, diarrhea, abdominal pain, flu-like symptoms, psychiatric reactions (depression, irritability, anxiety), injection site reaction
Rare (8%–5%)
Impaired concentration, diaphoresis, dry mouth, nausea, vomiting

■ **Serious Reactions**
- Serious, acute hypersensitivity reactions, such as urticaria, angioedema, bronchoconstriction, and anaphylaxis, may occur. Other rare reactions include pancreatitis, colitis, endocrine disorders (e.g., diabetes mellitus), hyperthyroidism or hypothyroidism, ophthalmologic, neuropsychiatric, autoimmune, ischemic, infectious, and pulmonary disorders.

Special Considerations
- Weekly administration of peginterferon alfa-2a equivalent to 3 times weekly administration of interferon alfa-2a for hepatitis C
- Sustained viral response rates substantially better when combined with ribavirin (genotype 1: 40%-50%; genotype 2 or 3: 70%-80% for combination therapy; overall response rate 40% for monotherapy)

■ **Patient/Family Education**
- The drug's therapeutic effect should appear in 1 to 3 mo
- Flu-like symptoms tend to diminish with continued therapy
- Immediately notify the physician if depression or suicidal thoughts occur
- Avoid performing tasks requiring mental alertness or motor skills until response to the drug has been established

■ **Monitoring Parameters**
- Availability of expert consultation for management of toxicity is essential

- *Baseline tests*: CBC, hepatic function, pregnancy test, TSH, renal function, uric acid, HCV RNA level. Exclusions to treatment: platelet count <90,000 cells/mm³ (as low as 75,000 cells/mm³ in patients with cirrhosis); absolute neutrophil count <1,500 cells/mm³; serum creatinine concentration >1.5 × upper limit of normal; abnormal thyroid function
- CBC q2weeks
- ALT, bilirubin q4weeks; if ALT rises persistently above baseline values, reduce dose to 135 μg per week; if ALT increases are progressive despite dose reduction or accompanied by increased bilirubin or evidence of hepatic decompensation, therapy should be immediately discontinued
- TSH q12weeks
- Depression, evaluated q2weeks for weeks 1-8 of treatment; may require dose reduction
- All patients should receive an eye examination at baseline; patients with preexisting ophthalmologic disorders (e.g., diabetic or hypertensive retinopathy) should receive periodic ophthalmologic exams during interferon alpha treatment
- HCV RNA (early virologic response defined as HCV RNA undetectable or >2 $\log_{10}$ lower than baseline at 12 weeks and 24 weeks); for patients who lack an early viral response at 12 weeks, chance of sustained viral response is 13%; for patients who lack an early viral response at 24 weeks, chance of sustained viral response is near zero; in consultation with experts, consider stopping peginterferon therapy if virologic response absent at 12-24 weeks

■ **Geriatric side effects at a glance:**
   ☑ CNS   ☑ Bowel Dysfunction   ☐ Bladder Dysfunction   ☐ Falls

■ **U.S. Regulatory Considerations**
   ☑ FDA Black Box
Interferons may cause or aggravate neuropsychiatric (depression), autoimmune, ischemic, and infectious disorders.
   ☐ OBRA regulated in U.S. Long Term Care

penbutolol sulfate

(pen-byoo'-toe-lole sul'-fate)

■ **Brand Name(s):** Levatol
   Chemical Class: β-Adrenergic blocker, nonselective

■ **Clinical Pharmacology:**
   Mechanism of Action: An antihypertensive that possesses nonselective beta-blocking. Has moderate intrinsic sympathomimetic activity. **Therapeutic Effect:** Reduces cardiac output, decreases blood pressure (BP), increases airway resistance, and decreases myocardial ischemia severity.
   Pharmacokinetics: Rapidly and extensively absorbed from the gastrointestinal (GI) tract. Protein binding: 80%-90%. Metabolized in liver. Excreted primarily via urine. **Half-life:** 17-26 hr.

■ **Available Forms:**
  - *Tablets*: 20 mg.

■ **Indications and Dosages:**
  Hypertension: PO Initially, 10 mg/day.

■ **Contraindications:** Bronchial asthma or related bronchospastic conditions, cardiogenic shock, pulmonary edema, second- or third-degree atrioventricular (AV) block, severe bradycardia, overt cardiac failure, hypersensitivity to penbutolol or any component of the formulation

■ **Side Effects**
  Frequent
  Decreased sexual ability, drowsiness, trouble sleeping, unusual tiredness/weakness
  Occasional
  Diarrhea, bradycardia, depression, cold hands/feet, constipation, anxiety, nasal congestion, nausea, vomiting
  Rare
  Altered taste, dry eyes, itching, numbness of fingers, toes, scalp

■ **Serious Reactions**
  - Abrupt withdrawal may result in sweating, palpitations, headache, and tremulousness.
  - Hypoglycemia may occur in patients with previously controlled diabetes.

Special Considerations
  - Exacerbation of ischemic heart disease following abrupt withdrawal due to rebound sensitivity to catecholamines possible
  - Comparative trials indicate that penbutolol is as effective as propranolol and atenolol in the treatment of hypertension; may have fewer adverse CNS effects than propranolol

■ **Patient/Family Education**
  - The full antihypertensive effect of penbutolol will be noted in 1 to 2 weeks
  - Do not abruptly discontinue penbutolol; compliance with the therapy regimen is essential to control hypertension
  - Avoid tasks that require mental alertness or motor skills until response to the drug is established
  - Notify the physician if excessive fatigue or prolonged dizziness occurs
  - Do not take nasal decongestants and OTC cold preparations, especially those containing stimulants, without physician approval
  - Limit alcohol and salt intake

■ **Monitoring Parameters**
  - Blood pressure, pulse
  - ECG for arrhythmias
  - Daily bowel activity and stool consistency
  - Skin for rash

■ **Geriatric side effects at a glance:**
  ❏ CNS   ❏ Bowel Dysfunction   ❏ Bladder Dysfunction   ❏ Falls

U.S. Regulatory Considerations

☑ FDA Black Box

In patients using <u>orally administered</u> beta-blockers, abrupt withdrawal may precipitate angina or lead to myocardial infarction or ventricular arrhythmias.

❑ OBRA regulated in U.S. Long Term Care

penciclovir

(pen-sye'-kloe-veer)

Brand Name(s): Denavir

Chemical Class: Acyclic purine nucleoside analog

Clinical Pharmacology:

Mechanism of Action: Penciclovir triphosphate inhibits HSV polymerase competitively with deoxyguanosine triphosphate. Consequently, herpes viral DNA synthesis and, therefore, replication are selectively inhibited. **Therapeutic Effect:** An antiviral compound that has inhibitory activity against herpes simplex virus types 1 (HSV-1) and 2 (HSV-2).

Pharmacokinetics: Measurable penciclovir concentrations were not detected in plasma or urine. The systemic absorption of penciclovir following topical administration has not been evaluated.

Available Forms:

• Cream: 10 mg/g

Indications and Dosages:

Herpes labialis (cold sores): Topical   Penciclovir should be applied every 2 hours during waking hours for a period of 4 days. Treatment should be started as early as possible (i.e., during the prodrome or when lesions appear).

Unlabeled Uses: Varicella-zoster virus

Contraindications: Hypersensitivity to penciclovir or any of its components.

Side Effects

Frequent

Headache

Occasional

Change in sense of taste; decreased sensitivity of skin, particularly to touch; redness of the skin; skin rash (maculopapular, erythematous), local edema, skin discoloration; pruritus; hypoesthesia; paresthesias; parosmia; urticaria; oral/pharyngeal edema

Rare

Mild pain, burning, or stinging

Special Considerations

• In clinical trials, shortened the duration of lesions by approximately ½ day compared to placebo (4½ vs. 5 days); duration of pain was also shortened by approximately ½ day

- **Patient/Family Education**
  - Avoid exposure of cold sores to direct sunlight

- **Monitoring Parameters**
  - Therapeutic response

- **Geriatric side effects at a glance:**
  - ❑ CNS ❑ Bowel Dysfunction ❑ Bladder Dysfunction ❑ Falls

- **U.S. Regulatory Considerations**
  - ❑ FDA Black Box ❑ OBRA regulated in U.S. Long Term Care

penicillamine

(pen-i-sill'-a-meen)

- **Brand Name(s):** Cuprimine, Depen
  Chemical Class: Thiol derivative

- **Clinical Pharmacology:**
  Mechanism of Action: A heavy metal antagonist that chelates copper, iron, mercury, lead to form complexes, promoting excretion of copper. Combines with cystine-forming complex, thus reducing concentration of cystine to below levels for formation of cystine stones. Exact mechanism for rheumatoid arthritis is unknown. May decrease cell-mediated immune response. May inhibit collagen formation. **Therapeutic Effect:** Promotes excretion of copper, prevents renal calculi, dissolves existing stones, acts as anti-inflammatory drug.
  Pharmacokinetics: Moderately absorbed from the gastrointestinal (GI) tract. Protein binding: 80% to albumin. Metabolized in small amounts in liver. Excreted unchanged in urine. **Half-life:** 1.7-3.2 hr.

- **Available Forms:**
  - *Capsules*: 125 mg, 250 mg (Cuprimine).
  - *Tablets*: 250 mg (Depen).

- **Indications and Dosages:**
  Wilson's disease: PO Initially, 250 mg 4 times/day (some pts may begin at 250 mg/day; gradually increase). Dosages of 750-1,500 mg/day that produce initial 24-hr cupruresis >2 mg should be continued for 3 mo. Maintenance: Based on serum-free copper concentration (<10 mcg/dl indicative of adequate maintenance). Maximum: 2 g/day.
  Cystinuria: PO Initially, 250 mg/day. Gradually increase dose. Maintenance: 2 g/day. Range: 1-4 g/day.
  Rheumatoid arthritis: PO Initially, 125-250 mg/day. May increase by 125-250 mg/day at 1-3 mo intervals. Maintenance: 500-750 mg/day. After 2-3 mo with no improvement or toxicity, may increase by 250 mg/day at 2-3 mo intervals until remission or toxicity. Maximum: 1g up to 1.5 g/day.

- **Unlabeled Uses:** Treatment of rheumatoid vasculitis, heavy metal toxicity.

- **Contraindications:** History of penicillamine-related aplastic anemia or agranulocytosis, rheumatoid arthritis patients with history or evidence of renal insufficiency

- **Side Effects**

  Frequent

  Rash (pruritic, erythematous, maculopapular, morbilliform), reduced/altered sense of taste (hypogeusia), GI disturbances (anorexia, epigastric pain, nausea, vomiting, diarrhea), oral ulcers, glossitis

  Occasional

  Proteinuria, hematuria, hot flashes, drug fever

  Rare

  Alopecia, tinnitus, pemphigoid rash (water blisters)

- **Serious Reactions**

  - Aplastic anemia, agranulocytosis, thrombocytopenia, leukopenia, myasthenia gravis, bronchiolitis, erythematouslike syndrome, evening hypoglycemia, skin friability at sites of pressure/trauma producing extravasation or white papules at venipuncture, surgical sites reported.
  - Iron deficiency may develop.

Special Considerations

  - Because penicillamine can cause severe adverse reactions, restrict its use in rheumatoid arthritis to patients who have severe, active disease and who have failed to respond to an adequate trial of conventional therapy

- **Patient/Family Education**

  - Should be administered on empty stomach, ½-1 hr before meals or at least 2 hr after meals
  - Urine may become discolored (red)
  - Patients with cystinuria should drink large amounts of water
  - Therapeutic effect may take 1-3 mo

- **Monitoring Parameters**

  - Hepatic, renal studies: CBC, urinalysis, skin for rash
  - Urinary copper excretion
  - WBC

- **Geriatric side effects at a glance:**

  ❑ CNS ❑ Bowel Dysfunction ❑ Bladder Dysfunction ❑ Falls

- **U.S. Regulatory Considerations**

  ☑ FDA Black Box
  - Should be administered by an experienced physician

  ❑ OBRA regulated in U.S. Long Term Care

penicillin

(pen-i-sill'-in)

■ **Brand Name(s):** *Penicillin* G (*Aqueous Pen* G:) Pfizerpen

■ **Brand Name(s):** *Penicillin* G: Pentids

■ **Brand Name(s):** *Penicillin* V: (Phenoxy-methyl Penicillin), Beepen VK, Pen-V, Pen-Vee K, Truxcillin VK, Veetids

■ **Brand Name(s):** *Penicillin* G *Benzathine*: Bicillin L-A, Permapen

■ **Brand Name(s):** *Penicillin* G *Procaine*: Crysticillin, Wycillin

■ **Brand Name(s):** *Penicillin* G *Benzathine and Procaine combined*: Bicillin C-R

Combinations
Rx: amoxicillin, ampicillin, bacampicillin, carbenicillin, cloxacillin, dicloxacillin, flucloxacillin, methicillin, mezlocillin, nafcillin, oxacillin, penicillin G benzathine, penicillin G potassium, penicillin V potassium, piperacillin, pivampicillin, pivmecillinam, ticarcillin; Penicillin and beta-lactamase inhibitors: amoxicillin/clavulanate potassium, ampicillin/sulbactam sodium, piperacillin sodium/tazobactam sodium, ticarcillin disodium/clavulanate potassium
Chemical Class: Penicillin, natural

■ **Clinical Pharmacology:**
Mechanism of Action: Penicillins bind to bacterial cell wall, inhibiting bacterial cell wall synthesis. ***Therapeutic Effect:*** Inhibits bacterial cell wall synthesis. Beta-lactamase inhibitors: inhibit the action of bacterial beta-lactamase. ***Therapeutic Effect:*** Protects the penicillin from enzymatic degradation.
Pharmacokinetics: Penicillins are generally well absorbed from the gastrointestinal (GI) tract after oral administration. Widely distributed to most tissues and body fluids. Protein binding: 20%. Partially metabolized in liver. Primarily excreted in urine. **Half-life:** varies (half-life increased in reduced renal function).

■ **Available Forms:**
• Penicillins are available in tablets, chewable tablets, capsules, powder for oral suspension, powder for injection, prefilled syringes for injection, premixed dextrose solutions for injection, and solutions for infusion.

■ **Indications and Dosages:** Penicillins may be used to treat a large number of infections, including pneumonia and other respiratory diseases, urinary tract infections, septicemia, meningitis, intra-abdominal infections, gonorrhea, syphilis, and bone and joint infections.
Dosages: Doses vary depending on the drug used. In general, penicillins should be taken on an empty stomach. Patients with impaired renal function may require dose adjustment.

■ **Unlabeled Uses:** Some penicillins, such as amoxicillin, have been used in the treatment of Lyme disease and typhoid fever.

- **Contraindications:** Hypersensitivity to any penicillin, infectious mononucleosis

- **Side Effects**
  Frequent
  GI disturbances (mild diarrhea, nausea, or vomiting), headache, oral or vaginal candidiasis
  Occasional
  Generalized rash, urticaria

- **Serious Reactions**
  - Altered bacterial balance may result in potentially fatal superinfections and antibacterial-associated colitis as evidenced by abdominal cramps, watery or severe diarrhea, and fever.
  - Severe hypersensitivity reactions, including anaphylaxis and acute interstitial nephritis occur rarely.

Special Considerations
  - Cross-reactivity with cephalosporins is approximately 10%
  - Individualize treatment based on local susceptibility patterns.

- **Patient/Family Education**
  - Space doses evenly around the clock and continue taking the drug for the full course of treatment
  - Immediately notify the physician if bleeding, bruising, diarrhea, a rash, or any other new symptoms occur

- **Monitoring Parameters**
  - Intake and output, renal function, urinalysis for signs of nephrotoxicity
  - Severe diarrhea with abdominal pain, fever, and mucus or blood in stools may indicate antibiotic-associated colitis
  - Be alert for signs and symptoms of superinfection, including anal or genital pruritus, vaginal discharge, diarrhea, increased fever, nausea and vomiting, sore throat, and stomatitis
  - Check for signs of bleeding, including ecchymosis, overt bleeding, and swelling of tissue

- **Geriatric side effects at a glance:**
  ❑ CNS ☑ Bowel Dysfunction ❑ Bladder Dysfunction ❑ Falls

- **U.S. Regulatory Considerations**
  ❑ FDA Black Box ❑ OBRA regulated in U.S. Long Term Care

pentamidine isethionate

(pen-tam'-i-deen i-sah-thi'-oh-nate)

■ **Brand Name(s):** NebuPent, Pentam 300
   Chemical Class: Aromatic diamidine derivative

■ **Clinical Pharmacology:**
   Mechanism of Action: An anti-infective that interferes with nuclear metabolism and incorporation of nucleotides, inhibiting DNA, RNA, phospholipid, and protein synthesis. **Therapeutic Effect:** Produces antibacterial and ID-antiprotozoal effects.
   Pharmacokinetics: Well absorbed after IM administration; minimally absorbed after inhalation. Widely distributed. Primarily excreted in urine. Minimally removed by hemodialysis. **Half-life:** 6.5 hr (increased in impaired renal function).

■ **Available Forms:**
   • *Injection* (Pentam-300): 300 mg.
   • *Powder for Nebulization* (Nebupent): 300 mg.

■ **Indications and Dosages:**
   Pneumocystis carinii pneumonia (PCP): IV, IM   4 mg/kg/day once a day for 14-21 days.
   Prevention of PCP: Inhalation   300 mg once q4wk.

■ **Unlabeled Uses:** Treatment of African trypanosomiasis, cutaneous or visceral leishmaniasis

■ **Contraindications:** Concurrent use with didanosine

■ **Side Effects**
   Frequent
   Injection (greater than 10%): Abscess, pain at injection site
   Inhalation (greater than 5%): Fatigue, metallic taste, shortness of breath, decreased appetite, dizziness, rash, cough, nausea, vomiting, chills
   Occasional
   Injection (10%-1%): Nausea, decreased appetite, hypotension, fever, rash, altered taste, confusion
   Inhalation (5%-1%): Diarrhea, headache, anemia, muscle pain
   Rare
   Injection (less than 1%): Neuralgia, thrombocytopenia, phlebitis, dizziness

■ **Serious Reactions**
   • Rare reactions include life-threatening or fatal hypotension, arrhythmias, hypoglycemia, leukopenia, nephrotoxicity or renal failure, anaphylactic shock, Stevens-Johnson syndrome, and toxic epidural necrolysis.
   • Hyperglycemia and insulin-dependent diabetes mellitus (often permanent) may occur even months after therapy has stopped.

Special Considerations
   • Considered second line for *P. carinii* pneumonia, following cotrimoxazole (unresponsive to or intolerant of cotrimoxazole)

Patient/Family Education

- Remain flat in bed during pentamidine administration and get up slowly and with assistance only when blood pressure becomes stable
- Notify the health care provider immediately if light-headedness, palpitations, shakiness, or sweating occurs
- Drowsiness, decreased appetite, and increased thirst and urination may develop in the months following therapy
- Drink plenty of water to maintain adequate hydration
- Avoid consuming alcohol during therapy

Monitoring Parameters

- BUN, serum creatinine, blood glucose daily
- CBC and platelets; liver function tests, including bilirubin, alkaline phosphatase, AST, and ALT; and serum calcium before, during, and after therapy
- ECG at regular intervals
- Skin for rash

Geriatric side effects at a glance:

❑ CNS   ❑ Bowel Dysfunction   ❑ Bladder Dysfunction   ❑ Falls

U.S. Regulatory Considerations

❑ FDA Black Box   ❑ OBRA regulated in U.S. Long Term Care

pentazocine lactate

(pen-taz'-oh-seen)

Brand Name(s): Talwin

Combinations
Rx: with ASA (Talwin Compound); with APAP (Talacen); with naloxone (Talwin NX)
Chemical Class: Benzomorphan; opiate derivative

DEA Class: Schedule IV

Clinical Pharmacology:

Mechanism of Action: An opioid antagonist that binds with opioid receptors within CNS. **Therapeutic Effect:** Alters processes affecting pain perception, emotional response to pain.
Pharmacokinetics: Well absorbed after administration. Widely distributed including CSF. Metabolized in liver via oxidative and glucuronide conjugation pathways, extensive first-pass effect. Excreted in small amounts as unchanged drug. **Half-life:** 2-3 hr, (prolonged with hepatic impairment).

Available Forms:

- *Tablets:* 12.5 mg and 325 mg aspirin (Talwin Compound), 25 mg and 650 mg acetaminophen (Talacen), 50 mg pentazocine and 0.5 mg naloxone (Talwin NX), 50 mg (Talwin).

- *Injection*: 30 mg (Talwin).

■ **Indications and Dosages:**
    Analgesia: PO 50 mg q4h. IM 25 mg q4h.

■ **Contraindications:** Hypersensitivity to pentazocine or any component of the formulation

■ **Side Effects**
    Frequent
    Drowsiness, euphoria, nausea, vomiting
    Occasional
    Allergic reaction, histamine reaction (decreased BP, increased sweating, flushing, wheezing), decreased urination, altered vision, constipation, dizziness, dry mouth, headache, hypotension, pain/burning at injection site

■ **Serious Reactions**
- Overdosage results in severe respiratory depression, skeletal muscle flaccidity, cyanosis, extreme somnolence progressing to convulsions, stupor, and coma.
- Abrupt withdrawal after prolonged use may produce symptoms of narcotic withdrawal (abdominal cramps, rhinorrhea, lacrimation, nausea, vomiting, restlessness, anxiety, increased temperature, piloerection).

Special Considerations
- Naloxone 0.5 mg added to oral tablets to discourage misuse via parenteral inj
- Less effective compared to morphine, but less respiratory depression and opposite cardiovascular pharmacodynamics; increases pulmonary, arterial, and central venous pressure

■ **Patient/Family Education**
- Report any symptoms of CNS changes, allergic reactions
- Physical dependency may result when used for extended periods
- Change position slowly, orthostatic hypotension may occur
- Avoid hazardous activities if drowsiness or dizziness occurs
- Avoid alcohol, other CNS depressants unless directed by clinician

■ **Monitoring Parameters**
- Degree of pain relief

■ **Geriatric side effects at a glance:**
    ☑ CNS ☑ Bowel Dysfunction ☑ Bladder Dysfunction ☑ Falls

■ **U.S. Regulatory Considerations**
    ☑ FDA Black Box
    Oral use only, potentially fatal if injected
    ☐ OBRA regulated in U.S. Long Term Care

pentobarbital sodium

(pen-toe-bar'-bi-tal soe'-dee-um)

- **Brand Name(s):** Nembutal
  Chemical Class: Barbituric acid derivative

  DEA Class: Schedule II; Schedule III

- **Clinical Pharmacology:**
  Mechanism of Action: A barbiturate that binds at the GABA receptor complex, enhancing GABA activity. **Therapeutic Effect:** Depresses central nervous system (CNS) activity and reticular activating system.
  Pharmacokinetics: Well absorbed after PO, parenteral administration. Protein binding: 35%-55%. Rapidly, widely distributed. Metabolized in liver. Primarily excreted in urine. Removed by hemodialysis. **Half-life:** 15-48 hr.

- **Available Forms:**
  - *Capsules:* 50 mg, 100 mg.
  - *Injection:* 50 mg/ml.
  - *Suppositories:* 30 mg, 120 mg, 200 mg.

- **Indications and Dosages:**
  Preanesthetic: PO 100 mg. IM 150-200 mg.
  Hypnotic: PO 100 mg at bedtime. IM 150-200 mg at bedtime. IV 100 mg initially then, after 1 minute, may give additional small doses at 1-minute intervals, up to 500 mg total. Rectal 120-200 mg at bedtime.
  Anticonvulsant: IV 2-15 mg/kg loading dose given slowly over 1-2 hours. Maintenance infusion: 0.5-5 mg/kg/hr.

- **Unlabeled Uses:** Intracranial hypertension, psychiatric interviews, sedative withdrawal, drug abuse withdrawal

- **Contraindications:** Porphyria, hypersensitivity to barbiturates

- **Side Effects**
  Occasional
  Agitation, confusion, dizziness, somnolence
  Rare
  Confusion, paradoxical CNS excitement or restlessness

- **Serious Reactions**
  - Agranulocytosis, megaloblastic anemia, apnea, hypoventilation, bradycardia, hypotension, syncope, hepatic damage, and Stevens-Johnson syndrome occur rarely.
  - Abrupt withdrawal after prolonged therapy may produce effects ranging from markedly increased dreaming, nightmares or insomnia, tremor, sweating and vomiting, to hallucinations, delirium, seizures, and status epilepticus.
  - Skin eruptions appear as hypersensitivity reactions.

- Overdosage produces cold or clammy skin, hypothermia, severe CNS depression, cyanosis, and rapid pulse.

■ **Patient/Family Education**
- Avoid driving or other activities requiring alertness
- Avoid alcohol ingestion or CNS depressants
- Do not discontinue medication abruptly after long-term use
- Limit caffeine intake
- May be habit-forming
- Avoid tasks that require mental alertness or motor skills until response to the drug is established
- Notify the physician of feelings of depression or thoughts of suicide

■ **Monitoring Parameters**
- Excessive usage; hypnotic hangover
- Blood pressure, heart rate, respiratory rate
- Liver and renal function
- CNS status

■ **Geriatric side effects at a glance:**
☑ CNS ☐ Bowel Dysfunction ☐ Bladder Dysfunction ☑ Falls
Other: Withdrawal symptoms after long-term use

■ **Use with caution in older patients with:** Not recommended for use in older adults.

■ **U.S. Regulatory Considerations**
☐ FDA Black Box ☑ OBRA regulated in U.S. Long Term Care

■ **Other Uses in Geriatric Patient:** Anxiety disorders, sleep disorders, seizure disorders

■ **Side Effects:**
Of particular importance in the geriatric patient: Sedation, withdrawal symptoms when abruptly discontinued (e.g., during hospitalization) rather than tapered

■ **Geriatric Considerations - Summary:** Because barbiturates have a low therapeutic window, a wide range of drug interactions and rapid development of tolerance, great potential for abuse and dependence, these agents are not recommended for use in older adults.

■ **Reference:**
1. Hypnotic drugs. Med Lett Drugs Ther 2000;42:71-72.

pentosan polysulfate sodium

(pen-toe-san pol-ee-sul'-fate soe'-dee-um)

- **Brand Name(s):** Elmiron
  Chemical Class: Glycosaminoglycan, sulfated; heparin derivative

- **Clinical Pharmacology:**
  Mechanism of Action: A negatively charged synthetic sulfated polysaccharide with heparin-like properties that appears to adhere to bladder wall mucosal membrane, may act as a buffering agent to control cell permeability preventing irritating solutes in the urine. Has anticoagulant/GU-interstitial cystitis effects. **Therapeutic Effect:** Relieves bladder pain.
  Pharmacokinetics: Poorly and erratically absorbed from the gastrointestinal tract. Distributed in uroepithelium of GU tract with lesser amount found in the liver, spleen, lung, skin, periosteum, and bone marrow. Metabolized in liver and kidney (secondary). Eliminated in the urine. **Half-life:** 4.8 hr.

- **Available Forms:**
  - *Capsules:* 100 mg.

- **Indications and Dosages:**
  Interstitial cystitis: PO 100 mg 3 times/day.

- **Unlabeled Uses:** Urolithiasis

- **Contraindications:** Hypersensitivity to pentosan polysulfate sodium or structurally related compounds

- **Side Effects**
  Frequent
  Alopecia areata (a single area on the scalp), diarrhea, nausea, headache, rash, abdominal pain, dyspepsia.
  Occasional
  Dizziness, depression, increased liver function tests.

- **Serious Reactions**
  - Ecchymosis, epistaxis, gum hemorrhage have been reported (drug produces weak anticoagulant effect).
  - Overdose may produce liver function abnormalities.

- **Patient/Family Education**
  - Take with water
  - Notify the physician if any unusual bleeding occurs

- **Monitoring Parameters**
  - CBC, aPTT, PT, liver and renal function

- **Geriatric side effects at a glance:**
  - ☐ CNS ☑ Bowel Dysfunction ☐ Bladder Dysfunction ☐ Falls

- **U.S. Regulatory Considerations**
  - ☐ FDA Black Box ☐ OBRA regulated in U.S. Long Term Care

pentoxifylline

(pen-tox-i'-fi-leen)

- **Brand Name(s):** Pentopak, Pentoxil, Trental
  Chemical Class: Dimethylxanthine derivative

- **Clinical Pharmacology:**
  Mechanism of Action: A blood viscosity-reducing agent that alters the flexibility of RBCs; inhibits production of tumor necrosis factor, neutrophil activation, and platelet aggregation. **Therapeutic Effect:** Reduces blood viscosity and improves blood flow. **Pharmacokinetics:** Well absorbed after oral administration. Undergoes first-pass metabolism in the liver. Primarily excreted in urine. Unknown if removed by hemodialysis. **Half-life:** 24–48 min; metabolite, 60–90 min.

- **Available Forms:**
  - *Tablets (Controlled-Release [Pentopak, Pentoxil, Trental]):* 400 mg.

- **Indications and Dosages:**
  Intermittent claudication: PO 400 mg 3 times a day. Decrease to 400 mg twice a day if GI or CNS adverse effects occur. Continue for at least 8 wk.

- **Unlabeled Uses:** Diabetic neuropathy, gangrene, hemodialysis shunt thrombosis, septic shock, sickle cell syndrome, vascular impotence

- **Contraindications:** History of intolerance to xanthine derivatives, such as caffeine, theophylline, or theobromine; recent cerebral or retinal hemorrhage

- **Side Effects**
  Occasional (5%–2%)
  Dizziness; nausea; altered taste; dyspepsia, marked by heartburn, epigastric pain, and indigestion
  Rare (less than 2%)
  Rash, pruritus, anorexia, constipation, dry mouth, blurred vision, edema, nasal congestion, anxiety

- **Serious Reactions**
  - Angina and chest pain occur rarely and may be accompanied by palpitations, tachycardia, and arrhythmias.
  - Signs and symptoms of overdose, such as flushing, hypotension, nervousness, agitation, hand tremor, fever, and somnolence, appear 4–5 hr after ingestion and last for 12 hr.

- Statistically, but not always, clinically significant effects in intermittent claudication; however, other drugs less impressive; will not replace surgical options

■ **Patient/Family Education**
- Therapeutic effect may require 2-4 wk
- Stop smoking
- Avoid tasks requiring mental alertness or motor skills until response has been established
- Limit caffeine intake

■ **Monitoring Parameters**
- Assess for hand tremor
- Monitor the patient for relief of signs and symptoms of intermittent claudication. Symptoms generally occur while walking or exercising or with weight bearing in the absence of walking or exercising

■ **Geriatric side effects at a glance:**
 ❏ CNS ❏ Bowel Dysfunction ❏ Bladder Dysfunction ❏ Falls

■ **U.S. Regulatory Considerations**
 ❏ FDA Black Box ❏ OBRA regulated in U.S. Long Term Care

pergolide mesylate

(per'-go-lide mes'-sil-ate)

■ **Brand Name(s):** Permax
 Chemical Class: Ergoline derivative

■ **Clinical Pharmacology:**
 Mechanism of Action: A centrally active dopamine agonist that directly stimulates dopamine receptors. **Therapeutic Effect:** Decreases signs and symptoms of Parkinson's disease.
 Pharmacokinetics: Well absorbed from the GI tract. Protein binding: 90%. Undergoes extensive first-pass metabolism in the liver. Primarily excreted in urine. Unknown if removed by hemodialysis.

■ **Available Forms:**
- Tablets: 0.05 mg, 0.25 mg, 1 mg.

■ **Indications and Dosages:**
 Parkinsonism: PO Initially, 0.05 mg/day for 2 days. May increase by 0.1-0.15 mg/day every 3 days over the next 12 days; afterward may increase by 0.25 mg/day every 3 days. Range: 2-3 mg/day in 3 divided doses. Maximum: 5 mg/day.

■ **Unlabeled Uses:** Chronic motor or vocal tic disorder, Tourette's disorder

■ **Contraindications:** Hypersensitivity to other ergot derivatives

■ **Side Effects**
Frequent (24%-10%)
Nausea, dizziness, hallucinations, constipation, rhinitis, dystonia, confusion, somnolence
Occasional (9%-3%)
Orthostatic hypotension, insomnia, dry mouth, peripheral edema, anxiety, diarrhea, dyspepsia, abdominal pain, headache, abnormal vision, anorexia, tremor, depression, rash
Rare (less than 2%)
Urinary frequency, vivid dreams, neck pain, hypotension, vomiting

■ **Serious Reactions**
- Symptoms of overdose may vary from CNS depression, characterized by sedation, apnea, cardiovascular collapse, and death, to severe paradoxical reactions, such as hallucinations, tremor, and seizures.

Special Considerations
- Adjunct to levodopa/carbidopa in Parkinson's disease; longer acting than bromocriptine

■ **Patient/Family Education**
- Hypotensive cautions
- Avoid tasks that require mental alertness or motor skills until response to the drug has been established
- Avoid alcohol

■ **Monitoring Parameters**
- Blood pressure, ECG
- Assess the patient for relief of parkinsonian symptoms, such as improvement of masklike facial expression, muscular rigidity, shuffling gait, and resting tremors of the hands and head
- Overdose may require supportive measures to maintain BP. Plan to monitor cardiac function, obtain vital signs, and check ABG and serum electrolyte levels
- Activated charcoal may be more effective than emesis or lavage for overdose

■ **Geriatric side effects at a glance:**
  ❑ CNS ❑ Bowel Dysfunction ❑ Bladder Dysfunction ❑ Falls
  Other: Orthostatic hypotension, daytime somnolence, and sudden drowsiness.

■ **Use with caution in older patients with:** Preexisting psychotic symptoms

■ **U.S. Regulatory Considerations**
  ❑ FDA Black Box ❑ OBRA regulated in U.S. Long Term Care

■ **Other Uses in Geriatric Patient:** Restless legs syndrome

■ **Side Effects:**
  Of particular importance in the geriatric patient: Nausea/vomiting can result in weight loss

- **Geriatric Considerations - Summary:** Pergolide is a synthetic ergot dopamine agonist that causes potent and prolonged dopamine D_2 stimulation. If discontinued, pergolide should be slowly tapered because abrupt discontinuation can cause confusion, hallucinations, and a condition similar to neuroleptic malignant syndrome.

- **References:**

1. Miyasaki JM, Martin WRW, Suchowersky O, et al. Practice parameter: initiation of treatment for Parkinson's disease: an evidence based review. Neurology 2002;58:11-17.
2. Happe S, Berger K. The association of dopamine agonists with daytime sleepiness, sleep problems and quality of life in patients with Parkinson's disease: a prospective study. J Neurol 2001;248:1062-1067.

perindopril erbumine

(per-in'-doe-pril er-byoo'-meen)

- **Brand Name(s):** Aceon
  Chemical Class: Angiotensin-converting enzyme (ACE) inhibitor, nonsulfhydryl

- **Clinical Pharmacology:**
  Mechanism of Action: An ACE inhibitor that suppresses the renin-angiotensin-aldosterone system and prevents conversion of angiotensin I to angiotensin II, a potent vasoconstrictor; may also inhibit angiotensin II at local vascular and renal sites. **Therapeutic Effect:** Reduces peripheral arterial resistance and BP.
  Pharmacokinetics: Rapidly absorbed from the GI tract. Protein binding: 60%. Extensively metabolized in liver. Excreted in urine. **Half-life:** 0.8-1 hr.

- **Available Forms:**
  - *Tablets*: 2 mg, 4 mg, 8 mg.

- **Indications and Dosages:**
  Hypertension: PO 2-8 mg/day as single dose or in 2 divided doses. Maximum: 16 mg/day.

- **Unlabeled Uses:** Management of heart failure, hypertension and/or renal crisis in scleroderma

- **Contraindications:** History of angioedema from previous treatment with ACE inhibitors

- **Side Effects**
  Occasional (5%-1%)
  Cough, back pain, sinusitis, upper extremity pain, dyspepsia, fever, palpitations, hypotension, dizziness, fatigue, syncope

- **Serious Reactions**
  - Excessive hypotension ("first-dose syncope") may occur in patients with CHF and in those who are severely salt or volume depleted.

- Angioedema (swelling of face and lips) and hyperkalemia occur rarely.
- Agranulocytosis and neutropenia may be noted in those with collagen vascular disease, including scleroderma and systemic lupus erythematosus, and impaired renal function.
- Nephrotic syndrome may be noted in those with history of renal disease.
- Hypoglycemia may occur in patients with diabetes using glucose-lowering drugs.

■ Patient/Family Education
- Caution with salt substitutes containing potassium chloride
- Rise slowly to sitting/standing position to minimize orthostatic hypotension
- Dizziness, fainting, light-headedness may occur during first few days of therapy
- May cause altered taste perception or cough; persistent dry cough usually does not subside unless medication is stopped; notify clinician if these symptoms persist
- Warnings regarding angioedema (swelling of face, extremities, eyes, lips, tongue, hoarseness, or difficulty swallowing or breathing), especially following first dose
- Skipping doses or voluntarily discontinuing the drug may produce severe, rebound hypertension

■ Monitoring Parameters
- Baseline electrolytes, renal function tests, and urinalysis baseline and at least BUN, creatinine, potassium within 2 weeks after initiation of therapy (increased levels may indicate acute renal failure)
- Serial orthostatic blood pressures and pulse rates
- Pattern of daily bowel activity and stool consistency

■ Geriatric side effects at a glance:
☐ CNS ☐ Bowel Dysfunction ☐ Bladder Dysfunction ☐ Falls

■ U.S. Regulatory Considerations
☑ FDA Black Box
Although not relevant for geriatric patients, teratogenicity is associated with the use of ACE inhibitors.
☐ OBRA regulated in U.S. Long Term Care

permethrin

(per-meth'-rin)

■ Brand Name(s): Acticin, Elimite
OTC: A200 Lice, Nix, RID
Chemical Class: Pyrethroid derivative

■ Clinical Pharmacology:
Mechanism of Action: An antiparasitic agent that inhibits sodium influx through nerve cell membrane channels. **Therapeutic Effect:** Results in delayed repolarization, paralysis, and death of parasites.

Pharmacokinetics: Less than 2% absorption after topical application. Detected in residual amounts on hair for at least 10 days following treatment. Metabolized by liver to inactive metabolites. Excreted in urine.

■ **Available Forms:**
- *Cream:* 5% (Acticin).
- *Liquid, topical:* 1% (Nix).
- *Shampoo:* 0.33% (A200 Lice).
- *Solution:* 0.25% (Nix), 0.5% (A200 Lice, RID).

■ **Indications and Dosages:**
Head lice: Shampoo Shampoo hair, towel dry, apply to scalp, leave on for 10 minutes and rinse. Remove nits with nit comb. Repeat application if live lice present 7 days after initial treatment.
Scabies: Topical Apply from head to feet, leave on for 8-14 hr. Wash with soap and water. Repeat application if living mites present 14 days after initial treatment.

■ **Unlabeled Uses:** Demodicidosis, insect bite prophylaxis, leishmaniasis prophylaxis, malaria prophylaxis

■ **Contraindications:** Hypersensitivity to pyrethyroid, pyrethrin, chrysanthemums or any component of the formulation

■ **Side Effects**
Occasional
Burning, pruritus, stinging, erythema, rash, swelling

■ **Serious Reactions**
- Shortness of breath and difficulty breathing have been reported.

■ **Patient/Family Education**
- For external use only; shake well
- Avoid contact with eyes, mucous membranes
- Itching may be temporarily aggravated following application
- Do not repeat administration sooner than 1 wk
- Itching from allergic reaction caused by mite may persist for several weeks even though infestation is cured
- Disinfect clothing, bedding, combs, and brushes

■ **Monitoring Parameters**
- After treatment with permethrin, patients should be observed for the presence of live lice. If live lice are detected 14 days after the initial application of permethrin, retreatment is indicated
- Check skin for local burning, itching, and irritation

■ **Geriatric side effects at a glance:**
❑ CNS ❑ Bowel Dysfunction ❑ Bladder Dysfunction ❑ Falls

■ **U.S. Regulatory Considerations**
❑ FDA Black Box ❑ OBRA regulated in U.S. Long Term Care

perphenazine

(per-fen'-a-zeen)

■ **Brand Name(s):** Trilafon
  Chemical Class: Piperidine phenothiazine derivative

■ **Clinical Pharmacology:**
  Mechanism of Action: An antipsychotic agent and antiemetic that blocks postsynaptic dopamine receptor sites in the brain. **Therapeutic Effect:** Suppresses behavioral response in psychosis, and relieves nausea and vomiting.
  Pharmacokinetics: Well absorbed following oral administration. Protein binding: greater than 90%. Metabolized in liver. Excreted in urine. **Half-life:** 9-12 hr.

■ **Available Forms:**
  • *Oral Concentrate*: 16 mg/5 ml.
  • *Tablets*: 2 mg, 4 mg, 8 mg, 16 mg.

■ **Indications and Dosages:**
  Severe schizophrenia: PO Initially, 2-4 mg/day. May increase at 4-7 day intervals by 2-4 mg/day up to 32 mg/day.
  Severe nausea and vomiting: PO 8-16 mg/day in divided doses up to 24 mg/day.

■ **Contraindications:** Coma, myelosuppression, hypersensitivity to other piperazine phenothiazines, severe cardiovascular disease, severe CNS depression, subcortical brain damage

■ **Side Effects**
  Occasional
  Marked photosensitivity, somnolence, dry mouth, blurred vision, lethargy, constipation or diarrhea, nasal congestion, peripheral edema, urine retention
  Rare
  Ocular changes, altered skin pigmentation, hypotension, dizziness, syncope

■ **Serious Reactions**
  • Extrapyramidal symptoms appear to be dose-related and are divided into 3 categories: akathisia (characterized by inability to sit still, tapping of feet), parkinsonian symptoms (including mask-like face, tremors, shuffling gait, hypersalivation), and acute dystonias (such as torticollis, opisthotonos, and oculogyric crisis).
  • Tardive dyskinesia occurs rarely.
  • Abrupt withdrawal after long-term therapy may precipitate nausea, vomiting, gastritis, dizziness, and tremors.

■ **Patient/Family Education**
  • Arise slowly from reclining position
  • Do not discontinue abruptly

- Use a sunscreen during sun exposure to prevent burns, take special precautions to stay cool in hot weather
- Concentrate may be diluted just prior to administration with distilled water, acidified tap water, orange or grape juice
- Drowsiness generally subsides during continued therapy

■ **Monitoring Parameters**
- Observe closely for signs of tardive dyskinesia (abnormal involuntary movement scale)
- Periodic CBC with platelets, hepatic and renal function during prolonged therapy
- Blood pressure for hypotension
- Therapeutic response, such as increased ability to concentrate and interest in surroundings, improvement in self-care, and a relaxed facial expression

■ **Geriatric side effects at a glance:**
☑ CNS ☑ Bowel Dysfunction ☐ Bladder Dysfunction ☑ Falls
Other: Orthostatic hypotension, cardiac conduction disturbances, anticholinergic side effects

■ **Use with caution in older patients with:** Parkinson's disease (an atypical antipsychotic is recommended), seizure disorders, cardiovascular disease with conduction disturbance, hepatic encephalopathy, narrow-angle glaucoma

■ **U.S. Regulatory Considerations**
☐ FDA Black Box ☑ OBRA regulated in U.S. Long Term Care

■ **Other Uses in Geriatric Patient:** Behavior disturbances in the setting of dementia

■ **Side Effects:**
Of particular importance in the geriatric patient: Tardive dyskinesia, akathisia (may appear to exacerbate behavioral disturbances), anticholinergic effects, may increase risk of sudden death

■ **Geriatric Considerations - Summary:** Sink and colleagues' systematic review showed statistically significant improvements on neuropsychiatric and behavioral scales for some drugs, but improvements were small and unlikely to be clinically important. Because of documented risks, and uncertain benefits, these agents should be used with caution in demented elderly persons, with frequent monitoring for side effects and a low threshold for discontinuing use.

■ **References:**
1. Leipzig RM, Cumming RG, Tinetti ME. Drugs and falls in older people: a systematic review and meta-analysis: I. Psychotropic drugs. J Am Geriatr Soc 1999;47:30-39.
2. Sink KM, Holden KF, Yaffe K. Pharmacological treatment of neuropsychiatric symptoms of dementia: a review of the evidence. JAMA 2005;293:596-608.
3. Ray WA, Meredith S, Thapa PB, Meador KG, Hall K, Murray KT. Antipsychotics and the risk of sudden cardiac death. Arch Gen Psychiatry 2001;58:1161-1167.

phenazopyridine hydrochloride

(fen-az'-o-peer'-i-deen hye-droe-klor'-ide)

■ **Brand Name(s):** Azo-Gesic, Azo-Standard, Eridium, Prodium, Pyridiate, Pyridium, Uristat, Urodol, Urogesic

Combinations
Rx: with sulfamethoxazole (Azo-Gantanol); with sulfisoxazole (Azo-Gantrisin)
Chemical Class: Azo dye

■ **Clinical Pharmacology:**
Mechanism of Action: An interstitial cystitis agent that exerts topical analgesic effect on urinary tract mucosa. **Therapeutic Effect:** Relieves urinary pain, burning, urgency, and frequency.
Pharmacokinetics: Well absorbed from the GI tract. Partially metabolized in the liver. Primarily excreted in urine. **Half-life:** Unknown.

■ **Available Forms:**
- *Tablets:* 95 mg (Pyridium), 100 mg (Azo-Gesic, Azo-Standard, Prodium, Uristat), 200 mg (Azo-Gesic, Azo-Standard, Prodium, Uristat).

■ **Indications and Dosages:**
Urinary analgesic: PO 100–200 mg 3–4 times a day.
Dosage in renal impairment: Dosage interval is modified based on creatinine clearance.

Creatinine Clearance	Interval
50–80 ml/min	Usual dose q8–16h
less than 50 ml/min	Avoid use.

■ **Contraindications:** Hepatic or renal insufficiency

■ **Side Effects**
Occasional
Headache, GI disturbance, rash, pruritus

■ **Serious Reactions**
- Overdose may lead to hemolytic anemia, nephrotoxicity, or hepatotoxicity. Patients with renal impairment or severe hypersensitivity to the drug may also develop these reactions.
- A massive and acute overdose may result in methemoglobinemia.

■ **Patient/Family Education**
- May cause GI upset
- Take after meals

- May cause reddish-orange discoloration of urine; may stain fabric; may also stain contact lenses

■ **Monitoring Parameters**
  - Assess the patient for a therapeutic response: relief of urinary frequency, pain, and burning

■ **Geriatric side effects at a glance:**
  ❏ CNS   ❏ Bowel Dysfunction   ❏ Bladder Dysfunction   ❏ Falls

■ **U.S. Regulatory Considerations**
  ❏ FDA Black Box   ❏ OBRA regulated in U.S. Long Term Care

phendimetrazine tartrate

(fen-dye-me'-tra-zeen tar'-trate)

■ **Brand Name(s):** Adipost, Bontril PDM, Bontril Slow-Release, Melfiat, Obezine, Phendiet, Phendiet-105, Plegine, Prelu-2
  Chemical Class: Morpholine

  DEA Class: Schedule III; Schedule IV

■ **Clinical Pharmacology:**
  Mechanism of Action: A phenylalkylamine sympathomimetic with activity similar to amphetamines that stimulates the central nervous system (CNS) and elevates blood pressure (BP) most likely mediated via norepinephrine and dopamine metabolism. Causes stimulation of the hypothalamus. **Therapeutic Effect:** Decreases appetite. **Pharmacokinetics:** The pharmacokinetics of phendimetrazine tartrate has not been well established. Metabolized to active metabolite, phendimetrazine. Excreted in urine. **Half-life:** 2-4 hr.

■ **Available Forms:**
  - *Tablets*: 35 mg (Bontril PDM, Obezine, Phendiet, Plegine).
  - *Capsules (Extended-Release)*: 105 mg (Adipost, Bontril Slow-Release, Melfiat, Phendiet-105, Prelu-2).

■ **Indications and Dosages:**
  Obesity: PO 105 mg/day in the morning or before the morning meal (sustained-release); 35 mg 2-3 times/day (immediate-release). Maximum: 70 mg 3 times/day.

■ **Contraindications:** Advanced arteriosclerosis, agitated states, glaucoma, history of drug abuse, history of hypersensitivity to sympathomimetic amines, hyperthyroidism, moderate to severe hypertension, symptomatic cardiovascular disease, use within 14 days of discontinuing MAOI, hypersensitivity to phendimetrazine

Side Effects
Occasional
Constipation, nausea, diarrhea, dry mouth, dysuria, libido changes, flushing, hypertension, insomnia, nervousness, headache, dizziness, irritability, agitation, restlessness, palpitations, increased heart rate, sweating, tremor, urticaria

Serious Reactions
- Multivalvular heart disease, primary pulmonary hypertension and arrhythmias occur rarely.
- Overdose may produce flushing, arrhythmias, and psychosis.
- Abrupt withdrawal following prolonged administration of high doses may produce extreme fatigue and depression.

Patient/Family Education
- May cause insomnia; avoid taking late in the day
- Weight reduction requires strict adherence to caloric restriction
- Do not discontinue abruptly
- Swallow capsules whole
- Take 1 hr before meal, usually the first meal of the day
- Avoid performing tasks that require mental alertness or motor skills until response to the drug is established
- Notify the physician if palpitations, dizziness, dry mouth, or pronounced nervousness occurs

Monitoring Parameters
- Blood pressure, heart rate
- Weight
- CNS overstimulation

Geriatric side effects at a glance:
❑ CNS   ❑ Bowel Dysfunction   ❑ Bladder Dysfunction   ❑ Falls

U.S. Regulatory Considerations
❑ FDA Black Box   ❑ OBRA regulated in U.S. Long Term Care

phenelzine sulfate

(fen'-el-zeen sul'-fate)

Brand Name(s): Nardil
Chemical Class: Hydrazine derivative

Clinical Pharmacology:
Mechanism of Action: An MAOI that inhibits the activity of the enzyme monoamine oxidase at CNS storage sites, leading to increased levels of the neurotransmitters epinephrine, norepinephrine, serotonin, and dopamine at neuronal receptor sites. Therapeutic Effect: Relieves depression.

Pharmacokinetics: Well absorbed from GI tract. Metabolized in the liver. Primarily excreted in urine. **Half-life:** 1.2 hr.

■ Available Forms:
- *Tablets*: 15 mg.

■ Indications and Dosages:
Depression refractory to other antidepressants or electroconvulsive therapy: PO Initially, 7.5 mg/day. May increase by 7.5-15 mg/day q3-4wk up to 60 mg/day in divided doses.

■ Unlabeled Uses:
Treatment of panic disorder, selective mutism, vascular or tension headaches

■ Contraindications:
Cardiovascular or cerebrovascular disease, hepatic or renal impairment, pheochromocytoma

■ Side Effects
Frequent
Orthostatic hypotension, restlessness, GI upset, insomnia, dizziness, headache, lethargy, asthenia, dry mouth, peripheral edema
Occasional
Flushing, diaphoresis, rash, urinary frequency, increased appetite, transient impotence
Rare
Visual disturbances

■ Serious Reactions
- Hypertensive crisis occurs rarely and is marked by severe hypertension, occipital headache radiating frontally, neck stiffness or soreness, nausea, vomiting, diaphoresis, fever or chilliness, clammy skin, dilated pupils, palpitations, tachycardia or bradycardia, and constricting chest pain.
- Intracranial bleeding has been reported in association with severe hypertension.

■ Patient/Family Education
- Avoid tyramine-containing foods, beverages, and OTC products containing decongestants or dextromethorphan and products such as diet aids
- Avoid foods that require bacteria or molds for their preparation or preservation (such as yogurt and aged cheese)
- May cause drowsiness, dizziness, blurred vision
- Use caution driving or performing other tasks requiring alertness
- Arise slowly from reclining position
- Therapeutic effect may require 4-8 wk
- Notify the physician if headache or neck soreness or stiffness occurs

■ Monitoring Parameters
- Blood pressure, heart rate
- Weight
- Diet
- Behavior, level of interest, mood, and sleep pattern

- Monitor the patient for occipital headache radiating frontally and neck stiffness or soreness, which may be the first symptoms of an impending hypertensive crisis. If hypertensive crisis occurs, administer phentolamine 5-10 mg IV, as prescribed

■ **Geriatric side effects at a glance:**
  ❑ CNS ❑ Bowel Dysfunction ❑ Bladder Dysfunction ❑ Falls
  Other: Orthostatic hypotension

■ **Use with caution in older patients with:** None

■ **U.S. Regulatory Considerations**
  ☑ FDA Black Box
  - Because there is an increased risk of suicide in children and adolescents, older adults should also be closely monitored for suicide ideation.
  ☑ OBRA regulated in U.S. Long Term Care

■ **Other Uses in Geriatric Patient:** Depression refractory to other measures, anxiety symptoms and related disorders

■ **Side Effects:**
  Of particular importance in the geriatric patient: None

■ **Geriatric Considerations - Summary:** Because of the severe toxicity of these agents and the long list of potentially serious drug-drug and drug-food interactions, they are **not** recommended for routine treatment of depression in older adults. If prescribed, they require close monitoring by specialists.

■ **References:**
  1. Boyer EW, Shannon M. The serotonin syndrome. N Engl J Med 2005;352:1112-1120.
  2. Volz HP, Gleiter CH. Monoamine oxidase inhibitors. A perspective on their use in the elderly. Drugs Aging 1998;13:341-355.

phenobarbital

(fee-noe-bar'-bi-tal)

■ **Brand Name(s):** Luminal

  Combinations
  Rx: with atropine, hyoscyamine, scopolamine (Donnatal); with belladonna, ergotamine (Bellergal Spacetabs)
  Chemical Class: Barbituric acid derivative

  DEA Class: Schedule IV

■ **Clinical Pharmacology:**
  Mechanism of Action: A barbiturate that enhances the activity of gamma-aminobutyric acid (GABA) by binding to the GABA receptor complex. **Therapeutic Effect:** Depresses CNS activity.

Pharmacokinetics:

Route	Onset	Peak	Duration
PO	20-60 min	N/A	6-10 hr
IV	5 min	30 min	4-10 hr

Well absorbed after PO or parenteral administration. Protein binding: 35%-50%. Rapidly and widely distributed. Metabolized in the liver. Primarily excreted in urine. Removed by hemodialysis. **Half-life:** 53-118 hr.

■ **Available Forms:**
- *Elixir:* 15 mg/5 ml, 20 mg/5 ml.
- *Tablets:* 15 mg, 30 mg, 32.4 mg, 60 mg, 64.8 mg, 97.2 mg, 100 mg.
- *Injection:* 30 mg/ml, 60 mg/ml, 65 mg/ml, 130 mg/ml.

■ **Indications and Dosages:**
Status epilepticus: IV Initially, 300-800 mg, then 120-240 mg/dose at 20-min intervals until seizures are controlled or total dose of 1-2g administered.
Seizure control: PO, IV 1-3 mg/kg/day. Or 50-100 mg 2-3 times a day.
Sedation: PO, IM 30-120 mg/day in 2-3 divided doses.
Hypnotic: PO, IV, IM, Subcutaneous 100-320 mg at bedtime.

■ **Unlabeled Uses:** Management of sedative or hypnotic withdrawal

■ **Contraindications:** Hypersensitivity to other barbiturates, porphyria, preexisting CNS depression, severe pain, severe respiratory disease

■ **Side Effects**
Occasional (3%-1%)
Somnolence
Rare (less than 1%)
Confusion; paradoxical CNS reactions, such as excitement or restlessness (generally noted during first 2 weeks of therapy, particularly in presence of uncontrolled pain)

■ **Serious Reactions**
- Abrupt withdrawal after prolonged therapy may produce increased dreaming, nightmares, insomnia, tremor, diaphoresis, and vomiting, hallucinations, delirium, seizures, and status epilepticus.
- Skin eruptions may be a sign of a hypersensitivity reaction.
- Blood dyscrasias, hepatic disease, and hypocalcemia occur rarely.
- Overdose produces cold or clammy skin, hypothermia, severe CNS depression, cyanosis, tachycardia, and Cheyne-Stokes respirations.
- Toxicity may result in severe renal impairment.

■ **Patient/Family Education**
- Avoid driving or other activities requiring alertness
- Avoid alcohol ingestion or CNS depressants
- Do not discontinue medication abruptly after long-term use
- May be habit forming

■ **Monitoring Parameters**
- Periodic CBC, liver and renal function tests, serum folate, vitamin D during prolonged therapy

- Serum phenobarbital concentration (therapeutic range for seizure disorders: 20-40 mcg/ml)
- Blood pressure, heart rate, respiratory rate
- CNS status
- Seizure activity

■ **Geriatric side effects at a glance:**
☑ CNS ☐ Bowel Dysfunction ☐ Bladder Dysfunction ☑ Falls
Other: Withdrawal symptoms after long-term use

■ **Use with caution in older patients with:** Not recommended for use in older adults.

■ **U.S. Regulatory Considerations**
☐ FDA Black Box ☑ OBRA regulated in U.S. Long Term Care

■ **Other Uses in Geriatric Patient:** Anxiety disorders, sleep disorders, seizure disorders

■ **Side Effects:**
Of *particular importance in the geriatric patient*: Sedation, withdrawal symptoms when abruptly discontinued (e.g., during hospitalization) rather than tapered.

■ **Geriatric Considerations - Summary:** Because barbiturates have a low therapeutic window, a wide range of drug interactions and rapid development of tolerance, great potential for abuse and dependence, these agents are not recommended for use in older adults.

■ **Reference:**
1. Hypnotic drugs. Med Lett Drugs Ther 2000;42:71-72.

phenoxybenzamine hydrochloride

(fen-ox-ee-ben'-za-meen hye-droe-klor'-ide)

■ **Brand Name(s):** Dibenzyline
Chemical Class: Haloalkylamine derivative

■ **Clinical Pharmacology:**
Mechanism of Action: An antihypertensive that produces long-lasting noncompetitive alpha-adrenergic blockade of postganglionic synapses in exocrine glands and smooth muscles. Relaxes urethra and increases opening of the bladder. **Therapeutic Effect:** Controls hypertension.
Pharmacokinetics: Well absorbed from the gastrointestinal (GI) tract. Distributed into fatty tissue. Metabolized in liver. Eliminated in urine and feces. Not removed by hemodialysis. **Half-life:** 24 hr.

Available Forms:
- *Tablets*: 10 mg.

Indications and Dosages:
Pheochromocytoma: PO Initially, 10 mg twice daily. May increase dose every other day to 20-40 mg 2-3 times/day.

Unlabeled Uses:
Bladder instability, complex regional pain syndrome (CRPS), prostatic obstruction, Raynaud's disease

Contraindications:
Any condition compromised by hypotension, hypersensitivity to phenoxybenzamine or any component of the formulation

Side Effects
Frequent
Headache, lethargy, confusion, fatigue
Occasional
Nausea, postural hypotension, syncope, dry mouth
Rare
Palpitations, diarrhea, constipation, inhibition of ejaculation, weakness, altered vision, dizziness

Serious Reactions
- Overdosage produces severe hypotension, irritability, lethargy, tachycardia, dizziness and shock.

Patient/Family Education
- Avoid alcohol; avoid sudden changes in posture, dizziness may result
- Avoid cough, cold, or allergy medications containing sympathomimetics
- Avoid driving or other activities requiring alertness

Monitoring Parameters
- Blood pressure

Geriatric side effects at a glance:
☑ CNS ❑ Bowel Dysfunction ❑ Bladder Dysfunction ❑ Falls

U.S. Regulatory Considerations
❑ FDA Black Box ❑ OBRA regulated in U.S. Long Term Care

phentermine hydrochloride

(fen'-ter-meen hye-dro-klor'-ide)

- **Brand Name(s):** Adipex-P, Fastin, Ionamin, Oby-Cap, Phentercot, Pro-Fast HS, Pro-Fast SA, Pro-Fast SR, T-Diet, Teramine, Zantryl
  Chemical Class: Phenethylamine analog (amphetamine-like)

  DEA Class: Schedule IV

- **Clinical Pharmacology:**
  Mechanism of Action: A sympathomimetic amine structurally similar to dextroamphetamine and is most likely mediated via norepinephrine and dopamine metabolism. Causes stimulation of the hypothalamus. **Therapeutic Effect:** Decreased appetite.
  Pharmacokinetics: Well absorbed from the gastrointestinal (GI) tract; resin absorbed slower. Excreted unchanged in urine. **Half-life:** 20 hr.

- **Available Forms:**
  - *Capsules (as hydrochloride)*: 15 mg, 18.75 mg, 30 mg (Fastin), 37.5 mg (Adipex-P).
  - *Capsules (as resin complex)*: 15 mg (Ionamin), 30 mg (Ionamin).
  - *Tablets (as hydrochloride)*: 8 mg, 37.5 mg (Adipex-P).

- **Indications and Dosages:**
  Obesity: PO **Adipex-P**: 37.5 mg as a single daily dose or in divided doses. **Ionamin**: 15-37.5 mg/day before breakfast or 1-2 hr after breakfast. **Fastin**: 30 mg/day taken in the morning

- **Contraindications:** Advanced arteriosclerosis, agitated states, cardiovascular disease, concurrent use or within 14 days of discontinuation of MAOI therapy, glaucoma, history of drug abuse, hypertension (moderate-to-severe), hyperthyroidism, hypersensitivity to phentermine or sympathomimetic amines

- **Side Effects**
  Occasional
  Restlessness, insomnia, tremor, palpitations, tachycardia, elevation in blood pressure, headache, dizziness, dry mouth, unpleasant taste, diarrhea or constipation, changes in libido

- **Serious Reactions**
  - Primary pulmonary hypertension (PPH), psychotic episodes, and valvular heart disease rarely occur.
  - Anorectic agents have been associated with regurgitant multivalvular heart disease involving mitral, aortic, and/or tricuspid valves.
  - Prolonged use may cause physical or psychological dependence.

- **Patient/Family Education**
  - May cause insomnia, avoid taking late in the day
  - Weight reduction is facilitated by adherence to caloric restriction and exercise
  - Avoid tasks that require mental alertness or motor skills until response to the drug is established

- May be habit forming
- Notify the physician if fast, pounding, or irregular heartbeat occurs

Monitoring Parameters
- Blood pressure
- Weight

Geriatric side effects at a glance:
☑ CNS ❑ Bowel Dysfunction ❑ Bladder Dysfunction ❑ Falls

U.S. Regulatory Considerations
❑ FDA Black Box ❑ OBRA regulated in U.S. Long Term Care

phentolamine mesylate

(fen-tole'-a-meen mes'-sil-ate)

Brand Name(s): Regitine
Chemical Class: Imidazoline derivative

Clinical Pharmacology:
Mechanism of Action: An alpha-adrenergic blocking agent which produces peripheral vasodilation and cardiac stimulation. **Therapeutic Effect:** Decreases blood pressure (BP).
Pharmacokinetics: Poorly absorbed from the gastrointestinal (GI) tract. Protein binding: 72%. Metabolized in liver. Eliminated in urine and feces. Not removed by hemodialysis. **Half-life:** 19 min.

Available Forms:
- *Injection:* 5 mg/ml.

Indications and Dosages:
Extravasation - norepinephrine: SC Infiltrate area with a small amount (1 ml) of solution (made by diluting 5-10 mg in 10 ml of NS) within 12 hours of extravasation. Do not exceed 0.1-0.2 mg/kg or 5 mg total. If dose is effective, normal skin color should return to the blanched area within 1 hour.
Diagnosis of pheochromocytoma: IM, IV 5 mg as a single dose.
Surgery for pheochromocytoma: Hypertension IM, IV 5 mg given 1-2 hours before procedure and repeated as needed every 2-4 hours.
Hypertensive crisis: IV 5-20 mg as a single dose.

Unlabeled Uses: Treatment of pralidoxime-induced hypertension, arrhythmias, asthma, bladder instability, cardiac diseases, diabetes mellitus, erectile dysfunction, extravasation (dopamine and epinephrine), hyperhidrosis, myocardial infarction, Raynaud's phenomenon, surgery, sympathetic pain

Contraindications: Renal impairment; coronary or cerebral arteriosclerosis; concurrent use with phosphodiesterase-5 (PDE-5) inhibitors including sildenafil (>25 mg), tadalafil, or vardenafil; hypersensitivity to phentolamine or related compounds.

- ■ **Side Effects**
  Occasional
  Hypotension, tachycardia, arrhythmia, flushing, orthostatic hypotension, weakness, dizziness, nausea, vomiting, diarrhea, nasal congestion, pulmonary hypertension

- ■ **Serious Reactions**
  - Symptoms of overdosage include tachycardia, shock, vomiting, and dizziness.
  - Mixed agents, such as epinephrine, may cause more hypotension.

Special Considerations
  - Urinary catecholamines preferred over phentolamine for screening for pheochromocytoma

- ■ **Patient/Family Education**
  - Notify the physician if dizziness or palpitations occur
  - Avoid tasks that require mental alertness or motor skills until response to drug is established

- ■ **Monitoring Parameters**
  - Blood pressure

- ■ **Geriatric side effects at a glance:**
  ❑ CNS ❑ Bowel Dysfunction ❑ Bladder Dysfunction ❑ Falls

- ■ **U.S. Regulatory Considerations**
  ❑ FDA Black Box ❑ OBRA regulated in U.S. Long Term Care

phenylephrine (systemic)

(fen-ill-ef'-rin)

- ■ **Brand Name(s):** Neofrin; Neo-Synephrine Ophthalmic; Ocu-Phrin; Phenoptic; Rectasol

  Combinations
  Rx: with chlorpheniramine (Ed A-Hist, Prehist, Histatab); with brompheniramine (Dimetane); with chlorpheniramine, phenylpropanolamine (Hista-Vadrin); with chlorpheniramine, phenyltoloxamine (Comhist); with brompheniramine, phenylpropanolamine (Bromophen T.D., Tamine S.R.); with chlorpheniramine, phenyltoloxamine, phenylpropanolamine (Decongestabs, Naldecon, Nalgest, Tri-phen, Uni-decon); with chlorpheniramine, pyrilamine, phenylpropanolamine (Vanex, Histalet); with chlorpheniramine, pyrilamine (R-Tannate, Rhinatate, R-Tannamine, Rynatan, Tanoral, Triotann, Tritan, Tri-Tannate)
  Chemical Class: Substituted phenylethylamine

- ■ **Clinical Pharmacology:**
  Mechanism of Action: Phenylephrine is a powerful postsynaptic alpha-receptor stimulant with little effect on the beta receptors of the heart, lacking chronotropic and

inotropic actions on the heart. **Therapeutic Effect:** Vasoconstriction, decreases heart rate, increases stroke output, increases blood pressure

Pharmacokinetics: Phenylephrine is irregularly absorbed from and readily metabolized in the GI tract. After IV administration, a pressor effect occurs almost immediately and persists for 15-20 minutes. After IM administration, a pressor effect occurs within 10-15 minutes and persists for 50 minutes to 1 hour. After oral inhalation of phenylephrine in combination with isoproterenol, pulmonary effects occur within a few minutes and persist for about 3 hours. The pharmacologic effects of phenylephrine are terminated at least partially by the uptake of the drug into the tissues. Phenylephrine is metabolized in the liver and intestine by the enzyme monoamine oxidase (MAO). The metabolites and their route and rate of excretion have not been identified.

■ **Available Forms:**
- *Solution (Ophthalmic)*: 2.5%, 10%
- *Solution (Nasal)*: 0.125%, 0.16%, 0.25%, 0.5%
- *Solution (Injection)*: 10 mg/ml

■ **Indications and Dosages:**

Rhinitis, nasal congestion: Intranasal 2-3 drops or sprays of 0.25% or 0.5% solution into each nostril q4h as needed. Do not use longer than 3 days.

Mydriasis: Ophthalmic 1 drop of 2.5% or 10% solution to conjunctiva following a topical anesthetic.

Paroxysmal supraventricular tachycardia (PSVT): The initial dose, given by rapid IV injection, should not exceed 0.5 mg. Subsequent doses may be increased in increments of 0.1 to 0.2 mg. Maximum single dose is 1 mg IV.

Mild to moderate hypotension: SC, IM 2-5 mg (range 1-10 mg), repeated no more than every 10-15 minutes. Maximum initial dose: 5 mg. IV 0.2 mg (range 0.1 to 0.5 mg), given no more frequently than every 10-15 minutes. Maximum initial dose: 0.5 mg.

Severe hypotension, severe shock: IV Initially, 100-180 mcg/min IV infusion, with dose titration to the desired MAP and SVR. A maintenance infusion rate of 40-60 mcg/min IV is usually adequate after blood pressure stabilizes. If necessary to produce the desired pressor response, additional phenylephrine in increments of 10 mg or more may be added to the infusion solution and the rate of flow adjusted according to the response of the patient.

Hypotensive emergencies during spinal anesthesia: IV Initially, 0.2 mg IV. Subsequent doses should not exceed the previous dose by more than 0.1 to 0.2 mg. Maximum of 0.5 mg per dose.

Hypotension prophylaxis during spinal anesthesia: IM, SC 2-3 mg, 3 or 4 minutes before anesthesia. A dose of 2 mg is usually adequate with low spinal anesthesia; 3 mg may be necessary with high spinal anesthesia.

Vasoconstriction in regional anesthesia: IV The manufacturer states that the optimum concentration of phenylephrine HCl is 0.05 mg/ml (1:20,000). Solutions may be prepared for regional anesthesia by adding 1 mg of phenylephrine HCl to each 20 ml of local anesthesia solution. Some pressor response can be expected when at least 2 mg is injected.

Prolongation of spinal anesthesia: IV The addition of 2-5 mg added to the anesthetic solution increases the duration of motor block by as much as 50% without an increase in the incidence of complications such as nausea, vomiting, or blood pressure disturbances.

■ **Contraindications:** Phenylephrine HCl injection should not be used with patients with severe hypertension, ventricular tachycardia or fibrillation, acute myocardial infarction (MI), atrial flutter or fibrillation, cardiac arrhythmias, cardiac disease, cardiomyopathy, closed-angle glaucoma, coronary artery disease, patients who have a known hypersensitivity to phenylephrine, sulfites, or to any one of its components.

■ Side Effects

Occasional

Intranasal: Burning, stinging, sneezing, dryness of mucosa. Prolonged use may result in rebound congestion.

Systemic: Headache, reflex bradycardia, excitability, restlessness, and rarely arrhythmias.

Ophthalmic: Irritation, blurred vision, mydriasis

■ Serious Reactions

- Overdose may induce ventricular extrasystoles and short paroxysms of ventricular tachycardia, a sensation of fullness in the head, and tingling of the extremities. Should an excessive elevation of blood pressure occur, it may be immediately relieved by an α-adrenergic blocking agent, e.g., phentolamine.

Special Considerations

- *Antidote to extravasation:* 5-10 ml phentolamine in 10-15 ml saline infiltrated throughout ischemic area
- Not indicated for hypotension secondary to hypovolemia
- As not bioavailable orally (see pharmacokinetics), combination products essentially lack decongestant. Only available by prescription, as lack effectiveness data required by FDA OTC panels
- Manage rebound congestion by stopping phenylephrine: one nostril at a time, substitute systemic decongestant and/or inhaled steroid
- Ocular instillation of 10% solution may increase blood pressure

■ Patient/Family Education

- Immediately contact the physician and discontinue the drug if dizziness, feeling of irregular heartbeat, insomnia, tremor, or weakness occurs
- Discontinue and consult physician immediately if ocular pain or visual changes occur or if condition worsens or continues more than 72 hours.
- Do not use longer than 3 days.

■ Monitoring Parameters

- Blood pressure, heart rate

■ Geriatric side effects at a glance:

❑ CNS ❑ Bowel Dysfunction ❑ Bladder Dysfunction ❑ Falls

■ U.S. Regulatory Considerations

❑ FDA Black Box ☑ OBRA regulated in U.S. Long Term Care

phenylephrine (topical)

(fen-ill-ef'-rin)

■ **Brand Name(s):** AK-Dilate; Mydfrin; Neofrin; Neo-Synephrine Ophthalmic; Ocu-Phrin; Phenoptic; Rectasol

Combinations
Rx: (Nasal): with zinc (Zincfrin); with pheniramine (Dristan Nasal);
Rx: (Ophthalmic); with tropicamide (Diophenyl-t); with pyrilamine (Prefrin-A)
Chemical Class: Substituted phenylethylamine

■ **Clinical Pharmacology:**
Mechanism of Action: Phenylephrine HCl is an alpha-receptor sympathetic agonist used in local ocular disorders because of its vasoconstrictor and mydriatic action. It exhibits rapid and moderately prolonged action, and it produces little rebound vasodilatation. Systemic side effects are uncommon. **Therapeutic Effect:** Vasoconstriction and pupil dilation.
Pharmacokinetics: Some absorption systemically. The duration of action of intranasal administration ranges from 30 minutes to 4 hours. The duration of the mydriatic effect is roughly 3 hours after administration of the 2.5% solution but may be as long as 7 hours after the 10% solution.

■ **Available Forms:**
- *Solution (Ophthalmic):* 2.5%, 10%
- *Solution (Nasal):* 0.125%, 0.16%, 0.25%, 0.5%
- *Solution (Injection):* 10 mg/ml
- *Solution (Oral):* 5 mg/ml
- *Suppository (Rectal):* 0.25%

■ **Indications and Dosages:**
Mydriasis induction (ophthalmic): Topical Instill 1 or 2 drops of a 2.5% or 10% solution in eye before procedure. May be repeated in 10-60 minutes if needed. In general, the 2.5% solution is preferred in the elderly to avoid cardiac reactions.
Uveitis (posterior synechia): Topical Instill 1 drop of 10% solution in eye 3 or more times daily with atropine sulfate. In general, the 2.5% solution is preferred in elderly to avoid adverse cardiac reactions. Intranasal Apply 2-3 drops or 1-2 sprays of a 0.25% to 0.5% solution instilled in each nostril or a small quantity of 0.5% nasal jelly applied into each nostril. Apply every 4 hours as needed. The 1% solution may be used in patients with severe congestion.
Conjunctival congestion: Topical 1 to 2 drops of a 0.12% to 0.25% solution applied to the conjunctiva every 3 to 4 hours as needed. In general, the 2.5% solution is preferred in elderly to avoid cardiac reactions.
Postoperative malignant glaucoma: Topical Instill 1 drop of a 10% solution with 1 drop of a 1% to 4% solution 3 or more times per day. In general, the 2.5% solution is preferred in elderly to avoid cardiac reactions.
Vasoconstriction and pupil dilatation: Topical A drop of a suitable topical anesthetic may be applied, followed in a few minutes by 1 drop of the phenylephrine HCl 2.5% on the upper limbus.
Surgery: Topical When a short-acting mydriatic is needed for wide dilatation of the pupil before intraocular surgery, phenylephrine HCl 2.5% (or the 10%) may be applied topically from 30 to 60 minutes before the operation.

Cycloplegia: Topical One drop of the preferred cycloplegic is placed in each eye, followed in 5 minutes by one drop of phenylephrine HCl 2.5%.
Ophthalmoscopic examination: Topical One drop of phenylephrine HCl 2.5% is placed in each eye.
Blanching test: Topical One or two drops of phenylephrine HCl 2.5% should be applied to the injected eye.
Glaucoma: Topical In certain patients with glaucoma, temporary reduction of intraocular tension may be attained by producing vasoconstriction of the intraocular vessels; this may be accompanied by placing 1 drop of the 10% solution on the upper surface of the cornea. This treatment may be repeated as often as necessary.
Nasal congestion: Intranasal Use 2 or 3 drops or sprays of a 0.25 to 0.5% solution in the nose every 4 hours as needed

■ **Contraindications:** Ophthalmic solutions (both strengths) of phenylephrine HCl are contraindicated in patients with anatomically narrow angles or narrow-angle glaucoma, severe arteriosclerotic cardiovascular or cerebrovascular disease, use during intraocular operative procedures when the corneal epithelial barrier has been disturbed, and in persons with a known sensitivity to phenylephrine, sulfites, or any of its components including preservatives. The 10% solution is contraindicated in patients with aneurysms.

■ **Side Effects**
Frequent
Burning or stinging of eyes, headache or browache, sensitivity to light, watering of the eyes, increase in runny or stuffy nose, burning, stinging, dryness of inside the nose
Rare
Irritation, dizziness, fast and/or irregular and/or pounding heartbeat, increased sweating, increase in blood pressure, paleness, trembling, headache, nervousness, trouble sleeping

■ **Serious Reactions**
• There have been reports associating the use of phenylephrine HCl 10% ophthalmic solutions with the development of serious cardiovascular reactions, including ventricular arrhythmias and myocardial infarctions. These episodes, some ending fatally, have usually occurred in patients with preexisting cardiovascular diseases.

Special Considerations
• Do not administer for more than 3-5 days (nasal product) or 2-3 days (ocular product used as decongestant) due to rebound congestion

■ **Patient/Family Education**
• Burning or stinging of the eyes, headache, browache, sensitivity of eyes to light, and watering of eyes may occur

■ **Monitoring Parameters**
• Blood pressure, heart rate

■ **Geriatric side effects at a glance:**
❑ CNS ❑ Bowel Dysfunction ❑ Bladder Dysfunction ❑ Falls

■ **U.S. Regulatory Considerations**
❑ FDA Black Box ❑ OBRA regulated in U.S. Long Term Care

phenytoin/fosphenytoin

(fen'-i-toy-in / fos-fen'-i-toy-in)

- **Brand Name(s)—Phenytoin:** (Dilantin, Epamin)

- **Brand Name(s)—Phenytoin:** (Dilantin)

- **Brand Name(s)—Fosphenytoin:** (Cerebyx)
  Chemical Class: Hydantoin derivative

- **Clinical Pharmacology:**
  Mechanism of Action: An anticonvulsant agent that stabilizes neuronal membranes in motor cortex, and decreases abnormal ventricular automaticity. **Therapeutic Effect:** Limits spread of seizure activity. Stabilizes threshold against hyperexcitability. Decreases post-tetanic potentiation and repetitive discharge. Shortens refractory period, QT interval, and action potential duration.
  Pharmacokinetics:
  Phenytoin:
  Slowly, variably absorbed after PO administration; slow but completely absorbed after IM administration. Protein binding: 90%-95%. Widely distributed. Metabolized in liver. Primarily excreted in urine. Not removed by hemodialysis. **Half-life:** 22 hr.
  Fosphenytoin:
  Completely absorbed after IM administration. Protein binding: 95%-99%. After IM or IV administration, rapidly and completely hydrolyzed to phenytoin. Time of complete conversion to phenytoin: IM: 4 hr after injection; IV: 2 hr after the end of infusion. **Half-life** for conversion to phenytoin: 8-15 min.

- **Available Forms:**
  Phenytoin:
  - *Capsules:* 30 mg, 100 mg (Dilantin).
  - *Tablets (Chewable):* 50 mg (Dilantin).
  - *Oral Suspension:* 125 mg/5 ml (Dilantin).
  - *Injection, as sodium:* 50 mg/ml (Dilantin).
  Fosphenytoin:
  - *Injection:* 75 mg/ml, equivalent to 50 mg/ml phenytoin, or 50 mg phenytoin equivalent/ml (Cerebyx).

- **Indications and Dosages:**
  Status epilepticus (Phenytoin): IV Loading dose: 15-18 mg/kg. Maintenance dose: 300 mg/day in 2-3 divided doses.
  Status epilepticus (Fosphenytoin): IV Loading dose: 15-20 mg PE/kg infused at rate of 100-150 mg PE/min.
  Nonemergent seizures: IV Loading dose: 10-20 mg PE/kg. Maintenance: 4-6 mg PE/kg/day.
  Anticonvulsant: PO Loading dose: 15-20 mg/kg in 3 divided doses 2-4 hr apart. Maintenance dose: Same as above.
  Arrhythmias: IV Loading dose: 1.25 mg/kg q5min. May repeat up to total dose of 15 mg/kg. PO Maintenance dose: 250 mg 4 times/day for 1 day, then 250 mg 2 times/day for 2 days, then 300-400 mg/day in divided doses 1-4 times/day.

■ **Unlabeled Uses**
Phenytoin: Adjunct in treatment of tricyclic antidepressant toxicity, muscle relaxant in treatment of muscle hyperirritability, treatment of digoxin-induced arrhythmias and trigeminal neuralgia

■ **Contraindications:** Hydantoin hypersensitivity, seizures due to hypoglycemia, Adam-Stokes syndrome, second- and third-degree heart block, sinoatrial block, sinus bradycardia

■ **Side Effects**
Frequent
Drowsiness, lethargy, confusion, slurred speech, irritability, gingival hyperplasia, hypersensitivity reaction, including fever, rash, and lymphadenopathy, constipation, dizziness, nausea
Occasional
Headache, hair growth, insomnia, muscle twitching

■ **Serious Reactions**
- Abrupt withdrawal may precipitate status epilepticus.
- Blood dyscrasias, lymphadenopathy, and osteomalacia, caused by interference of vitamin D metabolism, may occur.
- Toxic phenytoin blood concentration of 25 mcg/ml may produce ataxia, characterized by muscular incoordination, nystagmus or rhythmic oscillation of eyes, and double vision. As level increases, extreme lethargy to comatose states occurs.

Special Considerations
- Prodrug, fosphenytoin rapidly converted to phenytoin in vivo: minimal activity before conversion; water soluble, thus more suitable for parenteral applications: does not require cardiac monitoring; can be administered at faster rate; no IV filter required; compatible with both saline and dextrose mixtures; requires refrigeration

■ **Patient/Family Education**
- Do not abruptly discontinue phenytoin after long-term use because doing so may precipitate seizures; strict maintenance of drug therapy is essential for control of seizures and arrhythmias
- IV injection may cause pain
- Maintain good oral hygiene, including gum massage and regular dental visits, to prevent gingival hyperplasia, marked by bleeding, swelling, and tenderness of gums
- Undergo a CBC every month for 1 year after the maintenance dose is established and every 3 mo thereafter
- Avoid tasks that require mental alertness or motor skills until response to the drug is established; drowsiness usually diminishes with continued therapy
- Notify the physician if fever, swollen glands, sore throat, a skin reaction, or signs of hematologic toxicity (such as a bleeding tendency, bruising, fatigue, or fever) occurs
- Avoid alcohol while taking phenytoin

■ **Monitoring Parameters**
- Therapeutic range 10-20 mcg/ml; nystagmus appears at 20 mcg/ml, ataxia at 30 mcg/ml, dysarthria and lethargy at levels above 40 mcg/ml; lethal dose 2-5g
- Blood pressure (with IV use), CBC, and renal and hepatic function

- Be alert for signs of IV phenytoin toxicity, such as cardiovascular collapse and CNS depression
- Signs of clinical improvement, such as a decrease in the frequency or intensity of seizures

■ Geriatric side effects at a glance:
☑ CNS ☐ Bowel Dysfunction ☐ Bladder Dysfunction ☐ Falls
Other: Osteoporosis

■ Use with caution in older patients with: Cognitive impairment, Hepatic impairment, End-stage renal disease, Hypoalbuminemia, Bradycardia, 2nd or 3rd degree heart block, Severe cardiovascular disease (when using IV), Osteoporosis, Unsteady gait, Urinary incontinence

■ U.S. Regulatory Considerations
☐ FDA Black Box ☐ OBRA regulated in U.S. Long Term Care

■ Other Uses in Geriatric Patient: Peripheral neuropathy

■ Side Effects:
Of particular importance in the geriatric patient: Delirium, confusion, cognitive impairment, amnesia, sedation, lethargy, ataxia, hypotension (with IV), osteomalacia, folate deficiency

■ Geriatric Considerations - Summary: Clearance may be reduced up to 20% in older adults; therefore lower doses are generally needed to achieve therapeutic serum concentrations. Nonlinear kinetics make dosing adjustments difficult, as small changes in dose can lead to large changes in serum concentration. When monitoring serum levels, correct for albumin levels if the patient's serum albumin is less than 4; monitoring the free fraction of phenytoin is preferred. Phenytoin may reduce bone mineral density by interfering with vitamin D catabolism. Calcium and vitamin D supplementation and monitoring of bone mineral density is recommended. Phenytoin is associated with numerous drug interactions and high incidence of CNS adverse effects. Comparative studies have shown that phenytoin has a greater effect on cognition than carbamazepine and valproic acid and may exacerbate preexisting cognitive deficits.

■ References:
1. Brodie M, Kwan P. Epilepsy in elderly people. BMJ 2005;331:1317-1322.
2. Ensrud KE, Walczak TS, Blackwell T, et. al. Antiepileptic drug use increases rates of bone loss in older women: a prospective study. Neurology 2004;62:2051-2057.
3. Arroyo S, Kramer G. Treating epilepsy in the elderly: safety considerations. Drug Saf 2001;24:991-1015.
4. Drugs that may cause cognitive disorders in the elderly. Med Let 2000;42:111-112.
5. Faught E. Epidemiolgy and drug treatment of epilepsy in elderly people. Drugs Aging 1999;15:255-269.

phosphorated carbohydrate solution

■ **Brand Name(s):** Emetrol
   Chemical Class: Hyperosmolar carbohydrate with phosphoric acid

■ **Clinical Pharmacology:**
   Mechanism of Action: An antiemetic whose mechanism of action has not been determined. Phosphorated carbohydrate solution consists of fructose, dextrose, and phosphoric acid, and may directly act on the wall of the gastrointestinal (GI) tract and reduce smooth muscle contraction and delay gastric emptying time through high osmotic pressure exerted by the solution of simple sugars. **Therapeutic Effect:** Relieves nausea and vomiting.
   Pharmacokinetics: *Fructose* Fructose is slowly absorbed from the GI tract. Metabolized in liver by phosphorylation and partly converted to liver glycogen and glucose. Excreted in urine.: *Dextrose* Dextrose is rapidly absorbed from GI tract. Distributed and stored throughout tissues. Metabolized in liver to carbon dioxide and water.

■ **Available Forms:**
   • *Solution*: 1.87g fructose/1.87g dextrose/21.5 mg phosphoric acid/5 ml (Emetrol).

■ **Indications and Dosages:**
   Antiemetic: PO 15-30 ml initially. May repeat dose every 15 minutes until distress subsides. Maximum: 5 doses in a 1-hr period

■ **Contraindications:** Symptoms of appendicitis or inflamed bowel, hereditary fructose intolerance, hypersensitivity to any component of the formulation

■ **Side Effects**
   Frequent
   Diarrhea, abdominal pain

■ **Serious Reactions**
   • Fructose intolerance includes symptoms of fainting, swelling of face, arms and legs, unusual bleeding, vomiting, weight loss, and yellow eyes and skin.

■ **Patient/Family Education**
   • Seek medical attention if symptoms are not relieved or recur frequently
   • Notify the physician if headache or persistent vomiting occurs

■ **Monitoring Parameters**
   • Bowel sounds for peristalsis; pattern of daily bowel activity and stool consistency

■ **Geriatric side effects at a glance:**
   ❑ CNS   ☑ Bowel Dysfunction   ❑ Bladder Dysfunction   ❑ Falls

physostigmine

(fi-zoe-stig'-meen)

■ **Brand Name(s):** Antilirium
   Chemical Class: Alkaloid; cholinesterase inhibitor; tertiary ammonium compound

■ **Clinical Pharmacology:**
   Mechanism of Action: A cholinergic that inhibits destruction of acetylcholine by enzyme acetylcholinesterase, thus enhancing impulse transmission across the myoneural junction. **Therapeutic Effect:** Improves skeletal muscle tone, stimulates salivary and sweat gland secretions.
   Pharmacokinetics: Penetrates blood-brain barrier. Rapidly hydrolyzed by cholinesterases. Small amount eliminated in urine; largely destroyed in body by hydrolysis. **Half-life:** Unknown.

■ **Available Forms:**
   • *Injection*: 1 mg/ml.

■ **Indications and Dosages:**
   To reverse CNS effects of anticholinergic drugs and tricyclic antidepressants: IV, IM Initially, 0.5–2 mg. If no response, repeat q20min until response or adverse cholinergic effects occur. If initial response occurs, may give additional doses of 1–4 mg q30-60min as life-threatening signs, such as arrhythmias, seizures, and deep coma, recur.

■ **Unlabeled Uses:** Treatment of hereditary ataxia

■ **Contraindications:** Active uveal inflammation, angle-closure glaucoma before iridectomy, asthma, cardiovascular disease, concurrent use of ganglionic-blocking agents, diabetes, gangrene, glaucoma associated with iridocyclitis, hypersensitivity to cholinesterase inhibitors or their components, mechanical obstruction of intestinal or urogenital tract, vagotonic state

■ **Side Effects**
   Expected
   Miosis, increased GI and skeletal muscle tone, bradycardia
   Occasional
   Marked drop in blood pressure (hypertensive patients)
   Rare
   Allergic reaction

■ **Serious Reactions**
   • Parenteral overdose produces a cholinergic crisis manifested as abdominal discomfort or cramps, nausea, vomiting, diarrhea, flushing, facial warmth, excessive salivation, diaphoresis, urinary urgency, and blurred vision. If overdose occurs, stop all anticholinergic drugs and immediately administer 0.6–1.2 mg atropine sulfate IM or IV.

* Atropine is antidote

■ **Patient/Family Education**
* The drug's adverse effects usually subside after the first few days of therapy
* Avoid driving at night and activities requiring visual acuity in dim light during physostigmine therapy

■ **Monitoring Parameters**
* Vital signs immediately before and every 15-30 min after physostigmine administration
* Monitor the patient for cholinergic reactions, such as abdominal pain, dyspnea, hypotension, arrhythmias, muscle weakness, and diaphoresis, after drug administration

■ **Geriatric side effects at a glance:**
❑ CNS ❑ Bowel Dysfunction ❑ Bladder Dysfunction ❑ Falls

■ **U.S. Regulatory Considerations**
❑ FDA Black Box ❑ OBRA regulated in U.S. Long Term Care

pilocarpine hydrochloride

(pye-loe-kar'-peen hye-droe-klor'-ide)

■ **Brand Name(s):** Adsorbocarpine, Akarpine, Isopto Carpine, Ocu-Carpine, Ocusert, Pilagan with C Cap, Pilocar, Pilopine-HS, Piloptic-HS, Piloptic-1, Piloptic-1/2, Piloptic-2, Piloptic-3, Piloptic-4, Piloptic-6, Pilostat, Salagen

Combinations
Rx: with epinephrine (E-Pilo-6)
Chemical Class: Choline ester

■ **Clinical Pharmacology:**
Mechanism of Action: A cholinergic parasympathomimetic that increases exocrine gland secretions by stimulating cholinergic receptors. Acts through direct stimulation of muscarinic neuroreceptors and smooth muscles such as the iris and secretory glands. Contracts the iris sphincter, causing increased tension on the scleral spur and opening of the trabecular meshwork spaces to facilitate outflow of aqueous humor.
Therapeutic Effect: Improves symptoms of dry mouth in patients with salivary gland hypofunction. Produces miosis. Lowers intraocular pressure (IOP).
Pharmacokinetics:

Route	Onset	Peak	Duration
PO	20 min	1 hr	3-5 hr
Ophthalmic	10-30 min	75 min - 2 hr	4-14 hr

Absorption decreased if taken with a high-fat meal. Inactivation of pilocarpine thought to occur at neuronal synapses and probably in plasma. Excreted in urine.
Half-life: 4-12 hr.

■ **Available Forms:**
- *Tablets (Salagen)*: 5 mg.
- *Ophthalmic Gel (Pilopine-HS)*: 4%.
- *Ophthalmic Solution*: 0.25% (Isopto Carpine), 0.5% (Ocu-Carpine, Pilostat, Piloptic-1/2, Pilocar), 1% (Ocu-Carpine, Pilocar, Piloptic-1, Pilostat), 2% (Akarpine, Ocu-Carpine, Pilocar, Piloptic-2), 3% (Ocu-Carpine, Pilocar, Piloptic-3, Pilostat), 4% (Akarpine, Isopto Carpine, Ocu-Carpine, Pilocar, Piloptic-4, Pilostat), 5% (Isopto Carpine, Ocu-Carpine), 6% (Isopto Carpine, Ocu-Carpine, Pilocar, Piloptic-6, Pilostat), 8% (Isopto Carpine).
- *Ophthalmic Solution, Nitrate (Pilagan with C Cap)*: 1%, 4%.

■ **Indications and Dosages:**
Dry mouth associated with radiation treatment for head and neck cancer: PO 5 mg three times a day. Range: 15-30 mg/day. Maximum: 2 tablets/dose.
Dry mouth associated with Sjögren's syndrome: PO 5 mg four times a day. Range: 20–40 mg/day.
Glaucoma: Ophthalmic 1-2 drops to affected eye(s) up to 4 times a day.
Miosis induction: Ophthalmic 1-2 drops to affected eye(s) up to 4 times a day.
Dosage in hepatic impairment: Dosage decreased to 5 mg twice a day for hepatic impairment.

■ **Contraindications:** Conditions in which miosis is undesirable, such as acute iritis and angle-closure glaucoma; uncontrolled asthma

■ **Side Effects**
Frequent
Oral: Diaphoresis
Ophthalmic: Stinging, burning
Occasional
Oral: Headache, dizziness, urinary frequency, flushing, dyspepsia, nausea, asthenia, lacrimation, visual disturbances
Ophthalmic: Blurred vision, itching of eye
Rare
Oral: Diarrhea, abdominal pain, peripheral edema, chills
Ophthalmic: Lens opacity

■ **Serious Reactions**
- Patients with diaphoresis who don't drink enough fluids may develop dehydration.
- Retinal detachment has been reported.

Special Considerations
- Antidote is atropine

■ **Patient/Family Education**
- Miotics cause poor dark adaptation; use caution with night driving
- Drink plenty of fluids
- Avoid tasks that require mental alertness or motor skills until response to the drug has been established

■ **Monitoring Parameters**
- Pattern of daily bowel activity and stool consistency
- Urinary frequency
- Monitor for signs of dehydration, such as decreased skin turgor, and dizziness

- **Geriatric side effects at a glance:**
  ☑ CNS ☐ Bowel Dysfunction ☐ Bladder Dysfunction ☐ Falls

- **U.S. Regulatory Considerations**
  ☐ FDA Black Box ☐ OBRA regulated in U.S. Long Term Care

pimecrolimus

(pim-e-kroe'-li-mus)

- **Brand Name(s):** Elidel
  Chemical Class: Ascomycin derivative

- **Clinical Pharmacology:**
  Mechanism of Action: An immunomodulator that inhibits release of cytokine, an enzyme that produces an inflammatory reaction. **Therapeutic Effect:** Produces anti-inflammatory activity.
  Pharmacokinetics: Minimal systemic absorption with topical application. Metabolized in liver. Excreted in feces.

- **Available Forms:**
  - Cream: 1% (Elidel).

- **Indications and Dosages:**
  Atopic dermatitis (eczema): Topical Apply to affected area twice daily for up to 3 weeks (up to 6 weeks in adolescents, children 2-17 yr). Rub in gently and completely.

- **Unlabeled Uses:** Allergic contact dermatitis, irritant contact dermatitis, psoriasis

- **Contraindications:** Hypersensitivity to pimecrolimus or any component of the formulation, Netherton's syndrome (potential for increased systemic absorption), application to active cutaneous viral infections.

- **Side Effects**
  Rare
  Transient application-site sensation of burning or feeling of heat

- **Serious Reactions**
  - Lymphadenopathy and phototoxicity occur rarely.

Special Considerations
  - May be associated with increased risk of varicella-zoster virus infection, herpes simplex virus infection, or eczema herpeticum

- **Patient/Family Education**
  - Do not use with occlusive dressings
  - Wash hands after application

- Minimize exposure to artificial sunlight or tanning beds

■ **Monitoring Parameters**
  - Therapeutic response

■ **Geriatric side effects at a glance:**
  ❑ CNS   ❑ Bowel Dysfunction   ❑ Bladder Dysfunction   ❑ Falls

■ **U.S. Regulatory Considerations**
  ❑ FDA Black Box   ❑ OBRA regulated in U.S. Long Term Care

pimozide

(pi'-moe-zide)

■ **Brand Name(s):** Orap
  Chemical Class: Diphenylbutylpiperidine derivative

■ **Clinical Pharmacology:**
  Mechanism of Action: A diphenylbutylpiperidine that blocks dopamine at postsynaptic receptor sites in the brain. **Therapeutic Effect:** Suppresses behavioral response in psychosis and decreases abnormal movements associated with Tourette's syndrome.

■ **Available Forms:**
  - *Tablets*: 1 mg, 2 mg.

■ **Indications and Dosages:**
  Tourette's syndrome: PO 1-2 mg/day in divided doses 3 times/day. Maximum: 10 mg/day.

■ **Contraindications:** Aggressive schizophrenics when sedation is required, concurrent administration of pemoline, methylphenidate or amphetamines, concurrent administration of dofetilide, sotalol, quinidine, other Class IA and III antiarrhythmics, mesoridazine, thioridazine, chlorpromazine, droperidol, sparfloxacin, gatifloxacin, moxifloxacin, halofantrine, mefloquine, pentamidine, arsenic trioxide, levomethadyl acetate, dolasetron mesylate, probucol, tacrolimus, ziprasidone, sertraline, macrolide antibiotics, drugs that cause QT prolongation, and less potent inhibitors of CYP3A, congenital or drug-induced long QT syndrome, doses greater than 10 mg daily, history of cardiac arrhythmias, Parkinson's disease, patients with known hypokalemia or hypomagnesemia, severe central nervous system depression, simple tics or tics not associated with Tourette's syndrome, hypersensitivity to pimozide or any of its components

■ **Side Effects**
  Occasional
  Akathisia, dystonic extrapyramidal effects, parkinsonian extrapyramidal effects, tardive dyskinesia, blurred vision, ocular changes, constipation, decreased sweating, dry mouth, nasal congestion, dizziness, drowsiness, orthostatic hypotension, urinary retention, somnolence

Rare
Rash, cholestatic jaundice, priapism

■ **Serious Reactions**
- Serious reactions such as blood dyscrasias, agranulocytosis, leukocytopenia, thrombocytopenia, cholestatic jaundice, neuroleptic malignant syndrome (NMS), constipation or paralytic ileus, priapism, QT prolongation and torsades de pointes, seizure, systemic lupus erythematosus-like syndrome, and temperature regulation dysfunction (heatstroke or hypothermia) occur rarely.
- Abrupt withdrawal following long-term therapy may precipitate nausea, vomiting, gastritis, dizziness, and tremors.

■ **Patient/Family Education**
- Notify the physician if fast or irregular heartbeat, fast breathing, fever, severe muscle stiffness, muscle spasms, twitching, or uncontrolled tongue or jaw movement occurs
- Do not abruptly discontinue the drug after long-term therapy
- Drowsiness usually subsides during continued therapy
- Avoid alcohol

■ **Monitoring Parameters**
- ECG
- Blood pressure

■ **Geriatric side effects at a glance:**
☑ CNS ☑ Bowel Dysfunction ☐ Bladder Dysfunction ☑ Falls
Other: Orthostatic hypotension, cardiac conduction disturbances, torsades de pointes, anticholinergic side effects

■ **Use with caution in older patients with:** Parkinson's disease (an atypical antipsychotic is recommended), seizure disorders, cardiovascular disease with conduction disturbance, hepatic encephalopathy, narrow-angle glaucoma, congenital prolonged Q-T syndrome or drugs which prolong Q-T interval.

■ **U.S. Regulatory Considerations**
☐ FDA Black Box ☑ OBRA regulated in U.S. Long Term Care

■ **Other Uses in Geriatric Patient:** Behavior disturbances in the setting of dementia

■ **Side Effects:**
Of particular importance in the geriatric patient: Tardive dyskinesia, akathisia (may appear to exacerbate behavioral disturbances), anticholinergic effects, may increase risk of sudden death

■ **Geriatric Considerations - Summary:** Sink and colleagues' systematic review showed statistically significant improvements on neuropsychiatric and behavioral scales for some drugs, but improvements were small and unlikely to be clinically important. Because of documented risks, and uncertain benefits, these agents should be used with caution in demented elderly persons, with frequent monitoring for side effects and a low threshold for discontinuing use.

References:
1. Leipzig RM, Cumming RG, Tinetti ME. Drugs and falls in older people: a systematic review and meta-analysis: I. Psychotropic drugs. J Am Geriatr Soc 1999;47:30-39.
2. Sink KM, Holden KF, Yaffe K. Pharmacological treatment of neuropsychiatric symptoms of dementia: a review of the evidence. JAMA 2005;293:596-608.
3. Ray WA, Meredith S, Thapa PB, et al. Antipsychotics and the risk of sudden cardiac death. Arch Gen Psychiatry 2001;58:1161-1167.

pindolol

(pin'-doe-loll)

■ **Brand Name(s):** Visken
  Chemical Class: β-Adrenergic blocker, nonselective

■ **Clinical Pharmacology:**
  Mechanism of Action: A nonselective beta-blocker that blocks $beta_1$- and $beta_2$-adrenergic receptors. **Therapeutic Effect:** Slows heart rate, decreases cardiac output, decreases blood pressure (BP), and exhibits antiarrhythmic activity. Decreases myocardial ischemia severity by decreasing oxygen requirements.
  Pharmacokinetics: Completely absorbed from GI tract. Metabolized in liver. Primarily excreted in urine. **Half-life:** 3-4 hr (half-life increased with imparied renal function, elderly).

■ **Available Forms:**
  • *Capsules*: 5 mg, 10 mg.

■ **Indications and Dosages:**
  Usual elderly dosage: PO Initially, 5 mg/day. May increase by 5 mg q3-4 wk.

■ **Unlabeled Uses:** Treatment of chronic angina pectoris, hypertrophic cardiomyopathy, tremors, and mitral valve prolapse syndrome. Increases antidepressant effect with fluoxetine and other SSRIs.

■ **Contraindications:** Bronchial asthma, COPD, uncontrolled cardiac failure, sinus bradycardia, heart block greater than first degree, cardiogenic shock, CHF (unless secondary to tachyarrhythmias)

■ **Side Effects**
  Frequent
  Decreased sexual ability, drowsiness, trouble sleeping, unusual tiredness/weakness
  Occasional
  Bradycardia, depression, cold hands/feet, diarrhea, constipation, anxiety, nasal congestion, nausea, vomiting
  Rare
  Altered taste, dry eyes, itching, numbness of fingers, toes, and scalp

993

■ Serious Reactions
- Overdosage may produce profound bradycardia and hypotension.
- Abrupt withdrawal may result in sweating, palpitations, headache, and tremulousness.
- May precipitate congestive heart failure or myocardial infarction in patients with heart disease; thyroid storm in those with thyrotoxicosis; or peripheral ischemia in those with existing peripheral vascular disease.
- Hypoglycemia may occur in previously controlled diabetics.
- Signs of thrombocytopenia, such as unusual bleeding or bruising, occur rarely.

Special Considerations
- Abrupt discontinuation may precipitate angina; taper over 1-2 wk
- Effective antihypertensive and probably antianginal agent (though not approved for this indication), especially for patients who develop symptomatic bradycardia with beta-blockade

■ Patient/Family Education
- Do not abruptly discontinue the drug
- Report excessive fatigue, headache, prolonged dizziness, shortness of breath or weight gain
- Avoid nasal decongestants or OTC cold preparations (stimulants) without physician approval
- Avoid salt and alcohol intake

■ Monitoring Parameters
- *Angina*: Reduction in nitroglycerin usage; frequency, severity, onset, and duration of angina pain; heart rate
- *Hypertension*: Blood pressure
- *Toxicity*: Blood glucose, bronchospasm, hypotension, bradycardia, depression, confusion, hallucination, sexual dysfunction

■ Geriatric side effects at a glance:
❑ CNS   ❑ Bowel Dysfunction   ❑ Bladder Dysfunction   ❑ Falls

■ U.S. Regulatory Considerations
☑ FDA Black Box
In patients using orally administered beta-blockers, abrupt withdrawal may precipitate angina or lead to myocardial infarction or ventricular arrhythmias.
❑ OBRA regulated in U.S. Long Term Care

pioglitazone hydrochloride

(pye-oh-gli'-ta-zone hye-droe-klor'-ide)

■ **Brand Name(s):** Actos
 Chemical Class: Thiazolidinedione

■ **Clinical Pharmacology:**
 Mechanism of Action: An antidiabetic that improves target-cell response to insulin without increasing pancreatic insulin secretion. Decreases hepatic glucose output and increases insulin-dependent glucose utilization in skeletal muscle. **Therapeutic Effect:** Lowers blood glucose concentration.
 Pharmacokinetics: Rapidly absorbed. Highly protein bound (99%), primarily to albumin. Metabolized in the liver. Excreted in urine. Unknown if removed by hemodialysis. **Half-life:** 16–24 hr.

■ **Available Forms:**
 • *Tablets*: 15 mg, 30 mg, 45 mg.

■ **Indications and Dosages:**
 Diabetes mellitus, combination therapy: PO With insulin: Initially, 15–30 mg once a day. Initially, continue current insulin dosage; then decrease insulin dosage by 10% to 25% if hypoglycemia occurs or plasma glucose level decreases to less than 100 mg/dl. Maximum: 45 mg/day. With sulfonylureas: Initially, 15–30 mg/day. Decrease sulfonylurea dosage if hypoglycemia occurs. With metformin: Initially, 15–30 mg/day. As monotherapy: Monotherapy is not to be used if patient is well controlled with diet and exercise alone. Initially, 15–30 mg/day. May increase dosage in increments until 45 mg/day is reached.

■ **Contraindications:** Active hepatic disease; diabetic ketoacidosis; increased serum transaminase levels, including ALT greater than 2.5 times normal serum level; type 1 diabetes mellitus

■ **Side Effects**
 Frequent (13%–9%)
 Headache, upper respiratory tract infection
 Occasional (6%–5%)
 Sinusitis, myalgia, pharyngitis, aggravated diabetes mellitus

■ **Serious Reactions**
 • Hepatotoxicity occurs rarely.

Special Considerations
 • Expected hypoglycemic effects: Decreases in serum glucose: 50-75 mg/dL; decreases in hemoglobin A_{1c}: 1.2-1.5%

■ **Patient/Family Education**
 • Caloric restriction, weight loss, and exercise are essential adjuvant therapy

- Blood draws for LFT monitoring along with routine diabetes mellitus labs. Review symptoms of hepatitis (unexplained nausea, vomiting, abdominal pain, fatigue, anorexia, or dark urine)
- Notify clinician for rapid increases in weight or edema or symptoms of heart failure (shortness of breath, nocturia)
- Review hypoglycemia risks and symptoms when added to other hypoglycemic agents
- Avoid alcohol
- The prescribed diet is a principal part of treatment

■ **Monitoring Parameters**
- Diabetes mellitus symptoms, periodic serum glucose and HbA_{1c} measurements; LFT (AST, ALT) prior to initiation of therapy and periodically thereafter; hemoglobin/hematocrit, signs and symptoms of heart failure

■ **Geriatric side effects at a glance:**
☐ CNS   ☐ Bowel Dysfunction   ☐ Bladder Dysfunction   ☐ Falls
Other: Edema

■ **Use with caution in older patients with:** CHF, CAD, NYHA Class III or IV, Hepatic impairment (avoid if ALT > 2.5 times the upper limit of normal)

■ **U.S. Regulatory Considerations**
☐ FDA Black Box   ☐ OBRA regulated in U.S. Long Term Care

■ **Other Uses in Geriatric Patient:** None

■ **Side Effects:**
Of particular importance in the geriatric patient: Edema, weight gain, anemia

■ **Geriatric Considerations - Summary:** Fluid retention may lead to mild CHF in patients with CAD and unrecognized or compensated heart failure. Discontinue drug with any sign of decline in cardiac function. Avoid in older adults with NYHA Class III or IV cardiac status. Demonstrated effectiveness in patients 65 years of age and older.

■ **References:**
1. Haas L. Management of diabetes mellitus medications in the nursing home. Drugs Aging 2005;22:209-218.
2. Rajagopalan R, Perez A, Ye Z, et. al. Pioglitazone is effective therapy for elderly patients with type 2 diabetes mellitus. Drugs Aging 2004;21:259-271.
3. Rosenstock J. Management of type 2 diabetes mellitus in the elderly: special considerations. Drugs Aging 2001;18:31-44.

piperacillin sodium/ tazobactam sodium

(pi-per'-a-sill-in soe'-dee-um/ta-zoe-bak'-tam soe'-dee-um)

■ **Brand Name(s):** *Piperacillin/tazobactam*: Zosyn; *Piperacillin*: Pipracil

■ **Brand Name(s):** *Piperacillin/tazobactam*: Zosyn
  Chemical Class: Penicillin derivative, extended-spectrum; β-lactamase inhibitor (tazobactam)

■ **Clinical Pharmacology:**
  Mechanism of Action: Piperacillin inhibits cell wall synthesis by binding to bacterial cell membranes. Tazobactam inactivates bacterial beta-lactamase. **Therapeutic Effect:** Piperacillin is bactericidal in susceptible organisms. Tazobactam protects piperacillin from enzymatic degradation, extends its spectrum of activity, and prevents bacterial overgrowth.
  Pharmacokinetics: Protein binding: 16%-30%. Widely distributed. Primarily excreted unchanged in urine. Removed by hemodialysis. **Half-life:** 0.7-1.2 hr (increased in hepatic cirrhosis and impaired renal function).

■ **Available Forms (piperacillin/tazobactam):**
  • *Alert* Piperacillin/tazobactam is a combination product in an 8:1 ratio of piperacillin to tazobactam.
  • *Powder for Injection*: 2.25 g, 3.375 g, 4.5 g.
  • *Premix Ready to Use*: 2.25 g, 3.375 g, 4.5 g.

■ **Indications and Dosages (piperacillin/tazobactam):**
  Severe infections: IV 4 g/0.5 g q8h or 3 g/0.375 g q6h. Maximum: 18 g/2.25 g daily.
  Moderate infections: IV 2 g/0.225g q6–8h.
  Dosage in renal impairment: Dosage and frequency are modified based on creatinine clearance.

Creatinine Clearance	Dosage
20-40 ml/min	8 g/1 g/day (2.25g q6h)
less than 20 ml/min	6 g/0.75 g/day (2.25g q8h)

  Dosage in hemodialysis patients: IV 2.25g q8h with additional dose of 0.75g after each dialysis session.

■ **Contraindications:** Hypersensitivity to any penicillin, cephalosporins, or beta-lactamase inhibitors

■ **Side Effects**
  Frequent
  Diarrhea, headache, constipation, nausea, insomnia, rash
  Occasional
  Vomiting, dyspepsia, pruritus, fever, agitation, candidiasis, dizziness, abdominal pain, edema, anxiety, dyspnea, rhinitis

- **Serious Reactions**
  - Antibiotic-associated colitis and other superinfections may result from altered bacterial balance.
  - Seizures and other neurologic reactions are more likely to occur in patients with renal impairment and those who have received an overdose.
  - Severe hypersensitivity reactions, including anaphylaxis, occur rarely.

Special Considerations
  - Preferred over mezlocillin, more effective against *Pseudomonas,* reserve for carbenicillin- or ticarcillin-resistant *P. aeruginosa* infections in combination with an aminoglycoside
  - Individualize treatment based on local susceptibility patterns.

- **Patient/Family Education**
  - Notify the physician if severe diarrhea occurs and avoid taking antidiarrheals until directed to do so
  - Notify the physician if pain, redness, or swelling occurs at the infusion site
  - Reduce salt intake because piperacillin contains sodium

- **Monitoring Parameters**
  - Electrolyte levels (especially potassium), intake and output, renal function test results, and urinalysis results
  - Pattern of daily bowel activity and stool consistency; mild GI effects may be tolerable, but severe symptoms may indicate the onset of antibiotic-associated colitis
  - Be alert for signs and symptoms of superinfection, including abdominal pain, moderate to severe diarrhea, severe anal or genital pruritus, and stomatitis

- **Geriatric side effects at a glance:**
  ☐ CNS ☑ Bowel Dysfunction ☐ Bladder Dysfunction ☐ Falls

- **U.S. Regulatory Considerations**
  ☐ FDA Black Box ☐ OBRA regulated in U.S. Long Term Care

pirbuterol acetate

(peer-byoo'-ter-ole ass'-eh-tayte)

- **Brand Name(s):** Maxair, Maxair Autohaler
  Chemical Class: Sympathomimetic amine; β_2-adrenergic agonist

- **Clinical Pharmacology:**
  Mechanism of Action: A sympathomimetic, adrenergic agonist, that stimulates beta$_2$-adrenergic receptors in the lungs, resulting in relaxation of bronchial smooth muscle.
  Therapeutic Effect: Relieves bronchospasm, reduces airway resistance.
  Pharmacokinetics: Absorbed from bronchi following inhalation. Metabolized in liver. Primarily excreted in urine. Unknown if removed by hemodialysis. **Half-life:** 2-3 hr.

- **Available Forms:**
  - *Oral Inhalation:* 0.2 mg/actuation (Maxair Autohaler).

- **Indications and Dosages:**
  Prevention of bronchospasm: Inhalation 2 inhalations q4-6h. Maximum: 12 inhalations daily.
  Treatment of bronchospasm: Inhalation 2 inhalations separated by at least 1-3 minutes, followed by a third inhalation. Maximum: 12 inhalations daily.

- **Contraindications:** History of hypersensitivity to pirbuterol, albuterol, or any of its components

- **Side Effects**
  Occasional (7%-1%)
  Nervousness, tremor, headache, palpitations, nausea, dizziness, tachycardia, cough

- **Serious Reactions**
  - Excessive sympathomimetic stimulation may produce palpitations, extrasystoles, tachycardia, chest pain, slight increases in BP followed by a substantial decrease, chills, sweating and blanching of skin.
  - Too frequent or excessive use may lead to loss of bronchodilating effectiveness and severe, paradoxical bronchoconstriction.

Special Considerations

- No significant advantage over other selective β_2-agonists

- **Patient/Family Education**
  - Initial and periodic reviews of metered dose inhaler technique
  - Increase fluid intake to decrease the viscosity of pulmonary secretions
  - Rinse mouth immediately after inhalation to prevent mouth and throat dryness
  - Avoid excessive use of caffeine derivatives, such as chocolate, cocoa, coffee, cola, and tea

- **Monitoring Parameters**
  - Depth, rate, rhythm, and type of respirations
  - Quality and rate of pulse

- **Geriatric side effects at a glance:**
  ❑ CNS ❑ Bowel Dysfunction ❑ Bladder Dysfunction ❑ Falls

- **U.S. Regulatory Considerations**
  ❑ FDA Black Box ❑ OBRA regulated in U.S. Long Term Care

piroxicam

(peer-ox'-i-kam)

■ **Brand Name(s):** Feldene
  Chemical Class: Oxicam derivative

■ **Clinical Pharmacology:**
  Mechanism of Action: An NSAID that produces analgesic and anti-inflammatory effects by inhibiting prostaglandin synthesis. **Therapeutic Effect:** Reduces inflammatory response and intensity of pain.
  Pharmacokinetics: Well absorbed following oral administration. Protein binding: 99%. Extensively metabolized in liver. Primarily excreted in urine; small amount eliminated in feces. **Half-life:** 50 hr.

■ **Available Forms:**
  • *Capsules:* 10 mg, 20 mg.

■ **Indications and Dosages:**
  Acute or chronic rheumatoid arthritis and osteoarthritis: PO Initially, 10–20 mg/day as a single dose or in divided doses. Some patients may require up to 30–40 mg/day.

■ **Unlabeled Uses:** Treatment of acute gouty arthritis, ankylosing spondylitis

■ **Contraindications:** Active peptic ulcer disease, chronic inflammation of the GI tract, GI bleeding or ulceration, history of hypersensitivity to aspirin or NSAIDs

■ **Side Effects**
  Frequent (9%–4%)
  Dyspepsia, nausea, dizziness
  Occasional (3%–1%)
  Diarrhea, constipation, abdominal cramps or pain, flatulence, stomatitis
  Rare (less than 1%)
  Hypertension, urticaria, dysuria, ecchymosis, blurred vision, insomnia, phototoxicity

■ **Serious Reactions**
  • Rare reactions with long-term use include peptic ulcer disease, GI bleeding, gastritis, severe hepatic reaction (cholestasis, jaundice), nephrotoxicity (dysuria, hematuria, proteinuria, nephrotic syndrome), hematologic sensitivity (anemia, leukopenia, eosinophilia, thrombocytopenia), and a severe hypersensitivity reaction (fever, chills, bronchospasm).

Special Considerations
  • Similar in efficacy to the other NSAIDs but has the advantage and disadvantage of an extended t½; high GI toxicity potential

■ **Patient/Family Education**
  • Take piroxicam with food, milk, or antacids if GI upset occurs

- Avoid tasks that require mental alertness or motor skills until response to the drug has been established
- Avoid alcohol and aspirin during piroxicam therapy because these substances increase the risk of GI bleeding

■ Monitoring Parameters
- Initial hematocrit and fecal occult blood test within 3 mo of starting regular chronic therapy; repeat every 6-12 mo (more frequently in high-risk patients (>65 years, peptic ulcer disease, concurrent steroids or anticoagulants); electrolytes, creatinine, and BUN within 3 mo of starting regular chronic therapy; repeat every 6-12 mo
- Therapeutic response, such as improved grip strength, increased joint mobility, and decreased pain, tenderness, stiffness, and swelling
- Pattern of daily bowel activity and stool consistency

■ Geriatric side effects at a glance:
☑ CNS   ❑ Bowel Dysfunction   ❑ Bladder Dysfunction   ❑ Falls
☑ Other: Gastropathy

■ Use with caution in older patients with: Renal impairment, Hepatic impairment, CHF, HTN, PUD, History of GI bleeding, GERD, Bleeding and platelet disorders, History of aspirin sensitivity reaction. Also use with caution in patients taking Anticoagulants, Aspirin, and Antihypertensive agents.

■ U.S. Regulatory Considerations
☑ FDA Black Box
- Cardiovascular risk
- Gastrointestinal risk
❑ OBRA regulated in U.S. Long Term Care

■ Other Uses in Geriatric Patient: Acute gout

■ Side Effects:
Of particular importance in the geriatric patient: Confusion, cognitive impairment, delirium, dizziness, dyspepsia, fluid retention, renal impairment

■ Geriatric Considerations - Summary: Use of NSAIDs in older adults increases the risk of GI complications including gastric ulceration, bleeding, and perforation. These complications are not necessarily preceded by less severe GI symptoms. Concomitant use of a proton pump inhibitor or misoprostol reduces the risk for gastric ulceration and bleeding, but may not prevent long-term GI toxicity.

■ References:
1. COX-2 alternatives and GI protection. Med Lett Drugs Ther 2004;46:91.
2. Drugs that may cause cognitive disorders in the elderly. Med Lett Drugs Ther 2000;42:111-112.

plicamycin

(plye-ka-mye'-sin)

- **Brand Name(s):** Mithracin
  Chemical Class: Crystalline aglycone

- **Clinical Pharmacology:**
  Mechanism of Action: An antibiotic that forms complexes with DNA, inhibiting DNA-directed RNA synthesis. May inhibit parathyroid hormone effect on osteoclasts and inhibit bone resorption. **Therapeutic Effect:** Lowers serum calcium and phosphate levels. Blocks hypercalcemic action of vitamin D and action of parathyroid hormone. Decreases serum calcium.
  Pharmacokinetics:

Route	Onset	Peak	Duration
IV	1-2 days	2-3 days	3-15 days

  Protein binding: None. Greatest concentrations in liver, kidney, and formed bone surfaces. Crosses the blood-brain barrier and enters CSF. Primarily excreted in urine.

- **Available Forms:**
  - *Powder for Injection*: 2,500 mcg.

- **Indications and Dosages:**
  Testicular tumors: IV 25-30 mcg/kg/day for 8-10 days. Repeat at monthly intervals.
  Hypercalcemia, hyperuricemia: IV 25 mcg/kg as a single dose; may repeat in 48 hr if no response occurs. Or give 25 mcg/kg/day for 3-4 days or 25-50 mcg/kg/dose every other day for 3-8 doses.
  Paget's disease: IV 15 mcg/kg/day for 10 days.

- **Unlabeled Uses:** Treatment of Paget's disease refractory to other therapy

- **Contraindications:** Preexisting coagulation disorders, thrombocytopathy, thrombocytopenia, impaired bone marrow function, or tendency to hemorrhage

- **Side Effects**
  Frequent
  Nausea, vomiting, anorexia, diarrhea, stomatitis
  Occasional
  Fever, drowsiness, weakness, lethargy, malaise, headache, depression, nervousness, dizziness, rash, acne

- **Serious Reactions**
  - The risk of hematologic toxicity (characterized by marked facial flushing, persistent nosebleeds, hemoptysis, purpura, ecchymosis, leukopenia, and thrombocytopenia) increases with administration of high dosages or more than 10 doses.
  - Electrolyte imbalances may occur.

Special Considerations
  - Effective but also toxic; use is therefore limited; additive with other calcium lowering therapies

Patient/Family Education
- Maintain fastidious oral hygiene
- Do not have immunizations without physician's approval (drug lowers body's resistance)
- Avoid crowds, those with infection
- Promptly report fever, sore throat, signs of local infection, easy bruising, and unusual bleeding from any site
- Contact physician if nausea/vomiting continues at home

Monitoring Parameters
- CBC, differential, platelet count qwk; withhold drug if WBC is <4000/mm^3 or platelet count is <50,000/mm^3
- Renal function studies: BUN, serum uric acid, urine CrCl, electrolytes, input and output ratio
- Liver function tests: bilirubin, AST, ALT, alk phosphatase before and during therapy
- Monitor for stomatitis (burning/erythema of oral mucosa at inner margin of lips, sore throat, difficulty swallowing, oral ulceration)
- Monitor for thrombocytopenia (bleeding from gums, tarry stool, petechiae, small subcutaneous hemorrhages)

Geriatric side effects at a glance:
❏ CNS ☑ Bowel Dysfunction ❏ Bladder Dysfunction ❏ Falls

U.S. Regulatory Considerations
❏ FDA Black Box ❏ OBRA regulated in U.S. Long Term Care

podofilox

(po-doe-fil'-ox)

Brand Name(s): Condylox
Chemical Class: Podophyllum derivative

Clinical Pharmacology:
Mechanism of Action: An active component of podophyllin resin that binds to tubulin to prevent formation of microtubules resulting in mitotic arrest. Exercises many biologic effects such as damages endothelium of small blood vessels, attenuates nucleoside transport, suppresses immune responses, inhibits macrophage metabolism, induces interleukin-1 and interleukin-2, decreases lymphocyte response to mitogens, and enhances macrophage growth. **Therapeutic Effect:** Removes genital warts.
Pharmacokinetics: Time to peak occurs in 1-2 hr. Some degree of absorption. **Half-life:** 1-4.5 hr.

Available Forms:
- **Gel:** 0.5% (Condylox).
- **Solution:** 0.5% (Condylox).

- **Indications and Dosages:**
  Anogenital warts: Topical Apply 0.5% gel for 3 days, then withhold for 4 days. Repeat cycle up to 4 times.
  Genital warts (condylomata acuminata): Topical Apply 0.5% solution or gel q12h in the morning and evening for 3 days, then withhold for 4 days. Repeat cycle up to 4 times.

- **Contraindications:** Bleeding warts, moles, birthmarks, or unusual warts with hair; diabetes; poor blood circulation; steroid use; hypersensitivity to podofilox or any component of its formulation

- **Side Effects**
  Occasional
  Erosion, inflammation, itching, pain, burning
  Rare
  Nausea, vomiting

- **Serious Reactions**
  - Nausea and vomiting occur rarely and usually after cumulative doses.

Special Considerations
  - Safety preferred over podophyllum resin

- **Patient/Family Education**
  - Use a small amount of solution on the warts with a dry cotton-tipped swab

- **Monitoring Parameters**
  - Skin for burning, itching, and irritation

- **Geriatric side effects at a glance:**
  ☐ CNS ☐ Bowel Dysfunction ☐ Bladder Dysfunction ☐ Falls

- **U.S. Regulatory Considerations**
  ☐ FDA Black Box ☐ OBRA regulated in U.S. Long Term Care

podophyllum resin

(pode-oh-fill'-um rez'-in)

- **Brand Name(s):** (Podocon-25, Pododerm)
  Chemical Class: Podophyllum derivative

- **Clinical Pharmacology:**
  Mechanism of Action: A cytotoxic agent that directly affects epithelial cell metabolism by arresting mitosis through binding to a protein subunit of spindle microtubules.
  Therapeutic Effect: Removes soft genital warts.

Pharmacokinetics: Topical podophyllum is systemically absorbed. Absorption may be increased if applied to bleeding, friable, or recently biopsied warts.

■ **Available Forms:**
- *Liquid*: 25% (Podocon-25, Pododerm).

■ **Indications and Dosages:**
Genital warts (condylomata acuminata): Topical Apply 10%-25% solution in compound benzoin tincture to dry surface. Use 1 drop at a time allowing drying between drops until area is covered. Total volume should be limited to less than 0.5 ml per treatment session.

■ **Unlabeled Uses:** Epitheliomatosis, laryngeal papilloma

■ **Contraindications:** Concomitant steroid therapy; circulation disorders; bleeding warts, moles, birthmarks, or unusual warts with hair growing from them; hypersensitivity to podophyllum resin preparations

■ **Side Effects**
Occasional (10%-1%)
Pruritus, nausea, vomiting, abdominal pain, diarrhea

■ **Serious Reactions**
- Paresthesia, polyneuritis, paralytic ileus, pyrexia, leukopenia, thrombocytopenia, coma, and death have been reported with podophyllum resin use.

Special Considerations
- Not to be dispensed to the patient; professional application only
- Because of the potential for toxicity, cryotherapy should be attempted first or podofilox substituted

■ **Patient/Family Education**
- Avoid contact with eyes
- Notify the physician if painful urination, dizziness, light-headedness, increased heart rate, constipation, or tingling in hands or feet occurs

■ **Monitoring Parameters**
- Electrolytes, serum calcium
- Hgb concentrations

■ **Geriatric side effects at a glance:**
❑ CNS ❑ Bowel Dysfunction ❑ Bladder Dysfunction ❑ Falls

■ **U.S. Regulatory Considerations**
❑ FDA Black Box ❑ OBRA regulated in U.S. Long Term Care

polymyxin B sulfate

(polly-mix-in B sul'-fate)

■ **Brand Name(s):** Aerosporin

Combinations
Rx: *Ophth*: with bacitracin (Polysporin); with dexamethasone, neomycin (Dexacidin, Maxitrol); with hydrocortisone, neomycin (Cortisporin); with neomycin, bacitracin (Neosporin, Ocutricin); with neomycin, gramicidin (Neosporin); with oxytetracycline (Terak); with prednisolone, neomycin (Poly-Pred); with trimethoprim (Polytrim). *Topical*: with bacitracin, hydrocortisone, neomycin (Cortisporin); with dexamethasone, neomycin (Dioptrol, Maxitrol); with hydrocortisone, neomycin (Cortisporin)
OTC: *Topical*: with bacitracin (Bacimyxin, Polysporin); with bacitracin, neomycin (Neosporin, Triple Antibiotic); with bacitracin, neomycin, lidocaine (Lanabiotic, Spectrocin); with gramicidin (Polysporin); with gramicidin, lidocaine (Lidosporin, Polysporin Burn Formula); with gramicidin, neomycin (Neosporin)
Chemical Class: Polymyxin derivative

■ **Clinical Pharmacology:**
Mechanism of Action: An antibiotic that alters cell membrane permeability in susceptible microorganisms. **Therapeutic Effect:** Bactericidal activity.
Pharmacokinetics: Negligible absorption. Protein binding: low. Excreted in urine. Poor removal in hemodialysis. **Half-life:** 6 hr.

■ **Available Forms:**
• *Powder*: 500,000 units/vials (Aerosporin).

■ **Indications and Dosages:**
Mild to moderate infections: IV 15,000-25,000 units/kg/day in divided doses q12h. IM 25,000-30,000 units/kg/day in divided doses q4-6h.
Usual irrigation dosage: Continuous Bladder Irrigation 1 ml urogenital concentrate (contains 200,000 units polymyxin B, 57 mg neomycin) added to 1,000 ml 0.9% NaCl. Give each 1,000 ml >24 hr for up to 10 days (may increase to 2,000 ml/day when urine output >2 L/day).
Usual ophthalmic dosage: Ophthalmic 1 drop q3-4h.

■ **Contraindications:** Hypersensitivity to polymyxin B or any component of the formulation

■ **Side Effects**
Frequent
Severe pain, irritation at IM injection sites, phlebitis, thrombophlebitis with IV administration
Occasional
Fever, urticaria

■ **Serious Reactions**
• Nephrotoxicity, especially with concurrent/sequential use of other nephrotoxic drugs, renal impairment, concurrent/sequential use of muscle relaxants.

- Superinfection, especially with fungi, may occur.

Special Considerations
- Generally replaced by the aminoglycosides or extended-spectrum penicillins for serious infections; still used for bladder irrigation and gut decontamination; used in combination with other antibiotics and/or corticosteroids topically to treat infections of the eye and skin

■ Patient/Family Education
- Continue for the full length of treatment
- Space doses evenly
- Discomfort may occur at IM injection site
- Report any increased irritation, inflammation, itching, or burning with ophthalmic therapy

■ Monitoring Parameters
- Intake and output, BUN, creatinine, urinalysis

■ Geriatric side effects at a glance:
❑ CNS ❑ Bowel Dysfunction ❑ Bladder Dysfunction ❑ Falls

■ U.S. Regulatory Considerations
☑ FDA Black Box
- Risk of nephrotoxicity and neurotoxicity with parenteral use.
- Parenteral use rarely indicated.
❑ OBRA regulated in U.S. Long Term Care

polythiazide

(polly-thi'-a-zide)

■ Brand Name(s): Renese

Combinations
Rx: with prazosin (Minizide); with reserpine (Renese-R)
Chemical Class: Sulfonamide derivative

■ Clinical Pharmacology:
Mechanism of Action: A sulfonamide derivative that acts as a thiazide diuretic and antihypertensive. As a diuretic blocks reabsorption of water, sodium and potassium at cortical diluting segment of distal tubule. As an antihypertensive it reduces plasma and extracellular fluid volume and decreases peripheral vascular resistance (PVR) by direct effect on blood vessels. *Therapeutic Effect:* Promotes diuresis, reduces blood pressure (BP).
Pharmacokinetics: Rapidly absorbed from the gastrointestinal (GI) tract. Primarily excreted unchanged in urine. Not removed by hemodialysis. *Half-life:* 25.7 hr.

■ **Available Forms:**
- *Tablets*: 1 mg, 2 mg, 4 mg (Renese).

■ **Indications and Dosages:**
Edema: PO 1-4 mg/day.
Hypertension: PO 2-4 mg/day.

■ **Unlabeled Uses:** Prevention of calcium-containing renal stones

■ **Contraindications:** Anuria, history of hypersensitivity to sulfonamides or thiazide diuretics, renal decompensation

■ **Side Effects**
Expected
Increase in urine frequency and volume
Frequent
Potassium depletion
Occasional
Postural hypotension, headache, GI disturbances, photosensitivity reaction

■ **Serious Reactions**
- Vigorous diuresis may lead to profound water loss and electrolyte depletion, resulting in hypokalemia, hyponatremia, and dehydration.
- Acute hypotensive episodes may occur.
- Hyperglycemia may be noted during prolonged therapy.
- GI upset, pancreatitis, dizziness, paresthesias, headache, blood dyscrasias, pulmonary edema, allergic pneumonitis, and dermatologic reactions occur rarely.
- Overdosage can lead to lethargy and coma without changes in electrolytes or hydration.

Special Considerations
- Doses above 1 mg provide no further blood pressure reduction, but are more likely to induce metabolic disturbance (hypokalemia, hyperuricemia, etc.)
- May protect against osteoporotic hip fractures
- Loop diuretics or metolazone more effective if CrCl <40-50 ml/min
- Although allergic cross-reactivity with sulfonamide antibiotics and sulfonamide nonantibiotics has not been demonstrated, use with caution in patients with a history of severe sulfa allergies.

■ **Patient/Family Education**
- Will increase urination temporarily (approx. 3 wk); take early in the day to prevent sleep disturbance
- May cause sensitivity to sunlight; avoid prolonged exposure to the sun and other ultraviolet light
- May cause gout attacks; notify clinician if sudden joint pain occurs
- Rise slowly from lying to sitting position and permit legs to dangle momentarily before standing to reduce the drug's hypotensive effect

■ **Monitoring Parameters**
- Weight, urine output, serum electrolytes, BUN, creatinine, CBC, uric acid, glucose, lipids
- Blood pressure

potassium acetate/potassium bicarbonate-citrate/ potassium chloride/ potassium gluconate

(poe-tass'-i-um)

■ **Brand Name(s):** (potassium bicarbonate-citrate) Effer K, Klor-Con EF, K-Lyte, K-Lyte DS

■ **Brand Name(s):** (potassium chloride) Cena K, Ed K+10, K+Care, K-8, K-10, Kaochlor, Kaon-Cl, Kaon-Cl 10, Kaon-Cl 20%, Kato, Kay Ciel, KCl-20, KCl-40, K-Dur, K-Dur 10, K-Dur 20, K-Lor, K-Lor-Con M 15, Klor-Con, Klor-Con 8, Klor-Con 10, Klor-Con/25, Klor-Con M10, Klor-Con M15, Klor-Con M20, Klotrix, K-Norm, K-Sol, K-Tab, Micro-K, Micro-K 10, Rum-K

■ **Brand Name(s):** (potassium gluconate) Kaon
Chemical Class: Monovalent cation

■ **Clinical Pharmacology:**
Mechanism of Action: An electrolyte that is necessary for multiple cellular metabolic processes. Primary action is intracellular. **Therapeutic Effect:** Needed for nerve impulse conduction and contraction of cardiac, skeletal, and smooth muscle; maintains normal renal function and acid-base balance.
Pharmacokinetics: Well absorbed from the GI tract. Enters cells by active transport from extracellular fluid. Primarily excreted in urine.

■ **Available Forms:**
Potassium Acetate:
• *Injection*: 2 mEq/ml.
Potassium Bicarbonate and Potassium Citrate:
• *Tablets for Solution*: 25 mEq (Klor-Con EF, Effer-K, K-Lyte), 50 mEq (K-Lyte DS).
Potassium Chloride:
• *Capsules (Controlled-Release [Micro-K])*: 8 mEq, 10 mEq.
• *Liquid*: 20 mEq/15 ml (Kaochlor), 40 mEq/15 ml (Kaon-Cl).
• *Powder for Oral Solution (K-Lor)*: 20 mEq.
• *Powder for Reconstitution (K+Care)*: 20 mEq.
• *Injection*: 2 mEq/ml.

- *Tablets (Extended-Release)*: 8 mEq (K-8, Klor-Con, Klor-Con 8, Klor-Con M10, Micro-K, Micro-K10), 10 mEq (K-8, Kaon-CL, Kaon-CL 10, K-Dur, Klor-Con, Klor-Con 8, Klor-Con M10, Klotrix, K-Tab, Micro-K, Micro-K 10), 20 mEq (K-Dur).

Potassium Gluconate:
- *Elixir (Kaon)*: 20 mEq/15 ml.

■ **Indications and Dosages:**
Prevention of hypokalemia (in patients on diuretic therapy): PO 20–40 mEq/day in 1–2 divided doses.
Treatment of hypokalemia: PO 40–80 mEq/day; further doses based on laboratory values. IV 5–10 mEq/hr. Maximum: 400 mEq/day.

■ **Contraindications:** Concurrent use of potassium-sparing diuretics, digitalis toxicity, heat cramps, hyperkalemia, postoperative oliguria, severe burns, severe renal impairment, shock with dehydration or hemolytic reaction, untreated Addison's disease

■ **Side Effects**
Occasional
Nausea, vomiting, diarrhea, flatulence, abdominal discomfort with distention, phlebitis with IV administration (particularly when potassium concentration of greater than 40 mEq/L is infused)
Rare
Rash

■ **Serious Reactions**
- Hyperkalemia (more common in elderly patients and those with impaired renal function) may be manifested as paresthesia, feeling of heaviness in the lower extremities, cold skin, grayish pallor, hypotension, confusion, irritability, flaccid paralysis, and cardiac arrhythmias.

Special Considerations
- Avoid use of compressed tablets or enteric-coated tablets (i.e., nonsustained release or effervescent tablets for sol) due to significant ulcerogenic tendency and propensity to cause significant local tissue destruction
- Solution, powder, and oral susp: dilute or dissove in 120 ml cold water or juice
- Extended-release caps and tabs: do not crush; take with food; swallow with full glass of liquid
- Injectable potassium products must be diluted prior to administration; direct inj of potassium concentrate may be fatal
- Central line preferable for IV infusions concentrated >40 mEq/L

■ **Patient/Family Education**
- Foods rich in potassium: apricots, avocados, bananas, beans, beef, broccoli, brussels sprouts, cantaloupe, chicken, dates, fish, ham, lentils, milk, molasses, potatoes, prunes, raisins, spinach, turkey, watermelon, veal, and yams
- Notify the physician if a feeling of heaviness in the lower extremities and paresthesia occurs

■ **Monitoring Parameters**
- ECG monitoring advisable for IV infusion rate >10 mEq/hr
- Normal serum potassium level 3.5-5.0 mEq/L
- Intake and output diligently for diuresis; be alert for decreased urine output, which may be an indication of renal insufficiency
- Pattern of daily bowel activity and stool consistency

- Be alert for signs and symptoms of hyperkalemia, including cold skin, feeling of heaviness in lower extremities, paresthesia, and skin pallor

■ **Geriatric side effects at a glance:**
  ❑ CNS   ❑ Bowel Dysfunction   ❑ Bladder Dysfunction   ❑ Falls

■ **U.S. Regulatory Considerations**
  ❑ FDA Black Box   ☑ OBRA regulated in U.S. Long Term Care

pralidoxime chloride

(pra-li-dox'-eem klor'-ide)

■ **Brand Name(s):** Protopam Chloride
  Chemical Class: Quaternary ammonium derivative

■ **Clinical Pharmacology:**
  Mechanism of Action: Reactivates cholinesterase activity by 2-formyl-1-methylpyridinium ion. **Therapeutic Effect:** Restores cholinesterase activity following organophosphate anticholinesterase poisoning.
  Pharmacokinetics: Onset of activity is 1 hr and duration of action is short, which may require readministration. Not protein bound. Excreted in urine. **Half-life:** 1.2-2.6 hr.

■ **Available Forms:**
  • *Injection, Powder for Reconstitution:* 1g.

■ **Indications and Dosages:**
  Anticholinesterase overdosage: IV 1-2g initially, followed by increments of 250 mg q5min until response is observed.
  Organophosphate poisoning: IV 1-2g initially in 100 ml 0.9 NaCl infused over 15-30 minutes or 5% solution in sterile water for injection over not less than 5 minutes. Repeat 1-2g in 1 hr if muscle weakness persists.

■ **Contraindications:** Use of aminophylline, morphine, theophylline, and succinylcholine; hypersensitivity to pralidoxime or any of its components

■ **Side Effects**
  Occasional
  Blurred vision, dizziness, headache, laryngospasm, hyperventilation, nausea, tachycardia, hypertension, pain at injection site
  Rare
  Rash, muscle rigidity, decreased renal function

■ **Serious Reactions**
  - Excessive doses may cause blurred vision, nausea, tachycardia, and dizziness.

■ **Patient/Family Education**
  - Avoid consuming an excessive amount of caffeine derivatives such as chocolate, cocoa, coffee, cola, or tea
  - Immediately report any new symptoms such as weakness, dizziness, nausea, or tachycardia

■ **Monitoring Parameters**
  - CBC; plasma cholinesterase activity may help confirm diagnosis and follow course of illness
  - Respiratory rate, heart rate

■ **Geriatric side effects at a glance:**
  ❑ CNS ❑ Bowel Dysfunction ❑ Bladder Dysfunction ❑ Falls

■ **U.S. Regulatory Considerations**
  ❑ FDA Black Box ❑ OBRA regulated in U.S. Long Term Care

pramipexole dihydrochloride

(pra-mi-pex′-ole dye-hye-droe-klor′-ide)

■ **Brand Name(s):** Mirapex
  Chemical Class: Benzothiazolamine derivative

■ **Clinical Pharmacology:**
  Mechanism of Action: An antiparkinson agent that stimulates dopamine receptors in the striatum. **Therapeutic Effect:** Relieves signs and symptoms of Parkinson's disease. **Pharmacokinetics:** Rapidly and extensively absorbed after PO administration. Protein binding: 15%. Widely distributed. Steady-state concentrations achieved within 2 days. Primarily eliminated in urine. Not removed by hemodialysis. **Half-life:** 8 hr (12 hr in patients older than 65 yr).

■ **Available Forms:**
  - *Tablets*: 0.125 mg, 0.25 mg, 0.5 mg, 1 mg, 1.5 mg.

■ **Indications and Dosages:**
  Parkinson's disease: PO Initially, 0.375 mg/day in 3 divided doses. Don't increase dosage more frequently than every 5-7 days. Maintenance: 1.5-4.5 mg/day in 3 equally divided doses.
  Dosage in renal impairment: Dosage and frequency are modified based on creatinine clearance.

Creatinine Clearance	Initial Dose	Maximum Dose
Greater than 60 ml/min	0.125 mg 3 times a day	1.5 mg 3 times a day
35-59 ml/min	0.125 mg twice a day	1.5 mg twice a day
15-34 ml/min	0.125 mg once a day	1.5 mg once a day

■ **Unlabeled Uses:** Depression (due to bipolar disorder), fibromyalgia, restless legs syndrome

■ **Contraindications:** History of hypersensitivity to pramipexole

■ **Side Effects**

Frequent

Early Parkinson's disease (28%-10%): Nausea, asthenia, dizziness, somnolence, insomnia, constipation

Advanced Parkinson's disease (53%-17%): Orthostatic hypotension, extrapyramidal reactions, insomnia, dizziness, hallucinations

Occasional

Early Parkinson's disease (5%-2%): Edema, malaise, confusion, amnesia, akathisia, anorexia, dysphagia, peripheral edema, vision changes, impotence

Advanced Parkinson's disease (10%-7%): Asthenia, somnolence, confusion, constipation, abnormal gait, dry mouth

Rare

Advanced Parkinson's disease (6%-2%): General edema, malaise, chest pain, amnesia, tremor, urinary frequency or incontinence, dyspnea, rhinitis, vision changes

■ **Serious Reactions**

• Vascular disease, MI, angina pectoris, atrial fibrillation, heart failure, arrhythmia, atrial arrhythmia, and pulmonary embolism have been reported.

Special Considerations

• At least as effective as bromocriptine in the treatment of advanced parkinsonian patients with levodopa-related motor fluctuations; adverse effects similar in incidence and severity; appears to lack some of the toxicity seen with bromocriptine, pergolide, and cabergoline (e.g., pleuropulmonary disease); may be a useful alternative in patients with intolerable adverse effects due to ergot derivatives

■ **Patient/Family Education**

• Take pramipexole with food if nausea is a problem
• Do not abruptly discontinue pramipexole
• The drug may cause hallucinations
• Orthostatic hypotension occurs more commonly during initial therapy
• Avoid tasks that require mental alertness or motor skills until response to the drug has been established

■ **Monitoring Parameters**

• United Parkinson Disease Rating Scale (UPDRS) useful for monitoring efficacy endpoints
• Relief of symptoms, such as improvement of masklike facial expression, muscular rigidity, shuffling gait, and resting tremors of the hands and head
• Assess for constipation

■ **Geriatric side effects at a glance:**

❑ CNS ❑ Bowel Dysfunction ❑ Bladder Dysfunction ❑ Falls

Other: Orthostatic hypotension, hallucinations, daytime somnolence, and sudden drowsiness.

■ **Use with caution in older patients with:** Preexsisting psychotic symptoms

■ **U.S. Regulatory Considerations**
  ❑ FDA Black Box ❑ OBRA regulated in U.S. Long Term Care

■ **Other Uses in Geriatric Patient:** Restless legs syndrome

■ **Side Effects:**
  Of particular importance in the geriatric patient: Nausea/vomiting can result in weight loss

■ **Geriatric Considerations - Summary:** Pramipexole is a nonergot dopamine agonist that directly stimulates dopamine D_2 receptors. It can be used in combination with levodopa or as monotherapy. If discontinued, pramipexole should be slowly tapered because abrupt discontinuation can cause confusion, hallucinations, and a condition similar to neuroleptic malignant syndrome.

■ **References:**
  1. Miyasaki JM, Martin WRW, Suchowersky O, et al. Practice parameter: initiation of treatment for Parkinson disease: an evidence based review. Neurology 2002;58:11-17.
  2. Happe S, Berger K. The association of dopamine agonists with daytime sleepiness, sleep problems and quality of life in patients with Parkinson disease: prospective study. J Neurol 2001;248:1062-1067.
  3. Guttman M, International Pramipexole-Bromocriptine Study Group. Double blind comparison of pramipexole and bromocriptine treatment with placebo in advanced Parkinson disease. Neurology 1997;49:1060-1063.

pramoxine hydrochloride

(pra-mox'-een hye-droe-klor'-ide)

■ **Brand Name(s):** Analpram-HC, Anusol, Enzone, Epifoam, Itch-X, Pramosome, Prax, ProctoCream, ProctoFoam NS, Rectocort, Tronolane, Zone-A
  Chemical Class: Morpholine derivative

■ **Clinical Pharmacology:**
  Mechanism of Action: A surface or local anesthetic which is not chemically related to the "caine" types of local anesthetics. Decreases the neuronal membrane permeability to sodium ions, blocking both initiation and conduction of nerve impulses, therefore inhibiting depolarization of the neuron. **Therapeutic Effect:** Temporarily relieves pain and itching associated with anogenital pruritus or irritation.
  Pharmacokinetics: Onset of action occurs within a few minutes of application. Peak effect is reached in 3-5 minutes. Duration is several days.

■ **Available Forms:**
  • *Foam:* 1% (ProctoFoam NS).
  • *Cream:* 1% (Tronolane).

- *Gel*: 1% (Itch-X).
- *Lotion*: 1% (Prax).
- *Ointment*: 1% (Anusol).
- *Solution*: 1% (Itch-X).
- *Suppository*: 1% (Tronolane).

■ **Indications and Dosages:**
Anogenital pruritus or irritation, dermatosis, minor burns, hemorrhoids: Topical Apply to affected area 3 or 4 times daily.

■ **Contraindications:** Hypersensitivity to any component of the product.

■ **Side Effects**
Occassional
Angioedema, contact dermatitis, burning, itching, irritation, stinging
Rare
Dryness, folliculitis, hypopigmentation, perioral dermatitis, maceration of the skin, secondary infection, skin atrophy, striae, miliaria.

■ **Serious Reactions**
- None known.

Special Considerations
- Cross-sensitization with other local anesthetics unlikely

■ **Patient/Family Education**
- Do not use near eyes or nose
- Contact clinician if condition fails to improve after 3-4 days, or worsens
- Do not apply to large areas
- Do not apply to unaffected areas
- Notify the physician if bleeding at affected area, hoarseness, hives, rash, severe itching, difficulty breathing or swallowing, or swelling of the face, throat, lips, eyes, hands, feet, or ankles occurs
- Wash hands before and after administration

■ **Monitoring Parameters**
- Therapeutic response
- Skin for irritation

■ **Geriatric side effects at a glance:**
❑ CNS ❑ Bowel Dysfunction ❑ Bladder Dysfunction ❑ Falls

■ **U.S. Regulatory Considerations**
❑ FDA Black Box ❑ OBRA regulated in U.S. Long Term Care

pravastatin sodium

(pra'-va-stat-in soe'-dee-um)

- **Brand Name(s):** Pravachol
  Chemical Class: Substituted hexahydronaphthalene

- **Clinical Pharmacology:**
  Mechanism of Action: An HMG-CoA reductase inhibitor that interferes with cholesterol biosynthesis by preventing the conversion of HMG-CoA reductase to mevalonate, a precursor to cholesterol. **Therapeutic Effect:** Lowers serum LDL and VLDL cholesterol and plasma triglyceride levels; increases serum HDL concentration.
  Pharmacokinetics: Poorly absorbed from the GI tract. Protein binding: 50%. Metabolized in the liver (minimal active metabolites). Primarily excreted in feces via the biliary system. Not removed by hemodialysis. **Half-life:** 2.7 hr.

- **Available Forms:**
  - *Tablets:* 10 mg, 20 mg, 40 mg, 80 mg.

- **Indications and Dosages:**
  Hyperlipidemia, primary and secondary prevention of cardiovascular events in patient with elevated cholesterol levels: PO Initially, 40 mg/day. Titrate to desired response. Range: 10–80 mg/day.
  Dosage in hepatic and renal impairment: Give 10 mg/day initially. Titrate to desired response.

- **Contraindications:** Active hepatic disease or unexplained, persistent elevations of liver function test results

- **Side Effects**
  Pravastatin is generally well tolerated. Side effects are usually mild and transient.
  Occasional (7%–4%)
  Nausea, vomiting, diarrhea, constipation, abdominal pain, headache, rhinitis, rash, pruritus
  Rare (3%–2%)
  Heartburn, myalgia, dizziness, cough, fatigue, flu-like symptoms

- **Serious Reactions**
  - Malignancy and cataracts may occur.
  - Hypersensitivity occurs rarely.
  - Myopathy and rhabdomyolysis have been reported.

Special Considerations
  - Statin selection based on lipid-lowering prowess, cost, and availability

- **Patient/Family Education**
  - Avoid prolonged exposure to sunlight and other UV light
  - Promptly report any unexplained muscle pain, tenderness, or weakness, especially if accompanied by fever or malaise

- Strictly adhere to low cholesterol diet
- Take daily doses in the evening for increased effect
- Periodic laboratory tests are an essential part of therapy
- Avoid tasks that require mental alertness or motor skills until response to the drug is established

■ Monitoring Parameters
- ALT and AST at baseline, and at 12 weeks of therapy. If no change at 12 weeks, no further monitoring necessary (discontinue if elevations persist at >3 times upper limit of normal)
- CPK in any patient complaining of diffuse myalgia, muscle tenderness, or weakness
- Fasting lipid profile
- Pattern of daily bowel activity and stool consistency
- Skin for rash
- Assess the patient for malaise and muscle cramping or weakness. If these conditions occur and are accompanied by fever, expect that pravastatin may be discontinued

■ Geriatric side effects at a glance:
❑ CNS   ❑ Bowel Dysfunction   ❑ Bladder Dysfunction   ❑ Falls

■ U.S. Regulatory Considerations
❑ FDA Black Box   ❑ OBRA regulated in U.S. Long Term Care

praziquantel

(pray-zih-kwon'-tel)

■ Brand Name(s): Biltricide
Chemical Class: Pyrazinoisoquinoline derivative

■ Clinical Pharmacology:
Mechanism of Action: An antihelmintic that increases cell permeability in susceptible helminths resulting in loss of intracellular calcium, massive contractions and paralysis of their musculature, followed by attachment of phagocytes to the parasites. **Therapeutic Effect:** Vermicidal. Dislodges the dead and dying worms.
Pharmacokinetics: Well absorbed from gastrointestinal (GI) tract. Protein binding: 80%. Widely distributed including CSF. Metabolized in liver. Primarily excreted in urine. Not removed by hemodialysis. **Half-life:** 4-5 hr.

■ Available Forms:
- *Tablets*: 600 mg.

■ Indications and Dosages:
Schistosomiasis: PO 3 doses of 20 mg/kg as 1-day treatment. Do not give doses less than 4 hours or more than 6 hours apart.
Clonorchiasis/opisthorchiasis: PO 3 doses of 25 mg/kg as 1-day treatment.

■ **Contraindications:** Ocular cysticercosis, hypersensitivity to praziquantel or any component of the formulation

■ **Side Effects**
Frequent
Headache, dizziness, malaise, abdominal pain
Occasional
Anorexia, vomiting, diarrhea, severe cramping, abdominal pain may occur within 1 hour of administration w/fever, sweating, bloody stools
Rare
Giddiness, urticaria

■ **Serious Reactions**
• Overdose should be treated with fast-acting laxative.

■ **Patient/Family Education**
• Swallow tablets unchewed with some liquid during meals
• May cause drowsiness
• Use caution driving or performing other tasks requiring alertness
• Take for the full course of therapy
• Notify the physician if symptoms do not improve in a few days

■ **Monitoring Parameters**
• Collect stool and urine specimens to monitor effectiveness
• Check hematology results for anemia

■ **Geriatric side effects at a glance:**
❑ CNS ☑ Bowel Dysfunction ❑ Bladder Dysfunction ❑ Falls

■ **U.S. Regulatory Considerations**
❑ FDA Black Box ❑ OBRA regulated in U.S. Long Term Care

prazosin hydrochloride

(pra'-zoe-sin hye-droe-klor'-ide)

■ **Brand Name(s):** Minipress

Combinations
Rx: with polythiazide (Minizide)
Chemical Class: Quinazoline derivative

■ **Clinical Pharmacology:**
Mechanism of Action: An antidote, antihypertensive, and vasodilator that selectively blocks alpha$_1$-adrenergic receptors, decreasing peripheral vascular resistance. *Ther-*

apeutic Effect: Produces vasodilation of veins and arterioles, decreases total peripheral resistance, and relaxes smooth muscle in bladder neck and prostate. **Pharmacokinetics:** Well absorbed following oral administration. Protein binding: 92%-97%. Metabolized in liver. Primarily excreted in feces. **Half-life:** 2-4 hr.

■ **Available Forms:**
- *Capsules:* 1 mg, 2 mg, 5 mg.

■ **Indications and Dosages:**
Mild to moderate hypertension: PO Initially, 1 mg 2–3 times a day. Maintenance: 3–15 mg/day in divided doses. Maximum: 20 mg/day.
Benign prostatic hyperplasia: PO Initially, 1 mg 2 times/day. First dose should be administered at bedtime to avoid orthostasis and syncope. Titrate to 2 mg twice a day.

■ **Unlabeled Uses:** Treatment of ergot alkaloid toxicity, pheochromocytoma, Raynaud's phenomenon

■ **Contraindications:** Hypersensitivity to quinazolines

■ **Side Effects**
Frequent (10%–7%)
Dizziness, somnolence, headache, asthenia (loss of strength, energy)
Occasional (5%–4%)
Palpitations, nausea, dry mouth, nervousness
Rare (less than 1%)
Angina, urinary urgency

■ **Serious Reactions**
- First-dose syncope (hypotension with sudden loss of consciousness) may occur 30 to 90 minutes following initial dose of more than 2 mg, a too-rapid increase in dosage, or addition of another antihypertensive agent to therapy. First-dose syncope may be preceded by tachycardia (pulse rate of 120–160 beats/minute).

Special Considerations
- The doxazosin arm of the ALLHAT study was stopped early; the doxazosin group had a 25% greater risk of combined cardiovascular disease events which was primarily accounted for by a doubled risk of CHF vs the chlorthalidone group; doxazosin was also found to be less effective at controlling systolic BP an average of 3 mm Hg; may want to consider primary antihypertensives in addition to α-blockers for BPH symptoms
- Use as single antihypertensive agent limited by tendency to cause sodium and water retention and increased plasma volume

■ **Patient/Family Education**
- Alert patients to the possibility of syncopal and orthostatic symptoms, especially with the first dose ("1st-dose syncope")
- Initial dose should be administered at bedtime in the smallest possible dose
- Avoid tasks that require mental alertness or motor skills until response to the drug is established
- Notify the physician if dizziness or palpitations become bothersome

■ **Monitoring Parameters**
- Blood pressure, pulse

- **Geriatric side effects at a glance:**
  ☑ CNS ☐ Bowel Dysfunction ☐ Bladder Dysfunction ☑ Falls
  Other: Orthostatic hypotension, worsening of urge or mixed urinary incontinence

- **Use with caution in older patients with:** Congestive heart failure, patients taking medications for impotence (e.g., vardenafil, sildenafil, or tadalafil).

- **U.S. Regulatory Considerations**
  ☑ FDA Black Box ☐ OBRA regulated in U.S. Long Term Care
  Do not use the fixed combination of prazosin/polythiazide in the initial management of hypertension.

- **Side Effects:**
  Of particular importance in the geriatric patient: Orthostatic hypotension, worsening of urge or mixed urinary incontinence

- **Geriatric Considerations - Summary:** Alpha-adrendergic blockers are modestly effective alone, and in combination with 5-alpha reductase inhibitors (e.g., finasteride) in the treatment of urinary obstructive symptoms related to benign prostatic hyperplasia. The main side effect of these agents is orthostatic hypotension, and in hypertensive patients, these agents may increase the risk of congestive heart failure as reported in the ALLHAT study.

- **References:**
  1. Lepor H, Williford WO, Barry MJ, et al. The efficacy of terazosin, finasteride, or both in benign prostatic hyperplasia. Veterans Affairs Cooperative Studies Benign Prostatic Hyperplasia Study Group. N Engl J Med 1996;335:533-539.
  2. McConnell JD, Roehrborn CG, Bautista OM, et al. The long-term effect of doxazosin, finasteride, and combination therapy on the clinical progression of benign prostatic hyperplasia. N Engl J Med 2003;349:2387-2398.
  3. Major cardiovascular events in hypertensive patients randomized to doxazosin vs chlorthalidone: the antihypertensive and lipid-lowering treatment to prevent heart attack trial (ALLHAT). ALLHAT Collaborative Research Group. JAMA 2000;283:1967-1975.

prednisolone

(pred-niss'-oh-lone)

- **Brand Name(s):** AK-Pred, Cotolone, Depo-Predate, Hydeltrasol, Inflamase Forte, Inflamase Mild, Key-Pred, Key-Pred SP, Orapred, Predacort 50, Predaject-50, Predate-50, Pred Forte, Pred-Ject-50, Pred Mild, Prednisolone Acetate, Prelone
  Chemical Class: Glucocorticoid, synthetic

- **Clinical Pharmacology:**
  Mechanism of Action: An adrenocortical steroid that inhibits accumulation of inflammatory cells at inflammation sites, phagocytosis, lysosomal enzyme release and synthesis, and release of mediators of inflammation. ***Therapeutic Effect:*** Prevents or suppresses cell-mediated immune reactions. Decreases or prevents tissue response to inflammatory process.

Pharmacokinetics: Well absorbed from the GI tract. Protein binding: 90%-95%. Widely distributed. Metabolized in the liver. Primarily excreted in urine. Not removed by hemodialysis. **Half-life:** 2.6-3 hr.

■ **Available Forms:**
- *Tablets:* 5 mg.
- *Syrup:* 5 mg/5 ml (Prelone), 15 mg/5 ml (Prednisolone Acetate, Prelone).
- *Oral Liquid, Sodium Phosphate:* 5 mg/5 ml (Orapred), 15 mg/5 ml (Orapred).
- *Injectable Solution, Sodium Phosphate* (**Hydeltrasol, Key-Pred** SP): 20 mg/ml.
- *Injectable Suspension, Acetate:* 25 mg/ml (Cotolone, Key-Pred), 40 mg/ml (Depo-Predate), 50 mg/ml (Cotolone, Predacort 50, Pred-Ject-50, Predate-50, Pred-Ject-50), 80 mg/ml (Depo-Predate).
- *Ophthalmic Solution, Sodium Phosphate:* 0.125% (Inflamase Mild), 1% (AK-Pred, Inflamase Forte).
- *Ophthalmic Suspension, Acetate:* 0.12% (Pred Mild), 1% (Pred Forte).

■ **Indications and Dosages:**
Substitution therapy for deficiency states: acute or chronic adrenal insufficiency, congenital adrenal hyperplasia, and adrenal insufficiency secondary to pituitary insufficiency; nonendocrine disorders: arthritis; rheumatic carditis; allergic, collagen, intestinal tract, liver, ocular, renal, skin diseases; bronchial asthma; cerebral edema; malignancies: PO 5–60 mg/day in divided doses. Intra-articular, Intralesional (acetate) 4-100 mg, repeated as needed. Intra-articular, Intralesional (sodium phosphate) 2-30 mg, repeated at 3-day to 3-week intervals, as needed. IM (acetate, sodium phosphate) 4-60 mg a day.
Treatment of conjunctivitis and corneal injury: Ophthalmic 1-2 drops every hr during day and q2h during night. After response, decrease dosage to 1 drop q4h, then 1 drop 3-4 times a day.

■ **Contraindications:** Acute superficial herpes simplex keratitis, systemic fungal infections, varicella

■ **Side Effects**
Frequent
Insomnia, heartburn, nervousness, abdominal distention, increased sweating, acne, mood swings, increased appetite, facial flushing, delayed wound healing, increased susceptibility to infection, diarrhea, or constipation
Occasional
Headache, edema, change in skin color, frequent urination
Rare
Tachycardia, allergic reaction (such as rash and hives), psychological changes, hallucinations, depression
Ophthalmic: stinging or burning, posterior subcapsular cataracts

■ **Serious Reactions**
- Long-term therapy may cause hypocalcemia, hypokalemia, muscle wasting (especially in the arms and legs), osteoporosis, spontaneous fractures, amenorrhea, cataracts, glaucoma, peptic ulcer disease, and CHF.
- Abruptly withdrawing the drug after long-term therapy may cause anorexia, nausea, fever, headache, severe or sudden joint pain, rebound inflammation, fatigue, weakness, lethargy, dizziness, and orthostatic hypotension.
- Suddenly discontinuing prednisolone may be fatal.

Patient/Family Education
- May cause GI upset
- Take single daily doses in AM
- Increased dose of rapidly acting corticosteroids may be necessary in patients subjected to unusual stress
- Signs of adrenal insufficiency include fatigue, anorexia, nausea, vomiting, diarrhea, weight loss, weakness, dizziness, and low blood sugar
- Avoid abrupt withdrawal of therapy following high-dose or long-term therapy. Relative insufficiency may exist for up to 1 yr after discontinuation
- Patients on chronic steroid therapy should wear medical alert bracelet
- Do not give live virus vaccines to patients on prolonged therapy
- Avoid exposure to chickenpox or measles
- Avoid alcohol and limit caffeine intake

Monitoring Parameters
- Potassium and blood sugar during long-term therapy
- Edema, blood pressure, cardiac symptoms, mental status, weight
- Check intraocular pressure and lens frequently during prolonged use of ophthalmic preparations
- Be alert to signs and symptoms of infection, such as fever, sore throat, and vague symptoms
- Check mouth for signs and symptoms of candidal infection, such as white patches and painful mucous membranes and tongue

Geriatric side effects at a glance:
☑ CNS   ❏ Bowel Dysfunction   ❏ Bladder Dysfunction   ❏ Falls

U.S. Regulatory Considerations
❏ FDA Black Box   ☑ OBRA regulated in U.S. Long Term Care

prednisone

(pred'-ni-sone)

Brand Name(s): Deltasone, Liquid Pred, Meticorten, Prednicen-M, Prednicot, Prednisone Intensol, Sterapred, Sterapred DS
Chemical Class: Glucocorticoid, synthetic

Clinical Pharmacology:
Mechanism of Action: An adrenocortical steroid that inhibits accumulation of inflammatory cells at inflammation sites, phagocytosis, lysosomal enzyme release and synthesis, and release of mediators of inflammation. **Therapeutic Effect:** Prevents or suppresses cell-mediated immune reactions. Decreases or prevents tissue response to inflammatory process.

Pharmacokinetics: Well absorbed from the GI tract. Protein binding: 70%–90%. Widely distributed. Metabolized in the liver and converted to prednisolone. Primarily excreted in urine. Not removed by hemodialysis. **Half-life:** 3.4–3.8 hr.

■ **Available Forms:**
- *Oral Concentrate (Prednisone Intensol):* 5 mg/ml.
- *Oral Solution (Liquid Pred):* 5 mg/5 ml.
- *Tablets:* 1 mg (Sterapred), 2.5 mg (Deltasone), 5 mg (Deltasone, Prednicen-M, Sterapred), 10 mg (Deltasone, Sterapred), 20 mg (Deltasone), 50 mg (Deltasone).

■ **Indications and Dosages:**
Substitution therapy in deficiency states: acute or chronic adrenal insufficiency, congenital adrenal hyperplasia, and adrenal insufficiency secondary to pituitary insufficiency; nonendocrine disorders: arthritis; rheumatic carditis; allergic, collagen, intestinal tract, liver, ocular, renal, skin diseases; bronchial asthma; cerebral edema; malignancies: PO 5–60 mg/day in divided doses.

■ **Contraindications:** Acute superficial herpes simplex keratitis, systemic fungal infections, varicella

■ **Side Effects**
Frequent
Insomnia, heartburn, nervousness, abdominal distention, increased sweating, acne, mood swings, increased appetite, facial flushing, delayed wound healing, increased susceptibility to infection, diarrhea, or constipation
Occasional
Headache, edema, change in skin color, frequent urination
Rare
Tachycardia, allergic reaction (including rash and hives), psychological changes, hallucinations, depression

■ **Serious Reactions**
- Long-term therapy may cause muscle wasting in the arms and legs, osteoporosis, spontaneous fractures, amenorrhea, cataracts, glaucoma, peptic ulcer disease, and CHF.
- Abruptly withdrawing the drug following long-term therapy may cause anorexia, nausea, fever, headache, sudden or severe joint pain, rebound inflammation, fatigue, weakness, lethargy, dizziness, and orthostatic hypotension.
- Suddenly discontinuing prednisone may be fatal.

■ **Patient/Family Education**
- May cause GI upset, teach patient to take with meals or snacks
- May mask infections
- Take single daily doses in AM
- Increased dose of rapidly acting corticosteroids may be necessary in patients subjected to unusual stress
- Signs of adrenal insufficiency include fatigue, anorexia, nausea, vomiting, diarrhea, weight loss, weakness, dizziness, and low blood sugar
- Avoid abrupt withdrawal of therapy following high-dose or long-term therapy; relative insufficiency may exist for up to 1 yr after discontinuation
- Patients on chronic steroid therapy should wear medical alert bracelet

- Do not give live virus vaccines to patients on prolonged therapy
- Avoid exposure to chickenpox or measles
- Avoid alcohol and limit caffeine intake

■ **Monitoring Parameters**
- Serum K and glucose
- Edema, blood pressure, CHF symptoms, mental status, weight
- Be alert to signs and symptoms of infection, such as fever, sore throat, and vague symptoms
- Check mouth for signs and symptoms of candidal infection, such as white patches and painful mucous membranes and tongue

■ **Geriatric side effects at a glance:**
    ☑ CNS   ❑ Bowel Dysfunction   ❑ Bladder Dysfunction   ❑ Falls

■ **U.S. Regulatory Considerations**
    ❑ FDA Black Box   ☑ OBRA regulated in U.S. Long Term Care

primaquine phosphate

(prim-a-kween)

■ **Brand Name(s):** Primaquine
    Chemical Class: 8-Aminoquinoline derivative

■ **Clinical Pharmacology:**
    Mechanism of Action: An antimalarial and antirheumatic that eliminates tissue exo-erythrocytic forms of **Plasmodium falciparum**. Disrupts mitochondria and binds to DNA.
    Therapeutic Effect: Inhibits parasite growth.
    Pharmacokinetics: Well absorbed. Metabolized in the liver to the active metabolite, carboxyprimaquine. Excreted in the urine in small amounts as unchanged drug. **Half-life:** 4-6 hr.

■ **Available Forms:**
    - **Tablets:** 26.3 mg (Primaquine phosphate).

■ **Indications and Dosages:**
    Treatment of malaria: PO 15 mg base daily for 14 days.
    Malaria prophylaxis: PO 30 mg base daily. Begin 1 day before departure and continue for 7 days after leaving malarious area.

■ **Contraindications:** Concomitant medications which cause bone marrow suppression, rheumatoid arthritis, lupus erythematosus, glucose-6-phosphate dehydrogenase (G-6-PD) deficiency, hypersensitivity to primaquine or any of its components

■ **Side Effects**
    Frequent
    Abdominal pain, nausea, vomiting

Rare

Leukopenia, hemolytic anemia, methemoglobinemia

■ **Serious Reactions**
- Leukopenia, hemolytic anemia, methemoglobinemia occur rarely.
- Overdosage includes symptoms of abdominal cramps, vomiting, burning epigastric distress, central nervous system and cardiovascular disturbances, cyanosis, methemoglobinemia, moderate leukocytosis or leukopenia, and anemia.
- Acute hemolysis occurs, but patients recover completely if the dosage is discontinued.

■ **Patient/Family Education**
- Take with food if GI upset occurs, notify clinician if GI distress continues
- Urine may turn brown
- Take for the full length of treatment
- Notify the physician if unexplained fever, sore throat, or weakness occurs

■ **Monitoring Parameters**
- CBC periodically during therapy, discontinue if marked darkening of urine or sudden decrease in hemoglobin concentrations or leukocyte count occurs

■ **Geriatric side effects at a glance:**
❑ CNS   ❑ Bowel Dysfunction   ❑ Bladder Dysfunction   ❑ Falls

■ **U.S. Regulatory Considerations**
❑ FDA Black Box   ❑ OBRA regulated in U.S. Long Term Care

primidone

(pri'-mi-done)

■ **Brand Name(s):** Mysoline
Chemical Class: Pyrimidinedione

DEA Class: Schedule IV

■ **Clinical Pharmacology:**
Mechanism of Action: A barbiturate that decreases motor activity from electrical and chemical stimulation and stabilizes the seizure threshold against hyperexcitability.
Therapeutic Effect: Reduces seizure activity.
Pharmacokinetics: Rapidly and usually completely absorbed following oral administration. Protein binding: 20%-30%. Extensively metabolized in liver to phenobarbital and phenylethylmalonamide (PEMA). Minimal excretion in urine. **Half-life:** 3.3-7 hr.

■ **Available Forms:**
  • *Tablets*: 50 mg, 250 mg.
  • *Oral Suspension*: 250 mg/5 ml.

■ **Indications and Dosages:**
  Seizure control: PO 125-150 mg/day at bedtime. May increase by 125-250 mg/day every 3-7 days. Maximum: 2 g/day.

■ **Unlabeled Uses:** Treatment of essential tremor

■ **Contraindications:** History of bronchopneumonia, hypersensitivity to phenobarbital, porphyria

■ **Side Effects**
  Frequent
  Ataxia, dizziness
  Occasional
  Anorexia, drowsiness, mental changes, nausea, vomiting, paradoxical excitement
  Rare
  Rash

■ **Serious Reactions**
  • Abrupt withdrawal after prolonged therapy may produce effects ranging from increased dreaming, nightmares, insomnia, tremor, diaphoresis, and vomiting to hallucinations, delirium, seizures, and status epilepticus.
  • Skin eruptions may be a sign of a hypersensitivity reaction.
  • Blood dyscrasias, hepatic disease, and hypocalcemia occur rarely.
  • Overdose produces cold or clammy skin, hypothermia, and severe CNS depression, followed by high fever and coma.

Special Considerations
  • Second-line anticonvulsant for treatment of generalized tonic-clonic seizures (or alternative to phenobarbital, which probably accounts for most of the anticonvulsant activity)
  • Most effective anti-essential tremor medication, but sedative side effects troublesome; usually used second line to β-adrenergic blocking agents (nonselective)

■ **Patient/Family Education**
  • Importance of adherence to regimen and risk associated with abrupt discontinuance of anticonvulsant
  • Sedative liabilities regarding driving and operating heavy machinery
  • Avoid alcohol

■ **Monitoring Parameters**
  • Therapeutic drug concentration for seizure control: 5-12 mcg/ml; serum concentrations should also include phenobarbital determinations (therapeutic: 20-40 mcg/ml)
  • Periodic CBC, liver and renal function tests, serum folate, vitamin D during prolonged therapy

■ **Geriatric side effects at a glance:**
  ❑ CNS ❑ Bowel Dysfunction ❑ Bladder Dysfunction ❑ Falls
  Other: Yes; see side effects, later.

- **Use with caution in older patients with:** Hepatic impairment, Renal impairment, Pulmonary dysfunction, Osteoporosis

- **U.S. Regulatory Considerations**
  - ❏ FDA Black Box   ❏ OBRA regulated in U.S. Long Term Care

- **Other Uses in Geriatric Patient:** Essential tremor

- **Side Effects:**
  Of particular importance in the geriatric patient: Delirium, confusion, cognitive impairment, amnesia, drowsiness, ataxia, behavioral changes, impotence

- **Geriatric Considerations - Summary:** Primidone is poorly tolerated in older adults; avoid use if possible. Dosage adjustments are required in renal impairment. Numerous drug interactions with primidone exist. Primidone may reduce bone mineral density by interfering with vitamin D catabolism. Calcium and vitamin D supplementation and monitoring of bone mineral density are recommended for older adults taking this drug.

- **References:**
  1. Arroyo S, Kramer G. Treating epilepsy in the elderly: safety considerations. Drug Saf 2001;24:991-1015.
  2. Drugs that may cause cognitive disorders in the elderly. Med Let 2000;42:111-112.

probenecid

(proe-ben'-e-sid)

- **Brand Name(s):** Probalan

  Combinations
  Rx: with colchicine (Colbenemid Proben-C); with ampicillin (Polycillin-PRB, Probampacin)
  Chemical Class: Sulfonamide derivative

- **Clinical Pharmacology:**
  Mechanism of Action: An antigout agent that competitively inhibits reabsorption of uric acid at the proximal convoluted tubule. Also, inhibits renal tubular secretion of weak organic acids, such as penicillins. **Therapeutic Effect:** Promotes uric acid excretion, reduces serum uric acid level, and increases plasma levels of penicillins and cephalosporins.
  Pharmacokinetics: Rapidly and completely absorbed following oral administration. Protein binding: High. Extensively metabolized in liver. Excreted in urine. Excretion is dependent upon urinary pH and is increased in alkaline urine. **Half-life:** 3-8 hr (dose-dependent).

- **Available Forms:**
  - *Tablets*: 500 mg.

■ Indications and Dosages:

Gout: PO Initially, 250 mg twice a day for 1 wk; then 500 mg twice a day. May increase by 500 mg q4wk. Maximum: 2–3 g/day. Maintenance: Dosage that maintains normal uric acid level.

■ Contraindications:
Blood dyscrasias, concurrent high-dose aspirin therapy, severe renal impairment, uric acid calculi

■ Side Effects

Frequent (10%–6%)

Headache, anorexia, nausea, vomiting

Occasional (5%–1%)

Lower back or side pain, rash, hives, itching, dizziness, flushed face, frequent urge to urinate, gingivitis

■ Serious Reactions

- Severe hypersensitivity reactions, including anaphylaxis, occur rarely and usually within a few hours after administration following previous use. If severe hypersensitivity reactions develop, discontinue the drug immediately and contact the physician.
- Pruritic maculopapular rash, possibly accompanied by malaise, fever, chills, arthralgia, nausea, vomiting, leukopenia, and aplastic anemias should be considered a toxic reaction.

■ Patient/Family Education

- Avoid aspirin or other salicylates
- Take with food or antacids
- Drink 48-64 oz water daily to prevent development of kidney stones
- Avoid alcohol
- Avoid eating high-purine foods, such as anchovies, kidneys, liver, meat extracts, sardines, and sweetbreads
- Full therapeutic response may take more than 1 wk
- Discontinue if rash or other evidence of an allergic reaction occurs

■ Monitoring Parameters

- Serum uric acid concentrations: continue the probenecid dose that maintains normal concentrations
- Renal function tests
- CBC
- Encourage the patient to maintain a high fluid intake (3,000 ml/day). Monitor the patient's intake and urine output. Output should be at least 2,000 ml/day
- Therapeutic response, including improved joint range of motion and reduced joint tenderness, redness, and swelling

■ Geriatric side effects at a glance:
❏ CNS ❏ Bowel Dysfunction ❏ Bladder Dysfunction ❏ Falls

■ U.S. Regulatory Considerations
❏ FDA Black Box ❏ OBRA regulated in U.S. Long Term Care

procainamide hydrochloride

(proe-kane'-a-mide hye-droe-klor'-ide)

■ **Brand Name(s):** Procanbid, Procan SR, Pronestyl, Pronestyl-SR
  Chemical Class: Para-aminobenzoic acid derivative

■ **Clinical Pharmacology:**
  Mechanism of Action: An antiarrhythmic that increases the electrical stimulation threshold of the ventricles and His-Purkinje system. Decreases myocardial excitability and conduction velocity and depresses myocardial contractility. Exerts direct cardiac effects. **Therapeutic Effect:** Suppresses arrhythmias.
  Pharmacokinetics: Rapidly, completely absorbed from the GI tract. Protein binding: 15%–20%. Widely distributed. Metabolized in the liver to active metabolite. Primarily excreted in urine. Removed by hemodialysis. **Half-life:** 2.5–4.5 hr; metabolite, 6 hr.

■ **Available Forms:**
  • *Capsules (Pronestyl):* 250 mg, 500 mg.
  • *Tablets (Pronestyl):* 250 mg, 375 mg, 500 mg.
  • *Tablets (Extended-Release [Pronestyl-SR]):* 500 mg.
  • *Tablest (Extended-Release [Procanbid]):* 500 mg, 750 mg, 1,000 mg.
  • *Injection (Pronestyl):* 100 mg/ml, 500 mg/ml.

■ **Indications and Dosages:**
  Maintenance of normal sinus rhythm after conversion of atrial fibrillation or flutter; treatment of premature ventricular contractions, paroxysmal atrial tachycardia, atrial fibrillation, and ventricular tachycardia: PO 250–500 mg of immediate-release tablets q3–6h. 0.5–1g of extended-release tablets q6h. 1–2g of Procanbid q12h. IV Loading dose: 50–100 mg. May repeat q5–10min or 15–18 mg/kg (maximum: 1–1.5 g). Then maintenance infusion of 3–4 mg/min. Range: 1–6 mg/min.
  Dosage in renal impairment: Dosage interval is modified based on creatinine clearance.

Creatinine Clearance	Dosage Interval
10–50 ml/min	q6–12h
less than 10 ml/min	q8–24h

■ **Unlabeled Uses:** Conversion and management of atrial fibrillation

■ **Contraindications:** Complete heart block, myasthenia gravis, preexisting QT prolongation, second-degree heart block, systemic lupus erythematosus, torsades de pointes

■ **Side Effects**
  Frequent
  PO: Abdominal pain or cramping, nausea, diarrhea, vomiting
  Occasional
  Dizziness, giddiness, weakness, hypersensitivity reaction (rash, urticaria, pruritus, flushing)
  IV: Transient, but at times, marked hypotension

Rare
Confusion, mental depression, psychosis

■ Serious Reactions
- Paradoxical, extremely rapid ventricular rate may occur during treatment of atrial fibrillation or flutter.
- Systemic lupus erythematosus–like syndrome (fever, myalgia, pleuritic chest pain) may occur with prolonged therapy.
- Cardiotoxic effects occur most commonly with IV administration and appear as conduction changes (50% widening of QRS complex, frequent ventricular premature contractions, ventricular tachycardia, and complete AV block).
- Prolonged PR and QT intervals and flattened T waves occur less frequently.

■ Patient/Family Education
- Strict compliance to dosage schedule imperative
- Empty wax core from sustained-release tablets may appear in stool; this is harmless
- Initiate therapy in facilities capable of providing continuous ECG monitoring and managing life-threatening dysrhythmias
- Do not abruptly discontinue the drug
- Do not take nasal decongestants or OTC cold preparations, especially those containing stimulants, without physician approval
- Avoid performing tasks that require mental alertness or motor skills until response to the drug is established

■ Monitoring Parameters
- CBC with differential and platelets qwk for first 3 mo, periodically thereafter
- ECG: R/O overdosage if QRS widens >25% or QT prolongation occurs; reduce dosage if QRS widens >50%
- ANA titer increases may precede clinical symptoms of lupoid syndrome
- Serum creatinine, urea nitrogen
- Plasma procainamide concentration (therapeutic range 3-10 mcg/ml; 10-30 mcg/ml N-acetyl procainamide)
- Check blood pressure every 5 to 10 minutes during IV infusion. If a fall in blood presure exceeds 15 mm Hg, discontinue infusion and contact the physician
- Pulse rate for quality and irregularity
- Intake and output
- Serum electrolyte levels, including chloride, potassium, and sodium
- Pattern of daily bowel activity and stool consistency
- Skin for hypersensitivity reaction, especially in patients receiving high-dose therapy

■ Geriatric side effects at a glance:
❏ CNS   ❏ Bowel Dysfunction   ❏ Bladder Dysfunction   ❏ Falls

■ U.S. Regulatory Considerations
☑ FDA Black Box
- Chronic administration may result in positive titers with or without symptoms of lupus erythematosus-like syndrome.
- Proarrhythmic effects limit the use of this drug to patients with life-threatening ventricular arrhythmias.

- Agranulocytosis, bone marrow depression, neutropenia, hypoplastic anemia, and thrombocytopenia have been reported and may occur within the first 12 wk of therapy at recommended doses. Caution should be used in patients with preexisting marrow failure or cytopenia.
- ❑ OBRA regulated in U.S. Long Term Care

procaine hydrochloride

(proe'-kane hye-droe-klor'-ide)

- **Brand Name(s):** Novocain, Mericaine
  Chemical Class: Benzoic acid derivative

- **Clinical Pharmacology:**
  Mechanism of Action: Procaine causes a reversible blockade of nerve conduction by decreasing nerve membrane permeability to sodium. **Therapeutic Effect:** Local anesthesia.
  Pharmacokinetics: Highly plasma protein-bound and distributed to all body tissues. Excreted in the urine (80%). **Half-life:** 40 ± 9 seconds in adults, 84 ± 30 seconds in neonates.

- **Available Forms:**
  - *Solution*: 0.25%, 0.5%, 10% (Novocain).

- **Indications and Dosages:**
  Spinal anesthesia: Intrathecal 0.5-1 ml of a 10% solution (50-100 mg) mixed with an equal volume of diluent injected into the third or fourth lumbar interspace (perineum and lower extremities). 2 ml of a 10% solution (200 mg) mixed with 1 ml of diluent injected into the second, third, or fourth interspace.
  Infiltration anesthesia, dental anesthesia, control of severe pain (post herpatic neuralgia, cancer pain, or burns): Topical A single dose of 350-600 mg using a 0.25 or 0.5% solution. Use 0.9% sodium chloride for dilution.
  Peripheral or sympathetic nerve block (regional anesthesia): Topical Up to 200 ml of a 0.5% solution (1 g), 100 ml of a 1% solution (1 g), or 50 ml of a 2% solution (1 g). The 2% solution should only be used when a small volume of anesthetic is required.

- **Unlabeled Uses:** Severe pain

- **Contraindications:** Hypersensitivity to ester local anesthetics, sulfites, PABA, patients on anticoagulant therapy, and in patients with coagulopathy, infection, thrombocytopenia. Should not be given via intra-arterial, intrathecal, or intravenous routes.

- **Side Effects**
  Frequent
  Numbness or tingling of the face or mouth, pain at the injection site, dizziness, drowsiness, light-headedness, nausea, vomiting, back pain, headache
  Rare
  Anxiety, restlessness, difficulty breathing, shortness of breath, seizures (convulsions), skin rash, itching (hives), slow irregular heartbeat (palpitations), swelling of the face or mouth, tremors, QT prolongation, PR prolongation, atrial fibrillation, sinus

bradycardia, hypotension, angina, cardiovascular collapse, fecal or urinary incontinence, loss of perineal sensation and sexual function, persistent motor, sensory, and/or autonomic (sphincter control) deficit

■ **Serious Reactions**
  • Procaine-induced CNS toxicity usually presents with symptoms of stimulation such as anxiety, apprehension, restlessness, nervousness, disorientation, confusion, dizziness, blurred vision, tremor, nausea/vomiting, shivering, or seizures. Subsequently, depressive symptoms can occur including drowsiness, unconsciousness, and respiratory arrest.
  • If higher concentrations are introduced into the bloodstream, depression of cardiac excitability and contractility may cause AV block, ventricular arrhythmias, or cardiac arrest. CNS toxicity including dizziness, tongue numbness, visual impairment and disturbances, and muscular twitching appear to occur before cardiotoxic effects.
  • **Alert** Procaine should be used with caution in patients who have asthma since there is the increased risk of anaphylactoid reactions including bronchospasm and status asthmaticus.

Special Considerations
  • Esther-type local anesthetic

■ **Patient/Family Education**
  • A burning sensation may occur at the site of injection

■ **Monitoring Parameters**
  • Blood pressure, pulse, respiration during treatment, ECG

■ **Geriatric side effects at a glance:**
  ❑ CNS ❑ Bowel Dysfunction ❑ Bladder Dysfunction ❑ Falls

■ **U.S. Regulatory Considerations**
  ❑ FDA Black Box ❑ OBRA regulated in U.S. Long Term Care

prochlorperazine

(proe-klor-per'-a-zeen)

■ **Brand Name(s):** Compazine, Compazine Spansule, Compro, Procot
  Chemical Class: Piperazine phenothiazine derivative

■ **Clinical Pharmacology:**
  Mechanism of Action: A phenothiazine that acts centrally to inhibit or block dopamine receptors in the chemoreceptor trigger zone and peripherally to block the vagus nerve in the GI tract. **Therapeutic Effect:** Relieves nausea and vomiting and improves psychotic conditions.

Pharmacokinetics:

Route	Onset	Peak	Duration
Tablets, oral solution	30-40 min	N/A	3-4 hr
Capsules (extended-release)	30-40 min	N/A	10-12 hr
Rectal	60 min	N/A	3-4 hr

Variably absorbed after PO administration. Widely distributed. Metabolized in the liver and GI mucosa. Primarily excreted in urine. Unknown if removed by hemodialysis. **Half-life:** 23 hr.

■ **Available Forms:**
- *Capsules (Extended-Release [Compazine Spansule])*: 10 mg, 15 mg.
- *Oral Solution (Compazine)*: 5 mg/5ml.
- *Tablets (Compazine)*: 5 mg, 10 mg.
- *Suppositories (Compazine)*: 2.5 mg, 5 mg, 25 mg.
- *Injection (Compazine, Procot)*: 5 mg/ml.

■ **Indications and Dosages:**
Nausea and vomiting: PO 5-10 mg 3-4 times a day. PO (Extended-Release) 10 mg twice a day or 15 mg once a day. IV 2.5-10 mg. May repeat q3-4h. IM 5-10 mg q3-4h. Rectal 25 mg twice a day.
Psychosis: PO 5-10 mg 3-4 times a day. Maximum: 150 mg/day. IM 10-20 mg q4h.

■ **Unlabeled Uses:** Behavior syndromes in dementia

■ **Contraindications:** Angle-closure glaucoma, CNS depression, coma, myelosuppression, severe cardiac or hepatic impairment, severe hypotension or hypertension

■ **Side Effects**
Frequent
Somnolence, hypotension, dizziness, fainting (commonly occurring after first dose, occasionally after subsequent doses, and rarely with oral form)
Occasional
Dry mouth, blurred vision, lethargy, constipation, diarrhea, myalgia, nasal congestion, peripheral edema, urine retention

■ **Serious Reactions**
- Extrapyramidal symptoms appear to be dose related and are divided into three categories: akathisia (marked by inability to sit still, tapping of feet), parkinsonian symptoms (including mask-like face, tremors, shuffling gait, hypersalivation), and acute dystonias (such as torticollis, opisthotonos, and oculogyric crisis). A dystonic reaction may also produce diaphoresis or pallor.
- Tardive dyskinesia, manifested as tongue protrusion, puffing of the cheeks, and puckering of the mouth, is a rare reaction that may be irreversible.
- Abrupt withdrawal after long-term therapy may precipitate nausea, vomiting, gastritis, dizziness, and tremors.
- Blood dyscrasias, particularly agranulocytosis and mild leukopenia, may occur.
- Prochlorperazine use may lower the seizure threshold.

■ **Patient/Family Education**
- Arise slowly from reclining position
- Do not discontinue abruptly

1033

- Use a sunscreen during sun exposure to prevent burns; take special precautions to stay cool in hot weather
- May cause drowsiness
- Avoid alcohol and limit caffeine intake
- Avoid tasks that require mental alertness or motor skills until response to the drug has been established

■ Monitoring Parameters
- Observe closely for signs of tardive dyskinesia
- Treat acute dystonic reactions with parenteral diphenhydramine (2 mg/kg to max 50 mg) or benztropine (2 mg)
- Periodic CBC with platelets during prolonged therapy
- Blood pressure for hypotension
- Therapeutic response, including improvement in self-care, increased ability to concentrate and interest in surroundings, and a relaxed facial expression

■ Geriatric side effects at a glance:
☑ CNS ☑ Bowel Dysfunction ❏ Bladder Dysfunction ☑ Falls
Other: Orthostatic hypotension, cardiac conduction disturbances, anticholinergic side effects

■ Use with caution in older patients with: Parkinson's disease (an atypical antipsychotic is recommended), seizure disorders, cardiovascular disease with conduction disturbance, hepatic encephalopathy, narrow-angle glaucoma

■ U.S. Regulatory Considerations
❏ FDA Black Box ☑ OBRA regulated in U.S. Long Term Care

■ Other Uses in Geriatric Patient: Behavior disturbances in the setting of dementia

■ Side Effects:
Of particular importance in the geriatric patient: Tardive dyskinesia, akathisia (may appear to exacerbate behavioral disturbances), anticholinergic effects, may increase risk of sudden death

■ Geriatric Considerations - Summary: Prochlorperazine is a phenothiazine derivative with strongly antihistaminic and anticholinergic effects. It is most often used as an antiemetic, but prescribers should be aware that the side-effect profile encompasses that seen in phenothiazines (e.g., akathisia) as well as anticholinergic drugs (e.g., urinary retention, visual changes, sedation, and delirium). In a comparative study, prochlorperazine was superior to promethazine in the treatment of emergency department patients with uncomplicated nausea and vomiting.

■ Reference:
1. Ernst AA, Weiss SJ, Park S, et al. Prochlorperazine versus promethazine for uncomplicated nausea and vomiting in the emergency department: a randomized, double-blind clinical trial. Ann Emerg Med 2000;36:89-94.

procyclidine hydrochloride

(proe-sye-kli-deen hye-droe-klor'-ide)

- **Brand Name(s):** Kemadrin
  Chemical Class: Tertiary amine

- **Clinical Pharmacology:**
  Mechanism of Action: An anticholinergic agent that exerts an atropine-like action and produces an antispasmodic effect on smooth muscle, is a potent mydriatic, and inhibits salivation. **Therapeutic Effect:** Relieves symptoms of Parkinson's disease and drug-induced extrapyramidal symptoms.
  Pharmacokinetics: Well absorbed from the gastrointestinal (GI) tract. Protein binding: extensive. Metabolized in liver and undergoes extensive first-pass effect. Primarily excreted in urine. Unknown if removed by hemodialysis. **Half-life:** 7.7-16.1 hr.

- **Available Forms:**
  - *Tablets:* 5 mg.

- **Indications and Dosages:**
  Drug-induced extrapyramidal reactions: PO Initially, 2.5 mg 3 times/day. May increase by 2.5 mg daily as needed. Maintenance: 10-20 mg/day in divided doses 3 times/day.
  Parkinson's disease: PO Initially, 2.5 mg 3 times/day after meals. Maintenance: 2.5-5 mg/day in divided doses 3 times/day after meals.
  Hepatic function impairment: PO 2.5-5 mg/day in divided doses twice a day after meals

- **Contraindications:** Angle-closure glaucoma

- **Side Effects**
  Frequent
  Blurred vision, mydriasis, disorientation, light-headedness, nausea, vomiting dry mouth, nose, throat, and lips

- **Serious Reactions**
  - Overdosage may vary from severe anticholinergic effects, such as unsteadiness, severe drowsiness, severe dryness of mouth, nose, or throat, tachycardia, shortness of breath, and skin flushing.
  - Also produces severe paradoxical reaction, marked by hallucinations, tremor, seizures, and toxic psychosis.

- **Patient/Family Education**
  - Do not discontinue this drug abruptly
  - Hard candy, frequent drinks, sugarless gum to relieve dry mouth
  - Take with or after meals to prevent GI upset
  - Use caution in hot weather, may increase susceptibility to heatstroke

- Avoid tasks that require mental alertness or motor skills until response to the drug is established
- Avoid alcohol

■ **Monitoring Parameters**
- Blood pressure
- Clinical reversal of symptoms, such as improvement of masklike facial expression, muscular rigidity, shuffling gait, and resting tremors of hands and head

■ **Geriatric side effects at a glance:**
  ☑ CNS ☑ Bowel Dysfunction ☑ Bladder Dysfunction ☐ Falls
  Other: Dry mouth, blurred vision, somnolence, confusion, psychoses

■ **Use with caution in older patients with:** Narrow-angle glaucoma, overflow incontinence, psychosis

■ **U.S. Regulatory Considerations**
  ☐ FDA Black Box ☑ OBRA regulated in U.S. Long Term Care

■ **Other Uses in Geriatric Patient:** Treatment of antipsychotic-induced adverse effects

■ **Side Effects:**
  Of particular importance in the geriatric patient: Anticholinergic effects

■ **Geriatric Considerations - Summary:** Procyclidine and related anticholinergics present significant risk to older adults. These drugs possess potent anticholinergic effects and can cause cognitive impairment, delirium, dry mouth, blurred vision, and increased risk of falls. The use of this drug and related compounds should be limited and when used, patients should be closely monitored.

■ **References:**
1. Vangala V, Tueth M. Chronic anticholinergic toxicity: identification and management in older patients. Geriatrics 2003;58:36-37.
2. Tune LE. Anticholinergic effects of medication in elderly patients. J Clin Psychiatry 2001;62(suppl 21):11-14.
3. Bamrah JS, Kumar V, Krska J, et al: Interactions between procyclidine and neuroleptic drugs: some pharmacological and clinical aspects. Br J Psychiatry 1986;149:726-733.

progesterone

(proe-jes'-ter-one)

■ **Brand Name(s):** Crinone, First Progesterone MC10, First Progesterone MC5, Prochieve, Prometrium
  Chemical Class: ENDO-progestin, natural

■ **Clinical Pharmacology:**
Mechanism of Action: A natural steroid hormone that promotes mammary gland development and relaxes uterine smooth muscle. **Therapeutic Effect:** Decreases abnormal uterine bleeding; transforms endometrium from proliferative to secretory in an estrogen-primed endometrium.
Pharmacokinetics: Oral: Maximum serum concentrations attained within 3 hours. Protein binding: 96%-99%. Metabolized in liver. Excreted in bile and urine. **Half-life:** 18.3 hr. IM: Rapidly absorbed. Undergoes rapid metabolism. **Half-life:** Few min. Long-acting form: Approximately 10 wk. Vaginal Gel: Rate limited by absorption rather than by elimination. Protein binding: 96%-99%. Undergoes both biliary and renal elimination. **Half-life:** 5-20 hr.

■ **Available Forms:**
- Capsules (Prometrium): 100 mg, 200 mg.
- Injection: 50 mg/ml.
- Vaginal Gel (Crinone, Prochieve): 4% (45 mg), 8% (90 mg).
- Topical Cream: 5% (First Progesterone MC5), 10% (First Progesterone MC10).

■ **Indications and Dosages:**
Abnormal uterine bleeding: IM 5–10 mg for 6 days. When estrogen given concomitantly, begin progesterone after 2 wk of estrogen therapy; discontinue when menstrual flow begins.
Prevention of endometrial hyperplasia: PO 200 mg in evening for 12 days per 28-day cycle in combination with daily conjugated estrogen.

■ **Unlabeled Uses:** Treatment of corpus luteum dysfunction

■ **Contraindications:** Allergy to peanut oil (oral), breast cancer, history of active cerebral apoplexy, thromboembolic disorders or thrombophlebitis, severe hepatic dysfunction, undiagnosed vaginal bleeding

■ **Side Effects**
Frequent
Breast tenderness
Gel: drowsiness
Occasional
Edema, weight gain or loss, rash, pruritus, photosensitivity, skin pigmentation
Rare
Pain or swelling at injection site, acne, depression, alopecia, hirsutism

■ **Serious Reactions**
- Thrombophlebitis, cerebrovascular disorders, retinal thrombosis, and pulmonary embolism occur rarely.

Special Considerations
- Gel provides enhanced uterine delivery compared with IM administration

■ **Patient/Family Education**
- Diabetic patients may note decreased glucose tolerance
- Notify clinician of abnormal or excessive bleeding, severe cramping, abnormal or odorous vaginal discharge
- Use sunscreen and wear protective clothing until tolerance to sunlight and ultraviolet light has been determined
- Stop smoking tobacco

■ **Monitoring Parameters**
- Weight
- Blood pressure
- Skin for rash

■ **Geriatric side effects at a glance:**
☐ CNS ☐ Bowel Dysfunction ☐ Bladder Dysfunction ☐ Falls

■ **U.S. Regulatory Considerations**
☐ FDA Black Box ☐ OBRA regulated in U.S. Long Term Care

promethazine hydrochloride

(proe-meth'-a-zeen hye-droe-klor'-ide)

■ **Brand Name(s):** Adgan, Anergan 50, Antinaus 50, Pentazine, Phenadoz, Phenergan, Phenoject-50, Promacot, Promethegan

Combinations
Rx: with codeine (Phenergan with Codeine Syrup); with dextromethorphan (Phenergan with Dextromethorphan Syrup)
Chemical Class: Ethylamine phenothiazine derivative

DEA Class: Schedule V

■ **Clinical Pharmacology:**
Mechanism of Action: A phenothiazine that acts as an antihistamine, antiemetic, and CNS-antipsychotic-typical-hypnotic. As an antihistamine, inhibits histamine at histamine receptor sites. As an antiemetic, diminishes vestibular stimulation, depresses labyrinthine function, and acts on the chemoreceptor trigger zone. As a sedative-hypnotic, produces CNS depression by decreasing stimulation to the brainstem reticular formation. **Therapeutic Effect:** Prevents allergic responses mediated by histamine, such as rhinitis, urticaria, and pruritus. Prevents and relieves nausea and vomiting.
Pharmacokinetics:

Route	Onset	Peak	Duration
PO	20 min	N/A	2–8 hr
IV	3–5 min	N/A	2–8 hr
IM	20 min	N/A	2–8 hr
Rectal	20 min	N/A	2–8 hr

Well absorbed from the GI tract after IM administration. Widely distributed. Metabolized in the liver. Primarily excreted in urine. Not removed by hemodialysis. **Half-life:** 16–19 hr.

■ **Available Forms:**
- *Syrup (Pentazine, Phenergan):* 6.25 mg/ml.
- *Tablets (Phenergan, Promacot):* 12.5 mg, 25 mg, 50 mg.

- *Injection*: 25 mg/ml (Phenergan), 50 mg/ml (Adgan, Anergan 50, Antinaus 50, Phenergan, Phenoject-50, Promacot).
- *Suppositories*: 12.5 mg (Phenergan, Promethegan), 25 mg (Phenadoz, Phenergan, Promethegan), 50 mg (Phenergan, Promethegan).

■ Indications and Dosages:
Allergic symptoms: PO 6.25–12.5 mg 3 times a day plus 25 mg at bedtime. IV, IM 25 mg. May repeat in 2 hr.
Motion sickness: PO 25 mg 30–60 min before departure; may repeat in 8–12 hr, then every morning on rising and before evening meal.
Prevention of nausea and vomiting: PO, IV, IM, Rectal 12.5–25 mg q4–6h as needed.
Preoperative and postoperative sedation; adjunct to analgesics: IV, IM 25–50 mg.
Sedative: PO, IV, IM, Rectal 25-50 mg/dose. May repeat q4-6h as needed.

■ Contraindications:
Angle-closure glaucoma, GI or GU obstruction, hypersensitivity to phenothiazines, severe CNS depression or coma

■ Side Effects
Expected
Somnolence, disorientation, hypotension, confusion, syncope
Frequent
Dry mouth, nose, or throat; urine retention; thickening of bronchial secretions
Occasional
Epigastric distress, flushing, visual disturbances, hearing disturbances, wheezing, paresthesia, diaphoresis, chills
Rare
Dizziness, urticaria, photosensitivity, nightmares

■ Serious Reactions
- Long-term therapy may produce extrapyramidal symptoms, such as dystonia (abnormal movements), pronounced motor restlessness, and parkinsonism.
- Blood dyscrasias, particularly agranulocytosis, occur rarely.

■ Patient/Family Education
- Avoid prolonged exposure to sunlight
- Drowsiness and dry mouth are expected side effects of the drug. Drinking coffee or tea may help reduce drowsiness and sipping tepid water and chewing sugarless gum may relieve dry mouth
- Avoid performing tasks that require mental alertness or motor skills until response to the drug has been established
- Notify the physician if visual disturbances occur
- Avoid alcohol

■ Monitoring Parameters
- Blood pressure, pulse
- Electrolytes

■ Geriatric side effects at a glance:
☑ CNS   ☑ Bowel Dysfunction   ☐ Bladder Dysfunction   ☑ Falls
Other: Orthostatic hypotension, cardiac conduction disturbances, anticholinergic side effects.

- **Use with caution in older patients with:** Not recommended for use in older alults.

- **U.S. Regulatory Considerations**
  ☑ FDA Black Box
  Although not relevant with older patients, dangerous to use in children younger than 2 years of age.
  ☑ OBRA regulated in U.S. Long Term Care

- **Other Uses in Geriatric Patient:** Allergic symptoms, motion sickness, antiemetic

- **Side Effects:**
  Of particular importance in the geriatric patient: Parkinson's disease (an atypical antipsychotic is recommended), seizure disorders, cardiovascular disease with conduction disturbance, hepatic encephalopathy, narrow-angle glaucoma, urinary retention.

- **Geriatric Considerations - Summary:** Promethazine is a phenothiazine derivative, with strongly antihistaminic and anticholinergic effects. It is most often used as an antiemetic, but prescribers should be aware that the side-effect profile encompasses that seen in phenothiazines (e.g., akathisia) as well as anticholinergic drugs (e.g., urinary retention, visual changes, sedation, and delirium). In a comparative study, prochlorperazine was superior to promethazine in the treatment of emergency department patients with uncomplicated nausea and vomiting.

- **Reference:**
  1. Ernst AA, Weiss SJ, Park S, et al. Prochlorperazine versus promethazine for uncomplicated nausea and vomiting in the emergency department: a randomized, double-blind clinical trial. Ann Emerg Med 2000;36:89-94.

propafenone hydrochloride

(proe-pa-feen'-one hye-droe-klor'-ide)

- **Brand Name(s):** Rythmol, Rythmol SR
  Chemical Class: 3-Phenylpropiophenone derivative

- **Clinical Pharmacology:**
  Mechanism of Action: An antiarrhythmic that decreases the fast sodium current in Purkinje or myocardial cells. Decreases excitability and automaticity; prolongs conduction velocity and the refractory period. **Therapeutic Effect:** Suppresses arrhythmias.
  Pharmacokinetics: Nearly completely absorbed following oral administration. Protein binding: 85%-97%. Metabolized in liver; undergoes first-pass metabolism. Primarily excreted in feces. **Half-life:** 2-10 hr.

- **Available Forms:**
  - *Tablets (Rythmol):* 150 mg, 225 mg, 300 mg.
  - *Capsules (Extended-Release [Rythmol SR]):* 225 mg, 325 mg, 425 mg.

■ **Indications and Dosages:**

Documented, life-threatening ventricular arrhythmias, such as sustained ventricular tachycardia: PO Initially, 150 mg q8h; may increase at 3- to 4-day intervals to 225 mg q8h, then to 300 mg q8h. Maximum: 900 mg/day. PO (Extended-Release) Initially, 225 mg q12h. May increase at 5-day intervals. Maximum: 425 mg q12h.

■ **Unlabeled Uses:** Treatment of supraventricular arrhythmias

■ **Contraindications:** Bradycardia; bronchospastic disorders; cardiogenic shock; electrolyte imbalance; sinoatrial, AV, and intraventricular impulse generation or conduction disorders, such as sick sinus syndrome or AV block, without the presence of a pacemaker; uncontrolled CHF

■ **Side Effects**

Frequent (13%–7%)

Dizziness, nausea, vomiting, altered taste, constipation

Occasional (6%–3%)

Headache, dyspnea, blurred vision, dyspepsia (heartburn, indigestion, epigastric pain)

Rare (less than 2%)

Rash, weakness, dry mouth, diarrhea, edema, hot flashes

■ **Serious Reactions**

- Propafenone may produce or worsen existing arrhythmias.
- Overdose may produce hypotension, somnolence, bradycardia, and atrioventricular conduction disturbances.

■ **Patient/Family Education**

- Signs of overdosage include hypotension, excessive drowsiness, decreased heart rate, or abnormal heartbeat
- Compliance is essential to control arrhythmias
- Altered taste sensation may occur
- Notify the physician if blurred vision or headache occurs
- Avoid tasks that require mental alertness or motor skills until response to the drug has been established

■ **Monitoring Parameters**

- ECG, consider dose reduction in patients with significant widening of the QRS complex or 2nd- or 3rd-degree AV block
- ANA, carefully evaluate abnormal ANA test, consider discontinuation if persistent or worsening ANA titers are detected
- Electrolytes
- Pattern of daily bowel activity and stool consistency
- Hepatic enzymes
- Therapeutic serum level, which is 0.06 to 1 mcg/ml

■ **Geriatric side effects at a glance:**

❑ CNS ❑ Bowel Dysfunction ❑ Bladder Dysfunction ❑ Falls

■ **U.S. Regulatory Considerations**

☑ FDA Black Box

Because of mortality risks noted for flecainide and/or encainide (type IC antiarrhythmics), this drug should be reserved for use in patients with life-threatening ventricular arrhythmias.
❑ OBRA regulated in U.S. Long Term Care

propantheline bromide

(proe-pan-the-leen broe'-mide)

■ **Brand Name(s):** Pro-Banthine
  Chemical Class: Quaternary ammonium derivative

■ **Clinical Pharmacology:**
  Mechanism of Action: A quaternary ammonium compound that has anticholinergic properties and that inhibits action of acetylcholine at postganglionic parasympathetic sites. **Therapeutic Effect:** Reduces gastric secretions and urinary frequency, urgency, and urge incontinence.
  Pharmacokinetics: Onset occurs within 90 min but less than 50% is absorbed from the gastrointestinal (GI) tract. Extensive hepatic metabolism. Excreted in the urine and feces. **Half-life:** 2.9 hr.

■ **Available Forms:**
  • **Tablets:** 7.5 mg, 15 mg.

■ **Indications and Dosages:**
  Peptic ulcer: PO 15 mg 3 times/day 30 min before meals and 30 mg at bedtime.

■ **Contraindications:** GI or genitourinary (GU) obstruction, myasthenia gravis, narrow-angle glaucoma, toxic megacolon, severe ulcerative colitis, unstable cardiovascular adjustment in acute hemorrhage, hypersensitivity to propantheline or other anticholinergics

■ **Side Effects**
  Frequent
  Dry mouth, decreased sweating, constipation
  Occasional
  Blurred vision, intolerance to light, urinary hesitancy, drowsiness, agitation, excitement
  Rare
  Confusion, increased intraocular pressure, orthostatic hypotension, tachycardia

■ **Serious Reactions**
  • Overdosage may produce temporary paralysis of ciliary muscle, pupillary dilation, tachycardia, palpitations, hot, dry, or flushed skin, absence of bowel sounds, hyperthermia, increased respiratory rate, ECG abnormalities, nausea, vomiting, rash over face or upper trunk, CNS stimulation, and psychosis, marked by agitation, restlessness, rambling speech, visual hallucinations, paranoid behavior, and delusions, followed by depression.

■ **Patient/Family Education**
- Avoid driving or other hazardous activities until stabilized on medication
- Avoid alcohol or other CNS depressants
- Avoid hot environments, heatstroke may occur
- Use sunglasses when outside to prevent photophobia, may cause blurred vision

■ **Monitoring Parameters**
- Blood pressure, body temperature
- Bowel sounds for peristalsis

■ **Geriatric side effects at a glance:**
☑ CNS   ☑ Bowel Dysfunction   ☑ Bladder Dysfunction   ❑ Falls
Other: Dry mouth, blurred vision, constipation

■ **Use with caution in older patients with:** Narrow-angle glaucoma, overflow incontinence,

■ **U.S. Regulatory Considerations**
❑ FDA Black Box   ❑ OBRA regulated in U.S. Long Term Care

■ **Other Uses in Geriatric Patient:** Urinary incontinence caused by detrusor hyperrflexia

■ **Side Effects:**
Of particular importance in the geriatric patient: Possibly less likely to antagonize cholinergic drug therapy in the treatment of Alzheimer's disease.

■ **Geriatric Considerations - Summary:** Propantheline is a peripheral anticholinergic drug that does not cross the blood-brain barrier so should cause less risk of psychosis and other central effects. Other anticholinergic side effects such as urinary retention and decreased bowel motility do occur and can limit the usefulness of this drug.

■ **References:**
1. Vangala V, Tueth M. Chronic anticholinergic toxicity: identification and management in older patients. Geriatrics 2003;58:36-37.
2. Tune LE. Anticholinergic effects of medication in elderly patients. J Clin Psychiatry 2001;62(suppl 21):11-14.

propoxyphene hydrochloride/ propoxyphene napsylate

(proe-pox'-i-feen hye-droe-klor'-ide/proe-pox'-i-feen nap'seh-late)

■ **Brand Name(s):** (propoxyphene hydrochloride) Darvon

■ **Brand Name(s):** (propoxyphene napsylate) Darvon-N

Combinations
Rx: with acetaminophen (Darvocet, Propacet, Wygesic)
Chemical Class: Diphenylheptane derivative; opiate derivative

DEA Class: Schedule IV

■ **Clinical Pharmacology:**
Mechanism of Action: An opioid agonist that binds with opioid receptors in the CNS.
Therapeutic Effect: Alters the perception of and emotional response to pain.
Pharmacokinetics:

Route	Onset	Peak	Duration
PO	15-60 min	N/A	4-6 hr

Well absorbed from the GI tract. Protein binding: High. Widely distributed. Metabolized in the liver. Primarily excreted in urine. Not removed by hemodialysis. **Half-life:** 6-12 hr; metabolite: 30-36 hr.

■ **Available Forms:**
  • *Capsules (Hydrochloride):* 65 mg.
  • *Tablets (Napsylate):* 100 mg.

■ **Indications and Dosages:**
Mild to moderate pain: PO (propoxyphene hydrochloride) 65 mg q4h as needed. Maximum: 390 mg/day. PO (propoxyphene napsylate) 100 mg q4h as needed. Maximum: 600 mg/day.

■ **Contraindications:** None known.

■ **Side Effects**
  Frequent
  Dizziness, somnolence, dry mouth, euphoria, hypotension (including orthostatic hypotension), nausea, vomiting, fatigue
  Occasional
  Allergic reaction (including decreased BP), diaphoresis, flushing, and wheezing), trembling, urine retention, vision changes, constipation, headache
  Rare
  Confusion, increased BP, depression, abdominal cramps, anorexia

Serious Reactions
- Overdose results in respiratory depression, skeletal muscle flaccidity, cold or clammy skin, cyanosis, and extreme somnolence progressing to seizures, stupor, and coma.
- Hepatotoxicity may occur with overdose of the acetaminophen component of fixed-combination products.
- The patient who uses propoxyphene repeatedly may develop a tolerance to the drug's analgesic effect and physical dependence.

Patient/Family Education
- May cause drowsiness, dizziness, or blurred vision
- Use caution driving or engaging in other activities requiring alertness
- Avoid alcohol
- Take propoxyphene before the pain fully returns, within prescribed intervals
- Do not abruptly discontinue the drug
- May be habit-forming

Monitoring Parameters
- Pattern of daily bowel activity and stool consistency
- Clinical improvement and onset of pain relief
- Though not used clinically, therapeutic serum level of propoxyphene is 100 to 400 ng/ml, and the toxic serum level is over 500 ng/ml

Geriatric side effects at a glance:
☑ CNS   ☑ Bowel Dysfunction   ☑ Bladder Dysfunction   ☑ Falls

U.S. Regulatory Considerations
☑ FDA Black Box
- Risk of CNS depression when used with other CNS depressants
- Do not use in suicidal or alcoholic patients
☐ OBRA regulated in U.S. Long Term Care

propranolol hydrochloride

(proe-pran'-oh-lole hye-droe-klor'-ide)

Brand Name(s): Inderal, Inderal LA, InnoPran XL, Propranolol Intensol

Combinations
Rx: with HCTZ (Inderide)
Chemical Class: β-Adrenergic blocker, nonselective

Clinical Pharmacology:
Mechanism of Action: An antihypertensive, antianginal, antiarrhythmic, and CV-antihypertensive-BB that blocks beta$_1$- and beta$_2$-adrenergic receptors. Decreases oxy-

1045

gen requirements. Slows AV conduction and increases refractory period in AV node. Large doses increase airway resistance. **Therapeutic Effect:** Slows sinus heart rate; decreases cardiac output, BP, and myocardial ischemia severity. Exhibits antiarrhythmic activity.
Pharmacokinetics:

Route	Onset	Peak	Duration
PO	1–2 hr	N/A	6 hr

Well absorbed from the GI tract. Protein binding: 93%. Widely distributed. Metabolized in the liver. Primarily excreted in urine. Not removed by hemodialysis. **Half-life:** 3–5 hr.

■ **Available Forms:**
- *Tablets (Inderal):* 10 mg, 20 mg, 40 mg, 60 mg, 80 mg.
- *Capsules (Extended-Release):* 60 mg (Inderal LA), 80 mg (Inderal LA, InnoPran XL), 120 mg (Inderal LA, InnoPran XL), 160 mg (Inderal LA).
- *Oral Solution (Inderal):* 20 mg/5 ml, 40 mg/5 ml.
- *Oral Concentrate (Propranolol Intensol):* 80 mg/ml.
- *Injection (Inderal):* 1 mg/ml.

■ **Indications and Dosages:**
Hypertension: PO Initially, 40 mg twice a day. May increase dose q3-7 days. Range: Up to 320 mg/day in divided doses. Maximum: 640 mg/day.
Angina: PO 80–320 mg/day in divided doses. (long acting): Initially, 80 mg/day. Maximum: 320 mg/day.
Arrhythmias: IV 1 mg/dose. May repeat q5min. Maximum: 5 mg total dose. PO Initially, 10–20 mg q6-8h. May gradually increase dose. Range: 40–320 mg/day.
Life-threatening arrhythmias: IV 0.5–3 mg. Repeat once in 2 min. Give additional doses at intervals of at least 4 hr.
Hypertrophic subaortic stenosis: PO 20–40 mg in 3–4 divided doses. Or 80–160 mg/day as extended-release capsule.
Adjunct to alpha-blocking agents to treat pheochromocytoma: PO 60 mg/day in divided doses with alpha-blocker for 3 days before surgery. Maintenance (inoperable tumor): 30 mg/day with alpha-blocker.
Migraine headache: PO 80 mg/day in divided doses. Or 80 mg once daily as extended-release capsule. Increase up to 160–240 mg/day in divided doses.
Reduction of cardiovascular mortality and reinfarction in patients with previous MI: PO 180–240 mg/day in divided doses.
Essential tremor: PO Initially, 40 mg twice a day increased up to 120–320 mg/day in 3 divided doses.

■ **Unlabeled Uses:** Treatment adjunct for anxiety, mitral valve prolapse syndrome, thyrotoxicosis, behavioral disturbance in dementia

■ **Contraindications:** Asthma, bradycardia, cardiogenic shock, chronic obstructive pulmonary disease (COPD), heart block, Raynaud's syndrome, uncompensated CHF

■ **Side Effects**
Frequent
Diminished sexual ability, drowsiness, difficulty sleeping, unusual fatigue or weakness
Occasional
Bradycardia, depression, sensation of coldness in extremities, diarrhea, constipation, anxiety, nasal congestion, nausea, vomiting
Rare
Altered taste, dry eyes, pruritus, paresthesia

■ Serious Reactions
- Overdose may produce profound bradycardia and hypotension.
- Abrupt withdrawal may result in sweating, palpitations, headache, and tremors.
- Propranolol administration may precipitate CHF and MI in patients with cardiac disease; thyroid storm in those with thyrotoxicosis; and peripheral ischemia in those with existing peripheral vascular disease.
- Hypoglycemia may occur in patients with previously controlled diabetes.

■ Patient/Family Education
- Do not discontinue abruptly, may require taper; rapid withdrawal may produce rebound hypertension or angina
- If a dose is missed, take the next scheduled dose and do not double the dose
- Rise slowly from a lying to sitting position and wait momentarily before standing, to avoid the drug's hypotensive effect
- Do not take nasal decongestants and OTC cold preparations, especially those containing stimulants, without physician approval
- Limit alcohol and salt intake

■ Monitoring Parameters
- *Angina*: Reduction in nitroglycerin usage; frequency, severity, onset, and duration of angina pain; heart rate
- *Arrhythmias*: Heart rate
- *Congestive heart failure*: Functional status, cough, dyspnea on exertion, paroxysmal nocturnal dyspnea, exercise tolerance, and ventricular function
- *Hypertension*: Blood pressure
- *Migraine headache*: Reduction in the frequency, severity, and duration of attacks
- *Postmyocardial infarction*: Left ventricular function, lower resting heart rate
- *Toxicity*: Blood glucose, bronchospasm, hypotension, bradycardia, depression, confusion, hallucination, sexual dysfunction

■ Geriatric side effects at a glance:
❑ CNS   ❑ Bowel Dysfunction   ❑ Bladder Dysfunction   ❑ Falls

■ U.S. Regulatory Considerations
☑ FDA Black Box
In patients using orally administered beta-blockers, abrupt withdrawal may precipitate angina or lead to myocardial infarction or ventricular arrhythmias.
❑ OBRA regulated in U.S. Long Term Care

propylthiouracil

(proe-pill-thye-oh-yoor'-a-sill)

Chemical Class: Thioamide derivative

■ **Clinical Pharmacology:**
Mechanism of Action: A thiourea derivative that blocks oxidation of iodine in the thyroid gland and blocks synthesis of thyroxine and triiodothyronine. **Therapeutic Effect:** Inhibits synthesis of thyroid hormone.
Pharmacokinetics: Readily absorbed from GI tract. Protein binding: 80%. Metabolized in liver. Excreted in urine. **Half-life:** 1-4 hr.

■ **Available Forms:**
- *Tablets:* 50 mg.

■ **Indications and Dosages:**
Hyperthyroidism: PO Initially: 300–450 mg/day in divided doses q8h. Maintenance: 100–150 mg/day in divided doses q8–12h.

■ **Contraindications:** None known.

■ **Side Effects**
Frequent
Urticaria, rash, pruritus, nausea, skin pigmentation, hair loss, headache, paresthesia
Occasional
Somnolence, lymphadenopathy, vertigo
Rare
Drug fever, lupus-like syndrome

■ **Serious Reactions**
- Agranulocytosis as long as 4 months after therapy, pancytopenia, and fatal hepatitis have occurred.

■ **Patient/Family Education**
- Notify clinician of fever, sore throat, unusual bleeding or bruising, rash, yellowing of skin, vomiting
- Space doses evenly around the clock
- Take resting pulse daily to monitor therapeutic results; report pulse rate of less than 60 beats/min
- Restrict consumption of iodine products and seafood

■ **Monitoring Parameters**
- CBC periodically during therapy (especially during initial 3 mo), TSH
- Pulse
- Weight
- Be alert to signs and symptoms of hepatitis, including somnolence, jaundice, nausea, and vomiting

- **Geriatric side effects at a glance:**
  - ❏ CNS ❏ Bowel Dysfunction ❏ Bladder Dysfunction ❏ Falls

- **U.S. Regulatory Considerations**
  - ❏ FDA Black Box ❏ OBRA regulated in U.S. Long Term Care

protamine sulfate

(proe'-ta-meen sul'-fate)

Chemical Class: Basic protein

- **Clinical Pharmacology:**
  Mechanism of Action: A protein that complexes with heparin to form a stable salt.
  Therapeutic Effect: Reduces anticoagulant activity of heparin.
  Pharmacokinetics: Metabolized by fibrinolysin. Half-life: 7.4 min.

- **Available Forms:**
  - Injection: 10 mg/ml.

- **Indications and Dosages:**
  Heparin overdose (antidote and treatment): IV 1-1.5 mg protamine neutralizes 100 units heparin. Heparin disappears rapidly from circulation, reducing the dosage demand for protamine as time elapses.

- **Unlabeled Uses:** Treatment of low-molecular-weight heparin toxicity

- **Contraindications:** None known.

- **Side Effects**
  Frequent
  Decreased BP, dyspnea
  Occasional
  Hypersensitivity reaction (urticaria, angioedema); nausea and vomiting, which generally occur in those sensitive to fish and seafood, vasectomized men, infertile men, those on isophane (NPH) insulin, or those previously on protamine therapy
  Rare
  Back pain

- **Serious Reactions**
  - Too-rapid IV administration may produce acute hypotension, bradycardia, pulmonary hypertension, dyspnea, transient flushing, and feeling of warmth.
  - Heparin rebound may occur several hours after heparin has been neutralized (usually 8–9 hr after protamine administration). Heparin rebound occurs most often after arterial or cardiac surgery.

Special Considerations
- Will not reliably inactivate low-molecular-weight heparin

- Activated partial thromboplastin time (aPTT) or protamine activated clotting time (ACT) 15 min after dose, then in several hr

■ **Patient/Family Education**
- Use an electric razor and soft toothbrush to prevent bleeding until coagulation studies normalize
- Report black or red stool, coffee-ground vomitus, dark or red urine, or red-speckled mucus from cough

■ **Monitoring Parameters**
- Activated clotting time, aPTT, BP, cardiac function, and other coagulation tests

■ **Geriatric side effects at a glance:**
❏ CNS ❏ Bowel Dysfunction ❏ Bladder Dysfunction ❏ Falls

■ **U.S. Regulatory Considerations**
❏ FDA Black Box ❏ OBRA regulated in U.S. Long Term Care

protriptyline hydrochloride

(proe-trip'-ti-leen hye-droe-klor'-ide)

■ **Brand Name(s):** Vivactil
Chemical Class: Dibenzocycloheptene derivative; secondary amine

■ **Clinical Pharmacology:**
Mechanism of Action: A tricyclic antidepressant that increases synaptic concentration of norepinephrine and/or serotonin by inhibiting their reuptake by presynaptic membranes. **Therapeutic Effect:** Produces antidepressant effect.
Pharmacokinetics: Well absorbed from the gastrointestinal (GI) tract. Protein binding: 92%. Widely distributed. Extensively metabolized in liver. Excreted in urine. Not removed by hemodialysis. **Half-life:** 54-92 hr.

■ **Available Forms:**
- *Tablets:* 5 mg, 10 mg.

■ **Indications and Dosages:**
Depression: PO 5 mg 3 times/day. May increase gradually.

■ **Unlabeled Uses:** Narcolepsy, sleep apnea, sleep hypoxemia

■ **Contraindications:** Acute recovery period after myocardial infarction, co-administration with cisapride, use of MAOIs within 14 days, hypersensitivity to protriptyline or any component of the formulation

■ **Side Effects**
Frequent
Drowsiness, weight gain, fatigue, dry mouth, blurred vision, constipation, delayed micturition, postural hypotension, diaphoresis, disturbed concentration, increased appetite, urinary retention

Occasional

GI disturbances, such as nausea, diarrhea, GI distress, metallic taste sensation

Rare

Paradoxical reaction, marked by agitation, restlessness, nightmares, insomnia, extrapyramidal symptoms, particularly fine hand tremor

■ **Serious Reactions**
- High dosage may produce confusion, seizures, severe drowsiness, arrhythmias, fever, hallucinations, agitation, shortness of breath, vomiting, and unusual tiredness or weakness.
- Abrupt withdrawal from prolonged therapy may produce severe headache, malaise, nausea, vomiting, and vivid dreams.

■ **Patient/Family Education**
- Therapeutic effects may take 2-3 wk
- Use caution in driving or other activities requiring alertness
- Avoid rising quickly from sitting to standing
- Avoid alcohol and other CNS depressants
- Do not discontinue abruptly after long-term use
- Wear sunscreen or large hat to prevent photosensitivity
- Chew sugarless gum for dry mouth

■ **Monitoring Parameters**
- CBC, weight, ECG, mental status (mood, sensorium, affect, suicidal tendencies)

■ **Geriatric side effects at a glance:**
   ☑ CNS   ☑ Bowel Dysfunction   ☑ Bladder Dysfunction   ☑ Falls
   Other: Orthostatic hypotension, cardiac conduction disturbances, anticholinergic side effects

■ **Use with caution in older patients with:** Cardiovascular disease, prostatic hyptertrophy or other conditions which increase the risk of urinary retention.

■ **U.S. Regulatory Considerations**
   ☑ FDA Black Box
- Because there is an increased risk of suicide in children and adolescents, older adults should also be closely monitored for suicide ideation.
   ☑ OBRA regulated in U.S. Long Term Care

■ **Other Uses in Geriatric Patient:** Neuropathic pain, urge urinary incontinence

■ **Side Effects:**
   Of particular importance in the geriatric patient: Anticholinergic effects

■ **Geriatric Considerations - Summary:** Although tricyclic antidepressants are effective in the treatment of major depression in older adults, the side-effect profile and low toxic-to-therapeutic ratio relegate them to second-line agents (after serotonin reuptake inhibitors) for most older patients. These agents are effective in the treatment of urge urinary incontinence and neuropathic pain, but must be monitored closely. Of the tricyclic antidepressants, imipramine and amitryptyline have the highest anticholinergic activity and may be best choice in this class for management of incontinence, but should otherwise be avoided.

■ References:

1. Leipzig RM, Cumming RG, Tinetti ME. Drugs and falls in older people: a systematic review and meta-analysis: I. Psychotropic drugs. J Am Geriatr Soc 1999;47:30-39.
2. Cadieux RJ. Antidepressant drug interactions in the elderly. Understanding the P-450 system is half the battle in reducing risks. Postgrad Med 1999;106:231-240, 245.
3. Ray WA, Meredith S, Thapa PB, et al. Cyclic antidepressants and the risk of sudden cardiac death. Clin Pharmacol Ther 2004;75:234-241.
4. Roose SP, Laghrissi-Thode F, Kennedy JS, et al. Comparison of paroxetine and nortriptyline in depressed patients with ischemic heart disease. JAMA 1998;279:287-291.

pseudoephedrine hydrochloride

(soo-doe-e-fed'-rin hye-droe-klor'-ide)

OTC: Biofed, Cenafed, Decofed, Decofed, Dimetapp Decongestant, Dimetapp 12 Hour Non-Drowsy Extentabs, Dimetapp Decongestant, Efidac Genaphed, Seudotabs, Sudafed, Sudafed 12 Hour Caplets, Sudafed 24 Hour

Combinations
Pseudoephedrine is available in many prescription and over-the-counter combinations; the following list is not all-inclusive.
Rx: with azatadine (Trinalin Repetabs); brompheniramine (Bromfed); carbinoxamine (Rondec); chlorpheniramine (Deconamine SR, Novafed A); codeine (Nucofed); guaifenesin and codeine (Novagest Expectorant); loratadine (Claritin-D)
OTC: with acetaminophen (Dristan Cold); chlorpheniramine (Chlor-Trimeton 12 Hour Relief); dexbrompheniramine (Drixoral Cold and Allergy); dextromethorphan (Thera-Flu Non-Drowsy Formula); diphenhydramine (Actifed Allergy); ibuprofen (Advil Cold & Sinus, Dristan Sinus); triprolidine (Actifed)
Chemical Class: Sympathomimetic amine

■ Clinical Pharmacology:
Mechanism of Action: A sympathomimetic that directly stimulates alpha-adrenergic and beta-adrenergic receptors. ***Therapeutic Effect:*** Produces vasoconstriction of respiratory tract mucosa; shrinks nasal mucous membranes; reduces edema and nasal congestion.

Pharmacokinetics:

Route	Onset	Peak	Duration
PO (tablets, syrup)	15–30 min	N/A	4–6 hr
PO (extended-release)	N/A	N/A	8–12 hr

Well absorbed from the GI tract. Partially metabolized in the liver. Primarily excreted in urine. Not removed by hemodialysis. ***Half-life:*** 9–16 hr (children, 3.1 hr).

Available Forms:
- *Gelcaps* (*Dimetapp Decongestant*): 30 mg.
- *Liquid*: 15 mg/5 ml.
- *Syrup* (*Biofed, Decofed*): 30 mg/5 ml.
- *Tablets* (*Genaphed, Sudafed*): 30 mg.
- *Tablets* (*Extended-Release*): 120 mg (Dimetapp 12 Hour Non-Drowsy Extentabs, Sudafed 12 Hour), 240 mg (Sudafed 24 Hour).

Indications and Dosages:
Decongestant: PO 30–60 mg q6h. Maximum: 240 mg/day. PO (Extended-Release) 120 mg q12h or 240 mg once daily.

Contraindications:
Coronary artery disease, severe hypertension, use within 14 days of MAOIs

Side Effects
Occasional (10%–5%)
Nervousness, restlessness, insomnia, tremor, headache
Rare (4%–1%)
Diaphoresis, weakness

Serious Reactions
- Large doses may produce tachycardia, palpitations (particularly in patients with cardiac disease), light-headedness, nausea, and vomiting.
- Overdose in patients older than 60 years may result in hallucinations, CNS depression, and seizures.

Patient/Family Education
- May cause wakefulness or nervousness
- Take last dose 4-6 hr prior to hs; notify clinician of insomnia, dizziness, weakness, tremor, or irregular heartbeat
- Swallow extended-release tablets whole, do not chew or crush them
- Discontinue therapy and notify the physician if dizziness, insomnia, irregular or rapid heartbeat, tremors, or other side effects occur

Monitoring Parameters
- Therapeutic response

Geriatric side effects at a glance:
☑ CNS   ☐ Bowel Dysfunction   ☑ Bladder Dysfunction   ☐ Falls

Use with caution in older patients with:
Hypertension, prostatic hypertrophy

U.S. Regulatory Considerations
☐ FDA Black Box   ☑ OBRA regulated in U.S. Long Term Care

Other Uses in Geriatric Patient:
Stress urinary incontinence

- **Side Effects:**
  Of particular importance in the geriatric patient: Insomnia, restlessness, increased blood pressure.

- **Geriatric Considerations - Summary:** Pseudoephedrine activates alpha-adrenergic receptors with the potential for CNS stimulation and increased blood pressure. Pseudoephedrine causes increased urethral tone which would benefit stress incontinence but could cause urinary retention in older males with prostate hypertrophy. Older adults may have a greater sensitivity to the CNS effects of pseudoephedrine.

- **Reference:**
  1. Chua SS, Benrimoj SI, Gordon RD, et al: A controlled clinical trial on the cardiovascular effects of single doses of pseudoephedrine in hypertensive patients. Br J Clin Pharmacol 1989;28:369-372.

psyllium

(sil'-i-yum)

OTC: Fiberall, Hydrocil, Konsyl, Metamucil, Perdiem

Combinations
OTC: with senna (Perdiem)
Chemical Class: Psyllium colloid

- **Clinical Pharmacology:**
  Mechanism of Action: A bulk-forming laxative that dissolves and swells in water providing increased bulk and moisture content in stool. ***Therapeutic Effect:*** Promotes peristalsis and bowel motility.
  Pharmacokinetics:

Route	Onset	Peak	Duration
PO	12–24 hr	2–3 days	N/A

  Acts in small and large intestines.

- **Available Forms:**
  - *Powder (Fiberall, Hydrocil, Konsyl, Metamucil).*
  - *Wafer (Metamucil):* 3.4 g/dose.
  - *Capsules (Metamucil):* 0.52 g.
  - *Granules (Perdiem):* 4 g/5 ml.

- **Indications and Dosages:**
  Constipation, irritable bowel syndrome: PO Alert 3.4g powder equals 1 rounded tsp, 1 packet, or 1 wafer. 2-5 capsules/dose 1-3 times a day. 1-2 tsp granules 1-2 times a day. 1 rounded tsp or 1 tbsp of powder 1-3 times a day. 2 wafers 1-3 times a day.

- **Contraindications:** Fecal impaction, GI obstruction, undiagnosed abdominal pain

- **Side Effects**
  Rare
  Some degree of abdominal discomfort, nausea, mild abdominal cramps, griping, faintness

Serious Reactions
- Esophageal or bowel obstruction may occur if administered less than 250 ml of liquid.

Patient/Family Education
- Maintain adequate fluid consumption
- Do not use in presence of abdominal pain, nausea, or vomiting
- Avoid inhaling dust from powder preparations; can cause runny nose, watery eyes, wheezing
- Institute measures to promote defecation such as increasing fluid intake, exercising, and eating a high-fiber diet

Monitoring Parameters
- Pattern of daily bowel activity and stool consistency; record time of evacuation
- Serum electrolyte levels

Geriatric side effects at a glance:
☐ CNS ☑ Bowel Dysfunction ☐ Bladder Dysfunction ☐ Falls

U.S. Regulatory Considerations
☐ FDA Black Box ☐ OBRA regulated in U.S. Long Term Care

pyrantel pamoate

(pi-ran'-tel pam'-oh-ate)

OTC: Antiminth, Pin-Rid, Pin-X, Reese's Pinworm
Chemical Class: Pyrimidine derivative

Clinical Pharmacology:
Mechanism of Action: A depolarizing neuromuscular blocking agent that causes the release of acetylcholine and inhibits cholinesterase. **Therapeutic Effect:** Results in a spastic paralysis of the worm and consequent expulsion from the host's intestinal tract.
Pharmacokinetics: Poorly absorbed through gastrointestinal (GI) tract. Time to peak occurs in 1-3 hr. Partially metabolized in liver. Primarily excreted in feces; minimal elimination in urine.

Available Forms:
- *Caplets:* 180 mg (Reese's Pinworm Caplets).
- *Capsules:* 180 mg (Pin-Rid).
- *Liquid:* 50 mg/ml (Reese's Pinworm Medicine).
- *Suspension, Oral:* 50 mg/ml (Antiminth, Pin-X).

■ **Indications and Dosages:**
   Enterobiasis vermicularis (pinworm): PO 11 mg base/kg once. Repeat in 2 wk. Maximum: 1 g/day.

■ **Contraindications:** Hypersensitivity to pyrantel or any of its components

■ **Side Effects**
   Occasional
   Nausea, vomiting, headache, dizziness, drowsiness, GI distress, weakness

■ **Serious Reactions**
   • Overdosage includes symptoms of anorexia, nausea, abdominal cramps, vomiting, diarrhea, and ataxia.

■ **Patient/Family Education**
   • Take with food or milk
   • Using a laxative to facilitate expulsion of worms is not necessary
   • All family members in close contact with patient should be treated
   • Strict hygiene is essential to prevent reinfection
   • Shake suspension well before pouring
   • Wash bedding and clothes to avoid being reinfected

■ **Monitoring Parameters**
   • Examine stool for presence of eggs or worms

■ **Geriatric side effects at a glance:**
   ☐ CNS   ☐ Bowel Dysfunction   ☐ Bladder Dysfunction   ☐ Falls

■ **U.S. Regulatory Considerations**
   ☐ FDA Black Box   ☐ OBRA regulated in U.S. Long Term Care

pyrazinamide

(peer-a-zin′-a-mide)

■ **Brand Name(s):** Pyrazinamide
   Chemical Class: Niacinamide derivative

■ **Clinical Pharmacology:**
   Mechanism of Action: An antitubercular whose exact mechanism of action is unknown. **Therapeutic Effect:** Either bacteriostatic or bactericidal, depending on the drug's concentration at the infection site and the susceptibility of infecting bacteria. **Pharmacokinetics:** Nearly completely absorbed from GI tract. Protein binding: 5%-10%. Excreted in urine. **Half-life:** 9-23 hr.

■ **Available Forms:**
- *Tablets*: 500 mg.

■ **Indications and Dosages:**
Tuberculosis (in combination with other antituberculars): PO 15-30 mg/kg/day in 1-4 doses. Maximum: 3 g/day.

■ **Contraindications:** Severe hepatic dysfunction

■ **Side Effects**
Frequent
Arthralgia, myalgia (usually mild and self-limiting)
Rare
Hypersensitivity reaction (rash, pruritus, urticaria), photosensitivity, gouty arthritis

■ **Serious Reactions**
- Hepatotoxicity, gouty arthritis, thrombocytopenia, and anemia occur rarely.

■ **Patient/Family Education**
- Compliance with full course is essential
- Notify clinician of fever, loss of appetite, malaise, nausea and vomiting, darkened urine, yellowish discoloration of skin and eyes, pain or swelling of joints
- Take with food to reduce GI upset
- Do not skip doses
- Follow-up physician office visits and laboratory tests are essential parts of treatment
- Avoid overexposure to the sun or ultraviolet light

■ **Monitoring Parameters**
- Liver function tests, serum uric acid at baseline and periodically throughout therapy
- Blood glucose levels, especially in patients with diabetes mellitus, because pyrazinamide administration may make diabetes management difficult
- Skin for rash
- CBC for anemia and thrombocytopenia

■ **Geriatric side effects at a glance:**
❑ CNS ❑ Bowel Dysfunction ❑ Bladder Dysfunction ❑ Falls

■ **U.S. Regulatory Considerations**
❑ FDA Black Box ❑ OBRA regulated in U.S. Long Term Care

pyridostigmine bromide

(peer-id-oh-stig'-meen broe'-mide)

■ **Brand Name(s):** Mestinon, Mestinon Timespan
   Chemical Class: Cholinesterase inhibitor; quaternary ammonium derivative

■ **Clinical Pharmacology:**
   Mechanism of Action: A cholinergic agent that prevents destruction of acetylcholine by inhibiting the enzyme acetylcholinesterase, thus enhancing impulse transmission across the myoneural junction. **Therapeutic Effect:** Produces miosis; increases intestinal, skeletal muscle tone; stimulates salivary and sweat gland secretions.
   Pharmacokinetics: Not protein bound. Excreted unchanged in urine. **Half-life:** Unknown.

■ **Available Forms:**
   • *Syrup* (Mestinon): 60 mg/5 ml.
   • *Tablets* (Mestinon): 60 mg.
   • *Tablets* (Extended-Release [Mestinon Timespan]): 180 mg.
   • *Injection* (Mestinon): 5 mg/ml.

■ **Indications and Dosages:**
   Myasthenia gravis: PO Initially, 60 mg 3 times a day. Dosage increased at 48-hr intervals. Maintenance: 60 mg –1.5g a day. PO (Extended-Release) 180-540 mg once or twice a day with at least a 6-hr interval between doses. IV, IM 2 mg q2–3h.
   Reversal of nondepolarizing neuromuscular blockade: IV 10–20 mg with, or shortly after, 0.6–1.2 mg atropine sulfate or 0.3–0.6 mg glycopyrrolate.

■ **Contraindications:** Mechanical GI or urinary tract obstruction, hypersensitivity to anticholinesterase agents

■ **Side Effects**
   Frequent
   Miosis, increased GI and skeletal muscle tone, bradycardia, constriction of bronchi and ureters, diaphoresis, increased salivation
   Occasional
   Headache, rash, temporary decrease in diastolic BP with mild reflex tachycardia, short periods of atrial fibrillation (in hyperthyroid patients), marked drop in BP (in hypertensive patients)

■ **Serious Reactions**
   • Overdose may produce a cholinergic crisis, manifested as increasingly severe muscle weakness that appears first in muscles involving chewing and swallowing and is followed by muscle weakness of the shoulder girdle and upper extremities, respiratory muscle paralysis, and pelvis girdle and leg muscle paralysis. If overdose occurs, stop all cholinergic drugs and immediately administer 1–4 mg atropine sulfate IV.

■ **Patient/Family Education**
   • Do not crush or chew sustained-release preparations

- Notify the physician if diarrhea, difficulty breathing, profuse salivation or sweating, irregular heartbeat, muscle weakness, severe abdominal pain, or nausea and vomiting occurs
- Keep a log of energy level and muscle strength to help guide drug dosing

■ Monitoring Parameters
- Therapeutic response: increased muscle strength, improved gait, absence of labored breathing (if severe)
- Appearance of side effects (narrow margin between first appearance of side effects and serious toxicity)
- Symptoms of increasing muscle weakness may be due to cholinergic crisis (overdosage) or myasthenic crisis (increased disease severity). If crisis is myasthenia, patient will improve after 1-2 mg edrophonium; if cholinergic, withdraw pyridostigmine and administer atropine

■ Geriatric side effects at a glance:
❑ CNS ☑ Bowel Dysfunction ❑ Bladder Dysfunction ❑ Falls

■ U.S. Regulatory Considerations
❑ FDA Black Box ❑ OBRA regulated in U.S. Long Term Care

pyridoxine hydrochloride (NUTR-vitamin B₆)

(peer-i-dox'-een hye-droe'-klor-ide)

■ Brand Name(s): Aminoxin, Beesix, Doxine, Nestrex, Pryi, Rodex, Vitabee 6, Vitamin B6
Chemical Class: NUTR-vitamin B complex

■ Clinical Pharmacology:
Mechanism of Action: Acts as a coenzyme for various metabolic functions, including metabolism of proteins, carbohydrates, and fats. Aids in the breakdown of glycogen and in the synthesis of gamma-aminobutyric acid in the CNS. **Therapeutic Effect:** Prevents pyridoxine deficiency. Increases the excretion of certain drugs, such as isoniazid, that are pyridoxine antagonists.
Pharmacokinetics: Readily absorbed primarily in jejunum. Stored in the liver, muscle, and brain. Metabolized in the liver. Primarily excreted in urine. Removed by hemodialysis. **Half-life:** 15–20 days.

■ Available Forms:
- *Capsules*: 250 mg.
- *Tablets*: 25 mg, 50 mg, 100 mg, 250 mg, 500 mg.
- *Tablets (Enteric-Coated [Aminoxin])*: 20 mg.
- *Injection (Vitamin B₆)*: 100 mg/ml.

■ **Indications and Dosages:**
   Dietary Supplement (RDA): PO *Males*: 1.7 mg/day. *Females*: 1.5 mg/day.
   Pyridoxine deficiency: PO Initially, 2.5–10 mg/day; then 2.5 mg/day when clinical signs are corrected.
   Drug-induced neuritis: PO (treatment) 100–300 mg/day in divided doses PO (prophylaxis) 25–100 mg/day.

■ **Contraindications:** None known.

■ **Side Effects**
   Occasional
   Stinging at IM injection site
   Rare
   Headache, nausea, somnolence; sensory neuropathy (paresthesia, unstable gait, clumsiness of hands) with high doses

■ **Serious Reactions**
   • Long-term megadoses (2-6g over more than 2 mo) may produce sensory neuropathy (reduced deep tendon reflexes, profound impairment of sense of position in distal limbs, gradual sensory ataxia). Toxic symptoms subside when drug is discontinued.
   • Seizures have occurred after IV megadoses.

■ **Patient/Family Education**
   • Avoid doses exceeding RDA unless directed by clinician
   • IM injection may cause discomfort
   • Eat foods rich in pyridoxine, including avocados, bananas, bran, carrots, eggs, organ meats, tuna, shrimp, hazelnuts, legumes, soybeans, sunflower seeds, and wheat germ

■ **Monitoring Parameters**
   • Respiratory rate, heart rate, blood pressure during large IV doses
   • Observe the patient for improvement of deficiency symptoms, including CNS abnormalities (anxiety, depression, insomnia, motor difficulty, paresthesia and tremors) and skin lesions (glossitis, seborrhea-like lesions around eyes, mouth, nose)

■ **Geriatric side effects at a glance:**
   ❑ CNS   ❑ Bowel Dysfunction   ❑ Bladder Dysfunction   ❑ Falls

■ **U.S. Regulatory Considerations**
   ❑ FDA Black Box   ❑ OBRA regulated in U.S. Long Term Care

pyrimethamine

(pye-ri-meth'-a-meen)

■ **Brand Name(s):** Daraprim

Combinations
Rx: with sulfadoxine (Fansidar)
Chemical Class: Aminopyrimidine derivative

■ **Clinical Pharmacology:**
Mechanism of Action: An antiprotozoal with blood and some tissue schizonticidal activity against malaria parasites of humans. Highly selective activity against plasmodia and *Toxoplasma gondii*. **Therapeutic Effect:** Inhibition of tetrahydrofolic acid synthesis.
Pharmacokinetics: Well absorbed, peak levels occurring between 2-6 hours following administration. Protein binding: 87%. Eliminated slowly. **Half-life:** approximately 96 hours.

■ **Available Forms:**
  • *Tablets:* 25 mg (Daraprim)

■ **Indications and Dosages:**
Toxoplasmosis: PO Initially, 50-75 mg daily, with 1-4g daily of a sulfonamide of the sulfapyrimidine type (e.g., sulfadoxine). Continue for 1-3 weeks, depending on response of patient and tolerance to therapy then reduce dose to one-half that previously given for each drug and continue for additional 4-5 weeks.
Acute malaria: PO *In combination with sulfonamide:* 25 mg daily for 2 days with a sulfonamide *Without concomitant sulfonamide:* 50 mg for 2 days
Chemoprophylaxis of malaria: PO 25 mg once weekly.

■ **Unlabeled Uses:** Prophylaxis for first episode and recurrence of *Pneumocystis carinii* pneumonia and *Toxoplasma gondii* in HIV-infected patients.

■ **Contraindications:** Hypersensitivity to pyrimethamine, megaloblastic anemia due to folate deficiency, monotherapy for treatment of acute malaria.

■ **Side Effects**
Frequent
Anorexia, vomiting
Occasional
Hypersensitivity reactions, Stevens-Johnson syndrome, toxic epidermal necrolysis, erythema multiforme, anaphylaxis, hyperphenylalaninemia, megaloblastic anemia, leukopenia, thrombocytopenia, pancytopenia, atrophic glossitis, hematuria, and disorders of cardiac rhythm
Rare
Pulmonary eosinophilia

■ **Serious Reactions**
  • None known.

- Discontinue if folate deficiency develops; administer leucovorin 5-15 mg IM qd for ≥3 days when recovery slow

■ **Patient/Family Education**
- Take with food
- Discontinue at 1st sign of rash
- Take each dose with a full glass of water

■ **Monitoring Parameters**
- CBC with platelets semi-weekly during therapy for toxoplasmosis, less frequently for malaria-related indications

■ **Geriatric side effects at a glance:**
❑ CNS ❑ Bowel Dysfunction ❑ Bladder Dysfunction ❑ Falls

■ **U.S. Regulatory Considerations**
❑ FDA Black Box ❑ OBRA regulated in U.S. Long Term Care

quazepam

(kway'-ze-pam)

■ **Brand Name(s):** Doral
Chemical Class: Benzodiazepine

DEA Class: Schedule IV

■ **Clinical Pharmacology:**
Mechanism of Action: A BZ-1 receptor selective benzodiazepine with sedative properties. **Therapeutic Effect:** Produces sedative effect from its central nervous system (CNS) depressant action.
Pharmacokinetics: Rapidly absorbed from gastrointestinal (GI) tract. Food increases absorption. Protein binding: 95%. Extensively metabolized in liver. Excreted in urine and feces. Unknown if removed by hemodialysis. **Half-life:** 25-41 hr.

■ **Available Forms:**
- **Tablets:** 7.5 mg, 15 mg.

■ **Indications and Dosages:**
Insomnia: PO Initially, 7.5-15 mg at bedtime. Adjust dose depending on initial response.

■ **Contraindications:** Sleep apnea, hypersensitivity to quazepam or any component of the formulation

■ **Side Effects**
Frequent
Muscular incoordination (ataxia), light-headedness, transient mild drowsiness, slurred speech

Occasional

Confusion, depression, blurred vision, constipation, diarrhea, dry mouth, headache, nausea

Rare

Behavioral problems such as anger, impaired memory; paradoxical reactions such as insomnia, nervousness, or irritability

- **Serious Reactions**
  - Abrupt or too-rapid withdrawal may result in pronounced restlessness, irritability, insomnia, hand tremors, abdominal and muscle cramps, sweating, vomiting, and seizures.
  - Overdosage results in somnolence, confusion, diminished reflexes, and coma.
  - Blood dyscrasias have been reported rarely.

- **Patient/Family Education**
  - Avoid alcohol and other CNS depressants
  - Do not discontinue abruptly after prolonged therapy
  - May cause daytime sedation, use caution while driving or performing other tasks requiring alertness
  - May be habit forming
  - Stop smoking

- **Monitoring Parameters**
  - Hepatic and renal function
  - Therapeutic response

- **Geriatric side effects at a glance:**
  ☑ CNS ☐ Bowel Dysfunction ☐ Bladder Dysfunction ☑ Falls
  Other: None

- **Use with caution in older patients with:** Concurrent treatment with potent CYP 3A4 inhibitors leads to increased plasma concentrations of quazepam; COPD; untreated sleep apnea

- **U.S. Regulatory Considerations**
  ☐ FDA Black Box ☑ OBRA regulated in U.S. Long Term Care

- **Other Uses in Geriatric Patient:** Anxiety symptoms and related disorders; dementia-related behavioral problems

- **Side Effects:**
  Of particular importance in the geriatric patient: Sedation

- **Geriatric Considerations - Summary:** Benzodiazepines are effective anxiolytic agents, and hypnotics. These drugs should be reserved for short-term use. SSRIs are preferred for long-term management of anxiety disorders in older adults, and sedating antidepressants (e.g., trazodone) or eszopiclone are preferred for long-term management of sleep problems. Long-acting benzodiazepines, including flurazepam, chlordiazepoxide, clorazepate, diazepam, clonazepam, and quazepam should generally be avoided in older adults as these agents have been associated with oversedation. On the other hand, short-acting benzodiazepines (e.g., triazolam) have been associated with a higher risk of withdrawal symptoms. When initiating therapy, benzodiazepines should be titrated carefully to avoid oversedation. In addition, many of the drugs in this class have been associated with severe withdrawal symptoms (e.g., anxiety and/or agitation, seizures) when discontinued abruptly.

■ **References:**
1. Leipzig RM, Cumming RG, Tinetti ME. Drugs and falls in older people: a systematic review and meta-analysis: I. Psychotropic drugs. J Am Geriatr Soc 1999;47:30-39.
2. Shorr RI, Robin DW. Rational use of benzodiazepines in the elderly. Drugs Aging 1994;4:9-20.
3. Shader RI, Greenblatt DJ. Use of benzodiazepines in anxiety disorders. N Engl J Med 1993;328:1398-1405.

quetiapine fumarate

(kwe-tye'-a-peen fyoo'-muh-rate)

■ **Brand Name(s):** Seroquel
  Chemical Class: Dibenzothiazepine derivative

■ **Clinical Pharmacology:**
  Mechanism of Action: A dibenzothiazepine derivative that antagonizes dopamine, serotonin, histamine, and alpha$_1$-adrenergic receptors. **Therapeutic Effect:** Diminishes manifestations of psychotic disorders. Produces moderate sedation, few extrapyramidal effects, and no anticholinergic effects.
  Pharmacokinetics: Well absorbed after PO administration. Protein binding: 83%. Widely distributed in tissues; CNS concentration exceeds plasma concentration. Undergoes extensive first-pass metabolism in the liver. Primarily excreted in urine. **Half-life:** 6 hr.

■ **Available Forms:**
  • *Tablets:* 25 mg, 100 mg, 200 mg, 300 mg.

■ **Indications and Dosages:**
  To manage manifestations of psychotic disorders: PO Initially, 25 mg twice a day, then 25-50 mg 2-3 times a day on the second and third days, up to 300-400 mg/day in divided doses 2-3 times a day by the fourth day. Further adjustments of 25-50 mg twice a day may be made at intervals of 2 days or longer. Maintenance: 300-800 mg/day (adults); 50-200 mg/day (elderly).
  Mania in bipolar disorder: PO Initially, 50 mg twice a day for 1 day. May increase in increments of 100 mg/day to 200 mg twice a day on day 4. May increase in increments of 200 mg/day to 800 mg/day on day 6. Range: 400-800 mg/day.
  Dosage in hepatic impairment, elderly or debilitated patients, and those predisposed to hypotensive reactions: These patients should receive a lower initial dose and lower dosage increases.

■ **Unlabeled Uses:** Autism

■ **Contraindications:** None known.

1064

■ **Side Effects**
  Frequent (19%-10%)
  Headache, somnolence, dizziness
  Occasional (9%-3%)
  Constipation, orthostatic hypotension, tachycardia, dry mouth, dyspepsia, rash, asthenia, abdominal pain, rhinitis
  Rare (2%)
  Back pain, fever, weight gain

■ **Serious Reactions**
  • Overdose may produce heart block, hypotension, hypokalemia, and tachycardia.

Special Considerations
  • Limited clinical experience, but similar to clozapine and risperidone; may be effective for negative symptoms of schizophrenia; so far no agranulocytosis reported with quetiapine

■ **Patient/Family Education**
  • Avoid alcohol
  • Take quetiapine as ordered; do not abruptly discontinue the drug or increase the dosage
  • Drowsiness generally subsides during continued therapy
  • Avoid tasks that require mental alertness or motor skills until response to the drug has been established
  • Change positions slowly to reduce the hypotensive effect of quetiapine
  • Drink lots of fluids, especially during physical activity

■ **Monitoring Parameters**
  • Blood pressure for hypotension and pulse rate for tachycardia, especially if the drug dosage has been increased rapidly
  • Pattern of daily bowel activity and stool consistency
  • Assess for evidence of a therapeutic response, such as improvement in self-care, increased interest in surroundings and ability to concentrate, and relaxed facial expression
  • Closely supervise suicidal patients during early therapy; as depression lessens, the patient's energy level improves, which increases the suicide potential

■ **Geriatric side effects at a glance:**
  ☑ CNS   ☑ Bowel Dysfunction   ❑ Bladder Dysfunction   ☑ Falls
  Other: Weight gain, glucose intolerance, diabetes, orthostatic hypotension, extrapyramidal symptoms

■ **Use with caution in older patients with:** Diabetes, glucose intolerance, cardiovascular disease

■ **U.S. Regulatory Considerations**
  ☑ FDA Black Box
  There is an increased risk of death in older patients with dementia. Although the causes of death were varied, most of the deaths appeared to be either cardiovascular (e.g., heart failure, sudden death) or infectious (e.g., pneumonia) in nature. This drug is not approved for treatment of patients with dementia-related psychosis.
  ☑ OBRA regulated in U.S. Long Term Care

- **Other Uses in Geriatric Patient:** Behavior disturbances in the setting of dementia

- **Side Effects:**
  Of particular importance in the geriatric patient: Weight gain, glucose intolerance, diabetes, increased risk of death (see FDA black box warning)

- **Geriatric Considerations - Summary:** Direct comparisons between older and newer antipsychotic drugs in demented elderly persons are scarce. Newer agents have the theoretical advantage of a lower incidence of tardive dyskinesia but may cause weight gain, impaired glycemic control, and increased risk for cardiovascular events. These agents should be used with caution in demented elderly persons, with frequent monitoring for side effects and a low threshold for discontinuing use. Indeed, the Food and Drug Administration has recently released an advisory about these medications outlining the risk for increased mortality.

- **References:**
  1. Sink KM, Holden KF, Yaffe K. Pharmacological treatment of neuropsychiatric symptoms of dementia: a review of the evidence. JAMA 2005;293:596-608.
  2. Alexopoulos GS, Streim J, Carpenter D, Docherty JP. Using antipsychotic agents in older patients. J Clin Psychiatry 2004;65 (Suppl 2):5-99.
  3. Cohen D. Atypical antipsychotics and new onset diabetes mellitus. An overview of the literature. Pharmacopsychiatry 2004;37:1-11.
  4. Deaths with antipsychotics in elderly patients with behavioral disturbances. Available at: www.fda.gov/cder/drug/advisory/antipsychotics.htm.
  5. Katz IR. Optimizing atypical antipsychotic treatment strategies in the elderly. J Am Geriatr Soc 2004;52:S272-S277.

quinapril hydrochloride

(kwin'-a-pril hye-droe-klor'-ide)

- **Brand Name(s):** Accupril
  Chemical Class: Angiotensin-converting enzyme (ACE) inhibitor, nonsulfhydryl

- **Clinical Pharmacology:**
  Mechanism of Action: An ACE inhibitor that suppresses the renin-angiotensin-aldosterone system and prevents the conversion of angiotensin I to angiotensin II, a potent vasoconstrictor; may also inhibit angiotensin II at local vascular and renal sites. **Therapeutic Effect:** Reduces peripheral arterial resistance, BP, and pulmonary capillary wedge pressure; improves cardiac output.
  Pharmacokinetics:

Route	Onset	Peak	Duration
PO	1 hr	N/A	24 hr

  Readily absorbed from the GI tract. Protein binding: 97%. Metabolized in the liver, GI tract, and extravascular tissue to active metabolite. Primarily excreted in urine. Minimal removal by hemodialysis. **Half-life:** 1-2 hr; metabolite, 3 hr (increased in those with impaired renal function).

- **Available Forms:**
  - *Tablets*: 5 mg, 10 mg, 20 mg, 40 mg.

- **Indications and Dosages:**

  Hypertension (monotherapy): PO Initially, 10-20 mg/day. May adjust dosage at intervals of at least 2 wk or longer. Maintenance: 20-80 mg/day as single dose or 2 divided doses. Maximum: 80 mg/day. *Elderly.* Initially, 2.5-5 mg/day. May increase by 2.5-5 mg q1-2wk.

  Hypertension (combination therapy): PO Initially, 2.5-5 mg/day. May increase by 2.5-5 mg q1-2wk.

  Adjunct to manage heart failure: PO Initially, 5 mg twice a day. Range: 20-40 mg/day.

  Dosage in renal impairment: Dosage is titrated to the patient's needs after the following initial doses:

Creatinine Clearance	Initial Dose
more than 60 ml/min	10 mg
30-60 ml/min	5 mg
10-29 ml/min	2.5 mg

- **Unlabeled Uses:** Treatment of hypertension and renal crisis in scleroderma, treatment of left ventricular dysfunction following MI

- **Contraindications:** Bilateral renal artery stenosis, history of angioedema from previous treatment with ACE inhibitors

- **Side Effects**

  Frequent (7%-5%)

  Headache, dizziness

  Occasional (4%-2%)

  Fatigue, vomiting, nausea, hypotension, chest pain, cough, syncope

  Rare (less than 2%)

  Diarrhea, cough, dyspnea, rash, palpitations, impotence, insomnia, drowsiness, malaise

- **Serious Reactions**
  - Excessive hypotension ("first-dose syncope") may occur in patients with CHF and in those who are severely salt or volume depleted.
  - Angioedema and hyperkalemia occur rarely.
  - Agranulocytosis and neutropenia may be noted in those with collagen vascular disease, including scleroderma and systemic lupus erythematosus, and impaired renal function.
  - Nephrotic syndrome may be noted in those with history of renal disease.
  - Hypoglycemia may occur in patients with diabetes using glucose-lowering drugs.

- **Patient/Family Education**
  - Caution with salt substitutes containing potassium chloride
  - Rise slowly to sitting/standing position to minimize orthostatic hypotension
  - Dizziness, fainting, light-headedness may occur during first few days of therapy
  - May cause altered taste perception or cough; persistent dry cough usually does not subside unless medication is stopped; notify clinician if these symptoms persist
  - Full therapeutic effect of quinapril may take 1-2 wk to appear

- Discontinuing the drug or skipping doses of quinapril may produce severe, rebound hypertension
- Avoid tasks that require mental alertness or motor skills until response to the drug has been established

■ **Monitoring Parameters**
- BUN, creatinine, potassium within 2 wk after initiation of therapy (increased levels may indicate acute renal failure), WBC count

■ **Geriatric side effects at a glance:**
  ❑ CNS ❑ Bowel Dysfunction ❑ Bladder Dysfunction ❑ Falls

■ **U.S. Regulatory Considerations**
  ☑ FDA Black Box
  Although not relevant for geriatric patients, teratogenicity is associated with the use of ACE inhibitors.
  ❑ OBRA regulated in U.S. Long Term Care

quinidine gluconate

(kwin'-i-deen glue'-kun-ate)

■ **Brand Name(s):** Apo-Quin-G, BioQuin Durules, Quinaglute Dura-Tabs, Quinidex Extentabs
  Chemical Class: Quinine isomer, dextrorotatory

■ **Clinical Pharmacology:**
  Mechanism of Action: An antiarrhythmic that decreases sodium influx during depolarization, potassium efflux during repolarization, and reduces calcium transport across the myocardial cell membrane. Decreases myocardial excitability, conduction velocity, and contractility. **Therapeutic Effect:** Suppresses arrhythmias.
  Pharmacokinetics: Almost completely absorbed after PO administration. Protein binding: 80%-90%. Metabolized in liver. Excreted in urine. Removed by hemodialysis. **Half-life:** 6-8 hr.

■ **Available Forms:**
- *Injection*: 80 mg/ml.
- *Tablets*: 200 mg, 300 mg.
- *Tablets (Extended-Release)*: 300 mg (Quinidex Extentabs), 324 mg (Quinaglute Dura-Tabs).

■ **Indications and Dosages:**
  Maintenance of normal sinus rhythm after conversion of atrial fibrillation or flutter; prevention of premature atrial, AV, and ventricular contractions; paroxysmal atrial tachycardia; paroxysmal AV junctional rhythm; atrial fibrillation; atrial flutter; paroxysmal ventricular tachycardia not associated with complete heart block: PO 100–600 mg q4–6h. (Long-acting): 324–972 mg q8–12h. IV 200–400 mg.

■ **Unlabeled Uses:** Treatment of malaria (IV only)

■ **Contraindications:** Complete AV block, development of thrombocytopenic purpura during prior therapy with quinidine or quinine, intraventricular conduction defects (widening of QRS complex)

■ **Side Effects**
Frequent
Abdominal pain and cramps, nausea, diarrhea, vomiting (can be immediate, intense)
Occasional
Mild cinchonism (ringing in ears, blurred vision, hearing loss) or severe cinchonism (headache, vertigo, diaphoresis, light-headedness, photophobia, confusion, delirium)
Rare
Hypotension (particularly with IV administration), hypersensitivity reaction (fever, anaphylaxis, photosensitivity reaction)

■ **Serious Reactions**
- Cardiotoxic effects occur most commonly with IV administration, particularly at high concentrations, and are observed as conduction changes (50% widening of QRS complex, prolonged QT interval, flattened T waves, and disappearance of P wave), ventricular tachycardia or flutter, frequent premature ventricular contractions (PVCs), or complete AV block.
- Quinidine-induced syncope may occur with the usual dosage.
- Severe hypotension may result from high dosages.
- Patients with atrial flutter and fibrillation may experience a paradoxical, extremely rapid ventricular rate that may be prevented by prior digitalization.
- Hepatotoxicity with jaundice due to drug hypersensitivity may occur.

Special Considerations
- 267 mg gluconate = 275 mg polygalacturonate = 200 mg sulfate

■ **Patient/Family Education**
- Take with food to decrease GI upset
- Do not crush or chew sustained-release tablets
- Notify the physician if fever, ringing in the ears, or visual disturbances occur
- Avoid direct sunlight or artificial light

■ **Monitoring Parameters**
- Plasma quinidine concentration (therapeutic range 2-6 mcg/ml)
- ECG
- Liver function tests during the 1st 4-8 wk
- CBC periodically during prolonged therapy
- Intake and output
- Renal function tests
- Serum potassium level

■ **Geriatric side effects at a glance:**
☑ CNS   ☐ Bowel Dysfunction   ☐ Bladder Dysfunction   ☐ Falls

■ **U.S. Regulatory Considerations**
☑ FDA Black Box

Because of mortality risks noted for flecainide and/or encainide (type IC antiarrhythmics), this drug should be reserved for use in patients with life-threatening ventricular arrhythmias.
❏ OBRA regulated in U.S. Long Term Care

quinine sulfate

(kwye'-nine sul'-fate)

■ **Brand Name(s):** Quinine
Chemical Class: Cinchona alkaloid

■ **Clinical Pharmacology:**
Mechanism of Action: A cinchona alkaloid that relaxes skeletal muscle by increasing the refractory period, decreasing excitability of motor end plates (curare-like), and affecting distribution of calcium with muscle fiber. Antimalaria: Depresses oxygen uptake, carbohydrate metabolism, elevates pH in intracellular organelles of parasites.
Therapeutic Effect: Relaxes skeletal muscle; produces parasite death.
Pharmacokinetics: Rapidly absorbed mainly from upper small intestine. Protein binding: 70%-95%. Metabolized in liver. Excreted in feces, saliva, and urine. **Half-life:** 8-14 hr (adults), 6-12 hr (children).

■ **Available Forms:**
• *Capsules*: 200 mg, 325 mg.
• *Tablets*: 260 mg.

■ **Indications and Dosages:**
Nocturnal leg cramps: PO 260-300 mg at bedtime as needed.
Treatment of malaria: PO 260-650 mg 3 times a day for 6-12 days.
Dosage in renal impairment:

Creatinine Clearance	Dosage Interval
10-50 ml/min	75% of normal dose or q12h
Less than 10 ml/min	30%-50% of normal dose or q24h

■ **Contraindications:** Hypersensitivity to quinine (possible cross-sensitivity to quinidine), G-6-PD deficiency, tinnitus, optic neuritis, history of thrombocytopenia during previous quinine therapy, blackwater fever

■ **Side Effects**
Frequent
Nausea, headache, tinnitus, slight visual disturbances (mild cinchonism)
Occasional
Extreme flushing of skin with intense generalized pruritus is most typical hypersensitivity reaction; also rash, wheezing, dyspnea, angioedema.
Prolonged therapy: cardiac conduction disturbances, decreased hearing

■ Serious Reactions
- Overdosage (severe cinchonism) may result in cardiovascular effects, severe headache, intestinal cramps w/vomiting and diarrhea, apprehension, confusion, seizures, blindness, and respiratory depression.
- Hypoprothrombinemia, thrombocytopenic purpura, hemoglobinuria, asthma, agranulocytosis, hypoglycemia, deafness, and optic atrophy occur rarely.

■ Patient/Family Education
- Take with food
- May cause blurred vision, use caution driving
- Discontinue drug if flushing, itching, rash, fever, stomach pain, difficult breathing, ringing in ears, visual disturbances occur
- Periodic lab tests are part of therapy

■ Monitoring Parameters
- Check for hypersensitivity: flushing, rash/urticaria, itching, dyspnea, wheezing
- Assess level of hearing, visual acuity, presence of headache/tinnitus, nausea and report adverse effects promptly (possible cinchonism)
- CBC results for blood dyscrasias; be alert to infection (fever, sore throat) and bleeding/bruising or unusual tiredness/weakness
- Pulse, ECG for arrhythmias
- Fasting blood sugar levels and watch for hypoglycemia (cold sweating, tremors, tachycardia, hunger, anxiety)

■ Geriatric side effects at a glance:
❑ CNS   ❑ Bowel Dysfunction   ❑ Bladder Dysfunction   ❑ Falls

■ U.S. Regulatory Considerations
❑ FDA Black Box   ❑ OBRA regulated in U.S. Long Term Care

quinupristin/dalfopristin

(kwin-yoo'-pris-tin/dal'-foh-pris-tin)

■ Brand Name(s): Synercid
Chemical Class: Streptogramin combination

■ Clinical Pharmacology:
Mechanism of Action: Two chemically distinct compounds that, when given together, bind to different sites on bacterial ribosomes, inhibiting protein synthesis. **Therapeutic Effect:** Bactericidal.
Pharmacokinetics: After IV administration, both are extensively metabolized in the liver, with dalfopristin to active metabolite. Protein binding: quinupristin, 23%-32%; dalfopristin, 50%-56%. Primarily eliminated in feces. **Half-life:** quinupristin, 0.85 hr; dalfopristin, 0.7 hr.

■ **Available Forms:**
- *Injection*: 500-mg vial (150 mg quinupristin/350 mg dalfopristin).

■ **Indications and Dosages:**
Infections due to vancomycin-resistant Enterococcus faecium: IV 7.5 mg/kg/dose q8h.
Skin and skin-structure infections: IV 7.5 mg/kg/dose q12h.

■ **Contraindications:** Hypersensitivity to pristinamycin, virginiamycin

■ **Side Effects**
Frequent
Mild erythema, pruritus, pain, or burning at infusion site (with doses greater than 7 mg/kg)
Occasional
Headache, diarrhea
Rare
Vomiting, arthralgia, myalgia

■ **Serious Reactions**
- Antibiotic-associated colitis and other superinfections may result from bacterial imbalance.
- Hepatic function abnormalities and severe venous pain and inflammation may occur.

Special Considerations
- Most appropriate use is when vancomycin-resistant *Enterococcus faecium* (VREF) infection is documented or strongly suspected, or for therapy of methicillin-resistant *Staphylococcus aureus* infection

■ **Patient/Family Education**
- Due to high chance of drug interactions through inhibition of CYP 3A4, use caution with any additional drugs
- Notify the physician if pain, redness, or swelling at the infusion site occurs
- Immediately notify the physician if severe diarrhea occurs and avoid taking antidiarrheals until instructed to do so

■ **Monitoring Parameters**
- CBC, ALT, AST, bilirubin, renal function
- Withhold the drug and promptly inform the physician if diarrhea occurs; diarrhea with abdominal pain, fever, and mucus or blood in stools may indicate antibiotic-associated colitis
- Evaluate the IV site for redness, vein irritation, burning, pruritus, mild erythema, and pain
- Be alert for signs and symptoms of superinfection, such as anal or genital pruritus, diarrhea, increased fever, nausea and vomiting, sore throat, and stomatitis

■ **Geriatric side effects at a glance:**
❑ CNS   ❑ Bowel Dysfunction   ❑ Bladder Dysfunction   ❑ Falls

■ **U.S. Regulatory Considerations**
☑ FDA Black Box
Approved for serious or life-threatening VREF bacteremia only.
❑ OBRA regulated in U.S. Long Term Care

rabeprazole sodium

(ra-be'-pray-zole soe'-dee-um)

■ **Brand Name(s):** Aciphex
  Chemical Class: Benzimidazole derivative

■ **Clinical Pharmacology:**
  Mechanism of Action: A proton pump inhibitor that converts to active metabolites that irreversibly bind to and inhibit hydrogen-potassium adenosine triphosphate, an enzyme on the surface of gastric parietal cells. Actively secretes hydrogen ions for potassium ions, resulting in an accumulation of hydrogen ions in gastric lumen. **Therapeutic Effect:** Increases gastric pH, reducing gastric acid production.
  Pharmacokinetics: Rapidly absorbed from the GI tract after passing through the stomach relatively intact. Protein binding: 96%. Metabolized extensively in the liver. Primarily excreted in urine. Unknown if removed by hemodialysis. **Half-life:** 1–2 hr (increased with hepatic impairment).

■ **Available Forms:**
  • *Tablets* (*Delayed-Release*): 20 mg.

■ **Indications and Dosages:**
  Gastroesophageal reflux disease: PO 20 mg/day for 4–8 wk. Maintenance: 20 mg/day.
  Duodenal ulcer: PO 20 mg/day after morning meal for 4 wk.
  NSAID-induced ulcer: PO 20 mg/day.
  Pathologic hypersecretory conditions: PO Initially, 60 mg once a day. May increase to 60 mg twice a day.
  Helicobacter pylori infection: PO 20 mg twice a day for 7 days (given with amoxicillin 1,000 mg and clarithromycin 500 mg)

■ **Contraindications:** None known.

■ **Side Effects**
  Rare (less than 2%)
  Headache, nausea, dizziness, rash, diarrhea, malaise

■ **Serious Reactions**
  • Hyperglycemia, hypokalemia, hyponatremia, and hyperlipidemia occur rarely.

Special Considerations
  • Symptomatic response does not rule out gastric malignancy

■ **Patient/Family Education**
  • Sustained-action tablets should be swallowed whole, do not chew, crush, or split the tablets
  • Notify the physician if headache occurs during rabeprazole therapy

■ **Monitoring Parameters**
  • Symptom relief, mucosal healing
  • Assess the patient for diarrhea, GI discomfort, headache, nausea, and skin rash

■ **Geriatric side effects at a glance:**
  ❑ CNS ❑ Bowel Dysfunction ❑ Bladder Dysfunction ❑ Falls

■ **U.S. Regulatory Considerations**
  ❑ FDA Black Box ❑ OBRA regulated in U.S. Long Term Care

raloxifene hydrochloride

(ral-ox'-i-feen hye-droe-klor'-ide)

■ **Brand Name(s):** Evista
  Chemical Class: Benzothiophene derivative

■ **Clinical Pharmacology:**
  Mechanism of Action: A selective estrogen receptor modulator that affects some receptors like estrogen. **Therapeutic Effect:** Like estrogen, prevents bone loss and improves lipid profiles.
  Pharmacokinetics: Rapidly absorbed after PO administration. Highly bound to plasma proteins (greater than 95%) and albumin. Undergoes extensive first-pass metabolism in liver. Excreted mainly in feces and, to a lesser extent, in urine. Unknown if removed by hemodialysis. **Half-life:** 27.7 hr.

■ **Available Forms:**
  • *Tablets*: 60 mg.

■ **Indications and Dosages:**
  Prevention or treatment of osteoporosis: PO 60 mg a day.

■ **Unlabeled Uses:** Prevention of fractures, treatment of breast cancer in postmenopausal women

■ **Contraindications:** Active or history of venous thromboembolic events, such as deep vein thrombosis (DVT), pulmonary embolism, and retinal vein thrombosis

■ **Side Effects**
  Frequent (25%–10%)
  Hot flashes, flu-like symptoms, arthralgia, sinusitis
  Occasional (9%–5%)
  Weight gain, nausea, myalgia, pharyngitis, cough, dyspepsia, leg cramps, rash, depression
  Rare (4%–3%)
  Vaginitis, UTI, peripheral edema, flatulence, vomiting, fever, migraine, diaphoresis

■ **Serious Reactions**
  • Pneumonia, gastroenteritis, chest pain, vaginal bleeding, and breast pain occur rarely.

- Shown to preserve bone mass, increase bone mineral density, and reduce fracture rate relative to calcium alone
- Ensure adequate dietary or supplemental calcium, vitamin D
- Not associated with endometrial proliferation; however, investigate uterine bleeding
- Risk of thromboembolic events greatest in first 4 mo, discontinue at least 72 hr prior to surgery involving immobilization. Resume when patient fully ambulatory

■ Patient/Family Education
- May be taken without regard to meals
- Engage in weight-bearing exercises; do not smoke or use alcohol excessively
- Report leg pain or swelling, sudden chest pain, shortness of breath, vision changes
- Avoid restrictions of movement during travel. Discontinue if at bed rest.
- Take supplemental calcium and vitamin D if daily intake is inadequate

■ Monitoring Parameters
- Bone density tests (e.g., DEXA scan)
- Platelet count, and serum levels of inorganic phosphate, calcium, total and LDL cholesterol, and protein

■ Geriatric side effects at a glance:
❑ CNS ❑ Bowel Dysfunction ❑ Bladder Dysfunction ❑ Falls

■ U.S. Regulatory Considerations
❑ FDA Black Box ❑ OBRA regulated in U.S. Long Term Care

ramipril

(ra-mi'-pril)

■ Brand Name(s): Altace
Chemical Class: Angiotensin-converting enzyme (ACE) inhibitor, nonsulfhydryl

■ Clinical Pharmacology:
Mechanism of Action: An ACE inhibitor that suppresses the renin-angiotensin-aldosterone system. Decreases plasma angiotensin II, increases plasma renin activity, and decreases aldosterone secretion. **Therapeutic Effect:** Reduces peripheral arterial resistance and BP.
Pharmacokinetics:

Route	Onset	Peak	Duration
PO	1-2 hr	3-6 hr	24 hr

Well absorbed from the GI tract. Protein binding: 73%. Metabolized in the liver to active metabolite. Primarily excreted in urine. Not removed by hemodialysis. **Half-life:** 5.1 hr.

Available Forms:
- *Capsules:* 1.25 mg, 2.5 mg, 5 mg, 10 mg.

Indications and Dosages:
Hypertension (monotherapy): PO Initially, 2.5 mg/day. Maintenance: 2.5-20 mg/day as single dose or in 2 divided doses.
Hypertension (in combination with other antihypertensives): PO Initially, 1.25 mg/day titrated to patient's needs.
CHF: PO Initially, 1.25-2.5 mg twice a day. Maximum: 5 mg twice a day.
Risk reduction for MI stroke: PO Initially, 2.5 mg/day for 7 days, then 5 mg/day for 21 days, then 10 mg/day as a single dose or in divided doses.
Dosage in renal impairment: Creatinine clearance equal to or less than 40 ml/min. 25% of normal dose. **Hypertension.** Initially, 1.25 mg/day titrated upward. **CHF.** Initially, 1.25 mg/day, titrated up to 2.5 mg twice a day.

Unlabeled Uses: Treatment of hypertension and renal crisis in scleroderma

Contraindications: Bilateral renal artery stenosis

Side Effects
Frequent (12%-5%)
Cough, headache
Occasional (4%-2%)
Dizziness, fatigue, nausea, asthenia (loss of strength)
Rare (less than 2%)
Palpitations, insomnia, nervousness, malaise, abdominal pain, myalgia

Serious Reactions
- Excessive hypotension ("first-dose syncope") may occur in patients with CHF and in those who are severely salt or volume depleted.
- Angioedema and hyperkalemia occur rarely.
- Agranulocytosis and neutropenia may be noted in those with collagen vascular disease, including scleroderma and systemic lupus erythematosus, and impaired renal function.
- Nephrotic syndrome may be noted in those with history of renal disease.
- Hypoglycemia may occur in patients with diabetes using glucose-lowering drugs.

Patient/Family Education
- Caution with salt substitutes containing potassium chloride
- Rise slowly to sitting/standing position to minimize orthostatic hypotension
- Dizziness, fainting, light-headedness may occur during first few days of therapy
- May cause altered taste perception or cough; persistent dry cough usually does not subside unless medication is stopped; notify clinician if these symptoms persist
- Do not discontinue the drug without physician approval
- Notify the physician if chest pain, cough, or palpitations occur
- Avoid tasks that require mental alertness or motor skills until response to the drug has been established

Monitoring Parameters
- BUN, creatinine, potassium within 2 wk after initiation of therapy (increased levels may indicate acute renal failure)
- Potassium levels, although hyperkalemia rarely occurs

- WBC count
- Assess the patient for cough
- Assess the patient with CHF for crackles and wheezing
- Monitor urinalysis for proteinuria

■ **Geriatric side effects at a glance:**
   ❑ CNS   ❑ Bowel Dysfunction   ❑ Bladder Dysfunction   ❑ Falls

■ **U.S. Regulatory Considerations**
   ☑ FDA Black Box
   Although not relevant for geriatric patients, teratogenicity is associated with the use of ACE inhibitors.
   ❑ OBRA regulated in U.S. Long Term Care

ranitidine hydrochloride/ ranitidine bismuth citrate

(ra-ni'-ti-deen hye-dro-klor'-ide/ra-ni'-ti-deen biz'-muth sit'-rate)

■ **Brand Name(s):** Zantac, Zantac-150, Zantac-150 Maximum Strength, Zantac-300, Zantac EFFERdose, Zantac-25 EFFERdose, Zantac-150 EFFERdose
OTC: Zantac 75
Chemical Class: Aminoalkyl furan derivative

■ **Clinical Pharmacology:**
Mechanism of Action: An H_2-blocker that inhibits histamine action at histamine$_2$ receptors of gastric parietal cells. **Therapeutic Effect:** Inhibits gastric acid secretion when fasting, at night, or when stimulated by food, caffeine, or insulin. Reduces volume and hydrogen ion concentration of gastric juice.
Pharmacokinetics: Rapidly absorbed from the GI tract. Protein binding: 15%. Widely distributed. Metabolized in the liver. Primarily excreted in urine. Not removed by hemodialysis. **Half-life:** PO, 2.5 hr; IV, 2–2.5 hr (increased with impaired renal function).

■ **Available Forms:**
- *Tablets (Effervescent):* 25 mg (Zantac-25 EFFERdose), 150 mg (Zantac-150 EFFERdose).
- *Capsules (Zantac):* 150 mg, 300 mg.
- *Granules (Zantac EFFERdose):* 150 mg.
- *Syrup (Zantac):* 15 mg/ml.
- *Tablets:* 75 mg (Zantac 75), 150 mg (Zantac-150, Zantac-150 Maximum Strength), 300 mg (Zantac-300).
- *Injection (Zantac):* 25 mg/ml.

■ **Indications and Dosages:**
Duodenal ulcers, gastric ulcers, gastroesophageal reflux disease: PO 150 mg twice a day or 300 mg at bedtime. Maintenance: 150 mg at bedtime.

Duodenal ulcers associated with Helicobacter pylori infection: PO 400 mg twice a day for 4 weeks in combination with clarithromycin 500 mg 2-3 times a day for the first 2 weeks.
Erosive esophagitis: PO 150 mg 4 times a day. Maintenance: 150 mg twice a day or 300 mg at bedtime.
Hypersecretory conditions: PO 150 mg twice a day. May increase up to 6 g/day.
OTC use: PO 75 mg 30-60 minutes before eating food or drinking beverages that cause heartburn. Maximum: 150 mg per 24-hr period and/or longer than 14 days.
Usual parenteral dosage: IV, IM 50 mg/dose q6-8h. Maximum: 400 mg/day.
Dosage in renal impairment: For patients with creatinine clearance less than 50 ml/min, give 150 mg PO q24h or 50 mg IV or IM q18-24h.

■ **Unlabeled Uses:** Prevention of aspiration pneumonia, treatment of recurrent postoperative ulcer, upper GI bleeding, prevention of acid aspiration pneumonitis during surgery, prevention of stress-induced ulcers.

■ **Contraindications:** History of acute porphyria

■ **Side Effects**
   Occasional (2%)
   Diarrhea
   Rare (1%)
   Constipation, headache (may be severe)

■ **Serious Reactions**
   • Reversible hepatitis and blood dyscrasias occur rarely.

Special Considerations
   • No advantage over other agents in this class; base selection on cost

■ **Patient/Family Education**
   • Stagger doses of ranitidine and antacids
   • Dissolve effervescent tablets and granules in 6-8 oz water before drinking
   • Smoking decreases the effectiveness of ranitidine
   • Do not take ranitidine within 1 hour of magnesium- or aluminum-containing antacids
   • Transient burning or itching may occur with IV administration
   • Avoid alcohol and aspirin, both of which may cause GI distress, during ranitidine therapy

■ **Monitoring Parameters**
   • Intragastric pH when used for stress ulcer prophylaxis; titrate dose to maintain pH >4
   • Serum alkaline phosphatase, bilirubin, AST and ALT levels

■ **Geriatric side effects at a glance:**
   ☑ CNS   ❏ Bowel Dysfunction   ❏ Bladder Dysfunction   ❏ Falls
   ❏ Other: Delirium

■ **Use with caution in older patients with:** Renal impairment, Cognitive impairment

■ **U.S. Regulatory Considerations**
   ❏ FDA Black Box   ❏ OBRA regulated in U.S. Long Term Care

- **Other uses in Geriatric Patient:** Acute allergic reactions, urticaria (in addition to antihistamine therapy)

- **Side Effects:**
  Of particular importance in the geriatric patient: Anticholinergic effects, delirium, confusion, dizziness, headache, constipation, diarrhea

- **Geriatric Considerations - Summary:** Adjust dose based on creatinine clearance. Not effective in preventing NSAID-induced gastric ulceration and bleeding; proton pump inhibitors should be used for this indication instead. Anticholinergic adverse effects have been observed in older adults taking ranitidine.

- **References:**
  1. Gawrich S, Shaker R. Medical management of nocturnal symptoms of gastro-oesophageal reflux disease in the elderly. Drugs Aging 2003;20:509-516.
  2. Tune LE. Anticholinergic effects of medication in elderly patients. J Clin Psychiatry 2001;62(suppl 21):11-14.
  3. Thomson ABR. Gastro-oesophageal reflux in the elderly. Role of drug therapy in management. Drugs Aging 2001;18:409-414.
  4. Drugs that may cause cognitive disorders in the elderly. Med Let 2000;42:111-112.

repaglinide

(re-pag'-lin-ide)

- **Brand Name(s):** Prandin
  Chemical Class: Meglitinide

- **Clinical Pharmacology:**
  Mechanism of Action: An antihyperglycemic that stimulates release of insulin from beta cells of the pancreas by depolarizing beta cells, leading to an opening of calcium channels. Resulting calcium influx induces insulin secretion. **Therapeutic Effect:** Lowers blood glucose concentration.
  Pharmacokinetics: Rapidly, completely absorbed from the GI tract. Protein binding: 98%. Metabolized in the liver to inactive metabolites. Excreted primarily in feces with a lesser amount in urine. Unknown if removed by hemodialysis. **Half-life:** 1 hr.

- **Available Forms:**
  - *Tablets:* 0.5 mg, 1 mg, 2 mg.

- **Indications and Dosages:**
  Diabetes mellitus: PO 0.5–4 mg 2–4 times a day. Maximum: 16 mg/day.

- **Contraindications:** Diabetic ketoacidosis, type 1 diabetes mellitus

- **Side Effects**
  Frequent (10%–6%)
  Upper respiratory tract infection, headache, rhinitis, bronchitis, back pain

Occasional (5%–3%)
Diarrhea, dyspepsia, sinusitis, nausea, arthralgia, UTI
Rare (2%)
Constipation, vomiting, paresthesia, allergy

■ **Serious Reactions**
  • Hypoglycemia occurs in 16% of patients.
  • Chest pain occurs rarely.

■ **Patient/Family Education**
  • Skip the dose of this medication if you skip a meal; take an extra dose with extra meal
  • Recognize and treat hypoglycemia; maintain ready supply of glucose (glucose tablets or gel)
  • The prescribed diet is a principal part of treatment
  • Be aware of the typical signs and symptoms of hypoglycemia and hyperglycemia
  • Wear medical alert identification stating that he or she has diabetes
  • Consult the physician when glucose demands are altered, such as with fever, heavy physical activity, infection, stress, or trauma
  • Diabetes mellitus requires lifelong control
  • Adhere to dietary instructions, a regular exercise program, and regular testing of urine or blood glucose
  • If the patient is taking repaglinide with insulin or a sulfonylurea, always have a source of glucose available to treat symptoms of low blood sugar

■ **Monitoring Parameters**
  • Blood glucose—biggest effect noted on postprandial values (50-75 mg/dl reductions expected); minimal effect on fasting blood glucose
  • Glycosylated hemoglobin (1% to 2% reductions expected)
  • Hyperglycemia/hypoglycemia signs and symptoms
  • Be alert to conditions that alter blood glucose requirements, such as fever, increased activity, stress, or a surgical procedure

■ **Geriatric side effects at a glance:**
  ❑ CNS   ❑ Bowel Dysfunction   ❑ Bladder Dysfunction   ❑ Falls
  Other: Hypoglycemia

■ **Use with caution in older patients with:** Hepatic impairment, Severe renal impairment

■ **U.S. Regulatory Considerations**
  ❑ FDA Black Box   ❑ OBRA regulated in U.S. Long Term Care

■ **Other Uses in Geriatric Patient:** None

■ **Side Effects:**
  Of particular importance in the geriatric patient: Hypoglycemia, headache, weight gain

■ **Geriatric Considerations - Summary:** Minimal renal clearance and metabolized to inactive metabolites, therefore may be safer in older adults with impaired renal function. Because of its short half-life and premeal administration, repaglinide can be held if the patient does not eat a meal in order to prevent hypoglycemia.

■ **References:**

1. Haas L. Management of diabetes mellitus medications in the nursing home. Drugs Aging 2005;22:209-218.
2. Chelliah A, Burge MR. Hypoglycemia in elderly patients with diabetes mellitus. Causes and strategies for prevention. Drugs Aging 2004;21:511-530.
3. Rosenstock J. Management of type 2 diabetes mellitus in the elderly: special considerations. Drugs Aging 2001;18:31-44.

reserpine

(reh-zer'-peen)

■ **Brand Name(s):** Serpalan

Combinations
Rx: with thiazide diuretics: i.e., bendroflumethazide (flumethiazide), chlorothiazide, chlorthalidone (Regreton), hydrochlorothiazide (Hydropres, Hydroserpalan, Hydroserpine, Mallopress), hydroflumethiazide (Salutensin), polythiazide (Reneese), quinethazone (Hydromox R), trichloromethiazide (Metatensin, Naquival), hydrochlorothiazide and hydralazine (Hyserp, Lo-Ten, Marpres, Ser-A-Gen, Seralazide, Ser-Ap-Es, Unipres, Uni-Serp)
Chemical Class: Rauwolfia alkaloid

■ **Clinical Pharmacology:**
Mechanism of Action: An antihypertensive that depletes stores of catecholamines and 5-hydroxytryptamine in many organs, including the brain and adrenal medulla. Depression of sympathetic nerve function results in a decreased heart rate and a lowering of arterial blood pressure. Depletion of catecholamines and 5-hydroxytryptamine from the brain is thought to be the mechanism of the sedative and tranquilizing properties. **Therapeutic Effects:** Decreases blood pressure and heart rate; sedation.
Pharmacokinetics: Characterized by slow onset of action and sustained effects. Both cardiovascular and central nervous system effects may persist for a period of time following withdrawal of the drug. Mean maximum plasma levels were attained after a median of 3.5 hours. Bioavailability was approximately 50% of that of a corresponding intravenous dose. Protein binding: 96%. **Half life:** 33 hours.

■ **Available Forms:**
• *Tablets*: 0.25 mg, 0.1 mg (reserpine).

■ **Indications and Dosages:**
Hypertension: PO Usual initial dosage 0.5 mg daily for 1 or 2 weeks. For maintenance, reduce to 0.1 to 0.25 mg daily.
Psychiatric disorders: PO Initial dosage 0.5 mg daily, may range from 0.1-1.0 mg. Adjust dosage upward or downward according to response.

- **Unlabeled Uses:** Cerebral vasospasm, migraines, Raynaud's syndrome, reflex sympathetic dystrophy, refractory depression, tardive dyskinesia, thyrotoxic crisis.

- **Contraindications:** Hypersensitivity, mental depression or history of mental depression (especially with suicidal tendencies), active peptic ulcer, ulcerative colitis, patients receiving electroconvulsive therapy.

- **Side Effects**
  Occasional
  Burning in the stomach, nausea, vomiting, diarrhea, dry mouth, nosebleed, stuffy nose, dizziness, headache, nervousness, nightmares, drowsiness, muscle aches, weight gain, redness of the eyes
  Rare
  Irregular heartbeat, difficulty breathing, heart problems, feeling faint, swelling, gynecomastia, decreased libido

- **Serious Reactions**
  - None known.

Special Considerations
  - Only remaining rauwolfia derivative available

- **Patient/Family Education**
  - May cause drowsiness or dizziness, use caution driving or participating in other activities requiring alertness
  - Therapeutic effect may take 2-3 wk
  - A low-salt diet should be followed
  - Notify physician immediately if depression, nightmares, fainting, slow heartbeat, chest pain, or swollen ankles and feet occur

- **Monitoring Parameters**
  - Blood pressure, edema, drowsiness, despondency or self-depreciation, early morning insomnia, CNS depression, hypothermia, extrapyradimal tract effects

- **Geriatric side effects at a glance:**
  ☑ CNS ❑ Bowel Dysfunction ❑ Bladder Dysfunction ❑ Falls

- **U.S. Regulatory Considerations**
  ❑ FDA Black Box ❑ OBRA regulated in U.S. Long Term Care

reteplase, recombinant

(re'-te-plays)

■ **Brand Name(s):** Retavase
  Chemical Class: Tissue plasminogen activator (tPA)

■ **Clinical Pharmacology:**
  Mechanism of Action: A tissue plasminogen activator that activates the fibrinolytic system by directly cleaving plasminogen to generate plasmin, an enzyme that degrades the fibrin of the thrombus. **Therapeutic Effect:** Exerts CV-thrombolytic action. **Pharmacokinetics:** Rapidly cleared from plasma. Eliminated primarily by the liver and kidney. **Half-life:** 13–16 min.

■ **Available Forms:**
  • *Powder for Injection:* 10.4 units (18.1 mg).

■ **Indications and Dosages:**
  Acute MI, CHF: IV Bolus 10 units over 2 min; repeat in 30 min.

■ **Unlabeled Uses:** Occluded catheters

■ **Contraindications:** Active internal bleeding, AV malformation or aneurysm, bleeding diathesis, history of cerebrovascular accident (CVA), intracranial neoplasm, recent intracranial or intraspinal surgery or trauma, severe uncontrolled hypertension

■ **Side Effects**
  Frequent
  Bleeding at superficial sites, such as venous injection sites, catheter insertion sites, venous cutdowns, arterial punctures, and sites of recent surgical procedures, gingival bleeding

■ **Serious Reactions**
  • Bleeding at internal sites may occur, including intracranial, retroperitoneal, GI, GU, and respiratory sites.
  • Lysis or coronary thrombi may produce atrial or ventricular arrhythmias and stroke.

Special Considerations
  • No other IV medications should be administered in the same line

■ **Patient/Family Education**
  • Use an electric razor and soft toothbrush to prevent bleeding during drug therapy
  • Report black or red stool, coffee-ground vomitus, dark or red urine, red-speckled mucus from cough, or other signs of bleeding
  • Immediately report chest pain, headache, palpitations, or shortness of breath

■ **Monitoring Parameters**
  • Carefully monitor all needle puncture sites and catheter insertion sites for bleeding

- Continuous cardiac monitoring for arrhythmias, blood pressure, and pulse and respiration rates until patient is stable
- Evaluate breath sounds and peripheral pulses
- Monitor for relief of chest pain

■ **Geriatric side effects at a glance:**
 ☐ CNS   ☐ Bowel Dysfunction   ☐ Bladder Dysfunction   ☐ Falls

■ **U.S. Regulatory Considerations**
 ☐ FDA Black Box   ☐ OBRA regulated in U.S. Long Term Care

ribavirin

(rye-ba-vye'-rin)

■ **Brand Name(s):** Rebetron

Combinations
Rx: with interferon alfa-2b (Rebetron); with peginterferon alfa-2b (PEG-Intron)
Chemical Class: Nucleoside analog

■ **Clinical Pharmacology:**
Mechanism of Action: A synthetic nucleoside that inhibits influenza virus RNA polymerase activity and interferes with expression of messenger RNA. **Therapeutic Effect:** Inhibits viral protein synthesis and replication of viral RNA and DNA.
Pharmacokinetics: Rapidly absorbed from the GI tract following oral administration. A small amount is systemically absorbed following inhalation. Primarily excreted in urine. **Half-life:** 298 hr (oral); 9.5 hr (inhalation).

■ **Available Forms:**
- *Capsules (Rebetol):* 200 mg.
- *Tablets (Copegus):* 200 mg.
- *Powder for Reconstitution (Aerosol):* 6 g.
- *Oral Solution (Rebetol):* 40 mg/ml.

■ **Indications and Dosages:**
Chronic hepatitis C: PO (capsule or oral solution in combination with interferon alfa-2b) 1,000-1,200 mg/day in 2 divided doses. PO (capsules in combination with peginterferon alfa-2b) 800 mg/day in 2 divided doses. PO (tablets in combination with peginterferon alfa-2b) 800-1,200 mg/day in 2 divided doses. Ribavirin with peginterferon alfa-2b requires individualized dosing.

■ **Unlabeled Uses:** Treatment of influenza A or B and west Nile virus

■ **Contraindications:** Autoimmune hepatitis, creatinine clearance less than 50 ml/min, hemoglobinopathies, hepatic decompensation, hypersensitivity to ribavirin products, pregnancy, significant or unstable cardiac disease

■ **Side Effects**
Frequent (greater than 10%)
Dizziness, headache, fatigue, fever, insomnia, irritability, depression, emotional labil-ity, impaired concentration, alopecia, rash, pruritus, nausea, anorexia, dyspepsia, vomiting, decreased hemoglobin, hemolysis, arthralgia, musculoskeletal pain, dys-pnea, sinusitis, flu-like symptoms
Occasional (1%-10%)
Nervousness, altered taste, weakness

■ **Serious Reactions**
- Cardiac arrest, apnea and ventilator dependence, bacterial pneumonia, pneumo-nia, and pneumothorax occur rarely.
- Anemia may occur if ribavirin therapy exceeds 7 days.

■ **Patient/Family Education**
- Female health care workers who are pregnant or may become pregnant should avoid exposure to ribavirin
- Immediately report difficulty breathing or itching, redness, or swelling of the eyes

■ **Monitoring Parameters**
- Hematocrit
- Blood pressure, respirations
- Intake and output
- Be alert for impaired ventilation and gas exchange resulting from drug precipitate
- Periodically assess breath sounds and check the skin for a rash

■ **Geriatric side effects at a glance:**
❑ CNS   ❑ Bowel Dysfunction   ❑ Bladder Dysfunction   ❑ Falls

■ **U.S. Regulatory Considerations**
☑ FDA Black Box   ❑ OBRA regulated in U.S. Long Term Care
Although not relevant for geriatric patients, ribavirin/interferon combinations are as-sociated with significant teratogenicity.

rifabutin

(rif'-a-byoo-tin)

■ **Brand Name(s):** Mycobutin
Chemical Class: Rifamycin S derivative

■ **Clinical Pharmacology:**
Mechanism of Action: An antitubercular that inhibits DNA-dependent RNA poly-merase, an enzyme in susceptible strains of *Escherichia coli* and *Bacillus subtilis*. Rifabutin has a broad spectrum of antimicrobial activity, including against mycobacteria such as *Mycobacterium avium* complex (MAC). **Therapeutic Effect:** Prevents MAC disease.

Pharmacokinetics: Readily absorbed from the GI tract (high-fat meals delay absorption). Protein binding: 85%. Widely distributed. Crosses the blood-brain barrier. Extensive intracellular tissue uptake. Metabolized in the liver to active metabolite. Excreted in urine; eliminated in feces. Unknown if removed by hemodialysis. **Half-life:** 16-69 hr.

■ **Available Forms:**
- *Capsules:* 150 mg.

■ **Indications and Dosages:**
Prevention of MAC disease (first episode): PO 300 mg as a single dose or in 2 divided doses if GI upset occurs.
Prevention of recurrent MAC disease: PO 300 mg/day (in combination)
Dosage in renal impairment: Dosage is modified based on creatinine clearance. If creatinine clearance is less than 30 ml/min, reduce dosage by 50%.

■ **Unlabeled Uses:** Part of multidrug regimen for treatment of MAC

■ **Contraindications:** Active tuberculosis; hypersensitivity to other rifamycins, including rifampin

■ **Side Effects**
Frequent (30%)
Red-orange or red-brown discoloration of urine, feces, saliva, skin, sputum, sweat, or tears
Occasional (11%-3%)
Rash, nausea, abdominal pain, diarrhea, dyspepsia, belching, headache, altered taste, uveitis, corneal deposits
Rare (less than 2%)
Anorexia, flatulence, fever, myalgia, vomiting, insomnia

■ **Serious Reactions**
- Hepatitis and thrombocytopenia occur rarely. Anemia and neutropenia may also occur.

Special Considerations
- Has liver enzyme-inducing properties similar to rifampin although less potent
- Unlike rifampin, does not appear to alter the acetylation of isoniazid

■ **Patient/Family Education**
- May discolor bodily secretions brown-orange, soft contact lenses may be permanently stained
- Avoid crowds until no longer contagious
- Notify the physician promptly if dark urine, flu-like symptoms, nausea or vomiting, unusual bleeding or bruising, or any visual disturbances occur

■ **Monitoring Parameters**
- Periodic CBC with differential and platelets
- Liver function tests
- Hgb and Hct
- Body temperature

■ **Geriatric side effects at a glance:**
❑ CNS ❑ Bowel Dysfunction ❑ Bladder Dysfunction ❑ Falls

rifampin

(rif-am'-pin)

■ **Brand Name(s):** Rifadin, Rifadin IV, Rimactane
Chemical Class: Rifamycin B derivative

■ **Clinical Pharmacology:**
Mechanism of Action: An antitubercular that interferes with bacterial RNA synthesis by binding to DNA-dependent RNA polymerase, thus preventing its attachment to DNA and blocking RNA transcription. **Therapeutic Effect:** Bactericidal in susceptible microorganisms.
Pharmacokinetics: Well absorbed from the GI tract (food delays absorption). Protein binding: 80%. Widely distributed. Metabolized in the liver to active metabolite. Primarily eliminated by the biliary system. Not removed by hemodialysis. **Half-life:** 3-5 hr (increased in hepatic impairment).

■ **Available Forms:**
• *Capsules:* 150 mg (Rifadin), 300 mg (Rifadin, Rimactane).
• *Injection, Powder for Reconstitution (Rifadin IV):* 600 mg.

■ **Indications and Dosages:**
Tuberculosis: PO, IV 10 mg/kg/day. Maximum: 600 mg/day.
Prevention of meningococcal infections: PO, IV 600 mg q12h for 2 days.
Staphylococcal infections: PO, IV 600 mg once a day.
Staphylococcus aureus infections (in combination with other anti-infectives): PO 300-600 mg twice a day.
Prevention of Haemophilus influenzae infection: PO 600 mg/day for 4 days

■ **Unlabeled Uses:** Prophylaxis of *Haemophilus influenzae* type b infection; treatment of atypical mycobacterial infection and serious infections caused by *Staphylococcus* species

■ **Contraindications:** Concomitant therapy with amprenavir, hypersensitivity to other rifamycins

■ **Side Effects**
Expected
Red-orange or red-brown discoloration of urine, feces, saliva, skin, sputum, sweat, or tears
Occasional (5%-2%)
Hypersensitivity reaction (such as flushing, pruritus, or rash)
Rare (2%-1%)
Diarrhea, dyspepsia, nausea, candida infection, evidenced by sore mouth or tongue

■ Serious Reactions
- Rare reactions include hepatotoxicity (risk is increased when rifampin is taken with isoniazid), hepatitis, blood dyscrasias, Stevens-Johnson syndrome, and antibiotic-associated colitis.

■ Patient/Family Education
- Take on empty stomach, at least 1 hr before or 2 hr after meals
- May cause reddish-orange discoloration of bodily secretions, may permanently discolor soft contact lenses
- Avoid consuming alcohol while taking this drug
- Do not take any other medications, including antacids, while taking rifampin without first consulting the physician; take rifampin at least 1 hour before taking an antacid
- Notify the physician immediately if fatigue, fever, flu-like symptoms, nausea, vomiting, unusual bleeding or bruising, weakness, yellow eyes and skin, or any other new symptoms occur

■ Monitoring Parameters
- Liver function tests at baseline and q2-4 wk during therapy
- CBC with differential and platelets at baseline and periodically throughout treatment
- Pattern of daily bowel activity and stool consistency

■ Geriatric side effects at a glance:
☐ CNS   ☑ Bowel Dysfunction   ☐ Bladder Dysfunction   ☐ Falls

■ U.S. Regulatory Considerations
☐ FDA Black Box   ☐ OBRA regulated in U.S. Long Term Care

rifapentine

(rif-a-pen'-teen)

■ Brand Name(s): Priftin
Chemical Class: Rifamycin B derivative

■ Clinical Pharmacology:
Mechanism of Action: An antitubercular that inhibits bacterial RNA synthesis by binding to DNA-dependent RNA polymerase in *Mycobacterium tuberculosis*. This action prevents the enzyme from attaching to DNA, thereby blocking RNA transcription. **Therapeutic Effect:** Bactericidal.
Pharmacokinetics: Rapidly and well absorbed from the GI tract. Protein binding: 97.7%. Metabolized in liver. Primarily eliminated in feces; partial excretion in urine. Not removed by hemodialysis. **Half-life:** 14-17 hr.

- **Available Forms:**
  - *Tablets*: 150 mg.

- **Indications and Dosages:**
  Tuberculosis: PO Intensive phase: 600 mg twice weekly for 2 mo (interval between doses no less than 3 days). Continuation phase: 600 mg weekly for 4 mo.

- **Contraindications:** History of hypersensitivity to any rifamycins (e.g., rifampin and rifabutin)

- **Side Effects**
  Rare (less than 4%)
  Red-orange or red-brown discoloration of urine, feces, saliva, skin, sputum, sweat, or tears; arthralgia, pain, nausea, vomiting, headache, dyspepsia, hypertension, dizziness, diarrhea

- **Serious Reactions**
  - Hyperuricemia, neutropenia, proteinuria, hematuria, and hepatitis occur rarely.

- **Patient/Family Education**
  - Avoid alcoholic beverages concurrently with this medication
  - Rifapentine causes urine, stool, saliva, sputum, sweat, and tears to turn reddish-orange to reddish-brown and may also permanently discolor soft contact lenses; avoid wearing soft contact lenses
  - Notify the physician if dark urine, decreased appetite, fever, nausea or vomiting, or pain or swelling of the joints occurs

- **Monitoring Parameters**
  - ALT, AST, alkaline phosphate, bilirubin, and CBC prior to treatment and monthly during treatment

- **Geriatric side effects at a glance:**
  ❏ CNS ❏ Bowel Dysfunction ❏ Bladder Dysfunction ❏ Falls

- **U.S. Regulatory Considerations**
  ❏ FDA Black Box ❏ OBRA regulated in U.S. Long Term Care

rifaximin

(rye-fax'-ih-min)

- **Brand Name(s):** Xifaxan
  Chemical Class: Semisynthetic rifamycin B derivative

- **Clinical Pharmacology:**
  Mechanism of Action: An anti-infective that inhibits bacterial RNA synthesis by binding to a subunit of bacterial DNA-dependent RNA polymerase. **Therapeutic Effect:** Bactericidal.
  Pharmacokinetics: Less than 0.4% absorbed after PO administration. Primarily eliminated in feces; minimal excretion in urine. **Half-life:** 5.85 hr.

- **Available Forms:**
  - *Tablets*: 200 mg.

- **Indications and Dosages:**
  Traveler's diarrhea: PO 200 mg 3 times a day for 3 days.
  Hepatic encephalopathy: PO 1,200 mg/day for 15-21 days.

- **Unlabeled Uses:** Treatment of hepatic encephalopathy

- **Contraindications:** Hypersensitivity to other rifamycin antibacterials

- **Side Effects**
  Occasional (11%-5%)
  Flatulence, headache, abdominal discomfort, rectal tenesmus, defecation urgency, nausea
  Rare (4%-2%)
  Constipation, fever, vomiting

- **Serious Reactions**
  - Hypersensitivity reactions, including dermatitis, angioneurotic edema, pruritus, rash, and urticaria may occur.
  - Superinfection occurs rarely.

Special Considerations
  - Has been used for diverticular disease and hepatic encephalopathy, but not FDA approved. Not effective for traveler's diarrhea due to bacteria other than enterotoxigenic *Escherichia coli*

- **Patient/Family Education**
  - Notify the physician if diarrhea worsens, a fever develops, or blood appears in the stool within 48 hours

- **Monitoring Parameters**
  - Bowel sounds for peristalsis; pattern of daily bowel activity and stool consistency

- **Geriatric side effects at a glance:**
  ❑ CNS ❑ Bowel Dysfunction ❑ Bladder Dysfunction ❑ Falls

- **U.S. Regulatory Considerations**
  ❑ FDA Black Box ❑ OBRA regulated in U.S. Long Term Care

riluzole

(ril'-yoo-zole)

- **Brand Name(s):** Rilutek
  Chemical Class: Benzothiazolamine derivative

- **Clinical Pharmacology:**
  Mechanism of Action: An amyotrophic lateral sclerosis (ALS) agent that inhibits presynaptic glutamate release in the CNS and interferes postsynaptically with the effects of excitatory amino acids. **Therapeutic Effect:** Extends survival of ALS patients.
  Pharmacokinetics: Well absorbed following PO administration. High-fat meals decrease absorption. Protein binding: 96%. Extensively metabolized in liver. Excreted in urine. **Half-life:** 12-14 hr.

- **Available Forms:**
  - *Tablets*: 50 mg.

- **Indications and Dosages:**
  ALS: PO 50 mg q12h.

- **Contraindications:** None known.

- **Side Effects**
  Frequent (greater than 10%)
  Nausea, asthenia, reduced respiratory function
  Occasional (10%–1%)
  Edema, tachycardia, headache, dizziness, somnolence, depression, vertigo, tremor, pruritus, alopecia, abdominal pain, diarrhea, anorexia, dyspepsia, vomiting, stomatitis, increased cough

- **Serious Reactions**
  - Cardiac arrest, neutropenia, jaundice, and respiratory depression have been reported.

- **Patient/Family Education**
  - Take riluzole at least 1 hr before or 2 hr after a meal and at the same times each day
  - Riluzole may cause drowsiness, dizziness, or vertigo
  - Avoid tasks requiring mental alertness or motor skills until response to the medication has been established
  - Avoid alcohol during therapy
  - Notify the physician if fever develops

- **Monitoring Parameters**
  - ALT, AST qmo for 3 mo, q3mo for 1 yr, then periodically thereafter; discontinue treatment if ALT or AST increases to >5 times upper limit of normal

■ **Geriatric side effects at a glance:**
  ☐ CNS ☐ Bowel Dysfunction ☐ Bladder Dysfunction ☐ Falls

■ **U.S. Regulatory Considerations**
  ☐ FDA Black Box ☐ OBRA regulated in U.S. Long Term Care

rimantadine hydrochloride

(ri-man'-ti-deen hye-droe-klor'-ide)

■ **Brand Name(s):** Flumadine
  Chemical Class: Tricyclic amine

■ **Clinical Pharmacology:**
  Mechanism of Action: An antiviral that appears to exert an inhibitory effect early in the viral replication cycle. May inhibit uncoating of the virus. **Therapeutic Effect:** Prevents replication of influenza A virus.
  Pharmacokinetics: Well absorbed following PO administration. Protein binding: 40%. Metabolized in liver. Excreted in urine. **Half-life:** 19-36 hr.

■ **Available Forms:**
  • *Syrup*: 50 mg/5 ml.
  • *Tablets*: 100 mg.

■ **Indications and Dosages:**
  Influenza A virus: PO 100 mg twice a day for 7 days. Nursing home patients, patients with severe hepatic or renal impairment: 100 mg once a day for 7 days.
  Prevention of influenza A virus: PO 100 mg twice a day for at least 10 days after known exposure (usually for 6-8 wk). Nursing home patients, patients with severe hepatic or renal impairment: 100 mg once a day.

■ **Contraindications:** Hypersensitivity to amantadine

■ **Side Effects**
  Occasional (3%-2%)
  Insomnia, nausea, nervousness, impaired concentration, dizziness
  Rare (less than 2%)
  Vomiting, anorexia, dry mouth, abdominal pain, asthenia, fatigue

■ **Serious Reactions**
  • None known.

■ **Precautions**
  • Resistant strains may develop during treatment (10%-30%)
  • Less CNS toxicity in at-risk populations

- **Patient/Family Education**
  - Avoid contact with people who are at high risk for developing influenza A because a rimantadine-resistant virus may be shed during therapy
  - Avoid performing tasks that require mental alertness or motor skills until response to the drug has been established
  - Do not take acetaminophen, aspirin, or compounds containing these drugs
  - Rimantadine may cause dry mouth

- **Monitoring Parameters**
  - Assess for anxiety, nervousness, and insomnia

- **Geriatric side effects at a glance:**
  ☑ CNS ☐ Bowel Dysfunction ☐ Bladder Dysfunction ☐ Falls

- **U.S. Regulatory Considerations**
  ☐ FDA Black Box ☐ OBRA regulated in U.S. Long Term Care

risedronate sodium

(rye-se-droe'-nate soe'-dee-um)

- **Brand Name(s):** Actonel
  Chemical Class: Pyrophosphate analog

- **Clinical Pharmacology:**
  Mechanism of Action: A bisphosphonate that binds to bone hydroxyapatite and inhibits osteoclasts. **Therapeutic Effect:** Reduces bone turnover (the number of sites at which bone is remodeled) and bone resorption.
  Pharmacokinetics: Rapidly absorbed following PO administration. Bioavailability is decreased when administered with food. Protein binding: 24%. Not metabolized. Excreted unchanged in urine and feces. Not removed by hemodialysis. **Half-life:** 1.5 hr (initial); 480 hr (terminal).

- **Available Forms:**
  - *Tablets:* 5 mg, 30 mg, 35 mg.

- **Indications and Dosages:**
  Paget's disease: PO 30 mg/day for 2 mo. Re-treatment may occur after 2-mo post-treatment observation period.
  Prevention and treatment of postmenopausal osteoporosis: PO 5 mg/day or 35 mg once weekly.
  Glucocorticoid-induced osteoporosis: PO 5 mg/day.

- **Contraindications:** Hypersensitivity to other bisphosphonates, including etidronate, tiludronate, risedronate, and alendronate; hypocalcemia; inability to stand or sit upright for at least 20 min; renal impairment when serum creatinine clearance is greater than 5 mg/dl

■ **Side Effects**
   Frequent (30%)
   Arthralgia
   Occasional (12%–8%)
   Rash, flu-like symptoms, peripheral edema
   Rare (5%–3%)
   Bone pain, sinusitis, asthenia, dry eye, tinnitus, osteonecrosis of the jaw

■ **Serious Reactions**
   • Overdose causes hypocalcemia, hypophosphatemia, and significant GI disturbances.

Special Considerations

   • A dental examination with appropriate preventive dentistry should be considered prior to treatment with bisphosphonates in patients with concomitant risk factors (e.g., cancer, chemotherapy, corticosteroid use, poor oral hygiene). While on bisphosphonate treatment, patients with concomitant risk factors should avoid invasive dental procedures if possible. For patients who develop osteonecrosis of the jaw while on bisphosphonate therapy, dental surgery may exacerbate the condition. For patients requiring dental procedures, there are no data available to suggest whether discontinuation of bisphosphonate treatment reduces the risk of osteonecrosis of the jaw.

■ **Patient/Family Education**
   • Administer 30 min before the first food/beverage/medication of the day, with 6-8 oz plain water
   • Taking risedronate with other beverages, including coffee, mineral water, and orange juice, significantly reduces the absorption of the drug
   • Consider beginning weight-bearing exercises and modifying behavioral factors, such as avoiding alcohol consumption and cigarette smoking
   • Inform your dentist if you are taking this drug.
   • If you develop jaw pain, loose teeth, or signs of oral infection, immediately inform your doctor.

■ **Monitoring Parameters**
   • Albumin-adjusted serum calcium; N-telopeptide, alkaline phosphatase, phosphorus, osteocalcin, DEXA scan, bone and joint pain, fractures on x-ray (osteoporosis, Paget's disease)
   • Serum electrolytes, BUN, intake and output
   • Serum creatinine in patients with renal impairment

■ **Geriatric side effects at a glance:**
   ❑ CNS ❑ Bowel Dysfunction ❑ Bladder Dysfunction ❑ Falls

■ **U.S. Regulatory Considerations**
   ❑ FDA Black Box ❑ OBRA regulated in U.S. Long Term Care

risperidone

(ris-per'-i-done)

■ **Brand Name(s):** Risperdal, Risperdal Consta, Risperdol M-Tabs
  Chemical Class: Benzisoxazole derivative

■ **Clinical Pharmacology:**
  Mechanism of Action: A benzisoxazole derivative that may antagonize dopamine and serotonin receptors. **Therapeutic Effect:** Suppresses psychotic behavior.
  Pharmacokinetics: Well absorbed from the GI tract; unaffected by food. Protein binding: 90%. Extensively metabolized in the liver to active metabolite. Primarily excreted in urine. **Half-life:** 3-20 hr; metabolite: 21-30 hr (increased in elderly).

■ **Available Forms:**
  • *Oral Solution (Risperdal):* 1 mg/ml.
  • *Tablets (Risperdal):* 0.25 mg, 0.5 mg, 1 mg, 2 mg, 3 mg, 4 mg.
  • *Tablets (Orally-Disintegrating [Risperdal M-Tabs]):* 0.5 mg, 1 mg, 2 mg.
  • *Injection (Risperdal Consta):* 25 mg, 37.5 mg, 50 mg.

■ **Indications and Dosages:**
  Psychotic disorder: PO Initially, 0.25-2 mg/day in 2 divided doses. May increase dosage slowly. Range: 2-6 mg/day. IM 25 mg q2wk. Maximum: 50 mg q2wk.
  Mania: PO Initially, 2-3 mg as a single daily dose. May increase at 24-hr intervals of 1 mg/day. Range: 2-6 mg/day.
  Dosage in renal impairment: Initial dosage is 0.25-0.5 mg twice a day. Dosage is titrated slowly to desired effect.

■ **Unlabeled Uses:** Behavioral symptoms associated with dementia, Tourette's disorder

■ **Contraindications:** None known.

■ **Side Effects**
  Frequent (26%-13%)
  Agitation, anxiety, insomnia, headache, constipation
  Occasional (10%-4%)
  Dyspepsia, rhinitis, somnolence, dizziness, nausea, vomiting, rash, abdominal pain, dry skin, tachycardia
  Rare (3%-2%)
  Visual disturbances, fever, back pain, pharyngitis, cough, arthralgia, angina, aggressive behavior, orthostatic hypotension, breast swelling

■ **Serious Reactions**
  • Rare reactions include tardive dyskinesia (characterized by tongue protrusion, puffing of the cheeks, and chewing or puckering of the mouth) and neuroleptic malignant syndrome (marked by hyperpyrexia, muscle rigidity, change in mental status, irregular pulse or BP, tachycardia, diaphoresis, cardiac arrhythmias, rhabdomyolysis, and acute renal failure).
  • Hyperglycemia, in some cases extreme and associated with ketoacidosis or hyperosmolar coma or death, has been reported.

■ **Patient/Family Education**
  - Risk of orthostatic hypotension, especially during the period of initial dose titration
  - Do not operate machinery during dose titration period
  - Notify the physician if altered gait, difficulty breathing, palpitations, pain or swelling in breasts, severe dizziness or fainting, trembling fingers, unusual movements, rash, or visual changes occur
  - Avoid alcohol during risperidone therapy

■ **Monitoring Parameters**
  - Blood pressure, heart rate, liver function test results, ECG, and weight
  - Observe the patient for fine tongue movement, which may be the first sign of irreversible tardive dyskinesia
  - Closely supervise suicidal patients during early therapy; as depression lessens, energy level improves, which increases the suicide potential
  - Therapeutic response, such as increased ability to concentrate and interest in surroundings, improvement in self-care, and relaxed facial expression
  - Monitor for signs of neuroleptic malignant syndrome, such as altered mental status, fever, irregular blood pressure or pulse, and muscle rigidity

■ **Geriatric side effects at a glance:**
  ☑ CNS ☑ Bowel Dysfunction ❏ Bladder Dysfunction ☑ Falls
  Other: Weight gain, glucose intolerance, diabetes, orthostatic hypotension, extrapyramidal symptoms

■ **Use with caution in older patients with:** Diabetes, glucose intolerance, cardiovascular disease

■ **U.S. Regulatory Considerations**
  ☑ FDA Black Box
  There is an increased risk of death in older patients with dementia. Although the causes of death were varied, most of the deaths appeared to be either cardiovascular (e.g., heart failure, sudden death) or infectious (e.g., pneumonia) in nature. This drug is not approved for treatment of patients with dementia-related psychosis.
  ☑ OBRA regulated in U.S. Long Term Care

■ **Other Uses in Geriatric Patient:** Behavior disturbances in the setting of dementia

■ **Side Effects:**
  Of particular importance in the geriatric patient: Weight gain, glucose intolerance, diabetes, increased risk of death (see FDA black box warning)

■ **Geriatric Considerations - Summary:** Direct comparisons between older and newer antipsychotic drugs in demented elderly persons are scarce. Newer agents have the theoretical advantage of a lower incidence of tardive dyskinesia but may cause weight gain, impaired glycemic control, and increased risk for cardiovascular events. These agents should be used with caution in demented elderly persons, with frequent monitoring for side effects and a low threshold for discontinuing use. Indeed, the Food and Drug Administration has recently released an advisory about these medications outlining the risk for increased mortality.

■ **References:**
1. Sink KM, Holden KF, Yaffe K. Pharmacological treatment of neuropsychiatric symptoms of dementia: a review of the evidence. JAMA 2005;293:596-608.
2. Alexopoulos GS, Streim J, Carpenter D, Docherty JP. Using antipsychotic agents in older patients. J Clin Psychiatry 2004;65 (Suppl 2):5-99.
3. Cohen D. Atypical antipsychotics and new onset diabetes mellitus. An overview of the literature. Pharmacopsychiatry 2004;37:1-11.
4. Deaths with antipsychotics in elderly patients with behavioral disturbances. Available at: www.fda.gov/cder/drug/advisory/antipsychotics.htm.

ritonavir

(ri-tone'-a-veer)

■ **Brand Name(s):** Norvir

    Combinations
    Rx: with lopinavir (Kaletra)
    Chemical Class: Protease inhibitor, HIV

■ **Clinical Pharmacology:**
    Mechanism of Action: Inhibits HIV-1 and HIV-2 proteases, rendering these enzymes incapable of processing the polypeptide precursors; this results in the production of noninfectious, immature HIV particles. **Therapeutic Effect:** Impedes HIV replication, slowing the progression of HIV infection.
    Pharmacokinetics: Well absorbed after PO administration (absorption increased with food). Protein binding: 98%-99%. Extensively metabolized in the liver to active metabolite. Primarily eliminated in feces. Unknown if removed by hemodialysis. **Half-life:** 2.7-5 hr.

■ **Available Forms:**
- *Oral Solution*: 80 mg/ml.
- *Soft Gelatin Capsules*: 100 mg.

■ **Indications and Dosages:**
    HIV infection: PO 600 mg twice a day. If nausea occurs at this dosage, give 300 mg twice a day for 1 day, 400 mg twice a day for 2 days, 500 mg twice a day for 1 day, then 600 mg twice a day thereafter.
    Dosage adjustments in combination therapy: *Amprenavir.* Amprenavir 1,200 mg and ritonavir 200 mg once a day or amprenavir 600 mg and ritonavir 100 mg twice a day. *Amprenavir and efavirenz.* Amprenavir 1,200 mg twice a day and ritonavir 200 mg twice a day with standard dose of efavirenz. *Indinavir.* Indinavir 800 mg twice a day and ritonavir 100-200 mg twice a day or indinavir 400 mg twice a day and ritonavir 400 mg twice a day. *Nelfinavir or saquinavir.* Ritonavir 400 mg twice a day. *Rifabutin.* Decrease rifabutin dosage to 150 mg every other day.

■ **Contraindications:** Concurrent use of amiodarone, astemizole, bepridil, bupropion, cisapride, clozapine, encainide, flecainide, meperidine, piroxicam, propafenone, propoxyphene, quinidine, rifabutin, or terfenadine (increased risk of serious or life-threatening drug interactions, such as arrhythmias, hematologic abnormalities, and seizures); concurrent use of alprazolam, clorazepate, diazepam, estazolam, flurazepam, midazolam, triazolam, or zolpidem (may produce extreme sedation and respiratory depression)

■ Side Effects
Frequent
GI disturbances (abdominal pain, anorexia, diarrhea, nausea, vomiting), circumoral and peripheral paresthesias, altered taste, headache, dizziness, fatigue, asthenia
Occasional
Allergic reaction, flu-like symptoms, hypotension
Rare
Diabetes mellitus, hyperglycemia

■ Serious Reactions
- Hepatitis and fatal cases of pancreatitis have been reported.

Special Considerations
- As with other protease inhibitors, ritonavir will predominantly be used in combination regimens; the ability of ritonavir (alone or in combinations) to modify clinical endpoints (e.g., time to first AIDS-defining illness or death) will be important in determining the ultimate role of this agent in HIV; potential for drug interaction is troublesome; as with other protease inhibitors, resistance has been problematic after several mo of treatment
- Always check updated treatment guidelines before initiating or changing antiretroviral therapy. (http://AIDSinfo.nih.gov)

■ Patient/Family Education
- Store capsules in the refrigerator until dispensed; refrigeration of capsules by patient not required if used within 30 days and stored below 77°F; store oral solution at room temperature, do not refrigerate, shake well; avoid exposure to excessive heat
- Take with food
- Space ritonavir doses evenly around the clock and continue taking the drug for the full course of treatment
- Notify the physician if abdominal pain, frequent urination, increased thirst, nausea, or vomiting occurs
- Ritonavir is not a cure for HIV infection, nor does it reduce the risk of transmitting HIV to others

■ Monitoring Parameters
- Therapeutic: serum HIV-1 RNA, and CD4+ cell counts (every 2-4 wk)
- Toxicity: complete blood counts, routine blood chemistry, liver function tests, and serum lipid and lipoprotein profiles
- Closely monitor for signs and symptoms of GI or neurologic disturbances, particularly paresthesias

■ Geriatric side effects at a glance:
☑ CNS ☑ Bowel Dysfunction ☐ Bladder Dysfunction ☐ Falls

■ U.S. Regulatory Considerations
☑ FDA Black Box

Ritonavir is a potent inhibitor of cytochrome P450 3A. Drug interactions may result in serious or life-threatening adverse events.
❑ OBRA regulated in U.S. Long Term Care

rivastigmine tartrate

(riv-a-stig'-meen tar'-trate)

■ **Brand Name(s):** Exelon
Chemical Class: Carbamate derivative; cholinesterase inhibitor

■ **Clinical Pharmacology:**
Mechanism of Action: An agent that inhibits the enzyme acetylcholinesterase, thus increasing the concentration of acetylcholine at cholinergic synapses and enhancing cholinergic function in the CNS. **Therapeutic Effect:** Slows the progression of symptoms of Alzheimer's disease.
Pharmacokinetics: Rapidly and completely absorbed. Protein binding: 60%. Widely distributed throughout the body. Rapidly and extensively metabolized. Primarily excreted in urine. **Half-life:** 1.5 hr.

■ **Available Forms:**
- *Capsules:* 1.5 mg, 3 mg, 4.5 mg, 6 mg.
- *Oral Solution:* 2 mg/ml.

■ **Indications and Dosages:**
Alzheimer's disease: PO Initially, 1.5 mg twice a day. May increase at intervals of at least 2 wk to 3 mg twice a day, then 4.5 mg twice a day, and finally 6 mg twice a day. Maximum: 6 mg twice a day.

■ **Contraindications:** Hypersensitivity to other carbamate derivatives

■ **Side Effects**
Frequent (47%-17%)
Nausea, vomiting, dizziness, diarrhea, headache, anorexia
Occasional (13%-6%)
Abdominal pain, insomnia, dyspepsia (heartburn, indigestion, epigastric pain), confusion, UTI, depression
Rare (5%-3%)
Anxiety, somnolence, constipation, malaise, hallucinations, tremor, flatulence, rhinitis, hypertension, flu-like symptoms, weight loss, syncope

■ **Serious Reactions**
- Overdose may result in cholinergic crisis, characterized by severe nausea and vomiting, increased salivation, diaphoresis, bradycardia, hypotension, respiratory depression, and seizures.

■ **Patient/Family Education**
- Patient and caregiver should be advised of high incidence of gastrointestinal effects and directions for resource and resolution
- Take with morning and evening meals
- Swallow capsules whole; do not break, chew, or crush them
- If the patient is using the oral solution, explain that he or she should withdraw the prescribed amount of drug into the syringe and either sip it directly from the syringe or first mix it with a small glass of water, cold fruit juice, or soda and then stir and drink the mixture

■ **Monitoring Parameters**
- Cognitive function (e.g., ADAS, Mini-Mental Status Exam (MMSE)), activities of daily living, global functioning, blood chemistry, complete blood counts, heart rate, blood pressure
- Monitor for a cholinergic reaction, including diaphoresis, dizziness, excessive salivation, facial warmth, abdominal cramps or discomfort, lacrimation, pallor, and urinary urgency

■ **Geriatric side effects at a glance:**
☑ CNS ☑ Bowel Dysfunction ❑ Bladder Dysfunction ❑ Falls
Other: Anorexia, weight loss, bradycardia

■ **Use with caution in older patients with:** None

■ **U.S. Regulatory Considerations**
❑ FDA Black Box ❑ OBRA regulated in U.S. Long Term Care

■ **Other Uses in Geriatric Patient:** None

■ **Side Effects:**
Of particular importance in the geriatric patient: None

■ **Geriatric Considerations - Summary:** Rivastigmine, like other cholinesterase inhibitors, is modestly effective for treatment of cognitive decline associated with Alzheimer's disease. Compared to placebo, persons using rivastigmine have less decline in performance on cognitive tests, but most patients derive no clinical benefit, and there is no evidence the drug delays disability or institutionalization. Rivastigmine is expensive, and not cost-effective for this indication. Persons using drugs to treat Alzheimer's disease should be monitored closely, and prescribers should have a low threshold for discontinuing these agents if no clinical benefit is observed.

■ **References:**
1. Cummings JL. Alzheimer's disease. N Engl J Med 2004;351:56-67.
2. Kaduszkiewicz H, Zimmermann T, Beck-Bornholdt HP, et al. Cholinesterase inhibitors for patients with Alzheimer's disease: systematic review of randomised clinical trials. BMJ 2005;331:321-327.

rizatriptan benzoate

(rye-za-trip'-tan ben'-zoe-ate)

- **Brand Name(s):** Maxalt, Maxalt MLT
  Chemical Class: Serotonin derivative

- **Clinical Pharmacology:**
  Mechanism of Action: A serotonin receptor agonist that binds selectively to vascular receptors, producing a vasoconstrictive effect on cranial blood vessels. **Therapeutic Effect:** Relieves migraine headache.
  Pharmacokinetics: Well absorbed after PO administration. Protein binding: 14%. Crosses the blood-brain barrier. Metabolized by the liver to inactive metabolite. Eliminated primarily in urine and, to a lesser extent, in feces. **Half-life:** 2–3 hr.

- **Available Forms:**
  - *Tablets (Maxalt):* 5 mg, 10 mg.
  - *Tablets (Orally-Disintegrating [Maxalt-MLT]):* 5 mg, 10 mg.

- **Indications and Dosages:**
  Acute migraine attack: PO 5–10 mg. If headache improves, but then returns, dose may be repeated after 2 hr. Maximum: 30 mg/24 hr.

- **Contraindications:** Basilar or hemiplegic migraine, coronary artery disease, ischemic heart disease (including angina pectoris, history of MI, silent ischemia, and Prinzmetal's angina), uncontrolled hypertension, use within 24 hours of ergotamine-containing preparations or another serotonin receptor agonist, use within 14 days of MAOIs

- **Side Effects**
  Frequent (9%–7%)
  Dizziness, somnolence, paresthesia, fatigue
  Occasional (6%–3%)
  Nausea, chest pressure, dry mouth
  Rare (2%)
  Headache; neck, throat, or jaw pressure; photosensitivity

- **Serious Reactions**
  - Cardiac reactions (such as ischemia, coronary artery vasospasm, and MI) and non-cardiac vasospasm-related reactions (including hemorrhage and cerebrovascular accident [CVA]), occur rarely, particularly in patients with hypertension, diabetes, or a strong family history of coronary artery disease; obese patients; smokers; males older than 40 years; and postmenopausal women.

Special Considerations
  - Safety of treating, on average, more than 4 headaches in a 30-day period has not been established
  - Maxalt-MLT does not provide faster absorption or onset of effect because almost the entire dose is swallowed with saliva and absorbed in the GI tract

- Use only to treat migraine headache, not for prevention
- MLT, administration with liquid is not necessary; orally disintegrating tablet is packaged in a blister within an outer aluminum pouch, do not remove the blister from the outer pouch until just prior to dosing; blister pack should then be peeled open with dry hands and the orally disintegrating tablet placed on the tongue, where it will dissolve and be swallowed with the saliva
- Avoid tasks that require mental alertness or motor skills until response to the drug has been established
- Notify the physician immediately if palpitations, pain or tightness in the chest or throat, or pain or weakness in the extremities occurs
- Protect against exposure to sunlight and ultraviolet rays by using sunscreen and wearing protective clothing
- Do not smoke during rizatriptan therapy
- Lie down in a dark, quiet room for additional benefit after taking the drug

■ **Monitoring Parameters**
- Assess for relief of migraines and associated symptoms, including nausea and vomiting, photophobia, and phonophobia (sound sensitivity)

■ **Geriatric side effects at a glance:**
    ❑ CNS   ❑ Bowel Dysfunction   ❑ Bladder Dysfunction   ❑ Falls

■ **U.S. Regulatory Considerations**
    ❑ FDA Black Box   ❑ OBRA regulated in U.S. Long Term Care

ropinirole hydrochloride

(ro-pin'-i-role hye-droe-klor'-ide)

■ **Brand Name(s):** Requip
   Chemical Class: Dipropylaminoethyl indolone derivative

■ **Clinical Pharmacology:**
   Mechanism of Action: An antiparkinson agent that stimulates dopamine receptors in the striatum. **Therapeutic Effect:** Relieves signs and symptoms of Parkinson's disease. **Pharmacokinetics:** Rapidly absorbed after PO administration. Protein binding: 40%. Extensively distributed throughout the body. Extensively metabolized. Steady-state concentrations achieved within 2 days. Eliminated in urine. Unknown if removed by hemodialysis. **Half-life:** 6 hr.

■ **Available Forms:**
- **Tablets:** 0.25 mg, 0.5 mg, 1 mg, 2 mg, 3 mg, 4 mg, 5 mg.

■ **Indications and Dosages:**
   Parkinson's disease: PO Initially, 0.25 mg 3 times a day. May increase dosage every 7 days.

Restless legs syndrome: PO 0.25 mg for days 1 and 2; 0.5 mg for days 3-7; 1 mg for week 2; 1.5 mg for week 3; 2 mg for week 4; 2.5 mg for week 5; 3 mg for week 6; 4 mg for week 7. All doses to be given 1-3 hr before bedtime.

■ **Contraindications:** None known.

■ **Side Effects**
Frequent (60%–40%)
Nausea, dizziness, somnolence
Occasional (12%–5%)
Syncope, vomiting, fatigue, viral infection, dyspepsia, diaphoresis, asthenia, orthostatic hypotension, abdominal discomfort, pharyngitis, abnormal vision, dry mouth, hypertension, hallucinations, confusion
Rare (less than 4%)
Anorexia, peripheral edema, memory loss, rhinitis, sinusitis, palpitations, impotence

■ **Serious Reactions**
- Falling asleep without warning while engaged in activities of daily living, including driving motor vehicles, has been reported.

Special Considerations
- Domperidone 20 mg 1 hr prior to ropinirole prevents drug-induced postural effects
- Discontinue slowly over 1 wk

■ **Patient/Family Education**
- Take ropinirole with food if nausea is a problem
- Dizziness, drowsiness, and orthostatic hypotension are common initial responses to the drug; change positions slowly to help prevent orthostatic hypotension
- Avoid tasks that require mental alertness or motor skills until response to the drug has been established
- The drug may cause hallucinations

■ **Monitoring Parameters**
- Assess for relief of symptoms, such as improvement of masklike facial expression, muscular rigidity, shuffling gait, and resting tremors of the hands and head

■ **Geriatric side effects at a glance:**
❏ CNS   ❏ Bowel Dysfunction   ❏ Bladder Dysfunction   ❏ Falls
Other: Orthostatic hypotension, hallucinations, daytime somnolence, and sudden drowsiness.

■ **Use with caution in older patients with:** Preexisting psychotic symptoms

■ **U.S. Regulatory Considerations**
❏ FDA Black Box   ❏ OBRA regulated in U.S. Long Term Care

■ **Other Uses in Geriatric Patient:** Restless legs syndrome

■ **Side Effects:**
Of particular importance in the geriatric patient: Nausea/vomiting can result in weight loss

- **Geriatric Considerations - Summary:** Ropinirole is a nonergot dopamine agonist which directly stimulates dopamine D_2 receptors. It can be used in combination with levodopa or as monotherapy. If discontinued, ropinirole should be slowly tapered because abrupt discontinuation can cause confusion, hallucinations, and a condition similar to neuroleptic malignant syndrome.

- **References:**
  1. Miyasaki JM, Martin WRW, Suchowersky O, et al. Practice parameter: initiation of treatment for Parkinson's disease: an evidence based review. Neurology 2002;58:11-17.
  2. Happe S, Berger K. The association of dopamine agonists with daytime sleepiness, sleep problems and quality of life in patients with Parkinson's disease: a prospective study. J Neurol 2001;248:1062-1067.
  3. Whone AL, Watts RL, Stoessl AJ, et al. Slower progression of Parkinson's disease with ropinirole versus levodopa: the REAL-PET study. Ann Neurol 2003;54:93-101.

rosiglitazone maleate

(roz-ih-gli'-ta-zone mal'-ee-ate)

- **Brand Name(s):** Avandia

  Combinations
  Rx: with metformin (Avandamet)
  Chemical Class: Thiazolidinedione

- **Clinical Pharmacology:**
  Mechanism of Action: An antidiabetic that improves target-cell response to insulin without increasing pancreatic insulin secretion. Decreases hepatic glucose output and increases insulin-dependent glucose utilization in skeletal muscle. **Therapeutic Effect:** Lowers blood glucose concentration.
  Pharmacokinetics: Rapidly absorbed. Protein binding: 99%. Metabolized in the liver. Excreted primarily in urine, with a lesser amount in feces. Not removed by hemodialysis. **Half-life:** 3–4 hr.

- **Available Forms:**
  - **Tablets:** 2 mg, 4 mg, 8 mg.

- **Indications and Dosages:**
  Diabetes mellitus, combination therapy: PO (with sulfonylureas, metformin) Initially, 4 mg as a single daily dose or in divided doses twice a day. May increase to 8 mg/day after 12 wk of therapy if fasting glucose level is not adequately controlled. PO (with insulin) Initially, 4 mg/day in 1 or 2 doses and reduce insulin dose by 10%-25%. If hypoglycemia occurs or plasma glucose falls to less than 100 mg/dl, doses of rosiglitazone greater than 4 mg are not recommended.
  Diabetes mellitus, monotherapy: Initially, 4 mg as single daily dose or in divided doses twice a day. May increase to 8 mg/day after 12 wk of therapy.

- **Contraindications:** Active hepatic disease, diabetic ketoacidosis, increased serum transaminase levels, including ALT greater than 2.5 times the normal serum level, type I diabetes mellitus

■ **Side Effects**
   Frequent (9%)
   Upper respiratory tract infection
   Occasional (4%–2%)
   Headache, edema, back pain, fatigue, sinusitis, diarrhea

■ **Serious Reactions**
   • Hepatotoxicity occurs rarely.

Special Considerations

   • *Expected hypoglycemic effects*: Decreases in serum glucose: 50-75 mg/dl; decreases in HbA$_{1c}$ 1.2%-1.5%

■ **Patient/Family Education**
   • Caloric restriction, weight loss, and exercise essential adjuvant therapy
   • Blood draws for LFT monitoring along with routine diabetes mellitus labs; review symptoms of hepatitis (unexplained nausea, vomiting, abdominal pain, fatigue, anorexia, or dark urine)
   • Notify clinician of rapid increases in weight or edema or symptoms of heart failure (shortness of breath)
   • OK to take with food
   • Review hypoglycemia risks and symptoms when added to other hypoglycemic agents
   • Follow prescribed diet
   • Carry candy, sugar packets, or other sugar supplements for immediate response to hypoglycemia and wear medical alert identification stating he or she has diabetes
   • Avoid alcohol

■ **Monitoring Parameters**
   • "Poly" diabetes mellitus symptoms, periodic serum glucose and HbA$_{1c}$ measurements; LFT (AST, ALT) prior to initiation of therapy and periodically thereafter; hemoglobin/hematocrit, signs and symptoms of heart failure

■ **Geriatric side effects at a glance:**
   ❑ CNS   ❑ Bowel Dysfunction   ❑ Bladder Dysfunction   ❑ Falls
   Other: Edema, macular edema

■ **Use with caution in older patients with:** CHF, CAD, NYHA Class III or IV, Hepatic impairment (avoid if ALT > 2.5 times the upper limit of normal), Diabetic macular edema

■ **U.S. Regulatory Considerations**
   ❑ FDA Black Box   ❑ OBRA regulated in U.S. Long Term Care

■ **Other Uses in Geriatric Patient:** None

■ **Side Effects:**
   Of particular importance in the geriatric patient: Edema, weight gain, anemia, may precipitate or worsen diabetic macular edema

■ **Geriatric Considerations - Summary:** Fluid retention may lead to mild CHF in patients with CAD and unrecognized or compensated heart failure. Discontinue drug with any sign of decline in cardiac function. Avoid in older adults with NYHA Class III or IV cardiac status. Similar efficacy as in adults 65 years of age and older.

■ **References:**
1. Haas L. Management of diabetes mellitus medications in the nursing home. Drugs Aging 2005;22:209-218.
2. Rosenstock J. Management of type 2 diabetes mellitus in the elderly: special considerations. Drugs Aging 2001;18:31-44.
3. Beebe K, Patel J. Rosiglitazone is effective and well-tolerated in patients > 65 years with type 2 diabetes [abstract]. Diabetes 1999;42 (Suppl 1):A111.

rosuvastatin calcium

(roe-soo'-va-sta-tin kal'-see-um)

■ **Brand Name(s):** Crestor
Chemical Class: Substituted heptenoic acid derivative

■ **Clinical Pharmacology:**
Mechanism of Action: An antihyperlipidemic that interferes with cholesterol biosynthesis by inhibiting the conversion of the enzyme hydroxymethylglutaryl-CoA (HMG-CoA) to mevalonate, a precursor to cholesterol. **Therapeutic Effect:** Decreases LDL cholesterol, VLDL, and plasma triglyceride levels, increases HDL concentration.
Pharmacokinetics: Protein binding: 88%. Minimal hepatic metabolism. Primarily eliminated in the feces. **Half-life:** 19 hr (increased in patients with severe renal dysfunction).

■ **Available Forms:**
- *Tablets:* 5 mg, 10 mg, 20 mg, 40 mg.

■ **Indications and Dosages:**
Hyperlipidemia, dyslipidemia: PO 5 to 40 mg/day. Usual starting dosage is 10 mg/day, with adjustments based on lipid levels; monitor q2-4wk until desired level is achieved. Maximum: 40 mg/day.
Renal impairment (creatinine clearance less than 30 ml/min): PO 5 mg/day; do not exceed 10 mg/day.
Concurrent cyclosporine use: PO 5 mg/day.
Concurrent lipid-lowering therapy: PO 10 mg/day.

■ **Contraindications:** Active hepatic disease; unexplained, persistent elevations of serum transaminase levels

■ **Side Effects**
Rosuvastatin is generally well tolerated. Side effects are usually mild and transient.
Occasional (9%–3%)
Pharyngitis, headache, diarrhea, dyspepsia, including heartburn and epigastric distress, nausea
Rare (less than 3%)
Myalgia, asthenia or unusual fatigue and weakness, back pain

■ **Serious Reactions**
- Cases of rhabdomyolysis have been reported.
- Lens opacities may occur.

- Hypersensitivity reaction and hepatitis occur rarely.

Special Considerations
- Base statin selection on lipid-lowering prowess, cost, side effects, and availability of mortality reduction studies
- Rosuvastatin is the most potent statin on the market in its ability to decrease LDL with a significant reduction in total cholesterol, triglycerides, and increase in HDL; however, overall mortality rates are lacking
- Notable proteinuria (persistent) accompanies rosuvastatin use; clinical significance yet unknown; would hesitate to use as first-line statin
- Note: not dependent on metabolism by cytochrome P450 3A4 to a clinically significant extent

■ Patient/Family Education
- Report symptoms of myalgia, muscle tenderness, or weakness
- May be taken with or without food and regardless of the time of day
- Adjunctive to diet and exercise
- Periodic laboratory tests are an essential part of therapy

■ Monitoring Parameters
- *Efficacy*: Fasting lipid panel at 3-6 months
- AST/ALT at baseline, 12 weeks, following any elevation of dose, and then periodically (discontinue if elevations persist at >3 times upper limit of normal)
- CPK in patients complaining of unexplained diffuse myalgia, muscle tenderness, or muscle weakness
- Routine urinalysis for proteinuria; may need to reduce dose with persistent proteinuria

■ Geriatric side effects at a glance:
❑ CNS   ❑ Bowel Dysfunction   ❑ Bladder Dysfunction   ❑ Falls

■ U.S. Regulatory Considerations
❑ FDA Black Box   ❑ OBRA regulated in U.S. Long Term Care

salicylic acid

(sal-i-sill'-ik as'-id)

■ Brand Name(s): Compound W, Compound W One Step Wart Remover, DHS Sal, Dr. Scholl's Callus Remover, Dr. Scholl's Clear Away, DuoFilm, DuoPlant, Freezone, Fung-O, Gordofilm, Hydrisalic, Ionil, Ionil Plus, Keralyt, LupiCare Dandruff, LupiCare Psoriasis, LupiCare II, Mediplast, MG217 Sal-Acid, Mosco Corn and Callus Remover, NeoCeuticals Acne Spot Treatment, Neutrogena Acne Wash, Neutrogena Body Clear, Neutrogena Clear Pore, Neutrogena Clear Pore Shine Control, Neutrogena Healthy Scalp, Neutrogena Maximum Strength T/Sal, Neutrogena On The Spot Acne Patch, Occlusal-HP, Oxy Balance, Oxy Balance Deep Pore, Palmer's Skin Success

Acne Cleanser, Pedisilk, Propa pH, SalAc, Sal-Acid, Salactic, Sal-Plant, Stri-Dex, Stri-Dex Body Focus, Stri-Dex Facewipes To Go, Stri-Dex Maximum Strength, Tinamed, Tiseb, Trans-Ver-Sal, Wart-Off Maximum Strength, Zapzyt Acne Wash, Zapzyt Pore Treatment

Combinations
Rx: with sodium thiosulfate (Versiclear)
Chemical Class: Salicylate derivative

■ **Clinical Pharmacology:**
Mechanism of Action: A wart removal agent that produces desquamation of hyperkeratotic epithelium by dissolution of intercellular cement and causes the cornified tissue to swell, soften, macerate, and desquamate. *Therapeutic Effect:* Decreases acne, psoriasis and promotes wart removal
Pharmacokinetics: Absorption differs between formulations. Protein binding: 50%-80%. Bound to serum albumin. Metabolized to salicylate glucuronides and salicyluric acid. Excreted in urine.

■ **Available Forms:**
- *Cream*: 2% (Neutrogena Acne Wash), 2.5% (LupiCare Dandruff, LupiCare Psoriasis, LupiCare II).
- *Gel*: 0.5% (Neutrogena Clear Pore Shine Control), 2% (NeoCeuticals Acne Spot Treatment, Neutrogena Clear Pore, Oxy Balance, Stri-Dex Body Focus, Zapzyt Acne Wash, Zapzyt Pore Treatment), 6% (Hydrisalic, Keralyt), 17% (Compound W, DuoPlant, Sal-Plant).
- *Foam*: 2% (Neutrogena Acne Wash, SalAc).
- *Liquid*: 2% (NeoCeuticals Acne Spot Treatment, Neutrogena Acne Wash, Neutragena Body Clear, Propa pH, SalAc), 17% (Compound W, DuoFilm, Freezone, Fung-O, Gordofilm, Mosco Corn and Callus Remover, Occlusal-HP, Pedisilk, Salactic, Tinamed, Wart-Off).
- *Ointment*: 3% (MG217 Sal-Acid).
- *Pads*: 0.5% (Oxy Balance, Oxy Balance Deep Pore, Stri-Dex, Stri-Dex Facewipes To Go), 2% (Neutrogena Acne Wash, Stri-Dex Maximum Strength).
- *Patch*: 2% (Neutrogena On The Spot Acne Patch), 15% (Trans-Ver-Sal), 40% (Compound W, Dr. Scholl's Callus Remover, Dr. Scholl's Clear Away, DuoFilm).
- *Plaster*: 40% (Mediplast, Sal-Acid, Tinamed).
- *Shampoo*: 1.8% (Neutrogena Healthy Scalp), 2% (Ionil, Ionil Plus, LupiCare Dandruff, LupiCare Psoriasis, Tiseb), 3% (Neutrogena Maximum Strength T/Sal).
- *Soap*: 2%.
- *Solution*: 17% (Compound W).

■ **Indications and Dosages:**
Acne: Topical Apply cream, foam, gel, liquid, pads, patch, or soap 1-3 times/day.
Callus, corn, wart removal: Topical Apply gel, liquid, plaster, or patch to wart 1-2 times/day.
Dandruff, psoriasis, seborrheic dermatitis: Topical Apply cream, ointment, or shampoo 3-4 times/day.

■ **Unlabeled Uses:** Tinea pedis

■ **Contraindications:** Impaired circulation, hypersensitivity to salicylic acid or any of its components

■ **Side Effects**
Occasional
Burning, erythema, irritation, pruritus, stinging

Rare

Dizziness, nausea, vomiting, diarrhea, hypoglycemia

■ **Serious Reactions**
- Symptoms of salicylate toxicity include lethargy, hyperpnea, diarrhea, and psychic disturbances.

■ **Patient/Family Education**
- For external use only; avoid contact with face, eyes, genitals, mucous membranes, and normal skin surrounding warts
- May cause reddening or scaling of skin
- Soaking area in warm water for 5 min prior to application may enhance effect (remove any loose tissue with brush, washcloth, or emery board and dry thoroughly prior to application)

■ **Monitoring Parameters**
- Clinical improvement

■ **Geriatric side effects at a glance:**
❑ CNS ❑ Bowel Dysfunction ❑ Bladder Dysfunction ❑ Falls

■ **U.S. Regulatory Considerations**
❑ FDA Black Box ❑ OBRA regulated in U.S. Long Term Care

salmeterol xinafoate

(sal-me'-te-role zin-na'-foe-ate)

■ **Brand Name(s):** Serevent, Serevent Diskus

Combinations
Rx: with fluticasone (Advair)
Chemical Class: Sympathomimetic amine; β_2-adrenergic agonist

■ **Clinical Pharmacology:**
Mechanism of Action: An adrenergic agonist that stimulates $beta_2$-adrenergic receptors in the lungs, resulting in relaxation of bronchial smooth muscle. **Therapeutic Effect:** Relieves bronchospasm and reduces airway resistance.
Pharmacokinetics:

Route	Onset	Peak	Duration
Inhalation	10–20 min	3 hr	12 hr

Low systemic absorption; acts primarily in the lungs. Protein binding: 95%. Metabolized by hydroxylation. Primarily eliminated in feces. **Half-life:** 3–4 hr.

■ **Available Forms:**
  • *Powder for Oral Inhalation*: 50 mcg.

■ **Indications and Dosages:**
  Prevention and maintenance treatment of asthma: Inhalation (Diskus) 1 inhalation (50 mcg) q12h.
  Prevention of exercise-induced bronchospasm: Inhalation (Diskus) 1 inhalation at least 30 min before exercise.
  Chronic obstructive pulmonary disorder (COPD): Inhalation (Diskus) 1 inhalation q12h.

■ **Contraindications:** History of hypersensitivity to sympathomimetics

■ **Side Effects**
  Frequent (28%)
  Headache
  Occasional (7%–3%)
  Cough, tremor, dizziness, vertigo, throat dryness or irritation, pharyngitis
  Rare (3%)
  Palpitations, tachycardia, nausea, heartburn, GI distress, diarrhea

■ **Serious Reactions**
  • Salmeterol may prolong the QT interval, which may precipitate ventricular arrhythmias.
  • Hypokalemia and hyperglycemia may occur.

■ **Patient/Family Education**
  • Patients receiving salmeterol for asthma should normally also be receiving regular and adequate doses of an effective asthma controller medication, such as inhaled corticosteroid
  • Proper inhalation technique is vital
  • Notify clinician if no response to usual doses, or if palpitations, rapid heartbeat, chest pain, muscle tremors, dizziness, headache occur
  • **Do not use to treat acute symptoms or on an as-needed basis**
  • Keep the drug canister at room temperature because cold decreases the drug's effects
  • When the drug is used to prevent exercise-induced bronchospasm, administer the dose at least 30 to 60 minutes before exercising
  • Wait at least 1 full minute before the second inhalation
  • Do not abruptly discontinue the drug or exceed the recommended dosage
  • Avoid excessive consumption of caffeinated products, such as chocolate, cocoa, cola, coffee, and tea
  • Teach the patient how to measure peak flow readings and keep a log of measurements

■ **Monitoring Parameters**
  • Blood pressure, pulse rate and quality, and respiratory rate, depth, rhythm, and type
  • Periodically evaluate the serum potassium level

■ **Geriatric side effects at a glance:**
  ❑ CNS ❑ Bowel Dysfunction ❑ Bladder Dysfunction ❑ Falls

U.S. Regulatory Considerations
☑ FDA Black Box

May increase the risk of asthma-related death. This drug should be used as additional therapy for patients not adequately controlled on other antiasthma drugs.

❑ OBRA regulated in U.S. Long Term Care

salsalate

(sal'-sa-late)

- **Brand Name(s):** Amigesic, Disalcid, Mono-Gesic, Salflex, Salsitab
  Chemical Class: Salicylate derivative

- **Clinical Pharmacology:**
  Mechanism of Action: An NSAID that inhibits prostaglandin synthesis, reducing the inflammatory response and the intensity of pain stimuli reaching the sensory nerve endings. **Therapeutic Effect:** Produces analgesic and anti-inflammatory effects.
  Pharmacokinetics: Rapidly and completely absorbed from the GI tract. Food delays absorption of salsalate. Protein binding: High (to albumin). Metabolized in the liver. Excreted in urine. Removed by hemodialysis. **Half-life:** 1 hr.

- **Available Forms:**
  - *Tablets* (*Amigesic, Disalcid*): 500 mg, 750 mg.
  - *Tablets* (*Mono-Gesic, Salflex*): 750 mg.

- **Indications and Dosages:**
  Rheumatoid arthritis, osteoarthritis pain: PO Initially, 3 g/day in 2-3 divided doses. Maintenance: 2-4 g/day.

- **Contraindications:** Bleeding disorders, hypersensitivity to salicylates or NSAIDs

- **Side Effects**
  Occasional
  Nausea, dyspepsia (including heartburn, indigestion, and epigastric pain)

- **Serious Reactions**
  - There is an increased risk of cardiovascular events, including MI and cerebrovascular accident, and serious—potentially life-threatening—GI bleeding.
  - Tinnitus may be the first indication that the serum salicylic acid concentration is reaching or exceeding the upper therapeutic range.
  - Salsalate use may also produce vertigo, headache, confusion, drowsiness, diaphoresis, hyperventilation, vomiting, and diarrhea.
  - Severe overdose may result in electrolyte imbalance, hyperthermia, dehydration, and blood pH imbalance.
  - GI bleeding and peptic ulcer rarely occur.

- Consider for patients with GI intolerance to aspirin or patients in whom interference with normal platelet function by aspirin or other NSAIDs is undesirable

■ **Patient/Family Education**
- Take salsalate with food and use antacids to relieve upset stomach
- Notify the physician if persistent GI pain or ringing in ears occurs
- Avoid alcohol and NSAIDs during salsalate therapy

■ **Monitoring Parameters**
- AST, ALT, bilirubin, creatinine, CBC, hematocrit if patient is on long-term therapy
- Therapeutic response, such as improved grip strength, increased joint mobility, reduced joint tenderness, and relief of pain, stiffness, and swelling

■ **Geriatric side effects at a glance:**
   ☑ CNS   ❑ Bowel Dysfunction   ❑ Bladder Dysfunction   ❑ Falls
   ☑ Other: Gastropathy

■ **Use with caution in older patients with:** Renal impairment, Hepatic impairment, CHF, HTN, PUD, History of GI bleeding, GERD, Gout, Bleeding and platelet disorders, History of aspirin sensitivity reaction. Also use with caution in patients taking Anticoagulants, Aspirin, and Antihypertensive agents.

■ **U.S. Regulatory Considerations**
   ☑ FDA Black Box
- Increased cardiovascular risk
- Increased gastrointestinal risk
   ❑ OBRA regulated in U.S. Long Term Care

■ **Other Uses in Geriatric Patient:** None

■ **Side Effects:**
   Of particular importance in the geriatric patient: Confusion, cognitive impairment, delirium, dizziness, dyspepsia, fluid retention, renal impairment

■ **Geriatric Considerations - Summary:** As a nonacetylated salicylate, salsalate does not adversely affect platelet function and is associated with fewer adverse GI and renal effects. A preferred analgesic and anti-inflammatory agent for use in older adults. Use of NSAIDs in older adults increases the risk of GI complications including gastric ulceration, bleeding, and perforation. These complications are not necessarily preceded by less severe GI symptoms. Concomitant use of a proton pump inhibitor or misoprostol reduces the risk for gastric ulceration and bleeding, but may not prevent long-term GI toxicity.

■ **References:**
   1. COX-2 alternatives and GI protection. Med Lett Drugs Ther 2004;46:91.
   2. Drugs that may cause cognitive disorders in the elderly. Med Lett Drugs Ther 2000;42:111-112.

saquinavir

(sa-kwin'-a-veer)

- **Brand Name(s):** Fortovase, Invirase
  Chemical Class: Protease inhibitor, HIV

- **Clinical Pharmacology:**
  Mechanism of Action: Inhibits HIV protease, rendering the enzyme incapable of processing the polyprotein precursors needed to generate functional proteins in HIV-infected cells. **Therapeutic Effect:** Interferes with HIV replication, slowing the progression of HIV infection.
  Pharmacokinetics: Poorly absorbed after PO administration (absorption increased with high-calorie and high-fat meals). Protein binding: 99%. Metabolized in the liver to inactive metabolite. Primarily eliminated in feces. Unknown if removed by hemodialysis. **Half-life:** 13 hr.

- **Available Forms:**
  - *Capsules (Invirase):* 200 mg.
  - *Capsules, Gelatin (Fortovase):* 200 mg.
  - *Tablets (Invirase):* 500 mg.

- **Indications and Dosages:**
  HIV infection in combination with other antiretrovirals: PO (Fortovase) 1,200 mg 3 times a day or 1,000 mg twice a day in combination with ritonavir 100 mg twice a day. PO (Invirase) 1,000 mg (5×200 mg or 2×500 mg) twice a day in combination with ritonavir 100 mg twice a day. Dosage adjustments when given in combination therapy: *Delavirdine:* Fortovase 800 mg 3 times a day. *Lopinavir/ritonavir:* Fortovase 800 mg twice a day. *Nelfinavir:* Fortovase 800 mg 3 times a day or 1,200 mg twice a day. *Ritonavir:* Fortovase or Invirase 1,000 mg twice a day.

- **Contraindications:** Concurrent use with ergot medications, lovastatin, midazolam, simvastatin, or triazolam

- **Side Effects**
  Occasional
  Diarrhea, abdominal discomfort and pain, nausea, photosensitivity, stomatitis
  Rare
  Confusion, ataxia, asthenia, headache, rash

- **Serious Reactions**
  - Ketoacidosis occurs rarely.

Special Considerations

- Invirase and Fortovase not considered bioequivalent; no food effect on Invirase when taken with ritonavir; take Fortovase with large meal
- Fortovase is the recommended formulation
- Invirase should only be considered if it is to be combined with antiretrovirals that significantly inhibit saquinavir's metabolism

- Always check updated treatment guidelines before initiating or changing antiretroviral therapy. (http://AIDSinfo.nih.gov)

■ **Patient/Family Education**
- Take saquinavir within 2 hours after a full meal
- Space drug doses evenly around the clock and continue taking the drug for the full course of treatment
- Notify the physician if nausea or vomiting or persistent abdominal pain occurs
- Avoid grapefruit products while taking saquinavir
- Avoid exposure to artificial light sources and sunlight
- Saquinavir is not a cure for HIV infection, nor does it reduce the risk of transmitting HIV to others

■ **Monitoring Parameters**
- Blood chemistry and serum hepatic enzyme levels, CD4+ cell count and blood glucose, HIV RNA, and serum triglyceride levels
- Monitor for signs and symptoms of GI discomfort
- Assess pattern of daily bowel activity and stool consistency
- Inspect the patient's mouth for signs of mucosal ulceration
- If the patient experience severe toxicities, such as ketoacidosis, withhold the drug and notify the physician

■ **Geriatric side effects at a glance:**
  ❑ CNS ❑ Bowel Dysfunction ❑ Bladder Dysfunction ❑ Falls

■ **U.S. Regulatory Considerations**
  ❑ FDA Black Box ❑ OBRA regulated in U.S. Long Term Care

scopolamine

(skoe-pol'-a-meen)

■ **Brand Name(s):** Transdermal: Transderm Scōp

■ **Brand Name(s):** Ophth: Isopto Hyoscine

■ **Brand Name(s):** Oral: Scopace
  Chemical Class: Belladonna alkaloid

■ **Clinical Pharmacology:**
  Mechanism of Action: An anticholinergic that reduces excitability of labyrinthine receptors, depressing conduction in the vestibular cerebellar pathway. **Therapeutic Effect:** Prevents motion-induced nausea and vomiting.
  Pharmacokinetics: Well absorbed percutaneously. Crosses blood-brain barrier. Metabolized in liver. Excreted in urine. **Half-life:** 9.5 hr (transdermal).

■ **Available Forms:**
- *Transdermal System* (*Transderm Scōp*): 1.5 mg.

■ **Indications and Dosages:**
Prevention of motion sickness: Transdermal 1 system q72h.
Postoperative nausea or vomiting: Transdermal 1 system no sooner than 1 hr before surgery and removed 24 hr after surgery.

■ **Contraindications:** Angle-closure glaucoma, GI or GU obstruction, myasthenia gravis, paralytic ileus, tachycardia, thyrotoxicosis

■ **Side Effects**
Frequent (greater than 15%)
Dry mouth, somnolence, blurred vision
Rare (5%–1%)
Dizziness, restlessness, hallucinations, confusion, difficulty urinating, rash

■ **Serious Reactions**
- None known.

■ **Patient/Family Education**
- Avoid abrupt discontinuation (taper off over 1 wk)
- Wash hands thoroughly after handling transdermal patches before contacting eyes
- Avoid tasks requiring mental alertness or motor skills until response to the drug has been established

■ **Monitoring Parameters**
- BUN level; blood chemistry test results; and serum alkaline phosphatase, bilirubin, creatinine, AST (SGOT), and ALT (SGPT) levels to assess hepatic and renal function

■ **Geriatric side effects at a glance:**
☑ CNS ☑ Bowel Dysfunction ☑ Bladder Dysfunction ☑ Falls
Other: Dry mouth, blurred vision, confusion, psychoses

■ **Use with caution in older patients with:** Narrow-angle glaucoma, overflow incontinence, preexisting psychotic symptoms

■ **U.S. Regulatory Considerations**
☐ FDA Black Box ☑ OBRA regulated in U.S. Long Term Care

■ **Other Uses in Geriatric Patient:** Used to decrease salivation

■ **Side Effects:**
Of particular importance in the geriatric patient: Anticholinergic effects

■ **Geriatric Considerations - Summary:** Scopolamine and related anticholingerics have limited benefits in the treatment of nausea/vomiting and motion sickness and present significant risk to older adults. The use of the transdermal patch may be safer but can cause serious toxic effects. These drugs possess potent anticholinergic effects and can cause cognitive impairment, delirium, dry mouth, blurred vision, and increased risk of falls. The use of this drug and related compounds should be limited and when used, patients should be closely monitored.

■ **References:**
1. Vangala V, Tueth M. Chronic anticholinergic toxicity: identification and management in older patients. Geriatrics 2003;58:36-37.
2. Tune LE. Anticholinergic effects of medication in elderly patients. J Clin Psychiatry 2001;62(suppl 21):11-14.
3. Ziskind AA: Transdermal scopolamine-induced pyschosis. Postgrad Med 1988;84:73-76.

secobarbital sodium

(see-koe-bar'-bi-tal soe'-dee-um)

■ **Brand Name(s):** Seconal

Combinations
Rx: with amobarbital (Tuinal)
Chemical Class: Barbituric acid derivative

DEA Class: Schedule II

■ **Clinical Pharmacology:**
Mechanism of Action: A barbiturate that depresses the central nervous system (CNS) activity by binding to barbiturate site at the GABA-receptor complex enhancing GABA activity and depressing reticular activity system. ***Therapeutic Effect:*** Produces hypnotic effect due to CNS depression.
Pharmacokinetics: Well absorbed from the gastrointestinal (GI) tract. Protein binding: 52%-57%. Crosses blood-brain barrier. Widely distributed. Metabolized in liver by microsomal enzyme system to inactive and active metabolites. Primarily excreted in urine. Not removed by hemodialysis. ***Half-life:*** 15-40 hr.

■ **Available Forms:**
• *Capsules:* 50 mg (Seconal).

■ **Indications and Dosages:**
Insomnia: PO 100 mg at bedtime.
Preoperative sedation: PO 100-300 mg 1-2 hr before procedure.
Sedation, daytime: PO 30-50 mg 3-4 times/day.

■ **Unlabeled Uses:** Chemotherapy-induced nausea and vomiting

■ **Contraindications:** History of manifest or latent porphyria, marked liver dysfunction, marked respiratory disease in which dyspnea or obstruction is evident, and hypersensitivity to secobarbital or barbiturates

■ **Side Effects**
Frequent
Somnolence

Occasional

Agitation, confusion, hyperkinesia, ataxia, CNS depression, nightmares, nervousness, psychiatric disturbance, hallucinations, insomnia, anxiety, dizziness, abnormality in thinking, hypoventilation, apnea, bradycardia, hypotension, syncope, nausea, vomiting, constipation, headache

Rare

Hypersensitivity reactions, fever, liver damage, megaloblastic anemia

■ **Serious Reactions**
- Agranulocytosis, megaloblastic anemia, apnea, hypoventilation, bradycardia, hypotension, syncope, hepatic damage, and Stevens-Johnson syndrome rarely occur.
- Tolerance and physical dependence may occur with repeated use.

Special Considerations

- Compared to the benzodiazepine sedative-hypnotics, secobarbital is more lethal in overdosage, has a higher tendency for abuse and addiction, and is more likely to cause drug interactions via induction of hepatic microsomal enzymes; few advantages if any in safety or efficacy over benzodiazepines

■ **Patient/Family Education**
- Avoid driving and other dangerous activities
- Withdrawal insomnia may occur after short-term use; do not start using drug again, insomnia will improve in 1-3 nights
- May experience increased dreaming
- Avoid alcohol and limit caffeine intake

■ **Monitoring Parameters**
- Blood pressure, pulse, respiratory rate and rhythm

■ **Geriatric side effects at a glance:**
  ☑ CNS ☐ Bowel Dysfunction ☐ Bladder Dysfunction ☑ Falls
  Other: Withdrawal symptoms after long-term use

■ **Use with caution in older patients with:** Not recommeded for use in older adults.

■ **U.S. Regulatory Considerations**
  ☐ FDA Black Box ☑ OBRA regulated in U.S. Long Term Care

■ **Other Uses in Geriatric Patient:** Anxiety disorders, sleep disorders, seizure disorders

■ **Side Effects:**
  Of particular importance in the geriatric patient: Sedation, withdrawal symptoms when abruptly discontinued (e.g., during hospitalization) rather than tapered

■ **Geriatric Considerations - Summary:** Because barbiturates have a low therapeutic window, a wide range of drug interactions and rapid development of tolerance, great potential for abuse and dependence, these agents are not recommended for use in older adults.

■ **Reference:**
  1. Hypnotic drugs. Med Lett Drugs Ther 2000;42:71-72.

selegiline hydrochloride

(se-le'-ji-leen hye-droe-klor'-ide)

- **Brand Name(s):** Eldepryl
  Chemical Class: Phenethylamine derivative

- **Clinical Pharmacology:**
  Mechanism of Action: An antiparkinson agent that irreversibly inhibits the activity of monoamine oxidase type B, the enzyme that breaks down dopamine, thereby increasing dopaminergic action. **Therapeutic Effect:** Relieves signs and symptoms of Parkinson's disease.
  Pharmacokinetics: Rapidly absorbed from the GI tract. Crosses the blood-brain barrier. Metabolized in the liver to the active metabolites. Primarily excreted in urine.
  Half-life: 17 hr (amphetamine), 20 hr (methamphetamine).

- **Available Forms:**
  - *Capsules*: 5 mg.
  - *Tablets*: 5 mg.

- **Indications and Dosages:**
  Adjunctive treatment for parkinsonism: PO Initially, 5 mg in the morning. May increase up to 10 mg/day in divided doses, such as 5 mg at breakfast and lunch, given concomitantly with each dose of carbidopa and levodopa.

- **Unlabeled Uses:** Treatment of Alzheimer's disease, attention-deficit-hyperactivity disorder, depression, early Parkinson's disease, extrapyramidal symptoms, negative symptoms of schizophrenia

- **Contraindications:** Concurrent use with meperidine

- **Side Effects**
  Frequent (10%–4%)
  Nausea, dizziness, light-headedness, syncope, abdominal discomfort
  Occasional (3%–2%)
  Confusion, hallucinations, dry mouth, vivid dreams, dyskinesia
  Rare (1%)
  Headache, myalgia, anxiety, diarrhea, insomnia

- **Serious Reactions**
  - Symptoms of overdose may vary from CNS depression, characterized by sedation, apnea, cardiovascular collapse, and death, to severe paradoxical reactions, such as hallucinations, tremor, and seizures.
  - Other serious effects may include involuntary movements, impaired motor coordination, loss of balance, blepharospasm, facial grimaces, feeling of heaviness in the lower extremities, depression, nightmares, delusions, overstimulation, sleep disturbance, and anger.

- At low doses, irreversible type B MAOI; at higher doses is metabolized to amphetamine, inhibiting both A and B subtypes of MAO
- Several placebo-controlled studies have demonstrated a significant delay in the need to initiate levodopa therapy in patients who receive selegiline in the early phase of the disease
- May have significant benefit in slowing the onset of the debilitating consequences of Parkinson's disease

■ Patient/Family Education
- Dizziness, drowsiness, light-headedness, and dry mouth are common side effects of the drug but will diminish or disappear with continued treatment
- Change positions slowly and let legs dangle momentarily before standing to reduce the drug's hypotensive effect
- Avoid tasks that require mental alertness or motor skills until response to the drug has been established
- Avoid alcoholic beverages during therapy
- Avoid ingesting large amounts of caffeine or tyramine-rich foods, such as wine and aged cheese, to prevent a hypertensive reaction

■ Monitoring Parameters
- Monitor the patient for dyskinetic effects
- Assess the patient for clinical reversal of symptoms, including improvement of masklike facial expression, muscular rigidity, shuffling gait, and resting tremor of the hands and head
- Be alert for neurologic effects, including agitation, headache, lethargy, and confusion

■ Geriatric side effects at a glance:
☑ CNS   ❑ Bowel Dysfunction   ❑ Bladder Dysfunction   ❑ Falls
Other: None

■ Use with caution in older patients with: None

■ U.S. Regulatory Considerations
❑ FDA Black Box   ❑ OBRA regulated in U.S. Long Term Care

■ Other Uses in Geriatric Patient: None

■ Side Effects:
Of particular importance in the geriatric patient: None

■ Geriatric Considerations - Summary: Selegiline inhibits monoamine oxidase with a dose-dependent selectivity for MAO-B enzyme. This reduces the risk of dangerous drug or food interactions but this reduced risk of adverse effects is lost at doses greater than 10 mg daily. Selegiline is considered adjunctive therapy for Parkinson's disease. Selegiline is metabolized to amphetamine compounds which can cause decreased appetite, confusion, and agitation.

■ References:
1. Miyasaki JM, Martin WRW, Suchowersky O, et al. Practice parameter: initiation of treatment for Parkinson's disease: an evidence based review. Neurology 2002;58:11-17.

2. Gerlach M, Youdim MBH, Riederer P: Pharmacology of selegiline. Neurology 1996; 47(suppl 3):S137-S145.
3. Nutt JG, Wooten GF. Diagnosis and initial management of Parkinson's disease. N Engl J Med 2005;353:1021-1027.

senna

(sen'-na)

■ **Brand Name(s):** Ex-Lax, Senexon, Senna-Gen, Sennatural, Senokot, X-Prep
   Chemical Class: Anthraquinone derivative

■ **Clinical Pharmacology:**
   Mechanism of Action: A GI stimulant that has a direct effect on intestinal smooth musculature by stimulating the intramural nerve plexus. **Therapeutic Effect:** Increases peristalsis and promotes laxative effect.
   Pharmacokinetics:

Route	Onset	Peak	Duration
PO	6–12 hr	N/A	N/A
Rectal	0.5–2 hr	N/A	N/A

Minimal absorption after oral administration. Hydrolyzed to active form by enzymes of colonic flora. Absorbed drug metabolized in the liver. Eliminated in feces via biliary system.

■ **Available Forms:**
   • *Granules (Senokot):* 15 mg/tsp.
   • *Liquid (X-Prep):* 8.8 mg/5 ml.
   • *Syrup (Senokot):* 8.8 mg/5 ml.
   • *Tablets (Sennatural, Senokot, Senexon, Senna-Gen):* 8.6 mg, 15 mg.
   • *Tablets (Ex-Lax).*

■ **Indications and Dosages:**
   Constipation: PO (Tablets) 2 tablets at bedtime. Maximum: 4 tablets twice a day. PO (Syrup) 10–15 ml at bedtime. Maximum: 15 ml twice a day. PO (Granules) 1 tsp at bedtime. Maximum: 2 tsp twice a day.
   Bowel evacuation: PO 75 ml between 2 PM. and 4 PM. on day prior to procedure.

■ **Contraindications:** Abdominal pain, appendicitis, intestinal obstruction, nausea, vomiting

■ **Side Effects**
   Frequent
   Pink-red, red-violet, red-brown, or yellow-brown discoloration of urine
   Occasional
   Some degree of abdominal discomfort, nausea, mild cramps, griping, faintness

- **Serious Reactions**
  - Long-term use may result in laxative dependence, chronic constipation, and loss of normal bowel function.
  - Prolonged use or overdose may result in electrolyte and metabolic disturbances (such as hypokalemia, hypocalcemia, and metabolic acidosis or alkalosis), vomiting, muscle weakness, persistent diarrhea, malabsorption, and weight loss.

Special Considerations
  - Proposed laxative of choice for narcotic-induced constipation

- **Patient/Family Education**
  - Urine may turn pink-red, red-violet, red-brown, or yellow-brown
  - Institute measures to promote defecation, such as increasing fluid intake, exercising, and eating a high-fiber diet
  - Take other oral medications within 1 hour of taking senna because these substances may decrease the effectiveness of senna

- **Monitoring Parameters**
  - Bowel sounds for peristalsis
  - Pattern of daily bowel activity and stool consistency; record time of evacuation
  - Electrolytes

- **Geriatric side effects at a glance:**
  ☐ CNS ☑ Bowel Dysfunction ☐ Bladder Dysfunction ☐ Falls

- **U.S. Regulatory Considerations**
  ☐ FDA Black Box ☐ OBRA regulated in U.S. Long Term Care

sertraline hydrochloride

(ser'-tra-leen hy-droe-klor'-ide)

- **Brand Name(s):** Zoloft
  Chemical Class: Naphthalenamine derivative

- **Clinical Pharmacology:**
  Mechanism of Action: An antidepressant, anxiolytic, and obsessive-compulsive disorder adjunct that blocks the reuptake of the neurotransmitter serotonin at CNS neuronal presynaptic membranes, increasing its availability at postsynaptic receptor sites. **Therapeutic Effect:** Relieves depression, reduces obsessive-compulsive behavior, decreases anxiety.
  Pharmacokinetics: Incompletely and slowly absorbed from the GI tract; food increases absorption. Protein binding: 98%. Widely distributed. Undergoes extensive first-pass metabolism in the liver to active compound. Excreted in urine and feces. Not removed by hemodialysis. **Half-life:** 26 hr.

■ **Available Forms:**
- *Oral Concentrate*: 20 mg/ml.
- *Tablets*: 25 mg, 50 mg, 100 mg.

■ **Indications and Dosages:**
Depression: PO Initially, 25 mg/day. May increase by 25-50 mg/day at 7-day intervals up to 200 mg/day.
Obsessive-compulsive disorder: PO Initially, 25 mg/day. May increase by 25–50 mg/day at 7-day intervals. Maximum: 200 mg/day.
Panic disorder, posttraumatic stress disorder, social anxiety disorder: PO Adults, Elderly. Initially, 25 mg/day. May increase by 50 mg/day at 7-day intervals. Range: 50–200 mg/day. Maximum: 200 mg/day.

■ **Unlabeled Uses:** Eating disorders, generalized anxiety disorder (GAD), impulse control disorders

■ **Contraindications:** Use within 14 days of MAOIs

■ **Side Effects**
Frequent (26%–12%)
Headache, nausea, diarrhea, insomnia, somnolence, dizziness, fatigue, rash, dry mouth
Occasional (6%–4%)
Anxiety, nervousness, agitation, tremor, dyspepsia, diaphoresis, vomiting, constipation, abnormal ejaculation, visual disturbances, altered taste
Rare (less than 3%)
Flatulence, urinary frequency, paresthesia, hot flashes, chills

■ **Serious Reactions**
- None known.

Special Considerations
- SSRI of choice based on intermediate half-life, linear pharmacokinetics, absence of appreciable age effect on clearance, substantially less effect on P450 enzymes, reducing potential for drug interactions
- Oral concentrate contains 12% alcohol; dropper contains natural rubber, caution if latex allergy
- Splitting 100-mg tablets to yield 50-mg dose cuts costs

■ **Patient/Family Education**
- Oral concentrate must be diluted in water, ginger ale, lemon/lime soda, lemonade, or orange juice only, no other liquids should be used; do not mix in advance
- Avoid alcohol

■ **Geriatric side effects at a glance:**
❑ CNS   ☑ Bowel Dysfunction   ❑ Bladder Dysfunction   ☑ Falls
Other: Hyponatremia; weight gain (long term)

■ **Use with caution in older patients with:** None

■ **U.S. Regulatory Considerations**
☑ FDA Black Box
- Because there is an increased risk of suicide in children and adolescents, older adults should also be closely monitored for suicide ideation.

☑ OBRA regulated in U.S. Long Term Care

■ **Other Uses in Geriatric Patient:** Anxiety symptoms and related disorders

■ **Side Effects:**
Of particular importance in the geriatric patient: Hyponatremia, withdrawal symptoms when abruptly discontinued (e.g., during hospitalization) rather than tapered

■ **Geriatric Considerations - Summary:** Serotoninergic antidepressants are now considered by many the first-line therapy for treatment of depression in older adults. They are also effective in the management of symptoms of anxiety. Although these agents appear to have a more favorable side-effect profile than tricyclic antidepressants for most older adults, it is important to note that some of these agents have the potential for significant drug interactions, have been associated with falls, and require careful attention to electrolyte status. In addition, many of the drugs in this class have been associated with severe withdrawal symptoms (e.g., nausea and/or vomiting, dizziness, headaches, lethargy or light-headedness, anxiety and/or agitation) when discontinued abruptly.

■ **References:**
1. Cadieux RJ. Antidepressant drug interactions in the elderly. Understanding the P-450 system is half the battle in reducing risks. Postgrad Med 1999;106:231-240, 245.
2. Roose SP, Laghrissi-Thode F, Kennedy JS, et al. Comparison of paroxetine and nortriptyline in depressed patients with ischemic heart disease. JAMA 1998;279:287-291.
3. Thapa PB, Gideon P, Cost TW, et al. Antidepressants and the risk of falls among nursing home residents. N Engl J Med 1998;339:875-882.
4. Bouman WP, Pinner G, Johnson H. Incidence of selective serotonin reuptake inhibitor (SSRI) induced hyponatraemia due to the syndrome of inappropriate antidiuretic hormone (SIADH) secretion in the elderly. Int J Geriatr Psychiatry 1998;13:12-15.

sevelamer hydrochloride

(seh-vel'-ah-mer hye-droe-klor'-ide)

■ **Brand Name(s):** Renagel
Chemical Class: Allylamine

■ **Clinical Pharmacology:**
Mechanism of Action: An antihyperphosphatemia agent that binds with dietary phosphorus in the GI tract, thus allowing phosphorus to be eliminated through the normal digestive process and decreasing the serum phosphorus level. **Therapeutic Effect:** Decreases incidence of hypercalcemic episodes in patients receiving calcium acetate treatment.
Pharmacokinetics: Not absorbed systemically. Unknown if removed by hemodialysis.

■ **Available Forms:**
• *Capsules*: 403 mg.
• *Tablets*: 400 mg, 800 mg.

- **Indications and Dosages:**
  Hyperphosphatemia: PO 800–1,600 mg with each meal, depending on severity of hyperphosphatemia.

- **Contraindications:** Bowel obstruction, hypophosphatemia

- **Side Effects**
  Frequent (20%–11%)
  Infection, pain, hypotension, diarrhea, dyspepsia, nausea, vomiting
  Occasional (10%–1%)
  Headache, constipation, hypertension, thrombosis, increased cough

- **Serious Reactions**
  - Thrombosis occurs rarely.

Special Considerations
  - Has not been studied in ESRD patients not on hemodialysis
  - Compared to calcium acetate, may reduce the risk of developing hypercalcemia

- **Patient/Family Education**
  - A daily multivitamin supplement may prevent reduction in serum levels of vitamins D, E, K, and folic acid
  - Do not chew or take caps apart prior to administration
  - Space doses of sevelamer ≥1 hr before or 3 hr after concomitant medications
  - Take with food
  - Notify the physician if diarrhea, signs of hypotension (such as light-headedness), nausea or vomiting, or a persistent headache occurs

- **Monitoring Parameters**
  - Serum phosphorus, calcium, bicarbonate, and chloride levels

- **Geriatric side effects at a glance:**
  ☐ CNS ☑ Bowel Dysfunction ☐ Bladder Dysfunction ☐ Falls

- **U.S. Regulatory Considerations**
  ☐ FDA Black Box ☐ OBRA regulated in U.S. Long Term Care

sibutramine hydrochloride

(sih-byoo'-tra-meen hye-dro-klor'-ide)

- **Brand Name(s):** Meridia
  Chemical Class: Cyclobutanemethamine derivative

- **Clinical Pharmacology:**
  Mechanism of Action: A central nervous system (CNS) stimulant that inhibits reuptake of serotonin (enhancing satiety) and norepinephrine (raises metabolic rate) centrally. **Therapeutic Effect:** Induces and maintains weight loss.

Pharmacokinetics: Rapidly absorbed from the gastrointestinal (GI) tract. Protein binding: 95%-97%. Metabolized in liver, undergoes first-pass metabolism. Primarily excreted in urine, minimal elimination in feces. **Half-life:** 1.1 hr.

■ **Available Forms:**
- *Capsules*: 5 mg, 10 mg, 15 mg.

■ **Indications and Dosages:**
Weight loss: PO Initially, 10 mg/day. May increase up to 15 mg/day. Maximum: 20 mg/day.

■ **Contraindications:** Anorexia nervosa, concomitant MAOI use, concomitant use of centrally acting appetite suppressants, hypersensitivity to sibutramine or any component of the formulation

■ **Side Effects**
Frequent
Headache, dry mouth, anorexia, constipation, insomnia, rhinitis, pharyngitis
Occasional
Back pain, flu syndrome, dizziness, nausea, asthenia (loss of strength, energy), arthralgia, nervousness, dyspepsia, sinusitis, abdominal pain, anxiety
Rare
Depression, rash, cough, sweating, tachycardia, migraine, increased BP, paresthesia, altered taste

■ **Serious Reactions**
- Seizures, thrombocytopenia, and deaths have been reported.
- Serotonin syndrome can occur with concomitant use of drugs that increase serotonin.
- Large doses may produce extreme nervousness and tachycardia.

Special Considerations

- Primary pulmonary hypertension and cardiac valve disorders have been associated with other centrally acting weight loss agents that cause release of serotonin from nerve terminals; although sibutramine has not been associated with these effects in premarketing clinical studies, patients should be informed of the potential for these side effects and monitored closely for their occurrence
- Substantially increases blood pressure in some patients
- Maintenance of weight loss beyond 18 mo has not been studied

■ **Patient/Family Education**
- Avoid alcohol
- May be habit-forming
- Do not take OTC medications without first consulting the physician

■ **Monitoring Parameters**
- Regular blood pressure monitoring
- Heart rate, weight

■ **Geriatric side effects at a glance:**
☐ CNS ☐ Bowel Dysfunction ☐ Bladder Dysfunction ☐ Falls

sildenafil citrate

(sill-den'-a-fill sye'-trate)

■ **Brand Name(s):** Revatio, Viagra
Chemical Class: Cyclic GMP specific phosphodiesterase inhibitor

■ **Clinical Pharmacology:**
Mechanism of Action: An erectile dysfunction agent that inhibits phosphodiesterase type 5, the enzyme responsible for degrading cyclic guanosine monophosphate (cGMP) in the corpus cavernosum of the penis and pulmonary vascular smooth muscle, resulting in smooth muscle relaxation and increased blood flow. **Therapeutic Effects:** Facilitates an erection, produces pulmonary vasodilation.
Pharmacokinetics: Rapidly absorbed from the GI tract. Protein binding: greater than 96%. Metabolized in liver. Excreted primarily in the feces, urine, and semen. **Half-life:** 4 hr.

■ **Available Forms:**
• **Tablets:** 20 mg (Revatio), 25 mg (Viagra), 50 mg (Viagra), 100 mg (Viagra).

■ **Indications and Dosages:**
Erectile dysfunction: PO Consider starting dose of 25 mg 30 min-4 hr before sexual activity. Range: 25-100 mg. Maximum dosing frequency is once daily. Patients taking potent CYP3A4 inhibitors: starting dose of 25 mg.
Pulmonary arterial hypertension: PO 20 mg 3 times a day.

■ **Unlabeled Uses:** Treatment of diabetic gastroparesis, sexual dysfunction associated with the use of selective serotonin reuptake inhibitors

■ **Contraindications:** Concurrent use of sodium nitroprusside or nitrates in any form

■ **Side Effects**
Frequent
Headache (16%), flushing (10%)
Occasional (7%-3%)
Dyspepsia, nasal congestion, UTI, abnormal vision, diarrhea
Rare (2%)
Dizziness, rash

■ **Serious Reactions**
• Prolonged erections (lasting over 4 hr) and priapism (painful erections lasting over 6 hr) occur rarely.

Special Considerations
• Tablets are priced the same regardless of dose; 100-mg tablets can be broken in half

Patient/Family Education
- Sildenafil is not effective without sexual stimulation
- Seek treatment immediately if an erection lasts longer than 4 hr
- Avoid using nitrate drugs concurrently with sildenafil
- Avoid taking sildenafil within 4 hr of an alpha-blocker
- High-fat meals may affect the drug's absorption rate and effectiveness

Monitoring Parameters
- Blood pressure, heart rate

Geriatric side effects at a glance:
☑ CNS ☑ Bowel Dysfunction ☐ Bladder Dysfunction ☐ Falls

U.S. Regulatory Considerations
☐ FDA Black Box ☐ OBRA regulated in U.S. Long Term Care

silver nitrate

(sil'-ver ni'-trate)

Brand Name(s): Silver nitrate
Chemical Class: Heavy metal

Clinical Pharmacology:
Mechanism of Action: Free silver ions precipitate bacterial proteins by combining with chloride in tissue forming silver chloride; coagulates cellular protein to form an eschar or scab. The germicidal action is credited to precipitation of bacterial proteins by free silver ions. **Therapeutic Effect:** Inhibits growth of both gram-positive and gram-negative bacteria.

Pharmacokinetics: Minimal gastrointestinal (GI) tract and cutaneous absorption. Minimal excretion in urine.

Available Forms:
- *Applicator Sticks*: 75% silver nitrate and 25% potassium nitrate.
- *Ophthalmic Solution*: 1%.
- *Topical Solution*: 10%, 25%, 50%.

Indications and Dosages:
Exuberant granulations: Applicator Sticks Apply to mucous membranes and other moist skin surfaces only on area to be treated 2-3 times/wk for 2-3 wk. Topical Solution Apply a cotton applicator dipped in solution on the affected area 2-3 times/wk for 2-3 wk.

Contraindications: Broken skin, cuts, or wounds, hypersensitivity to silver nitrate or any of its components

Side Effects
Occasional
Ophthalmic: Chemical conjunctivitis
Topical: Burning, irritation, staining of the skin

Rare
Hyponatremia, methemoglobinemia

■ **Serious Reactions**
- Symptoms of overdose include blackening of skin and mucous membranes, pain and burning of the mouth, salivation, vomiting, diarrhea, shock, convulsions, coma, and death.
- Methemoglobinemia is caused by absorbed silver nitrate but occurs rarely.
- Cauterization of the cornea and blindness occur rarely.

■ **Patient/Family Education**
- Stains skin and utensils (removable with iodine tincture followed by sodium thiosulfate solution)
- Discontinue topical preparation if irritation or redness develops
- Do not use topical preparations near the eyes or abraded areas

■ **Monitoring Parameters**
- Skin for irritation, redness, and staining with application
- Methemoglobin levels with prolonged use

■ **Geriatric side effects at a glance:**
❏ CNS   ❏ Bowel Dysfunction   ❏ Bladder Dysfunction   ❏ Falls

■ **U.S. Regulatory Considerations**
❏ FDA Black Box   ❏ OBRA regulated in U.S. Long Term Care

silver sulfadiazine

(sil'ver sul-fa-dye'-a-zeen)

■ **Brand Name(s):** Silvadene, SSD, SSD AF, Thermazene
  Chemical Class: Sulfonamide derivative

■ **Clinical Pharmacology:**
  Mechanism of Action: An anti-infective that acts upon cell wall and cell membrane. Releases silver slowly in concentrations selectively toxic to bacteria. **Therapeutic Effect:** Produces bactericidal effect.
  Pharmacokinetics: Variably absorbed. Significant systemic absorption may occur if applied to extensive burns. Absorbed medication excreted unchanged in urine. **Half-life:** 10 hr (increased with impaired renal function).

■ **Available Forms:**
- **Cream:** 1% (Silvadene, SSD, SSD AF).

■ Indications and Dosages:
Burns: Topical   Apply 1-2 times daily.

■ Unlabeled Uses: Treatment of minor bacterial skin infection, dermal ulcer

■ Contraindications: Hypersensitivity to silver sulfadiazine or any component of the formulation

■ Side Effects
Side effects characteristic of all sulfonamides may occur when systemically absorbed, e.g. when used topically over large exposed areas, such as extensive burn areas. Anorexia, nausea, vomiting, headache, diarrhea, dizziness, photosensitivity, joint pain
Frequent
Burning feeling at treatment site
Occasional
Brown-gray skin discoloration, rash, itching
Rare
Increased sensitivity of skin to sunlight

■ Serious Reactions
- If significant systemic absorption occurs, less often but serious are hemolytic anemia, hypoglycemia, diuresis, peripheral neuropathy, Stevens-Johnson syndrome, agranulocytosis, disseminated lupus erythematosus, anaphylaxis, hepatitis, and toxic nephrosis.
- Fungal superinfections may occur.
- Interstitial nephritis occurs rarely.

Special Considerations
- Prior to application, burn wounds should be cleansed and debrided (following control of shock and pain)
- Use sterile glove and tongue blade to apply medication; apply a thin layer (1.5 mm) to completely cover wound; dressing as required only
- Continue until no chance of infection

■ Patient/Family Education
- Continue treatment until satisfactory healing has occurred, or until the burn site is ready for grafting

■ Monitoring Parameters
- Serum sulfa concentrations
- Renal function
- Urine for sulfa crystals

■ Geriatric side effects at a glance:
❑ CNS   ❑ Bowel Dysfunction   ❑ Bladder Dysfunction   ❑ Falls

■ U.S. Regulatory Considerations
❑ FDA Black Box   ❑ OBRA regulated in U.S. Long Term Care

simethicone

(sye-meth'-i-kone)

OTC: Alka-Seltzer Gas Relief, Gas-X, Genasyme, Mylanta Gas, Phazyme

Combinations
OTC: with calcium carbonate (Titralac Plus); with aluminum hydroxide, magnesium hydroxide (Mylanta Gelisil, Maalox Extra Strength); with calcium carbonate, magnesium hydroxide (Tempo, Rolaids); with Magaldrate, (Riopan Plus); with charcoal (Charcoal Plus, Flatulex)
Chemical Class: Siloxane polymer

■ Clinical Pharmacology:
Mechanism of Action: An antiflatulent that changes surface tension of gas bubbles, allowing easier elimination of gas. **Therapeutic Effect:** Drug dispersal, prevents formation of gas pockets in the GI tract.
Pharmacokinetics: Does not appear to be absorbed from GI tract. Excreted unchanged in feces.

■ Available Forms:
- *Softgel*: 125 mg (Alka-Seltzer Gas Relief, Gas-X, Mylanta Gas), 180 mg (Phazyme).
- *Tablets (Chewable)*: 80 mg (Gas-X, Genasyme, Mylanta Gas), 125 mg (Gas-X, Mylanta Gas).

■ Indications and Dosages:
Antiflatulent: PO 40–360 mg after meals and at bedtime. Maximum: 500 mg/day.

■ Unlabeled Uses: Adjunct to bowel radiography and gastroscopy

■ Contraindications: None known.

■ Side Effects
None known.

■ Serious Reactions
- None known.

Special Considerations
- Commonly prescribed, little evidence for any beneficial effect

■ Patient/Family Education
- Avoid carbonated beverages during simethicone therapy
- Chew tablets thoroughly before swallowing

■ Monitoring Parameters
- Therapeutic response (relief of abdominal bloating and flatulence)

■ Geriatric side effects at a glance:
❑ CNS ❑ Bowel Dysfunction ❑ Bladder Dysfunction ❑ Falls

- **U.S. Regulatory Considerations**
  ❑ FDA Black Box ❑ OBRA regulated in U.S. Long Term Care

simvastatin

(sim'-va-sta-tin)

- **Brand Name(s):** Zocor

  Combinations
  Rx: with ezetimibe (Vytorin)
  Chemical Class: Substituted hexahydronaphthalene

- **Clinical Pharmacology:**
  Mechanism of Action: A HMG-CoA reductase inhibitor that interferes with cholesterol biosynthesis by inhibiting the conversion of the enzyme HMG-CoA to mevalonate. **Therapeutic Effect:** Decreases serum LDL, cholesterol, VLDL, and plasma triglyceride levels; slightly increases serum HDL concentration.
  Pharmacokinetics:

Route	Onset	Peak	Duration
PO to reduce cholesterol	3 days	14 days	N/A

  Well absorbed from the GI tract. Protein binding: 95%. Undergoes extensive first-pass metabolism. Hydrolyzed to active metabolite. Primarily eliminated in feces. Unknown if removed by hemodialysis.

- **Available Forms:**
  - *Tablets:* 5 mg, 10 mg, 20 mg, 40 mg, 80 mg.

- **Indications and Dosages:**
  Prevention of cardiovascular events, hyperlipidemias: PO 20-40 mg once daily. Range: 5-80 mg/day.
  Homozygous familial hypercholesterol: PO 40 mg once daily in evening or 80 mg/day in divided doses.

- **Contraindications:** Active hepatic disease or unexplained, persistent elevations of liver function test results

- **Side Effects**
  Simvastatin is generally well tolerated. Side effects are usually mild and transient.
  Occasional (3%–2%)
  Headache, abdominal pain or cramps, constipation, upper respiratory tract infection
  Rare (less than 2%)
  Diarrhea, flatulence, asthenia (loss of strength and energy), nausea or vomiting

- **Serious Reactions**
  - Lens opacities may occur.
  - Hypersensitivity reaction and hepatitis occur rarely.

- Myopathy manifested as muscle pain, tenderness or weakness with elevated CK, sometimes taking the form of rhabdomyolysis fatalities, have occurred.

Special Considerations
- Superior to fibrates, cholestyramine, and probucol in lowering total and LDL cholesterol levels
- Statin selection based on lipid-lowering potency, cost, and availability

■ **Patient/Family Education**
- Report symptoms of myalgia, muscle tenderness, or weakness
- Take daily doses in the evening for increased effect
- Periodic laboratory tests are an essential part of therapy

■ **Monitoring Parameters**
- Cholesterol (maximum therapeutic response, 4-6 wk)
- LFTs (AST, ALT) at baseline and at 12 wk of therapy; if no change, no further monitoring necessary (discontinue if elevations persist at >3 × upper limit of normal)
- CPK at baseline and in patients complaining of diffuse myalgia, muscle tenderness, or weakness
- Pattern of daily bowel activity

■ **Geriatric side effects at a glance:**
  ☐ CNS ☐ Bowel Dysfunction ☐ Bladder Dysfunction ☐ Falls

■ **U.S. Regulatory Considerations**
  ☐ FDA Black Box ☐ OBRA regulated in U.S. Long Term Care

sirolimus

(sir-oh'-li-mus)

■ **Brand Name(s):** Rapamune
  Chemical Class: Macrolide derivative

■ **Clinical Pharmacology:**
  Mechanism of Action: An immunologic agent that inhibits T-lymphocyte proliferation induced by stimulation of cell surface receptors, mitogens, alloantigens, and lymphokines. Prevents activation of the enzyme target of rapamycin, a key regulatory kinase in cell cycle progression. **Therapeutic Effect:** Inhibits proliferation of T and B cells, essential components of the immune response; prevents organ transplant rejection.
  Pharmacokinetics: Rapidly absorbed from the GI tract. Protein binding: 92%. Extensively metabolized in liver. Primarily eliminated in feces; minimal excretion in urine.
  Half-life: 57-63 hr.

■ **Available Forms:**
  - *Oral Solution:* 1 mg/ml.
  - *Tablets:* 1 mg, 2 mg, 5 mg.

■ **Indications and Dosages:**
Prevention of organ transplant rejection: PO Loading dose: 6 mg. Maintenance: 2 mg/day.

■ **Unlabeled Uses:** Immunosuppression of other organ transplants

■ **Contraindications:** Malignancy

■ **Side Effects**
Occasional
Hypercholesterolemia, hyperlipidemia, hypertension, rash; with high doses (5 mg/day): anemia, arthralgia, diarrhea, hypokalemia, and thrombocytopenia
Rare
Peripheral edema, hypertension

■ **Serious Reactions**
• Pancytopenia and hepatotoxicity occur rarely.

Special Considerations
• Tablets and solution are not bioequivalent (tab has 27% > bioavailability); however, 2-mg tabs clinically equivalent to 2 mg oral sol; not known if higher doses of oral sol are clinically equivalent to higher doses of tabs
• Allows cyclosporine dose reduction
• Experience limited with use as rescue therapy
• Black patients had higher rejection rates (56% vs 13%) than non-blacks given same regimen; no significant differences in trough sirolimus concentrations at equal doses between blacks and non-blacks
• IV formulation is under development

■ **Patient/Family Education**
• Take medication the same each day with regard to timing of meals and other medications
• Limit UV/sunlight exposure, wear protective clothing, and use sunsreen due to increased risk of skin cancer
• Avoid grapefruit or grapefruit juice during therapy
• Avoid contact with people with colds or other infections

■ **Monitoring Parameters**
• Whole-blood sirolimus levels (drawn 1 hr prior to next dose), 5-7 days after initiation or dose change. Maintain levels at 10-15 ng/ml for first month, then consider increasing to 15-20 ng/ml, especially in patients receiving little cyclosporine
• CBC, platelets, lipids
• Liver function tests periodically

■ **Geriatric side effects at a glance:**
❑ CNS ❑ Bowel Dysfunction ❑ Bladder Dysfunction ❑ Falls

■ **U.S. Regulatory Considerations**
☑ FDA Black Box
• Should be administered by experienced personnel
• Increased susceptibility to infection and second malignancies
❑ OBRA regulated in U.S. Long Term Care

sodium bicarbonate

(soe'-dee-um bye-car'-bon-ate)

■ **Brand Name(s):** Neut

Combinations
OTC: with alginic acid (AlOH, Mg Trisilicate Gastrocote); with sodium citrate (Citro-carbonate)
Chemical Class: Monosodium salt of carbonic acid

■ **Clinical Pharmacology:**
Mechanism of Action: An alkalinizing agent that dissociates to provide bicarbonate ion. **Therapeutic Effect:** Neutralizes hydrogen ion concentration, raises blood and urinary pH.
Pharmacokinetics:

Route	Onset	Peak	Duration
PO	15 min	N/A	1–3 hr
IV	Immediate	N/A	8–10 min

After administration, sodium bicarbonate dissociates to sodium and bicarbonate ions. With increased hydrogen ion concentrations bicarbonate ions combine with hydrogen ions to form carbonic acid, which then dissociates to CO_2, which is excreted by the lungs.

■ **Available Forms:**
- *Tablets*: 325 mg, 650 mg.
- *Injection*: 0.5 mEq/ml (4%), 0.6 mEq/ml (5%), 0.9 mEq/ml (7.5%), 1 mEq/ml (8.4%).

■ **Indications and Dosages:**
Cardiac arrest: IV Initially, 1 mEq/kg (as 7.5%–8.4% solution). May repeat with 0.5 mEq/kg q10min during continued cardiopulmonary arrest. Use in the postresuscitation phase is based on arterial blood pH, partial pressure of carbon dioxide in arterial blood ($PaCO_2$) and base deficit calculation.
Metabolic acidosis (not severe): IV 2–5 mEq/kg over 4–8 hr. May repeat based on laboratory values.
Metabolic acidosis (associated with chronic renal failure): PO Initially, 20–36 mEq/day in divided doses.
Renal tubular acidosis (distal): PO 0.5–2 mEq/kg/day in 4–6 divided doses.
Renal tubular acidosis (proximal): PO 5–10 mEq/kg/day in divided doses.
Urine alkalinization: PO Initially, 4 g, then 1–2g q4h. Maximum: 16 g/day.
Antacid: PO 300 mg–2g 1–4 times a day.
Hyperkalemia: IV 1 mEq/kg over 5 minutes.

■ **Contraindications:** Excessive chloride loss due to diarrhea, diuretics, GI suctioning, or vomiting; hypocalcemia; metabolic or respiratory alkalosis, HTN, CHF

■ **Side Effects**
Frequent
Abdominal distention, flatulence, belching

- ■ **Serious Reactions**
  - Excessive or chronic use may produce metabolic alkalosis (characterized by irritability, twitching, paresthesias, cyanosis, slow or shallow respirations, headache, thirst, and nausea).
  - Fluid overload results in headache, weakness, blurred vision, behavioral changes, incoordination, muscle twitching, elevated BP, bradycardia, tachypnea, wheezing, coughing, and distended neck veins.
  - Extravasation may occur at the IV site, resulting in tissue necrosis and ulceration.

- ■ **Patient/Family Education**
  - Milk-alkali syndrome (may result from excessive antacid use): confusion, headache, nausea, vomiting, anorexia, urinary stones, hypercalcemia
  - To avoid drug interactions due to reduced absorption, separate intake by 2 hours
  - Check with the physician before taking OTC drugs because they may contain sodium
  - Patients with CHF or HTN should avoid taking antacids with sodium bicarbonate

- ■ **Monitoring Parameters**
  - Electrolytes, blood pH, PO_2, HCO_3, during treatment
  - ABGs frequently during emergencies
  - Serum calcium, phosphate, and uric acid levels
  - Signs and symptoms of fluid overload and metabolic alkalosis
  - Pattern of daily bowel activity and stool consistency
  - Relief of gastric distress
  - Clinical improvement of metabolic acidosis, including relief from disorientation, hyperventilation, and weakness

- ■ **Geriatric side effects at a glance:**
  - ❑ CNS ❑ Bowel Dysfunction ❑ Bladder Dysfunction ❑ Falls

- ■ **U.S. Regulatory Considerations**
  - ❑ FDA Black Box ❑ OBRA regulated in U.S. Long Term Care

sodium chloride

(soe'-dee-um klor'-ide)

OTC: Muro 128, Nasal Mist, Nasal Moist, Ocean, SalineX, SeaMist, Slo-Salt
Chemical Class: Monovalent cation

- ■ **Clinical Pharmacology:**
  Mechanism of Action: Sodium is a major cation of extracellular fluid that controls water distribution, fluid and electrolyte balance, and osmotic pressure of body fluids; it also maintains acid-base balance.
  Pharmacokinetics: Well absorbed from the GI tract. Widely distributed. Primarily excreted in urine.

■ **Available Forms:**
- *Tablets*: 1g
- *Injection (Concentrate)*: 23.4% (4 mEq/ml).
- *Injection*: 0.45%, 0.9%, 3%.
- *Irrigation*: 0.45%, 0.9%.
- *Nasal Gel (Nasal Moist)*: 0.65%.
- *Nasal Solution (OTC)*: 0.4% (SalineX), 0.65% (Nasal Moist, SeaMist).
- *Ophthalmic Solution (OTC [Muro 128])*: 5%.
- *Ophthalmic Ointment (OTC [Muro 128])*: 5%.

■ **Indications and Dosages:**
> *Prevention and treatment of sodium and chloride deficiencies; source of hydration:* IV 1–2 L/day 0.9% or 0.45% or 100 ml 3% or 5% over 1 hr; assess serum electrolyte levels before giving additional fluid.
> *Prevention of heat prostration and muscle cramps from excessive perspiration:* PO 1–2g 3 times a day.
> *Relief of dry and inflamed nasal membranes:* Intranasal Use as needed.
> *Diagnostic aid in ophthalmoscopic exam, treatment of corneal edema:* Ophthalmic solution Apply 1–2 drops q3–4h. Ophthalmic ointment Apply once a day or as directed.

■ **Contraindications:** Fluid retention, hypernatremia

■ **Side Effects**
Frequent
Facial flushing
Occasional
Fever; irritation, phlebitis, or extravasation at injection site
Ophthalmic: Temporary burning or irritation

■ **Serious Reactions**
- Too-rapid administration may produce peripheral edema, CHF, and pulmonary edema.
- Excessive dosage may cause hypokalemia, hypervolemia, and hypernatremia.

Special Considerations
- One g of sodium chloride provides 17.1 mEq sodium and 17.1 mEq chloride

■ **Patient/Family Education**
- Temporary burning or irritation after instillation of the ophthalmic drug may occur
- Discontinue the ophthalmic medication and notify the physician if acute redness of eyes, floating spots, severe eye pain or pain on exposure to light, a rapid change in vision (side and straight ahead), or headache occurs

■ **Monitoring Parameters**
- IV site for extravasation
- Fluid balance, acid-base balance, blood pressure, electrolytes
- Signs and symptoms of hypernatremia (edema, hypertension, and weight gain) and hyponatremia (dry mucous membranes, muscle cramps, nausea, and vomiting)

■ **Geriatric side effects at a glance:**
❑ CNS ❑ Bowel Dysfunction ❑ Bladder Dysfunction ❑ Falls

sodium oxybate

(soe'-dee-um ok'-si-bate)

■ **Brand Name(s):** Xyrem
  Chemical Class: Hydroxybutyrate

  DEA Class: Controlled Substance Schedule II

■ **Clinical Pharmacology:**
  Mechanism of Action: A naturally occurring inhibitory neurotransmitter that binds to gamma-aminobutyric acid (GABA)-B receptors and sodium oxybate specific receptors with its highest concentrations in the basal ganglia, which mediates sleep cycles, temperature regulation, cerebral glucose metabolism and blood flow, memory, and emotion control. **Therapeutic Effect:** Reduces the number of sleep episodes.
  Pharmacokinetics: Rapidly and incompletely absorbed. Absorption is delayed and decreased by a high fat meal. Protein binding: less than 1%. Widely distributed, including cerebrospinal fluid (CSF). Metabolized in liver. Excretion is less than 5% in the urine and negligible in feces. Unknown if removed by hemodialysis. **Half-life:** 20-53 min.

■ **Available Forms:**
  • *Oral Solution*: 500 mg/ml (Xyrem).

■ **Indications and Dosages:**
  Cataplexy of narcolepsy: PO 4.5 g/day in 2 equal doses of 2.25 g, the first taken at bedtime while in bed and the second 2.5-4 hr later. Maximum: 9 g/day in 2 weekly increments of 1.5 g/day.

■ **Unlabeled Uses:** Alcohol withdrawal

■ **Contraindications:** Metabolic/respiratory alkalosis, current treatment with sedative-hypnotics, succinic semialdehyde dehydrogenase deficiency, hypersensitivity to sodium oxybate or any component of the formulation

■ **Side Effects**
  Frequent
  Mild bradycardia
  Occasional
  Headache, vertigo, dizziness, restless legs, abdominal pain, muscle weakness
  Rare
  Dreamlike state of confusion

■ **Serious Reactions**
  • Agitation, excitation, increased blood pressure (BP), and insomnia may occur upon abrupt discontinuation of sodium oxybate.

- Sodium oxybate is effective and indicated for the treatment of cataplexy in patients with narcolepsy; it could also be effective for general anesthesia, narcolepsy, fibromyalgia syndrome, insomnia, alcoholism and opiate withdrawal, but its potential for abuse is unacceptable

■ **Patient/Family Education**
- Prepare both doses prior to bedtime; each dose must be diluted with 2 oz (60 ml) of water in the child-resistant dosing cups before ingestion
- The first dose is to be taken at bedtime while in bed and the second taken 2.5-4 hr later while sitting in bed; patients will probably need to set an alarm to awaken for the second dose
- The second dose must be prepared before ingesting the first dose, and should be placed in close proximity to the patient's bed
- After ingesting each dose the patient should then lie down and remain in bed
- Avoid tasks that require mental alertness or motor skills until response to the drug is established
- Avoid alcohol
- Avoid high-fat meals because it may delay the absorption of the drug

■ **Monitoring Parameters**
- History/physical exam: Review signs and symptoms for efficacy, toxicity and abuse, including tremor and coma
- Laboratory: Sodium and potassium plasma levels, hepatic functions, blood gas analysis

■ **Geriatric side effects at a glance:**
  ❏ CNS   ❏ Bowel Dysfunction   ❏ Bladder Dysfunction   ❏ Falls

■ **U.S. Regulatory Considerations**
  ☑ FDA Black Box   ❏ OBRA regulated in U.S. Long Term Care
- Abuse potential
- CNS side effects (seizures, respiratory depression, decreased level of consciousness, coma, death)

sodium polystyrene sulfonate

(soe'-dee-um po-lee-stye'-reen sul'-foe-nate)

■ **Brand Name(s):** Kayexalate, Kionex, SPS
  Chemical Class: Cation exchange resin

■ **Clinical Pharmacology:**
  Mechanism of Action: An ion exchange resin that releases sodium ions in exchange primarily for potassium ions. **Therapeutic Effect:** Moves potassium from the blood into the intestine so it can be expelled from the body.
  Pharmacokinetics: Not absorbed from GI tract. Not metabolized. Completely excreted in feces.

■ **Available Forms:**
- *Suspension* (SPS): 15 g/60 ml.
- *Powder for Suspension* (*Kayexalate*, *Kionex*): 454 g.
- *Rectal Enema*: 15 g/60 ml.

■ **Indications and Dosages:**
Hyperkalemia: PO 60 ml (15 g) 1–4 times a day. Rectal 30–50g as needed q6h.

■ **Contraindications:** Hypokalemia, hypernatremia, intestinal obstruction or perforation

■ **Side Effects**
Frequent
High dosage: Anorexia, nausea, vomiting, constipation
High dosage in elderly: Fecal impaction characterized by severe stomach pain with nausea or vomiting
Occasional
Diarrhea, sodium retention marked by decreased urination, peripheral edema, and increased weight

■ **Serious Reactions**
- Potassium deficiency may occur. Early signs of hypokalemia include confusion, delayed thought processes, extreme weakness, irritability, and ECG changes (including prolonged QT interval; widening, flattening, or inversion of T wave; and prominent U waves).
- Hypocalcemia, manifested by abdominal or muscle cramps, occurs occasionally.
- Arrhythmias and severe muscle weakness may be noted.

Special Considerations
- Exchange efficacy of resin is approximately 33%; 1g of resin (4.1 mEq of sodium) exchanges approximately 1 mEq of potassium
- Rectal route is less effective than oral administration
- Powder formulations very hydrophobic, difficult to mix. Pre-prepared suspensions in sorbitol preferable

■ **Patient/Family Education**
- Do not mix with orange juice
- Drink the entire amount of resin for best results
- When used rectally, try to retain the solution for several hours, if possible

■ **Monitoring Parameters**
- Serum K, Ca, Mg, Na, acid-base balance, bowel function, possibly ECG

■ **Geriatric side effects at a glance:**
❏ CNS ☑ Bowel Dysfunction ❏ Bladder Dysfunction ❏ Falls

■ **U.S. Regulatory Considerations**
❏ FDA Black Box ❏ OBRA regulated in U.S. Long Term Care

solifenacin succinate

(sol-i-fen'-a-cin suk'-si-nate)

- **Brand Name(s):** VESIcare
  Chemical Class: Antimuscarinic substituted amine

- **Clinical Pharmacology:**
  Mechanism of Action: A urinary antispasmodic that acts as a direct antagonist at muscarinic acetylcholine receptors in cholinergically innervated organs. Reduces tonus (elastic tension) of smooth muscle in the bladder and slows parasympathetic contractions. **Therapeutic Effect:** Decreases urinary bladder contractions, increases residual urine volume, and decreases detrusor muscle pressure.
  Pharmacokinetics: Well absorbed following PO administration. Protein binding: 98%. Metabolized by liver. Excreted in feces and urine. **Half-life:** 40-68 hr.

- **Available Forms:**
  - *Tablets*: 5 mg, 10 mg.

- **Indications and Dosages:**
  Overactive bladder: PO 5 mg/day; if tolerated, may increase to 10 mg/day.
  Dosage in renal or hepatic impairment: For patients with severe renal impairment or moderate hepatic impairment, maximum dosage is 5 mg/day.

- **Contraindications:** GI obstruction, uncontrolled angle-closure glaucoma, urine retention

- **Side Effects**
  Frequent (11%-5%)
  Dry mouth, constipation, blurred vision
  Occasional (5%-3%)
  UTI, dyspepsia, nausea
  Rare (2%-1%)
  Dizziness, dry eyes, fatigue, depression, edema, hypertension, upper abdominal pain, vomiting, urine retention, delirium

- **Serious Reactions**
  - Angioneurotic edema and GI obstruction occur rarely.
  - Overdose can result in severe central anticholinergic effects.

- **Geriatric side effects at a glance:**
  ☑ CNS   ☑ Bowel Dysfunction   ☑ Bladder Dysfunction   ☑ Falls
  Other: Dry mouth, blurred vision, dizziness, somnolence

- **Use with caution in older patients with:** Tachyarrythmias, overflow incontinence.

- **U.S. Regulatory Considerations**
  ❑ FDA Black Box   ❑ OBRA regulated in U.S. Long Term Care

- **Other Uses in Geriatric Patient:** None

Side Effects:

Of particular importance in the geriatric patient: Delirium, possible antagonism of cholinergic drug therapy in the treatment of Alzheimer's disease.

■ **Geriatric Considerations - Summary:** Solifenacin and other newer anticholinergic drugs are moderately effective in the treatment of urge urinary incontinence and offer the potential benefit of selective antagonism of muscarinic receptors with less potential for CNS adverse effects. The relative safety and efficacy of these agents, which are significantly more expensive, has not been well studied to determine if they are superior to longer-acting anticholinergic formulations. These newer drugs can produce anticholinergic adverse effects including cognitive impairment, dry mouth, blurred vision, and increased risk of falls.

■ **References:**

1. Hay-Smith J, Herbison P, Ellis G, Moore K. Anticholinergic drugs versus placebo for overactive bladder syndrome in adults. Cochrane Database System Rev 2003;3.
2. Cardozo L. Randomized, double-blind placebo controlled trial of once daily antimuscarinic agent solifenacin succinate in patients with overactive bladder. J Urol 2004;172:1919.
3. Tune LE. Anticholinergic effects of medication in elderly patients. J Clin Psychiatry 2001;62(suppl 21):11-14.
4. Ouslander JG. Management of overactive bladder. N Engl J Med 2004;350:786-799.

somatrem/somatropin

(soe'-ma-trem/soe-mah-troe'-pin)

■ **Brand Name(s):** (somatrem) Protopin

■ **Brand Name(s):** (somatropin) Genotropin, Genotropin Miniquick, Humatrope, Norditropin, Norditropin Cartridge, Nutropin, Nutropin AQ, Nutropin Depot, Saizen, Serostim, Zorbitive
Chemical Class: ENDO-growth hormone; recombinant human peptide

■ **Clinical Pharmacology:**
Mechanism of Action: A polypeptide hormone that stimulates cartilaginous growth areas of long bones, increases the number and size of skeletal muscle cells, influences the size of organs, and increases RBC mass by stimulating erythropoietin. Influences the metabolism of carbohydrates (decreases insulin sensitivity), fats (mobilizes fatty acids), minerals (retains phosphorus, sodium, potassium by promotion of cell growth), and proteins (increases protein synthesis). **Therapeutic Effect:** Stimulates growth.
Pharmacokinetics: Well absorbed after subcutaneous or IM administration. Localized primarily in the kidneys and liver. **Half-life:** IV, 20-30 min; subcutaneous, IM, 3-5 hr.

■ **Available Forms:**
- *Injection Powder for Reconstitution (somatrem [Protopin]):* 5 mg.
- *Injection Powder for Reconstitution (somatropin):* 0.4 mg (Genotropin Miniquick), 0.6 mg (Genotropin Miniquick), 0.8 mg (Genotropin Miniquick), 1 mg (Genotropin Miniquick), 1.2 mg (Genotropin Miniquick), 1.4 mg (Genotropin Miniquick), 1.5 mg

(Genotropin, Genotropin Miniquick), 1.6 mg (Genotropin Miniquick), 1.8 mg (Genotropin Miniquick), 2 mg (Genotropin Miniquick), 4 mg (Norditropin, Serostim, Zorbitive), 5 mg (Humatrope, Nutropin, Saizen, Serostim, Zorbitive), 5.8 mg (Genotropin), 6 mg (Humatrope, Serostim, Zorbitive), 8 mg (Norditropin), 8.8 mg (Saizen, Zorbitive), 10 mg (Nutropin), 12 mg (Humatrope), 13.5 mg (Nutropin Depot), 18 mg (Nutropin Depot), 22.5 mg (Nutropin Depot), 24 mg (Humatrope).
- *Solution for Injection (somatropin [Norditropin Cartridge])*: 15 mg/1.5 ml.
- *Injection Solution (somatropin [Nutropin AQ])*: 5 mg/ml.

■ **Indications and Dosages:**
   Growth hormone deficiency: Subcutaneous (Humatrope) 0.006 mg/kg once daily. Subcutaneous (Nutropin) 0.006 mg/kg once daily. Subcutaneous (Nutropin AQ) 0.006 mg/kg once daily. Subcutaneous (Genotropin) 0.04-0.08 mg/kg weekly divided into 6-7 equal doses/wk.
   AIDS-related wasting: Subcutaneous Weight > 55 *kg*. 6 mg once a day at bedtime. Weight 45-55 *kg*. 5mg once a day at bedtime. Weight 35-44*kg*. 4 mg once a day at bedtime. Weight < 35 *kg*. 0.1 mg/kg once a day at bedtime.
   Short bowel syndrome: Subcutaneous (Zorbitive) 0.1 mg/kg/day. Maximum: 8 mg/day.

■ **Contraindications:** Active neoplasia (either newly diagnosed or recurrent), critical illness, hypersensitivity to growth hormone

■ **Side Effects**
   Frequent
   Otitis media, other ear disorders (with Turner's syndrome)
   Occasional
   Carpal tunnel syndrome; gynecomastia; myalgia; swelling of hands, feet, or legs; fatigue; asthenia
   Rare
   Rash, pruritus, altered vision, headache, nausea, vomiting, injection site pain and swelling, abdominal pain, hip or knee pain

■ **Serious Reactions**
   - Glucose intolerance can occur with overdosage. Long-term overdosage with growth hormone could result in signs and symptoms of acromegaly.

■ **Monitoring Parameters**
   - Individualize doses for growth hormone inadequacy
   - Check for hypothyroidism, malnutrition, antibodies or opportunistic infections (AIDS patients) if no response to initial dose
   - TSH
   - Follow with funduscopy (papilledema)
   - Bone density, blood glucose level, serum calcium and phosphorus levels

■ **Geriatric side effects at a glance:**
   ❏ CNS ❏ Bowel Dysfunction ❏ Bladder Dysfunction ❏ Falls

■ **U.S. Regulatory Considerations**
   ❏ FDA Black Box ❏ OBRA regulated in U.S. Long Term Care

sorbitol

(sor'-bi-tole)

■ **Brand Name(s):** Sorbitol
  Chemical Class: Polyalcoholic sugar

■ **Clinical Pharmacology:**
  Mechanism of Action: A polyalcoholic sugar with osmotic cathartic actions. Specific mechanism unknown. **Therapeutic Effect:** Catharsis, urinary irrigation.
  Pharmacokinetics: Onset of action within 15-60 minutes. Poorly absorbed by both oral and rectal route. Metabolized in liver to primary metabolite, fructose.

■ **Available Forms:**
  • *Solution*: 3%

■ **Indications and Dosages:**
  Hyperosmotic laxative: PO 30-150 ml as a 70% solution Rectal 120 ml as a 25%-30% solution
  Transurethral surgical procedure: Topical 3%-3.3% as transurethral surgical procedure irrigation

■ **Contraindications:** Anuria

■ **Side Effects**
  Acidosis, electrolyte loss, marked diuresis, urinary retention, edema, dryness of mouth and thirst, dehydration, pulmonary congestion, hypotension, tachycardia, angina-like pains, blurred vision, convulsions, nausea, vomiting, diarrhea, rhinitis, chills, vertigo, backache, urticaria.

■ **Serious Reactions**
  • Life-threatening adverse reactions with IV sorbitol infusions have been reported in patients with fructose intolerance.

Special Considerations
  • Just as effective as lactulose as a laxative at reduced expense

■ **Patient/Family Education**
  • Notify the physician if dry mouth, nausea, vomiting, diarrhea, chills, dizziness, or backache occurs

■ **Monitoring Parameters**
  • Fluid and electrolytes
  • Blood glucose

■ **Geriatric side effects at a glance:**
  ❑ CNS ☑ Bowel Dysfunction ❑ Bladder Dysfunction ❑ Falls

sotalol hydrochloride

(soe'-ta-lole hye-droe-klor'-ide)

■ **Brand Name(s):** Betapace, Betapace AF, Sorine
  Chemical Class: β-Adrenergic blocker, nonselective

■ **Clinical Pharmacology:**
  Mechanism of Action: A beta-adrenergic blocking agent that prolongs action potential, effective refractory period, and QT interval. Decreases heart rate and AV node conduction; increases AV node refractoriness. **Therapeutic Effect:** Produces antiarrhythmic activity.
  Pharmacokinetics: Well absorbed from the GI tract. Protein binding: None. Widely distributed. Primarily excreted unchanged in urine. Removed by hemodialysis. **Half-life:** 12 hr (increased in the elderly and patients with impaired renal function).

■ **Available Forms:**
  • *Tablets*: 80 mg (Betapace, Betapace AF, Sorine), 120 mg (Betapace, Betapace AF, Sorine), 160 mg (Betapace, Betapace AF, Sorine), 240 mg (Betapace, Sorine).

■ **Indications and Dosages:**
  Documented, life-threatening arrhythmias: PO (Betapace, Sorine) Initially, 80 mg twice a day. May increase gradually at 2- to 3-day intervals. Range: 240–320 mg/day.
  Atrial fibrillation, atrial flutter: PO (Betapace AF) 80 mg twice a day.
  Dosage in renal impairment: Betapace, Sorine Dosage interval is modified based on creatinine clearance.
  Sorine

Creatinine Clearance	Dosage Interval
31-60 ml/min	24 hr
10-30 ml/min	36-48 hr
less than 10 ml/min	Individualized

  Betapace AF

Creatinine Clearance	Dosage Interval
greater than 60 ml/min	12 hr
40-60 ml/min	24 hr
less than 40 ml/min	Contraindicated

■ **Unlabeled Uses:** Maintenance of normal heart rhythm in chronic or recurring atrial fibrillation or flutter; treatment of anxiety, chronic angina pectoris, hypertension, hypertrophic cardiomyopathy, MI, mitral valve prolapse syndrome, pheochromocytoma, thyrotoxicosis, tremors

■ **Contraindications:** Bronchial asthma, cardiogenic shock, prolonged QT syndrome (unless functioning pacemaker is present), second- and third-degree heart block, sinus bradycardia, uncontrolled cardiac failure

■ Side Effects
Frequent
Diminished sexual function, drowsiness, insomnia, unusual fatigue or weakness
Occasional
Depression, cold hands or feet, diarrhea, constipation, anxiety, nasal congestion, nausea, vomiting
Rare
Altered taste, dry eyes, itching, numbness of fingers, toes, or scalp

■ Serious Reactions
- Bradycardia, CHF, hypotension, bronchospasm, hypoglycemia, prolonged QT interval, torsades de pointes, ventricular tachycardia, and premature ventricular complexes may occur.

■ Patient/Family Education
- Do not discontinue abruptly; may require taper; rapid withdrawal may produce rebound hypertension or angina
- Avoid tasks that require mental alertness or motor skills until response to the drug has been established
- Periodic laboratory tests and ECGs are a necessary part of therapy

■ Monitoring Parameters
- *Angina*: Reduction in nitroglycerin usage; frequency, severity, onset, and duration of angina pain; heart rate
- *Arrhythmias*: Heart rate and rhythm; monitor QT intervals (discontinue or reduce dose if QT >520 msec)
- *Congestive heart failure*: Functional status, cough, dyspnea on exertion, paroxysmal nocturnal dyspnea, exercise tolerance, and ventricular function
- *Hypertension*: Blood pressure
- *Toxicity*: Blood glucose, bronchospasm, hypotension, bradycardia, depression, confusion, hallucination, sexual dysfunction
- Because of prodysrhythmic risk, begin and increase drug in setting with cardiac rhythm monitoring

■ Geriatric side effects at a glance:
❑ CNS   ❑ Bowel Dysfunction   ❑ Bladder Dysfunction   ❑ Falls

■ U.S. Regulatory Considerations
☑ FDA Black Box
- To minimize the risk of induced arrhythmia, initiate or re-initiate therapy for > 3 days in a facility that can provide cardiac resuscitation and ECG monitoring.
- Dosage adjustment in renal impairment: Betapace is not approved for atrial fibrillation or flutter indication.
- Do not substitute Betapace for Betapace AF. Betapace does not have an atrial fibrillation indication or package insert information for patient.
- In patients using orally administered beta-blockers, abrupt withdrawal may precipitate angina or lead to myocardial infarction or ventricular arrhythmias.
❑ OBRA regulated in U.S. Long Term Care

spectinomycin hydrochloride

(spek-ti-noe-mye'-sin hye-droe-klor'-ide)

- **Brand Name(s):** Trobicin
  Chemical Class: Aminoglycoside derivative

- **Clinical Pharmacology:**
  Mechanism of Action: An anti-infective that inhibits protein synthesis of bacterial cells. **Therapeutic Effect:** Produces bacterial cell death.
  Pharmacokinetics: Rapid, complete absorption after intramuscular (IM) administration. Protein binding: Unknown. Widely distributed. Excreted unchanged in urine. Partially removed by hemodialysis. **Half-life:** 1.7 hr.

- **Available Forms:**
  - *Powder for Reconstitution*: 2g (Trobicin).

- **Indications and Dosages:**
  Treatment of acute gonococcal urethritis, proctitis in males, acute gonococcal cervicitis and proctitis in females: IM 2g once. In areas where ID-antibacterial resistance is known to be prevalent, 4g (10 ml) divided between 2 injection sites is preferred.

- **Unlabeled Uses:** Treatment of disseminated gonorrhea

- **Contraindications:** Hypersensitivity to spectinomycin or any component of the formulation

- **Side Effects**
  Frequent
  Pain at IM injection site
  Occasional
  Dizziness, insomnia
  Rare
  Decreased urine output

- **Serious Reactions**
  - Hypersensitivity reaction characterized as chills, fever, nausea, vomiting, urticaria, and anaphylaxis.

Special Considerations
  - Follow with doxycycline 100 mg bid for 7 days (erythromycin if pregnant or allergic)
  - Ineffective against syphilis and may mask symptoms
  - Give in gluteal muscle; dose >2g must be divided in 2 gluteal injections

- **Patient/Family Education**
  - IM injection may cause discomfort

- **Monitoring Parameters**
  - Observe patient 1 hour after injection due to potential for anaphylaxis

1146

- **Geriatric side effects at a glance:**
  - ☐ CNS ☐ Bowel Dysfunction ☐ Bladder Dysfunction ☐ Falls

- **U.S. Regulatory Considerations**
  - ☐ FDA Black Box ☐ OBRA regulated in U.S. Long Term Care

spironolactone

(speer-on-oh-lak'-tone)

- **Brand Name(s):** Aldactone

  Combinations
  Rx: with hydrochlorothiazide (Aldactazide)
  Chemical Class: Aldosterone antagonist

- **Clinical Pharmacology:**
  Mechanism of Action: A potassium-sparing diuretic that interferes with sodium reabsorption by competitively inhibiting the action of aldosterone in the distal tubule, thus promoting sodium and water excretion and increasing potassium retention. **Therapeutic Effect:** Produces diuresis; lowers BP; diagnostic aid for primary aldosteronism.
  Pharmacokinetics:

Route	Onset	Peak	Duration
PO	24–48 hr	48–72 hr	48–72 hr

  Well absorbed from the GI tract (absorption increased with food). Protein binding: 91%–98%. Metabolized in the liver to active metabolite. Primarily excreted in urine. Unknown if removed by hemodialysis. **Half-life:** 0–24 hr (metabolite, 13–24 hr).

- **Available Forms:**
  - *Tablets:* 25 mg, 50 mg, 100 mg.

- **Indications and Dosages:**
  Edema: PO 25–200 mg/day as a single dose or in 2 divided doses.
  Hypertension: PO 25-50 mg/day in 1-2 doses/day.
  Hypokalemia: PO 25-200 mg/day as a single dose or in 2 divided doses.
  Male hirsutism: PO 50-200 mg/day as a single dose or in 2 divided doses.
  Primary aldosteronism: PO 100–400 mg/day as a single dose or in 2 divided doses.
  CHF: PO 25 mg/day adjusted based on patient response and evidence of hyperkalemia.
  Dosage in renal impairment: Dosage interval is modified based on creatinine clearance.

Creatinine Clearance	Interval
10–50 ml/min	Usual dose q12–24h
less than 10 ml/min	Avoid use

- **Unlabeled Uses:** Female acne, hirsutism, polycystic ovary disease

■ **Contraindications:** Acute renal insufficiency, anuria, BUN and serum creatinine levels more than twice normal values, hyperkalemia

■ **Side Effects**
Frequent
Hyperkalemia (in patients with renal insufficiency and those taking potassium supplements), dehydration, hyponatremia, lethargy
Occasional
Nausea, vomiting, anorexia, abdominal cramps, diarrhea, headache, ataxia, somnolence, confusion, fever
Male: Gynecomastia, impotence, decreased libido
Female: Breast tenderness
Rare
Rash, urticaria, hirsutism

■ **Serious Reactions**
- Severe hyperkalemia may produce arrhythmias, bradycardia, and ECG changes (tented T waves, widening QRS complex, and ST segment depression). These may proceed to cardiac standstill or ventricular fibrillation.
- Cirrhosis patients are at risk for hepatic decompensation if dehydration or hyponatremia occurs.
- Patients with primary aldosteronism may experience rapid weight loss and severe fatigue during high-dose therapy.

■ **Patient/Family Education**
- Expect an increase in the frequency and volume of urination
- The drug's therapeutic effect takes several days to begin and can last for several days once the drug is discontinued (unless he or she is taking a potassium-losing drug concomitantly)
- Avoid consuming potassium supplements and foods high in potassium, including apricots, bananas, raisins, orange juice, potatoes, legumes, meat, and whole grains (such as cereals)
- Notify the physician if irregular heartbeat, diarrhea, muscle twitching, cold and clammy skin, confusion, drowsiness, dry mouth, or excessive thirst occurs
- Avoid performing tasks that require mental alertness or motor skills until response to the drug has been established

■ **Monitoring Parameters**
- When used for diagnosis of primary hyperaldosteronism, positive results are: (long test) correction of hyperkalemia and hypertension; (short test) serum potassium increases during administration, but falls upon discontinuation
- Blood pressure, edema, urine output, ECG (if hyperkalemia exists), urine electrolytes, BUN, creatinine, gynecomastia, impotence

■ **Geriatric side effects at a glance:**
❑ CNS ❑ Bowel Dysfunction ❑ Bladder Dysfunction ❑ Falls

■ **U.S. Regulatory Considerations**
☑ FDA Black Box
Spironolactone has been shown to be a tumorigen in chronic toxicity studies in rats.
❑ OBRA regulated in U.S. Long Term Care

stanozolol

(stan-oh'-zoe-lole)

- **Brand Name(s):** Winstrol
  Chemical Class: Anabolic steroid; testosterone derivative

  DEA Class: Schedule III

- **Clinical Pharmacology:**
  Mechanism of Action: A synthetic testosterone derivative that increases circulating levels of C1 INH and C4 through an increase in general protein anabolism, and more specifically, through an increase in the synthesis of messenger RNA. **Therapeutic Effect:** Decreases swelling of the face, extremities, genitalia, bowel wall, and upper respiratory tract
  Pharmacokinetics: Metabolized in liver. Primarily excreted in urine. Unknown if removed by hemodialysis.

- **Available Forms:**
  - *Tablets*: 2 mg.

- **Indications and Dosages:**
  Hereditary angioedema prophylaxis: PO Initially, 2 mg 2 times/day. Decrease at 1-3 month intervals. Maintenance: 2 mg/day.

- **Unlabeled Uses:** Antithrombin III deficiency, arterial occlusions, hemophilia A, lichen sclerosus et atrophicus, liposclerosis, necrobiosis lipoidica, osteoporosis, protein C deficiency, rheumatoid arthritis, thrombosis, urticaria

- **Contraindications:** Cardiac impairment, hypercalcemia, prostatic or breast cancer in males, severe liver or renal disease, hypersensitivity to stanozolol or its components

- **Side Effects**
  Frequent
  Gynecomastia, acne
  Females: Hirsutism deepening of voice, clitoral enlargement that may not be reversible when drug is discontinued
  Occasional
  Edema, nausea, insomnia, oligospermia, male pattern of baldness, bladder irritability, hypercalcemia in immobilized patients or those with breast cancer, hypercholesterolemia

- **Serious Reactions**
  - Peliosis hepatis (presence of blood-filled cysts in parenchyma of liver), hepatic neoplasms, and hepatocellular carcinoma have been associated with prolonged high dosage.

Special Considerations
- Anabolic steroids have potential for abuse

1149

Patient/Family Education
- Do not take more of the medicine than prescribed due to an increased risk of severe side effects
- Do not take any other medications, including OTC drugs, without first consulting the physician
- Notify the physician if acne, nausea, pedal edema, or vomiting occurs
- The female patient should promptly report deepening of voice, or hoarseness
- The male patient should report difficulty urinating, frequent erections, and gynecomastia

Monitoring Parameters
- LFTs, lipids
- Signs of virilization
- Blood Hgb and Hct periodically
- Electrolytes

Geriatric side effects at a glance:
❑ CNS ❑ Bowel Dysfunction ❑ Bladder Dysfunction ❑ Falls

U.S. Regulatory Considerations
❑ FDA Black Box ❑ OBRA regulated in U.S. Long Term Care

stavudine

(stav'-yoo-deen)

Brand Name(s): Zerit, Zerit XR
Chemical Class: Nucleoside analog

Clinical Pharmacology:
Mechanism of Action: Inhibits HIV reverse transcriptase by terminating the viral DNA chain. Also inhibits RNA- and DNA-dependent DNA polymerase, an enzyme necessary for HIV replication. **Therapeutic Effect:** Impedes HIV replication, slowing the progression of HIV infection.
Pharmacokinetics: Rapidly and completely absorbed after PO administration. Undergoes minimal metabolism. Excreted in urine. **Half-life:** 1.5 hr (increased in renal impairment).

Available Forms:
- *Capsules:* 15 mg, 20 mg, 30 mg, 40 mg.
- *Oral Solution:* 1 mg/ml.

Indications and Dosages:
HIV infection : PO *Weight 60 kg and more.* 40 mg q12h. *Weight < 60 kg.* 30 mg q12h.
Dosage in renal impairment: Dosage and frequency are modified based on creatinine clearance and patient weight.

Creatinine Clearance	Weight 60 kg or more	Weight less than 60 kg
greater than 50 ml/min	40 mg q12h	30 mg q12h
26–50 ml/min	20 mg q12h	15 mg q12h
10–25 ml/min	20 mg q24h	15 mg q24h

■ **Contraindications:** None known.

■ **Side Effects**
Frequent
Headache (55%), diarrhea (50%), chills and fever (38%), nausea and vomiting, myalgia (35%), rash (33%), asthenia (28%), insomnia, abdominal pain (26%), anxiety (22%), arthralgia (18%), back pain (20%), diaphoresis (19%), malaise (17%), depression (14%)
Occasional
Anorexia, weight loss, nervousness, dizziness, conjunctivitis, dyspepsia, dyspnea
Rare
Constipation, vasodilation, confusion, migraine, urticaria, abnormal vision

■ **Serious Reactions**
• Peripheral neuropathy (numbness, tingling, or pain in the hands and feet) occurs in 15% to 21% of patients.
• Ulcerative stomatitis (erythema or ulcers of oral mucosa, glossitis, gingivitis), pneumonia, and benign skin neoplasms occur occasionally.
• Pancreatitis, hepatomegaly, and lactic acidosis have been reported.

Special Considerations

• Always check updated treatment guidelines before initiating or changing antiretroviral therapy (http://AIDSinfo.nih.gov)

■ **Patient/Family Education**
• Report neuropathic symptoms (numbness, tingling, or pain in the feet or hands)
• Space doses evenly around the clock and continue taking the drug for the full course of treatment
• Do not take any other medications, OTC drugs, without first notifying the physician
• Stavudine is not a cure for HIV infection, nor does it reduce the risk of transmitting HIV to others

■ **Monitoring Parameters**
• CBC, SGOT, SGPT
• Weight
• Skin for rash
• Pattern of daily bowel activity and stool consistency
• Eyes for signs of conjunctivitis
• Monitor for signs and symptoms of peripheral neuropathy, such as numbness, pain, or tingling in the feet or hands. Be aware that these symptoms usually resolve promptly if stavudine therapy is discontinued, but they may worsen temporarily after the drug is withdrawn. If symptoms resolve completely, expect to resume drug therapy at a reduced dosage

■ **Geriatric side effects at a glance:**
☑ CNS ☐ Bowel Dysfunction ☐ Bladder Dysfunction ☐ Falls

■ **U.S. Regulatory Considerations**
☑ FDA Black Box
Pancreatitis and lactic acidosis.
❏ OBRA regulated in U.S. Long Term Care

streptokinase

(strep-toe-kin'-ace)

■ **Brand Name(s):** Kabikinase, Streptase
Chemical Class: Betahemolytic streptococcus filtrate, purified

■ **Clinical Pharmacology:**
Mechanism of Action: An enzyme that activates the fibrinolytic system by converting plasminogen to plasmin, an enzyme that degrades fibrin clots. Acts indirectly by forming a complex with plasminogen, which converts plasminogen to plasmin. Action occurs within the thrombus, on its surface, and in circulating blood. **Therapeutic Effect:** Destroys thrombi.
Pharmacokinetics: Rapidly cleared from plasma by antibodies and the reticuloendothelial system. Route of elimination unknown. Duration of action continues for several hours after drug has been discontinued. **Half-life:** 23 min.

■ **Available Forms:**
• *Powder for Injection* (*Kabikinase*, *Streptase*): 250,000 units, 750,000 units, 1.5 million units.

■ **Indications and Dosages:**
Acute evolving transmural MI (given as soon as possible after symptoms occur): IV Infusion (1.5 million units diluted to 45 ml). 1.5 million units infused over 60 min. Intracoronary Infusion (250,000 units diluted to 125 ml). Initially, 20,000 units (10-ml) bolus; then, 2,000 units/min for 60 min. Total dose: 140,000 units.
Pulmonary embolism, deep vein thrombosis (DVT), arterial thrombosis and embolism (given within 7 days of onset): IV Infusion (1.5 million units diluted to 90 ml). Initially, 250,000 units infused over 30 min; then, 100,000 units/hr for 24–72 hr for arterial thrombosis or embolism, and pulmonary embolism, 72 hr for DVT. Intra-arterial Infusion (1.5 million units diluted to 45 ml). Initially, 250,000 units infused over 30 min; then 100,000 units/hr for maintenance.

■ **Contraindications:** Carcinoma of the brain, cerebrovascular accident, internal bleeding, intracranial surgery, recent streptococcal infection, severe hypertension

■ **Side Effects**
Frequent
Fever, superficial bleeding at puncture sites, decreased BP
Occasional
Allergic reaction, including rash and wheezing; ecchymosis

■ **Serious Reactions**
• Severe internal hemorrhage may occur.
• Lysis of coronary thrombi may produce life-threatening arrhythmias.

Patient/Family Education
- Use an electric razor and soft toothbrush to prevent bleeding during drug therapy
- Report black or red stool, coffee-ground vomitus, dark or red urine, red-speckled mucus from cough, or other signs of bleeding
- Immediately report chest pain, headache, palpitations or shortness of breath

Monitoring Parameters
- Clinical response and vital signs
- Hgb and Hct, blood pressure, and platelet count; do not obtain blood pressure in lower extremities because a deep vein thrombus may be present
- aPTT, fibrinogen level, PT, and thrombin every 4 hr after therapy begins
- Stool for occult blood

Geriatric side effects at a glance:
❑ CNS   ❑ Bowel Dysfunction   ❑ Bladder Dysfunction   ❑ Falls

U.S. Regulatory Considerations
❑ FDA Black Box   ❑ OBRA regulated in U.S. Long Term Care

streptomycin sulfate

(strep-toe-mye'-sin sul'-fate)

Chemical Class: Aminoglycoside

Clinical Pharmacology:
Mechanism of Action: An aminoglycoside that binds directly to the 30S ribosomal subunits causing a faulty peptide sequence to form in the protein chain. **Therapeutic Effect:** Inhibits bacterial protein synthesis.
Pharmacokinetics: Protein binding: 34%-35%. Excreted in urine. **Half-life:** 2.5 hr.

Available Forms:
- *Injection:* 1 g.

Indications and Dosages:
Tuberculosis: IM 10 mg/kg/day. Maximum: 750 mg/day.
Dosage in renal impairment:

Creatinine Clearance	Dosage Interval
10–50 ml/min	q24–72h
less than 10 ml/min	q72–96h

Contraindications: Hypersensitivity to aminoglycosides

Side Effects
Occasional

Hypotension, drowsiness, headache, drug fever, paresthesia, rash, nausea, vomiting, anemia, arthralgia, weakness, tremor

■ Serious Reactions

- Nephrotoxicity (as evidenced by increased BUN and serum creatinine levels and decreased creatinine clearance) may be reversible if the drug is stopped at the first sign of nephrotoxic symptoms.
- Irreversible ototoxicity (manifested as tinnitus, dizziness, ringing or roaring in the ears, and impaired hearing) and neurotoxicity (as evidenced by headache, dizziness, lethargy, tremor, and visual disturbances) occur occasionally. Symptoms of ototoxicity, nephrotoxicity, and neuromuscular toxicity may occur.

Special Considerations

- Not usually used for long-term therapy secondary to nephrotoxicity and ototoxicity

■ Patient/Family Education

- Notify the physician if such symptoms as hearing loss, dizziness, or fullness or roaring in the ears occur

■ Monitoring Parameters

- Serum drug levels; therapeutic peak levels 20-30 mcg/ml, toxic peak levels (1 hr after IM administration) >50 mcg/ml
- Keep patient well hydrated
- Hearing
- Renal function

■ Geriatric side effects at a glance:

❑ CNS ❑ Bowel Dysfunction ❑ Bladder Dysfunction ❑ Falls

■ U.S. Regulatory Considerations

☑ FDA Black Box

Neurotoxicity (both auditory and vestibular ototoxicity) and nephrotoxicity. Risk increased in patients with impaired renal function and in those receiving high doses or prolonged therapy.

❑ OBRA regulated in U.S. Long Term Care

sucralfate

(soo'-kral-fate)

■ Brand Name(s): Carafate
Chemical Class: Aluminum complex of sulfated sucrose

■ Clinical Pharmacology:
Mechanism of Action: An antiulcer agent that forms an ulcer-adherent complex with proteinaceous exudate, such as albumin, at ulcer site. Also forms a viscous, adhesive barrier on the surface of intact mucosa of the stomach or duodenum. **Therapeutic Effect:** Protects damaged mucosa from further destruction by absorbing gastric acid, pepsin, and bile salts.

Pharmacokinetics: Minimally absorbed from the GI tract. Eliminated in feces, with small amount excreted in urine. Not removed by hemodialysis.

■ **Available Forms:**
  - *Oral Suspension:* 1 g/10 ml.
  - *Tablets:* 1 g.

■ **Indications and Dosages:**
  Active duodenal ulcers: PO 1g 4 times a day (before meals and at bedtime) for up to 8 wk.
  Maintenance therapy after healing of acute duodenal ulcers: PO 1g twice a day.

■ **Unlabeled Uses:** Prevention and treatment of stress-related mucosal damage, especially in acutely or critically ill patients; treatment of gastric ulcer and rheumatoid arthritis; relief of GI symptoms associated with NSAIDs; treatment of gastroesophageal reflux disease

■ **Contraindications:** None known.

■ **Side Effects**
  Frequent (2%)
  Constipation
  Occasional (less than 2%)
  Dry mouth, backache, diarrhea, dizziness, somnolence, nausea, indigestion, rash, hives, itching, abdominal discomfort

■ **Serious Reactions**
  - Bezoars (ingested compaction that does not pass into intestine) have been reported in patients treated with sucralfate.

■ **Patient/Family Education**
  - Take antacids prn for pain relief, but not within ½ hr before or after sucralfate
  - Take on an empty stomach
  - Take sips of tepid water and suck a hard candy to relieve dry mouth

■ **Monitoring Parameters**
  - Pattern of daily bowel activity and stool consistency

■ **Geriatric side effects at a glance:**
  ❑ CNS   ❑ Bowel Dysfunction   ❑ Bladder Dysfunction   ❑ Falls

■ **U.S. Regulatory Considerations**
  ❑ FDA Black Box   ❑ OBRA regulated in U.S. Long Term Care

sulfabenzamide / sulfacetamide / sulfathiazole

(sul-fa-ben'-za-mide/sul-fa-see'-ta-mide/sul-fa-thye'-a-zole)

■ **Brand Name(s):** V.V.S.
  Chemical Class: Sulfonamide derivative

■ **Clinical Pharmacology:**
  Mechanism of Action: Interferes with synthesis of folic acid that bacteria require for growth by inhibition of para-aminobenzoic acid metabolism. **Therapeutic Effect:** Prevents further bacterial growth.
  Pharmacokinetics: Absorption from vagina is variable and unreliable. Primarily metabolized by acetylation. Excreted in urine. **Half-life:** Unknown.

■ **Available Forms:**
  • *Vaginal Cream*: 3.7% sulfabenzamide, 2.86% sulfacetamide, 3.42% sulfathiazole (V.V.S).

■ **Indications and Dosages:**
  Treatment of Haemophilus vaginalis vaginitis: Vaginal Insert one applicatorful into vagina twice daily for 4-6 days. Dosage may then be decreased to 1/2 to 1/4 of an applicatorful twice daily.

■ **Contraindications:** Renal dysfunction, hypersensitivity to sulfabenzamide, sulfacetamide, sulfathiazole or any component of preparation

■ **Side Effects**
  Occasional
  Local irritation
  Rare
  Pruritus, urticaria, allergic reactions

■ **Serious Reactions**
  • Superinfection and Stevens-Johnson syndrome occur rarely.

■ **Patient/Family Education**
  • Insert high into vagina
  • Do not engage in vaginal intercourse during treatment
  • Complete the full course of therapy

■ **Monitoring Parameters**
  • Monitor the patient for skin rash or evidence of systemic toxicity; if these develop, discontinue medication

- **Geriatric side effects at a glance:**
  - ❑ CNS ❑ Bowel Dysfunction ❑ Bladder Dysfunction ❑ Falls

- **U.S. Regulatory Considerations**
  - ❑ FDA Black Box ❑ OBRA regulated in U.S. Long Term Care

sulfacetamide sodium

(sul-fa-see'-ta-mide soe'-dee-um)

- **Brand Name(s):** AK-Sulf, Bleph-10, Carmol, Isopto Cetamide, Klaron, Ocusulf-10, Ophthacet, Ovace, Sodium Sulamyd, Sulf-10, Sulfair

  Combinations
  Rx: with prednisolone (Blephamide, Dioptimyd, Metamyd, Vasocidin, Isopto Cetapred); with sulfur (Sulfacet-R); with sulfabenzamide (Sulfathiazole, Sulfa-Gyn, Sulnac, Trysul); with phenylephrine (Vasosulf); with fluorometholone (FML-S)
  Chemical Class: Sulfonamide derivative

- **Clinical Pharmacology:**
  Mechanism of Action: Interferes with synthesis of folic acid that bacteria require for growth. **Therapeutic Effect:** Prevents further bacterial growth. Bacteriostatic. **Pharmacokinetics:** Small amounts may be absorbed into the cornea. Excreted rapidly in urine. **Half-life:** 7-13 hr.

- **Available Forms:**
  - *Lotion*: 10% (Carmol, Klaron, Ovace).
  - *Ophthalmic Ointment*: 10% (AK-Sulf).
  - *Ophthalmic Solution*: 10% (Bleph-10, Ocusulf-10, Sulf-10).

- **Indications and Dosages:**
  Treatment of corneal ulcers, conjunctivitis and other superficial infections of the eye, prophylaxis after injuries to the eye/removal of foreign bodies, adjunctive therapy for trachoma and inclusion conjunctivitis: Ophthalmic Solution: 1-3 drops to lower conjunctival sac q2-3h. Seborrheic dermatitis, seborrheic sicca (dandruff), secondary bacterial skin infections Topical Ointment: Apply small amount in lower conjunctival sac 1-4 times/day and at bedtime.

- **Unlabeled Uses:** Treatment of bacterial blepharitis, blepharoconjunctivitis, bacterial keratitis, keratoconjunctivitis

- **Contraindications:** Hypersensitivity to sulfonamides or any component of preparation (some products contain sulfite), use in combination with silver-containing products

- **Side Effects**
  Frequent
  Transient ophthalmic burning, stinging

Occasional
Headache
Rare
Hypersensitivity (erythema, rash, itching, swelling, photosensitivity)

■ **Serious Reactions**
- Superinfection, drug-induced lupus erythematosus, and Stevens-Johnson syndrome occur rarely; nephrotoxicity with high dermatologic concentrations.

■ **Patient/Family Education**
- May cause sensitivity to bright light
- Do not touch tip of container to any surface
- May cause transient burning and stinging
- Notify the physician if swelling, itching, or rash occurs

■ **Monitoring Parameters**
- Monitor for signs of hypersensitivity reaction

■ **Geriatric side effects at a glance:**
❑ CNS ❑ Bowel Dysfunction ❑ Bladder Dysfunction ❑ Falls

■ **U.S. Regulatory Considerations**
❑ FDA Black Box ❑ OBRA regulated in U.S. Long Term Care

sulfasalazine

(sul-fa-sal'-a-zeen)

■ **Brand Name(s):** Azulfidine, Azulfidine EN-Tabs
Chemical Class: Salicylate derivative; sulfonamide derivative

■ **Clinical Pharmacology:**
Mechanism of Action: A sulfonamide that inhibits prostaglandin synthesis, acting locally in the colon. **Therapeutic Effect:** Decreases inflammatory response, interferes with GI secretion.
Pharmacokinetics: Poorly absorbed from the GI tract. Cleaved in colon by intestinal bacteria, forming sulfapyridine and mesalamine (5-ASA). Absorbed in colon. Widely distributed. Metabolized in the liver. Primarily excreted in urine. **Half-life:** Sulfapyridine, 6–14 hr; 5-ASA, 0.6–1.4 hr.

■ **Available Forms:**
- *Tablets (Azulfidine)*: 500 mg.
- *Tablets (Delayed-Release [Azulfidine EN-Tabs])*: 500 mg.

- ■ **Indications and Dosages:**
  Ulcerative colitis: PO 1g 3–4 times a day in divided doses q4–6h. Maintenance: 2 g/day in divided doses q6–12h. Maximum: 6 g/day.
  Rheumatoid arthritis: PO Initially, 0.5–1 g/day for 1 wk. Increase by 0.5 g/wk, up to 3 g/day.

- ■ **Unlabeled Uses:** Treatment of ankylosing spondylitis, collagenous colitis, Crohn's disease, psoriasis, psoriatic arthritis

- ■ **Contraindications:** Hypersensitivity to carbonic anhydrase inhibitors, local anesthetics, salicylates, sulfonamides, sulfonylureas, sunscreens containing PABA, or thiazide or loop diuretics; intestinal or urinary tract obstruction; porphyria; severe hepatic or renal dysfunction

- ■ **Side Effects**

  Frequent (33%)
  Anorexia, nausea, vomiting, headache, oligospermia (generally reversed by withdrawal of drug)

  Occasional (3%)
  Hypersensitivity reaction (rash, urticaria, pruritus, fever, anemia)

  Rare (less than 1%)
  Tinnitus, hypoglycemia, diuresis, photosensitivity

- ■ **Serious Reactions**
  - • Anaphylaxis, Stevens-Johnson syndrome, hematologic toxicity (leukopenia, agranulocytosis), hepatotoxicity, and nephrotoxicity occur rarely.

- ■ **Patient/Family Education**
  - • Adequate hydration and urinary output are essential to prevent crystalluria and stone formation
  - • Avoid prolonged exposure to sunlight
  - • Space drug doses around the clock and continue sulfasalazine therapy for the full course of treatment
  - • It is important to comply with follow-up and laboratory tests
  - • Inform the dentist or surgeon of sulfasalazine therapy if he or she will have dental or other surgical procedures

- ■ **Monitoring Parameters**
  - • *Inflammatory bowel disease:* Decrease in rectal bleeding or diarrhea in conjunction with mucosal healing
  - • *Rheumatoid arthritis:* Tender, swollen joints, visual analogue scale for pain; acute phase reactants (ESR, C-reactive protein), duration of early morning stiffness, preservation of function
  - • Baseline CBC with differential and liver function tests, then every second week during the first 3 months of therapy, monthly during the second 3 months of therapy, then every 3 months thereafter; urinalysis and renal function tests periodically
  - • Skin for rash

- ■ **Geriatric side effects at a glance:**
  ❑ CNS ❑ Bowel Dysfunction ❑ Bladder Dysfunction ❑ Falls

sulfinpyrazone

(sul-fin-pie'-ra-zone)

■ **Brand Name(s):** Anturane
Chemical Class: Pyrazolidine derivative

■ **Clinical Pharmacology:**
Mechanism of Action: A uricosuric that increases urinary excretion of uric acid, thereby decreasing blood urate levels. **Therapeutic Effect:** Promotes uric acid excretion and reduces serum uric acid levels.
Pharmacokinetics: Rapidly and completely absorbed from gastrointestinal (GI) tract. Widely distributed. Metabolized in liver to two active metabolite, p-hydroxy-sulfinpyrazone and a sulfide analog. Excreted primarily in urine. Not removed by hemodialysis. **Half-life:** 2.7-6 hr.

■ **Available Forms:**
• *Tablets:* 100 mg.

■ **Indications and Dosages:**
Gout: PO 100-200 mg 2 times/day. Maximum: 800 mg/day.

■ **Unlabeled Uses:** Mitral valve replacement, myocardial infarction

■ **Contraindications:** Active peptic ulcer, blood dyscrasias, GI inflammation, hypersensitivity to sulfinpyrazone, phenylbutazone, other pyrazoles, or any of its components

■ **Side Effects**
Frequent
Nausea, vomiting, stomach pain
Occasional
Flushed face, headache, dizziness, frequent urge to urinate, rash
Rare
Increased bleeding time, hepatic necrosis, nephrotic syndrome, uric acid stones

■ **Serious Reactions**
• Hematologic toxicity including anemia, leukopenia, agranulocytosis, thrombocytopenia, and aplastic anemia occur rarely.
• Overdose causes drowsiness, dizziness, anorexia, abdominal pain, hemolytic anemia, acidosis, jaundice, fever, and agranulocytosis.

■ **Patient/Family Education**
• Take with food, milk, or antacids to decrease stomach upset
• Avoid aspirin and other salicylate-containing products

- Drink plenty of fluids
- Report any unusual side effects

■ **Monitoring Parameters**
- Serum uric acid concentrations, renal function, CBC
- Therapeutic response such as reduced joint tenderness, limitation of motion, redness and swelling

■ **Geriatric side effects at a glance:**
❏ CNS ❏ Bowel Dysfunction ❏ Bladder Dysfunction ❏ Falls

■ **U.S. Regulatory Considerations**
❏ FDA Black Box ❏ OBRA regulated in U.S. Long Term Care

sulindac

(sul-in'-dak)

■ **Brand Name(s):** Clinoril
Chemical Class: Acetic acid derivative

■ **Clinical Pharmacology:**
Mechanism of Action: An NSAID that produces analgesic and anti-inflammatory effects by inhibiting prostaglandin synthesis. **Therapeutic Effect:** Reduces inflammatory response and intensity of pain.
Pharmacokinetics:

Route	Onset	Peak	Duration
PO (Antirheumatic)	7 days	2–3 wk	N/A

Well absorbed from the GI tract. Metabolized in liver to active metabolite. Primarily excreted in urine. Not removed by hemodialysis. **Half-life:** 7.8 hr; metabolite: 16.4 hr.

■ **Available Forms:**
- *Tablets:* 150 mg, 200 mg.

■ **Indications and Dosages:**
Rheumatoid arthritis, osteoarthritis, ankylosing spondylitis: PO Initially, 150 mg twice a day; may increase up to 400 mg/day.
Acute shoulder pain, gouty arthritis, bursitis, tendinitis: PO 200 mg twice a day.

■ **Contraindications:** Active peptic ulcer disease, chronic inflammation of GI tract, GI bleeding or ulceration, history of hypersensitivity to aspirin or NSAIDs

■ **Side Effects**
Frequent (9%–4%)
Diarrhea or constipation, indigestion, nausea, maculopapular rash, dermatitis, dizziness, headache

Occasional (3%–1%)
Anorexia, abdominal cramps, flatulence

■ **Serious Reactions**
  • Rare reactions with long-term use include peptic ulcer disease, GI bleeding, gastritis, nephrotoxicity (glomerular nephritis, interstitial nephritis, nephrotic syndrome), severe hepatic reactions (cholestasis, jaundice), and severe hypersensitivity reactions (fever, chills, and joint pain).

Special Considerations
  • No significant advantage over other NSAIDs; cost should govern use

■ **Patient/Family Education**
  • Avoid aspirin and alcoholic beverages
  • Take with food, milk, or antacids to decrease GI upset
  • Antirheumatic action may not be apparent for several weeks
  • Avoid performing tasks that require mental alertness or motor skills until response to the drug has been established

■ **Monitoring Parameters**
  • Initial hematocrit and fecal occult blood test within 3 mo of starting regular chronic therapy; repeat every 6-12 mo (more frequently in high-risk patients, e.g., >65 years, peptic ulcer disease, concurrent steroids or anticoagulants); electrolytes, creatinine, and BUN within 3 mo of starting regular chronic therapy; repeat every 6-12 mo

■ **Geriatric side effects at a glance:**
  ☑ CNS   ❑ Bowel Dysfunction   ❑ Bladder Dysfunction   ❑ Falls
  ☑ Other: Gastropathy

■ **Use with caution in older patients with:** Renal impairment, Hepatic impairment, CHF, HTN, PUD, History of GI bleeding, GERD, Bleeding and platelet disorders, History of aspirin sensitivity reaction. Also use with caution in patients taking Anticoagulants, Aspirin, and Antihypertensive agents.

■ **U.S. Regulatory Considerations**
  ☑ FDA Black Box
  • Increased cardiovascular risk
  • Increased gastrointestinal risk
  ❑ OBRA regulated in U.S. Long Term Care

■ **Other Uses in Geriatric Patient:** Acute gout

■ **Side Effects:**
  Of particular importance in the geriatric patient: Confusion, cognitive impairment, delirium, dizziness, dyspepsia, fluid retention, renal impairment

■ **Geriatric Considerations - Summary:** Use of NSAIDs in older adults increases the risk of GI complications including gastric ulceration, bleeding, and perforation. These complications are not necessarily preceded by less severe GI symptoms. Concomitant use of a proton pump inhibitor or misoprostol reduces the risk for gastric ulceration and bleeding, but may not prevent long-term GI toxicity.

■ **References:**
1. COX-2 alternatives and GI protection. Med Lett Drugs Ther 2004;46:91.
2. Drugs that may cause cognitive disorders in the elderly. Med Lett Drugs Ther 2000;42:111-112.

sumatriptan succinate

(soo-ma-trip'-tan suk'-si-nate)

■ **Brand Name(s):** Imitrex, Imitrex Nasal, Imitrex Statdose, Imitrex Statdose Refill
Chemical Class: Serotonin derivative

■ **Clinical Pharmacology:**
Mechanism of Action: A serotonin receptor agonist that binds selectively to vascular receptors, producing a vasoconstrictive effect on cranial blood vessels. **Therapeutic Effect:** Relieves migraine headache.
Pharmacokinetics:

Route	Onset	Peak	Duration
Nasal	15 min	N/A	24-48 hr
PO	30 min	2 hr	24-48 hr
Subcutaneous	10 min	1 hr	24-48 hr

Rapidly absorbed after subcutaneous administration. Absorption after PO administration is incomplete, with significant amounts undergoing hepatic metabolism, resulting in low bioavailability (about 14%). Protein binding: 10%-21%. Widely distributed. Undergoes first-pass metabolism in the liver. Excreted in urine. **Half-life:** 2 hr.

■ **Available Forms:**
- *Tablets* (Imitrex): 25 mg, 50 mg, 100 mg.
- *Injection* (Imitrex, Imitrex Statdose): 6 mg/0.5 ml.
- *Nasal Spray* (Imitrex Nasal): 5 mg, 20 mg.

■ **Indications and Dosages:**
Acute migraine attack: PO 25-50 mg. Dose may be repeated after at least 2 hr. Maximum: 100 mg/single dose; 200 mg/24 hr. Subcutaneous 6 mg. Maximum: Two 6-mg injections/24 hr (separated by at least 1 hr). Intranasal 5-20 mg; may repeat in 2 hr. Maximum: 40 mg/24 hr.

■ **Contraindications:** Cerebrovascular accident (CVA), ischemic heart disease (including angina pectoris, history of MI, silent ischemia, and Prinzmetal's angina), severe hepatic impairment, transient ischemic attack, uncontrolled hypertension, use within 14 days of MAOIs, use within 24 hr of ergotamine preparations

■ **Side Effects**
Frequent
Oral (10%-5%): Tingling, nasal discomfort

Subcutaneous (greater than 10%): Injection site reactions, tingling, warm or hot sensation, dizziness, vertigo
Nasal (greater than 10%): Bad or unusual taste, nausea, vomiting
Occasional
Oral (5%-1%): Flushing, asthenia, visual disturbances
Subcutaneous (10%-2%): Burning sensation, numbness, chest discomfort, drowsiness, asthenia
Nasal (5%-1%): Nasopharyngeal discomfort, dizziness
Rare
Oral (less than 1%): Agitation, eye irritation, dysuria
Subcutaneous (less than 2%): Anxiety, fatigue, diaphoresis, muscle cramps, myalgia
Nasal (less than 1%): Burning sensation

■ **Serious Reactions**
- Excessive dosage may produce tremor, red extremities, reduced respirations, cyanosis, seizures, and paralysis.
- Serious arrhythmias occur rarely, especially in patients with hypertension, diabetes, or a strong family history of coronary artery disease; obese patients; and smokers.

Special Considerations
- First inj should be administered under medical supervision

■ **Patient/Family Education**
- Use only to treat migraine headache; not for prevention
- Inject the medication and discard the syringe
- Inject the drug into an area with adequate subcutaneous tissue because the needle will penetrate the skin and adipose tissue as deeply as 6 mm
- Do not administer more than two subcutaneous injections during any 24-hour period and allow at least 1 hour between injections
- Notify the physician immediately if palpitations, a rash, wheezing, pain or tightness in the chest or throat, or facial edema occurs
- Lie down in dark, quiet room for additional benefit after taking sumatriptan

■ **Monitoring Parameters**
- Evaluate the patient for relief of migraines and associated symptoms, including nausea and vomiting, photophobia, and phonophobia (sound sensitivity)

■ **Geriatric side effects at a glance:**
❑ CNS   ❑ Bowel Dysfunction   ❑ Bladder Dysfunction   ❑ Falls

■ **U.S. Regulatory Considerations**
❑ FDA Black Box   ❑ OBRA regulated in U.S. Long Term Care

synthetic conjugated estrogens, B

(ess'-troe-jenz)

- **Brand Name(s):** Enjuvia

- **Clinical Pharmacology:**
  Mechanism of Action: An estrogen that increases synthesis of DNA, RNA, and various proteins in responsive tissues. Reduces release of gonadotropin-releasing hormone, reducing levels of follicle-stimulating hormone (FSH) and luteinizing hormone (LH). **Therapeutic Effect:** Promotes vasomotor stability, maintains genitourinary function and normal growth and development of female sex organs. Prevents accelerated bone loss by inhibiting bone resorption and restoring balance of bone resorption and formation. Inhibits LH production; decreases serum concentration of testosterone. **Pharmacokinetics:** Well absorbed from the gastrointestinal (GI) tract. Widely distributed. Protein binding: 50%-80%. Metabolized in liver. Primarily excreted in urine. **Half-life:** 11-14 hr.

- **Available Forms:**
  - *Tablets:* 0.625 mg, 1.25 mg (Enjuvia).

- **Indications and Dosages:**
  Vasomotor symptoms associated with menopause: PO 0.625-1.25 mg/day.

- **Contraindications:** Breast cancer with some exceptions, hepatic disease, thrombophlebitis, undiagnosed vaginal bleeding

- **Side Effects**
  Frequent
  Breast pain or tenderness; gynecomastia
  Occasional
  Headache, hypertension, intolerance to contact lenses
  Rare
  Loss of scalp hair, depression

- **Serious Reactions**
  - Prolonged administration may increase risk of gallbladder and thromboembolic disease and risk of breast, cervical, vaginal, endometrial, and liver carcinoma.

- **Geriatric side-effects at a glance:**
  ❑ CNS ❑ Bowel Dysfunction ❑ Bladder Dysfunction ❑ Falls

- **U.S. Regulatory Considerations**
  ❑ FDA Black Box ❑ OBRA regulated in U.S. Long Term Care

tacrine hydrochloride

(tak'-reen hye-droe-klor'-ide)

■ **Brand Name(s):** Cognex
Chemical Class: Cholinesterase inhibitor; monoamine acridine derivative

■ **Clinical Pharmacology:**
Mechanism of Action: An agent that inhibits the enzyme acetylcholinesterase, thus increasing the concentration of acetylcholine at cholinergic synapses and enhancing cholinergic function in the CNS. **Therapeutic Effect:** Slows the progression of Alzheimer's disease.
Pharmacokinetics: Rapidly absorbed following PO administration. Protein binding: 55%. Extensively metabolized in liver. Negligible amounts excreted in urine. **Half-life:** 2-4 hr.

■ **Available Forms:**
 • *Capsules*: 10 mg, 20 mg, 30 mg, 40 mg.

■ **Indications and Dosages:**
Alzheimer's disease: PO Initially, 10 mg 4 times a day for 6 wk, followed by 20 mg 4 times a day for 6 wk, 30 mg 4 times a day for 12 wk, then 40 mg 4 times a day if needed.
Dosage in hepatic impairment: For patients with ALT greater than 3-5 times normal, decrease the dose by 40 mg/day and resume the normal dose when ALT returns to normal. For patients with ALT greater than 5 times normal, stop treatment and resume it when ALT returns to normal.

■ **Contraindications:** Known hypersensitivity to tacrine, patients previously treated with tacrine who developed jaundice

■ **Side Effects**
Frequent (28%-11%)
Headache, nausea, vomiting, diarrhea, dizziness
Occasional (9%-4%)
Fatigue, chest pain, dyspepsia, anorexia, abdominal pain, flatulence, constipation, confusion, agitation, rash, depression, ataxia, insomnia, rhinitis, myalgia
Rare (less than 3%)
Weight loss, anxiety, cough, facial flushing, urinary frequency, back pain, tremor

■ **Serious Reactions**
 • Overdose can cause cholinergic crisis, marked by increased salivation, lacrimation, bradycardia, respiratory depression, hypotension, and increased muscle weakness. Treatment usually consists of supportive measures and an anticholinergic such as atropine.

Special Considerations
 • Transaminase elevation is the most common reason for withdrawal of drug (8%); monitor ALT qwk for first 18 wk, then decrease to q3 mo; when dose is increased, monitor qwk for 6 wk

- If elevations occur, modify dose as follows: ALT $\leq$3 times upper limit normal (ULN), continue current dose; ALT >3 to $\leq$5 times ULN, reduce dose by 40 mg qd and resume dose titration when within normal limits; ALT >5 times ULN, stop treatment; rechallenge may be tried if ALT is <10 times ULN
- Do not rechallenge if clinical jaundice develops
- Improvement in symptoms of dementia statistically, but perhaps not clinically significant; discontinue therapy if improvement not evident to family members and clinician

■ Patient/Family Education
- Take tacrine at regular intervals, between meals; take the drug with meals if GI upset occurs
- Do not abruptly discontinue tacrine or adjust the drug dosage
- Avoid smoking during tacrine therapy because smoking reduces the drug's blood level
- Tacrine is not a cure for Alzheimer disease but may slow the progression of its symptoms
- Refer the patient's family to the local chapter of the Alzheimer Disease Association for a guide to available services

■ Monitoring Parameters
- AST (SGOT) and ALT (SGPT) levels every other week for the first 4 months, then every other month thereafter
- Periodically monitor the ECG and rhythm strips of patients with underlying arrhythmias
- Assess for signs of GI distress
- Monitor behavioral, cognitive, and functional status

■ Geriatric side effects at a glance:
☑ CNS ☑ Bowel Dysfunction ❏ Bladder Dysfunction ❏ Falls
Other: Anorexia, weight loss, bradycardia

■ Use with caution in older patients with: None

■ U.S. Regulatory Considerations
❏ FDA Black Box ❏ OBRA regulated in U.S. Long Term Care

■ Other Uses in Geriatric Patient: None

■ Side Effects:
Of particular importance in the geriatric patient: None

■ Geriatric Considerations - Summary: Tacrine, like newer cholinesterase inhibitors, is modestly effective for treatment of cognitive decline associated with Alzheimer's disease. It is rarely used because of significant hepatotoxicity.

■ References:
1. Cummings JL. Alzheimer's disease. N Engl J Med 2004;351:56-67.
2. Kaduszkiewicz H, Zimmermann T, Beck-Bornholdt HP, et al. Cholinesterase inhibitors for patients with Alzheimer's disease: systematic review of randomised clinical trials. BMJ 2005;331:321-327.

tacrolimus

(ta-kroe'-li-mus)

■ **Brand Name(s):** Prograf, Protopic
  Chemical Class: Macrolide derivative

■ **Clinical Pharmacology:**
  Mechanism of Action: An immunologic agent that inhibits T-lymphocyte activation by binding to intracellular proteins, forming a complex, and inhibiting phosphatase activity. **Therapeutic Effect:** Suppresses the immunologically mediated inflammatory response; prevents organ transplant rejection.
  Pharmacokinetics: Variably absorbed after PO administration (food reduces absorption). Protein binding: 75%–97%. Extensively metabolized in the liver. Excreted in urine. Not removed by hemodialysis. **Half-life:** 11.7 hr.

■ **Available Forms:**
  • *Capsules (Prograf):* 0.5 mg, 1 mg, 5 mg.
  • *Injection (Prograf):* 5 mg/ml.
  • *Ointment (Protopic):* 0.03%, 0.1%.

■ **Indications and Dosages:**
  Prevention of liver transplant rejection: PO 0.1-0.15 mg/kg/day in 2 divided doses 12 hr apart. IV 0.03–0.15 mg/kg/day as a continuous infusion.
  Prevention of kidney transplant rejection: PO 0.2 mg/kg/day in 2 divided doses 12 hr apart IV 0.03-0.15 mg/kg/day as continuous infusion.
  Atopic dermatitis: Topical Apply 0.03% ointment to affected area twice a day. 0.1% ointment may be used in adults and the elderly. Continue until 1 wk after symptoms have cleared.

■ **Unlabeled Uses:** Prevention of organ rejection in patients receiving allogeneic bone marrow, heart, pancreas, pancreatic island cell, or small-bowel transplant, treatment of autoimmune disease, severe recalcitrant psoriasis

■ **Contraindications:** Concurrent use with cyclosporine (increases the risk of nephrotoxicity), hypersensitivity to HCO-60 polyoxyl 60 hydrogenated castor oil (used in solution for injection)

■ **Side Effects**
  Frequent (greater than 30%)
  Headache, tremor, insomnia, paresthesia, diarrhea, nausea, constipation, vomiting, abdominal pain, hypertension
  Occasional (29%–10%)
  Rash, pruritus, anorexia, asthenia, peripheral edema, photosensitivity

■ **Serious Reactions**
  • Nephrotoxicity (characterized by increased serum creatinine level and decreased urine output), neurotoxicity (including tremor, headache, and mental status changes), and pleural effusion are common adverse reactions.

- Thrombocytopenia, leukocytosis, anemia, atelectasis, sepsis, and infection occur occasionally.

Special Considerations
- Black patients may need higher doses in kidney transplant
- Also known as FK 506

■ Patient/Family Education
- Take the capsules on an empty stomach and do not mix them with grapefruit juice
- Take the drug at the same time each day and notify the physician if a dose is missed
- Avoid crowds and people with infections
- Notify the physician if chest pain, dizziness, headache, decreased urination, rash, respiratory infection, or unusual bleeding or bruising occurs
- Avoid exposure to sunlight and artificial light because this may cause a photosensitivity reaction

■ Monitoring Parameters
- Regularly assess serum creatinine, potassium, and fasting glucose
- Whole blood tacrolimus concentrations as measured by ELISA may be helpful in assessing rejection and toxicity, median trough concentrations measured after the second week of therapy ranged from 9.8 to 19.4 mg/ml
- CBC weekly during the first month of therapy, twice monthly during the second and third months of treatment, then monthly for the rest of the first year; liver function test results
- Intake and output

■ Geriatric side effects at a glance:
❏ CNS   ❏ Bowel Dysfunction   ❏ Bladder Dysfunction   ❏ Falls

■ U.S. Regulatory Considerations
☑ FDA Black Box
Increased susceptibility to infection and secondary malignancy
❏ OBRA regulated in U.S. Long Term Care

tadalafil

(tah-da'-la-fil)

■ Brand Name(s): Cialis
Chemical Class: Cyclic GMP specific phosphodiesterase inhibitor

■ Clinical Pharmacology:
Mechanism of Action: An erectile dysfunction agent that inhibits phosphodiesterase type 5, the enzyme responsible for degrading cyclic guanosine monophosphate (cGMP) in the corpus cavernosum of the penis, resulting in smooth muscle relaxation and increased blood flow. **Therapeutic Effect:** Facilitates an erection.

Pharmacokinetics:

Route	Onset	Peak	Duration
PO	16 min	2 hr	36 hr

Rapidly absorbed after PO administration. Drug has no effect on penile blood flow without sexual stimulation. **Half-life:** 17.5 hr.

■ Available Forms:
- *Tablets*: 5 mg, 10 mg, 20 mg.

■ Indications and Dosages:
Erectile dysfunction: PO 10 mg 30 min before sexual activity. Dose may be increased to 20 mg or decreased to 5 mg, based on patient tolerance. Maximum dosing frequency is once daily.

Dosage in renal impairment: For patients with a creatinine clearance of 31-50 ml/min, the starting dose is 5 mg before sexual activity once a day and the maximum dose is 10 mg no more frequently than once q48h. For patients with a creatinine clearance of less than 31 ml/min, the starting dose is 5 mg before sexual activity once a day.

Dosage in mild or moderate hepatic impairment: Patients with Child-Pugh Class A or B hepatic impairment should take no more than 10 mg once a day.

■ Contraindications:
Concurrent use of alpha-adrenergic blockers (other than the minimum dose tamsulosin), concurrent use of sodium nitroprusside or nitrates in any form, severe hepatic impairment

■ Side Effects
Occasional

Headache, dyspepsia, back pain, myalgia, nasal congestion, flushing

■ Serious Reactions
- Prolonged erections (lasting over 4 hr) and priapism (painful erections lasting over 6 hr) occur rarely.
- Angina, chest pain, and MI have been reported.

■ Patient/Family Education
- Sexual stimulation is required for an erection to occur after taking tadalafil
- Erectile function improved up to 36 hr following dose
- Seek treatment immediately if an erection lasts longer than 4 hr
- Avoid using nitrate drugs and alpha-adrenergic blockers concurrently with tadalafil

■ Monitoring Parameters
- Cardiovascular status

■ Geriatric side effects at a glance:
❑ CNS ❑ Bowel Dysfunction ❑ Bladder Dysfunction ❑ Falls

■ U.S. Regulatory Considerations
❑ FDA Black Box ❑ OBRA regulated in U.S. Long Term Care

tamoxifen citrate

(ta-mox'-i-fen sit'-trate)

- **Brand Name(s):** Nolvadex
  Chemical Class: Estrogen agonist-antagonist; triphenylethylene derivative

- **Clinical Pharmacology:**
  Mechanism of Action: A nonsteroidal antiestrogen that competes with estradiol for estrogen-receptor binding sites in the breasts, uterus, and vagina. **Therapeutic Effect:** Inhibits DNA synthesis and estrogen response.
  Pharmacokinetics: Well absorbed from the GI tract. Metabolized in the liver. Primarily eliminated in feces by biliary system. **Half-life:** 7 days.

- **Available Forms:**
  - *Tablets* (Nolvadex): 10 mg, 20 mg.

- **Indications and Dosages:**
  Adjunctive treatment of breast cancer: PO 20-40 mg/day. Give doses greater than 20 mg/day in divided doses.
  Prevention of breast cancer in high-risk women: PO 20 mg/day.

- **Unlabeled Uses:** Treatment of mastalgia, gynecomastia, pancreatic carcinoma, ovulation induction

- **Contraindications:** Concomitant coumarin-type therapy when used in the treatment of breast cancer in high-risk women, history of deep vein thrombosis or pulmonary embolism in high-risk women

- **Side Effects**
  Frequent
  Women (*greater than* 10%): Hot flashes, nausea, vomiting
  Occasional
  Women (9%-1%): Genital itching, vaginal discharge, endometrial hyperplasia or polyps
  Men: Impotence, decreased libido
  Men and women: Headache, nausea, vomiting, rash, bone pain, confusion, weakness, somnolence

- **Serious Reactions**
  - Retinopathy, corneal opacity, and decreased visual acuity have been noted in patients receiving extremely high dosages (240-320 mg/day) for longer than 17 mo.
  - There have been an increased number of incidences of endometrial changes, thromboembolic events, and uterine malignancies while using tamoxifen.

Special Considerations
  - Treatment duration >5 yr may provide no further benefit and increase risk of endometrial cancer for some women; reevaluate the need for continued therapy

- The Gail Model Risk Assessment Tool is available to health care professionals by calling (800) 456-3669 (ext. 3838)

■ **Patient/Family Education**
  - Notify the physician if leg cramps, weakness, weight gain, or vaginal bleeding, itching, or discharge occurs
  - May initially cause an increase in bone and tumor pain, which appears to indicate a good tumor response to tamoxifen
  - Notify the physician if nausea and vomiting continue at home

■ **Monitoring Parameters**
  - Endometrial biopsy indicated for abnormal vaginal bleeding
  - Intake and output
  - Weight
  - Be alert for reports of increased bone pain and provide adequate pain relief as ordered
  - Assess the patient for signs and symptoms of hypercalcemia, including constipation, deep bone or flank pain, excessive thirst, hypotonicity of muscles, increased urine output, nausea and vomiting, and renal calculi

■ **Geriatric side effects at a glance:**
  ❑ CNS ❑ Bowel Dysfunction ❑ Bladder Dysfunction ❑ Falls

■ **U.S. Regulatory Considerations**
  ☑ FDA Black Box
  For women with ductal carcinoma in situ (DCIS) and women at high risk for breast cancer: increased risk for uterine malignancies, stroke, and pulmonary embolism.
  ❑ OBRA regulated in U.S. Long Term Care

tamsulosin hydrochloride

(tam-soo-lo'-sin hye-droe-klor'-ide)

■ **Brand Name(s):** Flomax
  Chemical Class: Quinazoline

■ **Clinical Pharmacology:**
  Mechanism of Action: An alpha$_1$-antagonist that targets receptors around bladder neck and prostate capsule. **Therapeutic Effect:** Relaxes smooth muscle and improves urinary flow and symptoms of prostatic hyperplasia.
  Pharmacokinetics: Well absorbed and widely distributed. Protein binding: 94%-99%. Metabolized in the liver. Primarily excreted in urine. Unknown if removed by hemodialysis. **Half-life:** 9-13 hr.

■ **Available Forms:**
  - *Capsules:* 0.4 mg.

- **Indications and Dosages:**
  Benign prostatic hyperplasia: PO 0.4 mg once a day, approximately 30 min after same meal each day. May increase dosage to 0.8 mg if inadequate response in 2-4 wk.

- **Contraindications:** Concurrent use of sildenafil, tadalafil, or vardenafil

- **Side Effects**
  Frequent (9%-7%)
  Dizziness, somnolence
  Occasional (5%-3%)
  Headache, anxiety, insomnia, orthostatic hypotension
  Rare (less than 2%)
  Nasal congestion, pharyngitis, rhinitis, nausea, vertigo, impotence

- **Serious Reactions**
  - First-dose syncope (hypotension with sudden loss of consciousness) may occur within 30 to 90 min after administration of initial dose and may be preceded by tachycardia (pulse rate of 120-160 beats/min).

- **Patient/Family Education**
  - Consider administration of first dose at bedtime; caution following first 12 hr after initiation or reinitiation of therapy for "first dose phenomenon"
  - Use caution when getting up from a sitting or lying position
  - Avoid tasks that require mental alertness or motor skills until response to the drug has been established

- **Monitoring Parameters**
  - Blood pressure, pulse

- **Geriatric side effects at a glance:**
  ☑ CNS ☐ Bowel Dysfunction ☐ Bladder Dysfunction ☑ Falls
  Other: Orthostatic hypotension, worsening of urge or mixed urinary incontinence

- **Use with caution in older patients with:** Congestive heart failure, patients taking medications for impotence (e.g., vardenafil, sildenafil, or tadalafil)

- **U.S. Regulatory Considerations**
  ☐ FDA Black Box ☐ OBRA regulated in U.S. Long Term Care

- **Other Uses in Geriatric Patient:** Symptoms related to benign prostatic hypertrophy

- **Side Effects:**
  Of particular importance in the geriatric patient: Orthostatic hypotension, worsening of urge or mixed urinary incontinence, ejaculatory dysfunction

- **Geriatric Considerations-Summary:** Alpha-adrendergic blockers are modestly effective alone, and in combination with 5-alpha reductase inhibitors (e.g., finasteride) in the treatment of urinary obstructive symptoms related to benign prostatic hyperplasia. Tamsulosin is a "uroselective" alpha-blocker which appears to cause less orthostatic hypotension than nonselective alpha-blockers such as terazosin, prazosin, and doxazosin.

■ **References:**
1. McConnell JD, Roehrborn CG, Bautista OM, et al. The long-term effect of doxazosin, finasteride, and combination therapy on the clinical progression of benign prostatic hyperplasia. N Engl J Med 2003;349:2387-2398.
2. Lowe FC. Role of the newer alpha$_1$-adrenergic-receptor antagonists in the treatment of benign prostatic hyperplasia-related lower urinary tract symptoms. Clin Ther 2004;26:1701-1713.
3. Alfuzosin (Uroxatral)—another alpha$_1$-blocker for benign prostatic hyperplasia. Med Lett Drugs Ther 2004;46:1-2.

tazarotene

(ta-zare'-oh-teen)

■ **Brand Name(s):** Avage, Tazorac
Chemical Class: Retinoid prodrug; vitamin A derivative

■ **Clinical Pharmacology:**
Mechanism of Action: Modulates differentiation and proliferation of epithelial tissue, binds selectively to retinoic acid receptors. **Therapeutic Effect:** Restores normal differentiation of the epidermis and promotes reduction of epidermal inflammation.
Pharmacokinetics: Minimal systemic absorption occurs through the skin. Binding to plasma proteins is greater than 99%. Metabolism is in the skin and liver. Elimination occurs through the fecal and renal pathways. **Half-life:** 18 hr.

■ **Available Forms:**
- **Gel:** 0.05%, 0.1% (Tazorac)
- **Cream:** 0.05%, 0.1% (Tazorac)

■ **Indications and Dosages:**
Psoriasis: Topical   Thin film applied once daily in the evening; cover only the lesions, and area should be dry before application
Acne vulgaris: Topical   Thin film applied to affected areas once daily in the evening, after face is gently cleansed and dried.
Fine facial wrinkles, facial mottled hyperpigmentation (liver spots), hypopigmentation associated with photoaging: Topical   Thin film applied to affected areas once daily in the evening, after face is gently cleansed and dried.

■ **Contraindications:** Hypersensitivity to tazarotene, benzyl alcohol, or any one of its components.

■ **Side Effects**
Frequent
Desquamation, burning or stinging, dry skin, itching, erythema, worsening of psoriasis, irritation, skin pain, pruritis, xerosis, photosensitivity
Occasional
Irritation, skin pain, fissuring, localized edema, skin discoloration, rash, desquamation, contact dermatitis, skin inflammation, bleeding, dry skin, hypertriglyceridemia, peripheral edema, acne vulgaris, cheilitis

- Attractive alternative to oral retinoid therapy in psoriasis (e.g., etretinate), primarily due to less toxicity. Structural changes to the basic retinoid structure (e.g., conformational rigidity) are claimed to enhance therapeutic efficacy and reduce the local toxicity associated with topical tretinoin (retinoic acid). However, place in therapy should await direct comparisons vs standard regimens in terms of efficacy, toxicity, and cost

■ **Patient/Family Education**
- Burning or stinging after application, dryness, itching, peeling, or redness of the skin may occur during tazarotene therapy
- Avoid direct exposure to sunlight

■ **Monitoring Parameters**
- Therapeutic response to medication

■ **Geriatric side effects at a glance:**
  ❑ CNS ❑ Bowel Dysfunction ❑ Bladder Dysfunction ❑ Falls

■ **U.S. Regulatory Considerations**
  ❑ FDA Black Box ❑ OBRA regulated in U.S. Long Term Care

tegaserod maleate

(te-gas'-a-rod mal'-ee-ate)

■ **Brand Name(s):** Zelnorm
  Chemical Class: Pentylcarbazimidamide derivative

■ **Clinical Pharmacology:**
  Mechanism of Action: An anti-irritable bowel syndrome (IBS) agent that binds to 5-HT$_4$ receptors in the GI tract. **Therapeutic Effect:** Triggers a peristaltic reflex in the gut, increasing bowel motility.
  Pharmacokinetics: Rapidly absorbed. Widely distributed. Protein binding: 98%. Metabolized by hydrolysis in the stomach and by oxidation and conjugation of the primary metabolite. Primarily excreted in feces. **Half-life:** 11 hr.

■ **Available Forms:**
- **Tablets:** 2 mg, 6 mg.

■ **Indications and Dosages:**
  IBS: PO 6 mg twice a day for 4–6 wk.
  Chronic constipation: PO 6 mg twice a day.

■ **Contraindications:** Abdominal adhesions, diarrhea, history of bowel obstruction, moderate to severe hepatic impairment, severe renal impairment, suspected sphincter of Oddi dysfunction, symptomatic gallbladder disease

1175

Side Effects
Frequent (greater than 5%)
Headache, abdominal pain, diarrhea, nausea, flatulence
Occasional (5%–2%)
Dizziness, migraine, back pain, extremity pain

Serious Reactions
- Ischemic colitis, mesenteric ischemia, gangrenous bowel, rectal bleeding, syncope, hypotension, hypovolemia, electrolyte disorders, suspected sphincter of Oddi spasm, bile duct stone, cholecystitis with elevated transaminases, and hypersensitivity reaction including rash, urticaria, pruritus, and serious allergic type I reactions have been reported.

Patient/Family Education
- Take before a meal
- Consult prescriber if severe diarrhea or diarrhea accompanied by cramping, abdominal pain, or dizziness occurs

Monitoring Parameters
- Therapeutic response (relief from abdominal discomfort, bloating, cramping, and urgency)

Geriatric side effects at a glance:
❑ CNS ☑ Bowel Dysfunction ❑ Bladder Dysfunction ❑ Falls

U.S. Regulatory Considerations
❑ FDA Black Box ❑ OBRA regulated in U.S. Long Term Care

telithromycin

(tell-ith'-roe-my-sin)

Brand Name(s): Ketek, Ketek Pak
Chemical Class: Macrolide derivative

Clinical Pharmacology:
Mechanism of Action: A ketolide that blocks protein synthesis by binding to ribosomal receptor sites on the bacterial cell wall. **Therapeutic Effect:** Bactericidal.
Pharmacokinetics: Protein binding: 60%-70%. More of drug is concentrated in WBCs than in plasma, and drug is eliminated more slowly from WBCs than from plasma. Partially metabolized by the liver. Minimally excreted in feces and urine. **Half-life:** 10 hr.

Available Forms:
- *Tablets* (*Ketek, Ketek Pak*): 400 mg.

■ **Indications and Dosages:**
Chronic bronchitis, sinusitis: PO 800 mg once a day for 5 days.
Community-acquired pneumonia: PO 800 mg once a day for 7-10 days.

■ **Unlabeled Uses:** Treatment of tonsillitis and pharyngitis due to *Streptococcus pyogenes*

■ **Contraindications:** Hypersensitivity to macrolide antibacterials, concurrent use of cisapride or pimozide

■ **Side Effects**
Occasional (11%-4%)
Diarrhea, nausea, headache, dizziness
Rare (3%-2%)
Vomiting, loose stools, altered taste, dry mouth, flatulence, visual disturbances

■ **Serious Reactions**
• Hepatic dysfunction, severe hypersensitivity reaction, and atrial arrhythmias occur rarely.
• Antibiotic-associated colitis and other superinfections may result from altered bacterial balance.

Special Considerations
• Individualize treatment based on local susceptibility patterns.

■ **Patient/Family Education**
• May take without regard to meals; swallow tabs whole.
• Do not take if you or a close relative has a rare heart condition called prolongation of the QT interval. Notify provider if you faint while on this medication
• Do not take with diuretics or if you have low blood potassium or magnesium levels
• Telithromycin may produce difficulty focusing that may last several hours after the first or second dose
• Avoid tasks that require mental alertness or motor skills until response to the drug has been established

■ **Monitoring Parameters**
• Pattern of daily bowel activity and stool consistency
• Hepatic function

■ **Geriatric side effects at a glance:**
❑ CNS ❑ Bowel Dysfunction ❑ Bladder Dysfunction ❑ Falls

■ **U.S. Regulatory Considerations**
❑ FDA Black Box ❑ OBRA regulated in U.S. Long Term Care

telmisartan

(tel-mi-sar'-tan)

■ **Brand Name(s):** Micardis
Chemical Class: Angiotensin II receptor antagonist

■ **Clinical Pharmacology:**
Mechanism of Action: An angiotensin II receptor, type AT_1, antagonist that blocks vasoconstrictor and aldosterone-secreting effects of angiotensin II, inhibiting the binding of angiotensin II to the AT_1 receptors. **Therapeutic Effect:** Causes vasodilation, decreases peripheral resistance, and decreases BP.
Pharmacokinetics: Rapidly and completely absorbed after PO administration. Protein binding: greater than 99%. Undergoes metabolism in the liver to inactive metabolite. Excreted in feces. Unknown if removed by hemodialysis. **Half-life:** 24 hr.

■ **Available Forms:**
  • *Tablets*: 20 mg, 40 mg, 80 mg.

■ **Indications and Dosages:**
Hypertension: PO 40 mg once a day. Range: 20-80 mg/day.

■ **Unlabeled Uses:** Treatment of CHF

■ **Contraindications:** None known.

■ **Side Effects**
Occasional (7%-3%)
Upper respiratory tract infection, sinusitis, back or leg pain, diarrhea
Rare (1%)
Dizziness, headache, fatigue, nausea, heartburn, myalgia, cough, peripheral edema

■ **Serious Reactions**
  • Overdosage may manifest as hypotension and tachycardia. Bradycardia occurs less often.
  • Hypoglycemia may occur in patients with diabetes using glucose-lowering drugs.

Special Considerations
  • Potentially as or more effective than angiotensin-converting enzyme inhibitors, without cough; no evidence for reduction in morbidity and mortality as first-line agents in hypertension, yet; whether they provide the same cardiac and renal protection also still tentative; like ACE inhibitors, less effective in black patients

■ **Patient/Family Education**
  • Call your clinician immediately if note following side effects: wheezing; lip, throat, or face swelling; hives or rash
  • Drink fluids to maintain proper hydration
  • Avoid excessive exertion during hot weather because of the risks of dehydration and hypotension

Monitoring Parameters

- Baseline electrolytes, urinalysis, blood urea nitrogen and creatinine with recheck at 2-4 wk after initiation (sooner in volume-depleted patients); monitor sitting blood pressure; watch for symptomatic hypotension, particularly in volume-depleted patients

Geriatric side effects at a glance:

❏ CNS ❏ Bowel Dysfunction ❏ Bladder Dysfunction ❏ Falls

U.S. Regulatory Considerations

☑ FDA Black Box

Although not relevant for geriatric patients, teratogenicity is associated with the use of angiotensin II receptor antagonists.

❏ OBRA regulated in U.S. Long Term Care

temazepam

(te-maz'-e-pam)

Brand Name(s): Restoril
Chemical Class: Benzodiazepine

DEA Class: Schedule IV

Clinical Pharmacology:

Mechanism of Action: A benzodiazepine that enhances the action of the inhibitory neurotransmitter gamma-aminobutyric acid, resulting in CNS depression. **Therapeutic Effect:** Induces sleep.

Pharmacokinetics: Well absorbed from the GI tract. Protein binding: 96%. Widely distributed. Crosses the blood-brain barrier. Metabolized in the liver. Primarily excreted in urine. Not removed by hemodialysis. **Half-life:** 4-18 hr.

Available Forms:

- Capsules: 7.5 mg, 15 mg, 22.5 mg, 30 mg.

Indications and Dosages:

Insomnia: PO 7.5-15 mg at bedtime.

Unlabeled Uses: Treatment of anxiety, depression, panic attacks

Contraindications: Angle-closure glaucoma; CNS depression; severe, uncontrolled pain; sleep apnea

Side Effects

Frequent

Somnolence, sedation, rebound insomnia (may occur for 1-2 nights after drug is discontinued), dizziness, confusion, euphoria

Occasional
Asthenia, anorexia, diarrhea
Rare
Paradoxical CNS excitement or restlessness

■ **Serious Reactions**
- Abrupt or too-rapid withdrawal may result in pronounced restlessness, irritability, insomnia, hand tremor, abdominal or muscle cramps, vomiting, diaphoresis, and seizures.
- Overdose results in somnolence, confusion, diminished reflexes, respiratory depression, and coma.

Special Considerations
- Good benzodiazepine choice for elderly and patients with liver disease (phase II metabolism and lack of active metabolites)

■ **Patient/Family Education**
- Withdrawal symptoms may occur if administered chronically and discontinued abruptly; symptoms include dysphoria, abdominal and muscle cramps, vomiting, sweating, tremor, and seizure
- May cause impairment the day following administration, exercise caution with hazardous tasks and driving
- Take temazepam about 30 min before bedtime
- Avoid alcohol and other CNS depressants during therapy

■ **Monitoring Parameters**
- Cardiovascular, mental, and respiratory status
- Therapeutic response, such as a decrease in the number of nocturnal awakenings and a longer duration of sleep
- Assess patients for paradoxical reactions, particularly during early therapy

■ **Geriatric side effects at a glance:**
☑ CNS ☐ Bowel Dysfunction ☐ Bladder Dysfunction ☑ Falls
Other: Withdrawal symptoms after long-term use

■ **Use with caution in older patients with:** COPD; untreated sleep apnea

■ **U.S. Regulatory Considerations**
☐ FDA Black Box ☑ OBRA regulated in U.S. Long Term Care

■ **Other Uses in Geriatric Patient:** Hypnotic

■ **Side Effects:**
Of particular importance in the geriatric patient: Sedation, withdrawal symptoms when abruptly discontinued (e.g., during hospitalization) rather than tapered

■ **Geriatric Considerations - Summary:** Benzodiazepines are effective anxiolytic agents, and hypnotics. These drugs should be reserved for short-term use. SSRIs are preferred for long-term management of anxiety disorders in older adults, and sedating antidepressants (e.g., trazodone) or eszopiclone are preferred for long-term management of sleep problems. Long-acting benzodiazepines, including flurazepam, chlordiazepoxide, clorazepate, diazepam, clonazepam, and quazepam should generally be avoided in older adults as these agents have been associated with oversedation. On the other hand, short-acting benzodiazepines (e.g., triazolam) have been associated with a higher risk of withdrawal symptoms. When initiating therapy, benzodiazepines should be titrated carefully to avoid oversedation. In addition, many of the drugs in this class have been associated with severe withdrawal symptoms (e.g., anxiety and/or agitation, seizures) when discontinued abruptly.

■ **References:**

1. Leipzig RM, Cumming RG, Tinetti ME. Drugs and falls in older people: a systematic review and meta-analysis: I. Psychotropic drugs. J Am Geriatr Soc 1999;47:30-39.
2. Shorr RI, Robin DW. Rational use of benzodiazepines in the elderly. Drugs Aging 1994;4:9-20.
3. Shader RI, Greenblatt DJ. Use of benzodiazepines in anxiety disorders. N Engl J Med 1993;328:1398-1405.

tenofovir disoproxil fumarate

(te-noe'-fo-veer dye-soe-prox'-il fyoo'-mar-ate)

■ **Brand Name(s):** Viread

Combinations
Rx: with emtricitabine (Truvada)
Chemical Class: Nucleotide analog

■ **Clinical Pharmacology:**
Mechanism of Action: A nucleotide analog that inhibits HIV reverse transcriptase by being incorporated into viral DNA, resulting in DNA chain termination. **Therapeutic Effect:** Slows HIV replication and reduces HIV RNA levels (viral load).
Pharmacokinetics: Bioavailability in fasted patients is approximately 25%. High-fat meals increase the bioavailability. Protein binding: 0.7%-7.2%. Excreted in urine. Removed by hemodialysis. **Half-life:** Unknown.

■ **Available Forms:**
• *Tablets:* 300 mg.

■ **Indications and Dosages:**
HIV infection (in combination with other antiretrovirals): PO 300 mg once a day.
Dosage in renal impairment:

Creatinine Clearance	Dosage
30-49 ml/min	300 mg q48h
10-29 ml/min	300 mg twice a wk
less than 10 ml/min	Not recommended

■ **Contraindications:** None known.

- **Side Effects**
  Occasional
  GI disturbances (diarrhea, flatulence, nausea, vomiting)

- **Serious Reactions**
  - Lactic acidosis and hepatomegaly with steatosis occur rarely, but may be severe.

Special Considerations
  - Always check updated treatment guidelines before initiating or changing antiretroviral therapy (http://AIDSinfo.nih.gov)

- **Patient/Family Education**
  - When co-administered with didanosine or lopinavir/ritonavir, take tenofovir 2 hours before or 1 hour after taking them
  - Take tenofovir with a meal to increase the drug's absorption
  - Continue drug therapy for the full course of treatment
  - Notify the physician of nausea, vomiting, or persistent abdominal pain
  - Tenofovir is not a cure for HIV infection, nor does it reduce the risk of transmitting HIV to others

- **Monitoring Parameters**
  - CBC with platelet count, renal function, liver enzymes
  - CD4+ cell count, Hgb and HIV RNA plasma levels, and reticulocyte count
  - Pattern of daily bowel activity and stool consistency

- **Geriatric side effects at a glance:**
  ❑ CNS   ❑ Bowel Dysfunction   ❑ Bladder Dysfunction   ❑ Falls

- **U.S. Regulatory Considerations**
  ☑ FDA Black Box
  - Lactic acidosis and hepatomegaly reported with steatosis.
  - Tenofovir is not indicated for chronic hepatitis B virus (HBV) infection. Safety and efficacy have not been established in patients with HBV and HIV. Severe acute exacerbation of HBV infection has been reported in co-infected patients.
  ❑ OBRA regulated in U.S. Long Term Care

terazosin hydrochloride

(ter-a'-zoe-sin hye-droe-klor'-ide)

- **Brand Name(s):** Hytrin
  Chemical Class: Quinazoline derivative

- **Clinical Pharmacology:**
  Mechanism of Action: An antihypertensive and benign prostatic hyperplasia agent that blocks alpha-adrenergic receptors. Produces vasodilation, decreases peripheral

resistance, and targets receptors around bladder neck and prostate. **Therapeutic Effect:** In hypertension, decreases BP. In benign prostatic hyperplasia, relaxes smooth muscle and improves urine flow.

Pharmacokinetics:

Route	Onset	Peak	Duration
PO	15 min	1-2 hr	12-24 hr

Rapidly, completely absorbed from the GI tract. Protein binding: 90%-94%. Metabolized in the liver to active metabolite. Primarily eliminated in feces via biliary system; excreted in urine. Not removed by hemodialysis. **Half-life:** 12 hr.

■ **Available Forms:**
- *Capsules:* 1 mg, 2 mg, 5 mg, 10 mg.
- *Tablets:* 1 mg, 2 mg, 5 mg, 10 mg.

■ **Indications and Dosages:**
Mild to moderate hypertension: PO Initially, 1 mg at bedtime. Slowly increase dosage to desired levels. Range: 1–5 mg/day as single or 2 divided doses. Maximum: 20 mg.
Benign prostatic hyperplasia: PO Initially, 1 mg at bedtime. May increase up to 10 mg/day. Maximum: 20 mg/day.

■ **Contraindications:** None known.

■ **Side Effects**
Frequent (9%-5%)
Dizziness, headache, unusual tiredness
Rare (less than 2%)
Peripheral edema, orthostatic hypotension, myalgia, arthralgia, blurred vision, nausea, vomiting, nasal congestion, somnolence

■ **Serious Reactions**
- First-dose syncope (hypotension with sudden loss of consciousness) may occur 30 to 90 minutes after initial dose of 2 mg or more, a too-rapid increase in dosage, or addition of another antihypertensive agent to therapy. First-dose syncope may be preceded by tachycardia (pulse rate of 120-160 beats/minute).

Special Considerations
- The doxazosin arm of the ALLHAT study was stopped early; the doxazosin group had a 25% greater risk of combined cardiovascular disease events which was primarily accounted for by a doubled risk of CHF vs the chlorthalidone group; doxazosin was also found to be less effective at controlling systolic BP an average of 3 mm Hg; may want to consider primary antihypertensives in addition to α-blockers for BPH symptoms
- Use as a single antihypertensive agent limited by tendency to cause sodium and water retention and increased plasma volume

■ **Patient/Family Education**
- Alert patients to the possibility of syncopal and orthostatic symptoms, especially with the first dose ("1st dose syncope"); initial dose should be administered at bedtime in the smallest possible dose
- Nasal congestion may occur
- Full therapeutic effect of terazosin may not occur for 3 to 4 weeks
- Use caution when driving, performing tasks requiring mental alertness, and rising from a sitting or lying position

- Notify the physician if dizziness or palpitations occur

■ **Monitoring Parameters**
- Blood pressure, pulse

■ **Geriatric side effects at a glance:**
☑ CNS ☐ Bowel Dysfunction ☐ Bladder Dysfunction ☑ Falls
Other: Orthostatic hypotension, worsening of urge or mixed urinary incontinence

■ **Use with caution in older patients with:** Congestive heart failure, patients taking medications for impotence (e.g., vardenafil, sildenafil, or tadalafil).

■ **U.S. Regulatory Considerations**
☐ FDA Black Box ☐ OBRA regulated in U.S. Long Term Care

■ **Other Uses in Geriatric Patient:** Symptoms related to benign prostatic hypertrophy

■ **Side Effects:**
Of particular importance in the geriatric patient: Orthostatic hypotension, worsening of urge or mixed urinary incontinence

■ **Geriatric Considerations - Summary:** Alpha-adrenergic blockers are modestly effective alone, and in combination with 5-alpha reductase inhibitors (e.g., finasteride) in the treatment of urinary obstructive symptoms related to benign prostatic hyperplasia. The main side effect of these agents is orthostatic hypotension, and in hypertensive patients, these agents may increase the risk of congestive heart failure as reported in the ALLHAT study.

■ **References:**
1. Lepor H, Williford WO, Barry MJ, et al. The efficacy of terazosin, finasteride, or both in benign prostatic hyperplasia. Veterans Affairs Cooperative Studies Benign Prostatic Hyperplasia Study Group. N Engl J Med 1996;335:533-539.
2. McConnell JD, Roehrborn CG, Bautista OM, et al. The long-term effect of doxazosin, finasteride, and combination therapy on the clinical progression of benign prostatic hyperplasia. N Engl J Med 2003;349:2387-2398.
3. Major cardiovascular events in hypertensive patients randomized to doxazosin vs chlorthalidone: the antihypertensive and lipid-lowering treatment to prevent heart attack trial (ALLHAT). ALLHAT Collaborative Research Group. JAMA 2000;283:1967-1975.

terbinafine hydrochloride

(ter-bin'-a-feen hye-droe-klor'-ide)

■ **Brand Name(s):** Lamisil, Lamisil AT
Chemical Class: Allylamine derivative

■ **Clinical Pharmacology:**
Mechanism of Action: A fungicidal antifungal that inhibits the enzyme squalene epoxidase, thereby interfering with fungal biosynthesis. **Therapeutic Effect:** Results in death of fungal cells.

Pharmacokinetics: Well absorbed following PO administration. Protein binding: 99%. Metabolized by liver. Primarily excreted in urine; minimal elimination in feces. **Half-life:** (oral): 36 hr, (topical): 22-26 hr.

- ■ **Available Forms:**
  - • *Tablets (Lamisil):* 250 mg.
  - • *Cream (Lamisil AT):* 1%.
  - • *Topical Solution (Lamisil, Lamisil AT):* 1% .
  - • *Topical Spray (Lamisil AT):* 1%.

- ■ **Indications and Dosages:**

  Tinea pedis: Topical Apply twice a day until signs and symptoms significantly improve.

  Tinea cruris, tinea corporis: Topical Apply 1-2 times a day until signs and symptoms significantly improve.

  Onychomycosis: PO 250 mg/day for 6 wk (fingernails) or 12 wk (toenails).

  Tinea versicolor: Topical Solution Apply to the affected area twice a day for 7 days.

  Systemic mycosis: PO 250-500 mg/day for up to 16 mo.

- ■ **Contraindications:** None known.

- ■ **Side Effects**

  Frequent (13%)

  Oral: Headache

  Occasional (6%-3%)

  Oral: Diarrhea, rash, dyspepsia, pruritus, taste disturbance, nausea, abdominal pain, flatulence, urticaria, visual disturbance

  Topical: Irritation, burning, pruritus, dryness

- ■ **Serious Reactions**
  - • Hepatobiliary dysfunction (including cholestatic hepatitis), serious skin reactions, and severe neutropenia occur rarely.
  - • Ocular lens and retinal changes have been noted.

- ■ **Patient/Family Education**
  - • Optimal clinical effect in onychomycosis may not be apparent for several months following completion of therapy
  - • Rub topical terbinafine well into the affected and surrounding areas and do not cover the treated area with an occlusive dressing
  - • Keep the affected area clean and dry and wear light clothing to promote ventilation
  - • Separate personal items that come in contact with the affected area
  - • Do not let topical forms come in contact with eyes, mouth, nose, or other mucous membranes
  - • Notify the physician if diarrhea or skin irritation occurs

- ■ **Monitoring Parameters**
  - • Topical terbinafine should be used for at least 1 week but no more than 4 weeks
  - • Assess for signs of a therapeutic response
  - • Discontinue the drug and notify the physician if a local reaction (such as blistering, burning, irritation, pruritus, oozing, erythema, or edema) occurs

■ **Geriatric side effects at a glance:**
  ☑ CNS ☐ Bowel Dysfunction ☐ Bladder Dysfunction ☐ Falls

■ **U.S. Regulatory Considerations**
  ☐ FDA Black Box ☐ OBRA regulated in U.S. Long Term Care

terbutaline sulfate

(ter-byoo'-ta-leen sul'-fate)

■ **Brand Name(s):** Brethine
  Chemical Class: Sympathomimetic amine; β_2-adrenergic agonist

■ **Clinical Pharmacology:**
  Mechanism of Action: An adrenergic agonist that stimulates beta$_2$-adrenergic receptors, resulting in relaxation of uterine and bronchial smooth muscle. **Therapeutic Effect:** Relieves bronchospasm and reduces airway resistance. Also inhibits uterine contractions.
  Pharmacokinetics: Partially absorbed in GI tract following oral administration. Protein binding: 14%-25%. Metabolized in liver. Excreted in feces and urine. **Half-life:** 3-4 hr.

■ **Available Forms:**
  • *Tablets*: 2.5 mg, 5 mg.
  • *Injection*: 1 mg/ml.

■ **Indications and Dosages:**
  Bronchospasm: PO Initially, 2.5 mg 3–4 times a day. Maintenance: 2.5–5 mg 3 times a day q6h while awake. Maximum: 15 mg/day. Subcutaneous Initially, 0.25 mg. Repeat in 15–30 min if substantial improvement does not occur. Maximum: 0.5 mg/4 hr.

■ **Contraindications:** History of hypersensitivity to sympathomimetics

■ **Side Effects**
  Frequent (23%–18%)
  Tremor, anxiety
  Occasional (11%–10%)
  Somnolence, headache, nausea, heartburn, dizziness
  Rare (3%–1%)
  Flushing, asthenia, mouth and throat dryness or irritation (with inhalation therapy)

■ **Serious Reactions**
  • Too-frequent or excessive use may lead to decreased drug effectiveness and severe, paradoxical bronchoconstriction.
  • Excessive sympathomimetic stimulation may cause palpitations, extrasystoles, tachycardia, chest pain, a slight increase in BP followed by a substantial decrease, chills, diaphoresis, and blanching of skin.

Patient/Family Education
- Notify the physician if chest pain, difficulty breathing, dizziness, flushing, headache, muscle tremors, or palpitations occur
- May cause anxiety, nervousness, and shakiness
- Avoid excessive consumption of caffeinated products, such as chocolate, cocoa, cola, coffee, and tea

Monitoring Parameters
- Pulse rate and quality and respiratory rate, depth, rhythm, and type
- Breath sounds for rhonchi and wheezing
- Serum potassium level
- ABG levels
- Observe the patient's fingernails and lips for a blue or dusky color in light-skinned patients and a gray color in dark-skinned patients, which are signs of hypoxemia
- Clinical improvement, such as cessation of clavicular retractions, quieter and slower respirations, and a relaxed facial expression

Geriatric side effects at a glance:
☑ CNS   ☐ Bowel Dysfunction   ☐ Bladder Dysfunction   ☐ Falls

U.S. Regulatory Considerations
☐ FDA Black Box   ☑ OBRA regulated in U.S. Long Term Care

terconazole

(ter-kon'-a-zole)

Brand Name(s): Terazol 3, Terazol 7
Chemical Class: Triazole derivative

Clinical Pharmacology:
Mechanism of Action: An antifungal that disrupts fungal cell membrane permeability.
Therapeutic Effect: Produces antifungal activity.
Pharmacokinetics: Extent of systemic absorption after vaginal administration may be dependent on presence of a uterus: 5%-8% in women who had a hysterectomy versus 12%-16% in nonhysterectomized women.

Available Forms:
- *Suppository*: 80 mg (Terazol 3).
- *Cream*: 0.4 % (Terazol 7), 0.8% (Terazol 3).

Indications and Dosages:
Vulvovaginal candidiasis: Intravaginal Suppository: 1 vaginally at bedtime for 3 days .Cream: 1 applicatorful at bedtime for 7 days (0.4% cream) or for 3 days (0.8% cream).

- **Contraindications:** Hypersensitivity to terconazole or any component of the formulation

- **Side Effects**
  Frequent
  Headache, vulvovaginal burning
  Occasional
  Pain in female genitalia, abdominal pain, fever, itching
  Rare
  Chills

- **Serious Reactions**
  - Flu-like syndrome has been reported.

Special Considerations

- No significant advantage over less expensive OTC products

- **Patient/Family Education**
  - Insert the vaginal form high into the vagina
  - Complete for the full course of therapy
  - Notify the physician if itching or burning occurs

- **Monitoring Parameters**
  - Watch for local irritation

- **Geriatric side effects at a glance:**
  ❏ CNS   ❏ Bowel Dysfunction   ❏ Bladder Dysfunction   ❏ Falls

- **U.S. Regulatory Considerations**
  ❏ FDA Black Box   ❏ OBRA regulated in U.S. Long Term Care

teriparatide (rDNA origin)

(ter-i-par'-a-tide)

- **Brand Name(s):** Forteo
  Chemical Class: Recombinant human ENDO-parathyroid hormone (rDNA origin)

- **Clinical Pharmacology:**
  Mechanism of Action: A synthetic polypeptide hormone that acts on bone to mobilize calcium; also acts on kidney to reduce calcium clearance, increase phosphate excretion. **Therapeutic Effect:** Promotes an increased rate of release of calcium from bone into blood, stimulates new bone formation.

- **Available Forms:**
  - *Injection:* 3 ml prefilled pen containing 750 mcg teriparatide (Forteo).

- **Indications and Dosages:**
  Osteoporosis: SC 20 mcg once daily into the thigh or abdominal wall.

- **Contraindications:** Serum calcium above normal level, those at increased risk for osteosarcoma (Paget's disease, unexplained elevations of alkaline phosphatase, open epiphyses, prior radiation therapy that included the skeleton), hypercalcemic disorder (e.g., hyperparathyroidism), hypersensitivity to teriparatide or any of the components of the formulation

- **Side Effects**
  Occasional
  Leg cramps, nausea, dizziness, headache, orthostatic hypotension, increased heart rate

- **Serious Reactions**
  - None known.

Special Considerations

  - Treatment not recommended beyond 2 yr as safety and efficacy not established
  - Postural hypotension, if it occurs, happens within 4 hr and with the first several doses; does not preclude continued treatment
  - Inform patients teriparatide caused osteosarcoma in rats; clinical relevance in humans unknown
  - Maximal serum calcium levels occur 4-6 hr post dose

- **Patient/Family Education**
  - Initially administer lying down (postural hypotension)
  - Inject into thigh or abdominal wall
  - Refrigerate, minimize time out of refrigerator
  - Recap pen to protect from light
  - Discard if not used within 28 days
  - Notify provider of nausea, vomiting, constipation, lethargy, muscle weakness (possible hypercalcemia)

- **Monitoring Parameters**
  - Bone mineral density, parathyroid hormone level, and urinary and serum calcium levels
  - Blood pressure for hypotension and pulse rate for tachycardia
  - Signs and symptoms of hypercalcemia

- **Geriatric side effects at a glance:**
  ❑ CNS ❑ Bowel Dysfunction ❑ Bladder Dysfunction ❑ Falls

- **U.S. Regulatory Considerations**
  ☑ FDA Black Box
  There is an increased risk of osteosarcoma. Avoid in Paget's disease and other conditions which increase the risk of osteosarcoma.
  ❑ OBRA regulated in U.S. Long Term Care

testosterone

(tes tos' ter one)

- **Brand Name(s):** Androderm, AndroGel, Delatestryl, Depandro 100, Depo-Testoster-one, FIRST-Testosterone, FIRST-Testosterone MC, Striant, Testim, Testoderm, Testo-derm TTS, Testopel, Testro AQ, Testro-L.A.
  Chemical Class: Androgen

  DEA Class: Schedule III

- **Clinical Pharmacology:**
  Mechanism of Action: A primary endogenous androgen that promotes growth and development of male sex organs and maintains secondary sex characteristics in androgen-deficient males. **Therapeutic Effect:** Helps relieve androgen deficiency.
  Pharmacokinetics: Well absorbed after IM administration. Protein binding: 98%. Undergoes first-pass metabolism in the liver. Primarily excreted in urine. Unknown if removed by hemodialysis. **Half-life:** 10–20 min.

- **Available Forms:**
  - Cypionate Injection (Depo-Testosterone): 100 mg/ml, 200 mg/ml.
  - Ethanate Injection (Andro LA 200, Delatestryl, Testro-L.A.): 200 mg/ml.
  - Propionate Injection Solution (Depandro 100): 100 mg/ml.
  - Intramuscular Solution: 50 mg/ml (Testro AQ), 100 mg/ml (Testro AQ).
  - Subcutaneous Pellets (Testopel): 75 mg.
  - Topical Gel: 25 mg/2.5 g (AndroGel), 50 mg/5 g (AndroGel, Testim).
  - Topical Cream (FIRST-Testosterone MC): 2%.
  - Topical Ointment (FIRST-Testosterone): 2%.
  - Transdermal Patch: 2.5 mg/day (Androderm), 4 mg/day (Testoderm), 5 mg/day (Androderm), 6 mg/day (Testoderm).
  - Buccal (Striant): 30 mg.

- **Indications and Dosages:**
  Male hypogonadism: IM 50-400 mg q2-4wk. Subcutaneous (Pellets) 150-450 mg q3-6mo. Transdermal (Patch [Testoderm]) Start therapy with 6 mg/day patch. Apply patch to scrotal skin. Transdermal (Patch [Testoderm TTS]) Apply TTS patch to arm, back, or upper buttocks Transdermal (Patch [Androderm]) Start therapy with 5 mg/day patch applied at night. Apply patch to abdomen, back, thighs, or upper arms. Transdermal (Gel [AndroGel]) Initial dose of 5 mg delivers 50 mg testosterone and is applied once daily to the abdomen, shoulders, or upper arms. May increase to 7.5 g, then to 10 g, if necessary. Transdermal (Gel [Testim]) Initial dose of 5g delivers 50 mg testosterone and is applied once a day to the shoulders or upper arms. May increase to 10 g. Buccal System (Striant) 30 mg q12h.
  Breast carcinoma: IM (testosterone aqueous) 50–100 mg 3 times a week. IM (testosterone cypionate or testosterone ethanate) 200–400 mg q2–4wk. IM (testosterone propionate) 50–100 mg 3 times a week.

- **Contraindications:** Cardiac impairment, hypercalcemia, prostate or breast cancer in males, severe hepatic or renal disease

Side Effects

Frequent

Gynecomastia, acne

Females: Hirsutism, deepening of voice, clitoral enlargement that may not be reversible when drug is discontinued

Occasional

Edema, nausea, insomnia, oligospermia, priapism, male-pattern baldness, bladder irritability, hypercalcemia (in immobilized patients or those with breast cancer), hypercholesterolemia, inflammation and pain at IM injection site

Transdermal: Pruritus, erythema, skin irritation

Rare

Polycythemia (with high dosage), hypersensitivity

Serious Reactions

- Peliosis hepatis (presence of blood-filled cysts in parenchyma of liver), hepatic neoplasms, and hepatocellular carcinoma have been associated with prolonged high-dose therapy.
- Anaphylactic reactions occur rarely.

Patient/Family Education

- Apply the patch to a clean, dry, hairless area of the skin, avoiding bony prominences
- Do not take any other medications, including OTC drugs, without first consulting the physician
- Consume a diet high in calories and protein; food may be better tolerated if he or she eats small, frequent meals
- Weigh oneself every day and report to the physician weight gain of 5 lb or more per week
- Notify the physician if acne, nausea, vomiting, or foot swelling occurs
- The female patient should promptly report deepening of the voice and hoarseness
- The male patient should report difficulty urinating, frequent erections, and gynecomastia
- Regular monitoring tests and visits to the physician are important

Monitoring Parameters

- LFTs, lipids, Hct and Hgb
- Blood pressure
- Weight
- Intake and output
- Electrolytes
- Signs of virilization

Geriatric side effects at a glance:

❏ CNS   ❏ Bowel Dysfunction   ❏ Bladder Dysfunction   ❏ Falls

U.S. Regulatory Considerations

❏ FDA Black Box   ❏ OBRA regulated in U.S. Long Term Care

tetracaine hydrochloride

(tet'-ra-cane hye-droe-klor'-ide)

- **Brand Name(s):** AK-T Caine, Opticaine, Pontocaine
  OTC: Cepacol, Viractin
  Chemical Class: Benzoic acid derivative

- **Clinical Pharmacology:**
  Mechanism of Action: Tetracaine causes a reversible blockade of nerve conduction by decreasing nerve membrane permeability to sodium. **Therapeutic Effect:** Local anesthetic.
  Pharmacokinetics: Systemic absorption of tetracaine is variable. Metabolized by plasma pseudocholinesterase. Excreted in the urine.

- **Available Forms:**
  - *Solution for injection*: 0.2%, 0.3%, 1%, 2% (Pontocaine)
  - *Cream*: 1%
  - *Ointment*: 0.5%

- **Indications and Dosages:**
  Anesthesia of the lower abdomen: Spinal 3-4 ml (9-12 mg) of a 0.3% solution
  Anesthesia of the perineum: Spinal 1-2 ml (3-6 mg) of a 0.3% solution
  Anesthesia of the upper abdomen: Spinal 5 ml (15 mg) of a 0.3% solution
  Anesthesia of the perineum: Intrathecal 0.5 ml (5 mg) of a 1% solution, diluted with equal amount of CSF or 10% dextrose injection.
  Anesthesia of the perineum and lower extremities: Intrathecal 1 ml (10 mg) as a 1% solution, diluted with equal amount of CSF or 10% dextrose injection.
  Anesthesia up to the costal margin: Intrathecal 1.5-2 ml (15-20 mg) of a 1% solution, diluted with equal amount of CSF.
  Topical anesthesia: Topical Apply to the affected areas as needed. Maximum dosage: 28g/24 hr.
  Topical anesthesia of nose and throat, abolish laryngeal and esophageal reflexes prior to diagnostic procedure: Topical Direct application of a 0.25% or 0.5% topical solution or by oral inhalation of a nebulized 0.5% solution. Total dose should not exceed 20 mg.
  Mild pain, burning and/or pruritus associated with herpes labialis (cold sores or fever blisters): Topical Apply to the affected area no more than 3-4 times a day.
  Ophthalmic anesthesia: Topical 1-2 drops of a 0.5% solution.

- **Contraindications:** Hypersensitivity to esther local anesthetics, sulfites, PABA, infection or inflammation at the injection site, bacteremia, platelet abnormalities, thrombocytopenia, increased bleeding time, uncontrolled coagulopathy, anticoagulant therapy, sulfonamide therapy.

- **Side Effects**
  Frequent
  Burning, stinging, or tenderness, skin rash, itching, redness, or inflammation, numbness or tingling of the face or mouth, pain at the injection site, sensitivity to light, swelling of the eye or eyelid, watering or the eyes, acute ocular pain and ocular irritation (burning, stinging, or redness)

Occasional

Paresthesias, weakness and paralysis of lower extremity, hypotension, high or total spinal block, urinary retention or incontinence, fecal incontinence, headache, back pain, septic meningitis, meningismus, arachnoiditis, shivering cranial nerve palsies due to traction on nerves from loss of CSF, and loss of perineal sensation and sexual function

Rare

Anxiety, restlessness, difficulty breathing, shortness of breath, dizziness, drowsiness, light-headedness, nausea, vomiting, seizures (convulsions), slow, irregular heartbeat (palpitations), swelling of the face or mouth, skin rash, itching (hives), tremors, visual impairment.

- ■ **Serious Reactions**
  - Tetracaine-induced CNS toxicity usually presents with symptoms of CNS stimulation such as anxiety, apprehension, restlessness, nervousness, disorientation, confusion, dizziness, tinnitus, blurred vision, tremor, and/or seizures. Subsequently, depressive symptoms may occur including drowsiness, respiratory arrest, or coma.
  - Depression or cardiac excitability and contractility may cause AV block, ventricular arrhythmias, or cardiac arrest. Symptoms of local anesthetic CNS toxicity, such as dizziness, tongue numbness, visual impairment or disturbances, and muscular twitching appear to occur before cardiotoxic effects. Cardiotoxic effects include angina, QT prolongation, PR prolongation, atrial fibrillation, sinus bradycardia, hypotension, palpitations, and cardiovascular collapse.
  - *Alert* Tetracaine is more likely than any other topical anesthetic to cause contact reactions, including skin rash (unspecified), mucous membrane irritation, erythema, pruritus, urticaria, burning, stinging, edema, or tenderness.

Special Considerations

- Previously used as component of "Magic Numbing Solution" or TAC Sol (epinephrine 1:2,000, tetracaine 0.5%, cocaine 11.8%) and LET Sol (lidocaine 4%, epinephrine 0.1%, tetracaine 0.5%), which are used as topical anesthesia for repair of minor lacerations. Topical tetracain solutions no longer available

- ■ **Patient/Family Education**
  - Notify the physician of any trouble breathing

- ■ **Monitoring Parameters**
  - Assess the effectiveness of anesthesia

- ■ **Geriatric side effects at a glance:**
  - ❏ CNS ❏ Bowel Dysfunction ❏ Bladder Dysfunction ❏ Falls

- ■ **U.S. Regulatory Considerations**
  - ❏ FDA Black Box ❏ OBRA regulated in U.S. Long Term Care

tetracycline hydrochloride

(tet-ra-sye'-kleen hye-droe-klor'-ide)

- **Brand Name(s):** Ala-Tet, Panmycin, Sumycin, Tetracon
  Chemical Class: Tetracycline

- **Clinical Pharmacology:**
  Mechanism of Action: A tetracycline antibacterial that inhibits bacterial protein synthesis by binding to ribosomes. **Therapeutic Effect:** Bacteriostatic.
  Pharmacokinetics: Readily absorbed from the GI tract. Protein binding: 30%-60%. Widely distributed. Excreted in urine; eliminated in feces through biliary system. Not removed by hemodialysis. **Half-life:** 6-11 hr (increased in impaired renal function).

- **Available Forms:**
  - *Capsules:* 250 mg (Ala-Tet, Panmycin, Sumycin, Tetracon), 500 mg (Sumycin, Tetracon).
  - *Oral Suspension (Sumycin):* 125 mg/5 ml.
  - *Tablets (Sumycin):* 250 mg, 500 mg.
  - *Topical Solution.* 2.2 mg/ml.
  - *Topical Ointment:* 3%.

- **Indications and Dosages:**
  Inflammatory acne vulgaris, Lyme disease, mycoplasmal disease, Legionella infections, Rocky Mountain spotted fever, chlamydial infections in patients with gonorrhea: PO 250-500 mg q6-12h.
  Helicobacter pylori infections: PO 500 mg 2-4 times a day (in combination). Topical Apply twice a day (once in the morning, once in the evening).
  Dosage in renal impairment: Dosage interval is modified based on creatinine clearance.

Creatinine Clearance	Dosage Interval
50-80 ml/min	Usual dose q8-12h
10-50 ml/min	Usual dose q12-24h
less than 10 ml/min	Usual dose q24h

- **Contraindications:** Hypersensitivity to sulfites

- **Side Effects**
  Frequent
  Dizziness, light-headedness, diarrhea, nausea, vomiting, abdominal cramps, possibly severe photosensitivity
  Topical: Dry, scaly skin; stinging or burning sensation
  Occasional
  Pigmentation of skin or mucous membranes, rectal or genital pruritus, stomatitis
  Topical: Pain, redness, swelling, or other skin irritation.

- **Serious Reactions**
  - Superinfection (especially fungal), anaphylaxis, and benign intracranial hypertension may occur.

  • Individualize treatment based on local susceptibility patterns.

■ **Patient/Family Education**
  • Avoid milk products, antacids, or separate by 2 hr; take with a full glass of water
  • Side effects noted for systemic administration not observed with topical formulations
  • Take oral tetracycline on an empty stomach
  • Space drug doses evenly around the clock and continue taking tetracycline for the full course of treatment
  • Notify the physician if diarrhea, rash, or any other new symptoms occur
  • Avoid overexposure to the sun or ultraviolet light to prevent photosensitivity reactions
  • Do not take any other medications, including OTC drugs, without consulting the physician
  • Topical tetracycline may turn skin yellow but washing removes the solution; fabrics may be stained by heavy topical application
  • Do not apply topical tetracycline to deep or open wounds
  • Avoid performing tasks that require mental alertness or motor skills until response to the drug has been established

■ **Monitoring Parameters**
  • Skin for rash
  • Blood pressure
  • Daily bowel activity and stool consistency. Although mild GI effects may be tolerable, severe symptoms may indicate the onset of antibiotic-associated colitis.
  • Signs and symptoms of superinfection include abdominal pain or cramping, anal or genital pruritus or discharge, moderate to severe diarrhea, severe mouth or tongue soreness, and new or increased fever.

■ **Geriatric side effects at a glance:**
  ☑ CNS ☐ Bowel Dysfunction ☐ Bladder Dysfunction ☐ Falls

■ **U.S. Regulatory Considerations**
  ☐ FDA Black Box ☐ OBRA regulated in U.S. Long Term Care

tetrahydrozoline hydrochloride

(tet-ra-hye-droz'-a-leen hye-droe-klor'-ide)

■ **Brand Name(s):** Tyzine
  OTC: Visine
  Chemical Class: Sympathomimetic amine

- **Clinical Pharmacology:**
  Mechanism of Action: A vasoconstrictor that stimulates alpha-adrenergic receptors in sympathetic nervous system. Constricts arterioles. **Therapeutic Effect:** Reduces redness, irritation, and congestion.
  Pharmacokinetics: May be systemically absorbed. Metabolic, elimination rates unknown.

- **Available Forms:**
  - *Nasal Solution*: 0.05%, 0.1% (Tyzine).
  - *Ophthalmic Solution*: 0.05% (Visine).

- **Indications and Dosages:**
  Conjunctivitis: Ophthalmic 1-2 drops 2-4 times/day.
  Rhinitis: Intranasal 2-4 drops (0.1% solution) to each nostril q4-6h (no sooner than q3h).

- **Contraindications:** Narrow-angle glaucoma or other serious eye diseases, hypersensitivity to tetrahydrozoline or any component of the formulation

- **Side Effects**
  Occasional
  Intranasal: Transient burning, stinging, sneezing, dryness of mucosa. Prolonged use may result in rebound congestion.
  Ophthalmic: Irritation, blurred vision, mydriasis
  Systemic sympathomimetic effects may occur with either route: headache, hypertension, weakness, sweating, palpitations, tremors.

- **Serious Reactions**
  - Large doses may produce tachycardia, hypertension, arrhythmias, palpitations, light-headedness, nausea, and vomiting.
  - Overdosage may produce hallucinations, CNS depression, and seizures.

Special Considerations
  - Manage rebound congestion by stopping tetrahydrozoline: one nostril at a time, substitute systemic decongestant and/or substitute inhaled steroid

- **Patient/Family Education**
  - Do not use for >3-5 days or rebound congestion may occur
  - Discontinue and consult physician immediately if ocular pain or visual changes occur or if condition worsens or continues for more than 72 hr

- **Geriatric side effects at a glance:**
  ❑ CNS ❑ Bowel Dysfunction ❑ Bladder Dysfunction ❑ Falls

- **U.S. Regulatory Considerations**
  ❑ FDA Black Box ❑ OBRA regulated in U.S. Long Term Care

thalidomide

(tha-li'-doe-mide)

■ **Brand Name(s):** Thalomid
   Chemical Class: Glutamic acid derivative

■ **Clinical Pharmacology:**
   Mechanism of Action: An immunomodulator whose exact mechanism is unknown. Has sedative, anti-inflammatory, and immunosuppressive activity, which may be due to selective inhibition of the production of tumor necrosis factor-alpha. **Therapeutic Effect:** Improves muscle wasting in HIV patients; reduces local and systemic effects of leprosy.
   Pharmacokinetics: Protein binding: 55%. Metabolism and elimination are not known.
   Half-life: 5-7 hr.

■ **Available Forms:**
- *Capsules*: 50 mg, 100 mg, 200 mg.

■ **Indications and Dosages:**
   AIDS-*related muscle wasting*: PO 100–300 mg a day.
   Leprosy: PO Initially, 100-300 mg/day as single bedtime dose, at least 1 hr after the evening meal. Continue until active reaction subsides, then reduce dose q2-4wk in 50-mg increments.

■ **Unlabeled Uses:** Prevention and treatment of discoid lupus erythematosus, erythema multiforme, graft vs host reactions following bone marrow transplantation, rheumatoid arthritis; treatment of Behçet's syndrome, Crohn's disease, GI bleeding, multiple myeloma, pruritus, recurrent aphthous ulcers in HIV patients, wasting syndrome associated with HIV or cancer

■ **Contraindications:** Neutropenia, peripheral neuropathy

■ **Side Effects**
   Frequent
   Somnolence, dizziness, mood changes, constipation, dry mouth, peripheral neuropathy
   Occasional
   Increased appetite, weight gain, headache, loss of libido, edema of face and limbs, nausea, alopecia, dry skin, rash, hypothyroidism

■ **Serious Reactions**
- Neutropenia, peripheral neuropathy, and thromboembolism occur rarely.

■ **Patient/Family Education**
- Teratogenic in human whether taken by male or female
- Sedation common; usually taken at bedtime

- Avoid consuming alcohol or using other drugs that cause drowsiness during thalidomide therapy
- Avoid performing tasks that require mental alertness or motor skills until response to the drug has been established

■ **Monitoring Parameters**
- ALT, AST
- CBC
- Signs and symptoms of peripheral neuropathy

■ **Geriatric side effects at a glance:**
☑ CNS ❏ Bowel Dysfunction ❏ Bladder Dysfunction ❏ Falls

■ **U.S. Regulatory Considerations**
☑ FDA Black Box
- Restricted distribution program requiring registered prescribers and pharmacists in the S.T.E.P.S. program (System for Thalidomide Education and Prescribing Safety).
- Male patients must always use a latex condom during sexual contact with women of childbearing potential even if a successful vasectomy has been performed. Thalidomide is present in the semen of patients taking the drug. Report suspected fetal exposure to thalidomide to FDA (1-800-FDA-1088).
- The use of Thalomid (thalidomide) in multiple myeloma results in an increased risk of venous thromboembolic events, such as deep venous thrombosis and pulmonary embolus. This risk increases significantly when thalidomide is used in combination with standard chemotherapeutic agents including dexamethasone. Patients and physicians are advised to be observant for the signs and symptoms of thromboembolism. Patients should be instructed to seek medical care if they develop symptoms such as shortness of breath, chest pain, or arm or leg swelling. Preliminary data suggest that patients who are appropriate candidates may benefit from concurrent prophylactic anticoagulation or aspirin treatment.
❏ OBRA regulated in U.S. Long Term Care

theophylline

(thee-off'-i-lin)

■ **Brand Name(s):** Elixophyllin, Slo-Bid Gyrocaps, Quibron-T, Theochron, Theo-Dur, Theolair, Theo-Time, Theolair SR, T-Phyl, Truxophyllin, Uni-Dur, Uniphyl

Combinations
Rx: with guaifenesin (Elixophyllin-GG, Quibron); with potassium iodide (Elixophylline KI)
Chemical Class: Xanthine derivative

■ **Clinical Pharmacology:**
Mechanism of Action: An antiasthmatic medication with two distinct actions in the airways of patients with reversible obstruction: smooth muscle relaxation and sup-

pression of the response of airways to stimuli. Mechanisms of action are not known with certainty. It is known theophylline increases force of contraction of diaphragmatic muscles by enhancing calcium uptake through adenosine-mediated channels. **Therapeutic Effect:** Causes bronchodilation and decreased airway reactivity.

Pharmacokinetics: The pharmacokinetics of theophylline vary widely among similar patients and cannot be predicted by age, sex, body weight, or other demographic characteristics. Rapidly and completely absorbed after oral administration in solution or immediate-release solid oral dosage form. Distributed freely into fat-free tissues. Extensively metabolized in liver. **Half-life:** 4-8 hr.

■ Available Forms:
- *Capsule, Extended-Release*: 100mg, 125mg, 200mg, 300mg (Slo-Bid Gyrocaps)
- *Elixir*: 80mg/15mL (Elixophyllin)
- *Solution, Intravenous*: 40mg/100mL, 80mg/100mL, 160mg/100mL, 200mg/100mL, 200mg/50mL, 320mg/100mL, 400mg/100mL
- *Solution, Oral*: 80mg/15mL (Truxophyllin)
- *Tablet*: 100mg
- *Tablet, Extended-Release*: 100mg (Theo-Dur, Theochron, Theo-Time); 200mg (Theo-Dur, Theochron, Theo-Time); 300mg (Theo-Dur, Theochron, Theo-Time); 400mg (Uni-Dur); 450mg (Theochron)

■ Indications and Dosages:
Chronic asthma/lung diseases: PO Acute symptoms: 5 mg/kg as a loading dose, maintenance 3 mg/kg every 8 hours (non-smokers), 3 mg/kg every 6 hours (smokers), 2 mg/kg every 8 hours (older patients), 1-2 mg/kg every 12 hours (CHF); IV 5 mg/kg load over 20 minutes, maintenance 0.2 mg/kg/hour (CHF, elderly), 0.43 mg/kg/hour (non-smokers). *Slow titration:* Initial dose 16 mg/kg/day or 400mg daily, whichever is less, doses divided every 6-8 hours. *Dosage adjustment after serum theophylline measurement:* Serum level 5-10 mcg/ml, maintain dose by 25%, recheck level in 3 days. Serum level 10-20 mcg/ml, maintain dosage if tolerated, recheck level every 6-12 months. Serum level 20-25 mcg/ml, decrease dose by 10%, recheck level in 3 days. Serum level 25-30 mcg/ml, skip next dose, decrease dose by 25%, recheck level in 3 days. Serum level > 30 mcg/ml, skip next 2 doses, decrease dose by 50%, recheck level in 3 days.

■ Contraindications:
Hypersensitivity to theophylline or any component of the formulation, active peptic ulcer disease, underlying seizure disorders unless receiving appropriate anticonvulsant medication.

■ Side Effects
Anxiety, dizziness, headache, insomnia, light-headedness, muscle twitching, restlessness, seizures, dysrhythmias, fluid retention with tachycardia, hypotension, palpitations, pounding heartbeat, sinus tachycardia, anorexia, bitter taste, diarrhea, dyspepsia, gastroesophageal reflux, nausea, vomiting, urinary frequency, increased respiratory rate, flushing, urticaria

■ Serious Reactions
- Severe toxicity from theophylline overdose is a relatively rare event.

■ Patient/Family Education
- Contents of beaded capsules may be sprinkled over food

- Avoid excessive amounts of caffeine as well as extremes in dietary protein and carbohydrates
- Charbroiled foods may increase elimination and reduce the half-life
- Nervousness, restlessness, and increased heart rate may occur during theophylline therapy

■ Monitoring Parameters
- Blood levels; therapeutic level is 10-20 mcg/ml; toxicity may occur with small increase above 20 mcg/ml and occasionally at levels below this; obtain serum levels 1-2 hr after administration for immediate-release products and 5-9 hr after the AM dose for sustained-release formulations
- Recent evidence indicates that blood levels of 8-12 mcg/ml may provide adequate therapeutic effect with a lower risk of adverse events
- Signs of toxicity include nausea, vomiting, anxiety, insomnia, seizures, ventricular dysrhythmias

■ Geriatric side effects at a glance:
☑ CNS ❑ Bowel Dysfunction ❑ Bladder Dysfunction ❑ Falls
Other: Tachycardia, Psychosis, Tremor

■ Use with caution in older patients with:
Cardiovascular disease (CVD), especially angina, arrhythmias, or CHF, cor pulmonale, hepatic dysfunction, active peptic ulcer disease, GERD, anxiety, seizure disorders, migraine headaches, hyperthyroidism

■ U.S. Regulatory Considerations
❑ FDA Black Box ☑ OBRA regulated in U.S. Long Term Care

■ Side Effects:
Of particular importance in the geriatric patient: Anticholinergic effects, psychosis, confusion, nervousness, tachycardia, palpitations, PVCs, tremor, nausea, loss of appetite, hyperuricemia

■ Geriatric Considerations - Summary:
Increased risk of side effects in patients with CVD and hepatic dysfunction. Theophylline has a narrow therapeutic index and is associated with numerous drug interactions. Target serum concentrations are 5-20 mg/L, with adverse effects increasing between 15-20 mg/L. Hepatic metabolism and renal excretion declines with age and the half-life of theophylline increases by 3 to 9 hours in older adults. Smoking induces theophylline metabolism; therefore, if a patient stops smoking, empiric dosage reduction may be indicated and follow serum concentrations closely.

■ References:
1. Drugs that may cause cognitive disorders in the elderly. Med Let 2000;42:111-112.
2. Tune LE. Anticholinergic effects of medication in elderly patients. J Clin Psychiatry 2001;62(suppl 21):11-14.
3. Ohnishi A, Kato M, Kojima J, et al. Differential pharmacokinetics of theophylline in elderly patients. Drugs Aging 2003;20:71-84.
4. Ohta K, Fukuchi Y, Grouse L, et al. A prospective clinical study of theophylline safety in 3810 elderly with asthma or COPD. Resp Med 2004;98:1016-1024.
5. Newnham DM. Asthma medications and their potential adverse effects in the elderly: recommendations for prescribing. Drug Saf 2001;24:1065-1080.

thiabendazole

(thye-a-ben'-da-zole)

- **Brand Name(s):** Mintezol
  Chemical Class: Benzimidazole derivative

- **Clinical Pharmacology:**
  Mechanism of Action: An anthelmintic agent that inhibits helminth-specific mitochondrial fumarate reductase. **Therapeutic Effect:** Suppresses parasite production. **Pharmacokinetics:** Rapidly and well absorbed from the gastrointestinal (GI) tract. Rapidly metabolized in liver. Primarily excreted in urine; partially eliminated in feces. **Half-life:** 1.2 hr.

- **Available Forms:**
  - *Suspension*: 500 mg/5 ml (Mintezol).
  - *Tablets*: 500 mg (Mintezol).

- **Indications and Dosages:** Dose is based on patient's body weight.
  Cutaneous larva migrans (creeping eruption): PO 50 mg/kg/day q12h for 2 days. Maximum: 3 g/day.
  Intestinal roundworms: PO 50 mg/kg/day q12h for 2 days. Maximum: 3 g/day.
  Strongyloidiasis (threadworms): PO 50 mg/kg/day q12h for 2 days. Maximum: 3 g/day.
  Trichinosis: PO 50 mg/kg/day q12h for 2-4 days. Maximum: 3 g/day.
  Visceral larva migrans: PO 50 mg/kg/day q12h for 7 days. Maximum: 3 g/day.

- **Unlabeled Uses:** Angiostrongyliasis, capillaria infestations, dracunculus infestations, pediculosis capitis, tinea infections

- **Contraindications:** Prophylactic treatment of pinworm infestation, hypersensitivity to thiabendazole or its components

- **Side Effects**
  Occasional
  Dizziness, drowsiness, nausea, vomiting, diarrhea
  Rare
  Erythema multiforme, liver damage

- **Serious Reactions**
  - Overdose includes symptoms of altered mental status and visual problems.
  - Erythema multiforme, liver damage, and Stevens-Johnsons syndrome occur rarely.

- **Patient/Family Education**
  - Take after meals; chew before swallowing
  - Proper hygiene after bowel movement, including handwashing technique; change bed linen
  - Urine may turn red-brown or dark brown during drug therapy

- Avoid tasks that require mental alertness or motor skills until response to the drug is established

■ **Monitoring Parameters**
- Renal and hepatic function

■ **Geriatric side effects at a glance:**
❑ CNS   ❑ Bowel Dysfunction   ❑ Bladder Dysfunction   ❑ Falls

■ **U.S. Regulatory Considerations**
❑ FDA Black Box   ❑ OBRA regulated in U.S. Long Term Care

thiamine hydrochloride (vitamin B₁)

(thy'-a-min hye-droe-klor'-ide)

■ **Brand Name(s):** (Betaxin[CAN], Thiamilate, Vitamin B₁)

■ **Clinical Pharmacology:**
Mechanism of Action: The water-soluble vitamins are widely distributed in both plants and animals. They are absorbed in humans by both diffusion and active transport mechanisms. These vitamins are structurally diverse (derivatives of sugar, pyridine, purines, pyrimidine, organic acid complexes, and nucleotide complex) and act as coenzymes, as oxidation-reduction agents, or possibly as mitochondrial agents. Metabolism is rapid, and the excess is excreted in the urine. Thiamine is distributed in all tissues. The highest concentrations occur in liver, brain, kidney, and heart. When thiamine intake is greatly in excess of need, tissue stores increase 2-3 times. If intake is insufficient, tissues become depleted of their vitamin content. Absorption of thiamine following intramuscular administration is rapid and complete. Thiamine combines with adenosine triphosphate (ATP) to form thiamine pyrophosphate, also known as carboxylase, a coenzyme. Its role in carbohydrate metabolism is the decarboxylation of pyruvic acid and alpha-ketoacids to acetaldehyde and carbon dioxide. Increased levels of pyruvic acid in the blood indicate vitamin B₁ deficiency. The requirement for thiamine is greater when the carbohydrate content of the diet is raised. Body depletion of vitamin B₁ can occur after approximately 3 weeks of total abscence of thiamine in the diet. **Therapeutic Effect:** Prevents and reverses thiamine deficiency.
Pharmacokinetics: Metabolized to thiamine pyrophosphate (active) in the liver. At dietary levels thiamine is completely distributed to tissues. At pharmacologic doses, excess thiamine is excreted in urine.

■ **Available Forms:**
- *Capsules*: 50 mg.
- *Tablets*: 25 mg, 50 mg, 100 mg, 250 mg, 500 mg.
- *Enteric-Coated Tablet*: 20 mg.
- *Injection (Vitamin B₁)*: 100 mg/ml.

Indications and Dosages:
Dietary supplement (RDA): PO *Males*: 1.2 mg/day. *Females*: 1.1 mg/day.
Beriberi (thiamine deficiency): PO 5–10 mg 3 times/day up to 300 mg/day for severe deficiency. IV, IM 10-20 mg IM or slow IV infusion 3 times/day for up to 2 wk, followed by oral maintenance.
Alcohol withdrawal syndrome (acute): IV 100 mg per 25g of glucose; concurrent administration with IV glucose.
Wernicke's encephalopathy: IM, IV 100 mg IM or slow IV infusion for 3 days, up to 1,000 mg may be necessary in the first 12 hr, then 50-100 mg IM daily until adequate oral intake occurs.

Contraindications: None known.

Side Effects
Frequent
IM: Tenderness, induration
PO: Feeling of warmth, mild nausea, skin rash
IV: Sensitivity or intolerance to thiamine may develop with repeated IV administration

Serious Reactions
- IV administration may result in a rare, severe hypersensitivity reaction marked by a feeling of warmth, pruritus, urticaria, weakness, diaphoresis, nausea, restlessness, tightness in throat, angioedema, cyanosis, pulmonary edema, GI tract bleeding, and cardiovascular collapse.

thiethylperazine maleate

(thye-eth-il-per'-azeen mal'-ee-ate)

Brand Name(s): Torecan
Chemical Class: Piperazine phenothiazine derivative

Clinical Pharmacology:
Mechanism of Action: A piperazine phenothiazine that acts centrally to block dopamine receptors in chemoreceptor trigger zone in central nervous system (CNS). **Therapeutic Effect:** Relieves nausea and vomiting.

Available Forms:
- *Injection*: 5 mg/ml (Torecan).
- *Tablets*: 10 mg (Torecan).

Indications and Dosages:
Nausea or vomiting: PO, Rectal, IM 10 mg 1-3 times/day.

Contraindications: Comatose states, severe CNS depression, hypersensitivity to phenothiazines

Side Effects
Frequent
Drowsiness, dizziness

Occasional

Blurred vision, decreased color/night vision, fever, headache, orthostatic hypotension, rash, ringing in ears, constipation, dry mouth, decreased sweating.

■ **Serious Reactions**
- Extrapyramidal symptoms manifested as torticollis (neck muscle spasm), oculogyric crisis (rolling back of eyes), and akathisia (motor restlessness, anxiety) occur rarely.

Special Considerations
- Effective antiemetic agent for the treatment of postoperative nausea and vomiting, nausea and vomiting secondary to mildly emetic chemotherapeutic agents, and vomiting secondary to radiation therapy and toxins
- No comparisons with prochlorperazine
- More extrapyramidal reactions than chlorpromazine and promazine; thiethylperazine would be less desirable than these agents in patients where the occurrence of a dystonic reaction would be hazardous (i.e., head and neck surgery patients, patients with severe pulmonary disease, patients with a history of dyskinetic reactions)

■ **Patient/Family Education**
- Avoid hazardous activities, activities requiring alertness
- Notify the physician of any visual disturbances

■ **Monitoring Parameters**
- Respiratory status initially
- Blood pressure
- Intake and output

■ **Geriatric side effects at a glance:**
☑ CNS   ☐ Bowel Dysfunction   ☑ Bladder Dysfunction   ☐ Falls

■ **U.S. Regulatory Considerations**
☐ FDA Black Box   ☐ OBRA regulated in U.S. Long Term Care

thioridazine hydrochloride

(thye-or-rid'-a-zeen hye-droe-klor'-ide)

■ **Brand Name(s):** Mellaril, Thioridazine Intensol
  Chemical Class: Piperazine phenothiazine derivative

■ **Clinical Pharmacology:**
  Mechanism of Action: A phenothiazine that blocks dopamine at postsynaptic receptor sites. Possesses strong anticholinergic and sedative effects. **Therapeutic Effect:** Suppresses behavioral response in psychosis; reduces locomotor activity and aggressiveness.

■ Available Forms:
- *Oral Solution* (*Concentrate* [*Thioridazine Intensol*]): 30 mg/ml.
- *Tablets* (*Melleril*): 10 mg, 15 mg, 25 mg, 50 mg, 100 mg, 150 mg, 200 mg.

■ Indications and Dosages:
Psychosis: PO Initially, 25-100 mg 3 times a day; dosage increased gradually. Maximum: 800 mg/day.

■ Unlabeled Uses:
Treatment of behavioral problems associated with dementia, depressive neurosis

■ Contraindications:
Angle-closure glaucoma, blood dyscrasias, cardiac arrhythmias, cardiac or hepatic impairment, concurrent use of drugs that prolong QT interval, severe CNS depression

■ Side Effects
Occasional
Drowsiness during early therapy, dry mouth, blurred vision, lethargy, constipation or diarrhea, nasal congestion, peripheral edema, urine retention
Rare
Ocular changes, altered skin pigmentation (in those taking high doses for prolonged periods), photosensitivity, darkening of urine

■ Serious Reactions
- Prolonged QT interval may produce torsades de pointes, a form of ventricular tachycardia, and sudden death.

Special Considerations
- Phenothiazine with weak potency, low incidence of EPS, but high incidence of sedation, anticholinergic effects, and cardiovascular effects

■ Patient/Family Education
- Arise slowly from reclining position
- Avoid abrupt withdrawal
- Use a sunscreen during sun exposure
- Caution with activities requiring complete mental alertness (e.g., driving); may cause sedation
- Provide full information on risks of tardive dyskinesia
- Full therapeutic effect may take up to 6 wk to appear
- Notify the physician of any visual disturbances
- Avoid alcohol and exposure to artificial light and sunlight during thioridazine therapy

■ Monitoring Parameters
- Blood pressure, CBC, ECG, serum potassium level, and liver function test results, including serum alkaline phosphatase, bilirubin, AST (SGOT), and ALT (SGPT) levels
- Therapeutic response, such as improvement in self-care and ability to concentrate, increased interest in surroundings, and relaxed facial expression
- Therapeutic serum level for thioridazine is 0.2 to 2.6 mcg/ml, and the toxic serum level is not established

- **Geriatric side effects at a glance:**
  ☑ CNS ☑ Bowel Dysfunction ☑ Bladder Dysfunction ☑ Falls
  Other: Orthostatic hypotension, cardiac conduction disturbances, torsades de pointes, anticholinergic side effects

- **Use with caution in older patients with:** Parkinson's disease (an atypical antipsychotic is recommended), seizure disorders, cardiovascular disease with conduction disturbance, hepatic encephalopathy, narrow-angle glaucoma

- **U.S. Regulatory Considerations**
  ☑ FDA Black Box
  QTc prolongation dose-related; risk of torsades de pointes and sudden death
  ☑ OBRA regulated in U.S. Long Term Care

- **Other Uses in Geriatric Patient:** Behavior disturbances in the setting of dementia

- **Side Effects:**
  Of particular importance in the geriatric patient: Tardive dyskinesia, akathisia (may appear to exacerbate behavioral disturbances), anticholinergic effects, may increase risk of sudden death

- **Geriatric Considerations - Summary:** Sink and colleagues' systematic review showed statistically significant improvements on neuropsychiatric and behavioral scales for some drugs, but improvements were small and unlikely to be clinically important. Because of documented risks, and uncertain benefits, antipsychotic drugs should be used with caution in demented elderly persons, with frequent monitoring for side effects and a low threshold for discontinuing use.

- **References:**
  1. Leipzig RM, Cumming RG, Tinetti ME. Drugs and falls in older people: a systematic review and meta-analysis: I. Psychotropic drugs. J Am Geriatr Soc 1999;47:30-39.
  2. Sink KM, Holden KF, Yaffe K. Pharmacological treatment of neuropsychiatric symptoms of dementia: a review of the evidence. JAMA 2005;293:596-608.
  3. Ray WA, Meredith S, Thapa PB, et al. Antipsychotics and the risk of sudden cardiac death. Arch Gen Psychiatry 2001;58:1161-1167.

thiothixene

(thye-oh-thix'-een)

- **Brand Name(s):** Navane
  Chemical Class: Thioxanthene derivative

- **Clinical Pharmacology:**
  Mechanism of Action: An antipsychotic that blocks postsynaptic dopamine receptor sites in brain. Has alpha-adrenergic blocking effects, and depresses the release of hypothalamic and hypophyseal hormones. **Therapeutic Effect:** Suppresses psychotic behavior.

Pharmacokinetics: Well absorbed from the GI tract after IM administration. Widely distributed. Metabolized in the liver. Primarily excreted in urine. Unknown if removed by hemodialysis. **Half-life:** 34 hr.

■ **Available Forms:**
- *Capsules* (Navane): 1 mg, 2 mg, 5 mg, 10 mg, 20 mg.
- *Oral Concentrate* (Navane): 5 mg/ml.
- *Injection* (Navane): 5 mg of thiothixene and 59.6 mg of mannitol per ml when reconstituted with 2.2 ml of sterile water for injection.

■ **Indications and Dosages:**
Mild to moderate psychosis: PO 2 mg 3 times a day up to 20-30 mg/day.
Severe psychosis: PO Initially, 5 mg twice a day. May increase gradually up to 60 mg/day.
Rapid tranquilization of agitated patient: PO 5-10 mg q15-30min. Total dose: 15-30 mg.

■ **Contraindications:** Blood dyscrasias, circulatory collapse, CNS depression, coma, history of seizures

■ **Side Effects**
Expected
Hypotension, dizziness, syncope (occur frequently after first injection, occasionally after subsequent injections, and rarely with oral form)
Frequent
Transient drowsiness, dry mouth, constipation, blurred vision, nasal congestion
Occasional
Diarrhea, peripheral edema, urine retention, nausea
Rare
Ocular changes, altered skin pigmentation (in those taking high doses for prolonged periods), photosensitivity

■ **Serious Reactions**
- The most common extrapyramidal reaction is akathisia, characterized by motor restlessness and anxiety. Akinesia, marked by rigidity, tremor, increased salivation, mask-like facial expression, and reduced voluntary movements, occurs less frequently. Dystonias, including torticollis, opisthotonos, and oculogyric crisis, occur rarely.
- Tardive dyskinesia, characterized by tongue protrusion, puffing of the cheeks, and chewing or puckering of the mouth, occurs rarely but may be irreversible. Female patients have a greater risk of developing this reaction.
- Grand mal seizures may occur in epileptic patients, especially those receiving the drug by IM administration.
- Neuroleptic malignant syndrome occurs rarely.

Special Considerations
- High-potency antipsychotic with a relatively high incidence of EPS, but a low incidence of sedation, anticholinergic effects, and cardiovascular effects

■ **Patient/Family Education**
- Informed consent regarding risks of tardive dyskinesia, orthostatic hypotension
- Full therapeutic effect may take up to 6 wk to appear
- Avoid tasks that require mental alertness or motor skills until response to the drug has been established; drowsiness generally subsides during continued therapy

- Avoid alcohol and artificial light or direct sunlight
- Take sips of tepid water and chew sugarless gum to relieve dry mouth

■ Monitoring Parameters
- Blood pressure hypotension
- Pattern of daily bowel activity and stool consistency
- Monitor the patient for extrapyramidal reactions and early signs of tardive dyskinesia and potentially fatal neuroleptic malignant syndrome (such as altered mental status, fever, irregular pulse or blood pressure, and muscle rigidity)
- Therapeutic response, such as improvement in self-care and ability to concentrate, increased interest in surroundings, and relaxed facial expression

■ Geriatric side effects at a glance:
☑ CNS ☑ Bowel Dysfunction ☐ Bladder Dysfunction ☑ Falls
Other: Orthostatic hypotension, cardiac conduction disturbances, anticholinergic side effects

■ Use with caution in older patients with: Parkinson's disease (an atypical antipsychotic is recommended), seizure disorders, cardiovascular disease with conduction disturbance, hepatic encephalopathy, narrow-angle glaucoma

■ U.S. Regulatory Considerations
☐ FDA Black Box ☑ OBRA regulated in U.S. Long Term Care

■ Other Uses in Geriatric Patient: Behavior disturbances in the setting of dementia

■ Side Effects:
Of *particular importance in the geriatric patient*: Tardive dyskinesia, akathisia (may appear to exacerbate behavioral disturbances), anticholinergic effects, may increase risk of sudden death

■ Geriatric Considerations - Summary: Sink and colleagues' systematic review showed statistically significant improvements on neuropsychiatric and behavioral scales for some drugs, but improvements were small and unlikely to be clinically important. Because of documented risks, and uncertain benefits, antipsychotic drugs should be used with caution in demented elderly persons, with frequent monitoring for side effects and a low threshold for discontinuing use.

■ References:
1. Leipzig RM, Cumming RG, Tinetti ME. Drugs and falls in older people: a systematic review and meta-analysis: I. Psychotropic drugs. J Am Geriatr Soc 1999;47:30-39.
2. Sink KM, Holden KF, Yaffe K. Pharmacological treatment of neuropsychiatric symptoms of dementia: a review of the evidence. JAMA 2005;293:596-608.
3. Ray WA, Meredith S, Thapa PB, et al. Antipsychotics and the risk of sudden cardiac death. Arch Gen Psychiatry 2001;58:1161-1167.

thyroid

(thye'-roid)

■ **Brand Name(s):** Armour Thyroid, Nature-Throid NT, Westhroid
Chemical Class: ENDO-thyroid hormone in natural state

■ **Clinical Pharmacology:**
Mechanism of Action: A natural hormone derived from animal sources, usually beef or pork, that is involved in normal metabolism, growth, and development, especially the central nervous system (CNS) of infants. Possesses catabolic and anabolic effects. Provides both levothyroxine and liothyronine hormones. **Therapeutic Effect:** Increases basal metabolic rate, enhances gluconeogenesis, stimulates protein synthesis.
Pharmacokinetics: Partially absorbed from the gastrointestinal (GI) tract. Protein binding: 99%. Widely distributed. Metabolized in liver to active, liothyronine (T_3), and inactive, reverse triiodothyronine (rT_3), metabolites. Eliminated by biliary excretion. **Half-life:** 2-7 days.

■ **Available Forms:**
- **Capsules:** 15 mg, 30 mg, 60 mg, 90 mg, 120 mg, 180 mg, 240 mg, 300 mg.
- **Tablets:** 15 mg, 30 mg, 32.5 mg, 60 mg, 65 mg, 90 mg, 120 mg, 130 mg, 180 mg, 195 mg, 240 mg, 300 mg.

■ **Indications and Dosages:**
Hypothyroidism: PO Initially, 15-30 mg. May increase by 15-mg increments q2-4wk. Maintenance: 60-120 mcg/day. Use 15 mg in patients with cardiovascular disease or myxedema.

■ **Contraindications:** Uncontrolled adrenal cortical insufficiency, untreated thyrotoxicosis, treatment of obesity, uncontrolled angina, uncontrolled hypertension, uncontrolled myocardial infarction, and hypersensitivity to any component of the formulations

■ **Side Effects**
Rare
Dry skin, GI intolerance, skin rash, hives, severe headache

■ **Serious Reactions**
- Excessive dosage produces signs and symptoms of hyperthyroidism including weight loss, palpitations, increased appetite, tremors, nervousness, tachycardia, hypertension, headache, insomnia, and menstrual irregularities.
- Cardiac arrhythmias occur rarely.

Special Considerations
- Although used traditionally, natural hormones are less clinically desirable due to varying potencies, inconsistent clinical effects, and more adverse stimulatory effects; synthetic derivatives (i.e., levothyroxine) preferred

■ **Patient/Family Education**
- Do not discontinue the drug
- Follow-up office visits and thyroid function tests are essential
- Take drug at the same time each day, preferably in the morning
- Notify the physician if chest pain, insomnia, nervousness, tremors, or weight loss occurs

■ **Monitoring Parameters**
- TSH yearly

■ **Geriatric side effects at a glance:**
❑ CNS   ❑ Bowel Dysfunction   ❑ Bladder Dysfunction   ❑ Falls

■ **U.S. Regulatory Considerations**
☑ FDA Black Box
Should not be used in the treatment of obesity.
❑ OBRA regulated in U.S. Long Term Care

tiagabine hydrochloride

(tye-ah'-gah-been hye-droe-klor'-ide)

■ **Brand Name(s):** Gabitril
Chemical Class: Nipecotic acid derivative

■ **Clinical Pharmacology:**
Mechanism of Action: An anticonvulsant that enhances the activity of gamma-aminobutyric acid, the major inhibitory neurotransmitter in the CNS. **Therapeutic Effect:** Inhibits seizures.
Pharmacokinetics: Rapidly and nearly completely absorbed after PO administration. Protein binding: 96%. Metabolized in liver. Eliminated in urine and feces. Not removed by hemodialysis. **Half-life:** 7-9 hr.

■ **Available Forms:**
- **Tablets:** 2 mg, 4 mg, 12 mg, 16 mg.

■ **Indications and Dosages:**
Adjunctive treatment of partial seizures: PO Initially, 4 mg once a day. May increase by 4-8 mg/day at weekly intervals. Maximum: 56 mg/day.

■ **Unlabeled Uses:** Bipolar disorder

■ **Contraindications:** None known.

■ **Side Effects**
Frequent (34%-20%)
Dizziness, asthenia, somnolence, nervousness, confusion, headache, infection, tremor

1210

Occasional

Nausea, diarrhea, abdominal pain, impaired concentration

■ Serious Reactions

- Overdose is characterized by agitation, confusion, hostility, and weakness. Full recovery occurs within 24 hr.

Special Considerations

- Patients should exercise caution with initiation and dosage titration when driving, operating hazardous machinery, or other activities requiring mental concentration; patients should be advised to take the medication with food, to delay peak effects to avoid many CNS adverse effects

■ Patient/Family Education

- Change position slowly from recumbent to sitting position before standing if he or she experiences dizziness
- Avoid tasks that require mental alertness or motor skills until response to the drug is established
- Avoid alcohol while taking tiagabine

■ Monitoring Parameters

- Perform periodic CBCs and blood chemistry tests to assess hepatic and renal function
- Signs of clinical improvement, such as a decrease in the frequency or intensity of seizures

■ Geriatric side effects at a glance:

❑ CNS ❑ Bowel Dysfunction ❑ Bladder Dysfunction ❑ Falls

Other: Tremor

■ Use with caution in older patients with: Hepatic impairment, cognitive impairment, unsteady gait, parkinsonism, tremors, urinary incontinence

■ U.S. Regulatory Considerations

❑ FDA Black Box ❑ OBRA regulated in U.S. Long Term Care

■ Side Effects:

Of particular importance in the geriatric patient: Anticholinergic effects

■ Geriatric Considerations - Summary: Not well-studied in older adults. Few drug interactions.

■ References:

1. Brodie M, Kwan P. Epilepsy in elderly people. BMJ 2005;331:1317-1322.
2. Arroyo S, Kramer G. Treating epilepsy in the elderly: safety considerations. Drug Saf 2001;24:991-1015.
3. Drugs that may cause cognitive disorders in the elderly. Med Let 2000;42:111-112.
4. Willmore LJ. Choice and use of newer anticonvulsant drugs in older patients. Drugs Aging 2000;17:441-452.

ticarcillin disodium/ clavulanate potassium

(tye-car-sill'-in dye-soe'-dee-um/klav'-yoo-lan-ate poe-tas'-e-um)

- **Brand Name(s):** Timentin
  Chemical Class: Penicillin derivative, extended-spectrum

- **Clinical Pharmacology:**
  Mechanism of Action: Binds to bacterial cell walls, inhibiting cell wall synthesis. Clavulanate inhibits the action of bacterial beta-lactamase. **Therapeutic Effect:** Ticarcillin is bactericidal in susceptible organisms. Clavulanate protects ticarcillin from enzymatic degradation.
  Pharmacokinetics: Widely distributed. Protein binding: ticarcillin 45%-60%, clavulanate 9%-30%. Minimally metabolized in the liver. Primarily excreted unchanged in urine. Removed by hemodialysis. **Half-life:** 1-1.2 hr (increased in impaired renal function).

- **Available Forms:**
  - ADD-*Vantage Vial* (*Timentin*): 3.1 g.
  - *Powder for Injection* (*Timentin*): 3.1 g.
  - *Premixed Solution for Infusion* (*Timentin*): 3.1 g/100 ml.

- **Indications and Dosages:**
  Skin and skin-structure, bone, joint, and lower respiratory tract infections; septicemia; endometriosis: IV 3.1g (3g ticarcillin) q4-6h. Maximum: 18-24 g/day.
  UTIs: IV 3.1g q6-8h.
  Dosage in renal impairment: Dosage interval is modified based on creatinine clearance.

Creatinine Clearance	Dosage Interval
10-30 ml/min	Usual dose q8h
less than 10 ml/min	Usual dose q12h

- **Contraindications:** Hypersensitivity to any penicillin or clavulanic acid

- **Side Effects**
  Frequent
  Phlebitis or thrombophlebitis (with IV dose), rash, urticaria, pruritus, altered smell or taste
  Occasional
  Nausea, diarrhea, vomiting
  Rare
  Headache, fatigue, hallucinations, bleeding or ecchymosis

- **Serious Reactions**
  - Overdosage may produce seizures and other neurologic reactions.
  - Antibiotic-associated colitis and other superinfections may result from bacterial imbalance.

- Severe hypersensitivity reactions, including anaphylaxis, occur rarely.

Special Considerations
- Synergistic with aminoglycosides
- Sodium content, 5.2 mEq/g ticarcillin
- For reliable activity against *Pseudomonas*, must be dosed q4h
- Individualize treatment based on local susceptibility patterns.

■ **Patient/Family Education**
- Notify the physician of pain, redness, or swelling at infusion site

■ **Monitoring Parameters**
- Electrolytes
- Daily bowel activity and stool consistency. Although mild GI effects may be tolerable, severe symptoms may indicate the onset of antibiotic-associated colitis.
- Signs and symptoms of superinfection include abdominal pain or cramping, anal or genital pruritus or discharge, moderate to severe diarrhea, severe mouth or tongue soreness, and new or increased fever.

■ **Geriatric side effects at a glance:**
   ❏ CNS   ❏ Bowel Dysfunction   ❏ Bladder Dysfunction   ❏ Falls

■ **U.S. Regulatory Considerations**
   ❏ FDA Black Box   ❏ OBRA regulated in U.S. Long Term Care

ticlopidine hydrochloride

(tye-kloe'-pi-deen hye-droe-klor'-ide)

■ **Brand Name(s):** Ticlid
   Chemical Class: Thienopyridine derivative

■ **Clinical Pharmacology:**
   Mechanism of Action: An aggregation inhibitor that inhibits the release of adenosine diphosphate from activated platelets, which prevents fibrinogen from binding to glycoprotein IIb/IIIa receptors on the surface of activated platelets. **Therapeutic Effect:** Inhibits platelet aggregation and thrombus formation.
   Pharmacokinetics: Rapidly absorbed following PO administration. Protein binding: 98%. Extensively metabolized in liver. Primarily excreted in urine; partially eliminated in feces. **Half-life:** 12.6 hr.

■ **Available Forms:**
- *Tablets*: 250 mg.

■ **Indications and Dosages:**
   Prevention of stroke: PO 250 mg twice a day.

■ **Unlabeled Uses:** Prevention of postoperative deep vein thrombosis (DVT), protection of aortocoronary bypass grafts, reduction of graft loss after renal transplant, treatment of intermittent claudication, sickle cell disease, subarachnoid hemorrhage, diabetic microangiopathy, ischemic heart disease

■ **Contraindications:** Active pathologic bleeding, such as bleeding peptic ulcer and intracranial bleeding; hematopoietic disorders, including neutropenia and thrombocytopenia; presence of hemostatic disorder; severe hepatic impairment

■ **Side Effects**
Frequent (13%–5%)
Diarrhea, nausea, dyspepsia, including heartburn, indigestion, GI discomfort, and bloating
Rare (2%–1%)
Vomiting, flatulence, pruritus, dizziness

■ **Serious Reactions**
- Neutropenia occurs in approximately 2% of patients.
- Thrombotic thrombocytopenic purpura, agranulocytosis, hepatitis, cholestatic jaundice, and tinnitus occur rarely.

Special Considerations
- Due to the risk of life-threatening neutropenia or agranulocytosis and cost, ticlopidine should be reserved for patients intolerant to aspirin or who fail aspirin

■ **Monitoring Parameters**
- CBC q2wk for first 3 mo of therapy, then periodically thereafter
- Pattern of daily bowel activity and stool consistency
- Heart sounds
- Blood pressure for hypotension
- Skin for erythema and rash
- Hepatic enzyme levels
- Observe for signs of bleeding

■ **Geriatric side effects at a glance:**
❑ CNS ❑ Bowel Dysfunction ❑ Bladder Dysfunction ❑ Falls

■ **U.S. Regulatory Considerations**
❑ FDA Black Box
- Life-threatening hematologic events have occurred among persons using ticlopidine including neutropenia, agranulocytosis, TTP, and aplastic anemia.
- Requires close monitoring—CBC every 2 wk for the first 3 mo of therapy. If drug is discontinued in the first 3 mo, continue to monitor CBC an additional 2 wk.
❑ OBRA regulated in U.S. Long Term Care

tiludronate disodium

(tye-loo-droe'-nate dye-soe'-dee-um)

- **Brand Name(s):** Skelid
  Chemical Class: Pyrophosphate analog

- **Clinical Pharmacology:**
  Mechanism of Action: A calcium regulator that inhibits functioning osteoclasts through disruption of cytoskeletal ring structure and inhibition of osteoclastic proton pump. **Therapeutic Effect:** Inhibits bone resorption.
  Pharmacokinetics: Well absorbed following PO administration. Protein binding: 90%. Not metabolized in liver. **Half-life:** 150 hr.

- **Available Forms:**
  - *Tablets*: 200 mg.

- **Indications and Dosages:**
  Paget's disease: PO 400 mg once a day for 3 mo. Must take with 6–8 oz plain water. Do not give within 2 hr of food intake. Avoid giving aspirin, calcium supplements, mineral supplements, or antacids within 2 hr of tiludronate administration.

- **Contraindications:** GI disease, such as dysphagia and gastric ulcer, impaired renal function

- **Side Effects**
  Frequent (9%–6%)
  Nausea, diarrhea, generalized body pain, back pain, headache
  Occasional
  Rash, dyspepsia, vomiting, rhinitis, sinusitis, dizziness
  Rare
  Osteonecrosis of the jaw

- **Serious Reactions**
  - Dysphagia, esophagitis, esophageal ulcer, and gastric ulcer occur rarely.

Special Considerations

- Studies needed to assess place in therapy with other bisphosphonates
- Inhibition of bone loss in osteoporosis may persist up to 2 yr after 6 mo of treatment and discontinuation of drug
- A dental examination with appropriate preventive dentistry should be considered prior to treatment with bisphosphonates in patients with concomitant risk factors (e.g., cancer, chemotherapy, corticosteroid use, poor oral hygiene). While on bisphosphonate treatment, patients with concomitant risk factors should avoid invasive dental procedures if possible. For patients who develop osteonecrosis of the jaw while on bisphosphonate therapy, dental surgery may exacerbate the condition. For patients requiring dental procedures, there are no data available to suggest whether discontinuation of bisphosphonate treatment reduces the risk of osteonecrosis of the jaw.

■ Patient/Family Education
- Take with 6-8 oz plain water; do not take within 2 hr of food or other medications
- Consult the physician to determine if he or she needs calcium and vitamin D supplements
- Inform your dentist if you are taking this drug.
- If you develop jaw pain, loose teeth, or signs of oral infection, immediately inform your doctor.

■ Monitoring Parameters
- Adjusted serum calcium, serum alkaline phosphatase, osteocalcin, and urinary hydroxyproline levels to assess the effectiveness of tiludronate

■ Geriatric side effects at a glance:
❏ CNS ❏ Bowel Dysfunction ❏ Bladder Dysfunction ❏ Falls

■ U.S. Regulatory Considerations
❏ FDA Black Box ❏ OBRA regulated in U.S. Long Term Care

timolol

(tim'-oh-lol)

■ Brand Name(s): Betimol, Blocadren, Istalol, Timolol Ophthalmic, Timoptic, Timoptic OccuDose, Timoptic Ocumeter, Timoptic Ocumeter Plus, Timoptic XE

Combinations
Rx: Ophthalmic with dorzol amide (Cosopt)
Chemical Class: β-Adrenergic blocker, nonselective

■ Clinical Pharmacology:
Mechanism of Action: An antihypertensive, antimigraine, and antiglaucoma agent that blocks $beta_1$- and $beta_2$-adrenergic receptors. **Therapeutic Effect:** Reduces intraocular pressure (IOP) by reducing aqueous humor production, lowers BP, slows the heart rate, and decreases myocardial contractility.
Pharmacokinetics:

Route	Onset	Peak	Duration
PO	15-45 min	0.5-2.5 hr	4 hr
Ophthalmic	30 min	1-2 hr	12-24 hr

Well absorbed from the GI tract. Protein binding: 60%. Minimal absorption after ophthalmic administration. Metabolized in the liver. Primarily excreted in urine. Not removed by hemodialysis. **Half-life:** 4 hr. Systemic absorption may occur with ophthalmic administration.

■ Available Forms:
- *Tablets (Blocadren):* 5 mg, 10 mg, 20 mg.
- *Ophthalmic Gel (Timoptic-XE):* 0.25%, 0.5%.

- *Ophthalmic Solution (Betimol, Timoptic, Timoptic OccuDose, Timoptic Ocumeter, Timoptic Ocumeter Plus)*: 0.25%, 0.5%.

■ Indications and Dosages:

Mild to moderate hypertension: PO Initially, 10 mg twice a day, alone or in combination with other therapy. Gradually increase at intervals of not less than 1 wk. Maintenance: 20-60 mg/day in 2 divided doses.

Reduction of cardiovascular mortality in definite or suspected acute MI: PO 10 mg twice a day, beginning 1-4 wk after infarction.

Migraine prevention: PO Initially, 10 mg twice a day. Range: 10-30 mg/day.

Reduction of IOP in open-angle glaucoma, aphakic glaucoma, ocular hypertension, and secondary glaucoma: Ophthalmic 1 drop of 0.25% solution in affected eye(s) twice a day. May be increased to 1 drop of 0.5% solution in affected eye(s) twice a day. When IOP is controlled, dosage may be reduced to 1 drop once a day. If patient is switched to EYE-glaucoma-topical-BB from another antiglaucoma agent, administer concurrently for 1 day. Discontinue other agent on following day. Ophthalmic (Timoptic XE) 1 drop/day Ophthalmic (Istalol) Apply once daily.

■ Unlabeled Uses:
Systemic: Treatment of anxiety, cardiac arrhythmias, chronic angina pectoris, hypertrophic cardiomyopathy, migraine, pheochromocytoma, thyrotoxicosis, tremors

Ophthalmic: To decrease IOP in acute or chronic angle-closure glaucoma, treatment of angle-closure glaucoma during and after iridectomy, malignant glaucoma, secondary glaucoma

■ Contraindications:
Bronchial asthma, cardiogenic shock, CHF unless secondary to tachyarrhythmias, chronic obstructive pulmonary disease (COPD), patients receiving MAOI therapy, second- or third-degree heart block, sinus bradycardia, uncontrolled cardiac failure

■ Side Effects

Frequent
Diminished sexual function, drowsiness, difficulty sleeping, unusual tiredness or weakness
Ophthalmic: Eye irritation, visual disturbances

Occasional
Depression, cold hands or feet, diarrhea, constipation, anxiety, nasal congestion, nausea, vomiting

Rare
Altered taste, dry eyes, itching, numbness of fingers, toes, or scalp

■ Serious Reactions
- Overdose may produce profound bradycardia, hypotension, and bronchospasm.
- Abrupt withdrawal may result in diaphoresis, palpitations, headache, and tremors.
- Timolol administration may precipitate CHF and MI in patients with cardiac disease; thyroid storm in those with thyrotoxicosis; and peripheral ischemia in those with existing peripheral vascular disease.
- Hypoglycemia may occur in patients with previously controlled diabetes.
- Ophthalmic overdose may produce bradycardia, hypotension, bronchospasm, and acute cardiac failure.

Special Considerations
- Currently available β-blockers appear to be equally effective; cardioselective or combined α- and β-adrenergic blockade are less likely to cause undesirable effects and may be preferred

■ **Patient/Family Education**
- Do not discontinue abruptly; may require taper; rapid withdrawal may produce rebound hypertension or angina
- Avoid tasks that require mental alertness or motor skills until response to the drug has been established
- Notify the physician if excessive fatigue, prolonged dizziness or headache, or shortness of breath occurs
- Do not use nasal decongestants and OTC cold preparations, especially those containing stimulants, without physician approval
- Limit alcohol and salt intake

■ **Monitoring Parameters**
- *Angina*: Reduction in nitroglycerin usage; frequency, severity, onset, and duration of angina pain; heart rate
- *Arrhythmias*: Heart rate
- *Congestive heart failure*: Functional status, cough, dyspnea on exertion, paroxysmal nocturnal dyspnea, exercise tolerance, and ventricular function
- *Hypertension*: Blood pressure
- *Migraine headache*: Reduction in the frequency, severity, and duration of attacks
- *Post myocardial infarction*: Left ventricular function, lower resting heart rate
- *Toxicity*: Blood glucose, bronchospasm, hypotension, bradycardia, depression, confusion, hallucination, sexual dysfunction

■ **Geriatric side effects at a glance:**
❑ CNS   ❑ Bowel Dysfunction   ❑ Bladder Dysfunction   ❑ Falls
Other: Cardiovascular and CNS effects

■ **Use with caution in older patients with:** Cardiovascular disease, 2nd or 3rd degree heart block, sinus bradycardia, respiratory disease (asthma, COPD), diabetes, myasthenia gravis

■ **U.S. Regulatory Considerations**
☑ FDA Black Box
In patients using <u>orally administered</u> beta-blockers, abrupt withdrawal may precipitate angina or lead to myocardial infarction or ventricular arrhythmias.
❑ OBRA regulated in U.S. Long Term Care

■ **Other Uses in Geriatric Patient:** None (ophthalmic)

■ **Side Effects:**
Of particular importance in the geriatric patient: Due to systemic absorption: bradycardia, arrhythmias, hypotension, dizziness, fatigue, somnolence, confusion, hallucinations, psychosis, headaches, bronchospasm, alopecia, arthralgia, impotence; due to topical administration: stinging, tearing, blurred vision, light sensitivity/photophobia, dryness, decreased visual acuity

■ **Geriatric Considerations - Summary:** Timolol Ophthalmic decreases intraocular pressure on average 20%-35% and is considered the gold standard against which other agents for the treatment of glaucoma are measured. Systemic absorption of ophthalmic drugs may occur and cause adverse effects in older adults. Since timolol is a nonselective beta-blocker, older adults may be more sensitive to the cardiovascular, CNS, and respiratory effects of the drug. Timolol may be less efficacious in patients with dark irises due to drug binding to iris melanin. Tachyphylaxis may occur after long-term therapy.

■ **References:**
1. Marquis RE, Whitson JT. Management of glaucoma: focus on pharmacological therapy. Drugs Aging 2005;22:1-22.
2. Camras CB, Toris CB, Tamesis RR. Efficacy and adverse effects of medications used in the treatment of glaucoma. Drugs Aging 1999;15:377-388.
3. Backlund M, Kirvela M, Lindgren L: Cardiac failure aggravated by timolol eye drops: preoperative improvement by changing to pilocarpine. Acta Anaesthesiol Scand 1996; 40:379-381.
4. Fraunfelder FT, Meyer SM, Menacker SJ: Alopecia possibly secondary to topical ophthalmic beta blockers (letter). JAMA 1990; 263:1493-1494.

tinidazole

(tin-nid'-ah-zole)

■ **Brand Name(s):** Tindamax
Chemical Class: Nitroimidazole derivative

■ **Clinical Pharmacology:**
Mechanism of Action: A nitroimidazole derivative that is converted to the active metabolite by reduction of cell extracts of **Trichomonas**. The active metabolite causes DNA damage in pathogens. **Therapeutic Effect:** Produces antiprotozoal effect.
Pharmacokinetics: Rapidly and completely absorbed. Protein binding: 12%. Distributed in all body tissues and fluids; crosses blood-brain barrier. Significantly metabolized. Primarily excreted in urine; partially eliminated in feces. **Half-life:** 12-14 hr.

■ **Available Forms:**
• **Tablets:** 250 mg, 500 mg.

■ **Indications and Dosages:**
Intestinal amebiasis: PO 2 g/day for 3 days.
Amebic hepatic abscess: PO 2 g/day for 3-5 days.
Giardiasis: PO 2g as a single dose.
Trichomoniasis: PO 2g as a single dose.

■ **Contraindications:** Hypersensitivity to nitroimidazole derivatives

■ **Side Effects**
Occasional (4%-2%)
Metallic or bitter taste, nausea, weakness, fatigue or malaise
Rare (less than 2%)
Epigastric distress, anorexia, vomiting, headache, dizziness, red-brown or darkened urine

■ **Serious Reactions**
• Peripheral neuropathy, characterized by paresthesia, is usually reversible if tinidazole treatment is stopped as soon as neurologic symptoms appear.
• Superinfection, hypersensitivity reaction, and seizures occur rarely.

- Also effective for bacterial vaginosis, but not FDA approved

■ **Patient/Family Education**
- For trichomoniasis, treat sexual partner; tinidazole may induce candidiasis
- Take with food
- May turn urine red-brown or darken it
- Avoid alcoholic beverages and alcohol-containing preparations (such as cough syrups) during therapy and for 3 days afterward
- Avoid performing tasks that require mental alertness or motor skills if dizziness occurs as a side effect of tinidazole use

■ **Monitoring Parameters**
- CBC with WBC differential if retreatment is necessary
- Be alert for neurologic symptoms, including dizziness and paresthesia of the extremities
- Assess for nausea and vomiting and initiate appropriate measures
- Observe for evidence of superinfection, such as anal or genital pruritus, furry tongue, stomatitis, and vaginal discharge

■ **Geriatric side effects at a glance:**
☐ CNS ☐ Bowel Dysfunction ☐ Bladder Dysfunction ☐ Falls

■ **U.S. Regulatory Considerations**
☑ FDA Black Box
Carcinogenicity has been seen in mice and rats treated chronically with mitronidazole, another agent in the nitroimidazole class. Although such data have not been reported with tinidazole, unnecessary use of this drug should be avoided.
☐ OBRA regulated in U.S. Long Term Care

tinzaparin sodium

(tin-za'-pa-rin soe'-dee-um)

■ **Brand Name(s):** Innohep
Chemical Class: Heparin derivative, depolymerized; low-molecular-weight heparin

■ **Clinical Pharmacology:**
Mechanism of Action: A low-molecular-weight heparin that inhibits factor Xa. Causes less inactivation of thrombin, inhibition of platelets, and bleeding than standard heparin. Does not significantly influence bleeding time, PT, aPTT. **Therapeutic Effect:** Produces anticoagulation.
Pharmacokinetics: Well absorbed after subcutaneous administration. Primarily eliminated in urine. **Half-life:** 3–4 hr.

■ **Available Forms:**
- Injection: 20,000 antifactor Xa international units/ml.

■ Indications and Dosages:
Deep vein thrombosis (DVT): Subcutaneous 175 antifactor Xa international units/kg once a day. Continue for at least 6 days and until patient is sufficiently anticoagulated with warfarin (INR of 2 or more for 2 consecutive days).

■ Contraindications:
Active major bleeding; concurrent heparin therapy; hypersensitivity to heparin, sulfites, benzyl alcohol, or pork products; thrombocytopenia associated with positive in vitro test for antiplatelet antibody

■ Side Effects
Frequent (16%)
Injection site reaction, such as inflammation, oozing, nodules, and skin necrosis
Rare (less than 2%)
Nausea, asthenia, constipation, epistaxis

■ Serious Reactions
- Overdose may lead to bleeding complications ranging from local ecchymoses to major hemorrhage. Antidote: Dose of protamine sulfate (1% solution) should be equal to dose of tinzaparin injected. One mg protamine sulfate neutralizes 100 units of tinzaparin. A second dose of 0.5 mg tinzaparin per 1 mg protamine sulfate may be given if aPTT tested 2–4 hr after the initial infusion remains prolonged.

Special Considerations
- Cannot be used interchangeably with unfractionated heparin or other low-molecular-weight heparin products

■ Patient/Family Education
- Administer by deep SC inj into abdominal wall; alternate inj sites
- Do not rub inj site after completion of the inj
- Report any unusual bruising or bleeding to clinician

■ Monitoring Parameters
- Periodic CBC with platelets
- Monitoring aPTT is not required
- Consider antifactor Xa monitoring in patients with impaired renal function and in very small or obese patients
- Assess signs of bleeding, including bleeding at injection or surgical sites or from gums, blood in stool, bruising, hematuria, and petechiae

■ Geriatric side effects at a glance:
❑ CNS ❑ Bowel Dysfunction ❑ Bladder Dysfunction ❑ Falls

■ U.S. Regulatory Considerations
☑ FDA Black Box
Increased risk of spinal/epidural hematomas with neuraxial anesthesia or spinal puncture. Risk is further increased by use of indwelling spinal catheters, repeated/traumatic epidural/spinal puncture, or use of drugs affecting hemostasis (NSAIDs, anticoagulants, platelet inhibitors).
❑ OBRA regulated in U.S. Long Term Care

tioconazole

(tye-oh-kon'-a-zole)

OTC: Vagistat-1, Monistat-1
Chemical Class: Imidazole derivative

■ **Clinical Pharmacology:**
Mechanism of Action: An imidazole derivative that inhibits synthesis of ergosterol (vital component of fungal cell formation). **Therapeutic Effect:** Damaging fungal cell membrane. Fungistatic.
Pharmacokinetics: Negliglble absorption from vaginal application.

■ **Available Forms:**
 • **Vaginal Ointment:** 6.5% (Monistat-1, Vagistat).

■ **Indications and Dosages:**
Vulvovaginal candidiasis: Intravaginal 1 applicatorful just before bedtime as a single dose.

■ **Contraindications:** Hypersensitivity to tioconazole or other imidazole antifungal agents

■ **Side Effects**
Frequent (25%)
Headache
Occasional (6%-1%)
Burning, itching
Rare (less than 1%)
Irritation, vaginal pain, dysuria, dryness of vaginal secretions, vulvar edema/ swelling

■ **Serious Reactions**
 • None reported.

Special Considerations
 • Similar in efficacy to miconazole, econazole, and clotrimazole for the topical management of fungal skin infections; choice determined by cost and availability; additional efficacy vs. trichomoniasis with longer course of therapy

■ **Patient/Family Education**
 • Avoid contact with eyes
 • Separate personal items that come in contact with affected areas
 • Avoid using condoms or diaphragms within 72 hr of administration of tioconazole

■ **Monitoring Parameters**
 • Assess the patient for vaginal irritation

■ **Geriatric side effects at a glance:**
 ❑ CNS   ❑ Bowel Dysfunction   ❑ Bladder Dysfunction   ❑ Falls

tiopronin

(tye-o-pro'-nin)

■ **Brand Name(s):** Thiola
   Chemical Class: Thiol derivative

■ **Clinical Pharmacology:**
   Mechanism of Action: A sulfhydryl compound with similar properties to those of penicillamine and glutathione that undergoes thiol-disulfide exchange with cysteine to form tiopronin-cysteine, a mixed disulfide. This disulfide is water soluble, unlike cysteine, and does not crystallize in the kidneys. May break disulfide bonds present in bronchial secretions and break the mucus complexes. **Therapeutic Effect:** Decreases cysteine excretion.
   Pharmacokinetics: Moderately absorbed from the gastrointestinal (GI) tract. Primarily excreted in urine. Following oral administration, up to 48% of dose appears in urine during the first 4 hr and up to 78% by 72 hr. **Half-life:** 53 hr.

■ **Available Forms:**
   • *Tablets*: 100 mg (Thiola).

■ **Indications and Dosages:**
   Crystinuria: PO Initially, 800 mg in 3 divided doses. Adjust and maintain crystine concentration below its solubility limit (usually less than 250 mg/L).

■ **Unlabeled Uses:** Cataracts, epilepsy, hepatitis, rheumatoid arthritis

■ **Contraindications:** History of agranulocytosis, aplastic anemia, or thrombocytopenia while on tiopronin, hypersensitivity to tiopronin or its components

■ **Side Effects**
   Frequent
   Pain, swelling, tenderness of skin, rash, hives, itching, oral ulcers
   Occasional
   GI upset, taste or smell impairment, bloody or cloudy urine, chills, difficulty in breathing, high blood pressure, hoarseness, joint pain, swelling of feet or lower legs, tenderness of glands
   Rare
   Chest pain, cough, difficulty in chewing, talking, swallowing, double vision, general feeling of discomfort, illness, weakness, muscle weakness, spitting up blood, swelling of lymph glands

■ **Serious Reactions**
   • Hematologic abnormalities, including myelosupression, unusual bleeding, drug fever, renal complications, and lupus erythematous-like reaction including fever, arthralgia, and lymphadenopathy rarely occur.

- May be associated with fever and less severe adverse reactions than D-penicilla-mine

■ **Patient/Family Education**
- Take on an empty stomach
- Increase fluid intake to at least 3 L of fluid

■ **Monitoring Parameters**
- CBC
- Liver function
- Urinary cystine

■ **Geriatric side effects at a glance:**
   ❑ CNS   ❑ Bowel Dysfunction   ❑ Bladder Dysfunction   ❑ Falls

■ **U.S. Regulatory Considerations**
   ❑ FDA Black Box   ❑ OBRA regulated in U.S. Long Term Care

tiotropium bromide

(tee-oh-tro'-pee-um bro'-mide)

■ **Brand Name(s):** Spiriva
   Chemical Class: Quaternary ammonium compound

■ **Clinical Pharmacology:**
   Mechanism of Action: An anticholinergic that binds to recombinant human muscarinic receptors at the smooth muscle, resulting in long-acting bronchial smooth-muscle relaxation. **Therapeutic Effect:** Relieves bronchospasm.
   Pharmacokinetics:

Route	Onset	Peak	Duration
Inhalation	N/A	N/A	24-36 hr

   Binds extensively to tissue. Protein binding: 72%. Metabolized by oxidation. Excreted in urine. **Half-life:** 5-6 days.

■ **Available Forms:**
- *Powder for Inhalation*: 18 mcg/capsule (in blister packs containing 6 capsules with inhaler).

■ **Indications and Dosages:**
   Chronic obstructive pulmonary disease (COPD): Inhalation 18 mcg (1 capsule)/day via HandiHaler inhalation device.

■ **Contraindications:** History of hypersensitivity to atropine or its derivatives, including ipratropium

1224

- **Side Effects**
  Frequent (16%-6%)
  Dry mouth, sinusitis, pharyngitis, dyspepsia, UTI, rhinitis
  Occasional (5%-4%)
  Abdominal pain, peripheral edema, constipation, epistaxis, vomiting, myalgia, rash, oral candidiasis

- **Serious Reactions**
  - Angina pectoris, depression, and flu-like symptoms occur rarely.

Special Considerations

- Compared to ipratropium is more expensive, but once-daily administration will likely improve adherence with therapy

- **Patient/Family Education**
  - Capsules should **not** be swallowed; use only 1 capsule for inhalation at a time
  - Refer to product information for instructions on how to administer tiotropium via the HandiHaler device
  - Should **not** be used for immediate relief of breathing problems, i.e., as a rescue medication
  - Do **not** store capsules in the HandiHaler
  - Rinse the mouth with water immediately after inhalation to prevent mouth and throat dryness and oral candidiasis
  - Drink plenty of fluids to decrease the thickness of lung secretions
  - Avoid excessive consumption of caffeine products, such as chocolate, cocoa, cola, coffee, and tea

- **Monitoring Parameters**
  - Improvement in symptoms; such as cessation of clavicular retractions, quieter and slower respirations, and a relaxed facial expression; reduction in the need for rescue short-acting beta$_2$-agonists
  - Pulse rate and quality and respiratory rate, depth, rhythm, and type
  - ABG levels
  - Examine lips and fingernails for signs of cyanosis, such as a blue or gray color in light-skinned patients and a gray color in dark-skinned patients

- **Geriatric side effects at a glance:**
  ❏ CNS   ❏ Bowel Dysfunction   ❏ Bladder Dysfunction   ❏ Falls

- **U.S. Regulatory Considerations**
  ❏ FDA Black Box   ❏ OBRA regulated in U.S. Long Term Care

tipranavir

(ti-pran'-ah-veer)

■ **Brand Name(s):** Aptivus

■ **Clinical Pharmacology:**
Mechanism of Action: A nonpeptide HIV-1 protease inhibitor that inhibits the virus-specific processing of polyproteins and HIV-1 infected cells. **Therapeutic Effect:** Prevents formation of mature viral cells.
Pharmacokinetics: Readily absorbed after PO administration. Protein binding: 98%-99%. Metabolized in liver. Excreted in urine. **Half-life:** 4.8-6 hr.

■ **Available Forms:**
  • *Capsules*: 250 mg.

■ **Indications and Dosages:**
HIV-1 infection (concurrent therapy with ritonavir): PO 500 mg (2 capsules) administered with 200 mg of ritonavir twice a day.

■ **Contraindications:** Moderate or severe hepatic insufficiency, hypersensitivity to tipranavir or any component of the formulation

■ **Side Effects**
Occasional
Diarrhea, nausea, fever, fatigue, vomiting, abdominal pain, headache, bronchitis, depression
Rare
Asthenia, insomnia, cough

■ **Serious Reactions**
  • Hepatic failure, rash, increased bleeding in patients with hemophilia, diabetes mellitus, increased lipid levels, and changes in body fat have been reported.

Special Considerations
  • Always check updated treatment guidelines before initiating or changing antiretroviral therapy (http://AIDSinfo.nih.gov)

■ **Geriatric side effects at a glance:**
  ❑ CNS   ❑ Bowel Dysfunction   ❑ Bladder Dysfunction   ❑ Falls

■ **U.S. Regulatory Considerations**
  ☑ FDA Black Box
  • Tipranavir co-administered with ritonavir (200 mg) has been associated with reports of both fatal and nonfatal intracranial hemorrhage.
  • Tipranavir co-administered with ritonavir (200 mg) has been associated with reports of clinical hepatitis and hepatic decompensation including some fatalities. Extra vigilance is warranted in patients with chronic hepatitis B or hepatitis C co-infection, as these patients have an increased risk of hepatotoxicity.
  ❑ OBRA regulated in U.S. Long Term Care

tirofiban hydrochloride

(tye-roe-fye'-ban hye-droe-klor'-ide)

- **Brand Name(s):** Aggrastat
  Chemical Class: Glycoprotein (GP) IIb/IIIa inhibitor

- **Clinical Pharmacology:**
  Mechanism of Action: An antiplatelet and antithrombotic agent that binds to platelet receptor glycoprotein IIb/IIIa, preventing binding of fibrinogen. **Therapeutic Effect:** Inhibits platelet aggregation and thrombus formation.
  Pharmacokinetics: Poorly bound to plasma proteins; unbound fraction in plasma: 35%. Limited metabolism. Primarily eliminated in the urine (65%) and, to a lesser amount, in the feces. Removed by hemodialysis. **Half-life:** 2 hr. Clearance is significantly decreased in severe renal impairment (creatinine clearance less than 30 ml/min).

- **Available Forms:**
  - *Injection* Premix: 12.5 mg/250 ml (50 mcg/ml); 25 mg/500 ml (50 mcg/ml).
  - *Vial:* 250 mcg/ml.

- **Indications and Dosages:**
  Inhibition of platelet aggregation: IV Initially, 0.4 mcg/kg/min for 30 min; then continue at 0.1 mcg/kg/min through procedure and for 12–24 hr after procedure.
  Severe renal insufficiency (creatinine clearance less than 30 ml/min): Half the usual rate of infusion.

- **Contraindications:** Active internal bleeding or a history of bleeding diathesis within previous 30 days, arteriovenous malformation or aneurysm, history of intracranial hemorrhage, history of thrombocytopenia after prior exposure to tirofiban, intracranial neoplasm, major surgical procedure within previous 30 days, severe hypertension, stroke

- **Side Effects**
  Occasional (6%–3%)
  Pelvis pain, bradycardia, dizziness, leg pain
  Rare (2%–1%)
  Edema and swelling, vasovagal reaction, diaphoresis, nausea, fever, headache

- **Serious Reactions**
  - Signs and symptoms of overdose include generally minor mucocutaneous bleeding and bleeding at the femoral artery access site.
  - Thrombocytopenia occurs rarely.

Special Considerations

- When bleeding cannot be controlled with pressure, discontinue INF

- Most major bleeding occurs at arterial access site for cardiac catheterization; prior to pulling femoral artery sheath, discontinue heparin for 3-4 hr and document activated clotting time (ACT) <180 sec or aPTT <45 sec; achieve sheath hemostasis ≥4 hr before discharge
- In clinical studies, patients received ASA unless it was contraindicated
- Tirofiban, eptifibitide, and abciximab can all decrease the incidence of cardiac events associated with acute coronary syndromes; direct comparisons are needed to establish which, if any, is superior; for angioplasty, until more data become available, abciximab appears to be the drug of choice

■ **Patient/Family Education**
- It may take longer to stop bleeding during tirofiban therapy
- Report unusual bleeding
- The patient should notify his or her dentist and other physicians of tirofiban therapy before surgery is scheduled or new drugs are prescribed

■ **Monitoring Parameters**
- Platelet count, hemoglobin, hematocrit, PT/aPTT (baseline, within 6 hr following bolus dose, then daily thereafter)
- Closely monitor the patient for bleeding, particularly at other arterial and venous puncture sites and IM injection sites

■ **Geriatric side effects at a glance:**
  ❑ CNS ❑ Bowel Dysfunction ❑ Bladder Dysfunction ❑ Falls

■ **U.S. Regulatory Considerations**
  ❑ FDA Black Box ❑ OBRA regulated in U.S. Long Term Care

tizanidine hydrochloride

(tye-zan'-i-deen hye-droe-klor'-ide)

■ **Brand Name(s):** Zanaflex
  Chemical Class: Imidazoline derivative

■ **Clinical Pharmacology:**
  Mechanism of Action: A skeletal muscle relaxant that increases presynaptic inhibition of spinal motor neurons mediated by alpha$_2$-adrenergic agonists, reducing facilitation to postsynaptic motor neurons. **Therapeutic Effect:** Reduces muscle spasticity.
  Pharmacokinetics:

Route	Onset	Peak	Duration
PO	N/A	1-2 hr	3-6 hr

Well absorbed following PO administration. Protein binding: 30%. Extensive first-pass metabolism. Metabolized in the liver. Partially excreted in urine; minimal elimination in feces. **Half-life:** 4-8 hr.

- **Available Forms:**
  - *Tablets*: 2 mg, 4 mg.

- **Indications and Dosages:**
  Muscle spasticity: PO Initially 2-4 mg, gradually increased in 2- to 4-mg increments and repeated q6-8h. Maximum: 3 doses/day or 36 mg/24 hr.

- **Unlabeled Uses:** Low back pain, spasticity associated with multiple sclerosis or spinal cord injury, tension headaches, trigeminal neuralgia

- **Contraindications:** None known.

- **Side Effects**
  Frequent (49%-41%)
  Dry mouth, somnolence, asthenia
  Occasional (16%-4%)
  Dizziness, UTI, constipation
  Rare (3%)
  Nervousness, amblyopia, pharyngitis, rhinitis, vomiting, urinary frequency

- **Serious Reactions**
  - Hypotension (a reduction in either diastolic or systolic BP) may be associated with bradycardia, orthostatic hypotension and, rarely, syncope. The risk of hypotension increases as dosage increases; BP may decrease within 1 hr after administration.

- **Patient/Family Education**
  - Arise slowly from a reclining position
  - Tizanidine may cause low blood pressure, impaired coordination, and sedation
  - Avoid tasks that require mental alertness or motor skills until response to the drug has been established
  - Change positions slowly to help prevent dizziness

- **Monitoring Parameters**
  - Perform periodic liver and renal function tests
  - Evaluate the patient for a therapeutic response, such as decreased stiffness, tenderness, and intensity of skeletal muscle pain and improved mobility

- **Geriatric side effects at a glance:**
  ☑ CNS ☐ Bowel Dysfunction ☐ Bladder Dysfunction ☑ Falls
  Other: Dry mouth, somnolence

- **Use with caution in older patients with:** Orthostatic hypotension

- **U.S. Regulatory Considerations**
  ☐ FDA Black Box ☐ OBRA regulated in U.S. Long Term Care

- **Other Uses in Geriatric Patient:** None

- **Side Effects:**
  Of particular importance in the geriatric patient: None

- **Geriatric Considerations - Summary:** The alpha$_2$-adrenergic agonist effect of tizanidine lowers blood pressure in a manner similar to clonidine but is less potent. Older adults are at risk of hypotension and when discontinued, this drug should be tapered to avoid hypertensive rebound.

- **Reference:**

1. Wagstaff AJ, Bryson HM: Tizanidine: a review of its pharmacology, clinical efficacy and tolerability in the management of spasticity associated with cerebral and spinal disorders. Drugs 1997;53(3):435-452.

tobramycin sulfate

(toe-bra-mye'-sin sul'-fate)

- **Brand Name(s):** AK-Tob, Nebcin, PMS-Tobramycin, TOBI, Tobrex

  Combinations
  Rx: Ophthalmic: with dexamethasone (Tobradex)
  Chemical Class: Aminoglycoside

- **Clinical Pharmacology:**
  Mechanism of Action: An aminoglycoside antibacterial that irreversibly binds to protein on bacterial ribosomes. **Therapeutic Effect:** Interferes with protein synthesis of susceptible microorganisms.
  Pharmacokinetics: Rapid, complete absorption after IM administration. Protein binding: less than 30%. Widely distributed (doesn't cross the blood-brain barrier; low concentrations in cerebrospinal fluid (CSF). Excreted unchanged in urine. Removed by hemodialysis. **Half-life:** 2-4 hr (increased in impaired renal function and neonates; decreased in cystic fibrosis and febrile or burn patients).

- **Available Forms:**
  - *Injection Solution (Nebcin)*: 40 mg/ml.
  - *Injection Powder for Reconstitution (Nebcin)*: 1.2 g.
  - *Ophthalmic Ointment (Tobrex)*: 0.3%.
  - *Ophthalmic Solution (AK-Tob, Tobrex)*: 0.3%.
  - *Nebulization Solution (TOBI)*: 60 mg/ml.

- **Indications and Dosages:**
  Usual parenteral dosage: IV 3-6 mg/kg/day in 3 divided doses. Once daily dosing: 4-7 mg/kg every 24 hr.
  Superficial eye infections, including blepharitis, conjunctivitis, keratitis, and corneal ulcers: Ophthalmic Ointment Usual dosage, apply a thin strip to conjunctiva q8-12h (q3-4h for severe infections). Ophthalmic Solution Usual dosage, 1-2 drops in affected eye q4h (2 drops/hr for severe infections).
  Dosage in renal impairment: Dosage and frequency are modified based on the degree of renal impairment and the serum drug concentration. After a loading dose of 1-2 mg/kg, the maintenance dose and frequency are based on serum creatinine levels and creatinine clearance.

- **Contraindications:** Hypersensitivity to other aminoglycosides (cross-sensitivity) and their components

- **Side Effects**
  Occasional
  IM: Pain, induration
  IV: Phlebitis, thrombophlebitis
  Topical: Hypersensitivity reaction (fever, pruritus, rash, urticaria)
  Ophthalmic: Tearing, itching, redness, eyelid swelling
  Rare
  Hypotension, nausea, vomiting

- **Serious Reactions**
  - Nephrotoxicity (as evidenced by increased BUN and serum creatinine levels and decreased creatinine clearance) may be reversible if the drug is stopped at the first sign of nephrotoxic symptoms.
  - Irreversible ototoxicity (manifested as tinnitus, dizziness, ringing or roaring in ears, and hearing loss) and neurotoxicity (manifested as headache, dizziness, lethargy, tremor, and visual disturbances) occur occasionally. The risk of these reactions increases with higher dosages or prolonged therapy and when the solution is applied directly to the mucosa.
  - Superinfections, particularly fungal infections, may result from bacterial imbalance with any administration route.
  - Anaphylaxis may occur.

Special Considerations

  - Gentamicin is first-line aminoglycoside of choice; differences in toxicity between gentamicin and tobramycin not likely to be clinically important in most patients with normal renal function given short courses of treatment; consider tobramycin in patients who are more likely to develop toxicity (prolonged and/or recurrent aminoglycoside therapy, those with renal failure) and in patients infected with *Pseudomonas aeruginosa* because of increased antibacterial activity

- **Patient/Family Education**
  - Notify the physician if any balance, hearing, urinary, or vision problems develop, even after therapy is completed
  - The patient using ophthalmic tobramycin should know that irritation, redness, blurred vision, or tearing may occur briefly after application
  - Notify the physician if these symptoms persist

- **Monitoring Parameters**
  - Serum Ca, Mg, Na; serum concentrations, peak (30 min following IV INF or 1 hr after IM inj) and trough (just prior to next dose); prolonged concentrations above 12 mcg/ml or trough levels above 2 mcg/ml may indicate tissue accumulation; such accumulation, advanced age, and cumulative dosage may contribute to ototoxicity and nephrotoxicity; perform serum concentration assays after 2 or 3 doses, so that the dosage can be adjusted if necessary, and at 3- to 4-day intervals during therapy; in the event of changing renal function, more frequent serum concentrations should be obtained and the dosage or dosage interval adjusted according to more detailed guidelines

- **Geriatric side effects at a glance:**
  ❑ CNS   ❑ Bowel Dysfunction   ❑ Bladder Dysfunction   ❑ Falls

    ☑ FDA Black Box
    Neurotoxicity, both auditory and vestibular ototoxicity, and nephrotoxicity can occur.
    Risk for both is greater in patients with impaired renal function and in those who re-
    ceive high doses or prolonged therapy.
    ❏ OBRA regulated in U.S. Long Term Care

tocainide hydrochloride

(toe-kay'-nide hye-droe-klor'-ide)

■ **Brand Name(s):** Tonocard
    Chemical Class: Lidocaine derivative

■ **Clinical Pharmacology:**
    Mechanism of Action: An amide-type local anesthetic that shortens the action poten-
    tial duration and decreases the effective refractory period and automaticity in the His-
    Purkinje system of the myocardium by blocking sodium transport across myocardial
    cell membranes. **Therapeutic Effect:** Suppresses ventricular arrhythmias.
    Pharmacokinetics: Very rapidly and completely absorbed following PO administra-
    tion. Protein binding: 10%. Metabolized in liver. Excreted in urine. **Half-life:** 15 hr.

■ **Available Forms:**
    • *Tablets*: 400 mg, 600 mg.

■ **Indications and Dosages:**
    Suppression and prevention of ventricular arrhythmias: PO Initially, 400 mg q8h.
    Maintenance: 1.2-1.8 g/day in divided doses q8h. Maximum: 2,400 mg/day.

■ **Unlabeled Uses:** Trigeminal neuralgia

■ **Contraindications:** Hypersensitivity to local anesthetics, second- or third-degree AV
    block

■ **Side Effects**
    Tocainide is generally well tolerated.
    Frequent (10%-3%)
    Minor, transient light-headedness, dizziness, nausea, paresthesia, rash, tremor
    Occasional (3%-1%)
    Clammy skin, night sweats, myalgia
    Rare (less than 1%)
    Restlessness, nervousness, disorientation, mood changes, ataxia (muscular incoor-
    dination), visual disturbances

■ **Serious Reactions**
    • High dosage may produce bradycardia or tachycardia, hypotension, palpitations,
      increased ventricular arrhythmias, premature ventricular contractions (PVCs),
      chest pain, and exacerbation of CHF.

- Can be considered oral lidocaine; antidysrhythmic drugs have not been shown to improve survival in patients with ventricular dysrhythmias; class I antidysrhythmic drugs (e.g., tocainide) have increased the risk of death when used in patients with non-life-threatening dysrhythmias
- Initiate therapy in facilities capable of providing continuous ECG monitoring and managing life-threatening dysrhythmias

■ Patient/Family Education

- Avoid tasks that require mental alertness or motor skills until response to the drug has been established
- Notify the physician of any breathing difficulties, palpitations, or tremor
- May be taken with food

■ Monitoring Parameters

- Blood concentrations (therapeutic concentrations 4-10 mcg/ml)
- Monitor the patient's ECG for changes, particularly shortening of the QT interval; notify the physician of significant interval changes
- Fluid status and serum electrolyte levels
- Intake and output
- Weight
- Assess the patient's hand movements for tremor, which is usually the first sign that the maximum dose is being reached
- Monitor the patient for numbness or tingling in the feet or hands
- Assess the patient's skin for clamminess and rash
- Observe the patient for CNS disturbances, including disorientation, incoordination, mood changes, and restlessness
- Assess the patient for signs and symptoms of CHF, including distended neck veins, dyspnea (particularly on exertion or lying down), night cough, and peripheral edema

■ Geriatric side effects at a glance:

❑ CNS   ❑ Bowel Dysfunction   ❑ Bladder Dysfunction   ❑ Falls

■ U.S. Regulatory Considerations

☑ FDA Black Box

- An excessive mortality or nonfatal cardiac arrest rate was observed in patients with non-life-threatening ventricular arrhythmias who had a recent MI.
- Ventricular proarrhythmic effects have been observed in patients with atrial fibrillation/flutter. This drug is not recommended in patients with chronic atrial fibrillation.
- Agranulocytosis, aplastic anemia, bone marrow depression, hypoplastic anemia, leukopenia, neutropenia, and septic shock have been reported when used within therapeutic dose ranges, typically within the first 12 wk of therapy. Use with caution in patients with preexisting marrow failure or cytopenia.
- Pulmonary fibrosis, interstitial pneumonitis, fibrosing alveolitis, pulmonary edema, and pneumonitis have been reported.

❑ OBRA regulated in U.S. Long Term Care

tolazamide

(tole-az'-a-mide)

- **Brand Name(s):** Tolinase
  Chemical Class: Sulfonylurea (1st generation)

- **Clinical Pharmacology:**
  Mechanism of Action: A first-generation sulfonylurea that promotes release of insulin from beta cells of pancreas. **Therapeutic Effect:** Lowers blood glucose concentration. **Pharmacokinetics:** Well absorbed from the gastrointestinal (GI) tract. Extensively metabolized in liver to five metabolites, three of which are active. Primarily excreted in urine. Unknown if removed by hemodialysis. **Half-life:** 7 hr.

- **Available Forms:**
  - *Tablets*: 100 mg, 250 mg, 500 mg (Tolinase).

- **Indications and Dosages:**
  Diabetes mellitus: PO Initially, 100-250 mg once a day, with breakfast or first main meal. Maintenance: 100-1,000 mg once a day. May increase by increments of 100-250 mg at weekly intervals, based on blood glucose response. May increase by 100-250 mg/day at weekly intervals. Maximum: 1,000 mg/day. Doses more than 500 mg/day should be given in 2 divided doses with meals.

- **Unlabeled Uses:** None known.

- **Contraindications:** Diabetic complications, such as ketosis, acidosis, and diabetic coma, sole therapy for type 1 diabetes mellitus, hypersensitivity to tolazamide or its components

- **Side Effects**
  Frequent
  Altered taste sensation, dizziness, drowsiness, weight gain, constipation, diarrhea, heartburn, nausea, vomiting, stomach fullness, headache
  Occasional
  Increased sensitivity of skin to sunlight, peeling of skin, itching, rash

- **Serious Reactions**
  - Severe hypoglycemia may occur due to overdosage and insufficient food intake, especially with increased glucose demands.
  - GI hemorrhage, cholestatic hepatic jaundice, leukopenia, thrombocytopenia, pancytopenia, agranulocytosis, and aplastic or hemolytic anemia occurs rarely.

Special Considerations
  - Similar clinical effect as second-generation agents (e.g., glyburide, glipizide); usually less expensive
  - Although allergic cross-reactivity with sulfonamide antibiotics and sulfonamide nonantibiotics has not been demonstrated, use with caution in patients with a history of severe sulfa allergies.

1234

- **Patient/Family Education**
  - Home blood glucose monitoring
  - Multiple drug interactions, including alcohol and salicylates
  - Symptoms of hypoglycemia: tingling lips/tongue, nausea, confusion, fatigue, sweating, hunger, visual changes (spots)
  - Carry candy, sugar packets, or other sugar supplements for immediate reponse to hypoglycemia
  - Notify the physician when glucose demands are altered, such as with fever, heavy physical activity, infection, stress, or trauma

- **Monitoring Parameters**
  - Self-monitored blood glucoses; glycosylated hemoglobin q3-6 mo

- **Geriatric side effects at a glance:**
  ☐ CNS   ☐ Bowel Dysfunction   ☐ Bladder Dysfunction   ☐ Falls
  Other: Hypoglycemia

- **Use with caution in older patients with:** Hepatic impairment, renal impairment

- **U.S. Regulatory Considerations**
  ☐ FDA Black Box   ☐ OBRA regulated in U.S. Long Term Care

- **Other Uses in Geriatric Patient:** Hepatic impairment, renal impairment

- **Side Effects:**
  Of particular importance in the geriatric patient: Hypoglycemia, weight gain, drug-induced disulfiram-like reaction

- **Geriatric Considerations - Summary:** Metabolized in the liver to inactive and active metabolites that are renally eliminated. Not well-studied in older adults.

- **References:**
  1. Haas L. Management of diabetes mellitus medications in the nursing home. Drugs Aging 2005;22:209-218.
  2. Shorr RI, Ray WA, Daugherty JR, et al. Incidence and risk factors for serious hypoglycemia in older persons using insulin or sulfonylureas. Arch Intern Med 1997;157:1681-1686.
  3. Shorr RI, Ray WA, Daugherty JR, et al. Individual sulfonylureas and serious hypoglycemia in older people. J Am Geriatr Soc 1996;44:751-755.

tolbutamide

(tole-byoo'-ta-mide)

- **Brand Name(s):** Orinase, Orinase Diagnostic, Tol-Tab
  Chemical Class: Sulfonylurea (1st generation)

- **Clinical Pharmacology:**
  Mechanism of Action: A first-generation sulfonylurea that promotes the release of insulin from beta cells of pancreas. **Therapeutic Effect:** Lowers blood glucose concentration.

Pharmacokinetics:

Route	Onset	Peak	Duration
PO	1 hr	5-8 hr	12-24 hr
IV	N/A	30-45 min	90-181 min

Well absorbed from the gastrointestinal (GI) tract. Protein binding: 80%-99%. Extensively metabolized in liver to 2 inactive metabolites, primarily via oxidation. Excreted in urine. Removed by hemodialysis. **Half-life:** 4.5-6.5 hr.

■ **Available Forms:**
  • *Tablets*: 500 mg (Orinase, Tol-Tab).
  • *Injection, Powder for Reconstitution*: 1g (Orinase Diagnostic).

■ **Indications and Dosages:**
  Diabetes mellitus: PO Initially, 1g daily, with breakfast or first main meal, or in divided doses. Maintenance: 0.25-3g once a day. After dose of 2g is reached, dosage should be increased in increments of up to 2 mg q1-2wk, based on blood glucose response. Maximum: 3 g/day.
  Endocrine tumor diagnosis: IV 1g infused over 2-3 min.

■ **Contraindications:** Diabetic ketoacidosis with or without coma, sole therapy for type 1 diabetes mellitus, hypersensitivity to tolbutamide or any component of its formulation

■ **Side Effects**
  Frequent
  Increased sensitivity of skin to sunlight, peeling of skin, itching, rash, dizziness, drowsiness, weight gain, constipation, diarrhea, heartburn, nausea, headache, pain at injection site
  Occasional
  Altered taste sensation, constipation, vomiting, stomach fullness

■ **Serious Reactions**
  • Severe hypoglycemia may occur because of overdosage or insufficient food intake, especially with increased glucose demands.
  • Cardiovascular mortality has been reported higher in patients treated with tolbutamide.
  • GI hemorrhage, cholestatic hepatic jaundice, leukopenia, thrombocytopenia, pancytopenia, agranulocytosis, and aplastic or hemolytic anemia occurs rarely.

Special Considerations
  • Possible differences exist for tolbutamide (short duration of action, hepatic clearance), potential preferred choice in older patients with poor general physical status and renal impairment
  • Although allergic cross-reactivity with sulfonamide antibiotics and sulfonamide nonantibiotics has not been demonstrated, use with caution in patients with a history of severe sulfa allergies.

■ **Patient/Family Education**
  • Multiple drug interactions, including alcohol and salicylates
  • Symptoms of hypoglycemia: tingling lips/tongue, nausea, confusion, fatigue, sweating, hunger, visual changes (spots)
  • Carry candy, sugar packets, or other sugar supplements for immediate response to hypoglycemia

- Notify the physician when glucose demands are altered, such as with fever, heavy physical activity, infection, stress or trauma

■ **Monitoring Parameters**
  - Self-monitored blood glucoses; glycosylated hemoglobin q3-6 mo

■ **Geriatric side effects at a glance:**
  ❑ CNS ❑ Bowel Dysfunction ❑ Bladder Dysfunction ❑ Falls
  Other: Hypoglycemia

■ **Use with caution in older patients with:** Hepatic impairment, renal impairment

■ **U.S. Regulatory Considerations**
  ❑ FDA Black Box ❑ OBRA regulated in U.S. Long Term Care

■ **Other Uses in Geriatric Patient:** None

■ **Side Effects:**
  Of particular importance in the geriatric patient: Hypoglycemia

■ **Geriatric Considerations - Summary:** Tolbutamide is primarily metabolized in the liver to inactive metabolites and has a short half-life, therefore may be safer in older adults.

■ **References:**
  1. Haas L. Management of diabetes mellitus medications in the nursing home. Drugs Aging 2005;22:209-218.
  2. Shorr RI, Ray WA, Daugherty JR, et al. Incidence and risk factors for serious hypoglycemia in older persons using insulin or sulfonylureas. Arch Intern Med 1997;157:1681-1686.
  3. Shorr RI, Ray WA, Daugherty JR, et al. Individual sulfonylureas and serious hypoglycemia in older people. J Am Geriatr Soc 1996;44:751-755.

tolcapone

(tole'-ka-pone)

■ **Brand Name(s):** Tasmar
  Chemical Class: Catechol-O-methyl-tranferase (COMT) inhibitor; nitrocatechol

■ **Clinical Pharmacology:**
  Mechanism of Action: An antiparkinson agent that inhibits the enzyme catechol-O-methyltransferase (COMT), potentiating dopamine activity and increasing the duration of action of levodopa. **Therapeutic Effect:** Relieves signs and symptoms of Parkinson's disease.
  Pharmacokinetics: Rapidly absorbed after PO administration. Protein binding: 99%. Metabolized in the liver. Eliminated primarily in urine (60%) and, to a lesser extent, in feces (40%). Unknown if removed by hemodialysis. **Half-life:** 2-3 hr.

Available Forms:
- *Tablets*: 100 mg, 200 mg.

Indications and Dosages:
Adjunctive treatment of Parkinson's disease: PO Initially, 100-200 mg 3 times a day concomitantly with each dose of carbidopa and levodopa. Maximum: 600 mg/day.
Dosage in hepatic impairment: Patients with moderate to severe cirrhosis should not receive more than 200 mg tolcapone 3 times a day.

Contraindications: None known.

Side Effects
Alert Frequency of side effects increases with dosage. The following effects are based on a 200-mg dose.
Frequent (35%-16%)
Nausea, insomnia, somnolence, anorexia, diarrhea, muscle cramps, orthostatic hypotension, excessive dreaming
Occasional (11%-4%)
Headache, vomiting, confusion, hallucinations, constipation, diaphoresis, bright yellow urine, dry eyes, abdominal pain, dizziness, flatulence
Rare (3%-2%)
Dyspepsia, neck pain, hypotension, fatigue, chest discomfort

Serious Reactions
- Upper respiratory tract infection and UTI occur in 7%-5% of patients.
- Too-rapid withdrawal from therapy may produce withdrawal-emergent hyperpyrexia, characterized by fever, muscular rigidity, and altered level of consciousness (LOC).
- Dyskinesia and dystonia occur frequently.

Special Considerations
- Because of the risk of liver failure, use only in patients who are experiencing symptom fluctuations and are not responding to, or are not candidates for, other adjunctive therapies
- Withdraw drug from patients who fail to show substantial clinical benefit within 3 wk of initiation
- Consider having patients sign informed consent alerting them to potential risks and benefits of this drug

Patient/Family Education
- Monitor for signs of liver disease (clay-colored stools, jaundice, dark urine, right upper quadrant tenderness, pruritus, fatigue, appetite loss, lethargy)
- Take tolcapone with food if nausea occurs
- Dizziness, drowsiness, and nausea may occur initially but will diminish or disappear with continued treatment
- Orthostatic hypotension commonly occurs during initial therapy but changing positions slowly can help prevent or minimize this effect
- Avoid tasks that require mental alertness or motor skills until response to the drug has been established
- Hallucinations occur more often in elderly patients, typically within the first 2 wk of therapy
- Urine may turn bright yellow
- Report to the physician if frequent falls occur

■ **Monitoring Parameters**
  - ALT/AST at baseline then q2 wk for first yr of therapy, q4 wk for next 6 mo, then q8 wk thereafter; repeat this cycle if dose increased to 200 mg tid; **discontinue tolcapone if ALT or AST exceeds upper limit of normal or if clinical signs and symptoms suggest onset of hepatic failure**
  - Plan to reduce the levodopa dosage if the patient experiences hallucinations. Keep in mind that hallucinations are usually accompanied by confusion and, to a lesser extent, insomnia
  - Assess for relief of symptoms, such as improvement of masklike facial expression, muscular rigidity, shuffling gait, and resting tremors of the hands and head

■ **Geriatric side effects at a glance:**
  ❑ CNS   ❑ Bowel Dysfunction   ❑ Bladder Dysfunction   ❑ Falls
  Other: Gastrointestinal discomfort, urine discoloration

■ **Use with caution in older patients with:** Psychotic symptoms, orthostatic hypotension

■ **U.S. Regulatory Considerations**
  ☑ FDA Black Box
  Significant risk of liver failure; restrict to patients who do not respond to other therapies.
  ❑ OBRA regulated in U.S. Long Term Care

■ **Other Uses in Geriatric Patient:** None

■ **Side Effects:**
  Of particular importance in the geriatric patient: Dyskinesias, hallucinations

■ **Geriatric Considerations - Summary:** Tolcapone inhibits peripheral COMT and increases levodopa's effects. Its primary role is as adjunct therapy to prolong the beneficial effects of levodopa and to decrease end-of-dose fluctuations in response to treatment. Due to the potential to cause serious hepatotoxicity, tolcapone requires frequent liver function monitoring and because of this risk, is rarely used.

■ **References:**
  1. Kaakkola S. Clinical pharmacology, therapeutic use and potential of COMT inhibitors in Parkinson's disease. Drugs 2000;59:1233-1250.
  2. Assal F, Spahr L, Hadengue A, et al. Tolcapone and fulminant hepatitis. Lancet 1998; 352:958.

tolmetin sodium

(tole'-met-in soe'-dee-um)

- **Brand Name(s):** Tolectin, Tolectin DS
  Chemical Class: Acetic acid derivative

- **Clinical Pharmacology:**
  Mechanism of Action: A nonsteroidal anti-inflammatory that produces analgesic and anti-inflammatory effect by inhibiting prostaglandin synthesis. **Therapeutic Effect:** Reduces inflammatory response and intensity of pain stimulus reaching sensory nerve endings.
  Pharmacokinetics: Rapidly absorbed from the gastrointestinal (GI) tract. Metabolized in liver. Excreted in urine. Minimally removed by hemodialysis. **Half-life:** 5 hr.

- **Available Forms:**
  - *Tablets*: 200 mg, 600 mg (Tolectin).
  - *Capsules*: 400 mg (Tolectin DS).

- **Indications and Dosages:**
  Rheumatoid arthritis, osteoarthritis: PO Initially, 400 mg 3 times/day (including 1 dose upon arising, 1 dose at bedtime). Adjust dose at 1-2 wk intervals. Maintenance: 600-1,800 mg/day in 3-4 divided doses.

- **Unlabeled Uses:** Treatment of ankylosing spondylitis, psoriatic arthritis

- **Contraindications:** Severely incapacitated, bedridden, wheelchair bound, hypersensitivity to aspirin or other NSAIDs

- **Side Effects**
  Occasional
  Nausea, vomiting, diarrhea, abdominal cramping, dyspepsia (heartburn, indigestion, epigastric pain), flatulence, dizziness, headache, weight decrease or increase
  Rare
  Constipation, anorexia, rash, pruritus

- **Serious Reactions**
  - Peptic ulcer, GI bleeding, gastritis, and severe hepatic reaction (cholestasis, jaundice) occur rarely.
  - Nephrotoxicity (dysuria, hematuria, proteinuria, nephrotic syndrome) and severe hypersensitivity reaction (fever, chills, bronchospasm) occur rarely.

- **Patient/Family Education**
  - Therapeutic effect is usually noted in 1-3 wk
  - Avoid alcohol and aspirin during therapy
  - Take with food or milk if GI upset occurs
  - Notify the physician if headache or GI distress occurs

Monitoring Parameters
- Initial hematocrit and fecal occult blood test within 3 mo of starting regular chronic therapy; repeat every 6-12 mo (more frequently in high-risk patients [>65 years, peptic ulcer disease, concurrent steroids or anticoagulants]); electrolytes, creatinine, and BUN within 3 mo of starting regular chronic therapy; repeat every 6-12 mo

Geriatric side effects at a glance:
☑ CNS ☐ Bowel Dysfunction ☐ Bladder Dysfunction ☐ Falls
☑ Other: Gastropathy

Use with caution in older patients with:
Renal impairment, Hepatic impairment, CHF, HTN, PUD, History of GI bleeding, GERD, Bleeding and platelet disorders, History of aspirin sensitivity reaction. Also use with caution in patients taking Anticoagulants, Aspirin, and Antihypertensive agents.

U.S. Regulatory Considerations
☑ FDA Black Box
- Increased cardiovascular risk
- Increased gastrointestinal risk
☐ OBRA regulated in U.S. Long Term Care

Other Uses in Geriatric Patient: Acute gout

Side Effects:
Of particular importance in the geriatric patient: Confusion, cognitive impairment, delirium, dizziness, dyspepsia, fluid retention, renal impairment

Geriatric Considerations - Summary:
Use of NSAIDs in older adults increases the risk of GI complications including gastric ulceration, bleeding, and perforation. These complications are not necessarily preceded by less severe GI symptoms. Concomitant use of a proton pump inhibitor or misoprostol reduces the risk for gastric ulceration and bleeding, but may not prevent long-term GI toxicity.

References:
1. COX-2 alternatives and GI protection. Med Lett Drugs Ther 2004;46:91.
2. Drugs that may cause cognitive disorders in the elderly. Med Lett Drugs Ther 2000;42:111-112.

tolnaftate

(tole-naf'-tate)

Brand Name(s):
Aftate Antifungal, Fungi-Guard, Tinactin Antifungal, Tinactin Antifungal Jock Itch, Tinaderm, Ting
Chemical Class: Carbamothioic acid derivative

Clinical Pharmacology:
Mechanism of Action: An antifungal that distorts hyphae and stunts mycelial growth in susceptible fungi. **Therapeutic Effect:** Results in fungal cell death.

■ **Available Forms:**
- Aerosol, Liquid, Topical: 1% (Aftate Antifungal, Tinactin Antifungal, Ting).
- Aerosol, Powder, Topical: 1% (Aftate Antifungal, Tinactin Antifungal, Tinactin Antifungal Jock Itch, Ting).
- Cream: 1% (Fungi-Guard, Tinactin Antifungal, Tinactin Antifungal Jock Itch).
- Powder: 1% (Tinactin Antifungal).
- Solution, Topical: 1% (Tinaderm).

■ **Indications and Dosages:**
Tinea pedis, tinea cruris, tinea corporis: Topical Spray aerosol or apply 1-3 drops of solution or a small amount of cream, gel, or powder 2 times daily for 2-4 wk.

■ **Unlabeled Uses:** Onychomycosis

■ **Contraindications:** Nail and scalp infections, hypersensitivity to tolnaftate or any component of its formulation

■ **Side Effects**
Rare
Irritation, burning, pruritus, contact dermatitis

■ **Serious Reactions**
- None known.

Special Considerations
- Nonprescription topical antifungal agent not effective in the treatment of deeper fungal infections of the skin, nor is it reliable in the treatment of fungal infections involving the scalp or nail beds; *Candida* is resistant; useful for patients desiring self-medication of mild tinea infections; patients must be advised of limitations
- Powders generally used as adjunctive therapy, but may be acceptable as primary therapy in very mild cases

■ **Patient/Family Education**
- Keep affected areas clean and dry and wear light clothing to promote ventilation
- Separate personal items that come in contact with affected areas
- Avoid topical cream contact with eyes, mouth, nose, or other mucous membranes
- Rub topical form well into affected and surrounding area

■ **Monitoring Parameters**
- Therapeutic response

■ **Geriatric side effects at a glance:**
❑ CNS ❑ Bowel Dysfunction ❑ Bladder Dysfunction ❑ Falls

■ **U.S. Regulatory Considerations**
❑ FDA Black Box ❑ OBRA regulated in U.S. Long Term Care

tolterodine tartrate

(tol-tare'-oh-deen tar'-trate)

- **Brand Name(s):** Detrol, Detrol LA
  Chemical Class: Tertiary amine

- **Clinical Pharmacology:**
  Mechanism of Action: An antispasmodic that exhibits potent antimuscarinic activity by interceding via cholinergic muscarinic receptors, thereby inhibiting urinary bladder contraction. **Therapeutic Effect:** Decreases urinary frequency, urgency.
  Pharmacokinetics: Rapidly and well absorbed after PO administration. Protein binding: 96%. Extensively metabolized in the liver to active metabolite. Primarily excreted in urine. Unknown if removed by hemodialysis. **Half-life:** 1.9–3.7 hr.

- **Available Forms:**
  - *Tablets* (Detrol): 1 mg, 2 mg.
  - *Capsules* (Extended-Release [Detrol LA]): 2 mg, 4 mg.

- **Indications and Dosages:**
  Overactive bladder: PO 1–2 mg twice a day.
  Dosage in severe renal or hepatic impairment: PO 1 mg twice a day. PO (Extended-Release) 2–4 mg once a day.

- **Contraindications:** Gastric retention, uncontrolled angle-closure glaucoma, urine retention

- **Side Effects**
  Frequent (40%)
  Dry mouth
  Occasional (11%–4%)
  Headache, dizziness, fatigue, constipation, dyspepsia (heartburn, indigestion, epigastric discomfort), upper respiratory tract infection, UTI, dry eyes, abnormal vision (accommodation problems), nausea, diarrhea
  Rare (3%)
  Somnolence, chest or back pain, arthralgia, rash, weight gain, dry skin, delirium

- **Serious Reactions**
  - Overdose can result in severe anticholinergic effects, including abdominal cramps, facial warmth, excessive salivation or lacrimation, diaphoresis, pallor, urinary urgency, blurred vision, and prolonged QT interval.

- **Patient/Family Education**
  - Dry mouth occurs in 40% of treated patients at a dose of 2 mg bid; incidence is dose-dependent
  - May cause blurred vision, GI upset or constipation, and dry eyes

Monitoring Parameters
- Monitor the patient for incontinence and residual urine in the bladder
- Determine if the patient experiences a change in vision

Geriatric side effects at a glance:
☑ CNS   ☑ Bowel Dysfunction   ☑ Bladder Dysfunction   ☑ Falls
Other: Dry mouth, blurred vision, dizziness, somnolence

Use with caution in older patients with: Tachyarrythmias, overflow incontinence.

U.S. Regulatory Considerations
☐ FDA Black Box
☑ OBRA regulated in U.S. Long Term Care

Other Uses in Geriatric Patient: None

Side Effects:
Of *particular importance in the geriatric patient*: Delirium, possible antagonism of cholinergic drug therapy in the treatment of Alzheimer's disease.

Geriatric Considerations - Summary: Tolterodine and other newer anticholinergic drugs are moderately effective in the treatment of urge urinary incontinence and offer the potential benefit of selective antagonism of muscarinic receptors with less potential for CNS adverse effects. The relative safety and efficacy of these agents, which are significantly more expensive, has not been well studied to determine if they are superior to longer-acting anticholinergic formulations. These newer drugs can produce anticholinergic adverse effects including cognitive impairment, dry mouth, blurred vision, and increased risk of falls.

References:
1. Hay-Smith J, Herbison P, Ellis G, Moore K. Anticholinergic drugs versus placebo for overactive bladder syndrome in adults. Cochrane Database System Rev 2003;3.
2. Vangala V, Tueth M. Chronic anticholinergic toxicity: identification and management in older patients. Geriatrics 2003;58:36-37.
3. Tune LE. Anticholinergic effects of medication in elderly patients. J Clin Psychiatry 2001;62(suppl 21):11-14.
4. Solifenacin and drifenacin for overactive bladder. Med Let 2005;47:23-24.
5. Ouslander JG. Management of overactive bladder. N Engl J Med 2004;350:786-799.

topiramate

(toe-pyre'-a-mate)

Brand Name(s): Topamax
Chemical Class: Sulfamate-substituted monosaccharide derivative

■ Clinical Pharmacology:

Mechanism of Action: An anticonvulsant that blocks repetitive, sustained firing of neurons by enhancing the ability of gamma-aminobutyric acid to induce an influx of chloride ions into the neurons; may also block sodium channels. **Therapeutic Effect:** Decreases seizure activity.

Pharmacokinetics: Rapidly absorbed after PO administration. Protein binding: 13%-17%. Not extensively metabolized. Primarily excreted unchanged in urine. Removed by hemodialysis. **Half-life:** 21 hr.

■ Available Forms:

- *Capsules* (*Sprinkle*): 15 mg, 25 mg.
- *Tablets*: 25 mg, 50 mg, 100 mg, 200 mg.

■ Indications and Dosages:

Adjunctive treatment of partial seizures, Lennox-Gastaut syndrome, tonic-clonic seizures: PO Initially, 25-50 mg for 1 wk. May increase by 25-50 mg/day at weekly intervals. Maximum: 1,600 mg/day.

Monotherapy with partial, tonic-clonic seizures: PO Initially, 25 mg twice a day. Increase at weekly intervals up to 400 mg/day according to the following schedule:

- Week 1, 25 mg twice a day
- Week 2, 50 mg twice a day
- Week 3, 75 mg twice a day
- Week 4, 100 mg twice a day
- Week 5, 150 mg twice a day
- Week 6, 200 mg twice a day

Migraine prevention: PO Initially, 25 mg/day. May increase by 25 mg/day at 7-day intervals up to a total daily dose of 100 mg/day in 2 divided doses.

Dosage in renal impairment: Expect to reduce drug dosage by 50% in patients with tonic-clonic seizures who have a creatinine clearance of less than 70 ml/min.

■ Unlabeled Uses: Treatment of alcohol dependence

■ Contraindications: Bipolar disorder

■ Side Effects

Frequent (30%-10%)

Somnolence, dizziness, ataxia, nervousness, nystagmus, diplopia, paresthesia, nausea, tremor

Occasional (9%-3%)

Confusion, breast pain, dysmenorrhea, dyspepsia, depression, asthenia, pharyngitis, weight loss, anorexia, rash, musculoskeletal pain, abdominal pain, difficulty with coordination, sinusitis, agitation, flu-like symptoms

Rare (3%-2%)

Mood disturbances, such as irritability and depression; dry mouth; aggressive behavior

■ Serious Reactions

- Psychomotor slowing, impaired concentration, language problems (such as word-finding difficulties), and memory disturbances occur occasionally. These reactions are generally mild to moderate but may be severe enough to require discontinuation of drug therapy.

■ Patient/Family Education
- Drink plenty of fluids to prevent kidney stone formation
- Avoid breaking tablets to avoid their bitter taste
- Do not abruptly discontinue topiramate because this may precipitate seizures; strict maintenance of drug therapy is essential for seizure control
- May cause dizziness, drowsiness, or impaired thinking; avoid tasks that require mental alertness or motor skills until response to the drug is established; drowsiness usually diminishes with continued therapy
- Avoid alcohol and other CNS depressants while on topiramate therapy
- Notify the physician if blurred vision or other visual changes occur
- The patient should always carry an identification card or wear an identification bracelet that displays seizure disorder and anticonvulsant therapy

■ Monitoring Parameters
- Assess for clinical improvement, such as a decrease in the frequency and intensity of seizures
- Renal function test results, including BUN and serum creatinine levels

■ Geriatric side effects at a glance:
❑ CNS ❑ Bowel Dysfunction ❑ Bladder Dysfunction ❑ Falls

Other: Worsening cognitive impairment

■ Use with caution in older patients with: Cognitive impairment, renal impairment, unsteady gait, nephrolithiasis, urinary incontinence

■ U.S. Regulatory Considerations
❑ FDA Black Box ❑ OBRA regulated in U.S. Long Term Care

■ Other Uses in Geriatric Patient: Alcohol withdrawal, essential tremor, migraine prophylaxis

■ Side Effects:
Of particular importance in the geriatric patient: Delirium, confusion, cognitive impairment, ataxia, impaired concentration, dizziness, fatigue, paresthesias, slowed thinking and speech, worsening memory, nausea, anorexia, weight loss, renal stones (dose-related)

■ Geriatric Considerations - Summary: Adjust dosage for creatinine clearance less than 70ml/min. Use with caution in older adults due to effects on cognition, which are more prominent at higher doses. Slow titration is required and reduces the impact on cognitive function. Adults taking topiramate showed significant declines in attention, word fluency, and learning. Not considered first-line therapy due to potential adverse effects on cognition, attention, and learning.

■ References:
1. Brodie M, Kwan P. Epilepsy in elderly people. BMJ 2005;331:1317-1322.
2. Groselj J, Fuerrini R, Van Oene J, et al. Experience with topiramate monotherapy in elderly patients with recent-onset epilepsy. Acta Neurol Scand 2005;112:144-150.
3. Arroyo S, Kramer G. Treating epilepsy in the elderly: safety considerations. Drug Saf 2001;24:991-1015.
4. Drugs that may cause cognitive disorders in the elderly. Med Let 2000;42:111-112.

5. Willmore LJ. Choice and use of newer anticonvulsant drugs in older patients. Drugs Aging 2000;17:441-452.
6. Faught E. Epidemiolgy and drug treatment of epilepsy in elderly people. Drugs Aging 1999;15:255-269.

torsemide

(tore'-se-mide)

■ **Brand Name(s):** Demadex, Demadex I.V.
Chemical Class: Pyridine-sulfonamide derivative

■ **Clinical Pharmacology:**
Mechanism of Action: A loop diuretic that enhances excretion of sodium, chloride, potassium, and water at the ascending limb of the loop of Henle; also reduces plasma and extracellular fluid volume. **Therapeutic Effect:** Produces diuresis; lowers BP.
Pharmacokinetics:

Route	Onset	Peak	Duration
PO	1 hr	1–2 hr	6–8 hr
IV	10 min	1 hr	6–8 hr

Rapidly and well absorbed from the GI tract. Protein binding: 97%–99%. Metabolized in the liver. Primarily excreted in urine. Not removed by hemodialysis. **Half-life:** 3.3 hr.

■ **Available Forms:**
• *Tablets* (Demadex): 5 mg, 10 mg, 20 mg, 100 mg.
• *Injection* (Demadex I.V.): 10 mg/ml.

■ **Indications and Dosages:**
Hypertension: PO Initially, 2.5-5 mg/day. May increase to 10 mg/day if no response in 4–6 wk. If no response, additional antihypertensive added.
CHF: PO, IV Initially, 10–20 mg/day. May increase by approximately doubling dose until desired therapeutic effect is attained. Doses greater than 200 mg have not been adequately studied.
Chronic renal failure: PO, IV Initially, 20 mg/day. May increase by approximately doubling dose until desired therapeutic effect is attained. Doses greater than 200 mg have not been adequately studied.
Hepatic cirrhosis: PO, IV Initially, 5 mg/day given with aldosterone antagonist or potassium-sparing diuretic. May increase by approximately doubling dose until desired therapeutic effect is attained. Doses greater than 40 mg have not been adequately studied.

■ **Contraindications:** Anuria, hepatic coma, severe electrolyte depletion

■ **Side Effects**
Frequent (10%–4%)
Headache, dizziness, rhinitis
Occasional (3%–1%)
Asthenia, insomnia, nervousness, diarrhea, constipation, nausea, dyspepsia, edema, ECG changes, pharyngitis, cough, arthralgia, myalgia

Rare (less than 1%)
Syncope, hypotension, arrhythmias

■ **Serious Reactions**
- Ototoxicity may occur with high doses or a too-rapid IV administration.
- Overdose produces acute, profound water loss; volume and electrolyte depletion; dehydration; decreased blood volume; and circulatory collapse.

Special Considerations
- Offers potential advantages over other loop diuretics, including a longer duration of action and fewer adverse electrolyte and metabolic effects; available data not extensive or convincing enough at present to recommend replacement of standard loop diuretic (furosemide); considered alternative in refractory patients
- Although allergic cross-reactivity with sulfonamide antibiotics and sulfonamide nonantibiotics has not been demonstrated, use with caution in patients with a history of severe sulfa allergies.

■ **Patient/Family Education**
- Take torsemide in the morning to prevent nocturia
- Expect an increase in the frequency and volume of urination
- Notify the physician if cramps, dizziness, an irregular heartbeat, muscle weakness, nausea, or hearing abnormalities occur
- Do not take other medications, including OTC drugs, without first consulting the physician
- Eat foods high in potassium, including apricots, bananas, raisins, orange juice, potatoes, legumes, meat, and whole grains (such as cereals)

■ **Monitoring Parameters**
- Urine volume, creatinine clearance, BUN, electrolytes, reduction in edema, increased diuresis, decrease in body weight, reduction in blood pressure, glucose, uric acid, serum calcium (tetany), tinnitus, vertigo, hearing loss (especially in those at risk for ototoxicity—IV doses >120 mg; concomitant ototoxic drugs), renal disease)

■ **Geriatric side effects at a glance:**
❑ CNS   ❑ Bowel Dysfunction   ❑ Bladder Dysfunction   ❑ Falls

■ **U.S. Regulatory Considerations**
❑ FDA Black Box   ❑ OBRA regulated in U.S. Long Term Care

tramadol hydrochloride

(trah'-ma-doll hye-droe-klor'-ide)

■ **Brand Name(s):** Ultram
  Combinations
  Rx: with acetaminophen (Ultracet)
  Chemical Class: Cyclohexanol derivative

■ **Clinical Pharmacology:**
  Mechanism of Action: An analgesic that binds to mu-opioid receptors and inhibits re-uptake of norepinephrine and serotonin. Reduces the intensity of pain stimuli reaching sensory nerve endings. **Therapeutic Effect:** Alters the perception of and emotional response to pain.
  Pharmacokinetics:

Route	Onset	Peak	Duration
PO	less than 1 hr	2-3 hr	4-6 hr

  Rapidly and almost completely absorbed after PO administration. Protein binding: 20%. Extensively metabolized in the liver to active metabolite (reduced in patients with advanced cirrhosis). Primarily excreted in urine. Minimally removed by hemodialysis. **Half-life:** 6-7 hr.

■ **Available Forms:**
  • *Tablets*: 50 mg.
  • *Orally-Disintegrating Tablets*: 50 mg.
  • *Extended-Release Tablets*: 100 mg, 200 mg, 300 mg.

■ **Indications and Dosages:**
  Moderate to moderately severe pain: PO (Immediate-Release, Orally-Disintegrating) 50-100 mg q4-6h. Maximum: 400 mg/day for patients 75 yr and younger; 300 mg/day for patients older than 75 yr. PO (Extended-Release) 100-300 mg once daily.
  Dosage in renal impairment: For patients with creatinine clearance of less than 30 ml/min, increase dosing interval to q12h. Maximum: 200 mg/day.
  Dosage in hepatic impairment: Dosage is decreased to 50 mg q12h.

■ **Contraindications:** Acute alcohol intoxication; concurrent use of centrally acting analgesics, hypnotics, opioids, or psychotropic drugs; hypersensitivity to opioids

■ **Side Effects**
  Frequent (25%-15%)
  Dizziness or vertigo, nausea, constipation, headache, somnolence
  Occasional (10%-5%)
  Vomiting, pruritus, CNS stimulation (such as nervousness, anxiety, agitation, tremor, euphoria, mood swings, and hallucinations), asthenia, diaphoresis, dyspepsia, dry mouth, diarrhea
  Rare (less than 5%)
  Malaise, vasodilation, anorexia, flatulence, rash, blurred vision, urine retention or urinary frequency, menopausal symptoms

■ Serious Reactions
- Seizures have been reported in patients receiving tramadol within the recommended dosage range.
- Overdose results in respiratory depression and seizures.
- Tramadol may have a prolonged duration of action and cumulative effect in patients with hepatic or renal impairment.

Special Considerations
- Expensive, non-narcotic, "narcotic"-tricyclic antidepressant combination analgesic; potential use in chronic pain; demonstrated efficacy in a variety of pain syndromes; minimal cardiovascular and respiratory side effects
- Does not completely bind to opioid receptors; caution in addicted patients
- Has more potential for abuse than previously thought
- Tolerance and withdrawal symptoms milder than with opiates
- Not chemically related to opiates

■ Patient/Family Education
- Tramadol use may cause dependence
- Avoid alcohol and OTC drugs such as analgesics and sedatives during tramadol therapy
- Tramadol may cause blurred vision, dizziness, and drowsiness; avoid tasks requiring mental alertness or motor skills until reaction to the drug has been established
- Notify the physician about chest pain, difficulty breathing, excessive sedation, muscle weakness, palpitations, seizures, severe constipation, or tremors

■ Monitoring Parameters
- Blood pressure, pulse rate
- Pattern of daily bowel activity
- Clinical improvement, and record the onset of pain relief

■ Geriatric side effects at a glance:
❑ CNS ☑ Bowel Dysfunction ❑ Bladder Dysfunction ☑ Falls

■ U.S. Regulatory Considerations
❑ FDA Black Box ❑ OBRA regulated in U.S. Long Term Care

trandolapril

(tran-dole'-a-pril)

■ Brand Name(s): Mavik

Combinations
Rx: with verapamil (Tarka)
Chemical Class: Angiotensin-converting enzyme (ACE) inhibitor, nonsulfhydryl

■ Clinical Pharmacology:

Mechanism of Action: An angiotensin-converting enzyme (ACE) inhibitor that suppresses the renin-angiotensin-aldosterone system and prevents the conversion of angiotensin I to angiotensin II, a potent vasoconstrictor; may also inhibit angiotensin II at local vascular and renal sites. Decreases plasma angiotensin II, increases plasma renin activity, and decreases aldosterone secretion. **Therapeutic Effect:** Reduces peripheral arterial resistance and pulmonary capillary wedge pressure; improves cardiac output and exercise tolerance.

Pharmacokinetics: Slowly absorbed from the GI tract. Protein binding: 80%. Metabolized in the liver and GI mucosa to active metabolite. Primarily excreted in urine. Removed by hemodialysis. **Half-life:** 24 hr.

■ Available Forms:

- *Tablets* (Mavik): 1 mg, 2 mg, 4 mg.

■ Indications and Dosages:

Hypertension (without diuretic): PO Initially, 1 mg once a day in nonblack patients, 2 mg once a day in black patients. Adjust dosage at least at 7-day intervals. Maintenance: 2-4 mg/day. Maximum: 8 mg/day.

Heart failure or left ventricular dysfunction post MI: PO Initially, 0.5-1 mg, titrated to target dose of 4 mg/day.

■ Unlabeled Uses: Treatment of systolic CHF

■ Contraindications: History of angioedema from previous treatment with ACE inhibitors

■ Side Effects

Frequent (35%-23%)

Dizziness, cough

Occasional (11%-3%)

Hypotension, dyspepsia (heartburn, epigastric pain, indigestion), syncope, asthenia (loss of strength), tinnitus

Rare (less than 1%)

Palpitations, insomnia, drowsiness, nausea, vomiting, constipation, flushed skin

■ Serious Reactions

- Excessive hypotension ("first-dose syncope") may occur in patients with CHF and in those who are severely salt or volume depleted.
- Angioedema and hyperkalemia occur rarely.
- Agranulocytosis and neutropenia may be noted in those with collagen vascular disease, including scleroderma and systemic lupus erythematosus, and impaired renal function.
- Nephrotic syndrome may be noted in those with history of renal disease.
- Hypoglycemia may occur in patients with diabetes using glucose-lowering drugs.

■ Patient/Family Education

- Caution with salt substitutes containing potassium chloride
- Rise slowly to sitting/standing position to minimize orthostatic hypotension
- Dizziness, fainting, light-headedness may occur during first few days of therapy
- May cause altered taste perception or cough; persistent dry cough usually does not subside unless medication is stopped; notify clinician if these symptoms persist

- Do not abruptly discontinue the drug
- Notify the physician if chest pain, cough, diarrhea, difficulty swallowing, fever, palpitations, sore throat, swelling of the face, or vomiting occurs

■ Monitoring Parameters
- BUN, creatinine, potassium within 2 wk after initiation of therapy (increased levels may indicate acute renal failure)
- Intake and output and urinary frequency
- Urinalysis for proteinuria
- Pattern of daily bowel activity and stool consistency

■ Geriatric side effects at a glance:
❑ CNS   ❑ Bowel Dysfunction   ❑ Bladder Dysfunction   ❑ Falls

■ U.S. Regulatory Considerations
☑ FDA Black Box
Although not relevant for geriatric patients, teratogenicity is associated with the use of ACE inhibitors.
❑ OBRA regulated in U.S. Long Term Care

tranylcypromine sulfate

(tran-ill-sip'-roe-meen sul'-fate)

■ Brand Name(s): Parnate
Chemical Class: Cyclopropylamine, substituted; nonhydrazine derivative

■ Clinical Pharmacology:
Mechanism of Action: An MAOI that inhibits the activity of the enzyme monoamine oxidase at CNS storage sites, leading to increased levels of the neurotransmitters epinephrine, norepinephrine, serotonin, and dopamine at neuronal receptor sites. **Therapeutic Effect:** Relieves depression.
Pharmacokinetics: Well absorbed from GI tract. Metabolized in the liver. Primarily excreted in urine. Removed by hemodialysis. **Half-life:** 1.5-3.5 hr.

■ Available Forms:
- *Tablets:* 10 mg.

■ Indications and Dosages:
Depression refractory to or intolerant of other therapy: PO Initially, 10 mg twice a day. May increase by 10 mg/day at 1- to 3-wk intervals up to 60 mg/day in divided doses.

■ Unlabeled Uses: Post-traumatic stress disorder

■ Contraindications: CHF, pheochromocytoma, severe hepatic or renal impairment, uncontrolled hypertension

Side Effects

Frequent

Orthostatic hypotension, restlessness, GI upset, insomnia, dizziness, lethargy, weakness, dry mouth, peripheral edema

Occasional

Flushing, diaphoresis, rash, urinary frequency, increased appetite, transient impotence

Rare

Visual disturbances

Serious Reactions

- Hypertensive crisis occurs rarely and is marked by severe hypertension, occipital headache radiating frontally, neck stiffness or soreness, nausea, vomiting, diaphoresis, fever or chills, clammy skin, dilated pupils, palpitations, tachycardia or bradycardia, and constricting chest pain.
- Intracranial bleeding has been reported in association with severe hypertension.

Special Considerations

- Irreversible nonselective MAOI effective for typical and atypical depression; equal efficacy to other MAOIs with quicker onset of action, and an amphetamine-like activity with a higher potential for abuse; no anticholinergic or cardiac effects

Patient/Family Education

- Therapeutic effects may take 1-4 wk
- Avoid alcohol ingestion, CNS depressants, OTC medications (cold, weight loss, hay fever, cough syrup)
- Prodromal signs of hypertensive crisis are increased headache, palpitations; discontinue drug immediately
- Do not discontinue medication abruptly after long-term use
- Avoid high-tyramine foods (aged cheese, sour cream, beer, wine, pickled products, liver, raisins, bananas, figs, avocados, meat tenderizers, chocolate, yogurt)

Monitoring Parameters

- Blood pressure, temperature, weight
- Behavior, level of interest, mood, sleep pattern
- Evaluate the patient for an occipital headache radiating frontally and neck stiffness or soreness, which may be the first symptoms of an impending hypertensive crisis. If hypertensive crisis occurs, administer phentolamine 5-10 mg IV, as prescribed

Geriatric side effects at a glance:

❑ CNS ❑ Bowel Dysfunction ❑ Bladder Dysfunction ❑ Falls
Other: Orthostatic hypotension

Use with caution in older patients with: None

U.S. Regulatory Considerations

☑ FDA Black Box
- Because there is an increased risk of suicide in children and adolescents, older adults should also be closely monitored for suicide ideation.
☑ OBRA regulated in U.S. Long Term Care

Other Uses in Geriatric Patient: Depression refractory to other measures, anxiety symptoms and related disorders

- **Side Effects:**
  Of particular importance in the geriatric patient: None

- **Geriatric Considerations - Summary:** Because of the severe toxicity of these agents and the long list of potentially serious drug-drug and drug-food interactions, they are **not** recommended for routine treatment of depression in older adults. If prescribed, they require close monitoring by specialists.

- **References:**
  1. Boyer EW, Shannon M. The serotonin syndrome. N Engl J Med 2005;352:1112-1120.
  2. Volz HP, Gleiter CH. Monoamine oxidase inhibitors. A perspective on their use in the elderly. Drugs Aging 1998;13:341-355.

travoprost

(tra'-voe-prost)

- **Brand Name(s):** Travatan
  Chemical Class: Prostaglandin F_2-alpha analog

- **Clinical Pharmacology:**
  Mechanism of Action: An ophthalmic agent that is a prostanoid selective receptor agonist. **Therapeutic Effect:** Reduces intraocular pressure (IOP) by reducing aqueous humor production.
  Pharmacokinetics: Absorbed through the cornea and hydrolyzed to the active free acid form. Metabolized in cornea and liver. Metabolites are inactive. Excreted in urine.
  Half-life: 17-86 min.

- **Available Forms:**
  - *Ophthalmic Solution*: 0.004% (Travatan).

- **Indications and Dosages:**
  Open-angle glaucoma, ocular hypertension: Ophthalmic 1 drop in affected eye(s) once daily, in the evening.

- **Contraindications:** Hypersensitivity to travoprost or benzalkonium chloride, or any other component of the formulation

- **Side Effects**
  Frequent
  Ocular hyperemia
  Occasional
  Ocular pain, pruritus, eye discomfort, decreased visual acuity, foreign body sensation
  Rare
  Abnormal vision, cataract, conjunctivitis, dry eye, eye disorder, flare, iris discoloration, keratitis, lid margin crusting, photophobia, subconjunctival hemorrhage, and tearing

- **Serious Reactions**
  - Ocular adverse events, including accidental injury, angina pectoris, anxiety, arthritis, back pain, bradycardia, bronchitis, chest pain, cold syndrome, depression, dyspepsia, gastrointestinal disorder, headache, hypercholesterolemia, hypertension, hypotension, infection, pain, prostate disorder, sinusitis, urinary incontinence, and urinary tract infection, occur rarely.

- **Geriatric side effects at a glance:**
  - ❑ CNS ❑ Bowel Dysfunction ❑ Bladder Dysfunction ❑ Falls

- **U.S. Regulatory Considerations**
  - ❑ FDA Black Box ❑ OBRA regulated in U.S. Long Term Care

trazodone hydrochloride

(tray'-zoe-done hye-droe-klor'-ide)

- **Brand Name(s):** Desyrel, Desyrel Dividose
  Chemical Class: Triazolopyridine derivative

- **Clinical Pharmacology:**
  Mechanism of Action: An antidepressant that blocks the reuptake of serotonin at neuronal presynaptic membranes, increasing its availability at postsynaptic receptor sites. **Therapeutic Effect:** Relieves depression.
  Pharmacokinetics: Well absorbed from the GI tract. Protein binding: 85%-95%. Metabolized in the liver. Primarily excreted in urine. Unknown if removed by hemodialysis. **Half-life:** 5-9 hr.

- **Available Forms:**
  - **Tablets:** 50 mg (Desyrel), 100 mg (Desyrel), 150 mg (Desyrel Dividose), 300 mg (Desyrel Dividose).

- **Indications and Dosages:**
  Depression: PO Initially, 25-50 mg at bedtime. May increase by 25-50 mg every 3-7 days. Range: 75-150 mg/day in divided doses.

- **Unlabeled Uses:** Treatment of neurogenic pain

- **Contraindications:** None known.

- **Side Effects**
  Frequent (9%-3%)
  Somnolence, dry mouth, light-headedness, dizziness, headache, blurred vision, nausea, vomiting
  Occasional (3%-1%)
  Nervousness, fatigue, constipation, generalized aches and pains, mild hypotension

Rare
Photosensitivity reaction

■ **Serious Reactions**
- Priapism, diminished or improved libido, retrograde ejaculation, and impotence occur rarely.
- Trazodone appears to be less cardiotoxic than tricyclic antidepressants, although arrhythmias may occur in patients with preexisting cardiac disease.

Special Considerations
- Very sedating antidepressant with minimal anticholinergic effects; good choice for elderly patients in whom sedating properties would be desirable

■ **Patient/Family Education**
- Take with food
- Use caution driving or performing other tasks requiring alertness
- Take trazodone at bedtime if drowsiness occurs while taking the drug
- Change positions slowly to avoid the drug's hypotensive effect
- The male patient should notify the physician immediately if a painful, prolonged penile erection occurs
- Photosensitivity to sunlight may occur during trazodone therapy
- Notify the physician if visual disturbances occur
- Avoid alcohol while taking trazodone
- Take sips of tepid water or chew sugarless gum to relieve dry mouth

■ **Monitoring Parameters**
- Behavior, level of interest, mood, and sleep pattern
- Serum neutrophil and WBC counts
- ECG for arrhythmias

■ **Geriatric side effects at a glance:**
☑ CNS   ☑ Bowel Dysfunction   ☑ Bladder Dysfunction   ☑ Falls
Other: Priapism

■ **Use with caution in older patients with:** None

■ **U.S. Regulatory Considerations**
☑ FDA Black Box
- Because there is an increased risk of suicide in children and adolescents, older adults should also be closely monitored for suicide ideation.
☐ OBRA regulated in U.S. Long Term Care

■ **Other Uses in Geriatric Patient:** Sleep disturbance, neuropathic pain

■ **Side Effects:**
Of *particular importance in the geriatric patient*: None

■ **Geriatric Considerations - Summary:** Trazodone is an effective antidepressant, with less cardiotoxicity than other antidepressants. Because it is more likely than other antidepressants to cause sedation, it is often used as a hypnotic drug when needed for long-term use. Although one study found users of trazodone less likely to fall than users of other antidepressants, older adults using trazodone, like other psychotropic drugs, should still be carefully monitered for falls.

■ **Reference:**
1. Thapa PB, Gideon P, Cost TW, et al. Antidepressants and the risk of falls among nursing home residents. N Engl J Med 1998;339:875-882.

treprostinil sodium

(treh-prost'-tin-il)

■ **Brand Name(s):** Remodulin
 Chemical Class: Prostacyclin analog

■ **Clinical Pharmacology:**
 Mechanism of Action: An antiplatelet that directly dilates pulmonary and systemic arterial vascular beds, inhibiting platelet aggregation. **Therapeutic Effect:** Reduces symptoms of pulmonary arterial hypertension associated with exercise.
 Pharmacokinetics: Rapidly, completely absorbed after subcutaneous infusion; 91% bound to plasma protein. Metabolized by the liver. Excreted mainly in the urine with a lesser amount eliminated in the feces. **Half-life:** 2–4 hr.

■ **Available Forms:**
 • *Injection*: 1 mg/ml, 2.5 mg/ml, 5 mg/ml, 10 mg/ml.

■ **Indications and Dosages:**
 Pulmonary arterial hypertension: Continuous Subcutaneous Infusion, IV Infusion Initially, 1.25 ng/kg/min. Reduce infusion rate to 0.625 ng/kg/min if initial dose cannot be tolerated. Increase infusion rate in increments of no more than 1.25 ng/kg/min per week for the first 4 wk and then no more than 2.5 ng/kg/min per week for the duration of infusion.
 Hepatic impairment (mild to moderate): Decrease the initial dose to 0.625 ng/kg/min based on ideal body weight and increase cautiously.

■ **Contraindications:** None known.

■ **Side Effects**
 Frequent
 Infusion site pain, erythema, induration, rash
 Occasional
 Headache, diarrhea, jaw pain, vasodilation, nausea
 Rare
 Dizziness, hypotension, pruritus, edema

■ **Serious Reactions**
 • Abrupt withdrawal or sudden large reductions in dosage may result in worsening of pulmonary arterial hypertension symptoms.

■ **Patient/Family Education**
 • Patient must be able to administer drug via continuous subcutaneous INF and care for the infusion system

- Therapy may be required for prolonged periods of time
- Solutions should be administered without additional dilution
- Report signs of increased pulmonary artery pressure, such as dyspnea, cough, or chest pain

■ Monitoring Parameters
- Blood pressure, clinical symptoms
- BUN, hepatic enzyme, and serum creatinine levels

■ Geriatric side effects at a glance:
❑ CNS ❑ Bowel Dysfunction ❑ Bladder Dysfunction ❑ Falls

■ U.S. Regulatory Considerations
❑ FDA Black Box ❑ OBRA regulated in U.S. Long Term Care

tretinoin

(tret'-i-noyn)

■ Brand Name(s): Altinac, Avita, Renova, Retin-A, Retin-A Micro, Vesanoid

Combinations
Rx: with fluocinolone/hydroquinone (Tri-Luma)
Chemical Class: Retinoid; vitamin A derivative

■ Clinical Pharmacology:
Mechanism of Action: A retinoid that decreases cohesiveness of follicular epithelial cells. Increases turnover of follicular epithelial cells. Bacterial skin counts are not altered. Transdermal: Exerts its effects on growth and differentiation of epithelial cells. Antineoplastic: Induces maturation, decreases proliferation of acute promyelocytic leukemia (APL) cells. **Therapeutic Effect:** Causes expulsion of blackheads; alleviates fine wrinkles, hyperpigmentation; causes repopulation of bone marrow and blood by normal hematopoietic cells.
Pharmacokinetics: Topical: Minimally absorbed. Protein binding: 95%. Metabolized in liver. Primarily excreted in urine, minimal excretion in feces. **Half-life:** 0.5-2 hr.

■ Available Forms:
- **Cream:** 0.025% (Altinac, Avita, Retin-A), 0.02% (Renova), 0.05% (Altinac, Renova, Retin-A), 0.1% (Altinac, Retin-A).
- **Gel:** 0.01% (Retin-A), 0.025% (Avita, Retin-A), 0.04% (Retin-A Micro), 0.1% (Retin-A Micro).
- **Topical Liquid:** 0.05% (Retin-A).

■ Indications and Dosages:
Acne: Topical Apply once daily at bedtime. Transdermal Apply to face once daily at bedtime.

- **Unlabeled Uses:** Treatment of disorders of keratinization, including photo-aged skin (wrinkled skin), liver spots

- **Contraindications:** Sensitivity to parabens (used as preservative in gelatin capsule)

- **Side Effects**
  Expected
  Topical: Temporary change in pigmentation, photosensitivity, Local inflammatory reactions (peeling, dry skin, stinging, erythema, pruritus) are to be expected and are reversible with discontinuation of tretinoin

- **Serious Reactions**
  - Topical
  - Possible tumorigenic potential when combined with ultraviolet radiation.

- **Patient/Family Education**
  - Keep away from eyes, mouth, angles of nose, and mucous membranes
  - Avoid exposure to ultraviolet light
  - Acne may worsen transiently
  - Normal use of cosmetics is permissible

- **Geriatric side effects at a glance:**
  ☐ CNS ☐ Bowel Dysfunction ☐ Bladder Dysfunction ☐ Falls

- **U.S. Regulatory Considerations**
  ☐ FDA Black Box ☐ OBRA regulated in U.S. Long Term Care

triamcinolone/triamcinolone acetonide/triamcinolone diacetate/triamcinolone hexacetonide

(trye-am-sin'-oh-lone)

- **Brand Name(s):** (Triamcinolone) Aristocort

- **Brand Name(s):** (Triamcinolone acetonide) Acetocot, Aristocort, Aristocort A, Aristocort Forte, Aristospan Injection, Azmacort, Clinacort, Clinalog, Kenalog, Kenalog-10, Kenalog-40, Kenalog in Orabase, Ken-Jec 40, Nasacort AQ, Triam-A, Triamcot, Triam-Forte, Triamonide 40, Triderm, Tri-Nasal, U-Tri-Lone

- **Brand Name(s):** (Triamcinolone diacetate) Amcort. Aristocort Intralesional

■ **Brand Name(s):** (Triamcinolone hexacetonide) Aristospan
  Chemical Class: Glucocorticoid, synthetic

■ **Clinical Pharmacology:**
  Mechanism of Action: An adrenocortical steroid that inhibits accumulation of inflammatory cells at inflammation sites, phagocytosis, lysosomal enzyme release and synthesis, and release of mediators of inflammation. **Therapeutic Effect:** Prevents or suppresses cell-mediated immune reactions. Decreases or prevents tissue response to inflammatory process.
  Pharmacokinetics: Minimal absorption following nasal and topical administration. Moderate absorption from the lungs and GI tract following administration of inhaled form. Rapidly and almost completely absorbed following PO administration. Metabolized in liver. Excreted in urine. **Half-life:** Unknown.

■ **Available Forms:**
  • *Oral (Topical Paste [Kenalog in Orabase]):* 0.1% or 5 g.
  • *Tablets (Aristocort):* 4 mg, 8 mg.
  • *Inhalation (Oral [Azmacort]):* 100 mcg/actuation.
  • *Nasal Spray:* 50 mcg/inhalation (Tri-Nasal), 55 mcg/inhalation (Nasacort AQ).
  • *Cream :* 0.025% (Aristocort A), 0.05% (Aristocort A), 0.1% (Aristocort A, Kenalog, Triderm).
  • *Ointment (Aristocort A, Kenalog):* 0.025%, 0.1%.
  • *Injection (acetonide):* 10 mg/ml (Kenalog-10), 40 mg/ml (Acetocot, Clinalog, Kenalog-40, Ken-Jec 40, Triam-A, Triamcot, Triamonide 40, U-Tri-Lone).
  • *Injection (diacetate):* 25 mg/ml (Aristocort), 40 mg/ml (Aristocort Forte, Clinacort, Triam-Forte).
  • *Injection (hexacetonide [Aristospan Injection]):* 5 mg/ml, 20 mg/ml.

■ **Indications and Dosages:**
  Immunosuppression, relief of acute inflammation: PO 4–60 mg/day. IM (triamcinolone acetonide) Initially, 2.5–60 mg/day. IM (triamcinolone diacetate) 40 mg/wk. IM (triamcinolone hexacetonide) Initially, 2.5–40 mg up to 100 mg; 2–20 mg. Intra-articular, Intralesional 5–40 mg.
  Control of bronchial asthma: Inhalation 2 inhalations 3–4 times a day.
  Rhinitis: Intranasal Initially, 2 sprays (55 mcg/spray) in each nostril once daily. Maintenance: 1 spray in each nostril once daily.
  Relief of inflammation or pruritus associated with corticoid-responsive dermatoses: Topical 2–4 times a day. May give 1–2 times a day or as intermittent therapy.

■ **Contraindications:** Administration of live virus vaccines, especially smallpox vaccine; hypersensitivity to corticosteroids or tartrazine; peptic ulcer disease (except life-threatening situations); systemic fungal infection
  Topical: Marked circulation impairment

■ **Side Effects**
  Frequent
  Insomnia, dry mouth, heartburn, nervousness, abdominal distention, diaphoresis, acne, mood swings, increased appetite, facial flushing, delayed wound healing, increased susceptibility to infection, diarrhea or constipation
  Occasional
  Headache, edema, change in skin color, frequent urination
  Rare
  Tachycardia, allergic reaction (including rash and hives), mental changes, hallucinations, depression
  Topical: Allergic contact dermatitis

■ Serious Reactions
- Long-term therapy may cause muscle wasting in the arms or legs, osteoporosis, spontaneous fractures, amenorrhea, cataracts, glaucoma, peptic ulcer disease, and CHF.
- Abruptly withdrawing the drug following long-term therapy may cause anorexia, nausea, fever, headache, arthralgia, rebound inflammation, fatigue, weakness, lethargy, dizziness, and orthostatic hypotension.
- Anaphylaxis occurs rarely with parenteral administration.
- Suddenly discontinuing triamcinolone may be fatal.
- Blindness has occurred rarely after intralesional injection around face and head.

■ Patient/Family Education
- May cause GI upset, take with meals or snacks (systemic)
- Do not give live virus vaccines to patients on prolonged systemic therapy
- Take PO as single daily dose in AM
- Signs of adrenal insufficiency include fatigue, anorexia, nausea, vomiting, diarrhea, weight loss, weakness, dizziness, and low blood sugar
- Avoid abrupt withdrawal of therapy following high-dose or long-term therapy
- Increased dose of rapidly acting corticosteroids may be necessary in patients subjected to unusual stress
- To be used on a regular basis, not for acute symptoms (nasal and inhalation)
- Use bronchodilators before oral inhaler (for patients using both)
- Rinse mouth to prevent oral candidiasis
- Nasal sol may cause drying and irritation of nasal mucosa; clear nasal passages prior to use

■ Monitoring Parameters
- Serum K and glucose
- Blood pressure, intake and output, weight
- Be alert to signs and symptoms of infection such as fever, pharyngitis, and vague symptoms
- Evaluate the patient for signs and symptoms of hypocalcemia (such as cramps, muscle twitching, and positive Chvostek's or Trousseau's signs), or hypokalemia (such as ECG changes, irritability, muscle cramps and weakness, nausea and vomiting, and numbness and tingling in the lower extremities)

■ Geriatric side effects at a glance:
❑ CNS ❑ Bowel Dysfunction ❑ Bladder Dysfunction ❑ Falls

■ U.S. Regulatory Considerations
❑ FDA Black Box ❑ OBRA regulated in U.S. Long Term Care

triamterene

(try-am'-ter-een)

■ **Brand Name(s):** Dyrenium

    Combinations
    Rx: with hydrochlorothiazide (Dyazide, Maxzide)
    Chemical Class: Pteridine derivative

■ **Clinical Pharmacology:**
    Mechanism of Action: A potassium-sparing diuretic that inhibits sodium, potassium, ATPase. Interferes with sodium and potassium exchange in distal tubule, cortical collecting tubule, and collecting duct. Increases sodium and decreases potassium excretion. Also increases magnesium, decreases calcium loss. *Therapeutic Effect:* Produces diuresis and lowers BP.
    Pharmacokinetics:

Route	Onset	Peak	Duration
PO	2–4 hr	N/A	7–9 hr

    Incompletely absorbed from the GI tract. Widely distributed. Metabolized in the liver. Primarily eliminated in feces via biliary route. *Half-life:* 1.5–2.5 hr (increased in renal impairment).

■ **Available Forms:**
    • *Capsules:* 50 mg, 100 mg.

■ **Indications and Dosages:**
    Edema, hypertension: PO 25–100 mg/day as a single dose or in 2 divided doses. Maximum: 300 mg/day.

■ **Unlabeled Uses:** Treatment adjunct for hypertension, prevention and treatment of hypokalemia

■ **Contraindications:** Anuria, drug-induced or preexisting hyperkalemia, progressive or severe renal disease, severe hepatic disease

■ **Side Effects**
    Occasional
    Fatigue, nausea, diarrhea, abdominal pain, leg cramps, headache
    Rare
    Anorexia, asthenia, rash, dizziness

■ **Serious Reactions**
    • Triamterene use may result in hyponatremia (somnolence, dry mouth, increased thirst, lack of energy) or severe hyperkalemia (irritability, anxiety, heaviness of legs, paresthesia, hypotension, bradycardia, ECG changes [tented T waves, widening QRS complex, ST segment depression]), particularly in those with renal impairment or diabetes, the elderly, or severely ill patients.
    • Agranulocytosis, nephrolithiasis, and thrombocytopenia occur rarely.

- **Patient/Family Education**
  - Take with meals
  - Avoid prolonged exposure to sunlight
  - Take single daily doses in AM
  - The drug's therapeutic effect takes several days to begin and can last for several days after the drug is discontinued
  - Expect an increase in the frequency and volume of urination
  - Notify the physician if dry mouth, fever, headache, nausea and vomiting, persistent or severe weakness, sore throat, or unusual bleeding or bruising occurs
  - Avoid consuming salt substitutes and foods high in potassium

- **Monitoring Parameters**
  - Blood pressure, edema, urine output, urine electrolytes, BUN, creatinine, ECG (if hyperkalemic), gynecomastia, impotence, weight

- **Geriatric side effects at a glance:**
  - ❏ CNS ❏ Bowel Dysfunction ❏ Bladder Dysfunction ❏ Falls

- **U.S. Regulatory Considerations**
  - ❏ FDA Black Box ❏ OBRA regulated in U.S. Long Term Care

triazolam

(trye-ay'-zoe-lam)

- **Brand Name(s):** Halcion
  Chemical Class: Benzodiazepine

  DEA Class: Schedule IV

- **Clinical Pharmacology:**
  Mechanism of Action: A benzodiazepine that enhances the action of the inhibitory neurotransmitter gamma-aminobutyric acid, resulting in CNS depression. **Therapeutic Effect:** Induces sleep.
  Pharmacokinetics: Rapidly and completely absorbed from GI tract. Protein binding: 89%-94%. Metabolized in the liver. Primarily excreted in urine. **Half-life:** 1.5-5.5 hr.

- **Available Forms:**
  - *Tablets:* 0.125 mg, 0.25 mg.

- **Indications and Dosages:**
  Insomnia: PO 0.0625-0.125 mg at bedtime.

- **Contraindications:** Angle-closure glaucoma; CNS depression; hypersensitivity to other benzodiazepines; severe, uncontrolled pain; sleep apnea

■ **Side Effects**
Frequent
Somnolence, sedation, dry mouth, headache, dizziness, nervousness, light-headedness, incoordination, nausea, rebound insomnia (may occur for 1-2 nights after drug is discontinued)
Occasional
Euphoria, tachycardia, abdominal cramps, visual disturbances
Rare
Paradoxical CNS excitement or restlessness (particularly in elderly or debilitated patients)

■ **Serious Reactions**
• Abrupt or too-rapid withdrawal may result in pronounced restlessness, irritability, insomnia, hand tremors, abdominal or muscle cramps, vomiting, diaphoresis, and seizures.
• Overdose results in somnolence, confusion, diminished reflexes, respiratory depression, and coma.

Special Considerations

• Prescriptions should be written for short-term use (7-10 days); drug should not be prescribed in quantities exceeding a 1-mo supply

■ **Patient/Family Education**
• Avoid alcohol and other CNS depressants
• Do not discontinue abruptly after prolonged therapy
• May cause drowsiness or dizziness; use caution while driving or performing other tasks requiring alertness
• May be habit forming
• Avoid consuming grapefruit or grapefruit juice during triazolam therapy because grapefruit decreases the drug's absorption
• Smoking reduces the drug's effectiveness

■ **Monitoring Parameters**
• Sleep pattern
• Cardiovascular, mental, and respiratory status
• Hepatic function of patients on long-term therapy
• Assess for a paradoxical reaction, particularly during early therapy
• Therapeutic response, such as a decrease in the number of nocturnal awakenings and a longer duration of sleep

■ **Geriatric side effects at a glance:**
☑ CNS   ☐ Bowel Dysfunction   ☐ Bladder Dysfunction   ☑ Falls
Other: Withdrawal symptoms after long-term use, rebound insomnia

■ **Use with caution in older patients with:** Concurrent treatment with potent CYP 3A4 inhibitors (e.g., nefazodone) leads to increased plasma concentrations of triazolam; COPD; untreated sleep apnea

■ **U.S. Regulatory Considerations**
☐ FDA Black Box   ☑ OBRA regulated in U.S. Long Term Care

■ **Other Uses in Geriatric Patient:** Hypnotic

- **Side Effects:**
  Of particular importance in the geriatric patient: Sedation, withdrawal symptoms when abruptly discontinued (e.g., during hospitalization) rather than tapered

- **Geriatric Considerations - Summary:** Benzodiazepines are effective anxiolytic agents, and hypnotics. These drugs should be reserved for short-term use. SSRIs are preferred for long-term management of anxiety disorders in older adults, and sedating antidepressants (e.g., trazodone) or eszopiclone are preferred for long-term management of sleep problems. Long-acting benzodiazepines, including flurazepam, chlordiazepoxide, clorazepate, diazepam, clonazepam, and quazepam, should generally be avoided in older adults as these agents have been associated with oversedation. On the other hand, short-acting benzodiazepines (e.g., triazolam) have been associated with a higher risk of withdrawal symptoms. When initiating therapy, benzodiazepines should be titrated carefully to avoid oversedation. In addition, many of the drugs in this class have been associated with severe withdrawal symptoms (e.g., anxiety and/or agitation, seizures) when discontinued abruptly.

- **References:**
  1. Leipzig RM, Cumming RG, Tinetti ME. Drugs and falls in older people: a systematic review and meta-analysis: I. Psychotropic drugs. J Am Geriatr Soc 1999;47:30-39.
  2. Shorr RI, Robin DW. Rational use of benzodiazepines in the elderly. Drugs Aging 1994;4:9-20.
  3. Shader RI, Greenblatt DJ. Use of benzodiazepines in anxiety disorders. N Engl J Med 1993;328:1398-1405.
  4. Greenblatt DJ, Harmatz JS, Shapiro L, et al. Sensitivity to triazolam in the elderly. N Engl J Med 1991;324:1691-1698.

trientine hydrochloride

(trye-en'-teen hye-droe-klor'-ide)

- **Brand Name(s):** Syprine
  Chemical Class: Thiol derivative

- **Clinical Pharmacology:**
  Mechanism of Action: An oral chelating agent that forms complexes by binding metal ions, particularly copper. **Therapeutic Effect:** Binds to copper and induces cupruresis. **Pharmacokinetics:** None reported.

- **Available Forms:**
  - *Capsules:* 250 mg.

- **Indications and Dosages:**
  Wilson's disease: PO 750-1,250 mg/day in 2-4 divided doses. Maximum: 2 g/day.

- **Contraindications:** Hypersensitivity to trientine or its components

- **Side Effects**
  Occasional
  Contact dermatitis, dystonia, muscular spasm, myasthenia gravis

Serious Reactions
- Iron deficiency anemia and systemic lupus erythematosus rarely occur.

Patient/Family Education
- Take on empty stomach
- Swallow capsules whole
- Notify the physician if pale skin, swelling of lymph glands, skin rash, fever, joint pain, or general feeling of weakness occurs
- Maintain adequate fluid intake

Monitoring Parameters
- Free serum copper (goal is <10 mcg/dl); increase daily dose only when clinical response is not adequate or concentration of free serum copper is persistently above 20 mcg/dl (determine optimal long-term maintenance dosage at 6-12 mo intervals)
- 24-hr urinary copper analysis at 6-12 mo intervals (adequately treated patients will have 0.5-1 mg copper/24 hr collection of urine)
- Temperature

Geriatric side effects at a glance:
❑ CNS   ❑ Bowel Dysfunction   ❑ Bladder Dysfunction   ❑ Falls

U.S. Regulatory Considerations
❑ FDA Black Box   ❑ OBRA regulated in U.S. Long Term Care

trifluoperazine hydrochloride

(trye-floo-oh-per'-a-zeen hye-droe-klor'-ide)

Brand Name(s): Stelazine
Chemical Class: Piperidine phenothiazine derivative

Clinical Pharmacology:
Mechanism of Action: A phenothiazine derivative that blocks dopamine at postsynaptic receptor sites. Possesses strong extrapyramidal and antiemetic effects and weak anticholinergic and sedative effects. *Therapeutic Effect:* Suppresses behavioral response in psychosis; reduces locomotor activity and aggressiveness.
Pharmacokinetics: Readily absorbed following PO administration. Protein binding: 90%-99%. Metabolized in liver. Excreted in urine. *Half-life:* 24 hr.

Available Forms:
- *Tablets:* 1 mg, 2 mg, 5 mg, 10 mg.
- *Injection:* 2 mg/ml.

■ **Indications and Dosages:**
Psychotic disorders: PO Initially, 2-5 mg once or twice a day. Range: 15-20 mg/day. Maximum: 40 mg/day. IM 1 mg q4-6h. Maximum: 6 mg/24h.

■ **Contraindications:** Angle-closure glaucoma, circulatory collapse, myelosuppression, severe cardiac or hepatic disease, severe hypertension or hypotension

■ **Side Effects**

Frequent

Hypotension, dizziness, and syncope (occur frequently after first injection, occasionally after subsequent injections, and rarely with oral form)

Occasional

Drowsiness during early therapy, dry mouth, blurred vision, lethargy, constipation or diarrhea, nasal congestion, peripheral edema, urine retention

Rare

Ocular changes, altered skin pigmentation (in those taking high doses for prolonged periods), photosensitivity

■ **Serious Reactions**
- Extrapyramidal symptoms appear to be dose-related (particularly high doses) and are divided into 3 categories: akathisia (inability to sit still, tapping of feet), parkinsonian symptoms (such as mask-like face, tremors, shuffling gait, and hypersalivation), and acute dystonias (such as torticollis, opisthotonos, and oculogyric crisis). Dystonic reactions may also produce diaphoresis and pallor.
- Tardive dyskinesia, marked by tongue protrusion, puffing of the cheeks, and chewing or puckering of the mouth, occurs rarely but may be irreversible.
- Abrupt withdrawal after long-term therapy may precipitate nausea, vomiting, gastritis, dizziness, and tremors.
- Blood dyscrasias, particularly agranulocytosis, and mild leukopenia may occur.
- Trifluoperazine may lower the seizure threshold.

■ **Patient/Family Education**
- Arise slowly from reclining position
- Do not discontinue abruptly
- Use a sunscreen during sun exposure; take special precautions to stay cool in hot weather
- Avoid tasks requiring mental alertness or motor skills until response to the drug has been established
- Do not take antacids within 1 hr of trifluoperazine
- Avoid alcohol

■ **Monitoring Parameters**
- Observe closely for signs of tardive dyskinesia
- Periodic CBC with platelets during prolonged therapy
- WBC count for blood dyscrasias, such as anemia, neutropenia, pancytopenia, and thrombocytopenia
- Blood pressure for hypotension
- Therapeutic response, such as improvement in self-care and ability to concentrate, increased interest in surroundings, and relaxed facial expression

- **Geriatric side effects at a glance:**
  - ☑ CNS ☑ Bowel Dysfunction ☐ Bladder Dysfunction ☑ Falls

  Other: Orthostatic hypotension, cardiac conduction disturbances, anticholinergic side effects

- **Use with caution in older patients with:** Parkinson's disease (an atypical antipsychotic is recommended), seizure disorders, cardiovascular disease with conduction disturbance, hepatic encephalopathy, narrow-angle glaucoma

- **U.S. Regulatory Considerations**
  - ☐ FDA Black Box ☑ OBRA regulated in U.S. Long Term Care

- **Other Uses in Geriatric Patient:** Behavior disturbances in the setting of dementia

- **Side Effects:**

  Of particular importance in the geriatric patient: Tardive dyskinesia, akathisia (may appear to exacerbate behavioral disturbances), anticholinergic effects, may increase risk of sudden death

- **Geriatric Considerations - Summary:** Sink and colleagues' systematic review showed statistically significant improvements on neuropsychiatric and behavioral scales for some drugs, but improvements were small and unlikely to be clinically important. Because of documented risks, and uncertain benefits, antipsychotic drugs should be used with caution in demented elderly persons, with frequent monitoring for side effects and a low threshold for discontinuing use.

- **References:**
  1. Leipzig RM, Cumming RG, Tinetti ME. Drugs and falls in older people: a systematic review and meta-analysis: I. Psychotropic drugs. J Am Geriatr Soc 1999;47:30-39.
  2. Sink KM, Holden KF, Yaffe K. Pharmacological treatment of neuropsychiatric symptoms of dementia: a review of the evidence. JAMA 2005;293:596-608.
  3. Ray WA, Meredith S, Thapa PB, et al. Antipsychotics and the risk of sudden cardiac death. Arch Gen Psychiatry 2001;58:1161-1167.

trifluridine

(trye-flure'-i-deen)

- **Brand Name(s):** Viroptic

  Chemical Class: Nucleoside analog

- **Clinical Pharmacology:**

  Mechanism of Action: An antiviral agent that incorporates into DNS causing increased rate of mutation and errors in protein formation. **Therapeutic Effect:** Prevents viral replication.

  Pharmacokinetics: Intraocular solution is undetectable in serum. **Half-life:** 12 min.

- **Available Forms:**
  - *Ophthalmic Solution*: 1% (Viroptic).

- **Indications and Dosages:**
  Herpes simplex virus ocular infections: Ophthalmic 1 drop onto cornea q2h while awake. Maximum: 9 drops/day. Continue until corneal ulcer has completely reepithelialized; then, 1 drop q4h while awake (minimum: 5 drops/day) for an additional 7 days.

- **Contraindications:** Hypersensitivity to trifluridine or any component of the formulation

- **Side Effects**
  Frequent
  Transient stinging or burning with instillation
  Occasional
  Edema of eyelid
  Rare
  Hypersensitivity reaction

- **Serious Reactions**
  - Ocular toxicity may occur if used longer than 21 days.

- **Patient/Family Education**
  - Notify clinician if no improvement after 7 days
  - Report any itching, swelling, redness, or increased irritation
  - Avoid contact with eye

- **Monitoring Parameters**
  - Therapeutic response

- **Geriatric side effects at a glance:**
  ❑ CNS ❑ Bowel Dysfunction ❑ Bladder Dysfunction ❑ Falls

- **U.S. Regulatory Considerations**
  ❑ FDA Black Box ❑ OBRA regulated in U.S. Long Term Care

trihexyphenidyl hydrochloride

(trye-hex-ee-fen'-i-dill hye-droe-klor'-ide)

- **Brand Name(s):** Artane
  Chemical Class: Tertiary amine

- **Clinical Pharmacology:**
    Mechanism of Action: An anticholinergic agent that blocks central cholinergic receptors (aids in balancing cholinergic and dopaminergic activity). **Therapeutic Effect:** Decreases salivation, relaxes smooth muscle.
    Pharmacokinetics: Well absorbed from gastrointestinal (GI) tract. Primarily excreted in urine. **Half-life:** 3.3-4.1 hr.

- **Available Forms:**
    - *Elixir:* 2 mg/5ml (Artane).
    - *Tablets:* 2 mg, 5 mg (Artane).

- **Indications and Dosages:**
    Parkinsonism: PO Initially, 1 mg on first day. May increase by 2 mg/day at 3-5 day intervals up to 6-10 mg/day (12-15 mg/day in patients with postencephalitic parkinsonism).
    Drug-induced extrapyramidal symptoms: PO Initially, 1 mg/day. Range: 5-15 mg/day.

- **Contraindications:** Angle-closure glaucoma, GI obstruction, paralytic ileus, intestinal atony, severe ulcerative colitis, prostatic hypertrophy, myasthenia gravis, megacolon, hypersensitivity to trihexyphenidyl or any component of the formulation

- **Side Effects**
    Elderly tend to develop mental confusion, disorientation, agitation, psychotic-like symptoms
    Frequent
    Drowsiness, dry mouth
    Occasional
    Blurred vision, urinary retention, constipation, dizziness, headache, muscle cramps
    Rare
    Seizures, depression, rash

- **Serious Reactions**
    - Hypersensitivity reaction (eczema, pruritus, rash, cardiac disturbances, photosensitivity) may occur.
    - Overdosage may vary from CNS depression (sedation, apnea, cardiovascular collapse, death) to severe paradoxical reaction (hallucinations, tremor, seizures).

- **Patient/Family Education**
    - Do not discontinue abruptly
    - Use caution in hot weather; drug may increase susceptibility to heatstroke
    - Avoid alcohol
    - Chew sugarless gum or take sips of tepid water to relieve dry mouth
    - Avoid tasks requiring mental alertness or motor skills until response to the drug has been established

- **Monitoring Parameters**
    - Clinical reversal of symptoms

- **Geriatric side effects at a glance:**
    ☑ CNS   ☑ Bowel Dysfunction   ☑ Bladder Dysfunction   ☑ Falls
    Other: Dry mouth, blurred vision, somnolence, confusion, psychoses

- **Use with caution in older patients with:** Narrow-angle glaucoma, overflow incontinence, psychosis

- **U.S. Regulatory Considerations**
  - ❑ FDA Black Box ☑ OBRA regulated in U.S. Long Term Care

- **Other Uses in Geriatric Patient:** Treatment of antipsychotic-induced adverse effects

- **Side Effects:**
  Of particular importance in the geriatric patient: Anticholinergic effects

- **Geriatric Considerations - Summary:** Trihexyphenidyl and related anticholingerics present significant risk to older adults. These drugs possess potent anticholinergic effects and can cause cognitive impairment, delirium, dry mouth, blurred vision, and increased risk of falls. The use of this drug and related compounds should be limited and when used, patients should be closely monitored.

- **References:**
  1. Vangala V, Tueth M. Chronic anticholinergic toxicity: identification and management in older patients. Geriatrics 2003;58:36-37.
  2. Tune LE. Anticholinergic effects of medication in elderly patients. J Clin Psychiatry 2001;62(suppl 21):11-14.

trimethobenzamide hydrochloride

(trye-meth-oh-ben'-za-mide hye-droe-klor'-ide)

- **Brand Name(s):** Benzacot, Benzocaine-Trimethobenzamide Adult, Navogan, Tebamide, Tigan, Tigan Adult
  Chemical Class: Ethanolamine derivative

- **Clinical Pharmacology:**
  Mechanism of Action: An anticholinergic that acts at the chemoreceptor trigger zone in the medulla oblongata. **Therapeutic Effect:** Relieves nausea and vomiting.
  Pharmacokinetics:

Route	Onset	Peak	Duration
PO	10-40 min	N/A	3-4 hr
IM	15-30 min	N/A	2-3 hr

  Partially absorbed from the GI tract. Distributed primarily to the liver. Metabolic fate unknown. Excreted in urine. **Half-life:** 7-9 hr.

- **Available Forms:**
  - *Capsules (Tigan):* 250 mg, 300 mg.
  - *Injection (Benzacot, Tigan):* 100 mg/ml.

- *Suppositories*: 100 mg (Navogan, Tebamide), 200 mg (Benzocaine-Trimethobenzamide Adult, Tebamide, Tigan Adult).

■ **Indications and Dosages:**
Nausea and vomiting: PO 300 mg 3-4 times a day. IM 200 mg 3-4 times a day. Rectal 200 mg 3-4 times a day.

■ **Contraindications:** Hypersensitivity to benzocaine or similar local anesthetics

■ **Side Effects**
Frequent
Somnolence
Occasional
Blurred vision, diarrhea, dizziness, headache, muscle cramps
Rare
Rash, seizures, depression, opisthotonos, parkinsonian syndrome, Reye's syndrome (marked by vomiting, seizures)

■ **Serious Reactions**
- A hypersensitivity reaction, manifested as extrapyramidal symptoms (EPS) such as muscle rigidity and allergic skin reactions, occurs rarely.
- Overdose may produce CNS depression (manifested as sedation, apnea, cardiovascular collapse, and death) or severe paradoxical reactions (such as hallucinations, tremor, and seizures).

Special Considerations
- Less effective than phenothiazines

■ **Patient/Family Education**
- Relief from nausea or vomiting generally occurs within 30 min of drug administration
- Trimethobenzamide causes drowsiness; avoid tasks that require mental alertness or motor skills until response to the drug has been established

■ **Monitoring Parameters**
- Blood pressure, especially in elderly patients, who are at increased risk for hypotension
- Electrolytes
- Intake and output
- Hydration status

■ **Geriatric side effects at a glance:**
☑ CNS ☐ Bowel Dysfunction ☑ Bladder Dysfunction ☐ Falls

■ **U.S. Regulatory Considerations**
☐ FDA Black Box ☑ OBRA regulated in U.S. Long Term Care

trimethoprim

(trye-meth'-oh-prim)

■ **Brand Name(s):** Primsol, Proloprim, Trimpex

Combinations
Rx: with sulfamethoxazole (see co-trimoxazole monograph); with polymixin B sulfate (Polytrim Ophthalmic)
Chemical Class: Folate-antagonist, synthetic

■ **Clinical Pharmacology:**
Mechanism of Action: A folate antagonist that blocks bacterial biosynthesis of nucleic acids and proteins by interfering with the metabolism of folinic acid. **Therapeutic Effect:** Bacteriostatic.
Pharmacokinetics: Rapidly and completely absorbed from the GI tract. Protein binding: 42%-46%. Widely distributed, including to CSF. Metabolized in the liver. Primarily excreted in urine. Moderately removed by hemodialysis. **Half-life:** 8-10 hr (increased in impaired renal function and newborns; decreased in children).

■ **Available Forms:**
- *Oral Solution (Primsol):* 50 mg/5 ml.
- *Tablets (Trimpex, Proloprim):* 100 mg, 200 mg.

■ **Indications and Dosages:**
Acute, uncomplicated UTI: PO 100 mg q12h or 200 mg once a day for 10 days.
Dosage in renal impairment: Dosage and frequency are modified based on creatinine clearance.

Creatinine Clearance	Dosage Interval
greater than 30 ml/min	No change
15-29 ml/min	50 mg q12h

■ **Unlabeled Uses:** Prevention of bacterial UTIs, treatment of pneumonia caused by *Pneumocystis carinii*

■ **Contraindications:** Megaloblastic anemia due to folic acid deficiency

■ **Side Effects**
Occasional
Nausea, vomiting, diarrhea, decreased appetite, abdominal cramps, headache
Rare
Hypersensitivity reaction (pruritus, rash), methemoglobinemia (bluish fingernails, lips, or skin; fever; pale skin; sore throat; unusual tiredness), photosensitivity

■ **Serious Reactions**
- Stevens-Johnson syndrome, erythema multiforme, exfoliative dermatitis, and anaphylaxis occur rarely.
- Hematologic toxicity (thrombocytopenia, neutropenia, leukopenia, megaloblastic anemia) is more likely to occur in elderly, debilitated, or alcoholic patients; in patients with impaired renal function; and in those receiving prolonged high dosage.

- Good alternative to co-trimoxazole in patients taking warfarin
- Individualize treatment based on local susceptibility patterns.

■ Patient/Family Education

- Space drug doses evenly around the clock and complete the full course of trimethoprim therapy, which usually lasts 10-14 days
- Take trimethoprim with food if stomach upset occurs
- Avoid sun and ultraviolet light and use sunscreen and wear protective clothing when outdoors
- Immediately report bleeding, bruising, skin discoloration, fever, pallor, rash, sore throat, and tiredness

■ Monitoring Parameters

- Skin for rash
- Serum hematology reports
- Liver and renal function
- Signs and symptoms of hematologic toxicity, such as bleeding, ecchymosis, fever, malaise, pallor, and sore throat

■ Geriatric side effects at a glance:
❑ CNS ❑ Bowel Dysfunction ❑ Bladder Dysfunction ❑ Falls

■ U.S. Regulatory Considerations
❑ FDA Black Box ❑ OBRA regulated in U.S. Long Term Care

trimetrexate

(tri-me-trex'-ate)

■ Brand Name(s): Neutrexin
Chemical Class: Dihydrofolate reductase inhibitor; substituted quinazoline

■ Clinical Pharmacology:
Mechanism of Action: A folate antagonist that inhibits the enzyme dihydrofolate reductase (DHFR). **Therapeutic Effect:** Disrupts purine, DNA, RNA, protein synthesis, with consequent cell death.
Pharmacokinetics: Following IV administration, distributed readily into ascitic fluid. Metabolized in liver. Eliminated in urine. **Half-life:** 11-20 hr.

■ Available Forms:
- *Powder for Injection:* 25 mg (Neutrexin).

■ Indications and Dosages:
Pneumocystis carinii pneumonia (PCP) : IV Infusion Trimetrexate: 45 mg/m^2 once daily over 60-90 min. Leucovorin: 20 mg/m^2 over 5-10 min q6h for total daily dose of 80 mg/m^2, or orally as 4 doses of 20 mg/m^2 spaced equally throughout the day. Round up the oral dose to the next higher 25-mg increment. Recommended course of therapy: 21 days trimetrexate, 24 days leucovorin.

■ **Unlabeled Uses:** Treatment of non-small cell lung, prostate, and colorectal cancer

■ **Contraindications:** Clinically significant hypersensitivity to trimetrexate, leucovorin, or methotrexate

■ **Side Effects**
Occasional
Fever, rash, pruritus, nausea, vomiting, confusion
Rare
Fatigue

■ **Serious Reactions**
- Trimetrexate given without concurrent leucovorin may result in serious or fatal hematologic, hepatic, and/or renal complications, including bone marrow suppression, oral and GI mucosal ulceration, and renal and hepatic dysfunction.
- In event of overdose, stop trimetrexate and give leucovorin 40 mg/m^2 q6h for 3 days.
- Anaphylaxis occurs rarely.

Special Considerations
- Reserve for patients intolerant of or refractory to trimethoprim-sulfamethoxazole
- Randomized trials show trimetrexate is less effective than trimethoprim-sulfamethoxazole (failure rates 40% and 24%, respectively)

■ **Patient/Family Education**
- Use two forms of contraception during therapy
- Avoid persons with bacterial infections
- Notify the physician if fever, chills, cough or hoarseness, lower back or side pain, or painful urination occurs
- Report any unusual bleeding or bruising

■ **Monitoring Parameters**
- Check at least twice per week: CBC with platelets, hepatic and renal function

■ **Geriatric side effects at a glance:**
❑ CNS   ❑ Bowel Dysfunction   ❑ Bladder Dysfunction   ❑ Falls

■ **U.S. Regulatory Considerations**
☑ FDA Black Box
Concurrent leucovorin must be used to avoid potentially serious or life-threatening toxicities.
❑ OBRA regulated in U.S. Long Term Care

trimipramine maleate

(trye-mi'-pra-meen mal'-ee-ate)

■ **Brand Name(s):** Surmontil
  Chemical Class: Dibenzazepine derivative; tertiary amine

■ **Clinical Pharmacology:**
  Mechanism of Action: A tricyclic antidepressant that blocks the reuptake of neurotransmitters, such as norepinephrine and serotonin, at presynaptic membranes, increasing their concentration at postsynaptic receptor sites. **Therapeutic Effect:** Results in antidepressant effect. Anticholinergic effect controls nocturnal enuresis.
  Pharmacokinetics: Rapidly, completely absorbed after PO administration, and not affected by food. Protein binding: 95%. Metabolized in liver (significant first-pass effect). Primarily excreted in urine. Not removed by hemodialysis. **Half-life:** 16-40 hr.

■ **Available Forms:**
  • *Capsules*: 25 mg, 50 mg, 100 mg (Surmontil).

■ **Indications and Dosages:**
  Depression: PO Initially, 25 mg/day at bedtime. May increase by 25 mg q3-7days. Maximum: 100 mg/day.

■ **Contraindications:** Acute recovery period after myocardial infarction (MI), within 14 days of MAOI ingestion, hypersensitivity to trimipramine or any component of the formulation

■ **Side Effects**
  Frequent
  Drowsiness, fatigue, dry mouth, blurred vision, constipation, delayed micturition, postural hypotension, diaphoresis, disturbed concentration, increased appetite, urinary retention, photosensitivity.
  Occasional
  Gastrointestinal (GI) disturbances, such as nausea, and a metallic taste sensation.
  Rare
  Paradoxical reaction, marked by agitation, restlessness, nightmares, insomnia, extrapyramidal symptoms, particularly fine hand tremors.

■ **Serious Reactions**
  • High dosage may produce cardiovascular effects, such as severe postural hypotension, dizziness, tachycardia, palpitations, arrhythmias, and seizures. High dosage may also result in altered temperature regulation, including hyperpyrexia or hypothermia.
  • Abrupt withdrawal from prolonged therapy may produce headache, malaise, nausea, vomiting, and vivid dreams.

■ **Patient/Family Education**
  • Therapeutic effects may take 2-3 wk
  • Avoid rising quickly from sitting to standing

1276

- Do not discontinue abruptly after long-term use
- Take sips of tepid water and chew sugarless gum to relieve dry mouth

■ Monitoring Parameters
- CBC, ECG
- Blood pressure, pulse

■ Geriatric side effects at a glance:
☑ CNS ☑ Bowel Dysfunction ☑ Bladder Dysfunction ☑ Falls
Other: Orthostatic hypotension, cardiac conduction disturbances, anticholinergic side effects

■ Use with caution in older patients with: Cardiovascular disease, prostatic hyptertrophy or other conditions which increase the risk of urinary retention

■ U.S. Regulatory Considerations
☑ FDA Black Box
- Because there is an increased risk of suicide in children and adolescents, older adults should also be closely monitored for suicide ideation.
☐ OBRA regulated in U.S. Long Term Care

■ Other Uses in Geriatric Patient: Neuropathic pain, urge urinary incontinence

■ Side Effects:
Of particular importance in the geriatric patient: Sedation, urinary retention, dry mouth

■ Geriatric Considerations - Summary: Although tricyclic antidepressants are effective in the treatment of major depression in older adults, the side-effect profile and low toxic-to-therapeutic ratio relegate them to second-line agents (after serotonin re-uptake inhibitors) for most older patients. These agents are effective in the treatment of urge urinary incontinence and neuropathic pain, but must be monitored closely. Of the tricyclic antidepressants, imipramine and amitryptyline have the highest anticholinergic activity and may be best choice in this class for management of incontinence, but should otherwise be avoided.

■ References:
1. Leipzig RM, Cumming RG, Tinetti ME. Drugs and falls in older people: a systematic review and meta-analysis: I. Psychotropic drugs. J Am Geriatr Soc 1999;47:30-39.
2. Cadieux RJ. Antidepressant drug interactions in the elderly. Understanding the P-450 system is half the battle in reducing risks. Postgrad Med 1999;106:231-240, 245.
3. Ray WA, Meredith S, Thapa PB, et al. Cyclic antidepressants and the risk of sudden cardiac death. Clin Pharmacol Ther 2004;75:234-241.
4. Roose SP, Laghrissi-Thode F, Kennedy JS, et al. Comparison of paroxetine and nortriptyline in depressed patients with ischemic heart disease. JAMA 1998;279:287-291.

trioxsalen

(trye-ox'-sa-len)

- **Brand Name(s):** Trisoralen
  Chemical Class: Psoralen derivative

- **Clinical Pharmacology:**
  Mechanism of Action: A member of the family of psoralens that induces the process of melanogenesis by a mechanism that is not known. **Therapeutic Effect:** Enhances pigmentation.
  Pharmacokinetics: Rapidly absorbed from the gastrointestinal (GI) tract. **Half-life:** 2 hr (skin sensitivity to light remains for 8-12 hr).

- **Available Forms:**
  - *Tablets*: 5 mg (Trisoralen).

- **Indications and Dosages:**
  Pigmentation: PO 10 mg/day 2 hr before exposure to UVA light or sun exposure.
  Vitiligo: PO 10 mg/day 2-4 hr before exposure to UVA light.

- **Unlabeled Uses:** Polymorphous light eruption, psoriasis, sunlight sensitivity

- **Contraindications:** Concomitant disease states associated with photosensitivity (acute lupus erythematosus, porphyria, leukoderma of infectious origin), concomitant use of preparations with any internal or external photosensitizing capacity, hypersensitivity to trioxsalen or any component of the formulation

- **Side Effects**
  Occasional
  Gastric discomfort, photosensitivity, pruritus

- **Serious Reactions**
  - Overdose or overexposure may result in serious blistering and burning.

- **Patient/Family Education**
  - Do not sunbathe during 24 hr prior to ingestion and UVA exposure
  - Wear UVA-absorbing sunglasses for 24 hr following treatment to prevent cataract
  - Avoid sun exposure for at least 8 hr after ingestion
  - Avoid furocoumarin-containing foods (e.g., limes, figs, parsley, parsnips, mustard, carrots, celery)
  - Repigmentation may begin after 2-3 wk but full effect may require 6-9 mo

- **Monitoring Parameters**
  - Skin for therapeutic response

trospium chloride

(trose'-pee-um klor'-ide)

■ **Brand Name(s):** Sanctura
   Chemical Class: Antimuscarinic substituted amine

■ **Clinical Pharmacology:**
   Mechanism of Action: An anticholinergic that antagonizes the effect of acetylcholine on muscarinic receptors, producing parasympatholytic action. **Therapeutic Effect:** Reduces smooth muscle tone in the bladder.
   Pharmacokinetics: Minimally absorbed after PO administration. Protein binding: 50%-85%. Distributed in plasma. Excreted mainly in feces and, to a lesser extent, in urine. **Half life:** 20 hr.

■ **Available Forms:**
   • *Tablets*: 20 mg.

■ **Indications and Dosages:**
   Overactive bladder: PO *Younger than 75 yrs.* 20 mg twice a day. *75 yrs and older.* Titrate dosage down to 20 mg once a day, based on tolerance.
   Dosage in renal impairment: For patients with creatinine clearance less than 30 ml/min, dosage reduced to 20 mg once a day at bedtime.

■ **Contraindications:** Decreased GI motility, gastric retention, uncontrolled angle-closure glaucoma, urine retention

■ **Side Effects**
   Frequent (20%)
   Dry mouth
   Occasional (10%-4%)
   Constipation, headache, delirium, confusion
   Rare (less than 2%)
   Fatigue, upper abdominal pain, dyspepsia, flatulence, dry eyes, urine retention

■ **Serious Reactions**
   • Overdose may result in severe anticholinergic effects, such as abdominal pain, nausea and vomiting, confusion, depression, diaphoresis, facial flushing, hypertension, hypotension, respiratory depression, irritability, lacrimation, nervousness, and restlessness.
   • Supraventricular tachycardia and hallucinations occur rarely.

1279

- Studies have not shown that trospium is better than generically available drugs for the same purpose

■ **Patient/Family Education**
- May precipitate urinary retention or narrow-angle glaucoma
- Do not take trospium with high-fat meals because they may reduce drug absorption
- Notify the health care provider if increased salivation or sweating, an irregular heartbeat, nausea and vomiting, or severe abdominal pain occurs

■ **Monitoring Parameters**
- Intake and output
- Pattern of daily bowel activity
- Symptomatic relief

■ **Geriatric side effects at a glance:**
☑ CNS ☑ Bowel Dysfunction ☑ Bladder Dysfunction ☑ Falls
Other: Dry mouth, blurred vision, dizziness, somnolence

■ **Use with caution in older patients with:** Tachyarrythmias, overflow incontinence.

■ **U.S. Regulatory Considerations**
☐ FDA Black Box
☑ OBRA regulated in U.S. Long Term Care

■ **Other Uses in Geriatric Patient:** None

■ **Side Effects:**
Of *particular importance in the geriatric patient*: Delirium, possible antagonism of cholinergic drug therapy in the treatment of Alzheimer's disease.

■ **Geriatric Considerations - Summary:** Trospium and other newer anticholinergic drugs are moderately effective in the treatment of urge urinary incontinence and offer the potential benefit of selective antagonism of muscarinic receptors with less potential for CNS adverse effects. The relative safety and efficacy of these agents, which are significantly more expensive, has not been well studied to determine if they are superior to longer-acting anticholinergic formulations. These newer drugs can produce anticholinergic adverse effects including cognitive impairment, dry mouth, blurred vision and increased risk of falls.

■ **References:**
1. Hay-Smith J, Herbison P, Ellis G, Moore K. Anticholinergic drugs versus placebo for overactive bladder syndrome in adults. Cochrane Database System Rev 2003;3.
2. Vangala V, Tueth M. Chronic anticholinergic toxicity: identification and management in older patients. Geriatrics 2003;58:36-37.
3. Tune LE. Anticholinergic effects of medication in elderly patients. J Clin Psychiatry 2001;62(suppl 21):11-14.
4. Trospium chloride: another anticholinergic for overactive bladder. Med Let 2004;46:63-64.
5. Ouslander JG. Management of overactive bladder. N Engl J Med 2004;350:786-799.

trovafloxacin / alatrofloxacin

(troe'-va-flox-a-sin / a-lat-roe-flox'-a-sin)

■ **Brand Name(s):** Trovan

  Combinations
  Rx: with azithromycin (Trovan/Zithromax Compliance Pak)
  Chemical Class: Fluoroquinolone derivative

■ **Clinical Pharmacology:**
  Mechanism of Action: A fluoroquinolone that inhibits the DNA enzyme gyrase in susceptible microorganisms, interfering with bacterial DNA replication and repair. **Therapeutic Effect:** Produces bactericidal activity.
  Pharmacokinetics: Well absorbed from the gastrointestinal (GI) tract. Protein binding: 76%. Widely distributed including cerebrospinal fluid (CSF). Metabolized in liver by conjugation. Excreted in feces. Not removed by hemodialysis. **Half-life:** 9-13 hr.

■ **Available Forms:**
  • *Tablets*: 100 mg, 200 mg (Trovan).
  • *Injection*: 200 mg/40 ml, 300 mg/60 ml (Trovan).

■ **Indications and Dosages:**
  Pneumonia: PO, IV 200 mg q24h for 7-14 days.
  Skin and skin-structure infections: PO, IV 200 mg q24h for 10-14 days.
  Gynecologic infections: IV 300 mg q24h for 7-14 days. PO 100 mg q24h for 7-14 days.
  Abdominal infection: 300 mg q24h for 7-14 days.
  Bronchitis: PO 100 mg q24h for 7-10 days.

■ **Contraindications:** History of hypersensitivity to other fluoroquinolones

■ **Side Effects**
  Occasional
  Diarrhea, dizziness, drowsiness, headache, light-headedness, vaginal pain and discharge
  Rare
  Confusion, hallucinations, restlessness, seizures, tremors, rapid heartbeat, shortness of breath, abdominal pain, dark urine, fatigue, loss of appetite, nausea, vomiting, jaundice, pain at injection site, stomach cramps, diarrhea, tendon rupture, increased sensitivity of skin to sunlight

■ **Serious Reactions**
  • Pseudomembranous colitis as evidenced by severe abdominal pain and cramps, and severe watery diarrhea, and fever, may occur.
  • Superinfection, manifested as genital or anal pruritus, ulceration or changes in oral mucosa, and moderate to severe diarrhea, may occur.
  • Hypersensitivity reactions, including photosensitivity as evidenced by rash, pruritus, blistering, swelling, and the sensation of the skin burning, have occurred in patients receiving fluoroquinolone therapy.

- Tendon effects, including ruptures of shoulder, hand, Achilles tendon or other tendons, may occur. Risk increases with concomitant corticosteriod use, especially in the elderly.

Special Considerations

- Individualize treatment based on local susceptibility patterns.

■ Patient/Family Education

- Do not take antacids (aluminum, calcium, or magnesium-containing) or iron within 2 hr of taking trovafloxacin. Take at bedtime or with food to minimize dizziness associated with trovafloxacin. Avoid excessive sunlight during treatment
- Drink 6 to 8 glasses of fluid a day
- Avoid tasks that require mental alertness or motor skills until response to the drug is established
- Notify the physician if chest pain, difficulty breathing, palpitations, persistent diarrhea, swelling, or tendon pain occurs
- Your skin may be more sensitive to sunlight while taking this medication. Wear sunscreen when outdoors. Avoid sunlamps and tanning beds.

■ Monitoring Parameters

- Transaminases if given for more than 7 days
- Signs of hypersensitivity reactions
- Be alert for signs and symptoms of superinfection manifested as anal or genital pruritus, moderate to severe diarrhea, new or increased fever, and ulceration or changes in oral mucosa

■ Geriatric side effects at a glance:

☑ CNS ❑ Bowel Dysfunction ❑ Bladder Dysfunction ❑ Falls

■ U.S. Regulatory Considerations

☑ FDA Black Box

Severe hepatotoxicity leading to transplantation and death. Risk increased with longer than 2 weeks' duration. Use only in life-threatening infections and in inpatient facility. Should not be used when safer alternatives are available.

❑ OBRA regulated in U.S. Long Term Care

undecylenic acid

(un-de-sill-enn'-ik as'-id)

OTC: Caldesene Medicated Powder, Cruex Antifgungal Cream, Cruex Antifungal Powder, Cruex Antifungal Spray Powder, Decylenes Powder, Desenex Antifungal Cream, Desenex Antifungal Liquid, Desenex Antifungal Ointment, Desenex Antifungal Penetrating Foam, Desenex Antifungal Powder, Desenex Antifungal Spray Powder, Gordochom Solution

Chemical Class: Hendecenoic acid derivative

■ **Clinical Pharmacology:**
Mechanism of Action: An antifungal whose mechanism of action is not well understood. **Therapeutic Effect:** Fungistatic.

■ **Available Forms:**
- *Aerosol Powder:* 10% (Cruex Antifungal Spray Powder, Desenex Antifungal Spray Powder).
- *Aerosol Foam:* 10% (Desenex Antifungal Penetrating Foam).
- *Cream:* 20% (Cruex Antifungal Cream, Desenex Antifungal Cream).
- *Solution, Topical:* 10% (Desenex Antifungal Liquid), 25% (Gordochom Solution).
- *Ointment:* 20% (Desenex Antifungal Ointment).
- *Powder:* 10% (Caldesene Medicated Powder, Cruex Antifungal Powder, Decylenes Powder), 19% (Desenex Antifungal Powder).

■ **Indications and Dosages:**
Tinea pedis, tinea corporis: Topical Apply 2 times/day to affected area for 4 wk.

■ **Contraindications:** Hypersensitivity to undecylenic acid or any component of its formulation

■ **Side Effects**
Occasional
Skin irritation, rash

■ **Serious Reactions**
- Hypersensitivity reactions characterized by rash, facial swelling, pruritus, and a sensation of warmth occur.

Special Considerations
- Newer topical antifungals more effective
- Powders are generally used as adjunctive therapy, but may be useful for primary therapy in very mild cases

■ **Patient/Family Education**
- Avoid contact with the eyes
- Separate personal items that come in direct contact with affected area
- Rub the topical form well into the affected area

■ **Monitoring Parameters**
- Skin for itching, rash, and urticaria

■ **Geriatric side effects at a glance:**
❏ CNS ❏ Bowel Dysfunction ❏ Bladder Dysfunction ❏ Falls

■ **U.S. Regulatory Considerations**
❏ FDA Black Box ❏ OBRA regulated in U.S. Long Term Care

unoprostone isopropyl

(yoo-noh-prost'-ohn eye-se-pro'-pel)

■ **Brand Name(s):** Rescula

■ **Clinical Pharmacology:**
Mechanism of Action: An ophthalmic agent that increases the outflow of aqueous humor. **Therapeutic Effect:** Decreases intraocular pressure.
Pharmacokinetics: Peak response occurs in 4-8 wk. The duration of a single dose is about 10 hr. Hydrolyzed to unoprostone free acid form in the cornea. Rapidly eliminated from plasma. Excreted as metabolites in urine. **Half-life:** 14 min.

■ **Available Forms:**
- *Ophthalmic Solution*: 0.15% (Rescula).

■ **Indications and Dosages:**
Glaucoma, ocular hypertension: Ophthalmic Instill 1 drop in affected eye(s) 2 times/day.

■ **Contraindications:** Hypersensitivity to unoprostone isopropyl, benzalkonium chloride, or any other component of the formulation

■ **Side Effects**
Frequent (25%-10%)
Burning, stinging, dry eyes, itching, increased eyelash length, and redness.
Occasional (less than 10%)
Abnormal vision, eyelid disorder, foreign body sensation.

■ **Serious Reactions**
- Elevated intraocular pressure occurs rarely.

■ **Geriatric side effects at a glance:**
❑ CNS   ❑ Bowel Dysfunction   ❑ Bladder Dysfunction   ❑ Falls

■ **U.S. Regulatory Considerations**
❑ FDA Black Box   ❑ OBRA regulated in U.S. Long Term Care

urea

(yoor-ee'-a)

■ **Brand Name(s):** Carmol-40, Epimide 50, Gordon's Urea, Urea Rea, Vanamide
   OTC: Topical: Aqua Care, Carmol, Gormel, Lanaphilic, UltraMide, Ureacin
   Chemical Class: Carbonic acid diamide salt

■ **Clinical Pharmacology:**
   Mechanism of Action: A diuretic which rapidly increases blood tonicity causing a greater urea concentration gradient in the blood than in the extravascular fluid resulting in movement of fluid from the tissues, including the brain and cerebrospinal fluid into the blood. A keratolytic that dissolves the intercellular matrix and thereby softens hyperkeratotic areas by enhancing the shedding of scales. **Therapeutic Effect:** Decreases ocular hypertension and cerebral edema.
   Pharmacokinetics: None known

■ **Available Forms:**
   • **Cream**: 22% (Gordon's Urea); 40% (Gordon's Urea, Carmol-40, Vanamide)
   • **Gel**: 40% (Carmol-40)
   • **Lotion**: 40% (Carmol-40)
   • **Paste**: 50% (Epimide 50)
   • **Powder**: 100% (Urea Rea)

■ **Indications and Dosages:**
   Reduction in intracranial/intraocular pressure: 1-1.5 g/kg. Maximum 120g daily.
   Skin/nail debridement: Topical Apply urea cream, 40% to affected areas. If desired, cover with occlusive dressing. Keep dry and occlusive for 3-7 days.

■ **Unlabeled Uses:** None known.

■ **Contraindications:** Severely impaired renal function, active intracranial bleeding, marked dehydration, frank liver failure,

■ **Side Effects**
   Common
   Transient stinging, burning, itching, irritation, headaches, nausea, vomiting, infection at site of injection, venous thrombosis or phlebitis extending from site of injection, extravasation, hypervolemia.
   Occasional
   Syncope, disorientation
   Rare
   Transient agitated confusional state, chemical phlebitis and thrombosis near site of injection

■ **Serious Reactions**
   • No serious reactions have been noted when solutions have been infused slowly provided renal function is not seriously impaired or there is no evidence of active intracranial bleeding.
   • Signs of overdosage include unusually elevated blood urea nitrogen (BUN) levels.

- Do not infuse into lower extremity veins
- Monitor for extravasation, tissue necrosis may occur

■ **Patient/Family Education**
- Headaches, nausea and vomiting, occasionally syncope and disorientation may occur following intravenous administration
- If redness or irritation occurs with topical use, discontinue use
- Wash excess cream from unaffected skin areas thoroughly after contact

■ **Monitoring Parameters**
- BUN
- Serum and urine sodium concentrations
- Electrolytes

■ **Geriatric side effects at a glance:**
    ❑ CNS   ❑ Bowel Dysfunction   ❑ Bladder Dysfunction   ❑ Falls

■ **U.S. Regulatory Considerations**
    ❑ FDA Black Box   ❑ OBRA regulated in U.S. Long Term Care

urokinase

(yoor-oh-kin'-ace)

■ **Brand Name(s):** Abbokinase, Abbokinase Open-Cath (not for systemic administration)
Chemical Class: Renal enzyme

■ **Clinical Pharmacology:**
Mechanism of Action: A thrombolytic agent that activates fibrinolytic system by converting plasminogen to plasmin (enzyme that degrades fibrin clots). Acts indirectly by forming complex with plasminogen, which converts plasminogen to plasmin. Action occurs within thrombus, on its surface, and in circulating blood. **Therapeutic Effect:** Destroys thrombi.
Pharmacokinetics: Rapidly cleared from circulation by liver. Small amounts eliminated in urine and via bile. **Half-life:** 20 min.

■ **Available Forms:**
- *Powder for Injection* (*Abbokinase*): 250,000 IU/vial.

■ **Indications and Dosages:**
Pulmonary embolism: IV Initially, 4,400 IU/kg at rate of 90 ml/hr over 10 min; then, 4,400 IU/kg at rate of 15 ml/hr for 12 hr. Flush tubing. Follow with anticoagulant therapy.
Coronary artery thrombi: Intracoronary 6,000 IU/min for up to 2 hr.

Occluded IV catheter: Disconnect IV tubing from catheter; attach a 1-ml TB syringe with 5,000 U urokinase to catheter; inject urokinase slowly (equal to volume of catheter). Connect empty 5-ml syringe; aspirate residual clot. When patency is restored, irrigate with 0.9% NaCl; reconnect IV tubing to catheter.

■ **Contraindications:** Active internal bleeding, atrioventricular (AV) malformation or aneurysm, bleeding diathesis, intracranial neoplasm, intracranial or intraspinal surgery or trauma, recent (within the past 2 mo) cerebrovascular accident

■ **Side Effects**
Frequent
Superficial or surface bleeding at puncture sites (venous cutdowns, arterial punctures, surgical sites, IM sites, retroperitoneal/intracerebral sites); internal bleeding (GI/GU tract, vaginal).
Rare
Mild allergic reaction such as rash or wheezing

■ **Serious Reactions**
• Severe internal hemorrhage may occur. Lysis of coronary thrombi may produce atrial/ventricular arrhythmias

■ **Patient/Family Education**
• Follow measures to reduce the risk of bleeding, such as using an electric razor and a soft toothbrush
• Immediately report signs of bleeding, such as oozing from cuts or gums

■ **Monitoring Parameters**
• Before beginning therapy, obtain a hematocrit, platelet count, and a thrombin time (TT), activated partial thromboplastin time (aPTT), or prothrombin time (PT)
• Following the intravenous infusion before (re) instituting heparin, the TT or APTT should be less than twice the upper limits of normal
• Blood pressure, pulse rate

■ **Geriatric side effects at a glance:**
❑ CNS   ❑ Bowel Dysfunction   ❑ Bladder Dysfunction   ❑ Falls

■ **U.S. Regulatory Considerations**
❑ FDA Black Box   ❑ OBRA regulated in U.S. Long Term Care

ursodiol

(er'-soe-dye-ol)

- **Brand Name(s):** Actigall, Urso
  Chemical Class: Ursodeoxycholic acid

- **Clinical Pharmacology:**
  Mechanism of Action: A gallstone solubilizing agent that suppresses hepatic synthesis and secretion of cholesterol; inhibits intestinal absorption of cholesterol. **Therapeutic Effect:** Changes the bile of patients with gallstones from precipitating (capable of forming crystals) to cholesterol solubilizing (capable of being dissolved).
  Pharmacokinetics: Absorbed from the small bowel following PO administration. Protein binding: 70%. Metabolized in colon. Primarily excreted in feces; small amount eliminated in urine. **Half-life:** 3.5-5.8 days.

- **Available Forms:**
  - *Capsules (Actigall):* 300 mg.
  - *Tablets (Urso):* 250 mg.

- **Indications and Dosages:**
  Dissolution of radiolucent, noncalcified gallstones when cholecystectomy is not recommended; treatment of biliary cirrhosis: PO 8–10 mg/kg/day in 2–3 divided doses. Treatment may require months. Obtain ultrasound image of gallbladder at 6-mo intervals for first year. If gallstones have dissolved, continue therapy and repeat ultrasound within 1–3 mo.
  Prevention of gallstones: PO 300 mg twice a day.

- **Unlabeled Uses:** Prophylaxis of liver transplant rejection, treatment of alcoholic cirrhosis, biliary atresia, chronic hepatitis, gallstone formation, sclerosing cholangitis

- **Contraindications:** Allergy to bile acids, calcified cholesterol stones, chronic hepatic disease, radiolucent bile pigment stones, radiopaque stones

- **Side Effects**
  Occasional
  Diarrhea

- **Serious Reactions**
  - None significant.

Special Considerations
  - Complete dissolution may not occur; likelihood of success is low if partial stone dissolution not seen by 12 mo
  - Stones recur within 5 yr in 50% of patients

- **Patient/Family Education**
  - Administer with food to facilitate dissolution in the intestine
  - Therapy requires months
  - Avoid taking antacids within hours of taking ursodiol

- **Monitoring Parameters**
  - Liver function

- **Geriatric side effects at a glance:**
  - ❑ CNS ❑ Bowel Dysfunction ❑ Bladder Dysfunction ❑ Falls

- **U.S. Regulatory Considerations**
  - ❑ FDA Black Box ❑ OBRA regulated in U.S. Long Term Care

valacyclovir hydrochloride

(val-a-sye'-kloh-vir hye-droe-klor'-ide)

- **Brand Name(s):** Valtrex
  Chemical Class: Acyclic purine nucleoside analog; acyclovir derivative

- **Clinical Pharmacology:**
  Mechanism of Action: A virustatic antiviral that is converted to acyclovir triphosphate, becoming part of the viral DNA chain. **Therapeutic Effect:** Interferes with DNA synthesis and replication of herpes simplex virus and varicella-zoster virus.
  Pharmacokinetics: Rapidly absorbed after PO administration. Protein binding: 13%-18%. Rapidly converted by hydrolysis to the active compound acyclovir. Widely distributed to tissues and body fluids (including cerebrospinal fluid [CSF]). Primarily eliminated in urine. Removed by hemodialysis. **Half-life:** 2.5-3.3 hr (increased in impaired renal function).

- **Available Forms:**
  - **Caplets:** 500 mg, 1000 mg.

- **Indications and Dosages:**
  Herpes zoster (shingles): PO 1g 3 times a day for 7 days.
  Herpes simplex (cold sores): PO 2g twice a day for 1 day.
  Initial episode of genital herpes: PO 1g twice a day for 10 days.
  Recurrent episodes of genital herpes: PO 500 mg twice a day for 3 days.
  Prevention of genital herpes: PO 500-1,000 mg/day.
  Dosage in renal impairment: Dosage and frequency are modified based on creatinine clearance.

Creatinine Clearance	Herpes Zoster	Genital Herpes
50 ml/min or higher	1g q8h	500 mg q12h
30-49 ml/min	1g q12h	500 mg q12h
10-29 ml/min	1g q24h	500 mg q24h
less than 10 ml/min	500 mg q24h	500 mg q24h

- **Unlabeled Uses:** To reduce the risk of heterosexual transmission of genital herpes

- **Contraindications:** Hypersensitivity to or intolerance of acyclovir, valacyclovir, or their components

1289

■ **Side Effects**
Frequent
Herpes zoster (17%-10%): Nausea, headache
Genital herpes (17%): Headache
Occasional
Herpes zoster (7%-3%): Vomiting, diarrhea, constipation (50 yr or older), asthenia, dizziness (50 yr and older)
Genital herpes (8%-3%): Nausea, diarrhea, dizziness
Rare
Herpes zoster (3%-1%): Abdominal pain, anorexia
Genital herpes (3%-1%): Asthenia, abdominal pain

■ **Serious Reactions**
- Thrombotic thrombocytopenic purpura/hemolytic uremic syndrome (TTP/HUS) has occurred in patients with advanced HIV disease and also in allogeneic bone marrow transplant and renal transplant recipients taking valacyclovir at doses of 8 g/day.

Special Considerations
- Acyclovir 400 mg PO bid less expensive for chronic suppression of genital herpes

■ **Patient/Family Education**
- Drink adequate fluids
- Start valacyclovir treatment at the first sign of a recurrent episode of genital herpes or herpes zoster; treatment is most effective when started within 48 hr after symptoms first appear
- Do not touch lesions to avoid spreading the infection to new sites
- Space doses evenly around the clock and continue taking the drug for the full course of treatment
- Avoid sexual intercourse while lesions are present to prevent infecting his or her partner
- Notify the physician if lesions don't improve or if they recur

■ **Monitoring Parameters**
- CBC, liver and renal function test results, and urinalysis results
- Evaluate for cutaneous lesions

■ **Geriatric side effects at a glance:**
☑ CNS ❑ Bowel Dysfunction ❑ Bladder Dysfunction ❑ Falls

■ **U.S. Regulatory Considerations**
❑ FDA Black Box ❑ OBRA regulated in U.S. Long Term Care

valganciclovir hydrochloride

(val-gan-sye'-kloh-veer hye-droe-klor'-ide)

- **Brand Name(s):** Valcyte
  Chemical Class: Acyclic purine nucleoside analog; ganciclovir derivative

- **Clinical Pharmacology:**
  Mechanism of Action: A synthetic nucleoside that competes with viral DNA esterases and is incorporated directly into growing viral DNA chains. **Therapeutic Effect:** Interferes with DNA synthesis and viral replication.
  Pharmacokinetics: Well absorbed and rapidly converted to ganciclovir by intestinal and hepatic enzymes. Widely distributed. Slowly metabolized intracellularly. Primarily excreted unchanged in urine. Removed by hemodialysis. **Half-life:** 18 hr (increased in impaired renal function).

- **Available Forms:**
  - *Tablets:* 450 mg.

- **Indications and Dosages:**
  Cytomegalovirus (CMV) *retinitis in patients with normal renal function:* PO Initially, 900 mg (two 450-mg tablets) twice a day for 21 days. Maintenance: 900 mg once a day.
  Prevention of CMV *after transplant:* PO 900 mg once a day beginning within 10 days of transplant and continuing until 100 days post-transplant.
  Dosage in renal impairment: Dosage and frequency are modified based on creatinine clearance.

Creatinine Clearance	Induction Dosage	Maintenance Dosage
60 ml/min or higher	900 mg twice a day	900 mg once a day
40–59 ml/min	450 mg twice a day	450 mg once a day
25–39 ml/min	450 mg once a day	450 mg every 2 days
10–24 ml/min	450 mg every 2 days	450 mg twice a wk

- **Contraindications:** Hypersensitivity to acyclovir or ganciclovir

- **Side Effects**
  Frequent (16%-9%)
  Diarrhea, neutropenia, headache
  Occasional (8%-3%)
  Nausea, anemia, thrombocytopenia
  Rare (less than 3%)
  Insomnia, paresthesia, vomiting, abdominal pain, fever

- **Serious Reactions**
  - Hematologic toxicity, including severe neutropenia (most common), anemia, and thrombocytopenia, may occur.
  - Retinal detachment occurs rarely.
  - An overdose may result in renal toxicity.
  - Valganciclovir may decrease sperm production and fertility.

Patient/Family Education
- Take with food
- Men should use a condom during sexual activity while using this medicine for at least 3 mo after treatment ends because valganciclovir interferes with normal sperm formation

Monitoring Parameters
- CBC, platelet count, creatinine

Geriatric side effects at a glance:
☑ CNS ☑ Bowel Dysfunction ☐ Bladder Dysfunction ☐ Falls

U.S. Regulatory Considerations
☑ FDA Black Box
- Valganciclovir is metabolized to ganciclovir. Risk of granulocytopenia, anemia, and thrombocytopenia. Aspermatogenesis, carcinogenic, teratogenic in animals.
- Oral capsules of ganciclovir have been associated with the risk of rapid-rate CMV retinitis progression and should be used as a maintenance therapy only in patients who benefit from avoiding daily intravenous infusions.
☐ OBRA regulated in U.S. Long Term Care

valproic acid / valproate sodium / divalproex sodium

(val-proe'-ik as'-id/val-proe'-ate soe'-dee-um/di-val'-pro-eks soe'-dee-um)

- **Brand Name(s):** (valproic acid) Depakene

- **Brand Name(s):** (valproate sodium) Depakene syrup

- **Brand Name(s):** (divalproex sodium) Depacon, Depakote, Depakote ER, Depakote Sprinkle
  Chemical Class: Carboxylic acid derivative

Clinical Pharmacology:
Mechanism of Action: An anticonvulsant that directly increases concentration of the inhibitory neurotransmitter gamma-aminobutyric acid. **Therapeutic Effect:** Reduces seizure activity.
Pharmacokinetics: Well absorbed from the GI tract. Protein binding: 80%-90%. Metabolized in the liver. Primarily excreted in urine. Not removed by hemodialysis. **Half-life:** 6-16 hr (may be increased in hepatic impairment, the elderly, and children younger than 18 mo).

■ **Available Forms:**
- *Capsules (Depakene)*: 250 mg.
- *Syrup (Depakene)*: 250 mg/5 ml.
- *Tablets (Delayed-Release [Depakote])*: 125 mg, 250 mg, 500 mg.
- *Tablets (Extended-Release [Depakote ER])*: 250 mg, 500 mg.
- *Capsules Sprinkles (Depakote Sprinkle)*: 125 mg.
- *Injection (Depacon)*: 100 mg/ml.

■ **Indications and Dosages:**
Seizures: PO Initially, 10-15 mg/kg/day in 1-3 divided doses. May increase by 5-10 mg/kg/day at weekly intervals up to 30-60 mg/kg/day. Usual adult dosage: 1,000-2,500 mg/day. IV Same as oral dose but given q6h.
Manic episodes: PO Initially, 750 mg/day in divided doses. Maximum: 60 mg/kg/day.
Prevention of migraine headaches: PO (Extended-Release) Initially, 500 mg/day for 7 days. May increase up to 1,000 mg/day. PO (Delayed-Release) Initially, 250 mg twice a day. May increase up to 1,000 mg/day.

■ **Unlabeled Uses:** Prevention of migraine; treatment of behavior disorders in Alzheimer's disease; bipolar disorder; chorea, myoclonic, simple partial, and tonic-clonic seizures; organic brain syndrome; schizophrenia; status epilepticus; tardive dyskinesia

■ **Contraindications:** Active hepatic disease, urea cycle disorders

■ **Side Effects**
Frequent
E*pilepsy*: Abdominal pain, diarrhea, transient alopecia, indigestion, nausea, vomiting, tremors, weight gain or loss
Mania (22%-19%): Nausea, somnolence
Occasional
E*pilepsy*: Constipation, dizziness, drowsiness, headache, skin rash, unusual excitement, restlessness
Mania (12%–6%): Asthenia, abdominal pain, dyspepsia (heartburn, indigestion, epigastric distress), rash
Rare
E*pilepsy*: Mood changes, diplopia, nystagmus, spots before eyes, unusual bleeding or ecchymosis

■ **Serious Reactions**
- **Alert** Hepatotoxicity may occur, particularly in the first 6 mo of valproic acid therapy. It may be preceded by loss of seizure control, malaise, weakness, lethargy, anorexia, and vomiting rather than abnormal serum liver function test results.
- Blood dyscrasias may occur.

■ **Patient/Family Education**
- Administer with food to decrease GI side effects
- Do not administer with carbonated beverages or milk

■ **Monitoring Parameters**
- Therapeutic levels (draw just before next dose) 50-100 mcg/ml
- ALT, AST, coagulation studies, and platelet count prior to and during therapy, especially first 6 mo
- Minor elevations in ALT, AST are frequent and dose related

- **Geriatric side effects at a glance:**
  - ❏ CNS   ❏ Bowel Dysfunction   ❏ Bladder Dysfunction   ❏ Falls

  Other: Tremor, osteoporosis

- **Use with caution in older patients with:** Hepatic impairment, End-stage renal disease, Osteoporosis, Parkinsonism, Essential tremor, Unsteady gait, Urinary incontinence

- **U.S. Regulatory Considerations**
  - ☑ FDA Black Box

  Hepatotoxicity, pancreatitis, teratogenicity
  - ❏ OBRA regulated in U.S. Long Term Care

- **Other Uses in Geriatric Patient:** Bipolar Disorder, Mania, Agitation in Dementia

- **Side Effects:**

  Of particular importance in the geriatric patient: delirium, confusion, cognitive impairment, amnesia, somnolence, reduction in bone mineral density, alopecia, tremor, weight gain, reversible parkinsonism, thrombocytopenia

- **Geriatric Considerations - Summary:** Valproic acid is a first-line treatment for partial or generalized seizures in older adults. Elimination half-life is doubled in older adults due to a larger volume of distribution. Serum concentrations are not correlated with behavior response and poorly correlated with CNS side effects. Tremor and parkinsonism tend to be dose-dependent. Sedation and gait disturbances are more likely with rapid titration. Ataxia and cognitive impairment occur less frequently than with phenytoin or carbamazepine. Valproic acid may reduce bone mineral density by interfering with osteoblastic function. Calcium and vitamin D supplementation and monitoring of bone mineral density is recommended for older adults taking valproate. Divalproex formulation is generally better tolerated than valproic acid.

- **References:**
  1. Brodie M, Kwan P. Epilepsy in elderly people. BMJ 2005;331:1317-1322.
  2. Birnbaum AK, Hardie NA, Conway JM, et al. Valproic acid doses, concentrations, and clearances in elderly nursing home residents. Epilepsy Res 2004;62:157-162.
  3. Arroyo S, Kramer G. Treating epilepsy in the elderly: safety considerations. Drug Saf 2001;24:991-1015.
  4. Drugs that may cause cognitive disorders in the elderly. Med Let 2000;42:111-112.
  5. Faught E. Epidemiolgy and drug treatment of epilepsy in elderly people. Drugs Aging 1999;15:255-269.

valsartan

(val-sar'-tan)

- **Brand Name(s):** Diovan

    Combinations
    Rx: with hydrochlorothiazide (Diovan HCT)
    Chemical Class: Angiotensin II receptor antagonist

- **Clinical Pharmacology:**
    Mechanism of Action: An angiotensin II receptor, type AT_1, antagonist that blocks vasoconstrictor and aldosterone-secreting effects of angiotensin II, inhibiting the binding of angiotensin II to the AT_1 receptors. **Therapeutic Effect:** Causes vasodilation, decreases peripheral resistance, and decreases BP.
    Pharmacokinetics: Poorly absorbed after PO administration. Food decreases peak plasma concentration. Protein binding: 95%. Metabolized in the liver. Recovered primarily in feces and, to a lesser extent, in urine. Unknown if removed by hemodialysis.
    Half-life: 6 hr.

- **Available Forms:**
    - *Tablets:* 40 mg, 80 mg, 160 mg, 320 mg.

- **Indications and Dosages:**
    Hypertension: PO Initially, 80-160 mg/day in patients who are not volume depleted. May increase up to a maximum: 320 mg/day.
    CHF: PO Initially, 40 mg twice a day. May increase up to 160 mg twice a day. Maximum: 320 mg/day.
    Post heart attack: PO Initially, 20 mg twice a day. May increase within 7 days to 40 mg twice a day. May further increase up to target dose of 160 mg twice a day.

- **Unlabeled Uses:** Diabetic nephropathy

- **Contraindications:** Bilateral renal artery stenosis, biliary cirrhosis or obstruction, hypoaldosteronism, severe hepatic impairment

- **Side Effects**
    Rare (2%-1%)
    Insomnia, fatigue, heartburn, abdominal pain, dizziness, headache, diarrhea, nausea, vomiting, arthralgia, edema

- **Serious Reactions**
    - Overdosage may manifest as hypotension and tachycardia. Bradycardia occurs less often.
    - Viral infection and upper respiratory tract infection (cough, pharyngitis, sinusitis, rhinitis) occur rarely.
    - Hypoglycemia may occur in patients with diabetes using glucose-lowering drugs.

Special Considerations
    - Potentially as or more effective than angiotensin-converting enzyme inhibitors, without cough; no evidence for reduction in morbidity and mortality as first-line agents in hypertension, yet; whether they provide the same cardiac and renal protection also still tentative; like ACE inhibitors, less effective in black patients

Patient/Family Education

- Call your clinician immediately if note following side effects: wheezing; lip, throat, or face swelling; hives or rash
- Female patients should be aware of the consequences of second- and third-trimester exposure to valsartan
- Valsartan must be taken for the rest of his or her life to control hypertension
- Do not exercise outside during hot weather because of the risks of dehydration and hypotension

Monitoring Parameters

- Baseline electrolytes, urinalysis, BUN and creatinine with recheck at 2-4 wk after initiation (sooner in volume-depleted patients); monitor sitting blood pressure; watch for symptomatic hypotension, particularly in volume-depleted patients
- Assess for signs and symptoms of an upper respiratory tract infection

Geriatric side effects at a glance:

❑ CNS ❑ Bowel Dysfunction ❑ Bladder Dysfunction ❑ Falls

U.S. Regulatory Considerations

☑ FDA Black Box

Although not relevant for geriatric patients, teratogenicity is associated with the use of angiotensin II receptor antagonists.

❑ OBRA regulated in U.S. Long Term Care

vancomycin hydrochloride

(van-koe-mye'-sin hye-droe-klor'-ide)

■ **Brand Name(s):** Lyphocin, Vancocin, Vancocin HCl, Vancocin HCl Pulvules
  Chemical Class: Tricyclic glycopeptide derivative

■ **Clinical Pharmacology:**
  Mechanism of Action: A tricyclic glycopeptide antibacterial that binds to bacterial cell walls, altering cell membrane permeability and inhibiting RNA synthesis. **Therapeutic Effect:** Bactericidal.
  Pharmacokinetics: PO: Poorly absorbed from the GI tract. Primarily eliminated in feces. **Parenteral:** Widely distributed. Protein binding: 55%. Primarily excreted unchanged in urine. Not removed by hemodialysis. **Half-life:** 4-11 hr (increased in impaired renal function).

■ **Available Forms:**
  - *Capsules (Vancocin HCl Pulvules):* 125 mg, 250 mg.
  - *Powder for Oral Suspension (Vancocin):* 1g (provides 250 mg/5 ml after mixing).
  - *Powder for Injection (Lyphocin, Vancocin HCl):* 500 mg, 1 g, 5 g, 10 g.
  - *Infusion (Premix [Vancocin HCl]):* 500 mg/100 ml, 1 g/200 ml.

■ Indications and Dosages:

Treatment of bone, respiratory tract, skin and soft-tissue infections, endocarditis, perito-
nitis, and septicemia; prevention of bacterial endocarditis in those at risk (if penicillin is
contraindicated) when undergoing biliary, dental, GI, GU, or respiratory surgery or in-
vasive procedures: IV 500 mg q6h or 1g q12h.
Staphylococcal enterocolitis, ID-antibacterial-associated pseudomembranous colitis
caused by Clostridium difficile: PO 0.5-2 g/day in 3-4 divided doses for 7-10 days.
Dosage in renal impairment: After a loading dose, subsequent dosages and frequency
are modified based on creatinine clearance, the severity of the infection, and the serum concentration of the drug.

■ Unlabeled Uses:
Treatment of brain abscess, perioperative infections, staphylococcal
or streptococcal meningitis

■ Contraindications:
None known.

■ Side Effects

Frequent
PO: Bitter or unpleasant taste, nausea, vomiting, mouth irritation (with oral solution)
Rare
Parenteral: Phlebitis, thrombophlebitis, or pain at peripheral IV site; dizziness; vertigo;
tinnitus; chills; fever; rash; necrosis with extravasation
PO: Rash.

■ Serious Reactions

• Nephrotoxicity and ototoxicity may occur.
• "Red-neck" syndrome (redness on face, neck, arms, and back; chills; fever; tachycardia; nausea or vomiting; pruritus; rash; unpleasant taste) may result from too-rapid
injection.

Special Considerations

• Individualize treatment based on local susceptibility patterns.

■ Patient/Family Education

• Space drug doses evenly around the clock and continue vancomycin therapy for the
full course of treatment
• Notify the physician if a rash, tinnitus, or signs and symptoms of nephrotoxicity occur
• Laboratory tests are an important part of the therapy regimen

■ Monitoring Parameters

• Audiograms, BUN, creatinine, serum vancomycin concentrations
• Renal function
• Intake and output
• Vancomycin therapeutic peak serum level is 20-40 mcg/ml, and the trough level is
5-15 mcg/ml. The toxic peak serum level is greater than 40 mcg/ml, and the trough
level is greater than 15 mcg/ml

■ Geriatric side effects at a glance:

❏ CNS ❏ Bowel Dysfunction ❏ Bladder Dysfunction ❏ Falls

■ U.S. Regulatory Considerations

❏ FDA Black Box ❏ OBRA regulated in U.S. Long Term Care

vardenafil hydrochloride

(var-den'-a-fil hye-droe-klor'-ide)

- **Brand Name(s):** Levitra
  Chemical Class: Cyclic GMP specific phosphodiesterase inhibitor

- **Clinical Pharmacology:**
  Mechanism of Action: An erectile dysfunction agent that inhibits phosphodiesterase type 5, the enzyme responsible for degrading cyclic guanosine monophosphate (cGMP) in the corpus cavernosum of the penis, resulting in smooth muscle relaxation and increased blood flow. **Therapeutic Effect:** Facilitates an erection.
  Pharmacokinetics: Rapidly absorbed after PO administration. Extensive tissue distribution. Protein binding: 95%. Metabolized in the liver. Excreted primarily in feces; a lesser amount eliminated in urine. Drug has no effect on penile blood flow without sexual stimulation. **Half-life:** 4–5 hr.

- **Available Forms:**
  - *Tablets*: 2.5 mg, 5 mg, 10 mg, 20 mg.

- **Indications and Dosages:**
  Erectile dysfunction: PO 5 mg approximately 1 hr before sexual activity. Dose may be increased to 10-20 mg, based on patient tolerance. Maximum dosing frequency is once daily.
  Dosage in moderate hepatic impairment: PO For patients with Child-Pugh Class B hepatic impairment, dosage is 5 mg 60 min before sexual activity.
  Dosage with concurrent ritonavir: PO 2.5 mg in a 72-hr period.
  Dosage with concurrent ketoconazole or itraconazole (at 400 mg/day), or indinavir: PO 2.5 mg in a 24-hour period.
  Dosage with concurrent ketoconazole or itraconazole (at 200 mg/day), or erythromycin: PO 5 mg in a 24-hr period.

- **Contraindications:** Concurrent use of alpha-adrenergic blockers, sodium nitroprusside, or nitrates in any form

- **Side Effects**
  Occasional
  Headache, flushing, rhinitis, indigestion
  Rare (less than 2%)
  Dizziness, changes in color vision, blurred vision

- **Serious Reactions**
  - Prolonged erections (lasting over 4 hr) and priapism (painful erections lasting over 6 hr) occur rarely.

Special Considerations
  - Rates of erection sufficient for penetration were 65%, 75%, and 80% with 5-mg, 10-mg, and 20-mg doses, respectively
  - For diabetics, rates of erection sufficient for penetration were 61% and 64% with 10-mg and 20-mg doses, respectively

- For men after radical prostatectomy, rates of erection sufficient for penetration were 47% and 48% with 10-mg and 20-mg doses, respectively

■ **Patient/Family Education**
- Sexual stimulation is required for an erection to occur after taking vardenafil
- Take vardenafil approximately 60 min before sexual activity; fatty meal may reduce effect
- Seek treatment immediately if an erection lasts longer than 4 hr
- Avoid using nitrate drugs and alpha-adrenergic blockers concurrently with vardenafil

■ **Monitoring Parameters**
- Cardiovascular status

■ **Geriatric side effects at a glance:**
❑ CNS ❑ Bowel Dysfunction ❑ Bladder Dysfunction ❑ Falls

■ **U.S. Regulatory Considerations**
❑ FDA Black Box ❑ OBRA regulated in U.S. Long Term Care

vasopressin

(vay-soe-press'-in)

■ **Brand Name(s):** Pitressin
Chemical Class: Arginine vasopressin

■ **Clinical Pharmacology:**
Mechanism of Action: A posterior pituitary hormone that increases reabsorption of water by the renal tubules. Increases water permeability at the distal tubule and collecting duct. Directly stimulates smooth muscle in the GI tract. **Therapeutic Effect:** Causes peristalsis and vasoconstriction.
Pharmacokinetics:

Route	Onset	Peak	Duration
IV	N/A	N/A	0.5–1 hr
IM, Subcutaneous	1–2 hr	N/A	2–8 hr

Distributed throughout extracellular fluid. Metabolized in the liver and kidney. Primarily excreted in urine. **Half-life:** 10–20 min.

■ **Available Forms:**
- *Injection:* 20 units/ml.

■ **Indications and Dosages:**
Cardiac arrest: IV 40 U as a one-time bolus.
Diabetes insipidus: IV Infusion 0.5 mU/kg/hr. May double dose q30min. Maximum: 10 mU/kg/hr. IM, Subcutaneous 5–10 U 2–4 times a day. Range: 5–60 U/day.

Abdominal distention, Intestinal paresis: IM Initially, 5 U. Subsequent doses, 10 U q3–4h.
GI hemorrhage: IV Infusion Initially, 0.2–0.4 U/min progressively increased to 0.9 U/min.
Vasodilatory shock: IV Initially, 0.04 - 0.1 U/min. Titrate to desired effect.

■ **Unlabeled Uses:** Adjunct in treatment of acute, massive hemorrhage

■ **Contraindications:** None known.

■ **Side Effects**
Frequent
Pain at injection site (with vasopressin tannate)
Occasional
Abdominal cramps, nausea, vomiting, diarrhea, dizziness, diaphoresis, pale skin, circumoral pallor, tremors, headache, eructation, flatulence
Rare
Chest pain; confusion; allergic reaction, including rash or hives, pruritus, wheezing or difficulty breathing, facial and peripheral edema; sterile abscess (with vasopressin tannate)

■ **Serious Reactions**
- Anaphylaxis, MI, and water intoxication have occurred.
- The elderly are at higher risk for water intoxication.

Special Considerations
- For diabetes insipidus, vasopressin solution for injection may be administered intranasally on cotton pledgets, by nasal spray, or by dropper; dose must be individualized

■ **Patient/Family Education**
- Common adverse effects (skin blanching, abdominal cramps, and nausea) may be reduced by taking 1-2 glasses of water with the dose of vasopressin; self-limited in minutes
- Report chest pain, headache, shortness of breath, or other symptoms
- Avoid alcohol
- Monitor fluid intake and output

■ **Monitoring Parameters**
- ECG, fluid and electrolyte status, urine specific gravity
- Extravasation may cause tissue necrosis
- Blood pressure, pulse rate
- Intake and output

■ **Geriatric side effects at a glance:**
❏ CNS   ❏ Bowel Dysfunction   ❏ Bladder Dysfunction   ❏ Falls

■ **U.S. Regulatory Considerations**
❏ FDA Black Box   ❏ OBRA regulated in U.S. Long Term Care

venlafaxine hydrochloride

(ven'-la-fax-een hye-droe-klor'-ide)

■ **Brand Name(s):** Effexor, Effexor XR
  Chemical Class: Phenethylamine derivative

■ **Clinical Pharmacology:**
  Mechanism of Action: A phenethylamine derivative that potentiates CNS neurotransmitter activity by inhibiting the reuptake of serotonin, norepinephrine and, to a lesser degree, dopamine. **Therapeutic Effect:** Relieves depression.
  Pharmacokinetics: Well absorbed from the GI tract. Protein binding: 25%-30%. Metabolized in the liver to active metabolite. Primarily excreted in urine. Not removed by hemodialysis. **Half-life:** 3-7 hr; metabolite, 9-13 hr (increased in hepatic or renal impairment.

■ **Available Forms:**
  • *Capsules (Extended-Release [Effexor XR]):* 37.5 mg, 75 mg, 150 mg.
  • *Tablets (Effexor):* 25 mg, 37.5 mg, 50 mg, 75 mg, 100 mg.

■ **Indications and Dosages:**
  Depression: PO Initially, 75 mg/day in 2-3 divided doses with food. May increase by 75 mg/day at intervals of 4 days or longer. Maximum: 375 mg/day in 3 divided doses. PO (Extended-Release) 75 mg/day as a single dose with food. May increase by 75 mg/day at intervals of 4 days or longer. Maximum: 225 mg/day.
  Social anxiety disorder, generalized anxiety disorder: PO (Extended-Release) Initially, 37.5-75 mg/day. May increase by 75 mg/day at 4-day intervals up to 225 mg/day.
  Dosage in renal and hepatic impairment: Expect to decrease venlafaxine dosage by 50% in patients with moderate hepatic impairment, 25% in patients with mild to moderate renal impairment, and 50% in patients on dialysis (withhold dose until completion of dialysis).

■ **Unlabeled Uses:** Prevention of relapses of depression; chronic fatigue syndrome, obsessive-compulsive disorder

■ **Contraindications:** Use within 14 days of MAOIs

■ **Side Effects**
  Frequent (greater than 20%)
  Nausea, somnolence, headache, dry mouth
  Occasional (20%-10%)
  Dizziness, insomnia, constipation, diaphoresis, nervousness, asthenia, ejaculatory disturbance, anorexia
  Rare (less than 10%)
  Anxiety, blurred vision, diarrhea, vomiting, tremor, abnormal dreams, impotence, hypertension

■ **Serious Reactions**
  • A sustained increase in diastolic BP of 10-15 mm Hg occurs occasionally.

■ **Patient/Family Education**
- Take venlafaxine with food to minimize GI distress
- Do not abruptly discontinue the drug or decrease or increase the dosage
- Avoid tasks that require mental alertness or motor skills until response to the drug has been established
- Avoid alcohol while taking venlafaxine

■ **Monitoring Parameters**
- Blood pressure, weight
- Closely supervise the suicidal patient during early therapy; as depression lessens, the patient's energy level improves, increasing the suicide potential
- Assess appearance, behavior, level of interest, mood, and sleep patterns for evidence of a therapeutic response

■ **Geriatric side effects at a glance:**
☑ CNS ☑ Bowel Dysfunction ☐ Bladder Dysfunction ☑ Falls
Other: Hyponatremia, increased diastolic BP (rare)

■ **Use with caution in older patients with:** None

■ **U.S. Regulatory Considerations**
☑ FDA Black Box
- Because there is an increased risk of suicide in children and adolescents, older adults should also be closely monitored for suicide ideation.
☐ OBRA regulated in U.S. Long Term Care

■ **Other Uses in Geriatric Patient:** Anxiety symptoms and related disorders

■ **Side Effects:**
Of *particular importance in the geriatric patient*: Hyponatremia, withdrawal symptoms when abruptly discontinued (e.g., during hospitalization) rather than tapered

■ **Geriatric Considerations - Summary:** Although there is some eveidence that venlafaxine may be more effective for the treatment of depression than SSRIs, this has not been well established. One study in long-term care found that compared to sertraline, venlafaxine was less well tolerated and more often discontinued. Several of the drugs in this class have been associated with severe withdrawal symptoms (e.g., nausea and/or vomiting, dizziness, headaches, lethargy or light-headedness, anxiety and/or agitation) when discontinued abruptly. Venlafaxine has not been well studied with respect to falls.

■ **References:**
1. Oslin DW, Ten Have TR, Streim JE, et al. Probing the safety of medications in the frail elderly: evidence from a randomized clinical trial of sertraline and venlafaxine in depressed nursing home residents. J Clin Psychiatry 2003;64:875-882.
2. Is Effexor more effective for depression than an SSRI? Med Lett Drugs Ther 2004;46:15-16.
3. Kirby D, Harrigan S, Ames D. Hyponatraemia in elderly psychiatric patients treated with selective serotonin reuptake inhibitors and venlafaxine: a retrospective controlled study in an inpatient unit. Int J Geriatr Psychiatry 2002;17:231-237.

4. Degner D, Grohmann R, Kropp S, et al. Severe adverse drug reactions of antidepressants: results of the German multicenter drug surveillance program AMSP. Pharmacopsychiatry 2004;37 (Suppl 1):S39-S45.
5. Smith D, Dempster C, Glanville J, et al. Efficacy and tolerability of venlafaxine compared with selective serotonin reuptake inhibitors and other antidepressants: a meta-analysis. Br J Psychiatry 2002;180:396-404.

verapamil hydrochloride

(ver-ap'-a-mill hye-droe-klor'-ide)

■ **Brand Name(s):** Calan, Calan SR, Covera-HS, Isoptin, Isoptin I.V., Isoptin SR, Verelan, Verelan PM

Combinations
Rx: with trandolapril (Tarka)
Chemical Class: Phenylalkylamine

■ **Clinical Pharmacology:**
Mechanism of Action: An antihypertensive and antianginal, antiarrhythmic, and antihypertensive agent that inhibits calcium ion entry across cardiac and vascular smooth-muscle cell membranes. This action causes the dilation of coronary arteries, peripheral arteries, and arterioles. **Therapeutic Effect:** Decreases heart rate and myocardial contractility and slows SA and AV conduction. Decreases total peripheral vascular resistance by vasodilation.
Pharmacokinetics:

Route	Onset	Peak	Duration
PO	30 min	1-2 hr	6-8 hr
PO (Extended-release)	30 min	N/A	N/A
IV	1-2 min	3-5 min	10-60 min

Well absorbed from the GI tract. Protein binding: 90% (60% in neonates.) Undergoes first-pass metabolism in the liver to active metabolite. Primarily excreted in urine. Not removed by hemodialysis. **Half-life:** 2-8 hr.

■ **Available Forms:**
- *Caplet (Calan* SR): 120 mg, 180 mg, 240 mg.
- *Capsules (Extended-Release [Verelan* PM]): 100 mg, 200 mg, 300 mg.
- *Capsules (Sustained-Release [Verelan]):* 120 mg, 180 mg, 240 mg, 360 mg.
- *Tablets (Calan):* 40 mg, 80 mg, 120 mg.
- *Tablets (Extended-Release [Covera-HS]):* 180 mg, 240 mg.
- *Tablets (Sustained-Release [Isoptin* SR]): 120 mg, 180 mg, 240 mg.
- *Injection:* 2.5 mg/ml.

■ **Indications and Dosages:**
Supraventricular tachyarrhythmias (SVT): IV Initially, 2.5-5 mg over 2 min. May give 5-10 mg 30 min after initial dose. Maximum initial dose: 20 mg.

Arrhythmias, including prevention of recurrent paroxysmal supraventricular tachycardia and control of ventricular resting rate in chronic atrial fibrillation or flutter (with digoxin): PO 240-480 mg/day in 3-4 divided doses.

Vasospastic angina (Prinzmetal's variant), unstable (crescendo or preinfarction) angina, chronic stable (effort-associated) angina: PO Initially, 80-120 mg 3 times a day. For elderly patients and those with hepatic dysfunction, 40 mg 3 times a day. Titrate to optimal dose. Maintenance: 240-480 mg/day in 3-4 divided doses.

Hypertension: PO (Immediate-Release) 80 mg 3 times a day. Range: 80-320 mg/day in 2 divided doses. PO (Sustained-Release) 120-240 mg/day. Range: 120-360 mg/day as single dose or in 2 divided doses. PO (Extended-Release [Covera-HS]) 120-360 mg once daily at bedtime. PO (Extended-Release [Verelan PM]) 200-400 mg once daily at bedtime.

■ **Unlabeled Uses:** Treatment of bipolar disorder, hypertrophic cardiomyopathy, vascular headaches

■ **Contraindications:** Atrial fibrillation or flutter and an accessory bypass tract, cardiogenic shock, heart block, hypotension, sinus bradycardia, ventricular tachycardia

■ **Side Effects**
Frequent (7%)
Constipation
Occasional (4%-2%)
Dizziness, light-headedness, headache, asthenia (loss of strength, energy), nausea, peripheral edema, hypotension
Rare (less than 1%)
Bradycardia, dermatitis, or rash

■ **Serious Reactions**
- Rapid ventricular rate in atrial flutter or fibrillation, marked hypotension, extreme bradycardia, CHF, asystole, and second- and third-degree AV block occur rarely.

Special Considerations
- Dihydropyridine calcium-channel blockers preferred over verapamil and diltiazem in patients with sinus bradycardia, conduction disturbances, and for combination with a β-blocker
- Differentiate PSVT from narrow-complex ventricular tachycardia prior to IV administration; failure to do so has resulted in fatalities

■ **Patient/Family Education**
- Do not abruptly discontinue verapamil; compliance with the treatment regimen is essential to control anginal pain
- To avoid the orthostatic effects of verapamil, rise slowly from a lying to a sitting position and wait momentarily before standing
- Avoid tasks that require mental alertness or motor skills until response to the drug has been established
- Avoid consuming grapefruit or grapefruit juice and limit caffeine intake while taking verapamil
- Notify the physician if anginal pain is not reduced by the drug; if constipation, dizziness, irregular heartbeat, nausea, shortness of breath, or swelling of the hands and feet occur

■ **Monitoring Parameters**
- Pulse for rate, rhythm, and quality
- ECG for changes, particularly PR-interval prolongation

- Assess stool consistency and frequency
- Therapeutic serum level for verapamil is 0.08 to 0.3 mcg/ml

■ Geriatric side effects at a glance:
☐ CNS   ☑ Bowel Dysfunction   ☐ Bladder Dysfunction   ☐ Falls

■ U.S. Regulatory Considerations
☐ FDA Black Box   ☐ OBRA regulated in U.S. Long Term Care

voriconazole

(vohr-ih-kon'-uh-zohl)

■ Brand Name(s): Vfend
Chemical Class: Triazole derivative

■ Clinical Pharmacology:
Mechanism of Action: A triazole derivative that inhibits the synthesis of ergosterol, a vital component of fungal cell wall formation. **Therapeutic Effect:** Damages fungal cell wall membrane.
Pharmacokinetics: Rapidly and completely absorbed after PO administration. Widely distributed. Protein binding: 98%. Metabolized in the liver. Primarily excreted as a metabolite in urine. **Half-life:** 6 hr.

■ Available Forms:
- *Tablets:* 50 mg, 200 mg.
- *Injection Powder for Reconstitution:* 200 mg.
- *Powder for Oral Suspension:* 200 mg/5 ml.

■ Indications and Dosages:
Invasive aspergillosis, other serious fungal infections caused by Scedosporium apiospermum and Fusarium species: PO *Weight 40 kg and more.* Initially, 400 mg q12h for 2 doses on day 1. Maintenance: 200 mg q12h (may increase to 200 mg q12h). *Weight less than 40 kg.* Initially, 200 mg q12h for 2 doses on day 1. Maintenance: 100 mg q12h (may increase to 150 mg q12h).
Usual parenteral dosage: IV Initially, 6 mg/kg/dose q12h for 2 doses, then 4 mg/kg/dose q12h (may decrease to 3 mg/kg/dose if patient is unable to tolerate 4 mg/kg/dose).
Candidemia in non-neutropenic patients: PO 200 mg q12h. IV Initially, 6 mg/kg/dose q12h for 2 doses, then 3-4 mg/kg/dose q12h.
Esophageal candidiasis: PO *Weight 40 kg and more.* 200 mg q12h for minimum of 14 days, then at least 7 days following resolution of symptoms. *Weight less than 40 kg.* 100 mg q12h for minimum 14 days, then at least 7 days following resolution of symptoms.

■ Contraindications: Concurrent administration of carbamazepine; ergot alkaloids; pimozide or quinidine (may cause prolonged QT interval or torsades de pointes); rifabutin; rifampin; or sirolimus

■ **Side Effects**
Frequent (20%-5%)
Abnormal vision, fever, nausea, rash, vomiting
Occasional (5%-2%)
Headache, chills, hallucinations, photophobia, tachycardia, hypertension

■ **Serious Reactions**
- Hepatotoxicity (e.g., jaundice, hepatitis, hepatic failure, acute renal failure) has been observed in severely ill patients.

Special Considerations
- Do not take oral within 1 hr of meals
- Do not drive at night while taking voriconazole
- Avoid direct sunlight

■ **Monitoring Parameters**
- Visual acuity, field, and color perception if taken more than 28 days
- ALT, AST, alkaline phosphatase, bilirubin, electrolytes, renal function

■ **Geriatric side effects at a glance:**
❑ CNS ❑ Bowel Dysfunction ❑ Bladder Dysfunction ❑ Falls

■ **U.S. Regulatory Considerations**
❑ FDA Black Box ❑ OBRA regulated in U.S. Long Term Care

warfarin sodium

(war'-far-in soe'-dee-um)

■ **Brand Name(s):** Coumadin, Jantoven
Chemical Class: Coumarin derivative

■ **Clinical Pharmacology:**
Mechanism of Action: A coumarin derivative that interferes with hepatic synthesis of vitamin K–dependent clotting factors, resulting in depletion of coagulation factors II, VII, IX, and X. **Therapeutic Effect:** Prevents further extension of formed existing clot; prevents new clot formation or secondary thromboembolic complications.
Pharmacokinetics:

Route	Onset	Peak	Duration
PO	1.5–3 days	5–7 days	N/A

Well absorbed from the GI tract. Metabolized in the liver. Primarily excreted in urine. Not removed by hemodialysis. **Half-life:** 1.5–2.5 days.

■ **Available Forms:**
- *Tablets* (*Coumadin, Jantoven*): 1 mg, 2 mg, 2.5 mg, 3 mg, 4 mg, 5 mg, 6 mg, 7.5 mg, 10 mg.

- ■ **Indications and Dosages:**
  Anticoagulant: PO Initially, 2-5 mg/day for 2–5 days; then adjust based on INR. Maintenance: 2–10 mg/day.

- ■ **Unlabeled Uses:** Prevention of myocardial infarction, recurrent cerebral embolism; treatment adjunct in transient ischemic attacks

- ■ **Contraindications:** Neurosurgical procedures, open wounds, severe hypertension, severe hepatic or renal damage, spinal puncture, uncontrolled bleeding, ulcers

- ■ **Side Effects**
  Occasional
  GI distress, such as nausea, anorexia, abdominal cramps, diarrhea
  Rare
  Hypersensitivity reaction, including dermatitis and urticaria, especially in those sensitive to aspirin

- ■ **Serious Reactions**
  - Bleeding complications ranging from local ecchymoses to major hemorrhage may occur. Drug should be discontinued immediately and vitamin K or phytonadione administered. Mild hemorrhage: 2.5–10 mg PO, IM, or IV. Severe hemorrhage: 10–15 mg IV and repeated q4h, as necessary.
  - Hepatotoxicity, blood dyscrasias, necrosis, vasculitis, and local thrombosis occur rarely.

Special Considerations
- Avoid use of initial doses >5 mg
- INR during first 5 days of therapy does not correlate with degree of anticoagulation
- Anticoagulant effect of warfarin may be reversed by administration of vitamin K or fresh frozen plasma; should only use in situations where INR is severely elevated >10, or when patient is actively bleeding

- ■ **Patient/Family Education**
  - Strict adherence to prescribed dosage schedule is necessary
  - Avoid alcohol, salicylates, and drastic changes in dietary habits
  - Do not change from one brand to another without consulting clinician
  - Consult the physician before having dental work
  - Use an electric razor and soft toothbrush, to prevent bleeding during warfarin therapy
  - Do not take other medications, including OTC drugs, especially aspirin and NSAIDs, without physician approval
  - Report black stool, bleeding; brown, dark, or red urine; coffee-ground vomitus; or red-speckled mucus from cough

- ■ **Monitoring Parameters**
  - Dosage of anticoagulants must be individualized and adjusted according to INR determinations; it is recommended that INR determinations be performed prior to initiation of therapy, at 24-hr intervals while maintenance dosage is being established, then once or twice weekly for the following 3-4 wk, then at 1-4 wk intervals for the duration of treatment
  - Maintain INR at 2-3 (2.5-3.5 for mechanical valves, recurrent systemic thromboembolism)

- Hct, and stool and urine cultures for occult blood, regardless of administration route
- Blood pressure, pulse rate
- Assess the patient's gums for erythema and gingival bleeding, skin for ecchymosis and petechiae, and urine for hematuria
- Examine the patient for excessive bleeding from minor cuts or scratches

■ **Geriatric side effects at a glance:**
  ❏ CNS ❏ Bowel Dysfunction ❏ Bladder Dysfunction ❏ Falls
  Other: Hemorrhage

■ **Use with caution in older patients with:** Recent bleeding or hemorrhage (GI, intracranial or urinary); postsurgery

■ **U.S. Regulatory Considerations**
  ❏ FDA Black Box
  ❏ OBRA regulated in U.S. Long Term Care

■ **Other Uses in Geriatric Patient:** None

■ **Side Effects:**
  Of *particular importance in the geriatric patient*: Bleeding, hemorrhage, increased bruising, hematoma

■ **Geriatric Considerations - Summary:** Older adults generally require smaller doses of warfarin to achieve a therapeutic INR and may exhibit increased sensitivity to its therapeutic effects. Small dosage changes may result in significant INR changes. With appropriate monitoring, the benefits of warfarin therapy in atrial fibrillation generally outweigh the risk of bleeding complications. Numerous drug interactions with warfarin exist that require increased monitoring. Evaluate concurrent conditions, physical function, fall risk, and alcohol intake to assess bleeding risk.

■ **References:**
  1. Johnson CE, Lim WK, Workman BS. People aged over 75 in atrial fibrillation on warfarin: the rate of major hemorrhage and stroke in more than 500 patient-years of follow-up. J Am Geriatr Soc 2005;53:655-659.
  2. Sebastian JL, Tresch DD. Use of oral anticoagulants in older patients. Drugs Aging 2000;16:409-435.

xylometazoline

(zye-loe-met-az'-oh-leen)

OTC: Otrivin Measured-Dose Pump with Moisturizers, Otrivin Nasal Drops, Otrivin Nasal Spray, Otrivin Nasal Spray with Eucalyptol, Otrivin Nasal Spray with Moisturizers, Otrivin with Measured-Dose Pump
Chemical Class: Imidazoline derivative

■ Clinical Pharmacology:
Mechanism of Action: A sympathomimetic that directly acts on alpha-adrenergic receptors in arterioles of the nasal mucosa to produce vasoconstriction resulting in decreased blood flow. **Therapeutic Effect:** Decreased nasal congestion.
Pharmacokinetics: Onset of action occurs within 5-10 minutes for a duration of action of 5-6 hours. Well absorbed through nasal mucosa. May also be systemically absorbed from both nasal mucosa and gastrointestinal (GI) tract. **Half-life:** Unknown.

■ Available Forms:
- **Nasal Drops:** 0.1% (Otrivin Nasal Drops).
- **Nasal Spray:** 0.1% (Otrivin Nasal Spray).

■ Indications and Dosages:
Rhinitis: Intranasal 1-3 drops (0.1%) in each nostril q8-10h or 1 to 2 sprays (0.1%) in each nostril q8-10h. Maximum: 3 doses/day.

■ Contraindications: Narrow-angle glaucoma, rhinitis sicca, hypersensitivity to xylometazoline or other adrenergic agents

■ Side Effects
Occasional
Intranasal: Burning, stinging, drying nasal mucosa, sneezing. Prolonged use may result in rebound congestion.

■ Serious Reactions
- Large doses may produce tachycardia, palpitations, light-headedness, nausea, and vomiting.
- Overdosage may produce hallucinations, CNS depression, and seizures.

Special Considerations
- Manage rebound congestion by stopping xylometazoline: one nostril at a time, substitute systemic decongestant and/or substitute inhaled steroid

■ Patient/Family Education
- Do not use for >3-5 days or rebound congestion may occur
- Use caution when performing tasks that require visual acuity during therapy

■ Monitoring Parameters
- Therapeutic response

- **Geriatric side effects at a glance:**
  ❑ CNS   ❑ Bowel Dysfunction   ❑ Bladder Dysfunction   ❑ Falls

- **U.S. Regulatory Considerations**
  ❑ FDA Black Box   ❑ OBRA regulated in U.S. Long Term Care

yohimbine

(yo-him'-been hye'-droe-klor'-ide)

- **Brand Name(s):** Actibine, Aphrodyne, Dayto-Himbin, Yocon, Yohimbe, Yohimex, Yovital
  Chemical Class: Indolalkylamine derivative

- **Clinical Pharmacology:**
  Mechanism of Action: An herb that produces genital blood vessel dilation, improves nerve impulse transmission to genital area. Increases penile blood flow, central sympathetic excitation impulses to genital tissues. **Therapeutic Effect:** Improves sexual vigor, affects impotence.
  Pharmacokinetics: Rapidly absorbed. Extensive metabolism in liver and kidneys. Minimal excretion in urine as unchanged drug. **Half-life:** 36 min.

- **Available Forms:**
  • **Tablets:** 5 mg (Actibine), 5.4 mg (Aphrodyne, Dayto-Himbin, Yocon, Yovital, Yohimex).

- **Indications and Dosages:**
  Impotence: PO 5.4 mg 3 times/day.

- **Unlabeled Uses:** Treatment of SSRI-induced sexual dysfunction, weight loss, sympatholytic and mydriatic, aphrodisiac

- **Contraindications:** Renal disease, hypersensitivity to yohimbine or any component of the formulation

- **Side Effects**
  Excitement, tremors, insomnia, anxiety, hypertension, tachycardia, dizziness, headache, irritability, salivation, dilated pupils, nausea, vomiting, hypersensitivity reaction

- **Serious Reactions**
  • Paralysis, severe hypotension, irregular heartbeats, and cardiac failure may occur. Overdose can be fatal.

- **Patient/Family Education**
  • Do not use other medications, including OTC drugs, without first notifying the physician

- **Monitoring Parameters**
  - Blood pressure
  - Liver and renal function

- **Geriatric side effects at a glance:**
  - ☐ CNS ☐ Bowel Dysfunction ☐ Bladder Dysfunction ☐ Falls

- **U.S. Regulatory Considerations**
  - ☐ FDA Black Box ☐ OBRA regulated in U.S. Long Term Care

zafirlukast

(za-feer'-loo-kast)

- **Brand Name(s):** Accolate
  Chemical Class: Tolylsulfonyl benzamide derivative

- **Clinical Pharmacology:**
  Mechanism of Action: An antiasthmatic that binds to leukotriene receptors, inhibiting bronchoconstriction due to sulfur dioxide, cold air, and specific antigens, such as grass, cat dander, and ragweed. **Therapeutic Effect:** Reduces airway edema and smooth muscle constriction; alters cellular activity associated with the inflammatory process.
  Pharmacokinetics: Rapidly absorbed after PO administration (food reduces absorption). Protein binding: 99%. Extensively metabolized in the liver. Primarily excreted in feces. Unknown if removed by hemodialysis. **Half-life:** 10 hr.

- **Available Forms:**
  - *Tablets:* 10 mg, 20 mg.

- **Indications and Dosages:**
  Bronchial asthma: PO 20 mg twice a day.

- **Unlabeled Uses:** Exercise-induced bronchospasm

- **Contraindications:** None known.

- **Side Effects**
  Frequent (13%)
  Headache
  Occasional (3%)
  Nausea, diarrhea
  Rare (less than 3%)
  Generalized pain, asthenia, myalgia, fever, dyspepsia, vomiting, dizziness

- **Serious Reactions**
  - Concurrent administration of inhaled corticosteroids increases the risk of upper respiratory tract infection.

Patient/Family Education
- Take regularly, even during symptom-free periods
- Do not alter the dosage or abruptly discontinue other asthma medications
- Zafirlukast is not intended to treat acute asthma episodes
- Drink plenty of fluids to decrease the thickness of lung secretions
- Notify the physician if abdominal pain, nausea, flu-like symptoms, jaundice, or worsening of asthma occurs

Monitoring Parameters
- ALT, AST, CBC
- Pulse rate and quality and respiratory rate, depth, rhythm, and type
- Observe the patient's fingernails and lips for cyanosis, manifested as a blue or dusky color in light-skinned patients and a gray color in dark-skinned patients

Geriatric side effects at a glance:
❏ CNS ❏ Bowel Dysfunction ❏ Bladder Dysfunction ❏ Falls

U.S. Regulatory Considerations
❏ FDA Black Box ❏ OBRA regulated in U.S. Long Term Care

zalcitabine

(zal-site'-a-been)

Brand Name(s): Hivid
Chemical Class: Nucleoside analog

Clinical Pharmacology:
Mechanism of Action: A nucleoside reverse transcriptase inhibitor that inhibits viral DNA synthesis. **Therapeutic Effect:** Prevents replication of HIV-1.
Pharmacokinetics: Readily absorbed from the GI tract (absorption decreased by food). Protein binding: less than 4%. Undergoes phosphorylation intracellularly to the active metabolite. Primarily excreted in urine. Removed by hemodialysis. **Half-life:** 1-3 hr; metabolite, 2.6-10 hr (increased in impaired renal function).

Available Forms:
- *Tablets*: 0.375 mg, 0.75 mg.

Indications and Dosages:
HIV infection (in combination with other ID-antiretrovirals): PO 0.75 mg q8h.
Dosage in renal impairment: Dosage and frequency are modified based on creatinine clearance.

Creatinine Clearance	Dose
10-40 ml/min	0.75 mg q12h
less than 10 ml/min	0.75 mg q24h

1312

- **Contraindications:** Moderate or severe peripheral neuropathy

- **Side Effects**
  Frequent (28%-11%)
  Peripheral neuropathy, fever, fatigue, headache, rash
  Occasional (10%-5%)
  Diarrhea, abdominal pain, oral ulcers, cough, pruritus, myalgia, weight loss, nausea, vomiting
  Rare (4%-1%)
  Nasal discharge, dysphagia, depression, night sweats, confusion

- **Serious Reactions**
  - Peripheral neuropathy (characterized by numbness, tingling, burning, and pain in the lower extremities) occurs in 17% to 31% of patients. These symptoms may be followed by sharp, shooting pain and progress to a severe, continuous, burning pain that may be irreversible if the drug is not discontinued in time.
  - Pancreatitis, leukopenia, neutropenia, eosinophilia, and thrombocytopenia occur rarely.

Special Considerations

  - Consult the most recent guidelines for HIV antiviral therapy prior to prescribing
  - Always check updated treatment guidelines before initiating or changing antiretroviral therapy (http://AIDSinfo.nih.gov)

- **Patient/Family Education**
  - Notify the physician of any signs or symptoms of pancreatitis or peripheral neuropathy
  - Zalcitabine is not a cure for HIV, nor does it reduce the risk of transmitting HIV to others

- **Monitoring Parameters**
  - Periodic CBC, serum chemistry tests, transaminase levels
  - Serum amylase and triglyceride concentrations in patients with history of elevated amylase, pancreatitis, ethanol abuse, or receiving parenteral nutrition
  - Assess the patient for evidence of potentially fatal pancreatitis, including abdominal pain, nausea and vomiting, and increasing serum amylase and triglyceride levels. If the patient develops any of these signs or symptoms, particularly abdominal pain, withhold the drug.

- **Geriatric side effects at a glance:**
  ❏ CNS ❏ Bowel Dysfunction ❏ Bladder Dysfunction ❏ Falls

- **U.S. Regulatory Considerations**
  ☑ FDA Black Box
  - Risk for severe peripheral neuropathy; use with extreme caution in patients with preexisting neuropathy.
  - Risk for pancreatitis but rare occurrence.
  - Lactic acidosis and hepatomegaly have been reported with steatosis (including fatal cases).
  ❏ OBRA regulated in U.S. Long Term Care

zaleplon

(zal'-e-plon)

■ **Brand Name(s):** Sonata
Chemical Class: Pyrazolopyrimidine derivative

■ **Clinical Pharmacology:**
Mechanism of Action: A nonbenzodiazepine that enhances the action of the inhibitory neurotransmitter gamma-aminobutyric acid. **Therapeutic Effect:** Induces sleep.
Pharmacokinetics: Rapidly and almost completely absorbed following PO administration. Protein binding: 60%. Metabolized in liver. Primarily excreted in urine. Partially eliminated in feces. **Half-life:** 1 hr.

■ **Available Forms:**
• *Capsules:* 5 mg, 10 mg.

■ **Indications and Dosages:**
Insomnia: PO 5 mg at bedtime.

■ **Contraindications:** Severe hepatic impairment

■ **Side Effects**
Expected
Somnolence, sedation, mild rebound insomnia (on first night after drug is discontinued)
Frequent (28%-7%)
Nausea, headache, myalgia, dizziness
Occasional (5%-3%)
Abdominal pain, asthenia, dyspepsia, eye pain, paresthesia
Rare (2%)
Tremors, amnesia, hyperacusis (acute sense of hearing), fever

■ **Serious Reactions**
• Zaleplon may produce altered concentration, behavior changes, and impaired memory.
• Taking the drug while up and about may result in adverse CNS effects, such as hallucinations, impaired coordination, dizziness, and light-headedness.
• Overdose results in somnolence, confusion, diminished reflexes, and coma.

Special Considerations
• Because of the short half-life, agent best for problems with sleep latency, rather than duration of sleep or number of awakenings (e.g., shift workers)
• Abuse potential similar to benzodiazepines
• Advantage over triazolam, given big cost difference, difficult to justify, if used correctly

■ **Patient/Family Education**
  • *Timing of administration*: Immediately before bedtime or after the patient has gone to bed and has experienced difficulty falling asleep
  • Do not take with alcohol or OTC cimetidine
  • Avoid activities requiring mental alertness or motor skills until response to the drug has been established

■ **Monitoring Parameters**
  • Sleep latency, number of awakenings, daytime function (hangover effect), dizziness, confusion

■ **Geriatric side effects at a glance:**
  ☑ CNS ❑ Bowel Dysfunction ❑ Bladder Dysfunction ☑ Falls
  Other: Withdrawal symptoms after long-term use, rebound insomnia

■ **Use with caution in older patients with:** COPD; untreated sleep apnea

■ **U.S. Regulatory Considerations**
  ❑ FDA Black Box
  ☑ OBRA regulated in U.S. Long Term Care

■ **Other Uses in Geriatric Patient:** Hypnotic

■ **Side Effects:**
  Of particular importance in the geriatric patient: Sedation, withdrawal symptoms when abruptly discontinued (e.g., during hospitalization) rather than tapered

■ **Geriatric Considerations - Summary:** Zaleplon is similar in efficacy and side-effect profile to a short-acting benzodiazepine. Zaleplon should be reserved for short-term use. Sedating antidepressants (e.g., trazodone) or eszopiclone are preferred for long-term management of sleep problems. Although this agent may cause falls, this has not been well studied. Because zaleplon is a substrate of CYP C3A, it should be used with caution, especially with drugs such as nefazodone, clarithromycin, or amiodarone. When initiating therapy, zaleplon should be titrated carefully to avoid oversedation. In addition, zaleplon has the potential to induce withdrawal symptoms (e.g., anxiety and/or agitation) when discontinued abruptly.

■ **References:**
  1. Eszopiclone (Lunesta), a new hypnotic. Med Lett Drugs Ther 2005;47:17-19.
  2. McCall WV. Diagnosis and management of insomnia in older people. J Am Geriatr Soc 2005;53:S272-S277
  3. Barbera J, Shapiro C. Benefit-risk assessment of zaleplon in the treatment of insomnia. Drug Saf 2005;28:301-318.

zanamivir

(za-na'-mi-veer)

■ **Brand Name(s):** Relenza
Chemical Class: Carboxylic acid ethyl ester

■ **Clinical Pharmacology:**
Mechanism of Action: An antiviral that appears to inhibit the influenza virus enzyme neuraminidase, which is essential for viral replication. **Therapeutic Effect:** Prevents viral release from infected cells.
Pharmacokinetics: Systemically absorbed, approximately 4%-17%. Protein binding: Low. Not metabolized. Partially excreted unchanged in urine. **Half-life:** 1.6-5.1 hr.

■ **Available Forms:**
• *Powder for Inhalation*: 5 mg/blister.

■ **Indications and Dosages:**
Influenza virus: Inhalation 2 inhalations (one 5-mg blister per inhalation for a total dose of 10 mg) twice a day (approximately 12 hr apart) for 5 days.
Prevention of influenza virus: Inhalation 2 inhalations once a day for the duration of the exposure period.

■ **Unlabeled Uses:** Influenza prophylaxis

■ **Contraindications:** None known.

■ **Side Effects**
Occasional (3%-2%)
Diarrhea, sinusitis, nausea, bronchitis, cough, dizziness, headache
Rare (less than 1.5%)
Malaise, fatigue, fever, abdominal pain, myalgia, arthralgia, urticaria

■ **Serious Reactions**
• Neutropenia may occur.
• Bronchospasm may occur in those with a history of chronic obstructive pulmonary disease (COPD) or bronchial asthma.

Special Considerations
• Off-label use to prevent influenza in family members of influenza patients (N Engl J Med 2000 Nov 2;343(18):1282-1289): Attack rate reduced from 19% to 4%

■ **Patient/Family Education**
• Expected benefit of zanamivir is one day of shortening of overall symptoms
• Patients with less severe symptoms get less benefit from therapy
• Influenza vaccine remains the best way to prevent influenza and use of zanamivir should not affect the evaluation of individuals for annual influenza vaccination
• Patients scheduled to use an inhaled bronchodilator at the same time as zanamivir should use their bronchodilator before taking zanamivir

- Two doses should be taken on the first day of treatment whenever possible provided there is at least 2 hours between doses

■ **Monitoring Parameters**
  - Pattern of daily bowel activity and stool consistency

■ **Geriatric side effects at a glance:**
  ❑ CNS ☑ Bowel Dysfunction ❑ Bladder Dysfunction ❑ Falls

■ **U.S. Regulatory Considerations**
  ❑ FDA Black Box ❑ OBRA regulated in U.S. Long Term Care

zidovudine

(zye-doe'-vyoo-deen)

■ **Brand Name(s):** Retrovir

> Combinations
> **Rx:** with lamivudine (Combivir)
> **Chemical Class:** Nucleoside analog

■ **Clinical Pharmacology:**
  Mechanism of Action: A nucleoside reverse transcriptase inhibitor that interferes with viral RNA-dependent DNA polymerase, an enzyme necessary for viral HIV replication. **Therapeutic Effect:** Interferes with HIV replication, slowing the progression of HIV infection.
  Pharmacokinetics: Rapidly and completely absorbed from the GI tract. Protein binding: 25%-38%. Undergoes first-pass metabolism in the liver. Crosses the blood-brain barrier and is widely distributed, including to cerebrospinal fluid (CSF). Primarily excreted in urine. Minimal removal by hemodialysis. **Half-life:** 0.8-1.2 hr (increased in impaired renal function).

■ **Available Forms:**
  - *Capsules (Retrovir):* 100 mg.
  - *Syrup (Retrovir):* 50 mg/5 ml.
  - *Tablets (Retrovir):* 300 mg.
  - *Injection (Retrovir):* 10 mg/ml.

■ **Indications and Dosages:**
  HIV infection: PO 200 mg q8h or 300 mg q12h. IV 1-2 mg/kg/dose q4h.

■ **Unlabeled Uses:** Prophylaxis in health care workers at risk of acquiring HIV after occupational exposure

■ **Contraindications:** Life-threatening allergic reactions to zidovudine or its components

■ **Side Effects**
  Expected (46%-42%)
  Nausea, headache
  Frequent (20%-16%)
  Abdominal pain, asthenia, rash, fever, acne
  Occasional (12%-8%)
  Diarrhea, anorexia, malaise, myalgia, somnolence
  Rare (6%-5%)
  Dizziness, paresthesia, vomiting, insomnia, dyspnea, altered taste

■ **Serious Reactions**
  • Serious reactions include anemia, which occurs most commonly after 4-6 weeks of therapy, and granulocytopenia; both effects are more likely to occur in patients who have a low Hgb level or granulocyte count before beginning therapy.
  • Neurotoxicity (as evidenced by ataxia, fatigue, lethargy, nystagmus, and seizures) may occur.

Special Considerations
  • Consult the most recent guidelines for HIV antiviral therapy prior to prescribing
  • Always check updated treatment guidelines before initiating or changing antiretroviral therapy (http://AIDSinfo.nih.gov)

■ **Patient/Family Education**
  • Close monitoring of blood counts is extremely important; does not reduce risk of transmitting HIV to others through sexual contact or blood contamination
  • Space zidovudine doses evenly around the clock
  • Report bleeding from the gums, nose, or rectum to the physician immediately
  • Have dental work done before therapy or postpone it until blood counts return to normal, which may be weeks after therapy has stopped
  • Do not take any other medications without the physician's prior approval
  • Notify physician if difficulty breathing, headache, inability to sleep, muscle weakness, a rash, signs of infection, or unusual bleeding occurs

■ **Monitoring Parameters**
  • CBC with differential and platelets q2wk initially for 2 mo, then q4-8 wk
  • CD4+ cell count, Hgb and HIV RNA plasma levels, mean corpuscular volume, and reticulocyte count
  • Pattern of daily bowel activity and stool consistency
  • Skin for acne or a rash
  • Assess the patient for signs and symptoms of opportunistic infections, such as chills, cough, fever, and myalgia
  • Intake and output
  • Serum renal and liver function test results

■ **Geriatric side effects at a glance:**
  ☑ CNS   ☐ Bowel Dysfunction   ☐ Bladder Dysfunction   ☐ Falls

■ **U.S. Regulatory Considerations**
  ☑ FDA Black Box
  • Risk for neutropenia and severe anemia, particularly in patients with advanced HIV disease.
  • Myopathy associated with prolonged use.

- Lactic acidosis and hepatomegaly have been reported with steatosis (including fatal cases).
- ❑ OBRA regulated in U.S. Long Term Care

zileuton

(zi-loo'-ton)

- **Brand Name(s):** Zyflo
  Chemical Class: Urea derivative

- **Clinical Pharmacology:**
  Mechanism of Action: A leukotriene inhibitor that inhibits the enzyme responsible for producing inflammatory response. Prevents formation of leukotrienes (leukotrienes induce bronchoconstriction response), enhances vascular permeability, stimulates mucus secretion. **Therapeutic Effect:** Prevents airway edema, smooth muscle contraction, and the inflammatory process, relieving signs and symptoms of bronchial asthma.
  Pharmacokinetics: Rapidly absorbed from gastrointestinal (GI) tract. Protein binding: 93%. Metabolized in liver. Primarily excreted in urine. Unknown if removed by hemodialysis. **Half-life:** 2.1-2.5 hr.

- **Available Forms:**
  - **Tablets:** 600 mg (Zyflo).

- **Indications and Dosages:**
  Bronchial asthma: PO 600 mg 4 times/day. Total daily dosage: 2,400 mg.

- **Contraindications:** Active liver disease, impaired liver function, hypersensitivity to zileuton or any component of the formulation

- **Side Effects**
  Frequent
  Headache
  Occasional
  Dyspepsia, nausea, abdominal pain, asthenia (loss of strength), myalgia
  Rare
  Conjunctivitis, constipation, dizziness, flatulence, insomnia

- **Serious Reactions**
  - Liver dysfunction occurs rarely and may be manifested as right upper quadrant pain, nausea, fatigue, lethargy, pruritus, jaundice or flulike symptoms.

- **Patient/Family Education**
  - Must be taken regularly, even during symptom-free periods
  - Not a bronchodilator; do not use to treat acute episodes of asthma
  - Increase fluid intake

- **Monitoring Parameters**
  - CBC, renal function, and transaminase levels periodically during 1st year of prolonged therapy
  - Rate, depth, and rhythm of respirations, pulse rate

- **Geriatric side effects at a glance:**
  - ❑ CNS ❑ Bowel Dysfunction ❑ Bladder Dysfunction ❑ Falls

- **U.S. Regulatory Considerations**
  - ❑ FDA Black Box ❑ OBRA regulated in U.S. Long Term Care

zinc oxide/zinc sulfate

(zink'- ox'-eyed/zink'- sul'-fate)

- **Brand Name(s):** (zinc oxide) Balmex, Desitin

- **Brand Name(s):** (zinc sulfate) Orazinc
  Chemical Class: Divalent cation

- **Clinical Pharmacology:**
  Mechanism of Action: A mineral that acts as a cofactor for enzymes that are important for protein and carbohydrate metabolism. **Therapeutic Effect:** Zinc oxide acts as a mild astringent and skin protectant. Zinc sulfate helps maintain normal growth and tissue repair as well as skin hydration.

- **Available Forms:**
  Zinc Oxide:
  - Ointment: 10%, 20%, 40%.
  Zinc Sulfate:
  - Capsules: 110 mg, 220 mg.
  - Tablets: 110 mg.
  - Injection: 1 mg/ml.

- **Indications and Dosages:**
  Mild skin irritations and abrasions (such as chapped skin, diaper rash): Topical (zinc oxide) Apply as needed.
  Treatment and prevention of zinc deficiency, wound healing: PO (zinc sulfate) 220 mg 3 times a day.

- **Unlabeled Uses:** Zinc sulfate: Wilson's disease

- **Contraindications:** None known.

- **Side Effects**
  Frequency not defined:
  Nausea, vomiting, epigastric discomfort

- **Serious Reactions**
  - Hypotension, arrhythmias, anemia, and thrombocytopenia occur rarely.

- Acetate not recommended for initial therapy of symptomatic Wilson's disease (should be treated initially with chelating agents)

- **Patient/Family Education**
  - Take acetate on an empty stomach
  - Coffee and dairy products may decrease the absorption of oral zinc sulfate capsules and tablets
  - Notify the physician if the skin condition doesn't improve after 7 days of treatment

- **Geriatric side effects at a glance:**
  - ❑ CNS ❑ Bowel Dysfunction ❑ Bladder Dysfunction ❑ Falls

- **U.S. Regulatory Considerations**
  - ❑ FDA Black Box ❑ OBRA regulated in U.S. Long Term Care

ziprasidone

(zi-pray'-si-done)

- **Brand Name(s):** Geodon
  Chemical Class: Benzisothiazole derivative

- **Clinical Pharmacology:**
  Mechanism of Action: A piperazine derivative that antagonizes alpha-adrenergic, dopamine, histamine, and serotonin receptors; also inhibits reuptake of serotonin and norepinephrine. **Therapeutic Effect:** Diminishes symptoms of schizophrenia and depression.
  Pharmacokinetics: Well absorbed after PO administration. Food increases bioavailability. Protein binding: 99%. Extensively metabolized in the liver. Not removed by hemodialysis. **Half-life:** 7 hr.

- **Available Forms:**
  - *Capsules*: 20 mg, 40 mg, 60 mg, 80 mg.
  - *Injection*: 20 mg/ml.

- **Indications and Dosages:**
  Schizophrenia: PO Initially, 20 mg twice a day with food. Titrate at intervals of no less than 2 days. Maximum: 80 mg twice a day. IM 10 mg q2h or 20 mg q4h. Maximum: 40 mg/day.
  Mania in bipolar disorder: PO Initially, 40 mg twice a day. May increase to 60-80 mg twice a day on second day of treatment. Range: 40-80 mg twice a day.

- **Unlabeled Uses:** Tourette's syndrome

■ **Contraindications:** Conditions that prolong the QT interval, such as congenital long QT syndrome

■ **Side Effects**
   Frequent (30%-16%)
   Headache, somnolence, dizziness
   Occasional
   Rash, orthostatic hypotension, weight gain, restlessness, constipation, dyspepsia
   Rare
   Hyperglycemia, priapism

■ **Serious Reactions**
   • Prolongation of QT interval may produce torsades de pointes, a form of ventricular tachycardia. Patients with bradycardia, hypokalemia, or hypomagnesemia are at increased risk.

Special Considerations
   • Atypical agents with less risk of movement disorders best for: Patients resistant to standard antipsychotic agents; patients with therapy-limiting extrapyramidal symptoms, other adverse effects; comparisons with other atypical agents: shorter half-life and bid dosing requirement potential disadvantage, but perhaps less weight gain

■ **Patient/Family Education**
   • Review presentation of cardiac (prolonged QT, torsades de pointes) and movement disorders; avoid electrolyte disturbance and drug interactions
   • Take with food
   • Avoid tasks requiring mental alertness or motor skills until response to the drug has been established

■ **Monitoring Parameters**
   • Improvement of symptomatology (both positive and negative symptoms), complete blood counts, liver function tests, serum prolactin, routine chemistry (especially K^+, Mg^{2+} during prolonged therapy); signs/symptoms of akathisia, abnormal movements, persistent constipation
   • Weight

■ **Geriatric side effects at a glance:**
   ☑ CNS   ☑ Bowel Dysfunction   ☐ Bladder Dysfunction   ☑ Falls
   Other: QTc prolongation, weight gain, glucose intolerance, diabetes, orthostatic hypotension, extrapyramidal symptoms

■ **Use with caution in older patients with:** Diabetes, glucose intolerance, cardiovascular disease, especially with history of syncope

■ **U.S. Regulatory Considerations**
   ☑ FDA Black Box
   There is an increased risk of death in older patients with dementia. Although the causes of death were varied, most of the deaths appeared to be either cardiovascular (e.g., heart failure, sudden death) or infectious (e.g., pneumonia) in nature. This drug is not approved for treatment of patients with dementia-related psychosis.
   ☑ OBRA regulated in U.S. Long Term Care

■ **Other Uses in Geriatric Patient:** Behavior disturbances in the setting of dementia

■ **Side Effects:**
Of particular importance in the geriatric patient: Weight gain, glucose intolerance, diabetes, increased risk of death (see FDA black box warning)

■ **Geriatric Considerations - Summary:** Direct comparisons between older and newer antipsychotic drugs in demented elderly persons are scarce. Newer agents have the theoretical advantage of a lower incidence of tardive dyskinesia but may cause weight gain, impaired glycemic control, and increased risk for cardiovascular events. These agents should be used with caution in demented elderly persons, with frequent monitoring for side effects and a low threshold for discontinuing use. Indeed, the Food and Drug Administration has recently released an advisory about these medications outlining the risk for increased mortality.

■ **References:**
1. Sink KM, Holden KF, Yaffe K. Pharmacological treatment of neuropsychiatric symptoms of dementia: a review of the evidence. JAMA 2005;293:596-608.
2. Alexopoulos GS, Streim J, Carpenter D, Docherty JP. Using antipsychotic agents in older patients. J Clin Psychiatry 2004;65 (Suppl 2):5-99.
3. Cohen D. Atypical antipsychotics and new onset diabetes mellitus. An overview of the literature. Pharmacopsychiatry 2004;37:1-11.
4. Deaths with antipsychotics in elderly patients with behavioral disturbances. Available at: www.fda.gov/cder/drug/advisory/antipsychotics.htm.
5. Katz IR. Optimizing atypical antipsychotic treatment strategies in the elderly. J Am Geriatr Soc 2004;52:S272-S277.
6. Glassman AH, Bigger JT, Jr. Antipsychotic drugs: prolonged QTc interval, torsades de pointes, and sudden death. Am J Psychiatry 2001;158:1774-1782.

zoledronic acid

(zole-eh-drone'-ick as'-id)

■ **Brand Name(s):** Zometa
Chemical Class: Bisphosphonic acid

■ **Clinical Pharmacology:**
Mechanism of Action: A bisphosphonate that inhibits the resorption of mineralized bone and cartilage; inhibits increased osteoclastic activity and skeletal calcium release induced by stimulatory factors produced by tumors. **Therapeutic Effect:** Increases urinary calcium and phosphorus excretion; decreases serum calcium and phosphorus levels.
Pharmacokinetics: Protein binding: 22%. Not metabolized. More than 95% excreted in urine. **Half-life:** 167 hr.

■ **Available Forms:**
• *Injection Powder for Reconstitution*: 4 mg.
• *Injection Solution*: 4 mg/5 ml.

■ **Indications and Dosages:**

Hypercalcemia: IV Infusion 4 mg IV infusion given over no less than 15 min. Retreatment may be considered, but at least 7 days should elapse to allow for full response to initial dose.

Multiple myeloma, bone metastases of solid tumors: IV 4 mg q3-4wk.

■ **Unlabeled Uses:** Prevention of bone metastases from breast, prostate cancer, treatment of bone diseases

■ **Contraindications:** Hypersensitivity to other bisphosphonates, including alendronate, etidronate, pamidronate, risedronate, and tiludronate

■ **Side Effects**

Frequent (44%–26%)

Fever, nausea, vomiting, constipation

Occasional (15%–10%)

Hypotension, anxiety, insomnia, flu-like symptoms (fever, chills, bone pain, myalgia, and arthralgia)

Rare

Conjunctivitis, osteonecrosis of the jaw

■ **Serious Reactions**

• Renal toxicity may occur if IV infusion is administered in less than 15 min.

Special Considerations

• Reconstitute with 5 ml sterile water, then further diluted in 100 ml 0.9% sodium chloride or 5% dextrose; do not mix with calcium-containing infusion solutions (i.e., lactated Ringer's)

• Most potent bisphosphonate available

• A dental examination with appropriate preventive dentistry should be considered prior to treatment with bisphosphonates in patients with concomitant risk factors (e.g., cancer chemotherapy, corticosteroid, poor oral hygiene). While on bisphosphonate treatment patients with concomitant risk factors should avoid invasive dental procedures if possible. For patients who develop osteonecrosis of the jaw while on bisphosphonate therapy, dental surgery may exacerbate the condition. For patients requiring dental procedures, there are no data available to suggest whether discontinuation of bisphosphonate treatment reduces the risk of osteonecrosis of the jaw.

■ **Patient/Family Education**

• Avoid drugs containing calcium and vitamin D, such as antacids, because they might antagonize the effects of zoledronic acid

• Inform your dentist if you are taking this drug.

• If you develop jaw pain, loose teeth, or signs of oral infection, immediately inform your doctor.

■ **Monitoring Parameters**

• Serum creatinine, electrolytes, phosphate, magnesium, CBC

• Assess for fever

• Monitor fluid intake and output, especially in patients with impaired renal function

■ **Geriatric side effects at a glance:**

❑ CNS   ☑ Bowel Dysfunction   ❑ Bladder Dysfunction   ❑ Falls

zolmitriptan

(zohl-mi-trip'-tan)

■ **Brand Name(s):** Zomig, Zomig-ZMT
  Chemical Class: Serotonin derivative

■ **Clinical Pharmacology:**
  Mechanism of Action: A serotonin receptor agonist that binds selectively to vascular receptors, producing a vasoconstrictive effect on cranial blood vessels. **Therapeutic Effect:** Relieves migraine headache.
  Pharmacokinetics: Rapidly but incompletely absorbed after PO administration. Protein binding: 15%. Undergoes first-pass metabolism in the liver to active metabolite. Eliminated primarily in urine (60%) and, to a lesser extent, in feces (30%). **Half-life:** 3 hr.

■ **Available Forms:**
  • *Tablets (Zomig):* 2.5 mg, 5 mg.
  • *Tablets (Orally-Disintegrating [Zomig-ZMT]):* 2.5 mg, 5 mg.
  • *Nasal Spray (Zomig):* 5 mg/0.1 ml.

■ **Indications and Dosages:**
  Acute migraine attack: PO Initially, 2.5 mg or less. If headache returns, may repeat dose in 2 hr. Maximum: 10 mg/24 hr. Intranasal 5 mg. May repeat in 2 hr. Maximum: 10 mg/24hr.

■ **Contraindications:** Arrhythmias associated with conduction disorders, basilar or hemiplegic migraine, coronary artery disease, ischemic heart disease (including angina pectoris, history of MI, silent ischemia, and Prinzmetal's angina), uncontrolled hypertension, use within 24 hr of ergotamine-containing preparations or another serotonin receptor agonist, use within 14 days of MAOIs, Wolff-Parkinson-White syndrome

■ **Side Effects**
  Frequent (8%-6%)
  Oral: Dizziness; tingling; neck, throat, or jaw pressure; somnolence
  Nasal: Altered taste, paresthesia
  Occasional (5%-3%)
  Oral: Warm or hot sensation, asthenia, chest pressure
  Nasal: Nausea, somnolence, nasal discomfort, dizziness, asthenia, dry mouth
  Rare (2%-1%)
  Diaphoresis, myalgia, paresthesia

■ **Serious Reactions**
  • Cardiac reactions (including ischemia, coronary artery vasospasm, and MI) and noncardiac vasospasm-related reactions (such as hemorrhage and cerebrovascular accident |CVA|) occur rarely, particularly in patients with hypertension, diabetes, or a strong family history of coronary artery disease; obese patients; smokers; males older than 40 years; and postmenopausal women.

Special Considerations
  • Alternative to sumatriptan for the treatment of migraine headache; has not been compared head-to-head with sumatriptan; choice should be based on cost and availability
  • First dose should be administered in medical office in case cardiac symptoms occur; take great care to exclude the possibility of silent cardiovascular disease prior to prescribing
  • Doses >2.5 mg were not associated with more headache relief, but were associated with increased side effects; if no relief is obtained after first dose, a second dose is unlikely to provide any benefit

■ **Patient/Family Education**
  • Take a single dose of zolmitriptan as soon as migraine symptoms appear
  • Zolmitriptan is intended to relieve migraines, not to prevent them or reduce the number of attacks
  • Avoid tasks that require mental alertness or motor skills until response to the drug has been established
  • Notify the physician if blood in urine or stool, chest pain, palpitations, easy bruising, numbness or pain in the arms or legs, throat tightness, or swelling of the eyelids, face, or lips occurs
  • Lie down in dark, quiet room for additional benefit after taking zolmitriptan

■ **Monitoring Parameters**
  • Blood pressure, especially in patients with hepatic impairment
  • Assess the patient for relief of migraines and associated symptoms, including nausea and vomiting, photophobia, and phonophobia (sound sensitivity)

■ **Geriatric side effects at a glance:**
  ❑ CNS ❑ Bowel Dysfunction ❑ Bladder Dysfunction ❑ Falls

■ **U.S. Regulatory Considerations**
  ❑ FDA Black Box ❑ OBRA regulated in U.S. Long Term Care

zolpidem tartrate

(zole-pi'-dem tar'-trate)

- **Brand Name(s):** Ambien, Ambien CR
  Chemical Class: Imidazopyridine derivative

  DEA Class: Schedule IV

- **Clinical Pharmacology:**
  Mechanism of Action: A nonbenzodiazepine that enhances the action of the inhibitory neurotransmitter gamma-aminobutyric acid. **Therapeutic Effect:** Induces sleep and improves sleep quality.
  Pharmacokinetics:

Route	Onset	Peak	Duration
PO	30 min	N/A	6-8 hr

  Rapidly absorbed from the GI tract. Protein binding: 92%. Metabolized in the liver; excreted in urine. Not removed by hemodialysis. **Half-life:** 1.4-4.5 hr (increased in hepatic impairment).

- **Available Forms:**
  - *Tablets (Ambien):* 5 mg, 10 mg.
  - *Tablets (Extended-Release [Ambien CR]):* 6.25 mg, 12.5 mg.

- **Indications and Dosages:**
  Insomnia: PO 5 mg at bedtime. PO (Extended-Release) 6.25 mg.

- **Contraindications:** None known.

- **Side Effects**
  Occasional (7%)
  Headache
  Rare (less than 2%)
  Dizziness, nausea, diarrhea, muscle pain

- **Serious Reactions**
  - Overdose may produce severe ataxia, bradycardia, altered vision (such as diplopia), severe drowsiness, nausea and vomiting, difficulty breathing, and unconsciousness.
  - Abrupt withdrawal of the drug after long-term use may produce asthenia, facial flushing, diaphoresis, vomiting, and tremor.
  - Drug tolerance or dependence may occur with prolonged, high-dose therapy.

- **Patient/Family Education**
  - Take immediately prior to retiring
  - Avoid alcohol
  - Use caution driving or performing other tasks requiring alertness

- Do not abruptly stop zolpidem after long-term use
- Drug dependence or tolerance may occur with prolonged use of high doses

■ **Monitoring Parameters**
  - Assess sleep pattern, including time needed to fall asleep and number of nocturnal awakenings
  - Evaluate for therapeutic response, such as a decrease in the number of nocturnal awakenings and an increased duration of sleep

■ **Geriatric side effects at a glance:**
  ☑ CNS   ☐ Bowel Dysfunction   ☐ Bladder Dysfunction   ☑ Falls
  Other: Withdrawal symptoms after long-term use, rebound insomnia

■ **Use with caution in older patients with:** Concurrent treatment with potent CYP 3A4 inhibitors; COPD; untreated sleep apnea

■ **U.S. Regulatory Considerations**
  ☐ FDA Black Box   ☑ OBRA regulated in U.S. Long Term Care

■ **Other Uses in Geriatric Patient:** Hypnotic

■ **Side Effects:**
  Of particular importance in the geriatric patient: Sedation, withdrawal symptoms when abruptly discontinued (e.g., during hospitalization) rather than tapered

■ **Geriatric Considerations - Summary:** Zolpidem is similar in efficacy and side-effect profile to a short-acting benzodiazepine. Zolpidem should be reserved for short-term use. A sedating antidepressant (e.g., trazodone) or eszopiclone are preferred for long-term management of sleep problems. Because zolpidem is a substrate of CYP C3A, 1A1 and 2D6, it should be used with caution, especially with drugs such as nefazodone and clarithromycin or amiodarone. When initiating therapy, zolpidem should be titrated carefully to avoid oversedation. In addition, abrupt discontinuation of zolpidem has been associated with withdrawal symptoms (e.g., anxiety and/or agitation).

■ **References:**
  1. Mahoney JE, Webb MJ, Gray SL. Zolpidem prescribing and adverse drug reactions in hospitalized general medicine patients at a Veterans Affairs hospital. Am J Geriatr Pharmacother 2004;2(1):66-74.
  2. Swainston HT, Keating GM. Zolpidem: a review of its use in the management of insomnia. CNS Drugs 2005;19:65-89.
  3. Eszopiclone (Lunesta), a new hypnotic. Med Lett Drugs Ther 2005;47:17-19.

zonisamide

(zoh-nis'-a-mide)

- **Brand Name(s):** Zonegran
  Chemical Class: Sulfonamide derivative

- **Clinical Pharmacology:**
  Mechanism of Action: A succinimide that may stabilize neuronal membranes and suppress neuronal hypersynchronization by blocking sodium and calcium channels.
  Therapeutic Effect: Reduces seizure activity.
  Pharmacokinetics: Well absorbed after PO administration. Extensively bound to RBCs. Protein binding: 40%. Primarily excreted in urine. **Half-life:** 63 hr (plasma), 105 hr (RBCs).

- **Available Forms:**
  - *Capsules:* 25 mg, 50 mg, 100 mg.

- **Indications and Dosages:**
  Partial seizures: PO Initially, 100 mg/day for 2 wk. May increase by 100 mg/day at intervals of 2 wk or longer. Range: 100-600 mg/day.

- **Unlabeled Uses:** Treatment of binge eating disorder, bipolar disorder, obesity

- **Contraindications:** Allergy to sulfonamides

- **Side Effects**
  Frequent (17%-9%)
  Somnolence, dizziness, anorexia, headache, agitation, irritability, nausea
  Occasional (8%-5%)
  Fatigue, ataxia, confusion, depression, impaired memory or concentration, insomnia, abdominal pain, diplopia, diarrhea, speech difficulty
  Rare (4%-3%)
  Paresthesia, nystagmus, anxiety, rash, dyspepsia, weight loss

- **Serious Reactions**
  - Overdose is characterized by bradycardia, hypotension, respiratory depression, and coma.
  - Leukopenia, anemia, and thrombocytopenia occur rarely.

Special Considerations
  - Due to long t½, steady state achievable with stable dosing for 2 wk
  - Adjunctive therapy for wide variety of seizure disorders, especially those refractory to other drugs

- **Patient/Family Education**
  - Low threshold for discussing signs and symptoms related to skin rash, liver problems, or blood problems with clinician

1329

- Do not abruptly discontinue the drug after long-term use because this may precipitate seizures
- Avoid tasks that require mental alertness or motor skills until response to the drug is established
- Avoid alcohol and CNS depressants while taking zonisamide

■ **Monitoring Parameters**
- Frequency and severity of seizures, neurotoxicity, hypersensitivity reactions, serum creatinine, BUN

■ **Geriatric side effects at a glance:**
❑ CNS ❑ Bowel Dysfunction ❑ Bladder Dysfunction ❑ Falls
Other: Increases in serum creatinine

■ **Use with caution in older patients with:** Cognitive impairment, Unsteady gait, Renal impairment, Nephrolithiasis

■ **U.S. Regulatory Considerations**
❑ FDA Black Box ❑ OBRA regulated in U.S. Long Term Care

■ **Other Uses in Geriatric Patient:** None

■ **Side Effects:**
Of *particular importance in the geriatric patient*: Delirium, confusion, cognitive impairment, drowsiness, sedation, altered thinking, ataxia, fatigue, anorexia, increase in creatinine, renal stones

■ **Geriatric Considerations - Summary:** Not well-studied in older adults; however, a Japanese trial included older adults up to 85 years of age. Contraindicated in patients with creatinine clearance less than 50ml/min. Slow titration is required. Patients should maintain fluid intake to reduce the risk of renal stones. Restrictions for use in renal impairment prevent its use in many older adults.

■ **References:**
1. Brodie M, Kwan P. Epilepsy in elderly people. BMJ 2005;331:1317-1322.
2. Arroyo S, Kramer G. Treating epilepsy in the elderly: safety considerations. Drug Saf 2001;24:991-1015.
3. Drugs that may cause cognitive disorders in the elderly. Med Let 2000;42:111-112.
4. Willmore LJ. Choice and use of newer anticonvulsant drugs in older patients. Drugs Aging 2000;17:441-452.

Index

Entries can be identified as follows: generic name, Trade name.

Anthra-Derm, 84-85
anthralin, 84-85
Antilirium, 987-988
Antiminth, 1055-1056
Antinaus 50, 1038-1040
Antispas, 121-123
Antispasmodic, 121-123
Anti-Tuss, 577-578
Antivert, 734-735
Antizol, 531-533
Anturane, 1160-1161
Anucort-HC, 593-595
Anumed-HC, 593-595
Anusol, 1014-1015
Anusol-HC, 593-595
Anutone-HC, 593-595
Anzemat, 390-391
Apacet, 9-10
Aphrodyne, 1310-1311
Aphthasol, 62-63
Apo-Quin-G, 1068-1070
apraclonidine hydrochloride, 85-86
aprepitant, 86-87
Apresazide, 588-589, 590-591
Apresoline, 588-589
Aptivus, 1226
Aquachloral Supprettes, 242-243
Aqua Gem E, 889-890
AquaMEPHYTON, 890-891
Aquasol A, 886-887
Aquasol E, 889-890
Aquatensen, 782-783
Aquazide H, 590-591
Aqueous CharcoAid, 241-242
Aqwesine, 590-591
Aramine, 760-761
Aranesp, 328-329
Arava, 677-678
Arcet, 167-169
Aredia, 932-934
Arestin, 808-809
argatroban, 88-89
Aricept, 391-393
Aricept ODT, 391-393
Arimidex, 83-84
aripiprazole, 89-91
Aristocort, 1259-1261
Aristocort Forte, 1259-1261
Aristospan, 1260-1261
Aristospan Injection, 1259-1261
Arixtra, 534-535
Armour Thyroid, 1209-1210
Aromatic Cascara Fluid extract, 201-202
Artane, 1269-1271
Arthotec, 356-358
Arthritis Foundation Pain Reliever, 608-610
Arthritis Pain Formula, 9-10
Arthrotec, 813-814
Asacol, 754-755

Ascomp with Codeine No.3, 167-169
ascorbic acid, 91-92
Ascorbicap, 91-92
Ascor L 500, 91-92
Ascriptin, 93-94
Asendin, 67-69
Asmanex Twisthaler, 819-820
A-Spas S/L, 605-607
Aspergum, 93-94
aspirin/acetylsalicylic acid/ASA, 93-94
Aspirin Free Pain Relief, 9-10
Astelin (nasal), 110-112
AsthmaHaler Mist, 435-437
Asthma-Nefrin, 435-437
Astramorph PF, 824-827
Atacand, 182-184
Atamet, 193-195
Atarax, 603-605
atazanavir sulfate, 94-96
atenolol, 96-98
Ativan, 716-718
atomoxetine hydrochloride, 98-99
atorvastatin calcium, 100-101
atovaquone, 101-102
Atretol, 188-190
Atridox, 403-404
AtroPen Autoinjector, 102-104
Atropine Care, 102-104
atropine sulfate, 102-104
atropine sulfate; diphenoxylate
  hydrochloride, 104-105
Atropisol, 102-104
Atrosulf-1, 102-104
Atrovent, 642-643
Atrovent Nasal, 642-643
A/T/S, Akne-Mycin, EES, Emgel, E-Mycin,
  Eryc, Erycette, EryDerm, Erygel, EryPed,
  Erymax, Ery-Tab, Erythra-Derm, Erythrocin,
  PCE Dispertab, Romycin, Roymicin,
  Staticin, Theramycin, Theramycin Z, T-Stat,
  451-453
A200 Lice, 964-965
Augmentin, 70-71
Augmentin ES-600, 70-71
Augmentin XR, 70-71
Auralgan, 127-129
auranofin/aurothioglucose, 105-107
Auro Ear Drops, 191
aurothioglucose/gold sodium thiomalate,
  107-108
Auroto, 127-129
Avage, 1174-1175
Avalide, 590-591, 643-645
Avandamet, 763-765, 1104-1106
Avandia, 1104-1106
Avapro, 643-645
Avelox, 827-828
Avelox IV, 827-828
Aventyl, 884-886
Avinza, 824-827

---

bivalirudin, 148-149
Blephamide, 1157-1158
Bleph-10, 1157-1158
Blocadren, 1216-1219
Bluboro, 43-45
Bonine, 734-735
Boniva, 607-608
Bontril PDM, 969-970
Bontril Slow-Release, 969-970
Borofair, 14-15
bosentan, 149-150
B & O Suppositories, 906-907
B & O Supprettes 15-A, 123-124
B & O Supprettes 16-A, 123-124
Breonesin, 577-578
Brethine, 1186-1187
bretylium tosylate, 150-151
Bretylium Tosylate-Dextrose, 150-151
Brevibloc, 455-456
brimonidine tartrate, 152
brinzolamide, 153
Bromadine-DM, 156-158
Bromarest DX, 156-158
Bromatane DX, 156-158
Bromfed, 156-158, 1052-1054
Bromfed DM, 156-158
bromfenac, 154
bromocriptine mesylate, 155-156
Bromophen T.D., 978-980
Bromphen DX, 156-158
brompheniramine maleate, 156-158
Broncholate, 433-435
Bronkometer, 649-650
Bronkosol, 649-650
BröveX, 156-158
BröveX CT, 156-158
budesonide, 158-159
Bufferin, 93-94
bumetanide, 160-161
Bumex, 160-161
Buprenex, 161-162
buprenorphine, 161-162
bupropion hydrochloride, 163-164
BuSpar, 165-166
BuSpar Dividose, 165-166
buspirone hydrochloride, 165-166
Butacet, 167-169
butalbital compound, 167-169
Butalbital Compound with Codeine, 167-169
Butalgen, 167-169
butenafine hydrochloride, 169-170
Butibel, 121-123
Butinal with Codeine No.3, 167-169
butoconazole nitrate, 170-171
butorphanol tartrate, 171-172
Bydramine Cough, 379-381
Byetta, 481

C

cabergoline, 173-174
Caduet, 63-64, 100-101
Cafergot, 447-448
Caffedrine, 175-176
caffeine, 175-176
Caladryl, 379-381
Calan, 1303-1305
Calan SR, 1303-1305
Cal-Carb Forte, 180-182
Calcibind, 233-234
Calci-Chew, 180-182
Calciferol, 887-889
Calcijex, 178-179
Calcimar, 177-178
Calci-Mix, 180-182
Calcione, 180-182
calcipotriene, 176-177
Calciquid, 180-182
calcitonin, 177-178
Cal-Citrate, 180-182
calcitriol, 178-179
calcium acetate/calcium carbonate/calcium
    chloride/calcium citrate/calcium
    glubionate/calcium gluconate, 180-182
Calcium acetate: PhosLo, 180-182
Calcium carbonate: Amitone, 180-182
Calcium citrate: Citracal, 180-182
Calcium Disodium Versenate, 414-415
Calcium glubionate, 180-182
Caldecort, 593-595
Caldesene Medicated Powder, 1282-1283
Caltrate, 180-182
Caltrate 600, 180-182
Cam-ap-es, 590-591
Campral, 4-5
Canasa, 754-755
candesartan cilexetil, 182-184
Capastat, 184-185
Capex, 510-511
Capital, 300-301
Capitrol, 249-250
Capoten, 186-188
Capozide, 186-188, 590-591
capreomycin sulfate, 184-185
capsaicin, 185-186
captopril, 186-188
Carafate, 1154-1155
Carbacot, 773-775
carbamazepine, 188-190
carbamide peroxide, 191
Carbatrol, 188-190
carbenicillin, 952-953
carbenicillin indanyl sodium, 192-193
carbidopa; levodopa, 193-195
Cardene, 864-866
Cardene IV, 864-866
Cardene SR, 864-866
Cardizem, 374-376

Entries can be identified as follows: generic name, Trade name.

Dioptrol, 1006-1007
Diovan, 1295-1296
Diovan HCT, 590-591, 1295-1296
Dipentum, 899-900
Diphedryl, 379-381
Diphen, 379-381
Diphen Cough, 379-381
Diphenhist, 379-381
diphenhydramine hydrochloride, 379-381
dipivefrin hydrochloride, 381-382
Diprolene, 134-136
dipyridamole, 382-383
dirithromycin, 383-384
Disalcid, 1111-1112
disopyramide phosphate, 385-386
Disotate, 416-417
DisperMox, 69-70
Ditropan, 922-924
Ditropan XL, 922-924
Diucardin, 595-597
Diupres, 247-249
Diuril, 247-249
Diuril Sodium, 247-249
Diutensen-R, 782-783
divalproex sodium, 1292-1294
Dizac, 353-355
Doan's Original, 725-727
dobutamine hydrochloride, 386-387
docusate, 388-389
dofetilide, 389-390
DOK, 388-389
dolasetron mesylate, 390-391
Dolmar, 167-169
Dolobid, 366-368
Dolophine, 767-768
Domeboro, 43-45
donepezil hydrochloride, 391-393
Donnamar, 605-607
Donnapine, 121-123
Donnatal, 121-123, 972-974
Donnatal Extentabs, 121-123
dopamine hydrochloride, 393-394
Dopar, 690-691
Dopram, 396-397
Doral, 1062-1064
Dorcol Children's Cold Formula Liquid,
    250-251
Dormarex 2, 379-381
Doryx, 403-404
dorzolamide hydrochloride; timolol maleate,
    395
DOSS DSS, 388-389
Dostinex, 173-174
Dovonex, 176-177
doxapram hydrochloride, 396-397
doxazosin mesylate, 397-399
doxepin hydrochloride, 399-401
doxercalciferol, 401-403
Doxidan, 388-389
Doxine, 1059-1060

Doxy Caps, 403-404
Doxychel Hyclate, 403-404
doxycycline, 403-404
Doxy-100, 403-404
Dramamine, 376-377
Drisdol, 887-889
Dristan Cold, 1052-1054
Dristan Nasal, 981-982
Dristan Sinus, 1052-1054
Drithocreme, 84-85
Dritho-Scalp, 84-85
Drituss G, 577-578
Drixoral, 156-158
Drixoral Cold and Allergy, 1052-1054
Drixoral Cold & Flu, 9-10
dronabinol, 404-406
droperidol, 406-408
Drotic, 593-595
drotrecogin alfa, 408-409
Dr. Scholl's Callus Remover, 1108-1109
Dr. Scholl's Clear Away, 1108-1109
Drysol, 42-43
D-Tal, 121-123
Ducosoft-S, 388-389
Dulcolax, 142-143
Dull-C, 91-92
duloxetine hydrochloride, 410-411
DuoFilm, 1108-1109
Duo-Medihaler, 652-653
DuoPlant, 1108-1109
Durabolin, 844-845
Duraclon, 288-290
Duramorph PF, 824-827
Duranest with Epinephrine, 435-437
Duratuss G, 577-578
Duricef, 204-206
Duvoid, 138-139
Dyazide, 590-591, 1262-1263
Dycil, 358-359
Dynabac, 383-384
Dynabac D5-Pak, 383-384
Dynacin, 808-809
DynaCirc, 655-657
DynaCirc CR, 655-657
dyphylline, 412-413
Dyrenium, 1262-1263

E

EC-Naprosyn, 845-848
econazole nitrate, 413-414
Ecotrin, 93-94
Ecotrin Maximum Strength, 93-94
Ed A-Hist, 978-980
edetate calcium disodium (calcium EDTA),
    414-415
edetate disodium, 416-417
Edex, 39-40
Ed K+10, 1009-1011

Entries can be identified as follows: generic name, Trade name.

edrophonium chloride, 417-418
efalizumab, 418-419
efavirenz, 420-421
Effer K, 1009-1011
Effexor, 1301-1303
Effexor XR, 1301-1303
Efidac Genaphed, 1052-1054
eflornithine, 421-422
E-Gems, 889-890
8-Hour Bayer Extended Release, 93-94
8-MOP, 777-778
Elavil, 60-62
Eldepryl, 1118-1120
Eldopaque, 599-600
Eldopaque Forte, 599-600
Eldoquin, 599-600
eletriptan, 422-424
Elidel, 990-991
Eligard, 682-684
Elimite, 964-965
Elixophyllin, 54-56
Elixophyllin, 1198-1200
Elixophylline KI, 1198-1200
Elixophyllin-GG, 1198-1200
ElixSure Cough, 352-353
Elmiron, 959-960
Elocon, 819-820
Eloxatin, 911-913
Emcort, 593-595
Emend, 86-87
Emend 3-Day, 86-87
Emetrol, 986-987
EMLA, 696-698
Empirin, 93-94
Empirin no. 3, 300-301
Empirin no. 4, 300-301
emtricitabine, 424-425
Emtriva, 424-425
Emulsoil, 202-203
Enablex, 329-330
enalapril maleate, 425-427
Enalaprilat, 425-427
Enalaprit Novaplus, 425-427
Enbrel, 470-471
Endocet, 924-926
Endodan, 924-926
Endolor, 167-169
Endrate, 416-417
Enduron, 782-783
Enerjets, 175-176
enfuvirtide, 427-429
Enjuvia, 462-464, 1165
Enlon, 417-418
Enlon-Plus, 417-418
enoxaparin sodium, 429-430
entacapone, 431-432
Entaprin, 93-94
entecavir, 432-433
Entex LA, 577-578
Entocort EC, 158-159

Enulose, 669-670
Enzone, 1014-1015
ephedrine, 433-435
Ephex SR, 433-435
Epifoam, 1014-1015
Epifrin, 435-437
E-Pilo Ophthalmic, 435-437
E-Pilo-6, 988-990
Epimide 50, 1285-1286
epinephrine, 435-437
EpiPen, 435-437
EpiPen Auto Injector, 435-437
EpiPen 2-Pak, 435-437
EpiQuin Micro, 599-600
Epitol, 188-190
Epivir, 670-671
Epivir-HBV, 670-671
eplerenone, 437-438
epoetin alfa, 438-440
Epogen, 438-440
epoprostenol sodium, prostacyclin, 440-442
eprosartan mesylate, 442-443
eptifibatide, 444-445
Epzicom, 1-2, 670-671
Equetro, 188-190
Ercaf, 447-448
ergoloid mesylates, 445-447
Ergomar, 447-448
ergotamine tartrate/dihydroergotamine,
   447-448
Eridium, 968-969
erlotinib, 449
E•R•O Ear, 191
ertapenem, 450-451
erythromycin, 451-453
escitalopram oxalate, 453-455
Esclim, 460-462
Esgic, 9-10, 167-169
Esgic-Plus, 167-169
Esidrix, 590-591
Esidrix-K, 590-591
Esimil, 590-591
Eskalith, 704-707
esmolol hydrochloride, 455-456
esomeprazole, 457-458
Esoterica Regular, 599-600
estazolam, 458-459
Estinyl, 473-474
Estrace, 460-462
Estraderm, 460-462
estradiol, 460-462
Estragyn 5, 466-467
Estrasorb, 460-462
Estratab, 464-465
Estratest, 464-465
Estring, 460-462
Estro-A, 466-467
EstroGel, 460-462
Estrogenic, 466-467
Estrogens, 466-467

Entries can be identified as follows: generic name, Trade name.

Entries can be identified as follows: generic name, Trade name.

kanamycin sulfate, 660-661
Kantrex, 660-661
Kaochlor, 1009-1011
Kaon, 1009-1011
Kaon-Cl, 1009-1011
Kaon-Cl 10, 1009-1011
Kaon-Cl 20%, 1009-1011
Kaopectate, 143-144
Kato, 1009-1011
Kay Ciel, 1009-1011
Kayexalate, 1138-1139
K+Care, 1009-1011
KCl-20, 1009-1011
KCl-40, 1009-1011
K-Dur, 1009-1011
K-Dur 10, 1009-1011
K-Dur 20, 1009-1011
Keep Alert, 175-176
Keflex, 235-236
Keftab, 235-236
Kefurox (as sodium), 230-231
Kefzol, 207-208
Kemadrin, 1035-1036
Kenalog, 1259-1261
Kenalog-10, 1259-1261
Kenalog-40, 1259-1261
Kenalog in Orabase, 1259-1261
Ken-Jec 40, 1259-1261
Kepivance, 930-931
Keppra, 684-685
Keralyt, 1108-1109
Kerlone, 136-138
Kerr Insta-Char, 241-242
Kestrone 5, 466-467
Ketek, 1176-1177
Ketek Pak, 1176-1177
ketoconazole, 661-663
ketoprofen, 663-665
ketorolac tromethamine, 665-667
Key-E, 889-890
Key-E Kaps, 889-890
Keygesic-10, 725-727
Key-Pred, 1020-1022
Key-Pred SP, 1020-1022
Kineret, 82-83
Kionex, 1138-1139
Klaron, 1157-1158
Klonopin, 286-288
Klonopin Wafer, 286-288
K-Lor, 1009-1011
Klor-Con, 1009-1011
Klor-Con EF, 1009-1011
Klor-Con 8, 1009-1011
Klor-Con M15, 1009-1011
Klor-Con M20, 1009-1011
K-Lor-Con M 15, 1009-1011
Klor-Con M10, 1009-1011
Klor-Con 10, 1009-1011
Klor-Con/25, 1009-1011
Klotrix, 1009-1011

K-Lyte, 1009-1011
K-Lyte DS, 1009-1011
K-Norm, 1009-1011
Kondon's Nasal, 433-435
Konsyl, 1054-1055
Kristalose, 669-670
K-Sol, 1009-1011
K-Tab, 1009-1011
Kutrase, 934-936
Ku-Zyme, 934-936
Ku-Zyme, 934-936
Ku-Zyme HP, 934-936
Kytril, 574-575

L

labetalol hydrochloride, 667-668
Lac-Hydrin, 64-65
Lac-Hydrin Five, 64-65
Lac-Lotion, 64-65
Lacticare-HC, 593-595
lactulose, 669-670
Lamictal, 672-674
Lamictal CD, 672-674
Lamisil, 1184-1186
Lamisil AT, 1184-1186
lamivudine, 670-671
lamotrigine, 672-674
Lamprene, 282-283
Lanabiotic, 1006-1007
Lanacane, 127-129
Lanacort-5, 593-595
Lanaphilic, 1285-1286
Laniroif, 167-169
Lanorinal, 167-169
Lanoxicaps, 368-369
Lanoxin, 368-369
lansoprazole, 674-675
Lariam, 741-742
Larodopa, 690-691
Lasix, 546-547
latanoprost, 676-677
LA-12, 311-312
leflunomide, 677-678
Lente: Humulin L, 629-631
Lente Iletin II, 629-631
lepirudin, 678-679
Lescol, 527-528
Lescol XL, 527-528
letrozole, 679-680
leucovorin calcium (folinic acid, citrovorum factor), 681-682
leuprolide acetate, 682-684
Levaquin, 692-694
Levaquin Leva-Pak, 692-694
Levatol, 947-949
Levbid, 605-607
Levemir, 628
levetiracetam, 684-685

Entries can be identified as follows: generic name, Trade name.

methamphetamine hydrochloride, 768-769
methazolamide, 770-771
methenamine, 771-772
methicillin, 952-953
methimazole, 772-773
methocarbamol, 773-775
methotrexate sodium, 775-777
methoxsalen, 777-778
methscopolamine bromide, 779-780
methsuximide, 780-781
methyclothiazide, 782-783
methylcellulose, 783-784
Methylcotol, 789-790
Methylcotolone, 789-790
methyldopa, 784-786
Methyldopate, 784-786
methylene blue, 786-787
Methylin, 787-788
Methylin ER, 787-788
methylphenidate hydrochloride, 787-788
Methylpred DP, 789-790
methylprednisolone/methylprednisolone
   acetate/methylprednisolone sodium
   succinate, 789-790
methyltestosterone, 791-792
Meticorten, 1022-1024
metoclopramide hydrochloride, 792-794
metolazone, 794-795
metoprolol tartrate, 796-797
MetroCream, 798-800
MetroGel, 798-800
MetroGel-Vaginal, 798-800
Metro I.V., 798-800
MetroLotion, 798-800
metronidazole, 798-800
Metronidazole Benzoate, 798-800
metyrosine, 800-801
Mevacor, 720-721
mexiletine hydrochloride, 801-802
Mexitil, 801-802
mezlocillin, 952-953
Mg Trisilicate Gastrocote, 1134-1135
MG217 Sal-Acid, 1108-1109
Miacalcin, 177-178
Miacalcin Nasal, 177-178
Micanol, 84-85
Micardis, 1178-1179
Micatin, 802-804
miconazole, 802-804
Micro-K, 1009-1011
Micro-K 10, 1009-1011
Micronase, 567-569
microNefrin, 435-437
Microzide, 590-591
Midamor, 51-53
midazolam hydrochloride, 804-805
Midchlor, 9-10
midodrine hydrochloride, 806-807
Midol PMS, 9-10
Midrin, 9-10, 11-12

Migranal, 371-372, 447-448
Migratine, 11-12
Migrin-A, 11-12
milrinone lactate, 807-808
Miltown, 751-752
Minipress, 1018-1020
Minirin, 340-341
Minitran, 876-878
Minizide, 1007-1009, 1018-1020
Minocin, 808-809
minocycline hydrochloride, 808-809
minoxidil, 810-811
Mintezol, 1201-1202
Mirapex, 1012-1014
mirtazapine, 811-813
misoprostol, 813-814
Mithracin, 1002-1003
Mitran, 245-247
Moban, 817-819
Mobic, 743-745
Mobidin, 725-727
modafinil, 814-815
Modane, 142-143
Modane Soft, 388-389
Moduretic, 51-53, 590-591
moexipril hydrochloride, 816-817
molindone hydrochloride, 817-819
Mollifene Ear Wax Removing, 191
Momentum, 725-727
mometasone furoate monohydrate, 819-820
Monistat-Derm, 802-804
Monistat-1, 1222-1223
Monistat-7, 802-804
Monistat-3, 802-804
monobenzone, 821
Monodox, 403-404
Mono-Gesic, 1111-1112
Monoket, 654-655
Monopril, 541-543
montelukast sodium, 822-823
Monurol, 540-541
moricizine hydrochloride, 823-824
morphine sulfate, 824-827
Mosco Corn and Callus Remover, 1108-1109
Motion-Aid, 376-377
Motrin, 608-610
Motrin IB, 608-610
Motrin IB Sinus, 608-610
moxifloxacin hydrochloride, 827-828
Moxilin, 69-70
M-Oxy, 924-926
MS Contin, 824-827
MSIR, 824-827
MS/S, 824-827
Mucinex, 577-578
Mucobid-L.A., 577-578
Muco-Fen, 577-578
Muco-Fen 800, 577-578
Muco-Fen 1200, 577-578
Mucomyst, 15-16

mupirocin, 829-830
Murine Ear Drops, 191
Muro 128, 1135-1137
Muse, 39-40
Myambutol, 472-473
Mycasone, 891-893
Mycelex, 294-295
Mycelex OTC, 294-295
Mycelex-3 2%, 170-171
Myciguent, 857-858
Mycinettes, 127-129
Mycitracin, 857-858
Myco Biotic II, 891-893
Mycobutin, 1085-1087
Mycogen II, 891-893
Mycolog-II, 891-893
Mycomer, 891-893
mycophenolate mofetil, 830-831
Mycostatin, 891-893
Mycostatin Pastilles, 891-893
Mycostatin Topical, 891-893
Myco-Triacet II, 891-893
Myfortic, 830-831
Mykrox (rapid acting), 794-795
Mylanta, 180-182
Mylanta AR, 484-486
Mylanta Extra Strength Liquid, 43-45
Mylanta Gas, 1130-1131
Mylanta Gelisil, 1130-1131
Mylanta Liquid, 43-45
My-O-Den, 22-23
Myphetane DX, 156-158
Myrac, 808-809
Mysoline, 1025-1027
Mytelase, 47-48
Mytrex, 891-893
Mytussin, 577-578

N

nabumetone, 832-833
nadolol, 834-835
Nafcil, 836-837
nafcillin, 952-953
nafcillin sodium, 836-837
naftifine hydrochloride, 837-838
Naftin, 837-838
nalbuphine hydrochloride, 838-839
Naldecon, 978-980
Naldecon Senior EX, 577-578
Nalfon, 491-492
Nalgest, 978-980
Nallpen, 836-837
nalmefene hydrochloride, 840-841
naloxone hydrochloride, 841-842
naltrexone hydrochloride, 842-844
Namenda, 745-747
nandrolone decanoate, 844-845
NapraPAC, 674-675, 845-848

Naprelan, 845-848
Naprelan 375, 845-848
Naprelan 500 , 845-848
naproxen, 845-848
naproxen/naproxen sodium, 845-848
naproxen sodium, 845-848
Naquival, 1081-1082
naratriptan hydrochloride, 848-849
Narcan, 841-842
Nardil, 970-972
Nasahist B, 156-158
Nasal, 981-982
Nasalcrom, 308-309
Nasalide, 509-510
Nasal Mist, 1135-1137
Nasal Moist, 1135-1137
Nasarel, 509-510
Nascobal, 311-312
Nasonex, 819-820
Natacyn, 849-850
natamycin, 849-850
nateglinide, 850-852
Natrecor, 860-861
Nature's Remedy, 388-389
Nature-Throid NT, 1209-1210
Navane, 1206-1208
Navogan, 1271-1272
ND Stat, 156-158
Nebcin, 1230-1232
NebuPent, 954-955
nedocromil sodium, 852-853
nefazodone hydrochloride, 853-855
nelfinavir mesylate, 855-856
Nembutal, 957-958
NeoCeuticals Acne Spot Treatment, 1108-1109
NeoDecadron, 344-346
Neo-Fradin, 857-858
Neofrin; Neo-Synephrine Ophthalmic;
    Ocu-Phrin; Phenoptic; Rectasol, 978-980
neomycin sulfate, 857-858
Neopap, 9-10
Neoral, 317-319
Neo-Rx, 857-858
Neosar, 314-315
Neosol, 605-607
Neosporin, 115-116, 857-858, 1006-1007
Neosporin G.U. irrigant, 857-858
neostigmine bromide, 858-859
NeoStrata AHA, 599-600
Neostrata HQ, 599-600
Neo-Tab, 857-858
Neotricin HC—ophthalmic, 593-595
Nephro-Calci, 180-182
Nephro-Fer, 495-496
Nephron, 435-437
Neptazane, 770-771
nesiritide, 860-861
Nestrex, 1059-1060
Neulasta, 944-945
Neuroforte-R, 311-312

Entries can be identified as follows: generic name, Trade name.

Ocu-Carpine, 988-990
Ocu-Chlor, 244-245
Ocuclear, 926-927
Ocufen (ophthalmic), 522-523
Ocuflox, 895-896
Ocu-Mycin, 558-560
Ocupress, 197-199
Ocusert, 988-990
Ocusulf-10, 1157-1158
Ocu-Tracin, 115-116
Ocutricin, 1006-1007
Ocu-Tropine, 102-104
ofloxacin, 895-896
Ogen, 467-469
olanzapine, 897-899
olsalazine sodium, 899-900
Olux, 280-281
Omacor, 902-903
omalizumab, 900-902
Omedia, 127-129
omega-3-acid ethyl esters, 902-903
omeprazole, 903-904
Omnicef, 209-210
Omnipen, 75-76
Omnipen-N, 75-76
ondansetron hydrochloride, 905-906
Ophthacet, 1157-1158
Ophthalmic, 981-982
Ophth: Isopto Hyoscine, 1114-1116
opium tincture, 906-907
Opthocort, 244-245
Opticaine, 1192-1193
Opticrom, 308-309
Optivar (ophthalmic), 110-112
Orabase-B, 127-129
Orabase HCA, 593-595
Orajel, 127-129
Orajel Maximum Strength, 127-129
Orajel Perioseptic, 191
Oral: Scopace, 1114-1116
Oramorph SR, 824-827
Orap, 991-993
Orapred, 1020-1022
Orasol, 127-129
Orazinc, 1320-1321
Oretic, 590-591
Oreton Methyl, 791-792
Organidin NR, 577-578
Organ-1 NR, 577-578
Orinase, 1235-1237
Orinase Diagnositic, 1235-1237
orlistat, 908-909
Ornade, 250-251
Ortho-Est, 467-469
Orudis KT, 663-665
Oruvail, 663-665
Os-Cal-D, 180-182
Os-Cal 500, 180-182
oseltamivir phosphate, 909-910
Osmitrol, 727-728

Osmoglyn, 569-571
Otic Domeboro, 43-45
Otocain, 127-129
Otocort—otic, 593-595
Otricaine, 127-129
Otrivin Measured-Dose Pump with
   Moisturizers, 1309-1310
Otrivin Nasal Drops, 1309-1310
Otrivin Nasal Spray, 1309-1310
Otrivin Nasal Spray with Eucalyptol,
   1309-1310
Otrivin Nasal Spray with Moisturizers,
   1309-1310
Otrivin with Measured-Dose Pump, 1309-1310
Ovace, 1157-1158
oxacillin, 952-953
oxacillin sodium, 910-911
oxaliplatin, 911-913
Oxandrin, 913-914
oxandrolone, 913-914
oxaprozin, 914-916
oxazepam, 916-918
oxcarbazepine, 918-920
oxiconazole, 920-921
Oxistat, 920-921
Oxsoralen, 777-778
Oxsoralen-Ultra, 777-778
oxtriphylline, 921-922
Oxy Balance, 1108-1109
Oxy Balance Deep Pore, 1108-1109
oxybutynin, 922-924
oxycodone hydrochloride, 924-926
OxyContin, 924-926
Oxydose, 924-926
OxyFast, 924-926
OxyIR, 924-926
oxymetazoline, 926-927
oxymorphone hydrochloride, 927-929
oxytetracycline hydrochloride, 929-930
Oxytrol, 922-924
Oysco 500, 180-182
Oyst-Cal 500, 180-182
Oyster Calcium, 180-182

P

Pacaps, 167-169
Pacerone, 58-59
palifermin, 930-931
Palmer's Skin Success Acne Cleanser,
   1108-1109
Palmer's Skin Success Fade Cream, 599-600
Palmitate A, 886-887
palonosetron hydrochloride, 931-932
Pamelor, 884-886
pamidronate disodium, 932-934
Pamidronate Disodium Novaplus, 932-934
Pamine, 779-780
Pamprin, 9-10, 845-848

Entries can be identified as follows: generic name, Trade name.

Panadol, 9-10
Panase, 934-936
Pancrease, 934-936
Pancrease MT 20, 934-936
Pancrease MT 4, 934-936
Pancreatic EC, 934-936
Pancreatil-UL 12, 934-936
pancreatin, 934-936
Pancreatin, 934-936
pancreatin/pancrelipase, 934-936
Pancrecarb MS-4, 934-936
Pancrecarb MS-8, 934-936
pancrelipase, 934-936
Pandel, 593-595
Pangestyme CN 10, 934-936
Pangestyme CN 20, 934-936
Pangestyme EC, 934-936
Pangestyme MT 16, 934-936
Pangestyme NL 18, 934-936
Panmycin, 1194-1195
Panokase, 934-936
pantoprazole sodium, 936-937
Parafon Forte DSC, Remular, Remular-S,
    257-258
Parcopa, 193-195
paregoric, 937-938
paricalcitol, 938-940
Parlodel, 155-156
Parnate, 1252-1254
paromomycin sulfate, 940-941
paroxetine hydrochloride, 941-943
Paser, 56-57
Pathocil, 358-359
Paxeva, 941-943
Paxil, 941-943
Paxil CR, 941-943
Pedi-Boro, 43-45
Pedisilk, 1107-1109
pegaptanib sodium, 943-944
Pegasys, 945-947
pegfilgrastim, 944-945
peginterferon alfa-2a, 945-947
penbutolol sulfate, 947-949
penciclovir, 949-950
Penecort, 593-595
penicillamine, 950-951
penicillin, 952-953
Penicillin G, 952-953
penicillin G benzathine, 952-953
penicillin G potassium, 952-953
penicillin V potassium, 952-953
Penlac, 262-263
pentamidine isethionate, 954-955
Pentam 300, 954-955
Pentasa, 754-755
Pentazine, 1038-1040
pentazocine lactate, 955-956
Pentids, 952-953
pentobarbital sodium, 957-958
Pentopak, 960-961

pentosan polysulfate sodium, 959-960
pentoxifylline, 960-961
Pentoxil, 960-961
Pen-V, 952-953
Pen-Vee K, 952-953
Pep-Back, 175-176
Pepcid, 484-486
Pepcid AC, 484-486
Pepcid Complete, 484-486
Pepcid RPD, 484-486
Pepto-Bismol, 143-144
Percocet, 9-10, 924-926
Percodan, 93-94, 924-926
Percolone, 924-926
Perdiem, 1054-1055
pergolide mesylate, 961-963
Periactin, 319-320
Peri-Colace, 388-389
perindopril erbumine, 963-964
Periostat, 403-404
Permapen, 952-953
Permax, 961-963
permethrin, 964-965
Permitil, 516-518
perphenazine, 966-967
Persantine, 382-383
Pfizerpen, 952-953
Pharmagesic, 167-169
Phazyme, 1130-1131
Phenadoz, 1038-1040
Phenaphen, 300-301
Phenaphen No. 2,3,4, 9-10
phenazopyridine hydrochloride, 968-969
Phendiet, 969-970
Phendiet-105, 969-970
phendimetrazine tartrate, 969-970
Phendry, 379-381
phenelzine sulfate, 970-972
Phenerbel-S, 121-123
Phenergan, 1038-1040
Phenergan with Codeine Syrup, 1038-1040
Phenergan with Dextromethorphan Syrup,
    1038-1040
phenobarbital, 972-974
Phenoject-50, 1038-1040
phenoxybenzamine hydrochloride, 974-975
Phenoxy-methyl Penicillin, 952-953
Phentercot, 976-977
phentermine hydrochloride, 976-977
phentolamine mesylate, 977-978
phenylephrine (systemic), 978-980
phenylephrine (topical), 981-982
phenytoin/fosphenytoin, 983-985
phosphorated carbohydrate solution, 986-987
Phrenilin, 9-10, 167-169
Phrenilin Forte, 167-169
Phyllocontin, 54-56
physostigmine, 987-988
Pilagan with C Cap, 988-990
Pilocar, 988-990

pilocarpine hydrochloride, 988-990
Pilopine-HS, 988-990
Piloptic-1, 988-990
Piloptic-1/2, 988-990
Piloptic-2, 988-990
Piloptic-3, 988-990
Piloptic-4, 988-990
Piloptic-6, 988-990
Piloptic-HS, 988-990
Pilostat, 988-990
pimecrolimus, 990-991
pimozide, 991-993
pindolol, 993-994
Pink Bismuth, 143-144
Pin-Rid, 1055-1056
Pin-X, 1055-1056
pioglitazone hydrochloride, 995-996
piperacillin, 952-953
piperacillin sodium/tazobactam sodium,
    952-953, 997-998
Pipracil, 997-998
pirbuterol acetate, 998-999
piroxicam, 1000-1001
Pitressin, 1299-1300
pivampicillin, 952-953
pivmecillinam, 952-953
Plaquenil, 600-602
Plaretase, 934-936
Plavix, 290-291
Plegine, 969-970
Plendil, 486-488
Pletal, 265-266
plicamycin, 1002-1003
PMB, 462-464
PMS-Tobramycin, 1230-1232
Pneumomist, 577-578
Podocon-25, Pododerm, 1004-1005
podofilox, 1003-1004
podophyllum resin, 1004-1005
Polaramine, 346-348
Polaramine Expectorant, 347-348
Polaramine Repetabs, 346-348
Polycillin, 75-76
Polycillin-N, 75-76
Polycillin PRB, 75-76
Polycillin-PRB, 1027-1028
Polymox, 69-70
polymyxin B sulfate, 1006-1007
Poly-Pred, 1006-1007
Polysporin, 115-116, 1006-1007
Polysporin Burn Formula, 1006-1007
polythiazide, 1007-1009
Polytrim, 1006-1007
Polytrim Ophthalmic, 1273-1274
Ponstel, 739-741
Pontocaine, 1192-1193
potassium acetate/potassium
    bicarbonate-citrate/potassium
    chloride/potassium gluconate, 1009-1011
potassium bicarbonate-citrate, 1009-1011

potassium chloride, 1009-1011
potassium gluconate, 1009-1011
pralidoxime chloride, 1011-1012
pramipexole dihydrochloride, 1012-1014
Pramosome, 1014-1015
pramoxine hydrochloride, 1014-1015
Prandin, 1079-1081
Pravachol, 1016-1017
pravastatin sodium, 1016-1017
Prax, 1014-1015
praziquantel, 1017-1018
prazosin hydrochloride, 1018-1020
Precose, 5-7
Predacort 50, 1020-1022
Predaject-50, 1020-1022
Predate-50, 1020-1022
Pred Forte, 1020-1022
Pred-G, 558-560
Pred-Ject-50, 1020-1022
Pred Mild, 1020-1022
Prednicen-M, 1022-1024
Prednicot, 1022-1024
prednisolone, 1020-1022
Prednisolone Acetate, 1020-1022
prednisone, 1022-1024
Prednisone Intensol, 1022-1024
Prefrin-A, 981-982
Prehist, 978-980
Prelone, 1020-1022
Prelu-2, 969-970
Premarin, 462-464
Premarin Intravenous, 462-464
Premarin Vaginal, 462-464
Premarin with methyltestosterone, 462-464
Premphase (cycled product), 462-464
Prempro (daily product), 462-464
Preparation H Hydrocortisone, 593-595
Pre-Pen, 132-133
Pretz-D, 433-435
Prevacid, 674-675
Prevacid IV, 674-675
Prevacid Solu-Tab, 674-675
Prevalite, 259-260
Priftin, 1088-1089
Prilosec, 903-904
Prilosec OTC, 903-904
Primacor, 807-808
Primacor I.V., 807-808
Primaquine, 1024-1025
primaquine phosphate, 1024-1025
Primatene Mist, 435-437
Primaxin IM, 615-616
Primaxin IV, 615-616
primidone, 1025-1027
Primsol, 1273-1274
Principen, 75-76
Prinivil, 702-704
Prinzide, 590-591, 702-704
ProAmatine, 806-807
Probalan, 1027-1028

Entries can be identified as follows: generic name, Trade name.

R

rabeprazole sodium, 1073-1074
raloxifene hydrochloride, 1074-1075
ramipril, 1075-1077
ranitidine hydrochloride/ranitidine bismuth
  citrate, 1077-1079
Rapamune, 1132-1133
Rapid-Acting: Insulin Lispro (Humalog),
  629-631
Rapiflux, 513-515
Rapi-Ject, 824-827
Raptiva, 418-419
Razadyne, 550-551
Razadyne ER, 550-551
Rebetron, 1084-1085
Rebetron Combination Therapy, 631-634
Rebif, 636-638
Rectasol-HC, 593-595
Rectocort, 1014-1015
Rederm, 593-595
Reese's Pinworm, 1055-1056
Refludan, 678-679
Regitine, 977-978
Reglan, 792-794
Regranex, 118-119
Regreton, 1081-1082
Regroton, 256-257
Regular Iletin II, 629-631
Regular Short-Acting: Humulin R, 629-631
Regulax SS, 388-389
Relafen, 832-833
Relagard, 14-15
Relenza, 1316-1317
Relpax, 422-424
Remeron, 811-813
Remeron Soltab, 811-813
Remicade, 626-627
Remodulin, 1257-1258
Renagel, 1123-1124
Reneese, 1081-1082
Renese, 1007-1009
Renese-R, 1007-1009
Renova, 1258-1259
ReoPro, 2-4
repaglinide, 1079-1081
Repan, 167-169
Reposans-10, 245-247
Requip, 1102-1104
Resaid S.R., 250-251
Rescriptor, 332-333
Rescula, 1284
Resectisol, 727-728
reserpine, 1081-1082
Respa-GF, 577-578
Restasis, 317-319
Restoril, 1179-1181
Retavase, 1083-1084
reteplase, recombinant, 1083-1084
Retin-A, 1258-1259

Retin-A Micro, 1258-1259
Retre-Gel, 127-129
Retrovir, 1317-1319
Revatio, 1126-1127
Reversol, 417-418
Revex, 840-841
ReVia, 842-844
Reyataz, 94-96
Rheumatrex, 775-777
Rhinatate, 978-980
Rhinocort, 158-159
Rhinocort Aqua, 158-159
ribavirin, 1084-1085
RID, 964-965
Ridaura, 105-107
rifabutin, 1085-1087
Rifadin, 1087-1088
Rifadin IV, 1087-1088
Rifamate, 650-652
rifampin, 1087-1088
rifapentine, 1088-1089
Rifater, 650-652
rifaximin, 1089-1090
Rilutek, 1091-1092
riluzole, 1091-1092
Rimactane, 1087-1088
rimantadine hydrochloride, 1092-1093
Riomet, 763-765
Riopan, 724-725
Riopan Plus, 724-725, 1130-1131
risedronate sodium, 1093-1094
Risperdal, 1095-1097
Risperdal Consta, 1095-1097
Risperdal M-Tabs, 1095-1097
risperidone, 1095-1097
Ritalin, 787-788
Ritalin LA, 787-788
Ritalin SR, 787-788
ritonavir, 1097-1099
rivastigmine tartrate, 1099-1100
rizatriptan benzoate, 1101-1102
RMS, 824-827
Robaxin, 773-775
Robaxisal, 773-775
Robinul, 571-573
Robinul Forte, 571-573
Robitussin, 577-578
Robitussin AC, 300-301
Robitussin CoughGels, 352-353
Robitussin DM, 352-353
Robitussin Honey Cough, 352-353
Robitussin Maximum Strength Cough, 352-353
Rocaltrol, 178-179
Rocephin, 228-229
Rocephin IM Convenience Kit, 228-229
Rodex, 1059-1060
Roferon-A (alfa-2a), 631-634
Rogaine, 810-811
Rolaids, 180-182, 1130-1131
Romazicon, 507-508

Rondec, 1052-1054
ropinirole hydrochloride, 1102-1104
rosiglitazone maleate, 1104-1106
rosuvastatin calcium, 1106-1107
Rowasa, 754-755
Roxanol, 824-827
Roxanol-T, 824-827
Roxicet, 9-10, 924-926
Roxicodone, 924-926
Roxicodone Intensol, 924-926
Roxilox, 924-926
Roxiprin, 924-926
Rozex, 798-800
R-Tannamine, 978-980
R-Tannate, 978-980
Rum-K, 1009-1011
Rynatan, 978-980
Rynaton, 250-251
Rythmol, 1040-1042
Rythmol SR, 1040-1042

S

Saizen, 1141-1142
SalAc, 1107-1109
Sal-Acid, 1107-1109
Salactic, 1107-1109
Salagen, 988-990
Salflex, 1111-1112
salicylic acid, 1107-1109
SalineX, 1135-1137
salmeterol xinafoate, 1109-1111
Sal-Plant, 1107-1109
salsalate, 1111-1112
Salsitab, 1111-1112
Sal-Tropine, 102-104
Saluron, 595-597
Salutensin, 595-597, 1081-1082
Salutensin-Demi, 595-597
Sanctura, 1279-1280
Sandimmune, 317-319
Sandostatin, 893-894
Sandostatin LAR Depot, 893-894
Sani-Supp, 569-571
Sanorex, 730-731
saquinavir, 1113-1114
Sarafem, 513-515
Scalp-Aid, 593-595
scopolamine, 1114-1116
Scot-Tussin DM Cough Chasers, 352-353
SeaMist, 1135-1137
secobarbital sodium, 1116-1117
Seconal, 1116-1117
Sectral, 7-8
Sedapap-10, 167-169
see co-trimoxazole monograph, 1273-1274
selegiline hydrochloride, 1118-1120
Senexon, 1120-1121
senna, 1120-1121

Senna-Gen, 1120-1121
Sennatural, 1120-1121
Senokot, 1120-1121
Senokot-S, 388-389
Sensipar, 268-269
Septra, 297-299
Septra DS, 297-299
Ser-A-Gen, 590-591, 1081-1082
Seralazide, 590-591, 1081-1082
Ser-Ap-Es, 588-589, 590-591, 1081-1082
Serax, 916-918
Serentil, 757-758
Serevent, 1109-1111
Serevent Diskus, 1109-1111
Seromycin, 316-317
Seroquel, 1064-1066
Serostim, 1141-1142
Serpalan, 1081-1082
Serpex, 590-591
sertraline hydrochloride, 1121-1123
Serzone, 853-855
Seudotabs, 1052-1054
sevelamer hydrochloride, 1123-1124
sibutramine hydrochloride, 1124-1126
sildenafil citrate, 1126-1127
Silphen DM, 352-353
Silvadene, 1128-1129
silver nitrate, 1127-1128
silver sulfadiazine, 1128-1129
simethicone, 1130-1131
Simply Cough, 352-353
simvastatin, 1131-1132
Sinarest, 9-10
Sine-Aid IB, 608-610
Sinemet, 193-195, 690-691
Sinemet CR, 193-195, 690-691
Sine-Off, 9-10
Sinequan, 399-401
Sinex 12 Hour Long-Acting, 926-927
Singulair, 822-823
sirolimus, 1132-1133
Skelaxin, 761-762
Skelid, 1215-1216
Slo-bid Gyrocaps, 54-56, 1198-1200
Slo-Niacin, 863-864
Slo-Salt, 1135-1137
Slow-Fe, 495-496
sodium bicarbonate, 1134-1135
sodium chloride, 1135-1137
sodium oxybate, 1137-1138
sodium polystyrene sulfonate, 1138-1139
Sodium Sulamyd, 1157-1158
Solaquin, 599-600
Solaquin Forte, 599-600
Solaraze, 356-358
Solarcaine, 127-129, 696-698
Solganal, 105-107
Solganal; Myochrysine, 107-108
solifenacin succinate, 1140-1141
Solu-Cortef, 593-595

Entries can be identified as follows: generic name, Trade name.

Tarka, 1250-1252, 1303-1305
Tasmar, 1237-1239
Tavist Allergy, 275-277
Tavist Allergy/Sinus/Headache Tablets,
275-277
Tavist ND, 714-715
tazarotene, 1174-1175
Tazicef, 223-225
Tazidime, 223-225
Tazorac, 1174-1175
Taztia XT, 374-376
T-Diet, 976-977
Tebamide, 1271-1272
Tecnal, 167-169
Teczem, 374-376, 425-427
tegaserod maleate, 1175-1176
Tegretol, 188-190
Tegretol-XR, 188-190
Tegrin-HC, 593-595
telithromycin, 1176-1177
telmisartan, 1178-1179
temazepam, 1179-1181
Temovate, 280-281
Tempo, 1130-1131
Tencet, 167-169
Tenex, 580-581
tenofovir disoproxil fumarate, 1181-1182
Tenoretic, 96-98, 256-257
Tenormin, 96-98
Tensilon, 417-418
Tenuate, 363-364
Tenuate Dospan, 363-364
Tequin, 553-555
Tequin Teqpaq, 553-555
Terak, 1006-1007
Teramine, 976-977
Terazol 3, 1187-1188
Terazol 7, 1187-1188
terazosin hydrochloride, 1182-1184
terbinafine hydrochloride, 1184-1186
terbutaline sulfate, 1186-1187
terconazole, 1187-1188
Terek, 929-930
teriparatide (rDNA origin), 1188-1189
Terra-Cortril—ophthalmic, 593-595
Terramycin IM, 929-930
Tessalon, 129-130
Tessalon Perles, 129-130
Testim, 1190-1191
Testoderm, 1190-1191
Testoderm TTS, 1190-1191
Testopel, 1190-1191
testosterone, 1190-1191
Testred, 791-792
Testro AQ, 1190-1191
Testro-L.A., 1190-1191
tetracaine hydrochloride, 1192-1193
Tetracon, 1194-1195
tetracycline hydrochloride, 1194-1195
tetrahydrozoline hydrochloride, 1195-1196

Teveten, 442-443
Texacort, 593-595
thalidomide, 1197-1198
Thalitone, 256-257
Thalomid, 1197-1198
Theochron, 54-56, 1198-1200
Theo-Dur, 1198-1200
Theodur, 54-56
Theolair, 54-56, 1198-1200
Theolair SR, 1198-1200
Theolair-SR, 54-56
theophylline, 54-56, 1198-1200
Theo-Time, 1198-1200
Theo-24, 54-56
Thera-Flu Non-Drowsy Formula, 1052-1054
Thermazene, 1128-1129
thiabendazole, 1201-1202
thiamine hydrochloride (vitamin B_1),
1202-1203
thiethylperazine maleate, 1203-1204
Thiola, 1223-1224
thioridazine hydrochloride, 1204-1206
Thioridazine Intensol, 1204-1206
thiothixene, 1206-1208
Thorazine, 252-254
thyroid, 1209-1210
Thyrolar, 695-696, 701-702
tiagabine hydrochloride, 1210-1211
Tiazac, 374-376
ticarcillin disodium/clavulanate potassium,
952-953, 1212-1213
ticarcillin; penicillin and beta-lactamase
inhibitors; amoxicillin/clavulanate
potassium, 952-953
Ticlid, 1213-1214
ticlopidine hydrochloride, 1213-1214
Tigan, 1271-1272
Tigan Adult, 1271-1272
Tija, 929-930
Tikosyn, 389-390
Tilade, 852-853
tiludronate disodium, 1215-1216
Timentin, 1212-1213
Timolide, 590-591
timolol, 1216-1219
Timolol Ophthalmic, 1216-1219
Timoptic, 1216-1219
Timoptic OccuDose, 1216-1219
Timoptic Ocumeter, 1216-1219
Timoptic Ocumeter Plus, 1216-1219
Timoptic XE, 1216-1219
Tinactin Antifungal, 1241-1242
Tinactin Antifungal Jock Itch, 1241-1242
Tinaderm, 1241-1242
Tinamed, 1107-1109
Tindamax, 1219-1220
Ting, 1241-1242
tinidazole, 1219-1220
tinzaparin sodium, 1220-1221
tioconazole, 1222-1223

Entries can be identified as follows: generic name, Trade name.   1359

Truvada, 424-425, 1181-1182
Truxcillin VK, 952-953
Truxophyllin, 1198-1200
Trysul, 1157-1158
Tuinal, 65-67, 1116-1117
Tums, 180-182
Tums Ex, 180-182
Tussin, 577-578
Tussionex, 250-251
Two-Dyne, 167-169
Tylenol, 9-10
Tylenol no. 2, 300-301
Tylenol no. 3, 300-301
Tylenol no. 4, 300-301
Tylox, 9-10, 924-926
Tympagesic, 127-129
Tyzine, 1195-1196

U

Ultracet, 1249-1250
Ultram, 1249-1250
UltraMide, 1285-1286
Ultra Pep-Back, 175-176
Ultrase, 934-936
Ultrase MT 12, 934-936
Ultrase MT 18, 934-936
Ultrase MT 20, 934-936
Ultravate, 583-584
Unasyn, 77-78
undecylenic acid, 1282-1283
Uni-Bent Cough, 379-381
Uni-decon, 978-980
Uni-Dur, 1198-1200
Unipen, 836-837
Uniphyl, 54-56, 1198-1200
Unipres, 590-591, 1081-1082
Uniretic, 590-591, 816-817
Uni-Serp, 590-591, 1081-1082
Unisom with Pain Relief, 379-381
Unithroid, 695-696
Univasc, 816-817
unoprostone isopropyl, 1284
urea, 1285-1286
Urea Rea, 1285-1286
Ureacin, 1285-1286
Urecholine, 138-139
Urex, 771-772
Urispas, 500-501
Uristat, 968-969
Urobiotic-250, 929-930
Urodol, 968-969
Urogesic, 968-969
urokinase, 1286-1287
Urolene Blue, 786-787
Uroplus, 297-299
Uroplus DS, 297-299
Urotrol, 922-924
Uroxatral, 31-33

Urso, 1288-1289
ursodiol, 1288-1289
U-Tri-Lone, 1259-1261
Uvadex, 777-778

V

Vagifem, Vivelle, 460-462
Vagistat-1, 1222-1223
valacyclovir hydrochloride, 1289-1290
Valcyte, 1291-1292
valganciclovir hydrochloride, 1291-1292
Valium, 353-355
valproate sodium, 1292-1294
valproic acid, 1292-1294
valproic acid / valproate sodium / divalproex
    sodium, 1292-1294
valsartan, 1295-1296
Valtrex, 1289-1290
Vanadom, 195-196
Vanamide, 1285-1286
Vancenase, 119-121
Vancenase AQ, 119-121
Vancenase AQ DS, 119-121
Vanceril, 119-121
Vanceril DS, 119-121
Vancocin, 1296-1297
Vancocin HCl, 1296-1297
Vancocin HCl Pulvules, 1296-1297
vancomycin hydrochloride, 1296-1297
Vanex, 978-980
Vaniqa, 421-422
Vantin, 221-222
vardenafil hydrochloride, 1298-1299
Vascor, 133-134
Vaseretic, 425-427, 590-591
Vasocidin, 1157-1158
vasopressin, 1299-1300
Vasosulf, 1157-1158
Vasotate, 14-15
Vasotec, 425-427
Vectrin, 808-809
Veetids, 952-953
Velosef, 236-237
venlafaxine hydrochloride, 1301-1303
Venofer, 646-647
Ventavis, 612-613
Ventolin, 25-27
Ventolin HFA, 25-27
Ventolin Rotacaps, 25-27
Veracolate, 142-143
verapamil hydrochloride, 1303-1305
Verelan, 1303-1305
Verelan PM, 1303-1305
Vermox, 731-732
Versed, 804-805
Versiclear, 1108-1109
Vesanoid, 1258-1259
VESIcare, 1140-1141

Entries can be identified as follows: generic name, Trade name.

Vfend, 1305-1306
Viadur, 682-684
Viagra, 1126-1127
Vi-Atro, 104-105
Vibramycin, 403-404
Vibra-Tabs, 403-404
Vicks cough silencers, 352-353
Vicks Formula 44 cough control discs, 352-353
Vicks 44 Cough Relief , 352-353
Vicodin, 9-10
Vicoprofen, 608-610
Videx, 361-363
Videx-EC, 361-363
Vigamox, 827-828
Vioform-Hydrocortisone Cream, 279-280
Vioform-Hydrocortisone Mild Cream, 279-280
Vioform-Hydrocortisone Mild Ointment, 279-280
Vioform-Hydrocortisone Ointment, 279-280
Viokase, 934-936
Viokase 16, 934-936
Viokase 8, 934-936
Viracept, 855-856
Viractin, 1192-1193
Viramune, 861-862
Virbutal, 167-169
Viread, 1181-1182
Virilon, 791-792
Viroptic, 1268-1269
Visine, 1195-1196
Visken, 993-994
Vistacot, 603-605
Vistaject-50, 603-605
Vistaril, 603-605
Vistaril IM, 603-605
Vistide, 263-264
Vitabee 6, 1059-1060
Vitabee 12, 311-312
Vitamin B6, 1059-1060
Vitamin B-12, 311-312
Vitamin K1, 890-891
Vitarsert, 552-553
Vita #12, 311-312
Vitravene, 533-534
Vivactil, 1050-1052
Vivarin, 175-176
Vivelle-Dot, 460-462
Volmax, 25-27
Voltaren, 356-358
Voltaren Ophthalmic, 356-358
Voltaren XR, 356-358
voriconazole, 1305-1306
Vosol, 14-15
VoSol HC Otic, 14-15
VoSpire ER, 25-27
V.V.S., 1156-1157
Vytorin, 482-483, 1131-1132

W

warfarin sodium, 1306-1308
Wart-Off Maximum Strength, 1107-1109
Welchol, 303-304
Wellbutrin, 163-164
Wellbutrin SR, 163-164
Wellbutrin XL, 163-164
Wellcovorin, 681-682
WestCort, 593-595
Westhroid, 1209-1210
Wigraine, 447-448
Winstrol, 1149-1150
Wycillin, 952-953
Wygesic, 9-10, 1044-1045
Wymox), 69-70
Wytensin, 579-580

X

Xalatan, 676-677
Xanax, 37-39
Xanax XR, 37-39
Xenical, 908-909
Xerac AC, 42-43
Xibrom, 154
Xifaxan, 1089-1090
Xigris, 408-409
Xolair, 900-902
X-Prep, 1120-1121
Xylocaine, 696-698
Xylocaine with Epinephrine, 435-437, 696-698
xylometazoline, 1309-1310
Xyrem, 1137-1138

Y

Yocon, 1310-1311
Yodoxin, 640
Yohimbe, 1310-1311
yohimbine, 1310-1311
Yohimex, 1310-1311
Yovital, 1310-1311
YSP Aspirin, 93-94

Z

zafirlukast, 1311-1312
zalcitabine, 1312-1313
zaleplon, 1314-1315
Zanaflex, 1228-1230
zanamivir, 1316-1317
Zantac, 1077-1079
Zantac-150, 1077-1079
Zantac-150 EFFERdose, 1077-1079
Zantac-150 Maximum Strength, 1077-1079
Zantac-25 EFFERdose, 1077-1079

Entries can be identified as follows: generic name, Trade name.

Entries can be identified as follows: generic name, Trade name.

General Formulas

BODY SURFACE AREA (BSA)

NOMOGRAM: Place a straightedge from the patient's height in the left column to his or her weight in the right column. The point of intersection on the body surface area column indicates the body surface area (BSA). Reproduced from data of Boyd E, modified by West CD. In Behrman RE, and Vaugh VC, editors: *Nelson's textbook of pediatrics*, ed 15, Philadelphia, 1996, WB Saunders.

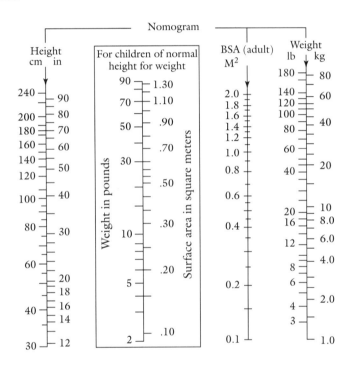

FORMULA (ADULT AND CHILD):
BSA (m^2) = Square root of {[height (inches) × weight (lb)]/3131}
BSA (m^2) = Square root of {[height (cm) × weight (kg)]/3600}